WHIPLASH AND RELATED HEADACHES

Bernard Swerdlow, M.D.

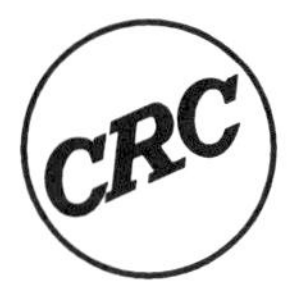

CRC Press
Boca Raton London New York Washington, D.C.

Library of Congress Cataloging-in-Publication Data

Swerdlow, Bernard.
Whiplash and related headaches / Bernard Swerdlow.
p. cm.
Includes bibliographical references and index.
ISBN 1-57444-232-5 (alk. paper)
1. Headache--etiology.. 2. Whiplash injuries. 3. Head--Wounds and Injuries--Complications.
I. Title
[DNLM: 1. Headache--etiology. 2. Headache--diagnosis. 3. Headache--psychology.
4. Whiplash Injuries--complications. 5. Head Injuries--complications. 6. Head Injuries--psychology.
7. Jurisprudence. WL342 S974W 1998]
RC392.S93 1998
DNLM/DLC
616.8 ' 491—dc21
for Library of Congress 98-41106
CIP

Direct all inquiries to CRC Press LLC, 2000 Corporate Blvd., N.W., Boca Raton, Florida 33431.

International Standard Book Number 1-57444-232-5
Library of Congress Card Number 98-41106
Printed in the United States of America 1 2 3 4 5 6 7 8 9 0
Printed on acid-free paper

Foreword

Whiplash and Related Headaches is an incredibly complete and massive undertaking. It has been written by Bernard Swerdlow, M.D., one of the foremost headache specialists in this country, and he has used a style and a format which makes it easy to read, easy to understand, and easy to follow. Difficult and complex issues are addressed, but Dr. Swerdlow puts them into language that is clear even to those readers who are not fundamentally grounded in the sciences.

Encouraged by his friends in the legal profession, Dr. Swerdlow began the book with the concept that it would be directed only towards lawyers. It is so well written, however, that it should be of equal interest to all patients who are headache sufferers, to paramedical personnel, and to medical students, as well as to physicians who have an interest in understanding more about the various headache problems experienced by their patients. In Part One he has addressed almost every variety of headache known to exist, and he has done this with clarity and a writing style that holds the reader's interest. The use of patient histories to give examples of each of these conditions gives the reader a feeling that she or he is right there as the patient gives the history to the doctor.

The emphasis of the book, however, is on whiplash and other forms of head trauma. Dr. Swerdlow has taken a complex subject, one which is often misunderstood, and often wrongly attributed to psychological problems or to malingerers who are exaggerating their problems in order to obtain financial rewards from the insurance industry, and makes it understandable.

When I went into practice many years ago, it was usual for patients who had a head injury, followed by headache, memory loss, impairment of concentration, depression, anxiety, anger outbursts, insomnia, personality changes, decreased sex drive, or any combination of these, to be considered to have these symptoms for psychological reasons. Therefore, they were likely to be sent for psychiatric management which led to minimal, if any, improvement in their status or well-being. Fortunately, as the scientific basis of medicine improved and research studies clearly showed that brain damage occurred when the head was subjected to injury (such as, but not limited to, acceleration/deceleration, and rotational movements of the head, popularly and medically as well, called whiplash), the pendulum has swung away from the psychological concept to one of an organic abnormality. That doesn't exclude a psychological overlay in some patients, but that is a far cry from concluding that psychological issues are the primary cause of the headache and other symptoms which are so frequently seen after injury to the head. All of these symptoms may have a tremendous impact on the patient's marriage, career, social life, and financial stability, and it should not be surprising that such devastating issues may lead to a disturbance in one's psychological makeup. They are all secondary to the underlying problem and cannot be considered the cause. The concept that "you would not have that headache if you didn't want it," or that green salve (money) will resolve all the symptoms that follow an injury, is no longer tenable. There is a need for physicians, lawyers, and those who make final decisions for third-party carriers to recognize the organicity behind headache-disabled patients.

Dr. Swerdlow has addressed all of these issues in this book in a way that makes it useful, not only for medically and legally oriented persons, the insurance industry, and the headache sufferer, but also for anyone who has a curiosity about headaches and why such headaches can totally disrupt the quality of life in some patients and, in time, to the point of total incapacitation.

William G. Speed, III, M.D.
Associate Professor of Medicine, Johns Hopkins School of Medicine
Fellow, American College of Physicians
Fellow, American Association for the Study of Headache
Diplomate, American Board of Internal Medicine
Past President, American Association for the Study of Headache
Founder and Director Emeritus of Speed Headache Associates, P.A.

Foreword

Dr. Swerdlow's book is really several books. It is a textbook on headaches generally and post traumatic headaches in particular. It is a book for headache sufferers who want to understand more about what is happening to them and perhaps in the process learn to manage their own pain and involvement with the medical community. It is a guide for lawyers presenting, evaluating, or defending claims involving headaches.

As I read, I found myself interested in the material on several levels, First, I have personal reasons for wanting to know more about headaches. My mother struggled with migraines all of her life. Second, I am a lawyer who often represents clients whose trauma-based physical and emotional problems include headaches and other symptoms of head or neck injury. Finally, again as a lawyer who understands the difficulty of evaluating claims based upon injuries of this nature, I appreciated Dr. Swerdlow's very specific and concrete approach to headache classification and diagnosis and the spotting of malingerers and other suspicious characters. I believe those who take the time to read this book also will find many ways to relate personally to the material.

The headache problem is big—very big. Putting aside headaches not related to trauma, eliminating those headaches from the statistics, the National Safety Council counted 12,800,000 auto accidents in 1989. Of these, 3,280,000 were rear end collisions and gave rise to 2,000,000 head and neck injuries . Many of the injured found their way to lawyer's offices pursuing claims against others involved in the collision, taking the position these others caused the accident and hence caused their neck injury. On the other side of these claims, insurance adjusters and lawyers for the insurance companies evaluated these claims and paid or resisted them. The issues are generally the same in these cases. Is the headache real? Is it really the result of the accident? Did it exist before the accident? What are the other symptoms? Are the other symptoms consistent with the diagnosis? The plaintiffs say they were fine before the accident and their troubles began immediately after the accident. The defendants say the accident never happened, the injury never happened, the plaintiff is making it all up, all the plaintiff's symptoms were there before the accident happened, and the complaints are subjective and impossible to demonstrate with objective proof.

In this ritual dance, it is necessary for a lawyer to understand headaches, especially post traumatic headaches and the syndromes they travel with. In evaluating and preparing a claim, it is important for the injured to understand headaches thoroughly. It is also important for them to organize their diagnosis and treatment around materials and concepts and to communicate them effectively to their clients, their lawyers, and in the cases which do not settle, to members of a jury. I believe these materials and concepts are contained in Dr. Swerdlow's book. As a plaintiff's lawyer, I would build my defense around this book. I believe the material is so well organized, so understandable, that in time it will alter the face of headache related litigation. In sum, it is a very important book for lawyers and their clients and their doctors.

Dr. Swerdlow takes a balanced approach in presenting the material. He does not seek to help plaintiff's lawyers more than defense lawyers. He seeks to bring out the reality of headaches, in the service of truth, not victory. The book will be a valuable resource to all who are involved in headache-related litigation. I don't think a headache case can be prepared, negotiated, or tried by anyone who has not taken the time to master the material which Dr. Swerdlow has so generously consumed and digested, interpreted, organized, and presented.

James N. Powers, J.D.
James N. Powers, P.A., Orlando, FL
Association of Trial Lawyers of America
Florida Academy of Trial Lawyers
American Bar Association

The Author

Bernard Swerdlow, M.D. is licensed and has been practicing medicine since 1965. He is board certified as a diplomate in psychiatry by the American Board of Psychiatry and Neurology (1976). He was psychiatric consultant to the Baptist Hospital Pain Treatment Center in Miami, Florida. From 1978 to 1982, he did additional training in neuroanatomy, neurology, and internal medicine at the University of Miami. He did further study in headache at the Montefiore Hospital Headache Clinic in the Bronx, New York; The Headache Research Foundation; The Faulkner Hospital, Boston, Massachusetts; The California Medical Clinic For Headaches, Los Angeles, California; and has attended many workshops on headache around the United States and Canada.

In 1985 he opened the only self-contained inpatient headache unit and was medical director of the Headache Treatment Center at Winter Park Memorial Hospital, Winter Park, Florida. This was the third inpatient headache facility to open in this country.

He became certified via examination by the American Academy of Thermology and The Academy of Neuro-Muscular Thermography.

He has published 15 scientific articles in this area and won The President's Award for the best scientific paper presented in 1986 at Johns Hopkins Medical Institutes. He has written many other papers, written and published *The Headache Handbook,* and has spoken at many scientific meetings around the U.S. and Canada.

He is Clinical Assistant Professor at The College of Health at the University of Central Florida. He has been asked by the Eisenhower, Citizen Ambassador Program, to speak in many of the iron curtain countries around the world on the subject of headache. He has appeared on television, radio, and has lectured to the lay population well over 100 times.

Over recent years, he has participated in the research of anti-migraine medications such as Imitrex, DHE, and anti-pain suppressor units.

From 1992 to the present he has been chosen by peer review to be listed in *The Best Doctors in America*, written by Steven Naifeh and Gregory White Smith, published by Woodward/White.

About the Contributing Authors

John N.I. Dieter, Ph.D. is a clinical psychologist who received his Ph.D. from Emory University. Dr. Dieter has had a diverse research and clinical career, spanning the fields of behavioral medical, psychophysiology, adult and pediatric neuropsychology, as well as individual psychotherapy. He has co-authored nearly fifty publications and conference presentations in the areas of chronic headache, biofeedback, psychophysiology, and premature infancy. Dr. Dieter is a recipient of a National Research Service Award from the National Institute of Mental Health (NIMH). This prestigious fellowship was awarded for his work in establishing supplemental treatment regimens directed towards ameliorating the neurobehavioral deficits associated with premature birth. Dr. Dieter's work with premature infants includes tenures as the director of the NICU Supplemental Stimulation Treatment Programs at both Grady Memorial Hospital in Atlanta and Jackson Memorial Hospital at the University of Miami School of Medicine. During his time at Jackson Memorial, Dr. Dieter was a Research Associate of the Touch Research Institute, under the direction of Dr. Tiffany Field. Dr. Dieter also completed his clinical psychology internship at Jackson, in the Department of Psychiatry and Behavioral Sciences.

Prior to his tenure at Emory, Dr. Dieter was a research and clinical associate of both the Headache Management Center and Headache Treatment Center at Winter Park Memorial Hospital, where he was also chief biofeedback technologist. It was during this period that Drs. Swerdlow and Dieter collaborated on research examining various physiological and behavioral components of chronic headache. Their work led to over a dozen published articles, numerous conference presentations, and several awards.

At present, Dr. Dieter's research focus is upon fetal development and early infancy. He is especially interested in the impact of the intrauterine environment on neuropsychological development. His clinical focus continues to be upon longer-term psychotherapy, and the etiology and treatment of severe personality disorder.

Dr. Dieter's clinical work has focused upon psychological and neuropsychological assessment, as well as longer-term individual psychotherapy. He was on the staff of the Neuropsychological Services at Crawford Long Memorial Hospital, under the direction of Dr. Eugene Emory. During this period, Dr. Dieter conducted numerous psychological and neuropsychological assessments of patients, including those who had experienced both minor and severe head injury. Dr. Dieter has particular expertise in personality assessment, especially through projective testing.

Thomas P. Hand, D.D.S. is a lifelong resident of Florida. He attended the University of Florida and graduated from Emory University School of Dentistry in 1959. He has practiced dentistry in the Orlando/Winter Park area for over 30 years.

Dr. Hand is a member of the American Dental Association, the Florida Dental Association, the Orange County Dental Society, the American Equilibration Society, an organization devoted to the study of temporomandibular joint disorders; and the American Prosthodontic Society, dedicated to the study of restorative and prosthetic dentistry.

He has served as president of the Orange County Dental Society, trustee and director of the L.D. Pankey Institute (the L.D. Pankey Institute is a graduate school that has trained over 14,000 practicing dentists worldwide), and as president of its International Alumni Association.

Dr. Hand is a fellow of the American College of Dentists, a prestigious honor given by his peers for leadership in dentistry. He has also been elected to the International College of Dentists, a worldwide dental leadership organization. This membership signifies international recognition for devoted services, contribution to the profession, and highest ethical standards.

Founder and chairman of the Facial Pain Center at Winter Park Memorial Hospital, Dr. Hand has served on the medical staff there and at Florida Hospital. He has conducted research projects on dental implants and has authored a chapter on temporomandibular joint dysfunction in *The Guide to Rehabilitation* utilized by the State of Florida.

Dr. Hand has presented programs on facial pain and restorative dentistry to dental societies nationally and has made presentations to the Orange County Bar Association. The Florida Biofeedback Society, and many hospital services. He has lectured at the University of California on temporomandibular joint dysfunction.

Dr. Hand's postgraduate training includes attendance at all courses of the L.D. Pankey Institute and all facial pain courses at the University of Florida. He has studied extensively in the fields of restorative and implant dentistry and facial pain over a 30-year period.

Don McKeever graduated from Florida State University in 1979. He attended Cumberland School of Law at Samford University and received his J.D. degree in 1983. In 1984, he opened his own practice and since that time has devoted his practice to only representing injured persons and their families.

His practice has involved litigated and nonlitigated matters. He has tried countless cases involving personal injury and wrongful death. His experience includes negotiation, arbitration, mediation, trial and appellate practice. In 1994, he obtained a personal injury verdict in excess of $9,000,000, which still stands as one of the highest ever rendered in Orange County, Florida.

He is a member of the Florida Academy of Trial Lawyers, Orange County Bar Association, Florida Bar Association, American Bar Association, and has been admitted to the District Court for Middle District of Florida.

In 1997, he founded the Law Firm of McKeever Albert and Barth. In addition to the above areas of practice, his firm has focused on the representation of health care providers in disputes against automobile insurance companies over payment for medical services.

Why This Book Was Written

I have spent 32 years practicing medicine and teaching, always in the area of chronic pain. Many of the patients I have treated and other professional colleagues encouraged me to record and share these experiences for the benefit of others. The combination of psychiatric training plus extensive study of the neurology of headache have given me a global view of this enormous problem.

During my residency in psychiatry, from 1964 to 1967, I found I was always interested in the mechanism of pain, both psychological and physiological. After spending 16 years in the practice of psychiatry, I decided to retrain in neurology and internal medicine exclusively in the area of headaches, and spent the next 16 years treating headache from a neurological discipline. This decision came after spending 6 years in the Pain Treatment Center at Baptist Hospital in Miami, Florida.

Although most of the patients there had low back problems, there was a significant number of headache patients. I observed the frustration the staff had with these patients and the same frustration the patients had with the staff. Most of the patients experienced headaches that were secondary to accidents and were now chronic sufferers. Many of these patients had compensation problems and many were in litigation. When these patients did not respond to our treatments, the staff would often come to the conclusion that secondary gain, financial or just attention seeking, was the reason they did not respond.

When working with workers compensation and litigation patients, all attempts are made to reduce or eliminate disability and the huge costs that are involved in their ongoing care, which can be lifelong. From a psychiatric approach, I felt that if I could devise a formula that could explain the breakdown of a happy productive human being to an angry dependent patient as a result of chronic pain from what appears to have been a relatively minor accident, then correcting that part of the formula should have a positive effect on the patient. What was left out of my formula was the enormous growth in information that has taken place over the past 25 years in the area of the physical causes of chronic pain.

I have taken the liberty of presenting this postulate of twenty-some years ago and hope the reader will understand my progress as they read the book.

In 1977, I presented a lecture in Miami to the Medical Institute for Attorneys, "Compensation and Traumatic Neurosis — Origin and Development, The Compensation Factor." I attempted mathematically to take all the elements involved to recompense the individual and set up an equation that would justify my postulates that a compensation factor exists and plays an important role in the possible change of personality during and perhaps even after litigation.

The foundation of thermodynamics has as its first law what is commonly known as the conservation of energy. Take one active, productive, employed person with the usual titer of anxiety and frustration, and reduce that person to the suspended state of partial invalidism and those energies create enormous tensions. Accentuate the tension with uncertainties as to the extent of disability or the economic stresses and be assured that the worries will take their toll.

$$\Delta P \cong T \times Cf$$

where ΔP = change in personality
T = trauma
Cf = compensation factor

$$Cf = \frac{ts \times u^2}{\Delta L} + \frac{a + l + \alpha}{e + s} + \frac{R}{P} + C$$

Cf	=	compensation factor
ts	=	time under stress
u^2	=	magnitude of uncertainty
L	=	change in lifestyle imposed by initial stress
a	=	angst (rage)
i	=	isolation (lack of communication from people he or she depends on for care)
α	=	abandonment (he/she senses from i plus other people in his/her personal world)
e	=	self esteem
s	=	sympathy (too much or too little)
R	=	regression
P	=	prognosis (maximum medical improvement)
C	=	patient's concept of compensation entitlement

There are four parts to this formula and this gives some clue as to the complexity of the dynamics.

1. The first component is the time of the stresses, times the magnitude squared over the change in lifestyle imposed by the initial stress.
2. The next expression is the rage or anger generated within the patient, plus the sense of isolation experienced or the lack of continued communication from the people on whom he or she depends for care and assistance and support, plus the sense of abandonment that the patient experiences divided by self esteem, plus sympathy that the patient receives. As one can see, the countervailing force of a strong sense of self esteem is preserved, or a strongly supported personal world can counter some very significant stresses. However, as so often is the case, the loss of self esteem, or contempt felt, magnifies isolation and frustration, and rage is experienced.
3. The next important element is the degree of regression and the inverse of the prognosis.
4. Finally, the significant element that can add meaningfully to the problems encountered in dealing with the patient's symptoms is the patient's concept of the compensation of the entitlement or how badly he feels he has been hurt or how much his hurt is due to negligence or the lack of concern of his employer.

Through the years, I recognized that this equation did not explain many of the problems I was encountering with the patients I was treating and with the explosion of information concerning pain in the past twenty years. I realized how top-heavy I was in the area of the psychology of pain and that I was not giving enough attention to physical mechanisms of pain. Of course, I realized that if there was to be a formula, it would have to include the pathophysiology as much as the pathopsychology.

Therefore, much of this book will be dedicated to the physical aspects of head and neck pain, with two chapters on the psychological consequences of head and neck injuries.

During the course of these years I have seen thousands of patients with headache caused by accidents, both automobile and other trauma, anywhere from blows to the head to what appears as minor stretching of the neck muscles. The puzzle was always, why do these accidents have such a devastating effect on these patients' lives? How much is "real" and how much is attributed to the gain of money or attention? Why did I feel I knew who was really suffering and who I felt was interested in secondary gain, and how accurate was I?

Were there any tests to substantiate my clinical impressions, or was this just intuition on my part?

Being a headache expert brought me in contact with many lawyers when I had to testify on behalf of their client, whether it be the patient or the insurance company. The obstacle in testifying was always the difficulty in having the lawyers and the jury understand the medical language and clinical symptoms that different headaches have. Making them understand that regardless of what causes the headache, the symptoms are really almost identical, is a very difficult concept for most people. That is, symptoms of a migraine attack, whether it is caused by stress, wine, lack of oxygen, high altitudes, menstrual periods, sensitivity to foods, infectious diseases, or whiplash, are the same. The biological mechanisms that cause the migraine syndrome are the same, only the triggering mechanisms are different. This would be the same for muscle tension or muscle contraction headaches.

Therefore, in order for the reader to understand the problems of whiplash headaches (acccel-eration/deceleration or flexion/extension headaches), it will be necessary to devote the first part of this book to headaches in general and the second part to post traumatic headaches. I will not discuss treatments in part one because there are many excellent books already published and I will make reference to them in the back of this book. Chapter 25 on Headache Treatments will also include many different treatments for the various types of headaches. After the reader understands the wide range of triggering mechanisms and the symptoms that come as a result of the different classification of headaches, the second part of the book will concern itself primarily with headaches that are a result of mechanical injury.

During the course of my practice, I have had to develop a method to make the lawyers representing either plaintiffs or insurance companies understand all the problems that relate to these injured patients. As a result of these demonstrations, these professionals asked if I would write a book, not only for them to understand, but also for the patients who are referred to different "specialists" and are constantly frustrated and angered that no one seems to understand their situation.

In the preparation of this book I have chosen three other specialists to write the chapters on TMJ (temporomandibular joint) injuries, the psychological aspects of post traumatic headache pain, and medical and legal problems in the court room.

Dr. Thomas Hand is a dentist who has spent decades studying TMJ injuries, and who has been not only a valuable asset to my practice but my mentor in understanding the complexities of the jaw and dental problems associated with flexion and extension injuries.

Dr. John Nathen Dieter was my research assistant for seven years and has written work on psychological testing on post traumatic injuries. His chapter covers the problems that we are confronted with in evaluating the enormous question of "Which came first, the chicken or the egg?" That is, how much of the symptoms are the result of the accident, the chronic pain, the disability, the legal stresses, or how much do we have to concern ourselves with litigation and secondary gain, a most difficult dilemma.

Mr. Don McKeever, Esq., who has a great deal of experience in personal injury, writes the chapter on medical and legal problems in the courtroom.

The enormity of how much headache affects our population and our economy is hard to measure. In 1988 a survey indicated that 158 million work days were lost. The amount of treatments given, the amount of medications, the legal expenses, etc., run into costs over 30 billion dollars. Headaches are a silent epidemic.

In writing this book, an effort was made to give actual case histories that will complement each diagnosis. Also, the method I used to diagnose these conditions will give the sufferers an opportunity to recognize their conditions. At the back of the book there will be blank history forms to fill out and headache logs that will help the patients measure their progress.

Over the past 12 years, the mortality from traumatic brain injury has exceeded the cumulative number of American battle deaths in all wars since the founding of our country. The number of head injuries is estimated from over 2 million to 7.5 million, and 500,000 to 1,000,000 require hospitalization. Approximately 80,000 to 240,000 each year face a lifelong disability. From 5,000 to 20,000 will develop epilepsy and 2,000 to 7,000 will live in a vegetative state. Fortunately, only 6% of these injuries are considered major injuries, and 90% of head trauma patients survive. About 80% achieve sufficient recovery to resume their pre-injury activities. Headaches from these injuries range from 44% to 80%.

Although the title *Whiplash Headaches* was used, an attempt will be made to use the diagnosis cervical acceleration/deceleration syndrome (CAD) or flexion/extension syndrome. Unfortunately, the term whiplash that was introduced by H.E. Crowe in 1928 to explain the biomechanics of the rear-ended accident has turned out to be for many "the manna for the plaintiff's attorney, pestilence for the defense attorney and a paid vacation for the unscrupulous patient." The term whiplash lent an evil connotation to the injury.

I do hope this book will bring credibility to a major medical condition that only research and objective reporting will eventually correct.

Bernard Swerdlow, M.D.

The case histories and stories in *Whiplash and Related Headaches* are medically accurate. Patient names, places, physicians' names have been deleted or changed in order to protect privacy. Any resemblance to persons living or dead is coincidental.

This book has been written to help educate the patient to understand his or her diagnosis. This should help the reader to select the best-suited clinician, and to reduce time and cost of suffering. This information is not intended to substitute for medical advice. No regimen of treatment should be instituted unless your physician feels that this treatment is suitable for you.

Every effort has been made to ensure that the care recommended herein, including diagnosis, drug choices, drug dosages and other treatments are in accord with standards and practice at the time of publication. Because there is constant change with research and regulation, it is recommended that the reader check the product information sheet in the package of each drug for recommended doses, warnings, and contraindications. There is inherent risk with all treatments with and without identification.

The purpose of this book is to inform and educate the reader, and it should not be employed as a substitute for professional diagnosis and treatment.

Acknowledgments

To Dr. Robert Lowenstein (Doc), high school teacher and mentor, for reviewing much of the work and for his suggestions.

To author and friend Philip Roth, for his guidance and help in bringing the manuscript from proposal to the press.

To Yvonne L. Allan, medical illustrator, for clarifying difficult concepts into understandable illustrations.

To Mary Ella Sears and Patricia N. Cole, librarians at Winter Park Memorial Hospital, for their help in gathering over six hundred references.

To René A. O'Connell, typist, whose energy, understanding, and ability and patience with the many drafts of this manuscript made its completion possible.

Dedication

I wish to dedicate this book to my grandchildren:

Sarah Ashley
Joshua Samuel

A special dedication to Clarnet and to the TransLife program at Florida Hospital; without them this book would never have been written.

On Sunday, October 3, 1994, I was in the final stages of end-stage renal disease. Florida Hospital's TransLife program in Orlando was doing everything possible to keep me alive with dialysis, to no avail. While I was so sick, a 14-year-old girl, living with her mother in a homeless shelter, died tragically of a cerebral hemorrhage. It was during this time of grief that the girl's mother made a generous and loving decision to donate organs and tissue for the benefit of others. On October 4, at 8 a.m., I was in the operating room, and 24 hours later this gray-black veil that covered me for well over a year was gone.

I know only this young girl's first name, Clarnet, but I shall always be grateful to her and to her mother for my gift of life.

Contents

* Written by Thomas P. Hand, D.D.S.
** Written by John N.I. Dieter, Ph.D.
*** Written by Don McKeever, Esq.

Part One

Chapter 1

An Old Problem

A day of watching television commercials leaves one with the impression that you have to be armed with at least a half dozen over-the-counter pills to fight your headache. You see hammers beating on your skull or people shouting at you or kids knocking their drinks all over your new carpet. Stress has become the key word for causing that terrible pain that interferes with your life. We all feel that being given an opportunity to go back to the good old days would save us so much head pain. After all, isn't it true that in this country alone we use at least 50 million pounds of aspirin, and that doesn't touch all the other types of medication that are available. It has been estimated that 70% of U.S. households have individuals who experience headaches. Approximately 60 to 80 million experience recurring headaches which are responsible for the loss of 160 million work days. Headache is the most frequent reason given by patients to visit doctors, and accounts for over 10 million office appointments with medical doctors (M.D.s) or doctors of osteopathy (D.O.s), and this does not include other health care professionals such as chiropractors, hypnotists, acupuncturists, psychologists, homeopaths, nutritionists, spiritualists, message therapists, ministers, priests, hair stylists, and the list continues. There are about 300 medical conditions that can cause headaches.

What if our president suffered chronic daily headaches and 40% of the time he was incapacitated? How might that affect decisions that concern our lives? How much did it affect the production of Thomas Jefferson, Sigmund Freud, Ulysses S. Grant, Karl Marx, Julius Caesar, Leo Tolstoy, Virginia Woolf, Edgar Allen Poe, Lewis Carrol, Tchaikovsky, Chopin, Charles Darwin, George Bernard Shaw, and many other notables who suffered severe migraine.[1,2,4]

Well, if you think going back to the good old days would solve your problems, think again. Lance[3] traces the history of headaches and documents that these problems go back as far as man existed. Lance observed in Java, where the pace has not quickened in a thousand years, that women working in the rice paddies wore cloth bands around their foreheads. These were not designed to keep sweat from their eyes, but were "headache bands," a traditional remedy for headaches. He spoke to Dr. Reuben Taureka, then a minister for education in Papua-New Guinea, who told Dr. Lance that it is common practice for tribes in the highlands to scarify their foreheads because of recurrent headaches.

He found that in primitive Melanesian communities on islands of the south Pacific, the custom of trepanning persisted until recently. Trepanning is an operation in which a hole is made in the skull with some sharp object to let the evil spirits out. Melanesians used this treatment for insanity, epilepsy, and chronic headache. Skulls found dating back to the Neolithic and Bronze ages in Europe, Mexico, and the American continent showed signs of trepanning. The skulls found in Europe were mostly oval, and the edges showed signs of healing, indicating that the operation had

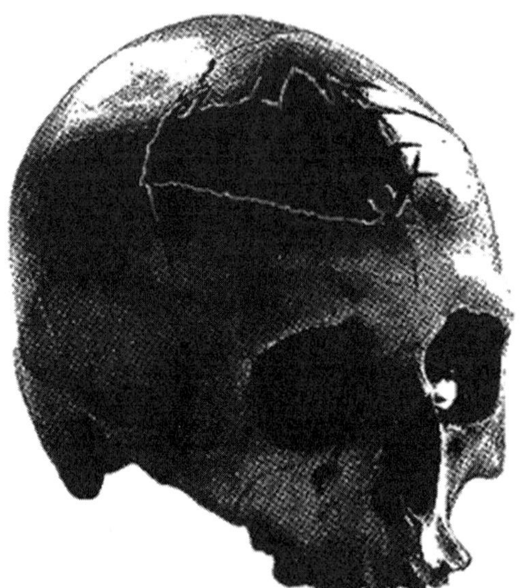

Figure 1.1 Trephination is a surgical procedure making a hole with a sharp object in the skull. In the cases of early history, it was used to let evil spirits out to reduce the migraine headache. Other than Peruvian Indians, who received some type of cocaine as an anesthetic, most of these surgical procedures were done without any anesthesia. The holes in the skull could be large or small, depending on the instrument used to cut them.

been carried out during life and that the patient had survived for some time afterward. This would give evidence dating back ten thousand years and certainly people had these symptoms long before then, and probably dating to the existence of the human species (Figure 1.1). An old joke finds Adam after marrying Eve asking God, "What is a headache?" The other joke is that at the same time, on the other side of the cave, Eve is asking God the same question.

Lance continues to trace the literature and finds in the Atharvaveda of India headache is mentioned in the book of knowledge of magic formulas written between 1500 and 800 B.C. Knowledge of medicine from Egypt comes from the Edwin Smith Papyrus (papyri are named after their discoverers), dating back to 3000–2500 B.C. It describes the appearance of the brain and types of paralysis following injury to the head. The Ebers Papyrus, written about 1600 B.C., and which probably originated more than a thousand years earlier, has written: "List of virtues of ricinus (castor oil plant): it was found in an ancient book concerning the things beneficial to mankind. If its peel is brayed in water and applied to a head that suffers, it will be cured immediately, as though it had never suffered."

From the Babylonian era there is an interesting poetic reference to headache dating 4000 to 3000 B.C.

Headache roameth over the desert, blowing like the wind,
Flashing like lightening, it is loosed above and below;
It cutteth off him who feareth not his god like a reed,
Like a stalk of henna it slitteth his thews.
It wasteth the flesh of him who hath no protecting goddess
Flashing like a heavenly star, it cometh like the dew;
It standeth hostile against the wayfarer, scorching him like the day,
This man it hath struck and
Like one with heart disease he staggereth,
Like one bereft of reason he is broken,

Like that which has been cast into the fire he is shriveled,
Like a wild ass... his eyes are full of cloud,
On himself he feedeth, bound in death;
Headache whose course like the dread windstorm none knoweth,
None knoweth its full time or its bond.

Another report comes from Hebrew medicine in the Bible (2 Kings 4: 19-20): "And he said unto his father, my head, my head. And he said to a servant, carry him to his mother. And when he had taken him, and brought him to his mother, he sat on her knees till noon and then died." The story continues with this fatal headache. Elisha, the prophet was summoned and was met with the news, "There was neither voice, nor hearing... the child is not awaked." Elisha "went up up, and lay upon the child, and put his mouth... and the flesh of the child waxed warm... the child sneezed seven times, and the child opened his eyes." Lance diagnoses this headache followed by loss of consciousness with recovery after mouth to mouth resuscitation. This provides a dramatic description of some form of cerebral hemorrhage or encephalitis.

Aesculapius, about 1259 B.C., starts Greek medicine. Aesculapius was so successful the supply of the souls to the underworld was dwindling. Pluto ordered Zeus to remove Aesculapius from the register of doctors with a thunderbolt. Aesculapius became regarded as a god and temples known as Asklepieia were devoted to the sick. There was one tablet at Epidaurus that described how headache was cured and how that cured Agestratos also of insomnia.

History goes on and Lance continues: Hippocrates was born on the island of Cos in 460 B.C. He described a headache which was probably migraine:

> Most of the time he seemed to see something shining before him like a light, usually in part of the right eye; at the moment, a violent pain supervened in the right temple, then in all the head and neck, where the head is attached to the spine... vomiting, when it became possible, was able to divert the pain and render it more moderate.

A detailed description of migraine was given by Aretaeus, who was born in Cappadocia in Asia Minor, now part of Turkey, about A.D. 81. He emphasized the fact that the pain commonly affects one side of the head, which he called heterocrania. His description then is still accurate today.

> In certain cases, the parts on the right side, or those on the left solely, so far that a separate temple, or ear, or one eyebrow, or one eye, or the nose which divides the face into two equal parts; and the does not pass this limit, but remains in the half of the head. This called heterocrania, an illness by no means mild, even though it intermits, and although it appears to be slight. For if at any time it set in acutely, it occasions unseemly and dreadful, spasm and distortion of the countenance takes place; the eyes either fixed intently like horns, or they are rolled inwardly to this side or to that; vertigo, deep seated pain of the eyes as far as the meninges; irrestrainable sweat; sudden pain of the tendons, as of one striking with a club; nausea, vomiting of bilious matters; collapse of the patient... there is much torpor, heaviness of the head, anxiety and ennui. For they flee the light; darkness soothes their disease: nor can they bear readily to look upon or hear anything agreeable; their sense of smell is vitiated, neither does anything agreeable to smell delight them, and they have also an aversion to fetid things: the patients, moreover, are weary of life and wish to die.

Galem (A.D 131-200) called a one-sided headache hemicrania, which is the origin of the Old English *megrim* and the French word *migraine* which is in common use today.

Further description of headache by Paul of Aegina (Greek) in A.D. 600 and Thomas Willis (1621-75) in London goes further in accurate descriptions of today's malady.

The Romans believed that headaches and other painful discomforts were punishments inflicted by the gods. The Latin word *poena,* from which the word pain derives, means penalty or punishment.[1] Many different methods were used to treat these headaches. Some medieval therapies are

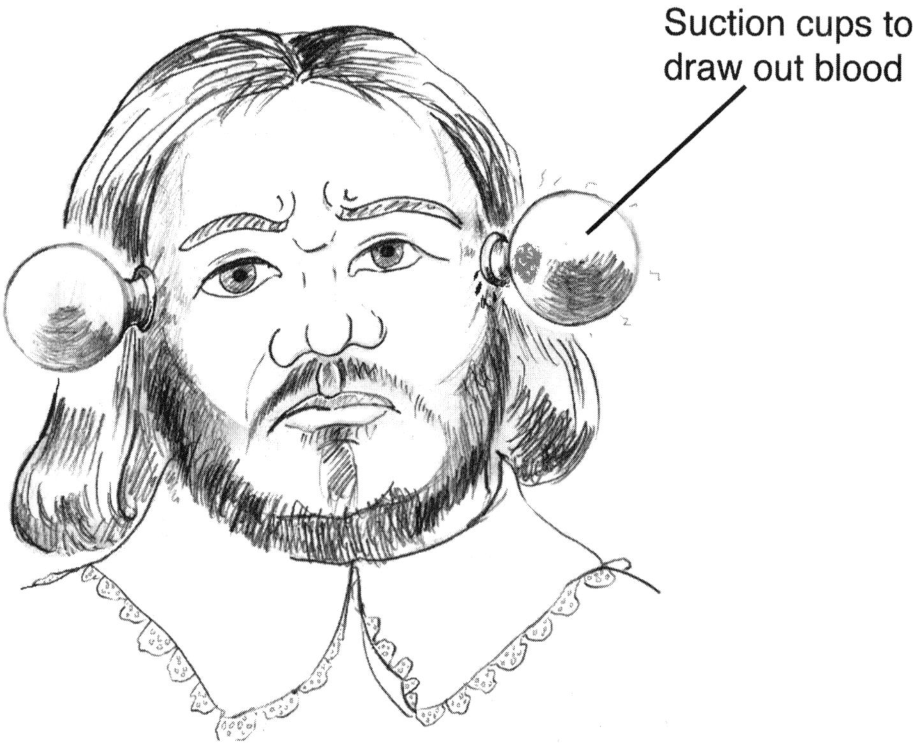

Figure 1.2 An illustration of another method used to treat headache often seen in the 1600s, and even later. Slight incisions were made near the temporals and heated cups were placed over the incisions and the temples. When the air cooled, this created a vacuum and drew out blood, which they hoped would ease the head pain. It was not uncommon that blood letting alone was used, even in this country, as a means of helping headache and other diseases. They thought that blood letting would help.

found in historical documents (Figure 1.2). Rags were soaked in vinegar and cow dung and applied to the area of pain; others dripped coca juice onto the painful area; and many painful parts were massaged with animal parts, including the genitalia. Interestingly, coca leaf has cocaine-like effects and the genitals of beavers have been found to have aspirin-like compounds.[1]

Other most interesting treatments include long religious pilgrimages to famous shrines. An Irish manuscript found instructed the headache sufferer to pray to the eye of Isaiah, tongue of Solomon, mind of Benjamin, heart of St. Paul, and faith of Abraham.[2]

After reviewing this past I'm no longer sure they were the "good old days" as far as headaches were concerned. It is now time to look at today and hopefully find a better prospect for tomorrow.

REFERENCES

1. Saper, J. R., *Help For Headaches,* Warner Books, 1987.
2. Saper, J. R., Magee, K. R., *Freedom From Headaches,* Simon and Schuster, New York, 1978.
3. Lance, J. W., *Headache — Understanding — Alleviation,* Charles Scribner's Sons, New York, 1975.
4. Swerdlow, B., *The Headache Handbook,* Mayfield Press, 1985.

Chapter 2

Classification of Headaches

Although headaches have been known for thousands of years, it wasn't until 1962 that a classification was done. It was done by an Ad Hoc Committee on the classification of headaches reported in *Archives of Neurology*, 1962; 6: 173-176 in the following manner.

The categories were divided into primary and secondary. Primary headaches are benign and are expressions of altered physiology where there doesn't seem to be any identifiable organic pathology. Secondary headaches are those that are caused by organic pathology. Examples of this would be some type of toxin, metabolic or structural changes, infections, trauma, and vascular disease.

Examples of these categories are shown in Table 2.1.

It was felt after 23 years that this classification was not adequate and, starting in 1985, the International Headache Society (IHS) appointed a committee from a number of countries to create a new system for the classification and diagnosis of headache disorders that would be less open to individual interpretation than the others. In 1988 IHS printed the new Classification and Diagnostic Criteria for Headache Disorders, Cranial Neuralgias and Facial Pain.[2] There are about 129 different diagnoses and some of these diagnoses have been challenged. In Part two of this book, which is devoted to post traumatic headache, I discuss the IHS classification of Headache Associated With Head Trauma and some of the differences I have with their classification.

In Part one of this book I select headache disorders that I feel are important for the reader to understand before reading the second part of this book. It is important for the reader to understand the basic diagnosis of vascular and muscle contraction headache to understand the kind of headaches someone will have after a head and neck trauma.

Although the following is a list of headaches as written by the Headache Classification Committee of the International Headache Society, the diagnostic criteria were felt to be too extensive for this book. The reader may research this material by referring to *Cephalalgia, An International Journal of Headache*, 1988.

Table 2.1

I. Primary vascular headaches[1]
  A. Migraine
    1. Classic migraine
      a) Hemiplegic/hemisensory migraine
      b) Ophthalmic (retinal) migraine
      c) Vertebrobasilar migraine
      d) Ophthalmoplegic migraine
      e) Complicated migraine
    2. Common migraine
  B. Carotidynia
  C. Cluster headache
    1. Episodic cluster headache
    2. Chronic cluster headache
    3. Chronic paroxysmal hemicrania
II. Secondary vascular headaches (Organic/Pathologic)
  A. Systemic infection and fever
  B. Hypoxia
  C. Cerebrovascular occlusive disease
  D. Arteritis (temporal arteritis, systemic lupus erythematosus, etc.)
  E. Carbon monoxide poisoning
  F. Nitrite/nitrate ingestion
  G. Postepileptic state
  H. Hypoglycemia
  I. Alcohol ingestion
  J. Hemodialysis
  K. Drug induced
  L. Rebound (toxic) headache

Headaches of muscular origin

I. Primary muscle contraction headache
II. Secondary muscle contraction headache (organic)
  A. Cervical arthritis
  B. Myositis
  C. Temporomandibular joint dysfunction
  D. Ocular disease
  E. Abnormalities of posture
  F. Congenital deformity of cervical or thoracic vertebrae
  G. Occipital/cervical disease

Traction headache (compression on intracranial structure)
  A. Intracranial mass lesions
  B. Increased intracranial pressure
  C. Post lumbar puncture headache
  D. Intracranial hemorrhage

Inflammatory or irrational headache

Cranial nerve (neuralgias) headache disorders

I. Trigeminal neuralgia
II. Glossopharyngeal neuralgia
III. Gradenigo syndrome
IV. Postherpetic neuralgia (5th and 7th cranial nerves)
V. Supraorbital neuralgia (a branch of the 5th cranial nerve)
VI. Occipital neuralgia

Table 2.1 (continued)

Psychogenic headaches
- A. Conversion cephalgia (hysterical headache)
- B. Delusion/hallucinatory headache (psychosis)
- C. Depression headache

Extracranial pain conditions
- A. Otolaryngological
- B. Ocular disease
- C. Central disease
- D. Others

Table 2.2 Classification – Headache Classification of the International Headache Society (IHS)

1. Migraine
   - 1.1 Migraine without aura
   - 1.2 Migraine with aura
     - 1.2.1 Migraine with typical aura
     - 1.2.2 Migraine with prolonged aura
     - 1.2.3 Familial hemiplegic migraine
     - 1.2.4 Basilar migraine
     - 1.2.5 Migraine aura without headache
     - 1.2.6 Migraine with acute onset aura
   - 1.3 Ophthalmoplegic migraine
   - 1.4 Retinal migraine
   - 1.5 Childhood periodic syndromes that may be precursors to or associated with migraine
     - 1.5.1 Benign paroxysmal vertigo of childhood
     - 1.5.2 Alternating hemiplegia of childhood
   - 1.6 Complications of migraine
     - 1.6.1 Status migrainous
     - 1.6.2 Migrainous infarction
   - 1.7 Migrainous disorder not fulfilling above criteria
2. Tension-type headache
   - 2.1 Episodic tension-type headache
     - 2.1.1 Episodic tension-type headache associated with disorder of pericranial muscles
     - 2.1.2 Episodic tension-type headache unassociated with disorder of pericranial muscles
   - 2.2 Chronic tension-type headache
     - 2.2.1 Chronic tension-type headache associated with disorder of pericranial muscles
     - 2.2.2 Chronic tension-type headache unassociated with disorder of pericranial muscles
   - 2.3 Headache of the tension type not fulfilling above criteria
3. Cluster headache and chronic paroxysmal hemicrania
   - 3.1 Cluster headache
     - 3.1.1 Cluster headache periodicity undetermined
     - 3.1.2 Episodic cluster headache
     - 3.1.3 Chronic cluster headache
       - 3.1.3.1 Unremitting from onset
       - 3.1.3.2 Evolved from episodic
   - 3.2 Chronic paroxysmal hemicrania
   - 3.3 Cluster headache-like disorder not fulfilling above criteria
4. Miscellaneous headaches unassociated with structural lesion
   - 4.1 Idiopathic stabbing headache
   - 4.2 External compression headache
   - 4.3 Cold stimulus headache
     - 4.3.1 External application of a cold stimulus
     - 4.3.2 Ingestion of a cold stimulus

Table 2.2 Classification – Headache Classification of the International Headache Society (IHS) (continued)

- 4.4 Benign cough headache
- 4.5 Benign exertional headache
- 4.6 Headache associated with sexual activity
  - 4.6.1 Dull type
  - 4.6.2 Explosive type
  - 4.6.3 Postural type

5. Headache associated with head trauma
   - 5.1 Acute post traumatic headache
     - 5.1.1 With significant head trauma and/or confirmatory signs
     - 5.1.2 With minor head trauma and no confirmatory signs
   - 5.2 Chronic post traumatic headache
     - 5.2.1 With significant head trauma and/or confirmatory signs
     - 5.2.2 With minor head trauma and no confirmatory signs
6. Headache associated with vascular disorders
   - 6.1 Acute ischemic cerebrovascular disease
     - 6.1.1 Transient ischemic attack (TIA)
     - 6.1.2 Thromboembolic stroke
   - 6.2 Intracranial hematoma
     - 6.2.1 Intracerebral hematoma
     - 6.2.2 Subdural hematoma
     - 6.2.3 Epidural hematoma
   - 6.3 Subarachnoid hemorrhage
   - 6.4 Unruptured vascular malformation
     - 6.4.1 Arteriovenous malformation
     - 6.4.2 Saccular aneurysm
   - 6.5 Arteritis
     - 6.5.1 Giant cell arteritis
     - 6.5.2 Other systemic arteritides
     - 6.5.3 Primary intracranial arteritis
   - 6.6 Carotid or vertebral artery pain
     - 6.6.1 Carotid or vertebral dissection
     - 6.6.2 Carotidynia (idiopathic)
     - 6.6.3 Post endarterectomy headache
   - 6.7 Venous thrombosis
   - 6.8 Arterial hypertension
     - 6.8.1 Acute pressor response to exogenous agent
     - 6.8.2 Pheochromocytoma
     - 6.8.3 Malignant (accelerated) hypertension
     - 6.8.4 Preeclampsia and eclampsia
   - 6.9 Headache associated with other vascular disorder
7. Headache associated with nonvascular intracranial disorder
   - 7.1 High cerebrospinal fluid pressure
     - 7.1.1 Benign intracranial hypertension
     - 7.1.2 High pressure hydrocephalus
   - 7.2 Low cerebrospinal fluid pressure
     - 7.2.1 Post lumbar puncture headache
     - 7.2.2 Cerebrospinal fluid fistula headache
   - 7.3 Intracranial infection
   - 7.4 Intracranial sarcoidosis and other noninfectious inflammatory diseases
   - 7.5 Headache related to intrathecal injections
     - 7.5.1 Direct effect
     - 7.5.2 Due to chemical meningitis
   - 7.6 Intracranial neoplasm
   - 7.7 Headache associated with other intracranial disorder
8. Headache associated with substances or their withdrawal
   - 8.1 Headache induced by acute substance use or exposure
     - 8.1.1 Nitrate/nitrate-induced headache
     - 8.1.2 Monosodium glutamate-induced headache

Table 2.2 Classification – Headache Classification of the International Headache Society (IHS) (continued)

8.1.3 Carbon monoxide-induced headache
8.1.4 Alcohol-induced headache
8.1.5 Other substances
8.2 Headache induced by chronic substance use or exposure
8.2.1 Ergotamine-induced headache
8.2.2 Analgesics abuse headache
8.2.3 Other substances
8.3 Headache from substance withdrawal (acute use)
8.3.1 Alcohol withdrawal headache (hangover)
8.3.2 Other substances
8.4 Headache from substance withdrawal (chronic use)
8.4.1 Ergotamine withdrawal headache
8.4.2 Caffeine withdrawal headache
8.4.3 Narcotics abstinence headache
8.4.4 Other substances
8.5 Headache associated with substances but with uncertain mechanism
8.5.1 Birth control pills or estrogens
8.5.2 Other substances
9. Headache associated with non-cephalic infection
9.1 Viral infection
9.1.1 Focal non-cephalic
9.1.2 Systemic
9.2 Bacterial infection
9.2.1 Focal non-cephalic
9.2.2 Systemic (septicemia)
9.3 Headache related to other infection
10. Headache associated with metabolic disorder
10.1 Hypoxia
10.1.1 High altitude headache
10.1.2 Hypoxic headache
10.1.3 Sleep apnea headache
10.2 Hypercapnia
10.3 Mixed hypoxia and hypercapnia
10.4 Hypoglycemia
10.5 Dialysis
10.6 Headache related to other metabolic abnormality
11. Headache or facial pain associated with disorder of cranium, neck, eyes, ears, nose, sinuses, teeth, mouth, or other facial or cranial structures
11.1 Cranial bone
11.2 Neck
11.2.1 Cervical spine
11.2.2 Retropharyngeal tendinitis
11.3 Eyes
11.3.1 Acute glaucoma
11.3.2 Refractive errors
11.3.3 Heterophoria or heterotropia
11.4 Ears
11.5 Nose and sinuses
11.5.1 Acute sinus headache
11.5.2 Other diseases of nose or sinuses
11.6 Teeth, jaws, and related structures
11.7 Temporomandibular joint disease
12. Cranial neuralgias, nerve trunk pain and deafferentation pain
12.1 Persistent (in contrast to tic-like) pain of cranial nerve origin
12.1.1 Compression or distortion of cranial nerves and second or third cervical roots
12.1.2 Demyelination of cranial nerves
12.1.2.1 Optic neuritis (retrobulbar neuritis)

Table 2.2 Classification – Headache Classification of the International Headache Society (IHS) (continued)

12.1.3 Infarction of cranial nerves
 12.1.3.1 Diabetic neuritis
12.1.4 Inflammation of cranial nerves
 12.1.4.1 Herpes zoster
 12.1.4.2 Chronic post-herpetic neuralgia
12.1.5 Tolosa-Hunt syndrome
12.1.6 Neck-tongue syndrome
12.1.7 Other causes of persistent pain of cranial nerve origin
12.2 Trigeminal neuralgia
 12.2.1 Idiopathic trigeminal neuralgia
 12.2.2 Symptomatic trigeminal neuralgia
  12.2.2.1 Compression of trigeminal root or ganglion
  12.2.2.2 Central lesions
12.3 Glossopharyngeal neuralgia
 12.3.1 Idiopathic glossopharyngeal neuralgia
 12.3.2 Symptomatic glossopharyngeal neuralgia
12.4 Nervus intermedius neuralgia
12.5 Superior laryngeal neuralgia
12.6 Occipital neuralgia
12.7 Central causes of head and facial pain other than tic douloureux
 12.7.1 Anesthesia dolorosa
 12.7.2 Thalamic pain
12.8 Facial pain not fulfilling criteria in groups 11 or 12
13. Headache not classifiable

REFERENCES

1. Saper, J.R., *Headache Disorder*, John Wright-PSG Inc., 1983.
2. *Cephalalgia Journal*, Norwegian University Press, 1988.

CHAPTER 3

Theories of Head Pain (Why Does Your Head Hurt?)

Anyone with a headache knows one thing, it hurts. The pain can be mild, moderate, severe, or incapacitating. Three words you will become familiar with are intensity, frequency, and duration. These words are important in making the diagnosis of the different types of headache. When we talk about intensity we will use the following descriptions: irritating, which is mild or annoying; interfering, which is moderate to severe; and incapacitating, which is exactly what it is — you are unable to function. Most vascular headaches are moderate to incapacitating and muscle tension headaches are irritating to moderate. However, we know now that these headaches are not that separate and vascular headaches have muscle tension, and muscle tension headaches will often have a vascular component. As a matter of fact, it has been demonstrated that migraine attacks have more muscle tension than muscle tension headaches. In any event, we will use these terms as a means of identifying and simplifying our understanding of pain. (It is advisable that the reader review Chapter 20, Introduction to Neuropsychology, Section II, Functional Neuroanatomy.)

One should know that when the head hurts the brain is not hurting. There are specific anatomical structures that have pain because certain nerves that carry the message of pain are attached to these structures. The two major nerves that carry the message of pain are the fifth cranial nerve or the trigeminal nerve, and the occipital nerves that come from the cervical nerves which are C-1, C-2, and C-3 (Figure 3.1). Other nerves that carry pain to a lesser extent are the seventh cranial nerve or the facial nerve, the ninth cranial nerve or the glossopharyngeal nerve, and the tenth cranial nerve or the vagus nerve. These pain fibers are attached to various structures around the brain that relay the pain. There are structures inside the skull that are pain sensitive and they are parts of the dura mater (the dura is one of the coverings of the brain), arteries of the dura mater, and the arteries of the base of the brain and their major branches. Also included are the cranial sinuses and the great venous sinuses. The structures outside the brain that convey pain are the skin, scalp, muscles around the scalp, and the tissues that attach the muscles to the scalp. Also sensitive are the tissues that are inside the mouth and the nose (the mucosa). The structures that are not pain sensitive are the brain itself, the ependyma (the coverings inside of the ventricles of the brain), the choroid plexus (the structure that manufactures the cerebral spinal fluid), some parts of the dura mater, and two other layers of the brain, the pia mater and the arachnoid membrane. The skull is only slightly sensitive (Figure 3.2).

Muscle tension or muscle contraction headache was considered due to increased muscle contraction around the skull and in the cervical (neck) musculature. Normally when a muscle contracts there is inhibition of the firing of the muscle spindle and there is a return to allow the muscle to relax. But if the system continues to fire because of the brain influences, or local irritation, the

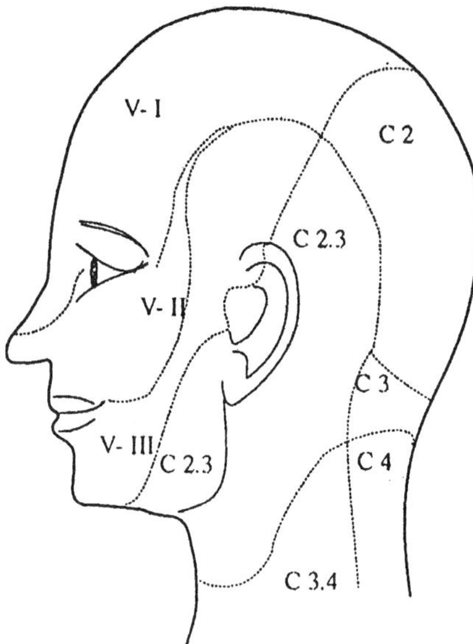

Figure 3.1 This illustration demonstrates the distribution of the pain in that particular area of the trigeminal or fifth cranial nerve (**V**). There are three divisions. One (**I**) is the ophthalmic division that relays information from the forehead, eyes, nose, temples, meninges, paranasal sinuses, and part of the nasal mucosa. Two (**II**) is the maxillary division, which delivers information from the upper jaw, teeth, lip, cheeks, hard palate, maxillary sinus, and nasal mucosa. Three (**III**) is the mandibular division, which delivers information from the lower jaw, teeth, lip, the buccal mucosa, tongue, and part of the external ear, auditory meatus, and meninges. The cervical nerves (**C**) are numbered for the particular vertebra from which they arise. Later on it will be shown how there is a way for messages from the cervical nerves to reach the trigeminal nerves, and vice versa.

muscle spindle remains tight and the muscle continues to contract until the contraction becomes painful and this becomes cyclic — spasm, tension, and pain; hence, muscle contraction headache. Unfortunately, recent studies do not support this mechanism as a primary cause of headache. Therefore, there must be a different neurological mechanism to explain this pain.

Vascular headaches include migraine, cluster, and many of the headaches listed in Chapter 2. These headaches are discussed in Chapters 6, 8, 11, 13, 14, and 19. The explanation of these headaches has changed a great deal in the last decade.

The hypotheses of these headaches have been the following: vascular, neural, neurovascular and disturbed serotonin activity.

The vascular hypothesis suggests that the headache pain of migraine is caused by dilatation of arteries outside of the brain and that any neurological symptoms are due to the initial constriction of these arteries. In 1938 Harold G. Wolff in his research suggested that vasoconstriction of these blood vessels caused the migraine aura (visual, sensory, motor, and neurological changes) because of a reduced blood supply. The pain is then caused by over-dilatation of these arteries with a release of chemicals that cause pain, which are called polypeptides. It was felt that this theory was accurate because there was pulsation of the superficial temporal artery and there was some relief when these arteries were compressed. Another indication was that the headache got worse with drugs that dilated the arteries and that the pain was reduced or eliminated with medications that constricted the arteries. A test done with transcranial Doppler sonography demonstrated, by reduction of the velocity of blood in the middle cranial arteries, that migraine is associated with intracranial arterial dilatation (Figure 3.3).

The neural hypothesis of migraine is that this vascular type of headache is due to neuronal dysfunction. The theory is that there is a low cerebral threshold and when precipitating factors exceed this threshold the attack occurs. This low threshold may be inherited. Other symptoms

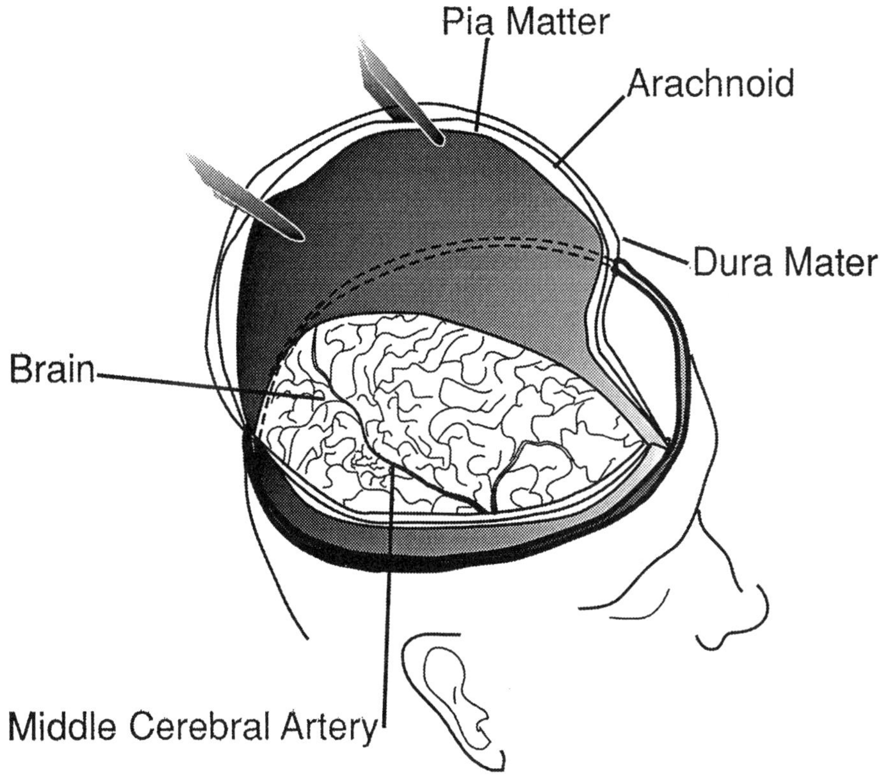

Figure 3.2 This illustration shows the layer covering the brain, called the *pia mater*; above that is the *arachnoid membrane.* Above that is the *dura mater.* Other than some parts of the dura mater, the rest are not pain sensitive; however, some of the large blood vessels traversing through these membranes can cause pain. The dura mater is a dense, fibrous structure with an inner and an outer layer. These layers are generally fused, except where they separate to provide space for the venous sinuses. The outer layer attaches to the inner surface of the cranial bones and sends vascular and fibrous extensions into the bone. The inner layer encloses some of the venous sinuses and forms partitions within the brain. The pia mater is a thin connective tissue membrane close to the brain and it carries blood vessels supplying the nervous tissues. It extends into the sulci and fissures throughout the brain. The arachnoid is a delicate nonvascular membrane between the dura and pia maters. It is separated from the overlying dura by a subdural space, and from the underlying pia mater by the subarachnoid space, which contains cerebrospinal fluid.

appear neural, such as prodromal symptoms that cannot be explained by the vascular theory. Prodromal symptoms often occur long before the attack. These symptoms may include euphoria, depression, hunger, loss of appetite, thirst, yawning, craving for certain foods, and many other symptoms. The aura, usually visual, must be neural. The vascular theory does not explain why the headaches are often unilateral or why, when taking a hot bath or exercising, which dilates the arteries, migrainers don't necessarily get headache attacks. The proponents of the neural theory question how the vascular proponents explain why dietary, hormonal, and stress factors and bright lights, loud noises, and strong odors cause these headaches. The neural theorists state that defects in motor movements, sensory activity, memory, language, visual and spatial perception must be neural.

If one looks at all the symptoms of migraine one has to come away with the concept that we seem to be dealing with a combined neurovascular hypothesis. That is, that there is a state of central neuronal hyperexcitability that sets off the vascular system.

In the last eight years, a great deal of work by distinguished scientists have begun to unravel some of the causes of what makes headache hurt. A particular neurotransmitter (a chemical that

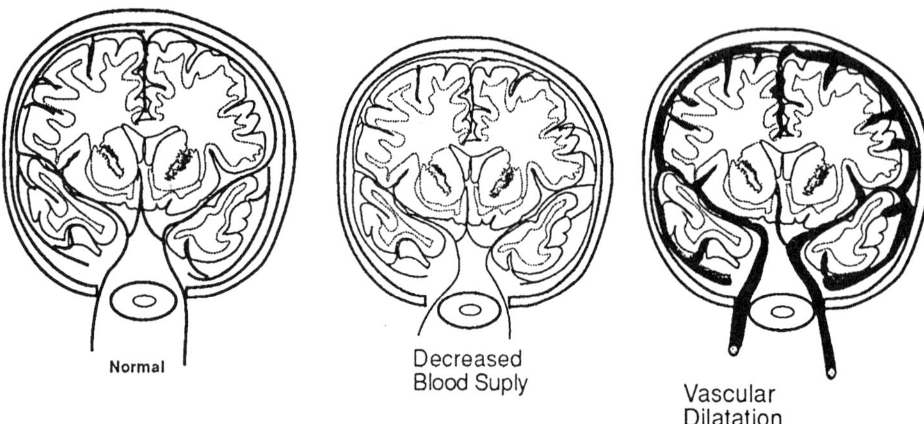

Figure 3.3 The vascular theory of migraine. (A) The normal vascular size, pre-headache; (B) the constriction phase (painless) prior to the dilation phase — this phase was considered the origin of the auras. (C) Represents the final stage of dilatation, which is responsible for the pain of migraine. The more recent neurovascular hypothesis has a different explanation for the mechanism of migraine and pain.

informs one nerve what the other nerve is thinking), called 5-hydroxytryptamine, or 5-HT or serotonin, seems to be very significant in the pathophysiology of migraine. The reason migraine is so important to notice is that many of the headaches that are associated with post trauma accidents are migraine-like headaches. Possible causes of migraine may be due to inadequate synthesis of 5-HT, or excessive breakdown of 5-HT. There may also be a formation of unstable 5-HT or an abnormality of 5-HT receptor function. It has been known for some time now that during a migraine attack blood levels of 5-HT decrease, while the breakdown products of 5-HT or 5-hydroxyindoleacetic acid increase in the urine. It is also known that drugs that deplete 5-HT (e.g., reserpine) may trigger a migraine attack. The administration of 5-HT intravenously could abort migraine, and some drugs used to treat migraine have a high affinity for 5-HT receptors.

The evidence to support the serotonin theory is the following. There is some evidence that gastrointestinal problems which some people experience with a migraine may be due to instability of serotonergic transmission in the nerves that innervate the stomach (myenteric plexus). The number of 5-HT receptors decreases with age, which may explain why migraine seems to diminish with age. In the brainstem there is an area that has a high concentration of serotonin called the dorsal raphe, and during sleep these cells seem to stop firing. This may explain why some patients can abort their attack by just going to sleep. Raskin[7] found that when electrodes to reduce pain from other causes were put into the brain near the dorsal raphe, even though the pain to the lower back was reduced some of these patients complained of migraine. The explanation for this is that the electrification of the dorsal rapha nucleus disturbed serotonergic neurotransmission. When Glaxo Pharmaceutical Co.[6] began its research on sumatriptan (Imitrex), a drug to abort migraine, it commissioned many researchers to investigate how this drug works. What they found is that there are many different types of serotonin (5-HT) receptor sites. This was extremely important because they found that different migraine medications work on different receptor sites. When a nerve sends an impulse to another nerve it transmits this message through a synapse, and therefore there is a presynaptic receptor site and a postsynaptic receptor site. They found that certain drugs, which are agonists, work on the prereceptor site, and some drugs, which are antagonists work on the postreceptor sites. It is interesting to observe that many of the drugs that are used to abort the migraine attack work on the prereceptor site and those used to prevent migraine attacks work on the postreceptor site.

The actual pathway of the pain fibers involves intricate actions of the nervous system (Figure 3.4). There are pain fiber pathways transmitting pain from the face, head, and neck regions. These

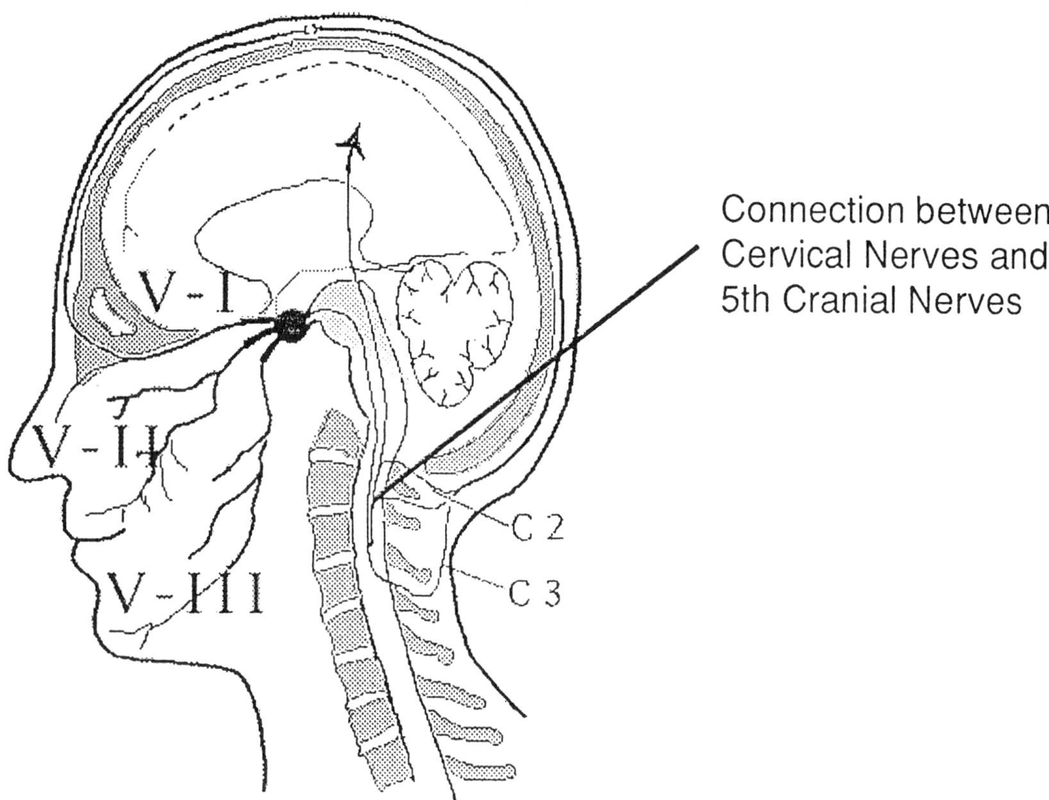

Figure 3.4 This illustration again demonstrates beneath the skin that the trigeminal or fifth cranial nerve (**V**) and its divisions I, II or III, plus irritation of the cervical nerves C1, C2, or C3, can send messages to the brain and the brain in turn will interpret the pain. There is also a connection between the cervical nerves in a lower segment of the trigeminal nerve that comes down to the first cervical vertebra, and this connection sends messages from the cervical nerves to the trigeminal nerve and vice versa. Therefore, someone who may be having irritation in the back of the neck may end up with pain in the front of the face as a result of these connections. This will be demonstrated in the chapters on whiplash and cervicogenic headache.

pain fibers are either small fibers that are covered with myelin, a fatty sheath, which transmit sharp pain, or larger and slower fibers that do not have this fatty sheath and which transmit pain that is aching and burning. These fibers terminate in a part of the spinal cord called the dorsal horn. After that, secondary fibers go from the dorsal horn of the spinal cord to the brain in an area called the thalmus. These travel by a tract called the spinal thalamic tract. The chemical that transmits the pain is a neuropeptide called substance P. This system also has a balance to inhibit pain. In the dorsal horn of thc spinal cord are interneurons that inhibit the action of the pain chemicals (substance P), and these chemicals are called enkephalins and to a lesser degree GABA or gamma-aminobutyric acid.

There are two pathways: one is called the serotonergic and the other is called the adrenergic pathway. They are pain controlling systems and, starting in the midbrain, they both have tracts that go to the upper brain and down to the spinal cord. The ascending serotonergic system starts in the brain and goes up to the thalmus and continues to the cortex of the brain. This system appears to be involved with cerebral blood flow, sleep, and neuroendocrine control. The descending serotonergic system starts in the midbrain (periaqueductal gray, PAG), travels through the pons, and connects (synapses) in the medulla (raphe magnus) and from there connects to the spinal cord (dorsal horn) of the first, second, and third cervical roots and to the spinal tract of the fifth cranial nerve (trigeminal nerve). The chemicals or neurotransmitters, norepinephrine, serotonin, and opiates

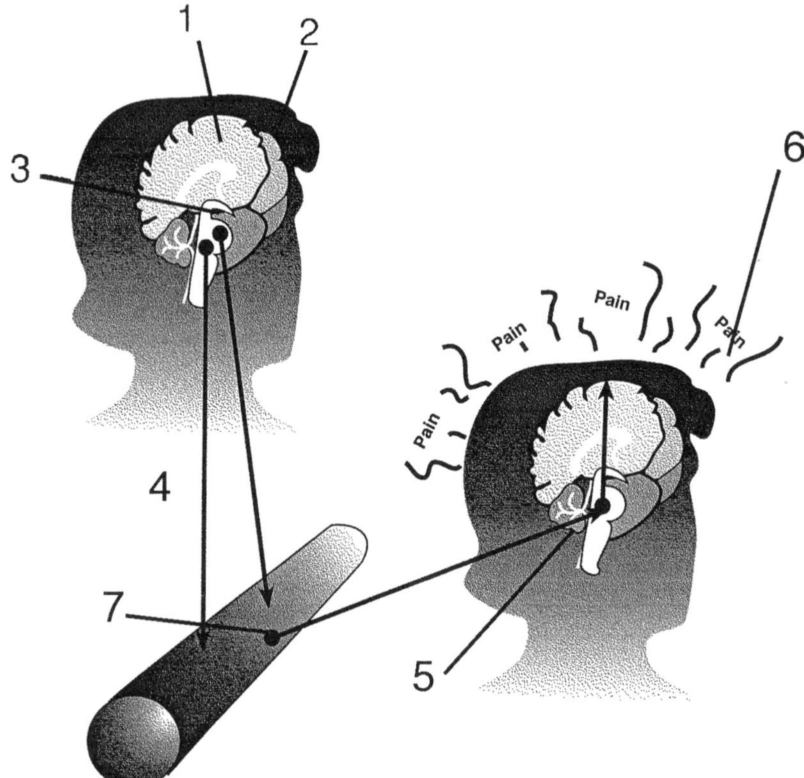

1. Triggering factors: hunger, fatigue, hormones, stress, senses
2. Threshold
3. Locus ceruleus and dorsal raphe nuclei
4. Activates neuro-inflammatory mediators.
5. Meninges
6. Awareness of pain
7. Pain chemicals

Figure 3.5 The neurovascular hypothesis of migraine or vascular headaches. (**1**) There are external or internal triggering factors that exceed (**2**) a threshold that different individuals have. When the threshold is exceeded, there is activation of (**3**) 5-HT (5-hydroxytryptamine) and norepinephrine-containing neurons in the locus ceruleus and dorsal raphe nuclei in the brainstem. (**4**) This activation alters the physiology of these neurons and eventually the blood cells, and generates pain-provoking chemicals (neuroinflammatory mediators) within the cerebral cortex and the supporting tissues. (**5**) These mediators activate pain receptors in the trigeminal vascular terminals within the coverings of the brain (meninges), which then stimulate neurons in the (**6**) brainstem and the thalamus and cerebral cortex that creates awareness of pain. (**7**) The activation by these pain chemicals, substance P, neurokinin A, and CGRP (calitonian gene-related piptide), causes a sterile inflammation that sensitizes nerve endings and causes dilatation of the arteries of the head and increased pain. If the migraine is not treated immediately, and these chemicals are permitted to stay around the nerve blood vessels, this may add to the length of time of the headache pain.

inhibit pain transmission from most regions of the head and neck. The adrenergic system also has ascending and descending pathways. The ascending system starts in the pons of the brain and travels to the cortex of the brain. The descending noradrenergic system starts in the pons of the brainstem (locus ceruleus) and travels through the medulla to the spinal cord.

Therefore, in this system there exist two ongoing processes, one to carry the message of pain and one to inhibit pain. What appears to take place (Figure 3.5) is that there are triggering factors that exceed the threshold that inhibits pain. This threshold maybe a genetic or inherited factor. The triggering factors vary and can be any one of many reasons that a migraine attack occurs. Some of these triggering factors are hunger, fatigue, hormones, stress, or any factor that can precipitate a migraine attack. Once the pain threshold is exceeded, the serotonergic (5-HT) and the adrenergic neurons are activated in the brainstem (locus cerulus and dorsal raphe). This activation alters the physiology of the neurons, the supporting tissue (glia) and blood vessels, and causes pain, provoking neuroinflammatory chemical mediators to react within the cerebral cortex and the supporting tissue. These chemical mediators activate the impulses of the nerve centers, giving rise to the sensations of pain (nociceptors) of the 5th cranial nerve (trigeminal nerve). The part of the trigeminal system that is affected is called the trigeminovascular afferent terminals in the meninges (the coverings of the brain), which in turn stimulate neurons in the brainstem, thalmus, and cerebral cortex to create the awareness of pain.

When these nerve centers are activated, various chemical mediators are released (substance P, neurokinin A, and CGRP [calcitonian gene-related peptide]) causing a sterile inflammatory process which sensitizes nerve endings, causes dilatation of the arteries of the head and increased pain (hyperalgesia), and this pain is sustained long after the initial trigger has disappeared. This is why the pain of migraine can last so long, and why it is important to abort this acute onset as soon as possible.[1-7]

Although this may seem to be a complicated chapter, many of the neuroanatomical, neurophysiological, and neurochemical terms have been avoided that would add more confusion and not clarify the point. What is important is that when cervical acceleration/deceleration syndrome (whiplash) is discussed in Part two of this book, the explanation of why headaches persist after head and neck trauma will be better understood.

REFERENCES

1. Lance, J.W., *Mechanism and Management of Headache*, 3rd ed., Butterworths, London, 1978.
2. Dalessio, D.J., *Wolff's Headache and Other Head Pain*, 4th ed., Oxford University Press, New York, 1980.
3. Diamond, S., Dalessio, D.J., *The Practicing Physician's Approach to Headache*, 4th ed., Williams & Wilkins, Baltimore, 1986.
4. Saper, J.R., Silberstein, S.D., Gordon, C.D., Hamel, R.L., *Handbook of Headache Management*, Williams & Wilkins, Baltimore, 1993.
5. Silberstein, S.D., Advances in understanding the pathophysiology of headache, *Neurology*, 42(3), Suppl. 2, 6-10, 1992.
6. Cerenex Pharmaceuticals, Slide Lecture Kit to Medical Profession, 1993.
7. Raskin, N.H., *Headache*, 2nd ed., Churchill Livingstone, New York, 1988.

Chapter 4

The Headache Intake Form

Without taking a proper headache history, it is almost impossible to make an accurate diagnosis. It cannot be over-emphasized how important the accuracy of this information is. This chapter will be devoted to the way I take a history and there will be blank forms at the back of the book for you to fill in. As you read the different chapters, I will use histories I have obtained from my patients that will give you an idea of how you can define your own problems. The first part of the book will be devoted to many types of headache problems and the second part will be devoted to the headaches caused by physical trauma. Again, as I have said earlier, you will find that headaches, regardless of the triggering mechanisms, are very similar and it will be important to differentiate between vascular (arteries), muscle, sinus, and intracranial pressure. The intake of nontrauma headaches requires less information concerning the actual event that precipitated the headache because of not having to deal with a legal format. Converting medical terminology into legal terminology at times becomes exasperating because there are some words and symptoms that when translated do not have the same meaning. This is why one has to be meticulous in the accuracy of the information given.

Age is important, because different ages give clues as to what may be happening to that individual. Many times women who have hormonal migraine may take on a totally different pattern of headaches after menopause. Older people may also experience a change in the character of their headaches or they may have been headache-free all their lives and all of a sudden they have daily headaches.

When children present with headaches, it is important to differentiate whether there is a problem at home or at school that is causing them to be in a stressful situation, or they are genetically predisposed to migraine at this time, or whether this calls our attention to a possible intracranial problem.

Gender or sex tells the examiner a great deal. As an example, women suffer migraine three to four times more than men because of hormonal influences. We ask about race because African Americans have a higher incidence of high blood pressure and kidney disease than Caucasians and this contributes to headache. I'm always interested in where a person was born and if they have moved a great deal, and if they have recently moved and if this was a positive move or has it created tension for them?

Occupation is obviously important. Is there stress or are there any occupational hazards, such as chemicals or other physical problems, that may precipitate headaches? It is important to find out if the patient was in the armed service and whether there was a medical discharge and if that was related to headaches. An accident history will help inform the examiner whether these headaches are accident related. If there were headaches before the accident, then fill out both the non-headache form and the intake form on post trauma headaches.

I have found that by simplifying the intake form it is much easier to assess the essential information and therefore easier to make a diagnosis. Most patients often start out describing their symptoms by giving you a diagnosis, which only confuses the examiner and the patient. The patient often starts the interview by saying, "My sinus headache started three years ago, and my stress headache started one year ago, and my cluster headache started six months ago, etc., etc." I have always been amazed how a simple approach to diagnosing the problem is complicated by misinformation. The approach I have is to break the pain into three categories:

Incapacitating (#3), or a number 3 headache: A no. 3 headache or incapacitating headache is the most severe headache you can have. A no. 3 headache means you cannot function (incapacitating). When a person has a no. 3 or incapacitating headache he or she must go to bed, stay frozen in a sitting position, pace, or position themselves in any way to reduce the amount of pain.

Interfering (#2), or a number 2 headache: A no. 2 headache or interfering headache is a moderate to severe headache. When this headache is in its moderate phase one can generally perform essential tasks with discomfort (sometimes using medications), but will not be able to do enjoyable things. When this headache is in the severe form, essential tasks are done with a great deal of difficulty and the person is very limited. This severe headache is a step away from becoming a no. 3 or incapacitating headache.

Irritating (#1), or a number 1 headache: A no. 1 headache or irritating headache is an annoying headache that is often relieved by over-the-counter medications or massaging. A more painful no. 1 headache is often a step before a no. 2 or interfering headache.

When filling out the *medical headache history* start with the:

Onset: Start with the headache that you are currently concerned about. How long ago did it start and how often do you get it (frequency)? Was there any other kind of headache that you had before and when did that start and what was the frequency? Again, mention as many different kinds of headaches as you think you had and when did they start and what was their frequency. If any of them started as a result of an accident or any other precipitating factor that you recall, such as menstruation, going on birth control pills, an infection, an allergic reaction, or any incident, it is important to make sure you include that in the history. *Again, break these down into categories of pain, incapacitating #3, interfering #2, and irritating #1.*

Current frequency: Whether you have one or more types of headaches, what is the current frequency? Have they increased, stayed the same, or decreased since their onset, and do you think they changed over time (biologically), or did they change because of treatment or any alterations that you have attempted to improve your problem? Any information that you have about frequency is important for the physician. Also, describe the number of headache attacks you have in one day: one, two, fifteen, etc. *Again, break these down into categories, #3, #2, and #1.*

Time of onset: When do you notice these headaches start? Is it in the morning, later in the day, after you get home from work, after your spouse gets home? Weekdays, weekends, holidays, entertaining friends at home, going to dress up for various functions, making a presentation at work, menstruation, ovulation, activity in sports, climbing upstairs, lifting heavy objects? List any relation to anything that goes on that starts your headache. Time of onset really means the time of day. Often the time that your headache starts can help in the diagnosis. The other information can be placed under the heading "Precipitating or Aggravating Factors" further down on the intake form. *Again, break these down into categories #3, #2, #1.*

Duration: How long does this intensity last without medication and with medication? What other conditions will reduce or increase the duration? Duration can be described in seconds, minutes, hours, or days. Are the attacks multiple or are they continuous? For example, are there twenty attacks a day lasting thirty seconds to a minute, or two attacks a day, each an hour to an hour and a half, or one headache that lasts two to six hours? Are there two or three types of headache, each having its own duration? These are important facts to know. Try to average these durations and not get too wordy. *Again, break these down into categories #3, #2, #1.*

Character: The character of the pain is extremely important and often is a lead in diagnosing the type of headache you have. There are many adjectives to describe pain; however, the physician would like to know if you feel the following: *throbbing, pulsating, stabbing, burning, ice pick, tight, dull, aching, exploding internal pressure, a hot poker*, or any word that best describes your pain. Too many words confuse the character of the headache and it is best to use one or two words that you feel initially. Remember, different classes of headache demonstrate different symptoms and if you just fill in a lot of words you distract the interviewer from the proper association. *Remember, incapacitating #3, interfering #2, and irritating #1.*

Prodrome or aura: Prodromes are warning signs that headache are going to start. Some people know one or two days before the headache starts. Symptoms such as diarrhea, frequent urination, queasy feelings, abdominal cramps, and giddiness, are signs that signal an upcoming headache attack. Most sufferers do not get any warning. Auras are seen with migraine about 15% of the time. Sometimes, auras are seen with headaches caused by a neurological problem. On occasion auras may exist with no headache pain. They generally appear thirty minutes before the headache and disappear when the pain starts. Some will continue through the attack and some rarely stay on after the pain goes into remission. They are seen as flashing lights, wavy lines, patterns like a fortress, distorted and colorful images, blind spots, etc. Some people will complain of tingling sensations in the face, arms, feet, and some will complain of weakness or a feeling of paralysis in their arms, hands, or feet. All these symptoms are important to report to your physician. These symptoms should be entered with the categories of pain, #3, #2, #1. Most of the time when a form is filled out and all the intensities are listed the auras appear in the #3 and rarely in the #2 categories.

Associating features: These are very important to identify to the interviewer. On the form, you will be asked to circle the following: nausea, vomiting, sensitivity to light, noise, odors. Do you get pale or flushed? Do your eyes get red or run? Does your nose get stuffy or run? Does your eyelid droop? Do you lie down? Do you have to sit, or do you have to pace? Any feature you are aware of or someone notices is important to note. List these features that are noticed with the headache. Make sure you put them in the intensity chart, #3, #2, #1.

Precipitating or aggravating factors: This is your opportunity to help your physician understand what you have kept in your secret store about what fears you have in daily living experiences that incapacitate you and make you miss days, weeks, and months each year. There is not enough room to list all these factors and now you will have a chance to make your own list. The following is an example of some of the factors that you have experienced. Does any kind of movement, such as climbing stairs, running, neck movements, or any type of exercise cause headache, including sex? Does any type of food or drink (aged cheese, hot dogs, bacon, any type of preservative, MSG [monosodium glutamate], sugar substitutes, alcohol of any type, etc.) cause headache? Do changes in weather, humidity, barometric pressure, temperature, or any other changes cause headache? Do things like pressure changes in airplanes, skiing, missing meals, menstrual periods, tension, fear, arguments, etc., trigger a headache? Any of these factors or others may trigger a headache and also contribute to the diagnosis and also the treatment. There was a patient of mine who would wake in the morning with a severe throbbing headache and miss enough work that her employer, though empathetic to her pain, was about to fire her. She was diagnosed with migraine and with careful evaluation of her history I found if she didn't eat at least every six hours she would get an attack. I had her set her alarm at 3:00 a.m. each morning seven days a week, and eat a few plain crackers and go back to sleep. After that, when she arose for work at 7:00 a.m. she was free of headaches 80% of the time!

Remember, whatever you do during the week you must do on the weekend. Once you set a biological rhythm that works during the week, continue this on the weekend and holidays. Yes, once again let the physician know if these factors happen in your #3, #2, or #1 categories.

Location of the headache: On the headache form later in this chapter you will see outlines of the head. Mark the locations of the pain for each intensity of the headache. Use a different color to indicate the different intensity. In our office, we used RED for the incapacitating or #3 headache, GREEN for the Interfering or #2 headache, and PURPLE or BLUE for the irritating or #1 headache.

This form is used for all our headache patients. When a post accident or injury patient is seen more information is gathered about the accident because litigation is involved. The biomechanics of the accident may be crucial in determining the reason for the headache.

The rest of the medical history is necessary to help the physician to understand if there has been any medical, physiological or psychological triggering mechanisms that cause or aggravate the headache problem.

The menstrual history is very important because women suffer migraine three to four times more than men.

Information about the birth of the patient informs us as to oxygen starvation or brain damage that leaves a permanent mark.

It is interesting that about 65% of migraine patients may have had the following problems prepuberty (preadolescence): bedwetting, motion or car sickness (motion sickness often continues into adult life), and abdominal cramps before puberty.

Any history of meningitis, encephalitis, scarlet fever, and rheumatic fever could leave an ongoing persistent headache problem into adult life.

A history of sensitivity to alcohol, smoke-filled rooms, and stimulants such as caffeine and mood elevators is a major problem for migraine sufferers.

The medical history is very important because there are about 300 different conditions that may cause headaches. It is also important that the physician is aware of all medical conditions and all medications the patient is on to avoid any interference with headache medication.

All surgical procedures are also important.

Psychiatric and psychological treatment and medications are very important to see how much these conditions trigger headache attacks.

About twelve years ago a very brilliant rocket engineer came to see me after leaving California where he worked on a secret space program. In his travels through seven states, he saw many doctors and was treated for an assortment of headaches. After a great deal of probing it became obvious that he could not stand the strain of his job and fled from his workplace. Because he was dealing with classified material, he thought the CIA was after him. I diagnosed him as a paranoid schizophrenic and felt his headaches were delusional as a means of dealing with his anxiety. He was sent to a psychiatrist and put on the proper medication for his nervous breakdown and his headaches went into remission.

Family history is very important, because a high percentage (more than 50%) of migraine sufferers have a family member who had severe headaches. It is also important to see if there is any disease that may run in the family. A marriage history with knowledge of the children will also help predict a family linkage to migraine headaches.

Stress factors are obvious to know about, again looking for triggering mechanisms.

Vegetative signs help the physician to recognize symptoms of depression. Depression alters serotonin and decreased serotonin in the brain could cause headaches.

It is imperative that the physician be aware of all the medications and any pharmaceuticals to which the patient is either allergic or hypersensitive. Attached to the medical history form is a list of many drugs that have been used for headache control.

The last sheet requests information on all the people who have treated you for headache and their professional titles and their specialty. All treatments and tests done are extremely important.

The physical and neurological examination will be done by the physician and any tests required will be determined, and then a diagnosis will be made and initial therapy that is agreeable to the patient will begin.

Medical Headache History

Name______________________________ **Date**____________________________

Referred by____________________________________ **Age** __________________

Date of Birth _________ **Sex** ___ **Birthplace** _________ **Education** ______________

Occupation ________________ **Armed Service & type of discharge** ________________

	Incapacitating #3	**Interfering #2**	**Irritating #1**
Onset: When did these start? Note if accident or incident started the headache or made a preexisting headache worse.			
Current Frequency: Compared with the frequency at onset, what is the frequency now?			
Time of Onset: Time of day, weekdays, weekends, menstrual time, end of the working day, etc.			
Duration: How long does this intensity last without medication? With medication? Seconds, minutes, hours, days, etc.			
Character: Throbbing, pulsating, stabbing, burning, ice pick, tight, dull, aching, exploding feeling or any words you want to use to describe your pain.			
Prodrome or Aura: Prodromes are warning signs that you are doing to get a headache (up to 24 hours before), like diarrhea, frequent urination, queasy feelings, nausea, etc. Auras are signals you get right before your headache, blind spots, light flashes, wavy lines, tingling, weakness in hands or feet, etc.			

Associating Features: Circle any features that you get with this type of headache.	Nausea; vomiting; sensitivity to light, noise, odors? Do you get pale or flush? Do your eyes or nose run or get stuffy? Does the white of your eyes get red? Does your eyelid droop? Do you pace or go to bed?	Nausea; vomiting; sensitivity to light, noise, odors? Do you get pale or flush? Do your eyes or nose run or get stuffy? Does the white of your eyes get red? Does your eyelid droop? Do you pace or go to bed?	Nausea; vomiting; sensitivity to light, noise, odors? Do you get pale or flush? Do your eyes or nose run or get stuffy? Does the white of your eyes get red? Does your eyelid droop? Do you pace or go to bed?
Precipitating or aggravating factors: Does anything make your headache worse? Any kind of movement? (climbing stairs, running, neck movements, etc.) Does food, alcohol (wines, etc.), weather, humidity, pressure changes in airplanes, skiing, missing meals, menstrual periods or anything else worsen or precipitate them?			
Location of the headache: You will be asked to mark the location for each type of headache with a different color pen. Incapacitating #3 = Red; Interfering #2= Green; Irritating #1=Blue.	LEFT RIGHT RIGHT LEFT LEFT RIGHT		

Menstrual History:

At what age did it begin? _____________ .
Were they regular or irregular? How are they related to your headache?
Are you or were you ever on Birth Control Pills and did they effect your headache?
Have you had a hysterectomy, partial or total, and why?
Are you in menopause, and if yes, how long?
Are you on hormones, and if yes, which ones?

Past History:

1. Did you have a normal birth? yes no
   a) forceps used? yes no
   b) Caesarean Section? yes no
2. Did you have problems with bedwetting? yes no
   a) If yes, age bedwetting stopped? __________
3. Were you car sick as a child (motion)?
   a) If yes, how severe? slight moderate severe

4. Did you have unexplained abdominal cramps as a child? yes no
5. Did you have any of the following illnesses in childhood?
   a) meningitis yes no
   b) encephalitis yes no
   c) scarlet fever yes no
   d) rheumatic fever yes no
6. Did you have any head injuries as a child? yes no
7. Were you treated for emotional illness as a child? yes no

Habits:

8. Do you drink alcohol? yes no
   a) If yes; what kind and how much? ____________________
   b) Does alcohol bring on or aggravate a headache? yes no
9. Do you smoke? yes no
   a) If yes, how much? ____________________
   b) Does smoking or smoke filled rooms cause or aggravate your headache? yes no
10. Do you drink caffeinated beverages? yes no
   a) If yes, how much? ____________________

Medical History:

Have you ever been or are you currently being treated for any of the following?
- a) high blood pressure yes no
- b) stomach ulcers yes no
- c) asthma yes no
- d) allergies yes no
- e) pneumonia yes no
- f) kidney problems yes no
- g) low blood sugar yes no
- h) glaucoma yes no
- i) diabetes yes no
- j) heart problems yes no

List all other medical problems you have had in the past. Include date diagnosed and any treatment. **DO NOT LIST OPERATIONS.**

____
____
____
____

Surgical History (List operations and date performed.)

____
____
____
____

Psychiatric History (List visits with counselors, psychologists, etc., and type of treatment)

____
____

____
____
____

Accidents in Adult Life: (Briefly describe any accident that caused any blow to the head or that you feel is related to your headache.)

____
____
____
____
____
____

Family History:

1) Is your father living? yes no
Age______
Cause of death________________________________
Was/is there a headache history? yes no

2) Is your mother living? yes no
Age__________
Cause of death?______________________________
Was/is there a headache history? yes no

3) Ages of brothers--Circle the ones with headache.

____

4) Ages of sisters---Circle the ones with headache.

____

5) List any other blood relatives with a history of severe headaches

____

Marital History:

List marriages:
1st marriage age______to______ Did spouse have headache? yes no
2nd marriage age______to______ Did spouse have headache? yes no
3rd marriage age______to______ Did spouse have headache? yes no
________ ________________ ________________________

Age of current spouse________________

List ages and sex of all children:

Age______ Sex ______ Headaches? yes no
Age______ Sex ______ Headaches? yes no
Age______ Sex ______ Headaches? yes no
Age______ Sex ______ Headaches? yes no
Age______ Sex ______ Headaches? yes no

Age______ Sex ______ Headaches? yes no

Stress Factors:

List any factors that may be affecting your headaches (money, loneliness, sexual problems, work, etc.)

____

____

____

____

Vegetative Signs:

1) Do you have trouble falling asleep?	yes	no
2) Do you have trouble staying asleep?	yes	no
3) Has you appetite decreased?	yes	no
4) Have you gained or lost weight in the past year?	yes	no
5) Have you felt tearful or depressed lately?	yes	no
6) Have you had any thoughts of wanting to die?	yes	no
7) Have you been forgetful lately?	yes	no
8) Any other changes in your normal day to day living?		

Please list any medications you are allergic or sensitive to:

____

____

Please List Medications you are currently taking (include dosages and frequency per day)

____

____

The following is a list of medications often given to headache patients. Circle the medications you have taken for headache treatment. *No list of medications is ever complete. Add any other medications you have taken.*

CHECK MEDICATIONS THAT YOU HAVE TAKEN FOR HEADACHE TREATMENT

BRAND NAME	GENERIC	EFFECTIVE	YES	NO
BETA BLOCKERS				
Inderal	Propranolol		☐	☐
Corgard	Nadolol		☐	☐
Lopressor	Metoprolol		☐	☐
Tenormin	Atenolol		☐	☐
Catapres	Clonidine		☐	☐
CALCIUM CHANNEL BLOCKERS				
Calan	Verapamil		☐	☐
Isoptin	Verapamil		☐	☐
Procardia	Nifedipine		☐	☐
Nimotop	Nimodipine		☐	☐
Cardene	Nicardipine		☐	☐
Cardizem	Diltiazem		☐	☐
LITHIUM				
Eskalith	Lithium carbonate		☐	☐
Lithobid	Lithium carbonate		☐	☐
Lithane	Lithium carbonate		☐	☐
ANTICONVULSANTS				
Dilantin	Phenytoin		☐	☐

BRAND NAME	GENERIC	EFFECTIVE	YES	NO
Tegretol	Carbamazepine		☐	☐
Depakote	Valproic acid		☐	☐
MUSCLE RELAXANTS				
Soma	Carisoprodol		☐	☐
Flexeril	Cyclobenzaprine		☐	☐
Norflex	Orphenadrine		☐	☐
Norgesic	Orphenadrine		☐	☐
Parafon Forte	Chlorzoxazone		☐	☐
Robaxin	Methocarbamol		☐	☐
Skelaxin	Metaxalone		☐	☐
MAO INHIBITORS				
Nardil	Phenelzine sulfate		☐	☐
Pamate	Tranylcypromine		☐	☐
SEROTONIN ACTIVE MEDICATIONS				
Elavil	Amitriptyline		☐	☐
Pamelor	Nortriptyline		☐	☐
Vivactil	Protriptyline		☐	☐
Sinequan	Doxepin		☐	☐
Adapin	Doxepin		☐	☐
Norpramin	Desipramine		☐	☐
Wellbutrin	Bupropion HCl		☐	☐

BRAND NAME	GENERIC	EFFECTIVE	YES	NO
Desyrel	Trazodone HCl		☐	☐
Tofranil	Imipramine		☐	☐
Ludiomil	Maprotiline		☐	☐
Ascendin	Amoxapine		☐	☐
Prozac	Fluoxetine		☐	☐
Zoloft	Sertraline		☐	☐
Luvox	Fluvoxamine		☐	☐
Paxil	Paroxetine		☐	☐
Effexor	Venlafaxine HCl		☐	☐
Periactin	Cyproheptadine HCl		☐	☐
ANXIOLYTICS / NEUROLEPTICS				
Librium	Chlordiazepoxide		☐	☐
Tranxene	Chlorazepate		☐	☐
Valium	Diazepam		☐	☐
Atarax	Hydroxyzine HCl		☐	☐
Ativan	Lorazepam		☐	☐
BuSpar	Buspirone HCl		☐	☐
Mellaril	Thioridazine HCl		☐	☐
Miltown	Meprobamate		☐	☐
Prolixin	Fluphenazine HCl		☐	☐
Serax	Oxazepam		☐	☐
Thorazine	Chlorpromazine		☐	☐
Triavil	Perphenazine/amitriptyline HCl		☐	☐

BRAND NAME	GENERIC	EFFECTIVE	YES	NO
Xanax	Alprazolam		☐	☐
NSAIDS				
Anaprox	Naproxen		☐	☐
Toradol	Ketorolac tromethamine		☐	☐
Orudis	Ketoprofen		☐	☐
Voltaren	Diclofenac sodium		☐	☐
Feldene	Piroxicam		☐	☐
Meclomen	Meclofenamate sodium		☐	☐
Motrin	Ibuprofen		☐	☐
Nalfon	Fenoprofen calcium		☐	☐
Indocin	Indomethacin		☐	☐
Clinoril	Sulindac		☐	☐
ANTIEMETICS				
Compazine	Prochlorperazine		☐	☐
Tigan	Trimethobenzamide HCl		☐	☐
Vistaril	Hydroxyzine		☐	☐
Reglan	Metoclopramide		☐	☐
Phenergan	Promethazine		☐	☐
Antivert	Meclizine HCl		☐	☐
Atarax	Hydroxyzine HCl		☐	☐
Benadryl	Diphenhydramine HCl		☐	☐
Bonine	Meclizine HCl		☐	☐

BRAND NAME	GENERIC	EFFECTIVE	YES	NO
Dramamine	Dimenhydrinate		☐	☐
ERGOTAMINES				
Bellergal-S	ergotamine/phenobarbital/bellafoline		☐	☐
Sansert	Methysergide		☐	☐
Cafergot tablets	ergotamine tartrate/caffeine		☐	☐
Cafergot suppositories	ergotamine tartrate/caffeine		☐	☐
Methergine	Methylergonovine		☐	☐
DHE 45	Dihydroergotamine mesylate		☐	☐
Imitrex	Sumatriptan succinate		☐	☐
Midrin	Isometheptene/dichloralphenazone/acetaminophen		☐	☐
COMPOUNDED ERGOTAMINES/ANALGESICS				
Ergo-Pac suppositories	Ergotamine/pentobarbital/atropine/caff.		☐	☐
Ergo-Pax + Pmz	Ergotamine/pentobarbital/atropine/caff./prometh		☐	☐
Ergo-Cap tablet	Ergotamine/pentobarbital/atropine/caff/prometh		☐	☐
Ergo-Cap + Pmz	Ergotamine/pentobarbital/atropine/caff/prometh		☐	☐
DHE Nasal Spray	Dihydroergotamine		☐	☐
DHE suppositories	Dihydroergotamine		☐	☐

BRAND NAME	GENERIC	EFFECTIVE	YES	NO
Oxycodone suppositories	Oxycodone		☐	☐
ANALGESICS				
Advil	Ibuprofen 200mg		☐	☐
Anexsia 5 & 7.5	Hydrocodone/acetaminophen		☐	☐
Axotal	Butalbital 50mg/ASA 650mg		☐	☐
Bancap HC	Hydrocodone 5mg/acetaminophen 500mg		☐	☐
Damason-P	Hydrocodone 5mg/ASA 500mg		☐	☐
Darvocet-N 100	Propoxyphene 100mg/acetaminophen 650mg		☐	☐
Darvocet-N 50	Propoxyphene 50mg/acetaminophen 325mg		☐	☐
Darvon Compound	Propoxyphene 32mg/ASA 389mg/caffeine 32mg		☐	☐
Darvon Compound-65	Propoxyphene 65mg/ASA 389mg/caffeine 32.4mg		☐	☐
Darvon-N	Propoxyphene napsylate		☐	☐
Darvon-N + ASA	Propoxyphene napsylate/ASA		☐	☐
Fioricet	Butalbital 50mg/acetominophen 325 mg/ caffeine 40mg		☐	☐
Fiorinal	Butalbital 50mg/ASA 325mg/caffeine 40mg		☐	☐
Fiorinal w/Codeine	Codeine phosphate 30mg/ASA 325mg/ caffeine 40mg/butalbital 50mg		☐	☐

BRAND NAME	GENERIC	EFFECTIVE YES	NO
Demerol	Meperidine HCl	☐	☐
Duocet	Hydrocodone 5mg/acetaminophen 500mg	☐	☐
Empirin	ASA 325mg	☐	☐
Empirin w/Codeine	ASA/codeine	☐	☐
Esgic	Butalbital/acetaminophen/caffeine	☐	☐
Esgic w/Codeine	Codeine/acetaminophen/caffeine	☐	☐
Lorcet	Hydrocodone bitartrate/acetaminophen	☐	☐
Medirim	Ibuprofen 200mg	☐	☐
Mepergan	Meperidine/promethazine	☐	☐
Nubaine	Nalbuphine HCl	☐	☐
Numorphan (inj./supp.)	Oxymorphone HCl	☐	☐
Percocet	Oxycodone HCl 5mg/acetaminophen 325mg	☐	☐
Percodan	Oxycodone HCl 4.5mg/oxycodone terephthalate 0.38mg/ASA 325mg	☐	☐
Percogesic	Phenyltoloxamine citrate;acetaminophen	☐	☐
Phenaphen w/codeine	Acetaminophen/codeine	☐	☐
Phrenilin	Butalbital/acetaminophen	☐	☐
Phrenilin w/codeine	Butalbital/codeine/acetaminophen	☐	☐
Stadol (inj. or nasal spray)	Butorphanol tartrate	☐	☐
Synalgos-DC	Dihydrocodeine bitartrate 16mg/ASA 356.4mg/caffeine 30mg	☐	☐
Talacen	Pentazocine HCl 25mg/acetaminophen 650mg	☐	☐

BRAND NAME	GENERIC	EFFECTIVE	YES	NO
Talwin Compound	Pentazocine HCl 12.5mg/aspirin 325mg		☐	☐
Talwin NX	Pentazocine HCl 50mg/naloxone 0.5mg		☐	☐
Tylox	Oxycodone 5mg/acetaminophen 500mg		☐	☐
Vicodin	Hydrocodone 5mg/acetaminophen 500mg		☐	☐
Zodone	Hydrocodone 5mg/acetaminophen 500mg		☐	☐

Previous Care:

1) List doctors who have treated you for headaches.

2) List any tests you have had for your headache (e.g. EEG, CT scan, MRI, X-ray, etc.)

3) List any other treatment you have had for your headache (e.g., biofeedback, acupuncture, chiropractic, or any other treatment you had.

The physical examination done by the physician will be done on this page.

PHYSICAL EXAMINATION - HEADACHE

Name____ Date______________________

T ____ P _______ R __ Ht. ______ Wt. ______ Visual ____ BP-R _____ BP-L __________

ALLERGIES ____

SCALP / FACE		CRANIAL NERVES	
asymmetry		I, II	smell, visual fields, fundi
lesions			
TMJ		III, IV, VI	strabismus, nystagmus, ptosis, pupil, e
vessel prominence			
		V	sensation, corneal reflex, jaw jerk
EYES			
conjunctiva		VII	facial movement, eyelid strength, smile wrinkle, frown
pupils			
fundi		VIII	vertigo, Weber, Rinne, tinnitus
bruits			
		IX, X	gagging, deglutination
NOSE			
		XI	sternocleidomastoid (turn head),, trapezius
EARS			
auditory canals		XII	tongue atrophy, deviation, strength
tympanic membranes			

MOUTH SINUSES NECK lymph nodes thyroid carotids LUNGS HEART ABDOMEN EXTREMITIES RECTAL / VAGINAL		Cerebellar: Romberg, finger to nose, diadochokinesis, heel-shin, tandem and heel toe walk Motor: atrophy, fasciculation, wasting, tremors muscle strength of arms, wrists, fingers toes Sensory: superficial tactile, pain and vibrations (wrists, elbows, knees, ankles), motion and positions of fingers, toes, 2-point discriminations Pulses: dorsalis pedis, posterior tibial and popliteal Reflexes: triceps, biceps, knee jerk, ankle jerk

COMMENTS:

Physician's Signature ______________________ Date__________

The following is additional information to be filled out for the person involved in an accident that may have caused a post trauma headache syndrome or a post headache whiplash syndrome.

Accidents: List all your accidents. Start with the most recent accident and then describe all other accidents working backwards. With all your accidents, describe whether there was any history of headache and neck pain and how long they lasted. When you describe the accident (if it involved an automobile), draw a description of how the vehicle was impacted and all the information concerning the speed and what happened to you after the vehicles collided. If possible, include the police report. **Use the headache intake forms to describe the headache and neck problems for each of the accidents described on the next page. Do Not Omit Any Accidents Or Previous Treatments For Headache.**

____

____

____

____

____

____

____

____

____

____

____

____

____

____

____

____

With these accidents, report the following:

1) Was there a loss of consciousness? Yes No

Were there any witnesses that saw you unconscious? Yes No

Do you think you were unconscious? Yes No

Explain:

____

____

____

2) Was there any loss of memory immediately before or after the accident? How do you know that? Yes No

____

____

____

3) Was there any alteration in your mental state at the time of the accident (feeling dazed, disoriented, confused, etc.)? Yes No

How do you know that?

____

____

____

4) Did you lose any sensation or movement in your face, neck, body, arms or legs? Yes No

Are there documents to support these claims?

____

____

____

5) Were/are any of the following symptoms a result of the accident and are they still present, or are they in a state of remission? *Unless you can document these symptoms or support these claims under cross examination, do not list them.*

			Which accident/s [dates]	**P**/for present	**R**/for remission
1. Headache	Yes	No			
2. Neck pain	Yes	No			
3. Lightheadedness	Yes	No			
4. Vertigo/dizziness	Yes	No			
5. Anxiety/nervousness	Yes	No			
6. Sleeping problems	Yes	No			
7. Depression	Yes	No			
8. Fatigue (mental/physical)	Yes	No			
9. Concentration problems	Yes	No			
10. Worries about health	Yes	No			
11. Impatience	Yes	No			
12. Restlessness	Yes	No			
13. Feeling disorganized	Yes	No			
14. Loss of interest	Yes	No			
15. Confusion	Yes	No			
16. Memory problems	Yes	No			

17. Sexual problems Yes No
18. Impotence Yes No
19. Light sensitivity Yes No
20. Noise sensitivity Yes No
21. Ringing in the ears Yes No
22. Outbursts of anger Yes No
22. Personality change Yes No
23. Intolerance to alcohol Yes No
24. Mood swings Yes No
25. Apathy Yes No
26. Arithmetic problems Yes No
27. Flashbacks Yes No
28. Nightmares Yes No
29. Tremors Yes No
30. Appetite change Yes No
31. Others Yes No
32. ____________ Yes No
33. ____________ Yes No
34. ____________ Yes No
35. ____________ Yes No

Explain any of the above symptoms in relationship with any of your accidents the best way you can in order for the examiner to understand the effect the accident had on you. Do not contrive symptoms for this report, because questionable symptoms will be held against you in your settlement.

____

____

____

This sheet will be filled out by your examiner:

Working Diagnosis and Discussion:

____

____

____

Recommended Tests:

____

____

____

Initial Therapy:

____

____

____

Final Diagnosis and Discussion:

____

____

____

We have now completed the headache intake form and will proceed with a discussion of the many diferent types of headaches.

CHAPTER 5

Muscle Contraction (Tension) Headache

There was a time not too long ago that the diagnosis of muscle tension or muscle contraction headache was easy to make. If it wasn't migraine, cluster, sinus, or caused by any other major medical problem, it was muscle tension headache. The thinking was that if the scalp muscles were tense and contracted around the skull (Figure 5.1) that was the cause of muscle contraction pain, and if you could relax these muscles the pain would go away. About ten years ago this whole concept began to change. What was considered to be an easy diagnosis has turned out to be much more complex and the treatment of these conditions is just as complex.

In 1962 the Ad Hoc Committee on Classification of Headache of the National Institute of Neurological Disease and Blindness (NINDB) defined muscle contraction or tension headache as follows: "ache or sensations of tightness, pressure, or constriction, varied in intensity, frequency and duration." These pains could be short or long lasting and were generally in the back of the head and neck (suboccipital), and were considered to be secondary to sustained contraction of the skeletal muscles. These muscle contractions were in the absence of any permanent structural change in the muscles and were generally considered to be a reaction to life stresses. Because of this classification, the headache was also called the stress headache, nervous headache, or tension headache, and was almost always referred to as a psychological problem.[1]

In 1988, The International Headache Society (IHS) developed and published a new classification on the diagnostic criteria of headache (see Chapter 2) and attempted to redefine this gray area of tension-type headache (see Table 5.1).

The difficulty of being accurate with this table is that one has to be dependent on subjective complaints and the lack of objective criteria. Before I mention the newer thinking on this mechanism, let's review what was always considered to be the plague of the tension headache.

It was always felt that, most of all, headache was muscle tension pain (Figure 5.1). The pain occurs on both sides of the head or anywhere around the head. It is described as band-like, or aching, pressing, tightening or dull. Many patients wake up with them, or they develop as the day goes on and often get worse. The headaches seem to wax and wane as the day progresses, and often if the headaches start as mild they become moderate to severe. Many patients complained that these headaches would usher in a migraine attack. Many of the symptoms that accompany migraine, such as throbbing, nausea, vomiting, light and noise sensitivity (photo- and sonophobia), etc., would not be associated with this tension headache. When these symptoms appeared we would diagnose these as two separate headaches, both tension and migraine. Tension headaches may start at any age and most childhood headaches were thought to be this type of headache. These symptoms may start in childhood and go into remission and disappear or they may reappear, or continue on

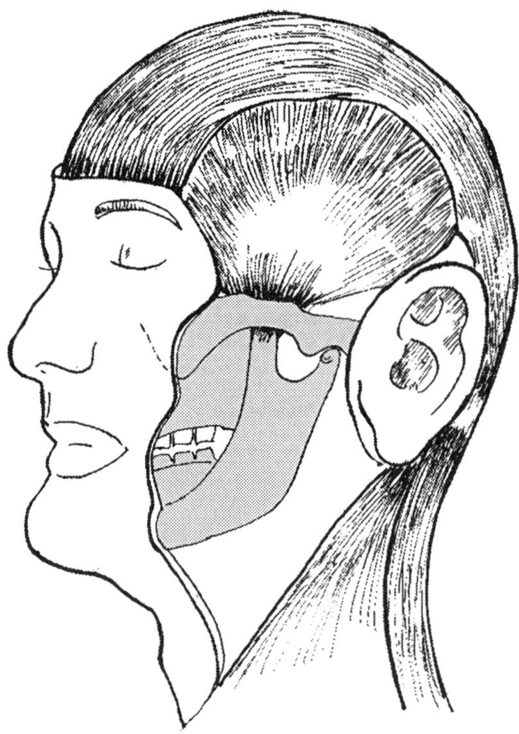

Figure 5.1 Muscles causing constriction and pain. There are many muscles around the skull and jaw and neck, both large and small, and it was always assumed that when these muscles spasmed or tightened a great deal, this was the origin of the muscle contraction/muscle tension headache. Studies have shown that there is more muscle contraction with migraine headaches than there are with muscle tension headaches. However, treatment to relax these muscles seems to be effective, although it is not certain specifically how these treatments work.

a daily basis. Many patients who have a combination of migraine and tension headaches may outgrow the migraine and continue with the tension type. The frequency of this problem varies, and some will have rare attacks while others could have them daily and the diagnosis would change from acute attacks to a chronic situation.

The terms tension and stress only contribute to the notion that muscle contraction headaches are all psychological, and that if you analyze the stress-provoking cause you can cure the headache. Unfortunately, this concept has prevented many people from seeking help for their misery. As we learn more about the mechanism of pain (see Chapter 3), we realize how many of these problems are physiological, chemical, neurological, and even genetic or inherited.[2,3]

As we learn more about the mechanism of headache pain, we are realizing that stress, tension, or anxiety are only a few of the many triggering factors that stimulate a headache. Most likely the brain has a predisposition for a low threshold that permits these triggering factors to start a neurophysiological course of headache pain.

At the present time we are focusing our attention on the serotonergic system, which is involved with sleep, dull pain, and emotions — both elation and depression. Many people with muscle contraction headaches also have associated problems with depression, insomnia, and panic attacks. However, some will get these same types of head pains with muscle spasm of the neck or back, carpal tunnel syndrome, muscle trigger points, poor posture, computer eye strain, arthritis in the

Table 5.1 International Headache Society Definition of Tension-Type Headache

2.1. Episodic tension-type headache
Previously used terms: tension headache, muscle contraction headache, psychomyogenic headache, stress headache, ordinary headache, essential headache, idiopathic headache, and psychogenic headache.
Diagnostic criteria:
- A. At least 10 previous headache episodes fulfilling criteria B-D listed below. Number of days with such headache <180/yr (<15/mo)
- B. Headache lasting from 30 minutes to 7 days
- C. At least two of the following pain characteristics:
  - 1) Pressing/tightening (non-pulsating) quality
  - 2) Mild or moderate intensity (may inhibit, but does not prohibit activities)
  - 3) Bilateral location
  - 4) No aggravation by walking stairs or similar routine physical activity
- D. Both of the following:
  - 1) No nausea or vomiting (anorexia may occur)
  - 2) Photophobia and phonophobia are absent, or one but not the other is present
- E. At least one of the following:
  - 1) History, physical, and neurologic examinations do not suggest one of the disorders listed in groups 5-11
  - 2) History and/or physical neurologic examinations do suggest such disorder, but it is ruled out by appropriate investigations
  - 3) Such disorder is present, but tension-type headache does not occur for the first time in close temporal relation to the disorder

2.1.2 Episodic tension-type headache associated with disorder of pericranial muscles
Previously used terms: muscle contraction headache
Diagnostic criteria:
- A. Fulfills criteria for 2.1
- B. At least one of the following:
  - 1) Increased tenderness of pericranial muscles demonstrated by manual palpation or pressure algometer
  - 2) Increased EMG (electromyogram) level of pericranial muscles at rest or during physiologic tests

2.1.3 Episodic tension-type headache unassociated with disorder of pericranial muscles
Previously used terms: idiopathic headache, essential headache, psychogenic headache
Diagnostic criteria:
- A. Fulfills criteria for 2.1
- B. No increased tenderness of pericranial muscles. If studied, EMG of pericranial muscles shows normal levels of activity

2.2 Chronic tension-type headache
Previously used terms: chronic daily headache
Diagnostic criteria:
- A. Average headache frequency >15 d/mo (180 d/yr) for >6 months fulfilling criteria B-D
- B. At least two of the following pain characteristics:
  - 1) Pressing/tightening quality
  - 2) Mild or moderate severity (may inhibit but does not prohibit activities)
  - 3) Bilateral location
  - 4) No aggravation by walking stairs or similar routine physical activity
- C. Both of the following:
  - 1) No vomiting
  - 2) No more than one of the following: nausea, photophobia, or phonophobia
- D. At least one of the following:
  - 1) History, physical, and neurologic examinations do not suggest one of the disorders listed in groups 5-11
  - 2) History and/or physical and/or neurologic examinations do suggest such disorder, but it is ruled out by appropriate investigations
  - 3) Such disorder is present, but tension-type headache does not occur for the first time in close temporal relation to the disorder

2.2.1 Chronic tension-type headache associated with disorder of pericranial muscles

2.2.2 Chronic tension-type headache unassociated with disorder of pericranial muscles

neck, and irritation to the nerves in the back of the head (occipital).[4,5] Most of the above issues are discussed in Part two of this book, where injury to the head and neck are discussed.

Currently, headache experts agree that tension headache is most likely a form or variant of migraine. Often these headaches, in their spectrum of intensities, have similar symptoms and respond to the same medications and non-medication therapies. Both headaches may have bilateral pain, and have nausea, photosensitivity, and similar male-to-female ratio and hereditary patterns. Another interesting point is that epidemiological studies could not distinguish tension headache from migraine on clinical or physiological grounds. This has led specialists to believe that both these types of headaches may have the same pathophysiology and therefore should not be considered separately. The likelihood is that these headaches just represent opposite poles of the same type of headache.[2,6]

Treatment of these headaches will not be discussed in Part one of this book and only those treatments that are related to the post traumatic types of headaches (similar to these headaches) are addressed. There are many excellent books that deal with the current approaches to the treatment of headaches and these are listed in the back of this book.

To summarize the tension-type headache, we categorize two areas, episodic tension-type headache and chronic tension-type headache. The chronic headache problem will be discussed in a separate chapter.

Episodic tension-type headache was previously described as tension headache, muscle contraction headache, psychomyogenic headache, stress headache, ordinary headache, essential headache, idiopathic headache, and psychogenic headache.

The International Headache Society feels before making this diagnosis there should have been at least 10 previous episodes of the following criteria:

- Headache lasting from 30 minutes to 7 days
- Pressing/tightening (non-pulsating/non-throbbing) quality
- Mild to moderate intensity (it should not stop normal activities)
- Bilateral location
- No aggravation by walking stairs or similar physical activity
- No nausea or vomiting
- May not have both photophobia and sonophobia, but may have one or the other
- That this headache does not have a neurological or medical condition that produces similar types of symptoms (Figure 5.2)

Another classification of this headache is episodic tension-type headache associated with disorder of pericranial muscles. This means that the headache fulfills the above criteria with the objective signs of muscle tenderness around the scalp that can be demonstrated by manual palpation or measured by pressure algometer or increased EMG (electromyogram) levels of the scalp muscles either at rest or during physiologic tests.

Most people with episodic tension-type headache do not seek medical attention. The pain is usually mild or moderate, felt as a dull pain or a cap around the head. Sometimes the pain includes the neck and or shoulders. Most of these headaches are infrequent, several times a year, month, or week. They do not exceed 15 or more times a month. The pain will last an hour to all day. Triggering mechanisms may be stress or biochemicals that accumulate as a result of muscle spasms. When these toxins accumulate faster than the body can eliminate them, the result can be another form of a triggering source.

At any rate, most people eliminate the pain by taking over-the-counter pain medication or recognizing the irritating influence and altering the source. Many times taking a break or going to sleep will "cure that headache." If this pain begins to interfere with the ability to function, then I

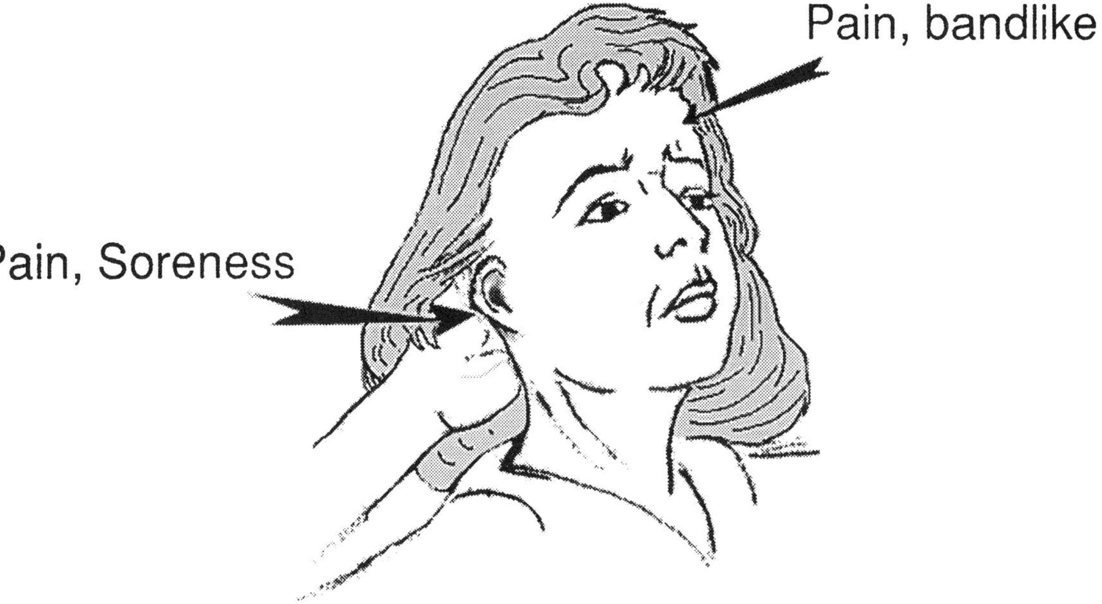

Figure 5.2 Muscle tension headaches are usually irritating (mild) or interfering (moderate). They can be intermittent, recurrent, or constant head pain, often in the forehead, temples, or the back of the head and neck, and are often described as "band-like," "tightness" or "vice-like." These headaches generally occur in the middle of the night, from 4:00 a.m. to 8:00 a.m. and can increase later in the day from 4:00 p.m. to 8:00 p.m. Most of the over-the-counter medicine that is purchased is for this type of headache.

would recommend seeing a physician who has an interest in headaches. In the back of the book there are references on organizations that will help you.

Some case histories have been included in this chapter (following the References).

REFERENCES

1. Rapoport, A.M., The diagnosis of migraine and tension type headache, then and now, *Neurology Journal*, 42 (3 Suppl. 2), 11–15, 1992.
2. Raskin, N.H., *Headache*, 2nd ed., Churchill Livingstone, New York, 1988.
3. Robbins, L., Lang, S.S., *Headache Help*, Houghton Mifflin, Boston, 1995.
4. Rapoport, A.M., Sheftel, F.D., *Headache Relief*, Simon and Schuster, New York, 1990.
5. Diamond, S., *Diagnosing and Managing Headaches*, 1st ed., Professional Communications, 1994.
6. Saper, J.R., Silberstein, S.D., Gordon, C.D., Hamel, R.L., *Handbook of Headache Management*, Williams & Wilkins, Baltimore, 1993.
7. Dieter, J.N., Swerdlow, B., A replicative investigation of the reliability of the MMPI in the classification of chronic headaches, *Headache Journal*, 28(3), 212–222, 1988.

CASE HISTORIES*

KEITH
Category: Tension-type headache

This is a 35-year-old man who came in complaining of incapacitating headaches and interfering headaches (moderate to severe). The incapacitating headaches began about two years ago. He does not recall having headaches prior to that. They occurred about twice a week, but he has not been experiencing this headache recently. He says that when he got the headache, it involved the entire head, worse in the back of the head, with sometimes pressure and throbbing. He would need to go to bed. He does not experience any nausea, vomiting, or being bothered by lights and noises. Sometimes changing his position will bring on more of a headache.

Interfering headaches (moderate to severe): These are the same as incapacitating headaches, but with less intensity. They occur almost every other day. They are also made worse by changing position. The patient states that ten years prior, while practicing karate, he might have had a whiplash injury, but there were no headaches after that.

The patient had cervical spine x-rays that were normal, and his medical and neurological examinations were essentially negative. He was diagnosed as having muscle tension headache, and possibly rule out an intracranial lesion because the headaches started back again. An MRI was done, which was normal.

He was started on some medication for this headache and in the following months reported a decrease in his headaches of approximately 44%. He would continue therapy.

* On the headache assessment forms that accompany these case histories, incapacitating headaches are indicated with solid black lines, interfering headaches with dotted lines, and irritating headaches with gray shading.

MEDICAL HEADACHE HISTORY

Name: Keith **Age:** 35 **Sex** M **Date:** 6/23/92

Date of Birth: 00/00/57 **Birthplace:** D.C. **Race:** C **Education:** 2 years college

Occupation: Fire Fighter **Accident:** N/A

Armed Services & Type of Discharge: N/A

PAST HISTORY:

1.	Did you have a normal birth?		**Yes**	No
	a) forceps used?		Yes	No
	b) cesarean section?		Yes	**No**
2.	Did you have problems with bedwetting?		Yes	**No**
	a) If yes, age bedwetting stopped		______	
3.	Were you car sick as a child (motion)?		Yes	**No**
	a) If yes, how severe?	Slight	Moderate	Severe
4.	Did you have unexplained abdominal cramps as a child?		Yes	**No**
5.	Did you have any of the following illnesses in childhood?			
	a) meningitis		Yes	**No**
	b) encephalitis		Yes	**No**
	c) scarlet fever		Yes	**No**
	d) rheumatic fever		Yes	**No**
6.	Did you have any head injuries as a child?		Yes	**No**
	a) If yes, please explain: ______			
7.	Were you treated for emotional illness as a child?		Yes	**No**

HABITS:

8.	Do you drink alcohol?	Yes	**No**
	a) If yes, what kind and how much? ______		
	b) Does alcohol bring on or aggravate a headache?	Yes	**No**
9.	Do you smoke?	Yes	**No**
	a) If yes, how much? ______		
	b) Does smoking or smoke-filled rooms cause or aggravate headaches?	Yes	**No**
10.	Do you drink caffeinated beverages?	**Yes**	No
	a) If yes, how much? 2 cups coffee, 1 cola, 2 to 3 glasses tea per day		

MENSTRUAL HISTORY:

At what age did menses begin? ______ Were they regular or irregular? ______

How were they related to your headache? ______

Are you or were you ever on Birth Control Pills? ______ Did they affect your headache? ______

Have you had a hysterectomy, partial or total, and why? ______

Are you in menopause, and if yes, how long? ______

Are you on hormones, and if yes, which ones? ______

HEADACHE ASSESSMENT FORM

HA PROFILE	INCAPACITATING #3	INTERFERING #2	IRRITATING #1
ONSET (Years ago and frequency)	2 years ago 2 per week	2 years ago 2 per week	N/A
CURRENT FREQUENCY	None now	Every other day	N/A
TIME OF ONSET	Anytime	Can awaken with	N/A
DURATION	All day	All day	N/A
CHARACTER	Throbbing, Pressure	Throbbing, Pressure	N/A
PRODROME OR AURA	N/A	N/A	N/A
ASSOCIATING FEATURES	Nausea; Vomiting; Sensitivity to Light? Noise? Odors? Do you get pale or flush? Do your eyes or nose run? Does your nose get stuffy? Does the white of your eyes get red? Does your eyelid droop? Do you pace, or go to bed?	Nausea; Vomiting; Sensitivity to Light? Noise? Odors? Do you get pale or flush? Do your eyes or nose run? Does your nose get stuffy? Does the white of your eyes get red? Does your eyelid droop? Do you pace, or go to bed?	Nausea; Vomiting; Sensitivity to Light? Noise? Odors? Do you get pale or flush? Do your eyes or nose run? Does your nose get stuffy? Does the white of your eyes get red? Does your eyelid droop? Do you pace, or go to bed?
PRECIPITATING OR AGGRAVATING FEATURES	Changing positions	Changing positions	N/A

LOCATION: Mark the location for each type of headache with a different color pen.
Incapacitating #3 is ——— Interfering #2 is ----------

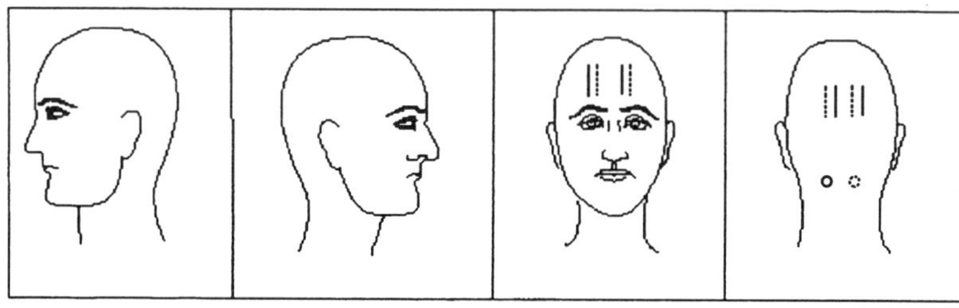

MEDICAL HISTORY:

Have you ever been or are you currently being treated for any of the following?

a) high blood pressure	Yes	No
b) stomach ulcers	Yes	No
c) asthma	Yes	No
d) allergies	Yes	No
e) pneumonia	Yes	No
f) kidney problems	Yes	No
g) low blood sugar	Yes	No
h) glaucoma	Yes	No
i) diabetes	Yes	No
j) heart problems	Yes	No

If you answered yes to any of the above, please describe: Environmental allergies.

List all other medical problems you have had in the past. Include date diagnosed and treatment.
DO NOT LIST OPERATIONS
Fractured orbit bone, 1980. Allergies to many things (shots for 2 years). Herpes II.

SURGICAL HISTORY (List operations and dates performed)
Packing of fractured orbit bone, 1980.

PSYCHIATRIC HISTORY (List visits with counselors, psychologists, etc., and type of treatment)

ACCIDENTS IN ADULT LIFE (Briefly describe any accident that caused any blow to the head or that you feel is related to your headache)
Hit in the nose; broken nose and fractured orbit bone.
Possible neck or whiplash during karate practice 10 years ago.

FAMILY HISTORY:

1. Is your father living? Yes No
   Age 67
   Cause of death ____
   Was there a headache history? Yes No

2. Is your mother living? Yes No
   Age 65
   Cause of death ______
   Was there a headache history? Yes No
3. Ages of brothers---Circle the ones with headache
   ______
4. Ages of sisters---Circle the ones with headache
   37
5. List any other blood relatives with a history of severe headaches.
   None

MARITAL HISTORY:

List marriages:

1st marriage age 31 to Present	Did spouse have headaches?	Yes	No
2nd marriage age ____ to ____	Did spouse have headaches?	Yes	No
3rd marriage age ____ to ____	Did spouse have headaches?	Yes	No

Age of current spouse: 27

List ages and sex of all children:

Age 18	Sex F	Headaches? Yes	No
Age ____	Sex ____	Headaches? Yes	No
Age ____	Sex ____	Headaches? Yes	No
Age ____	Sex ____	Headaches? Yes	No

STRESS FACTORS:

List any factors that may be affecting your headaches (money, loneliness, sexual problems, work, etc.)

______

______

VEGETATIVE SIGNS:

1. Do you have trouble falling asleep? Yes No
2. Do you have trouble staying asleep? Yes No
3. Has your appetite decreased? Yes No
4. Have you gained or lost weight in the past year? Yes No
5. Have you felt tearful or depressed lately? Yes No
6. Have you had any thoughts of wanting to die? Yes No
7. Have you been forgetful lately? Yes No
8. Any other changes in your normal day-to-day living? ______

Please list any medications you are allergic or sensitive to: None.

______

Please list any medications you are currently taking (including dosages and frequency per day):

Zovirax, 100 mg 1 a day.

______

PREVIOUS CARE:

1. List doctors who have treated you for headaches: Dr. S.

2. List any tests you have had for your headache (e.g., EEG, CT scan, MRI, X-Ray, etc.):
X-ray of neck. No problems found.

3. List any other treatment you have had for your headache (e.g., biofeedback, acupuncture, chiropractic, or any other treatment you had):
None.

ROBERT
Category: Tension-type headache

This 49-year-old man came in and complained of interfering headaches (moderate to severe) which started the beginning of the year that he came to see me. He was getting them every two or three days. Currently, he is getting them daily. They come at any time. It is constant, in his neck, and sometimes radiates to his temporal area. The character of the pain is soreness in his neck and sharp in the temporal area with movement. It is dull while he is sitting quietly. The pain is in the posterior cervical region (the back of the neck) radiating to the temporal region. There is no prodrome and no associated features. Changing positions, coughing, and sneezing sometimes can make the headache worse.

There is nothing significant in his past history or medical history related to his headaches. There is no headache history in his immediate family.

His neurological examination was essentially negative.

His diagnosis is chronic muscle tension headache. It was recommended that the patient have x-rays of the cervical spine, and also that a massage therapist teach his wife how to do massaging techniques, and stretch and spray techniques. He was also given a different non-steroidal medication. He was seen three times, and by the third visit, and after finding the proper anti-inflammatory medication, his headaches were reduced to one irritating headache a week, and he would be seen on an as-needed basis.

MEDICAL HEADACHE HISTORY

Name: Robert **Age:** 49 **Sex** M **Date:** 7/22/91

Date of Birth: 00/00/42 **Birthplace:** MD **Race:** C **Education:** B.A. Accounting

Occupation: CPA **Accident:** N/A

Armed Services & Type of Discharge: 1964-70 – Marines, Honorable Discharge

PAST HISTORY:

1.	Did you have a normal birth?	Yes	No
	a) forceps used?	Yes	No
	b) cesarean section?	Yes	No
2.	Did you have problems with bedwetting?	Yes	No
	a) If yes, age bedwetting stopped		
3.	Were you car sick as a child (motion)?	Yes	No
	a) If yes, how severe? Slight	Moderate	Severe
4.	Did you have unexplained abdominal cramps as a child?	Yes	No
5.	Did you have any of the following illnesses in childhood?		
	a) meningitis	Yes	No
	b) encephalitis	Yes	No
	c) scarlet fever	Yes	No
	d) rheumatic fever	Yes	No
6.	Did you have any head injuries as a child?	Yes	No
	a) If yes, please explain: Dove into pool and hit head on bottom; was unconscious		
7.	Were you treated for emotional illness as a child?	Yes	No

HABITS:

8.	Do you drink alcohol?	Yes	No
	a) If yes, what kind and how much? 1 to 2 drinks 3 to 4 times a week		
	b) Does alcohol bring on or aggravate a headache?	Yes	No
9.	Do you smoke?	Yes	No
	a) If yes, how much?		
	b) Does smoking or smoke-filled rooms cause or aggravate headaches?	Yes	No
10.	Do you drink caffeinated beverages?	Yes	No
	a) If yes, how much? 2 cups of coffee a day		

MENSTRUAL HISTORY:

At what age did menses begin?_______ Were they regular or irregular?____________________
How were they related to your headache?____
Are you or were you ever on Birth Control Pills?______ Did they affect your headache? _______
Have you had a hysterectomy, partial or total, and why?______________________________
Are you in menopause, and if yes, how long?_______________________________________
Are you on hormones, and if yes, which ones?______________________________________

HEADACHE ASSESSMENT FORM

HA PROFILE	INCAPACITATING #3	INTERFERING #2	IRRITATING #1
ONSET (Years ago and frequency)	N/A	6 to 8 months ago, every 2 to 3 days	N/A
CURRENT FREQUENCY	N/A	Every day	N/A
TIME OF ONSET	N/A	Anytime	N/A
DURATION	N/A	Constant in neck; 2 to 3 minutes in temple	N/A
CHARACTER	N/A	Soreness in neck; sharp in temple w/movement; very dull while sitting quietly	N/A
PRODROME OR AURA	N/A	N/A	N/A
ASSOCIATING FEATURES	Nausea; Vomiting; Sensitivity to Light? Noise? Odors? Do you get pale or flush? Do your eyes or nose run? Does your nose get stuffy? Does the white of your eyes get red? Does your eyelid droop? Do you pace, or go to bed?	Nausea; Vomiting; Sensitivity to Light? Noise? Odors? Do you get pale or flush? Do your eyes or nose run? Does your nose get stuffy? Does the white of your eyes get red? Does your eyelid droop? Do you pace, or go to bed?	Nausea; Vomiting; Sensitivity to Light? Noise? Odors? Do you get pale or flush? Do your eyes or nose run? Does your nose get stuffy? Does the white of your eyes get red? Does your eyelid droop? Do you pace, or go to bed?
PRECIPITATING OR AGGRAVATING FEATURES	N/A	Changing position, coughing, sneezing	N/A

LOCATION: Mark the location for each type of headache with a different color pen.

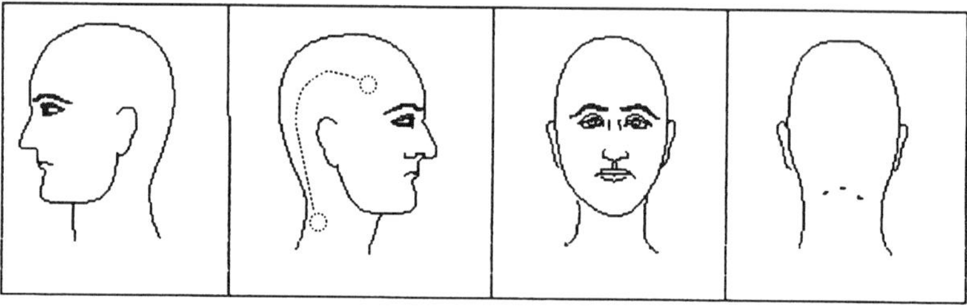

MEDICAL HISTORY:

Have you ever been or are you currently being treated for any of the following?

a) high blood pressure	Yes	No
b) stomach ulcers	Yes	No
c) asthma	Yes	No
d) allergies	Yes	No
e) pneumonia	Yes	No
f) kidney problems	Yes	No
g) low blood sugar	Yes	No
h) glaucoma	Yes	No
i) diabetes	Yes	No
j) heart problems	Yes	No

If you answered yes to any of the above, please describe:________________________

List all other medical problems you have had in the past. Include date diagnosed and treatment.
DO NOT LIST OPERATIONS

Possible Hiatal hernia, 1990 (Tagamet). Swollen testicle, 1990 (antibiotics). Headaches, 1991.

SURGICAL HISTORY (List operations and dates performed)

T&A, 1947. Appendectomy 1962. Collapsed lung injury, 1962.

PSYCHIATRIC HISTORY (List visits with counselors, psychologists, etc., and type of treatment)

Marriage counseling, 1987.

ACCIDENTS IN ADULT LIFE (Briefly describe any accident that caused any blow to the head or that you feel is related to your headache)

1958 – Hit bottom of swimming pool, hurt neck.

FAMILY HISTORY:

1.	Is your father living?	Yes	No
	Age 68		
	Cause of death________________		
	Was there a headache history?	Yes	No
2.	Is your mother living?	Yes	No
	Age 67		
	Cause of death________________		
	Was there a headache history?	Yes	No

3. Ages of brothers---Circle the ones with headache
   47 46 43
4. Ages of sisters---Circle the ones with headache
   29 27
5. List any other blood relatives with a history of severe headaches.
   N/A

MARITAL HISTORY:
List marriages:

1st marriage age 23 to 45	Did spouse have headaches?	Yes (underlined)	No
2nd marriage age 48 to Present	Did spouse have headaches?	Yes	No (underlined)
3rd marriage age ____ to ____	Did spouse have headaches?	Yes	No

Age of current spouse: 39

List ages and sex of all children:

Age 23 Sex F	Headaches?	Yes	No (underlined)
Age 17 Sex M	Headaches?	Yes	No (underlined)
Age ____ Sex ____	Headaches?	Yes	No
Age ____ Sex ____	Headaches?	Yes	No
Age ____ Sex ____	Headaches?	Yes	No

STRESS FACTORS:

List any factors that may be affecting your headaches (money, loneliness, sexual problems, work, etc.)
Money, Work, 3 businesses.

VEGETATIVE SIGNS:

1.	Do you have trouble falling asleep?	Yes	No (underlined)
2.	Do you have trouble staying asleep?	Yes	No (underlined)
3.	Has your appetite decreased?	Yes	No (underlined)
4.	Have you gained or lost weight in the past year?	Yes (underlined)	No
5.	Have you felt tearful or depressed lately?	Yes	No (underlined)
6.	Have you had any thoughts of wanting to die?	Yes	No (underlined)
7.	Have you been forgetful lately?	Yes	No (underlined)
8.	Any other changes in your normal day-to-day living? ____		

Please list any medications you are allergic or sensitive to: NK

Please list any medications you are currently taking (including dosages and frequency per day):
None

PREVIOUS CARE:

1. List doctors who have treated you for headaches: Dr. S.

2. List any tests you have had for your headache (e.g., EEG, CT scan, MRI, X-Ray, etc.):
CT scan, 5/91 (with and without contrast) – Saw 2 "large veins" (considered normal).

3. List any other treatment you have had for your headache (e.g., biofeedback, acupuncture, chiropractic, or any other treatment you had):

TIA
Category: Tension-type headache

This is a 19-year-old woman who came in complaining of interfering headaches (moderate to severe). They started as a child and she says that they were occasional. For the three weeks prior to her coming into the clinic, she was having them daily. Before that, she was having them once a month. They would last all day. The pain was a tight band and pressure around her head. There was no aura. Associated features were nausea, photophobia, sonophobia, and she would go to bed if possible. These associated features are often seen with migraine-like headaches.

The patient has two brothers who both have headaches. Her physical examination and neurological examination were negative. Her diagnosis would be tension-type headache with vascular components.

She was treated for both muscle tension headache and with medication for vascular headaches. Her symptoms decreased by 40% after the first visit.

MEDICAL HEADACHE HISTORY

Name: Tia **Age:** 19 **Sex** F **Date:** 10/9/91

Date of Birth: 00/00/71 **Birthplace:** NY **Race:** W **Education:** 1 year college

Occupation: Travel School **Accident:** N/A

Armed Services & Type of Discharge: N/A

PAST HISTORY:

1.	Did you have a normal birth?		<u>Yes</u>	No
	a) forceps used?		Yes	<u>No</u>
	b) cesarean section?		Yes	<u>No</u>
2.	Did you have problems with bedwetting?		Yes	<u>No</u>
	a) If yes, age bedwetting stopped		____	
3.	Were you car sick as a child (motion)?		<u>Yes</u>	No
	a) If yes, how severe?	<u>Slight</u>	Moderate	Severe
4.	Did you have unexplained abdominal cramps as a child?		Yes	<u>No</u>
5.	Did you have any of the following illnesses in childhood?			
	a) meningitis		Yes	<u>No</u>
	b) encephalitis		Yes	<u>No</u>
	c) scarlet fever		Yes	<u>No</u>
	d) rheumatic fever		Yes	<u>No</u>
6.	Did you have any head injuries as a child?		Yes	<u>No</u>
	a) If yes, please explain: ____			
7.	Were you treated for emotional illness as a child?		Yes	<u>No</u>

HABITS:

8.	Do you drink alcohol?	<u>Yes</u>	No
	a) If yes, what kind and how much? Maybe 3 beers a month		
	b) Does alcohol bring on or aggravate a headache?	Yes	<u>No</u>
9.	Do you smoke?	Yes	<u>No</u>
	a) If yes, how much? ____		
	b) Does smoking or smoke-filled rooms cause or aggravate headaches?	<u>Yes</u>	No
10.	Do you drink caffeinated beverages?	<u>Yes</u>	No
	a) If yes, how much? 2 cups of coffee a day		

MENSTRUAL HISTORY:

At what age did menses begin? 13 Were they regular or irregular? WNL
How were they related to your headache? N/A
Are you or were you ever on Birth Control Pills? Yes Did they affect your headache? No
Have you had a hysterectomy, partial or total, and why? No
Are you in menopause, and if yes, how long? No
Are you on hormones, and if yes, which ones? No

HEADACHE ASSESSMENT FORM

HA PROFILE	INCAPACITATING #3	INTERFERING #2	IRRITATING #1
ONSET (Years ago and frequency)	N/A	As a child, occasionally	N/A
CURRENT FREQUENCY	N/A	Every day for 3 weeks, before this, 1/month	N/A
TIME OF ONSET	N/A	Awaken with	N/A
DURATION	N/A	All day	N/A
CHARACTER	N/A	Tight band – pressure	N/A
PRODROME OR AURA	N/A	N/A	N/A
ASSOCIATING FEATURES	Nausea; Vomiting; Sensitivity to Light? Noise? Odors? Do you get pale or flush? Do your eyes or nose run? Does your nose get stuffy? Do the whites of your eyes get red? Does your eyelid droop? Do you pace, or go to bed?	Nausea; Vomiting; Sensitivity to Light? Noise? Odors? Do you get pale or flush? Do your eyes or nose run? Does your nose get stuffy? Do the whites of your eyes get red? Does your eyelid droop? Do you pace, or go to bed?	Nausea; Vomiting; Sensitivity to Light? Noise? Odors? Do you get pale or flush? Do your eyes or nose run? Does your nose get stuffy? Do the whites of your eyes get red? Does your eyelid droop? Do you pace, or go to bed?
PRECIPITATING OR AGGRAVATING FEATURES	N/A	N/A	N/A

LOCATION: Mark the location for each type of headache with a different color pen.

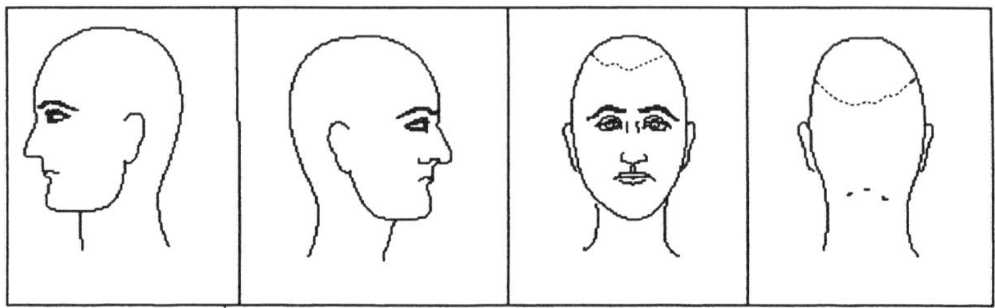

MEDICAL HISTORY:

Have you ever been or are you currently being treated for any of the following?

a) high blood pressure	Yes	No
b) stomach ulcers	Yes	No
c) asthma	Yes	No
d) allergies	Yes	No
e) pneumonia	Yes	No
f) kidney problems	Yes	No
g) low blood sugar	Yes	No
h) glaucoma	Yes	No
i) diabetes	Yes	No
j) heart problems	Yes	No

If you answered yes to any of the above, please describe: Asthma since age 3, still have occasional attacks

List all other medical problems you have had in the past. Include date diagnosed and treatment.
DO NOT LIST OPERATIONS
Blader infection, 1990.

SURGICAL HISTORY (List operations and dates performed)
Tonsillectomy, 1989. Finger, 1987. Moles removed, 1983.

PSYCHIATRIC HISTORY (List visits with counselors, psychologists, etc., and type of treatment)
5 times with a psychologist for very slight form of depression.

ACCIDENTS IN ADULT LIFE (Briefly describe any accident that caused any blow to the head or that you feel is related to your headache)

FAMILY HISTORY:

1.	Is your father living?	Yes	No
	Age 49		
	Cause of death ______		
	Was there a headache history?	Yes	No
2.	Is your mother living?	Yes	No
	Age 46		
	Cause of death ______		
	Was there a headache history?	Yes	No

3. Ages of brothers---Circle the ones with headache
(23) 21
4. Ages of sisters---Circle the ones with headache
None
5. List any other blood relatives with a history of severe headaches.
None that I'm aware of

MARITAL HISTORY:
List marriages:

1st marriage age _____ to _______	Did spouse have headaches?	Yes	No
2nd marriage age _____ to _______	Did spouse have headaches?	Yes	No
3rd marriage age _____ to _______	Did spouse have headaches?	Yes	No

Age of current spouse:__________

List ages and sex of all children:

Age ______ Sex ______	Headaches?	Yes	No
Age ______ Sex ______	Headaches?	Yes	No
Age ______ Sex ______	Headaches?	Yes	No

STRESS FACTORS:

List any factors that may be affecting your headaches (money, loneliness, sexual problems, work, etc.)
School

VEGETATIVE SIGNS:

1.	Do you have trouble falling asleep?	<u>Yes</u>	No
2.	Do you have trouble staying asleep?	<u>Yes</u>	No
3.	Has your appetite decreased?	<u>Yes</u>	No
4.	Have you gained or lost weight in the past year?	Yes	<u>No</u>
5.	Have you felt tearful or depressed lately?	Yes	<u>No</u>
6.	Have you had any thoughts of wanting to die?	Yes	<u>No</u>
7.	Have you been forgetful lately?	Yes	<u>No</u>
8.	Any other changes in your normal day-to-day living?__________		

Please list any medications you are allergic or sensitive to: None

Please list any medications you are currently taking (including dosages and frequency per day):
Propoxyphene for headaches, one before I go to sleep.

PREVIOUS CARE:

1. List doctors who have treated you for headaches: None.

2. List any tests you have had for your headache (e.g., EEG, CT scan, MRI, X-Ray, etc.):
CAT scan - 1991 (without contrast) – normal.

3. List any other treatment you have had for your headache (e.g., biofeedback, acupuncture, chiropractic, or any other treatment you had):
Blood tests – all normal.

ELIZABETH
Category: Tension-type headache

This is a 65-year-old woman who came in complaining of incapacitating headaches. They began at age 56. They were occasional with no known precipitating factors, and over recent months they have been coming on more frequently. She has been having them three to four times a week. She describes the pain as being over her forehead, and there is mild nausea.

There is nothing in her medical history that is associated with these headaches, and her medical and neurological examinations were negative. She would be diagnosed as having chronic tension-type headache.

MEDICAL HEADACHE HISTORY

Name: Elizabeth **Age:** 65 **Sex** F **Date:** 11/25/92

Date of Birth: 00/00/26 **Birthplace:** CN **Race:** W **Education:** Jr. college

Occupation: Homemaker **Accident:** N/A

Armed Services & Type of Discharge: N/A

PAST HISTORY:

1.	Did you have a normal birth?	?	Yes	No
	a) forceps used?	?	Yes	No
	b) cesarean section?		Yes	No
2.	Did you have problems with bedwetting?		Yes	No
	a) If yes, age bedwetting stopped			
3.	Were you car sick as a child (motion)?		Yes	No
	a) If yes, how severe?	Slight	Moderate	Severe
4.	Did you have unexplained abdominal cramps as a child?		Yes	No
5.	Did you have any of the following illnesses in childhood?			
	a) meningitis		Yes	No
	b) encephalitis		Yes	No
	c) scarlet fever		Yes	No
	d) rheumatic fever		Yes	No
6.	Did you have any head injuries as a child?		Yes	No
	a) If yes, please explain:			
7.	Were you treated for emotional illness as a child?		Yes	No

HABITS:

8.	Do you drink alcohol?	Yes	No
	a) If yes, what kind and how much?		
	b) Does alcohol bring on or aggravate a headache?	Yes	No
9.	Do you smoke?	Yes	No
	a) If yes, how much?		
	b) Does smoking or smoke-filled rooms cause or aggravate headaches?	Yes	No
10.	Do you drink caffeinated beverages?	Yes	No
	a) If yes, how much?		

MENSTRUAL HISTORY:

At what age did menses begin? 13 Were they regular or irregular? WNL

How were they related to your headache? N/A

Are you or were you ever on Birth Control Pills? Yes Did they affect your headache? N/A

Have you had a hysterectomy, partial or total, and why? No

Are you in menopause, and if yes, how long? Age 55

Are you on hormones, and if yes, which ones? No

HEADACHE ASSESSMENT FORM

HA PROFILE	INCAPACITATING #3	INTERFERING #2	IRRITATING #1
ONSET (Years ago and frequency)	Age 56, occasionally	N/A	Started this summer
CURRENT FREQUENCY	3 to 11 a month 3 to 4 a week	N/A	Can awaken with Daily
TIME OF ONSET	Awaken with	N/A	
DURATION	1 hour with Fiorinol	N/A	1 hour with Advil
CHARACTER	Constant ache	N/A	Steady pain
PRODROME OR AURA	N/A	N/A	N/A
ASSOCIATING FEATURES	Nausea; Vomiting; Sensitivity to Light? Noise? Odors? Do you get pale or flush? Do your eyes or nose run? Does your nose get stuffy? Does the white of your eyes get red? Does your eyelid droop? Do you pace, or go to bed?	Nausea; Vomiting; Sensitivity to Light? Noise? Odors? Do you get pale or flush? Do your eyes or nose run? Does your nose get stuffy? Does the white of your eyes get red? Does your eyelid droop? Do you pace, or go to bed?	Nausea; Vomiting; Sensitivity to Light? Noise? Odors? Do you get pale or flush? Do your eyes or nose run? Does your nose get stuffy? Does the white of your eyes get red? Does your eyelid droop? Do you pace, or go to bed?
PRECIPITATING OR AGGRAVATING FEATURES	N/A	N/A	N/A

LOCATION: Mark the location for each type of headache with a different color pen.

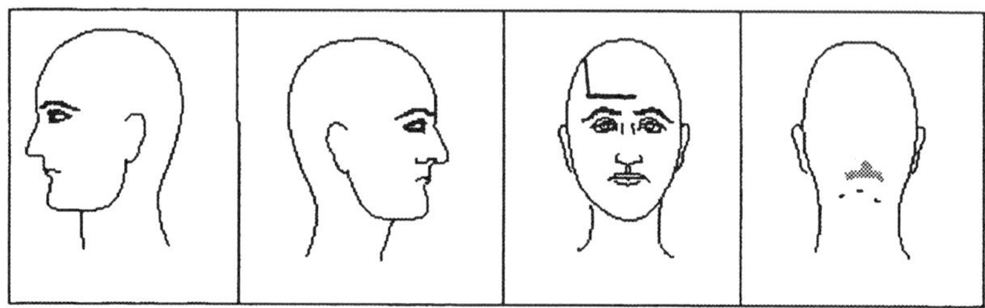

MEDICAL HISTORY:

Have you ever been or are you currently being treated for any of the following?

a) high blood pressure	Yes	No
b) stomach ulcers	Yes	No
c) asthma	Yes	No
d) allergies	Yes	No
e) pneumonia	Yes	No
f) kidney problems	Yes	No
g) low blood sugar	Yes	No
h) glaucoma	Yes	No
i) diabetes	Yes	No
j) heart problems	Yes	No

If you answered yes to any of the above, please describe: Ulcers diagnosed 5 years ago, take Zantac. Environmental allergies.

List all other medical problems you have had in the past. Include date diagnosed and treatment.
DO NOT LIST OPERATIONS

High cholesterol. Duodenal ulcer. Carpal tunnel syndrome, left hand. Ringing in ears.

SURGICAL HISTORY (List operations and dates performed)

Tonsillectomy & Adenoidectomy, 1945. Fusion of right hand, 1967. Umbilical hernia, 1972. Knee cap (R) scraped, 1972. Knee cap (R) removed, 1973. Fusion, left hand, 1974. Laminectomy L5, 1976. Total knee replacement (R), 1978. Cervical fusion C5-6, C6-7, 1981. Bunionectromy (R), 1990. Knee replacement (R), 1990.

PSYCHIATRIC HISTORY (List visits with counselors, psychologists, etc., and type of treatment)

1958-1959. Depression. Hospitalized for a month.

ACCIDENTS IN ADULT LIFE (Briefly describe any accident that caused any blow to the head or that you feel is related to your headache)

None.

FAMILY HISTORY:

1.	Is your father living?	Yes	No
	Age________		
	Cause of death Heart attack, age 60		
	Was there a headache history?	Yes	No
2.	Is your mother living?	Yes	No
	Age________		
	Cause of death Kidney problem, age 49		
	Was there a headache history?	Yes	No

3. Ages of brothers---Circle the ones with headache
   68 72

4. Ages of sisters---Circle the ones with headache
   N/A

5. List any other blood relatives with a history of severe headaches.
   ?

MARITAL HISTORY:

List marriages:

1st marriage age 22 to Present	Did spouse have headaches?	Yes	No (underlined)
2nd marriage age ____ to ____	Did spouse have headaches?	Yes	No
3rd marriage age ____ to ____	Did spouse have headaches?	Yes	No

Age of current spouse: 72

List ages and sex of all children:

Age 40	Sex M	Headaches? Yes	No
Age 36	Sex M	Headaches? Yes	No
Age 33	Sex M	Headaches? Yes	No
Age 31	Sex F	Headaches? Yes (underlined)	No
Age ____	Sex ____	Headaches? Yes	No

STRESS FACTORS:

List any factors that may be affecting your headaches (money, loneliness, sexual problems, work, etc.)

Restless, food, money

VEGETATIVE SIGNS:

1.	Do you have trouble falling asleep?	Yes	No (underlined)
2.	Do you have trouble staying asleep?	Yes	No (underlined)
3.	Has your appetite decreased?	Yes	No (underlined)
4.	Have you gained or lost weight in the past year?	Yes	No (underlined)
5.	Have you felt tearful or depressed lately?	Yes	No (underlined)
6.	Have you had any thoughts of wanting to die?	Yes	No (underlined)
7.	Have you been forgetful lately?	Yes	No (underlined)
8.	Any other changes in your normal day-to-day living? ____		

Please list any medications you are allergic or sensitive to: Dalmane; ASA; Norflex; Rabaxin; Tylox; Meprobamate; Prednisone; Sansert; Talwin; Tanderal; Indocin; Triavil; Tolectin; Butazoliden, Macrodantin

Please list any medications you are currently taking (including dosages and frequency per day):

Lopid, 600 mg 1 to 2 times a day; Butalbital, as needed; Zantac, as needed. Advil.

PREVIOUS CARE:

1. List doctors who have treated you for headaches: Dr. L.

2. List any tests you have had for your headache (e.g., EEG, CT scan, MRI, X-Ray, etc.):
None.

3. List any other treatment you have had for your headache (e.g., biofeedback, acupuncture, chiropractic, or any other treatment you had):
Chiropractic.

CHRISTY
Category: Tension-type headache

This is a 10-year-old girl who came in complaining about incapacitating headaches and interfering headaches (moderate to severe). The incapacitating headaches date back to when the patient was 4 years of age, until three months before she came into the clinic, and they began to reoccur. The headaches can last from 6 hours to a day, and she describes the pain as a squeezing-type pain "like something is too tight like a hat." There are no other warning signs that she is going to get a headache.

Interfering headaches (moderate to severe): These also began at age 4, and at that time the patient and her mother report that there was nausea and vomiting, which no longer occurs. It seems that since the beginning of the school year, they have been present on a daily basis. However, they can be present on weekends, as well as holidays.

There are no headaches in the family and the physical examination and neurological examination were within normal limits. She has had a CT scan, blood workup, EEGs in the past that all were normal.

Diagnosis: Chronic muscle tension headache in a child. The course of treatment for this child was biofeedback and an antihistamine to be taken twice a day. The treatment will be adjusted to the course of her therapy.

MEDICAL HEADACHE HISTORY

Name: Christy **Age:** 10 **Sex** F **Date:** 11/3/92

Date of Birth: 00/00/82 **Birthplace:** NJ **Race:** C **Education:** 5th grade

Occupation: Student **Accident:** N/A

Armed Services & Type of Discharge: N/A

PAST HISTORY:

1.	Did you have a normal birth?		Yes	No
	a) forceps used?		Yes	No
	b) cesarean section?		Yes	No
2.	Did you have problems with bedwetting?		Yes	No
	a) If yes, age bedwetting stopped		______	
3.	Were you car sick as a child (motion)?		Yes	No
	a) If yes, how severe?	Slight	Moderate	Severe
4.	Did you have unexplained abdominal cramps as a child?		Yes	No
5.	Did you have any of the following illnesses in childhood?			
	a) meningitis		Yes	No
	b) encephalitis		Yes	No
	c) scarlet fever		Yes	No
	d) rheumatic fever		Yes	No
6.	Did you have any head injuries as a child?		Yes	No
	a) If yes, please explain: ______			
7.	Were you treated for emotional illness as a child?		Yes	No

HABITS:

8.	Do you drink alcohol?	Yes	No
	a) If yes, what kind and how much? ______		
	b) Does alcohol bring on or aggravate a headache?	Yes	No
9.	Do you smoke?	Yes	No
	a) If yes, how much? ______		
	b) Does smoking or smoke-filled rooms cause or aggravate headaches?	Yes	No
10.	Do you drink caffeinated beverages?	Yes	No
	a) If yes, how much? ______		

MENSTRUAL HISTORY:

At what age did menses begin? N/A Were they regular or irregular? ______

How were they related to your headache? ______

Are you or were you ever on Birth Control Pills? ______ Did they affect your headache? ______

Have you had a hysterectomy, partial or total, and why? ______

Are you in menopause, and if yes, how long? ______

Are you on hormones, and if yes, which ones? ______

HEADACHE ASSESSMENT FORM

HA PROFILE	INCAPACITATING #3	INTERFERING #2	IRRITATING #1
ONSET (Years ago and frequency)	Age 4, every other day for 2 months, then occasionally	Age 4, occasionally	N/A
CURRENT FREQUENCY	1 to 2 a week since school started	Every day since school started	N/A
TIME OF ONSET	Can awaken with, but usually noon	Can awaken with, but usually noon	N/A
DURATION	6 hours to all day	Comes and goes all day	N/A
CHARACTER	Severe squeezing at temples	Same, but less intense	N/A
PRODROME OR AURA	N/A	N/A	N/A
ASSOCIATING FEATURES	Nausea; Vomiting; Sensitivity to Light? Noise? Odors? Do you get pale or flush? Do your eyes or nose run? Does your nose get stuffy? Does the white of your eyes get red? Does your eyelid droop? Do you pace, or go to bed?	Nausea; Vomiting; Sensitivity to Light? Noise? Odors? Do you get pale or flush? Do your eyes or nose run? Does your nose get stuffy? Does the white of your eyes get red? Does your eyelid droop? Do you pace, or go to bed?	Nausea; Vomiting; Sensitivity to Light? Noise? Odors? Do you get pale or flush? Do your eyes or nose run? Does your nose get stuffy? Does the white of your eyes get red? Does your eyelid droop? Do you pace, or go to bed?
PRECIPITATING OR AGGRAVATING FEATURES	N/A	N/A	N/A

LOCATION: Mark the location for each type of headache with a different color pen.

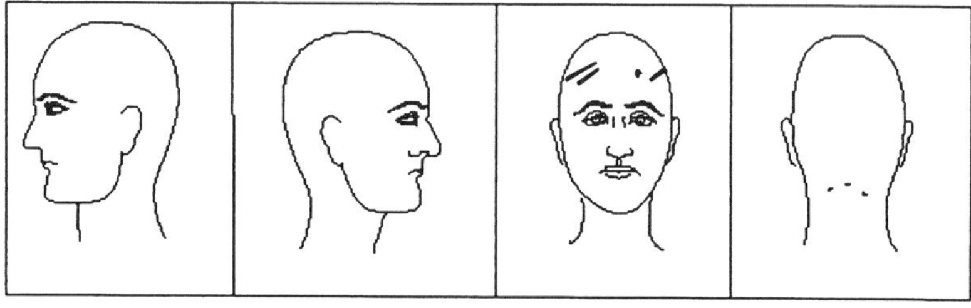

MEDICAL HISTORY:

Have you ever been or are you currently being treated for any of the following?

a) high blood pressure	Yes	No
b) stomach ulcers	Yes	No
c) asthma	Yes	No
d) allergies	Yes	No
e) pneumonia	Yes	No
f) kidney problems	Yes	No
g) low blood sugar	Yes	No
h) glaucoma	Yes	No
i) diabetes	Yes	No
j) heart problems	Yes	No

If you answered yes to any of the above, please describe: Asthma diagnosed at age 1-1/2. Allergies - Environmental.

List all other medical problems you have had in the past. Include date diagnosed and treatment.
DO NOT LIST OPERATIONS

Asthma since age 1-1/2. Allergies since age 3. Migraine headaches since age 4.

SURGICAL HISTORY (List operations and dates performed)

None.

PSYCHIATRIC HISTORY (List visits with counselors, psychologists, etc., and type of treatment)

None.

ACCIDENTS IN ADULT LIFE (Briefly describe any accident that caused any blow to the head or that you feel is related to your headache)

N/A

FAMILY HISTORY:

1.	Is your father living?	Yes	No
	Age 30		
	Cause of death ______		
	Was there a headache history?	Yes	No
2.	Is your mother living?	Yes	No
	Age 33		
	Cause of death ______		
	Was there a headache history?	Yes	No

3. Ages of brothers---Circle the ones with headache
   20 months (unknown)
4. Ages of sisters---Circle the ones with headache
   12
5. List any other blood relatives with a history of severe headaches.
   Paternal grandmother possibly.

MARITAL HISTORY:

List marriages:

1st marriage age ______ to ______ Did spouse have headaches?	Yes	No
2nd marriage age ______ to ______ Did spouse have headaches?	Yes	No
3rd marriage age ______ to ______ Did spouse have headaches?	Yes	No

Age of current spouse:___________

List ages and sex of all children:

Age _____ Sex ______ Headaches?	Yes	No
Age _____ Sex ______ Headaches?	Yes	No
Age _____ Sex ______ Headaches?	Yes	No

STRESS FACTORS:

List any factors that may be affecting your headaches (money, loneliness, sexual problems, work, etc.)

____

____

VEGETATIVE SIGNS:

1.	Do you have trouble falling asleep?	Yes (underlined)	No
2.	Do you have trouble staying asleep?	Yes (underlined)	No
3.	Has your appetite decreased?	Yes (underlined)	No
4.	Have you gained or lost weight in the past year?	Yes (underlined)	No
5.	Have you felt tearful or depressed lately?	Yes	No (underlined)
6.	Have you had any thoughts of wanting to die?	Yes	No (underlined)
7.	Have you been forgetful lately?	Yes	No (underlined)
8.	Any other changes in your normal day-to-day living?________________		

Please list any medications you are allergic or sensitive to: No known allergies.

____

____

Please list any medications you are currently taking (including dosages and frequency per day):

Periactin 4 mg twice a day.

____

PREVIOUS CARE:

1. List doctors who have treated you for headaches: Dr. A. Dr. G.

2. List any tests you have had for your headache (e.g., EEG, CT scan, MRI, X-Ray, etc.):
CAT scan 10/92 (without contrast) – normal. EEG at age 4 – normal. Blood work – normal.

3. List any other treatment you have had for your headache (e.g., biofeedback, acupuncture, chiropractic, or any other treatment you had):
N/A

MILDRED
Category: Tension-type headache

This is a 54-year-old woman who came in with a complaint of interfering headaches (moderate to severe). They started three months prior to her coming into the clinic, and she is having them daily. They can last half a day. She can get these headaches at any time if she doesn't take any medication, and she complains of a burning and tightness in the frontal part of her head and the occipital part of her head. There are associated features to these headaches, such as sonophobia, and she will go to bed if possible.

There is nothing in her medical history that would be associated with these headaches, and there is no headache history in the family. In the previous work-ups she has had CT scans and cervical spine x-rays, and all were normal. Physical examination and neurological examination were within normal limits.

She was diagnosed as having tension-type headache.

MEDICAL HEADACHE HISTORY

Name: Mildred **Age:** 54 **Sex** F **Date:** 10/17/90

Date of Birth: 00/00/35 **Birthplace:** TN **Race:** C **Education:** B.S. Ed.

Occupation: Middle School Teacher **Accident:** N/A

Armed Services & Type of Discharge: N/A

PAST HISTORY:

1.	Did you have a normal birth?		**Yes**	No
	a) forceps used?		Yes	No
	b) cesarean section?		Yes	**No**
2.	Did you have problems with bedwetting?		Yes	**No**
	a) If yes, age bedwetting stopped			
3.	Were you car sick as a child (motion)?		Yes	**No**
	a) If yes, how severe?	**Slight**	Moderate	Severe
4.	Did you have unexplained abdominal cramps as a child?		Yes	**No**
5.	Did you have any of the following illnesses in childhood?			
	a) meningitis		Yes	**No**
	b) encephalitis		Yes	**No**
	c) scarlet fever		Yes	**No**
	d) rheumatic fever		Yes	**No**
6.	Did you have any head injuries as a child?		Yes	**No**
	a) If yes, please explain:			
7.	Were you treated for emotional illness as a child?		Yes	**No**

HABITS:

8.	Do you drink alcohol?	Yes	**No**
	a) If yes, what kind and how much?		
	b) Does alcohol bring on or aggravate a headache?	Yes	**No**
9.	Do you smoke?	**Yes**	No
	a) If yes, how much? 1 pack daily		
	b) Does smoking or smoke-filled rooms cause or aggravate headaches?	Yes	**No**
10.	Do you drink caffeinated beverages?	**Yes**	No
	a) If yes, how much? 3 daily		

MENSTRUAL HISTORY:

At what age did menses begin? 14 Were they regular or irregular? WNL
How were they related to your headache? N/A
Are you or were you ever on Birth Control Pills? ______ Did they affect your headache? ______
Have you had a hysterectomy, partial or total, and why? '65 – partial (precancerous cells)
Are you in menopause, and if yes, how long? No
Are you on hormones, and if yes, which ones? Premarin 0.625 mg every day for 5 days, off 2 (not now)

HEADACHE ASSESSMENT FORM

HA PROFILE	INCAPACITATING #3	INTERFERING #2	IRRITATING #1
ONSET (Years ago and frequency)	N/A	3 months ago, every 2 days	N/A
CURRENT FREQUENCY	N/A	Every day	N/A
TIME OF ONSET	N/A	Anytime	N/A
DURATION	N/A	6 to 10 hours	N/A
CHARACTER	N/A	Burning and tightness	N/A
PRODROME OR AURA	N/A	N/A	N/A
ASSOCIATING FEATURES	Nausea; Vomiting; Sensitivity to Light? Noise? Odors? Do you get pale or flush? Do your eyes or nose run? Does your nose get stuffy? Do the whites of your eyes get red? Does your eyelid droop? Do you pace, or go to bed?	Nausea; Vomiting; Sensitivity to Light? Noise? Odors? Do you get pale or flush? Do your eyes or nose run? Does your nose get stuffy? Do the whites of your eyes get red? Does your eyelid droop? Do you pace, or go to bed?	Nausea; Vomiting; Sensitivity to Light? Noise? Odors? Do you get pale or flush? Do your eyes or nose run? Does your nose get stuffy? Do the whites of your eyes get red? Does your eyelid droop? Do you pace, or go to bed?
PRECIPITATING OR AGGRAVATING FEATURES	N/A	N/A	N/A

LOCATION: Mark the location for each type of headache with a different color pen.

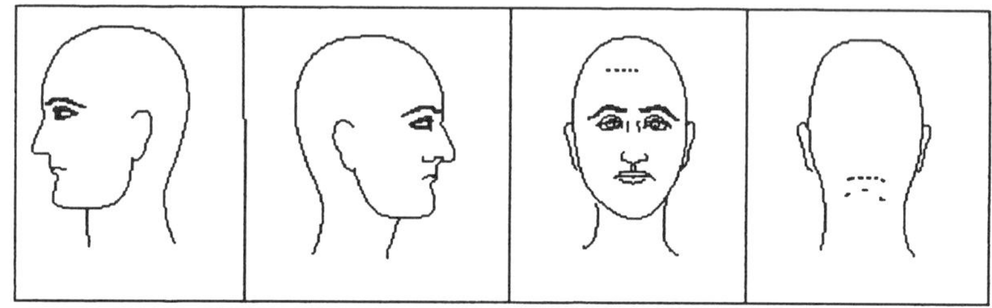

MEDICAL HISTORY:

Have you ever been or are you currently being treated for any of the following?

a) high blood pressure	<u>Yes</u>	No
b) stomach ulcers	Yes	<u>No</u>
c) asthma	Yes	<u>No</u>
d) allergies	Yes	<u>No</u>
e) pneumonia	Yes	<u>No</u>
f) kidney problems	Yes	<u>No</u>
g) low blood sugar	Yes	<u>No</u>
h) glaucoma	Yes	<u>No</u>
i) diabetes	Yes	<u>No</u>
j) heart problems	Yes	<u>No</u>

If you answered yes to any of the above, please describe: Hypertension diagnosed 6 years ago. Being treated with medication.

List all other medical problems you have had in the past. Include date diagnosed and treatment.
DO NOT LIST OPERATIONS

Cardiac catherization 1989 (normal). Thallium scan 1990 (negative).

SURGICAL HISTORY (List operations and dates performed)

Laminectomy 1970. Carpal tunnel syndrome 1974. Umbilical hernia repair 1990. Partial Hysterectomy 1965. Tonsillectomy & Adenoidectomy age 4.

PSYCHIATRIC HISTORY (List visits with counselors, psychologists, etc., and type of treatment)

N/A

ACCIDENTS IN ADULT LIFE (Briefly describe any accident that caused any blow to the head or that you feel is related to your headache)

N/A

FAMILY HISTORY:

1.	Is your father living?	Yes	<u>No</u>
	Age________		
	Cause of death Heart, age 70		
	Was there a headache history?	Yes	<u>No</u>
2.	Is your mother living?	<u>Yes</u>	No
	Age 84		
	Cause of death________		
	Was there a headache history?	Yes	<u>No</u>

3. Ages of brothers---Circle the ones with headache
   N/A
4. Ages of sisters---Circle the ones with headache
   N/A
5. List any other blood relatives with a history of severe headaches.
   N/A

MARITAL HISTORY:
List marriages:

1st marriage age 23 to 28	Did spouse have headaches?	Yes	No
2nd marriage age 29 to 35	Did spouse have headaches?	Yes	No
3rd marriage age 37 to 45	Did spouse have headaches?	Yes	No

Age of current spouse:__________

List ages and sex of all children:

Age 31	Sex M	Headaches?	Yes	No
Age 31	Sex M	Headaches?	Yes	No
Age 29	Sex M	Headaches?	Yes	No
Age 27	Sex M	Headaches?	Yes	No
Age ____	Sex ____	Headaches?	Yes	No

STRESS FACTORS:

List any factors that may be affecting your headaches (money, loneliness, sexual problems, work, etc.)
Problems with children.

VEGETATIVE SIGNS:

1.	Do you have trouble falling asleep?	Yes		No
2.	Do you have trouble staying asleep?	Yes		No
3.	Has your appetite decreased?	Yes		No
4.	Have you gained or lost weight in the past year?	Yes		No
5.	Have you felt tearful or depressed lately?	Yes		No
6.	Have you had any thoughts of wanting to die?	Yes	?	No
7.	Have you been forgetful lately?	Yes	?	No
8.	Any other changes in your normal day-to-day living?________			

Please list any medications you are allergic or sensitive to: Penicillin

Please list any medications you are currently taking (including dosages and frequency per day):
Maxzide and Calan-SR 240 mg once daily; Clorazepate 7.5 mg as needed; Methocarbamol 750 mg. 2 or 3 daily for the last 7 days; Doxepin 25 mg. ¾ of a tablet at bedtime.
Vicodin – 1 or 2 a day.

PREVIOUS CARE:

1. List doctors who have treated you for headaches: Dr. H.

2. List any tests you have had for your headache (e.g., EEG, CT scan, MRI, X-Ray, etc.):
CAT scan – brain (with and without contrast) 1990 – normal.
CAT scan – sinus 1990 – normal. CT – cervical spine.

3. List any other treatment you have had for your headache (e.g., biofeedback, acupuncture, chiropractic, or any other treatment you had):
None.

BERTHA
Category: Tension-type headache

This headache history is a good example of a muscle contraction headache. This is a 60-year-old woman who has been having headaches since age 30. She started having them twice a year; currently she is getting them every two weeks. It is aching. There might be some throbbing involved, and they are generally moderate-type headaches.

Patients in the age range of the late 50s and older, do not seem to respond as well as younger people to various medications. Oftentimes, different types of medications and forms of treatment can be used. Sometimes biofeedback and relaxation therapy are recommended to help this type of headache.

MEDICAL HEADACHE HISTORY

Name: Bertha **Age:** 60 **Sex** F **Date:** 2/1/84

Date of Birth: 00/00/23 **Birthplace:** NC **Race:** W **Education:** High school

Occupation: Accounting Clerk **Accident:** N/A

Armed Services & Type of Discharge: N/A

PAST HISTORY:

1.	Did you have a normal birth?	Yes	No
	a) forceps used?	Yes	No
	b) cesarean section?	Yes	No
2.	Did you have problems with bedwetting?	Yes	No
	a) If yes, age bedwetting stopped		
3.	Were you car sick as a child (motion)?	Yes	No
	a) If yes, how severe? Slight	Moderate	Severe
4.	Did you have unexplained abdominal cramps as a child?	Yes	No
5.	Did you have any of the following illnesses in childhood?		
	a) meningitis	Yes	No
	b) encephalitis	Yes	No
	c) scarlet fever	Yes	No
	d) rheumatic fever	Yes	No
6.	Did you have any head injuries as a child?	Yes	No
	a) If yes, please explain:		
7.	Were you treated for emotional illness as a child?	Yes	No

HABITS:

8.	Do you drink alcohol?	Yes	No
	a) If yes, what kind and how much? 1 glass of wine a week		
	b) Does alcohol bring on or aggravate a headache?	Yes	No
9.	Do you smoke?	Yes	No
	a) If yes, how much?		
	b) Does smoking or smoke-filled rooms cause or aggravate headaches?	Yes	No
10.	Do you drink caffeinated beverages?	Yes	No
	a) If yes, how much?		

MENSTRUAL HISTORY:

At what age did menses begin? 13 Were they regular or irregular? Irregular

How were they related to your headache? N/A

Are you or were you ever on Birth Control Pills? ______ Did they affect your headache? ______

Have you had a hysterectomy, partial or total, and why? Yes, age 40.

Are you in menopause, and if yes, how long? ______

Are you on hormones, and if yes, which ones? Premarin 0.625

HEADACHE ASSESSMENT FORM

HA PROFILE	INCAPACITATING #3	INTERFERING #2	IRRITATING #1
ONSET (Years ago and frequency)	N/A	Age 30 2 per year	N/A
CURRENT FREQUENCY	N/A	1 every 2 weeks	N/A
TIME OF ONSET	N/A	No pattern	N/A
DURATION	N/A	1 day to 1 week	N/A
CHARACTER	N/A	Aching, Throbbing	N/A
PRODROME OR AURA	N/A	N/A	N/A
ASSOCIATING FEATURES	Nausea; Vomiting; Sensitivity to Light? Noise? Odors? Do you get pale or flush? Do your eyes or nose run? Does your nose get stuffy? Does the white of your eyes get red? Does your eyelid droop? Do you pace, or go to bed?	Nausea; Vomiting; Sensitivity to Light? Noise? Odors? Do you get pale or flush? Do your eyes or nose run? Does your nose get stuffy? Does the white of your eyes get red? Does your eyelid droop? Do you pace, or go to bed?	Nausea; Vomiting; Sensitivity to Light? Noise? Odors? Do you get pale or flush? Do your eyes or nose run? Does your nose get stuffy? Does the white of your eyes get red? Does your eyelid droop? Do you pace, or go to bed?
PRECIPITATING OR AGGRAVATING FEATURES	N/A	N/A	N/A

LOCATION: Mark the location for each type of headache with a different color pen.

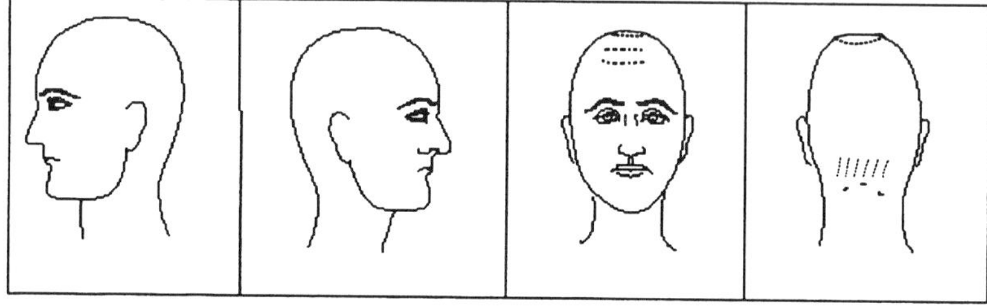

MEDICAL HISTORY:

Have you ever been or are you currently being treated for any of the following?

a) high blood pressure	Yes	No
b) stomach ulcers	Yes	No
c) asthma	Yes	No
d) allergies	Yes	No
e) pneumonia	Yes	No
f) kidney problems	Yes	No
g) low blood sugar	Yes	No
h) glaucoma	Yes	No
i) diabetes	Yes	No
j) heart problems	Yes	No

If you answered yes to any of the above, please describe:______________________________

List all other medical problems you have had in the past. Include date diagnosed and treatment.
DO NOT LIST OPERATIONS

Peptic ulcer, 30 years ago.

SURGICAL HISTORY (List operations and dates performed)

Hysterectomy 12 years ago, cyst on ovary. Tonsillectomy & Adenoidectomy 35 years ago

Appendectomy, years ago.

PSYCHIATRIC HISTORY (List visits with counselors, psychologists, etc., and type of treatment)

None

ACCIDENTS IN ADULT LIFE (Briefly describe any accident that caused any blow to the head or that you feel is related to your headache)

None

FAMILY HISTORY:

		Yes	No
1.	Is your father living?	Yes	No
	Age________		
	Cause of death___Age 55, cancer_______________		
	Was there a headache history?	Yes	No
2.	Is your mother living?	Yes	No
	Age________		
	Cause of death___Age 55, cancer_______________		
	Was there a headache history?	Yes	No
3.	Ages of brothers---Circle the ones with headache		
	____52_______________		
4.	Ages of sisters---Circle the ones with headache		
	____62 50 48_______________		
5.	List any other blood relatives with a history of severe headaches.		
	______None_______________		

MARITAL HISTORY:
List marriages:

1st marriage age __19__ to __28__	Did spouse have headaches?	Yes	No
2nd marriage age __40__ to __60__	Did spouse have headaches?	Yes	No
3rd marriage age ______ to ______	Did spouse have headaches?	Yes	No
_________ age ______ to ______	________________		

Age of current spouse:___62_______

List ages and sex of all children:

Age __39__ Sex __F__	Headaches?	Yes	No
Age ______ Sex ______	Headaches?	Yes	No
Age ______ Sex ______	Headaches?	Yes	No

STRESS FACTORS:

List any factors that may be affecting your headaches (money, loneliness, sexual problems, work, etc.)
____N/A____

____

VEGETATIVE SIGNS:

1.	Do you have trouble falling asleep?	Yes	No
2.	Do you have trouble staying asleep?	Yes	No
3.	Has your appetite decreased?	Yes	No
4.	Have you gained or lost weight in the past year?	Yes	No
5.	Have you felt tearful or depressed lately?	Yes	No
6.	Have you had any thoughts of wanting to die?	Yes	No
7.	Have you been forgetful lately?	Yes	No
8.	Any other changes in your normal day-to-day living?________________		

Please list any medications you are allergic or sensitive to:

Please list any medications you are currently taking (including dosages and frequency per day):
Premarin 0.625

PREVIOUS CARE:

1. List doctors who have treated you for headaches: Dr. Miller

2. List any tests you have had for your headache (e.g., EEG, CT scan, MRI, X-Ray, etc.):
None

3. List any other treatment you have had for your headache (e.g., biofeedback, acupuncture, chiropractic, or any other treatment you had):
Acupuncture

GAIL
Category: Tension-type headache

This patient complained of having had constant headaches for a year. Notice in her headache intake form that her #2 (interfering) headaches became an everyday occurrence and there was pressure and aching. Her #1 (irritating) headaches were occasional and 6 weeks prior to her seeing me, her incapacitating headaches started and they were daily. Notice the character of pain was a "tight band" and there was no nausea, vomiting, or throbbing seen in the vascular headache or migraine-like headache episodes.

The older diagnosis would label her as muscle contraction headache or tension headaches, and the new classification under the International Headache Society would label the diagnosis as Tension Type Headache 2.2, Chronic Tension Headache.

The patient was treated with various medications and biofeedback and eventually became headache-free.

MEDICAL HEADACHE HISTORY

Name: Gail **Age:** 52 **Sex** F **Date:** 6/10/87

Date of Birth: 00/00/34 **Birthplace:** AL **Race:** W **Education:** M.A.

Occupation: Teacher **Accident:** N/A

Armed Services & Type of Discharge: N/A

PAST HISTORY:

1.	Did you have a normal birth?	Yes (underlined)	No
	a) forceps used?	Yes	No
	b) cesarean section?	Yes	No
2.	Did you have problems with bedwetting?	Yes	No (underlined)
	a) If yes, age bedwetting stopped	______	
3.	Were you car sick as a child (motion)?	Yes	No (underlined)
	a) If yes, how severe? Slight	Moderate	Severe
4.	Did you have unexplained abdominal cramps as a child?	Yes	No (underlined)
5.	Did you have any of the following illnesses in childhood?		
	a) meningitis	Yes	No (underlined)
	b) encephalitis	Yes	No (underlined)
	c) scarlet fever	Yes (underlined)	No
	d) rheumatic fever	Yes	No (underlined)
6.	Did you have any head injuries as a child?	Yes	No (underlined)
	a) If yes, please explain: Scarlet fever in childhood.		
7.	Were you treated for emotional illness as a child?	Yes	No (underlined)

HABITS:

8.	Do you drink alcohol?	Yes (underlined)	No
	a) If yes, what kind and how much? Wine occasionally with dinner		
	b) Does alcohol bring on or aggravate a headache?	Yes	No (underlined)
9.	Do you smoke?	Yes	No (underlined)
	a) If yes, how much?		
	b) Does smoking or smoke-filled rooms cause or aggravate headaches?	Yes (underlined)	No
10.	Do you drink caffeinated beverages?	Yes	No
	a) If yes, how much? Rarely		

MENSTRUAL HISTORY:

At what age did menses begin? 14 Were they regular or irregular? WNL
How were they related to your headache? N/A
Are you or were you ever on Birth Control Pills? Yes Did they affect your headache? N/A
Have you had a hysterectomy, partial or total, and why? No
Are you in menopause, and if yes, how long? Yes, since 1986.
Are you on hormones, and if yes, which ones? Estraderm (increases headaches)

HEADACHE ASSESSMENT FORM

HA PROFILE	INCAPACITATING #3	INTERFERING #2	IRRITATING #1
ONSET (Years ago and frequency)	6 weeks ago	1986 – when started hormones	Adult life
CURRENT FREQUENCY	Daily	Every day constant	Occasionally
TIME OF ONSET	All day	There when awaken	Anytime
DURATION	Lasted 3 weeks	All day	1 hour with aspirin
CHARACTER	Tight band	Pressure, ache	Aching
PRODROME OR AURA	N/A	Occasional light-headedness, tinnitus, pressure in ears	N/A
ASSOCIATING FEATURES	Nausea; Vomiting; Sensitivity to Light? Noise? Odors? Do you get pale or flush? Do your eyes or nose run? Does your nose get stuffy? Do the whites of your eyes get red? Does your eyelid droop? Do you pace, or go to bed?	Nausea; Vomiting; Sensitivity to Light? Noise? Odors? Do you get pale or flush? Do your eyes or nose run? Does your nose get stuffy? Do the whites of your eyes get red? Does your eyelid droop? Do you pace, or go to bed?	Nausea; Vomiting; Sensitivity to Light? Noise? Odors? Do you get pale or flush? Do your eyes or nose run? Does your nose get stuffy? Do the whites of your eyes get red? Does your eyelid droop? Do you pace, or go to bed?
PRECIPITATING OR AGGRAVATING FEATURES	When told to move	Stress	Weather changes, stress

LOCATION: Mark the location for each type of headache with a different color pen.

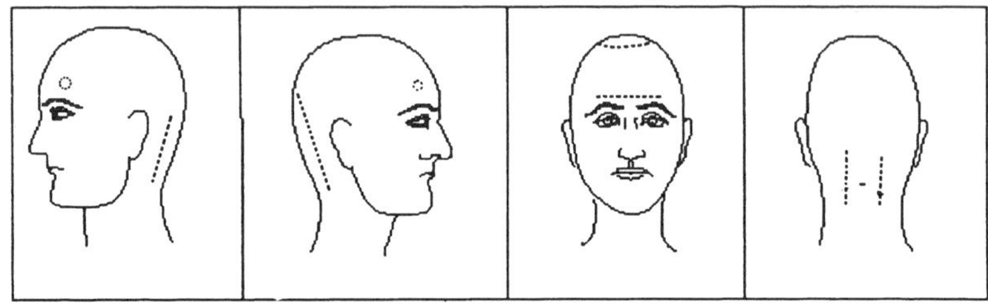

MEDICAL HISTORY:

Have you ever been or are you currently being treated for any of the following?

a) high blood pressure	Yes	<u>No</u>
b) stomach ulcers	Yes	<u>No</u>
c) asthma	Yes	<u>No</u>
d) allergies	Yes	<u>No</u>
e) pneumonia	<u>Yes</u>	No
f) kidney problems	Yes	<u>No</u>
g) low blood sugar	Yes	<u>No</u>
h) glaucoma	Yes	<u>No</u>
i) diabetes	Yes	<u>No</u>
j) heart problems	Yes	<u>No</u>

If you answered yes to any of the above, please describe:. Pneumonia 3 times as a child.

List all other medical problems you have had in the past. Include date diagnosed and treatment. DO NOT LIST OPERATIONS

Low thyroid at one time, 20-25 years ago. On medication for 3 years. Sinus infections with sore throats (last one in 1986, about every 5 years).

SURGICAL HISTORY (List operations and dates performed)

Removal of ovary and cyst – 1954. D&C - 1967 and 1986. Left knee surgery – 1987.

PSYCHIATRIC HISTORY (List visits with counselors, psychologists, etc., and type of treatment)

None.

ACCIDENTS IN ADULT LIFE (Briefly describe any accident that caused any blow to the head or that you feel is related to your headache)

Auto accident in 1983 which resulted in a broken jaw. Unconscious briefly.

FAMILY HISTORY:

1. Is your father living? Yes <u>No</u>

   Age_________

   Cause of death <u>Auto accident in early 20's</u>

   Was there a headache history? Yes <u>No</u>

2. Is your mother living? Yes <u>No</u>

   Age_________

   Cause of death <u>Many physical problems for 35 years</u>

   Was there a headache history? Don't know Yes No

3. Ages of brothers---Circle the ones with headache
   47 - Don't know
4. Ages of sisters---Circle the ones with headache
   42 - Don't know
5. List any other blood relatives with a history of severe headaches.
   Don't know

MARITAL HISTORY:

List marriages:

1st marriage age 21 to Present	Did spouse have headaches?	Yes	No
2nd marriage age _____ to ______	Did spouse have headaches?	Yes	No
3rd marriage age _____ to ______	Did spouse have headaches?	Yes	No

Age of current spouse: 53

List ages and sex of all children:

Age 29	Sex F	Headaches? Yes	No
Age 27	Sex M	Headaches? Yes	No
Age _____	Sex _____	Headaches? Yes	No
Age _____	Sex _____	Headaches? Yes	No

STRESS FACTORS:

List any factors that may be affecting your headaches (money, loneliness, sexual problems, work, etc.)
Responsibilities, not enough time to get things done or enough time for self; relocation decisions.

VEGETATIVE SIGNS:

1.	Do you have trouble falling asleep?	Yes	No
2.	Do you have trouble staying asleep?	Yes	No
3.	Has your appetite decreased?	Yes	No
4.	Have you gained or lost weight in the past year?	Yes	No
5.	Have you felt tearful or depressed lately?	Yes	No
6.	Have you had any thoughts of wanting to die?	Yes	No
7.	Have you been forgetful lately?	Yes	No
8.	Any other changes in your normal day-to-day living?______		

Please list any medications you are allergic or sensitive to: Novocaine

Please list any medications you are currently taking (including dosages and frequency per day):
Antihistamine, when I feel I need one. Hormones – Estraderm patch w/Provera 14-23 of month.

PREVIOUS CARE:

1. List doctors who have treated you for headaches: Dr. H. Dr. W.

2. List any tests you have had for your headache (e.g., EEG, CT scan, MRI, X-Ray, etc.):
1983 – Neck X-Ray (ok).

3. List any other treatment you have had for your headache (e.g., biofeedback, acupuncture, chiropractic, or any other treatment you had):
Counseling.

Chapter 6

Migraine

The subject of migraine can fill an entire book. As a matter of fact, in my personal library of 60 headache books, 12 are devoted only to migraine. I will attempt to blend the past theories and the current concepts of migraine. However, this attempt is primarily to introduce you to Part two of this book, where I explain how whiplash or acceleration/deceleration syndrome can cause a migraine or a migraine-like headache. Again, as I said in the last chapter on tension-like headaches, treatments will be discussed in part two of this book for post traumatic migraine-like headaches. There are many excellent books written on the treatment of migraine and at the end of this book there will be a list of some of them.

Aretaeus of Cappadocia in the 2nd century A.D. recognized this affliction of one side of the head (heterocrania) accompanied with gastrointestinal and visual symptoms. The term migraine is the French translation of the Greek word *hemikranios*, which Galen modified to "hemicrania." The Roman translation was "hemicranium" and the Old English translation became "megrim."[1]

Prior to 1988, when the International Headache Association reclassified headache disorders, the standard diagnosis of headaches that came from the 1962 Ad Hoc Committee on Classification of Headache of the National Institute of Neurological Disease and Blindness (NINDB) was used, and some still adhere to the old system (Table 6.1). That system divided vascular headaches into primary and secondary components.

Cluster headache will be discussed in Chapter 8.

In 1988, the journal *Cephalalgia, An International Journal of Headache*, published Volume 8, Supplement 7, titled "Classification and Diagnostic Criteria for Headache Disorders, Cranial Neuralgias and Facial Pain." The International Headache Society (IHS) formed committees and subcommittees of headache experts around the world and worked for three years to formulate a classification and operational diagnostic criteria for all headache disorders. A coding system was developed to make it possible to use the classification for those in routine practice. A more extensive system was also developed to be used by specialists and centers to accumulate data to become even more precise in identifying the pain problems. The reason for this extensive classification was to change what was considered to be just descriptions of migraine to more explicit definitions. The IHS wanted to alter what physicians would describe as symptoms that would appear to be common, often, or frequent into what would have to fulfill each type of headache category specifically.

Because patients may have different types of headaches within the same category, this type of classification would help identify the one or more types of migraine or any other type of headache. Therefore, if a patient's headache changes over time, the specific criteria would pick up the new type of headache. Also, as data are collected the ability to identify the different types of headache

Table 6.1

I. Primary Vascular Headaches
   A. Migraine
      1. Classic migraine: a biphasic migraine attack consisting of an aura (preheadache phase) of distinct neurological events, which is followed by the headache.
         a) Hemiplegic/hemisensory migraine: a migraine of classic subtype in which prodromal symptoms reflect neurological (motor and/or sensory) dysfunction.
         b) Ophthalmic (retinal) migraine: a migraine attack in which retinal impairment is present displaying photopsia (flashes or sparks of light) in one eye. This is followed by impairment of vision, generally preceding the headache.
         c) Vertebrobasilar migraine: there is a preheadache neurological set of symptoms that are a result of impairment of the vertebrobasilar arterial tree, which includes the brainstem, hypothalamus, thalmus, and occipital lobe. This headache is also called Bickerstaff's migraine and the symptoms include diplopia (double vision), vertigo, incoordination, ataxia (muscular uncoordination when attempting to walk), and dysarthria (stammering). Also seen with this headache is occasional fainting or sudden loss of consciousness.
         d) Ophthalmoplegic migraine: these symptoms can occur before the headache, during the headache and even after the headache, and have been reported to last days, weeks, and even became permanent after repeated attacks. There is often double vision and weakness of the extraocular muscles because it affects the 3rd cranial nerve (oculomotor).
         e) Complicated migraine: this is a migraine where the neurological symptoms outlast the pain by 24 hours or more. Sometimes these symptoms may last for a significant period of time.
         f) Facial migraine: sometimes known as "lower half headache," which describes recurrent pain below the level of the eyes. Although the pain is below the eyes, the other symptoms of migraine are the same. The pain is usually unilateral and the pain involves the nostril, cheek, gums, and teeth.
         g) Cardiac migraine: the term "cardiac migraine" was introduced by Leon-Sotomayer (1974) to demarcate a syndrome of classical migraine, with chest pain and functional hypoglycemia. During the prodrome of the attack, patients experience palpitations, anxiety symptoms, and chest pain, sometimes radiating to the inner aspect of the arm.
   B. Common migraine: This is a migraine attack without the distinct neurological symptoms discussed under (1) above.

II. Secondary vascular headaches are headaches of vascular origin but brought about as a consequence of a primary pathological or physiological process. These will be discussed in Chapter 10. Some examples are:
   A. Systemic infection and fever
   B. Hypoxia
   C. Cerebrovascular occlusive disease
   D. Arteritis
   E. Carbon monoxide poisoning
   F. Nitrite/nitrate ingestion
   G. Postepileptic state
   H. Hypoglycemia
   I. Alcohol ingestion
   J. Hemodialysis
   K. Drug induced
   L. Rebound (toxic) headache

From References 1 and 4.

would also help in the research needed desperately to make this a more scientific process, rather than an off-the-cuff "it's all in your head" type of diagnosis. When we have a better knowledge of the pathophysiology and the ability for objective testing, such as laboratory methods or imaging techniques, we will add more credibility to the diagnosis of headaches as exists in so many other areas of medical diseases.

The classification that is listed in *Cephalalgia* for migraine is ten pages long; only an abbreviated list is presented here.[5]

Although this is an abbreviated form of the classification of migraine, even the complete form cannot be exact and it will take much more investigation to eventually be complete.

Table 6.2 Classification of Migraine

1.1 Migraine without aura
- A. At least five attacks fulfilling B-D
- B. Headache attacks lasting 4–72 hours (untreated or unsuccessfully treated)
- C. Headache has at least two of the following characteristics:
  1. Unilateral location
  2. Pulsating quality
  3. Moderate to severe intensity
  4. Aggravation by walking stairs or similar routine physical activity
- D. During headache at least one of the following:
  1. Nausea and/or vomiting
  2. Photophobia and phonophobia

1.2 Migraine with aura
- A. At least two attacks fulfilling B
- B. At least three of the following four characteristics:
  1. One or more fully reversible aura symptoms indicating focal cerebral cortical and/or brainstem dysfunction
  2. At least one aura symptom develops gradually over more than 4 minutes, or two or more symptoms occur in succession
  3. No aura symptom lasts more than 60 minutes; if more than one aura symptom is present, accepted duration is proportionally increased
  4. Headache follows aura with a free interval of less than 60 minutes (it may also begin before or simultaneously with the aura)

1.2.1 Migraine with typical aura
- A Fulfills criteria for 1.2 including all four criteria under B.
- B. One or more aura symptoms of the following types:
  1. Homonymous (same side) visual disturbance
  2. Unilateral paresthesias and/or numbness
  3. Unilateral weakness
  4. Aphasia or unclassifiable speech difficulty

1.2.2 Migraine with prolonged aura
- A. Fulfills criteria for 1.2, but at least one symptom lasts more than 60 minutes and less than 7 days; If neuroimaging reveals relevant ischemic lesion, code 1.6.2, migrainous infarction, regardless of symptom duration

1.2.3 Familial hemiplegic migraine
- A. Fulfills criteria for 1.2
- B. The aura includes some degree of hemiparesis and may be prolonged
- C. At least one first degree relative has identical attacks

1.2.4 Basilar migraine
- A. Fulfills criteria 1.2
- B. Two or more aura symptoms of the following types:
  Visual symptoms in both the temporal and nasal fields of both eyes
  Dysarthria
  Vertigo
  Tinnitus
  Decreased hearing
  Double vision
  Ataxia
  Bilateral paresthesias
  Bilateral pareses
  Decreased level of consciousness

1.2.5 Migraine aura without headache
- A. Fulfills criteria for 1.2
- B. No headache

1.2.6 Migraine with acute onset aura
- A. Fulfills criteria for 1.2
- B. Neurological symptoms develop within 4 minutes
- C. Headache lasts 4–72 hours (untreated or unsuccessfully treated)

Table 6.2 Classification of Migraine (continued)

- D. Headache has at least two of the following characteristics:
  1. Unilateral location
  2. Pulsating quality
  3. Moderate or severe intensity
  4. Aggravation by walking stairs or similar routine physical activity
- E. During headache at least one of the following:
  1. Nausea and/or vomiting
  2. Photophobia and phonophobia
- F. Thromboembolic transient ischemic attack (TIA) and other intracranial lesion ruled out by appropriate investigations

1.3 Ophthalmoplegic migraine
- A. At least two attacks fulfilling B
- B. Headaches overlapping with paresis of one or more of cranial nerves III, IV, and VI
- C. Parasellar lesion ruled out by appropriate investigation

1.4 Retinal migraine
- A. At least two attacks fulfilling B-C
- B. Fully reversible monocular scotoma or blindness lasting less than 60 minutes and confirmed by examination during attack or (after proper instruction) by patient's drawing of monocular field defect during an attack
- C. Headache follows visual symptoms with a free interval of less than 60 minutes, but may precede them
- D. Normal ophthalmological examination outside of attack; embolism ruled out by appropriate investigations

1.5 Childhood periodic syndromes that may be precursors to or associated with migraine
- 1.5.1 Benign paroxysmal vertigo of childhood
  - A. Multiple, brief, sporadic episodes of disequilibrium, anxiety, and often nystagmus or vomiting
  - B. Normal neurological examination
  - C. Normal electroencephalogram
- 1.5.2 Alternating hemiplegia of childhood
  - A. Onset before 18 months of age
  - B. Repeated attacks of hemiplegia involving both sides of the body
  - C. Other paroxysmal phenomena, such as tonic spells, dystonic posturing, choreoathetoid movements, nystagmus or other ocular motor abnormalities, automatic disturbances associated with the bouts of hemiplegia or occurring independently
  - D. Evidence of mental or neurological deficits

1.6 Complications of migraine (code for previous migraine type plus the complications)
- 1.6.1 Status migrainosus
  - A. Fulfills criteria for 1.1 or 1.2
  - B. The present attack fulfills criteria for one form of migraine except that the headache lasts more than 72 hours whether treated or not
  - C. Headache is continuous throughout the attack or interrupted by headache-free intervals lasting less than 4 hours; interruption during sleep is disregarded
- 1.6.2 Migrainous infarction
  - A. Fulfills criteria for 1.2
  - B. The present attack is typical of previous attacks, but neurological deficits are not completely reversible within 7 days and/or neuroimaging demonstrates ischemic infarction in relevant area
  - C. Other causes of infarction ruled out by appropriate investigations

1.7 Migrainous disorder not fulfilling above criteria
- A. Fulfills all criteria but one for one or more forms of migraine (specify type[s])
- B. Does not fulfill criteria for tension-type headache

From *Cephalalgia*.[5]

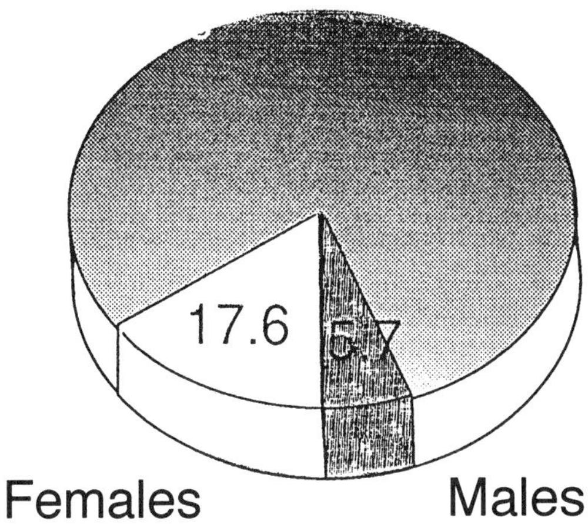

Figure 6.1 Distribution of migraine problems in the U.S. in millions. On the basis of a survey done by Stewart et al.,[6-8] it would appear the prevalence of migraine is approximately 18,000,000 females vs. almost 6,000,000 males. This is an extremely conservative number and most likely the prevalence of this problem is really much higher.

Stewart and Colleagues[6-8] have published an excellent study on the prevalence of migraine in the United States in 1992. They found that the prevalence of migraine increases with age to about age 40 and then decreases after age 40. Their conservative projections of the prevalence data to the national population indicates that 18 million women and about 5.6 million men suffer severe migraine headaches (Figure 6.1). They surveyed 15,000 households and the responses indicated that 8.7 million women and 2.6 million men were moderately to severely disabled by their migraine (see Chapter 4). They found, contrary to our belief, that migraine prevalence is considerably higher in groups with a low household income. The prevalence of migraine in households of incomes of less than $10,000 per year is more than 60% greater than in households in which the annual income is $30,000 or more. Females from age 30 to 49 years from lower income households have the highest risk of suffering migraine. Their data suggest these numbers because these people have inadequate medical care, poorer diets, greater problems, and there is always a downward drift of disability secondary to migraine which interferes with school and work, which may explain the cause of lower incomes. Their studies describe that diagnosed migraine is just the tip of the iceberg and that if 41% of the women have been diagnosed with migraine then there are 59% who are not diagnosed. If 29% of males are diagnosed, then 71% are not diagnosed (Figure 6.2).

This is attributed to several reasons. Some people do not consult a physician at all, while others fail to report their headache to their doctors. Other reasons may be that physicians may ignore complaints of headache, while some do not communicate effectively with patients with migraine, and others do not make the proper diagnosis. Men have a tendency not to see physicians about their headache problems; perhaps because of the myth that headache is a female disorder. Many think if they don't have an aura, or vomit, or are not disabled, they do not have a migraine. Because of poor public and physician education, there are vast numbers of people who are undiagnosed and untreated. There does not appear to be any significant difference of migraine regardless of race or urban or rural residence.

Their study has some interesting conclusions about medication use by migraine sufferers. For their migraines, men use 28.3% and women use 40.1% of prescription drugs. Persons who experience three or more disabling migraine attacks each month are generally considered candidates for preventive medication. With this concept of standard, 34% of females and 43% of males are not receiving prophylactic treatment. Where prescription medication could be used for symptomatic or abortive treatment of the migraine sufferer who experiences a moderate or severe disabling attack fewer than three times a month, 47% of women and 61% of males are not receiving proper treatment.

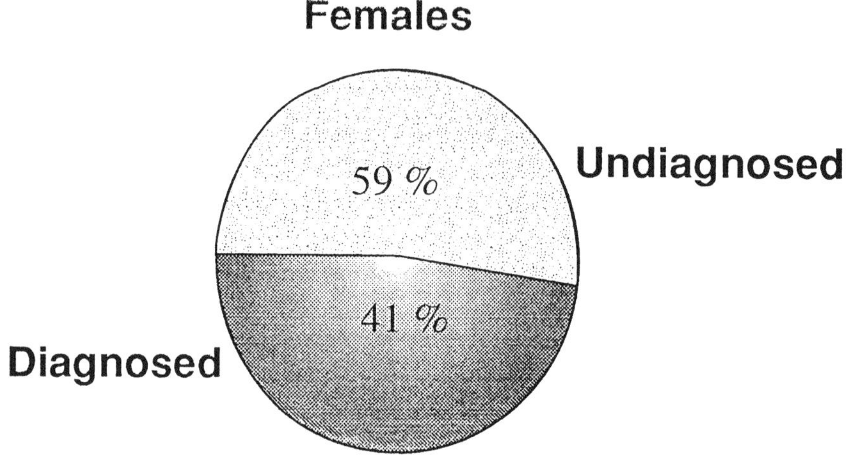

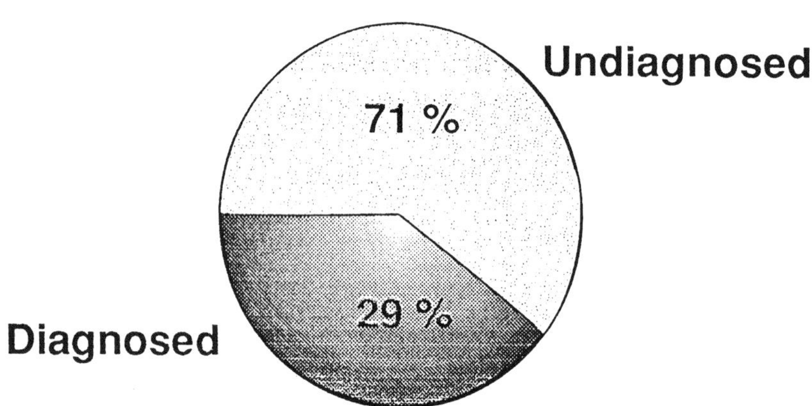

Figure 6.2 There is probably a much larger number of migraine sufferers who have not been diagnosed by a physician. Of the total population of migraine sufferers, Lipton et al.[6-8] estimate that approximately 59% of females have not been diagnosed, and approximately 71% of males have not been diagnosed.

Prescription medication increases with the following symptoms: vomiting (females 52%; males 38%), visual auras (females 48%; males 30%), frequent attacks, two to six times a week (females, 48%; males, 39%). The enormity of this problem is so great that a survey done by other sources in the mid-1980s shows that out of 550 million lost workdays, 157 million were due to headaches. Backaches caused 88 million lost workdays; muscle pains 58 million; joint pains 108 million; stomach pains 98 million; menstrual pains 24.5 million; and dental pains 15 million.

The question of whether migraine is inherited has always been an ongoing question. Fifty to sixty percent of patients with migraine report that one or both parents had migraine. Some studies report that 90% of patients with migraine have some member in the family who has reported headaches that appear to be migraine. The incidence of parental migraine indicates that there is a higher percentage with mothers than fathers, almost three to one. There have also been studies with

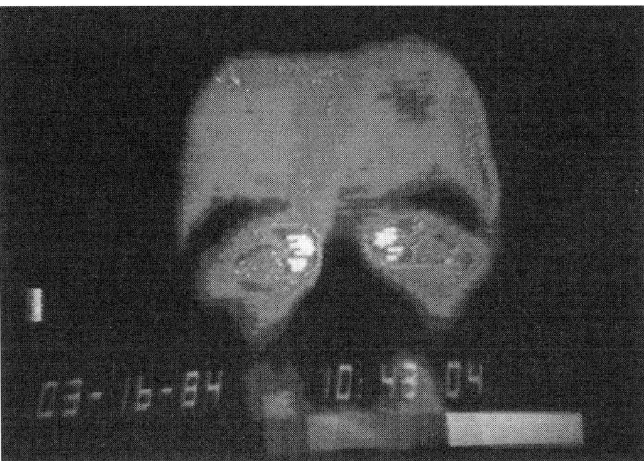

Figure 6.3 A vascular "cold patch" (right frontal region). This cold patch was demonstrated in 82% of migraine patients.

siblings and twins, both identical and fraternal. The evidence that there is a hereditary factor in migraine is substantial; what is not clear is the mode of inheritance.[9] Is there a specific gene for migraine or is there a genetic influence to lower the threshold that permits the pain process after some triggering factors are initiated? More recently, there have been studies that have identified some chromosomes that are related to familial hemiplegic migraine.

During the 1980s, Swerdlow and Dieter did numerous studies using thermography to identify a "cold patch" on the forehead that was statistically significant with migraine (Figure 6.3). We raised the question of whether there was a biological marker that may be inherent to migraine physiology. If there is a fixed thermographic pattern with migraine, then would this justify a consideration of a genetic factor?[10-16]

Women who suffer migraine, and their doctors, always believed that when the periods stopped (menopause), their headaches would stop. Unfortunately, there are no studies that verify this concept. At best some will get complete relief, most others may get less severe headaches, while others seem to get a different type of headache. Interestingly, some women who will report a total end to their headaches in their early adult lives will report a recurrence of headache in their sixties and seventies.

Most people report that their migraine headaches begin in the morning but many report that they can start anytime during the day or evening. Although cluster headaches (see Chapter 8) usually are nocturnal and will wake the patient from sleep, migraine does not appear to have the same characteristics. Although the word hemicrania, which the word migraine comes from, means one side of the head, the actual complaint of the patient is far from an only one-sided headache. Patients who characterize the location as one-sided will often say that the pain may be on one or the other side of their head. Others will state that the headache will start on one side and then move to the other side, while others may point out that they never know which side the headache may start out with. More than 50% of complaints will be frontal, one side or both, occipital (the back of the head), one side or both, the neck, or the whole head. Most of my patients will say that the headache will start at a certain location and move to another part of the head. For example, the patient may say that the pain may start on one side of the neck and then move forward to the side of the head and continue to the front part of the skull. Or one may complain that the pain starts in the front and moves to the side and then all the way to the neck. What is important is that location is not the best indicator of a migraine headache.

Untreated migraine attacks can last from hours to days and it is not uncommon that even treated migraines can last the same duration. Often, medications that work on some occasions do not help on others and patients will have to switch their medications to have effective treatments. Lying down in a dark room with little or no noise with something cool on their heads or going to sleep with the same conditions seems to be consistent. Also consistent is the complaint that movements that shake the head will increase the pain. The frequency of attacks also alters. Women who have migraine associated with hormonal changes will notice headaches one or two times a month. However, migraine attacks are reported from one to ten times a month and depending on the frequency of the assaults, medications may only be abortive or both abortive and preventive. In Chapter 7 on daily chronic headaches, we see how the distinct symptoms of migraine become clouded with symptoms of a muscle or tension type of headache or with symptoms of both types of headaches.

Most migraine sufferers feel that their pain will eventually become incapacitating even if it starts as dull or irritating. They often observe that if the headache starts as a dull pain, sudden movements such as bending over or walking up stairs, or sitting in the back of an automobile that is bouncing can change the nature of the pain and symptoms from aching and dull to severe and throbbing or pulsating. It is uncommon that someone with a migraine attack will be able to function or will be able to be productive at their minimal ability. It is truly a condition that is disabling.

Accompanying symptoms that are frequently associated with migraine are the following:

Gastrointestinal. Most patients will complain of nausea, either before or during the headache, and half of these patients will also mention that they vomit. Far fewer will complain of diarrhea. Nausea is a very important symptom to differentiate migraine from other types of headaches.

Neurological. Other very common symptoms are light sensitivity (photophobia), sensitivity to noise (sonophobia), and sensitivity to odors. One or more of these complaints are as frequent as the gastrointestinal symptoms. Often symptoms accompanying classical migraine or migraine with aura are scotomata or blind spots, teichopsia (fortification spectra or zigzag patterns resembling a fort) (Figure 6.4). Photopsia, flashes of lights, or visual or auditory hallucinations may be seen; Lewis Carroll drew these distortions in his book *Alice in Wonderland.* Other neurological symptoms that have been described in the classification of migraine are hemiplegia (paralysis of one half or one part of the body), hemiparesis (weakness or partial paralysis of one side of the body), dysarthria (difficulty in forming words in speech, or stammering), vertigo, tinnitus (ringing in the ear), double vision, ataxia (muscular incoordination), and rarely others. Whenever a patient presents with these symptoms it is essential that a complete neurological examination is done to rule out any significant neuropathological condition that may be causing these symptoms. If there are any convulsive movements, an examination must be done to access whether this is related to the severe pain or if this is seizure activity related to epilepsy.[18]

Edema. Some patients complain of swelling hours or days before the attack. They claim their rings or shoes or other clothing become tight. They have reported that there is a weight gain from 2 to 17 pounds. When the headache starts there is an associated polyuria (frequent urination) and most of the swelling goes away. Although measures are taken to prevent this swelling, it does not seem to prevent the migraine attack. It has therefore been suggested that these symptoms of edema are not a causal relationship to the migraine attack.[9]

Autonomic nervous system. Nasal stuffiness or nasal secretion is often reported. On occasion there is a drooping of the eyelid (ptosis) and dilatation of the pupil. Again if there is ever a dilatation of the pupil there must be a complete neurological examination to make sure there is no neuropathology present. Fever has been reported in some patients, especially children. There have also been reported rapid (tachycardia) and irregular heart beats (paroxysmal atrial tachycardia) (see Figure 6.5).

Figure 6.4 These illustrations demonstrate various auras. (a) On the left, lines that appear like a fort, and are called fortification spectra; (right) flashes of light in the center on the rooftops, or scintillating scotoma; (below) a blind spot, or negative scotoma, above the waterwheel. (b) A combination of fortification spectra and negative scotoma that a migraine sufferer may visualize while reading text. Often the sufferer may think this is associated with eye pathology. These auras are temporary and usually disappear when the headache starts.

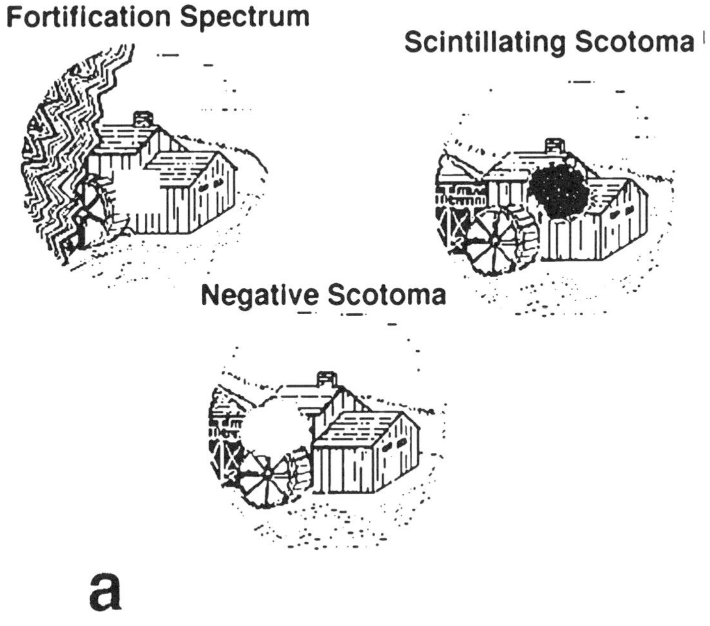

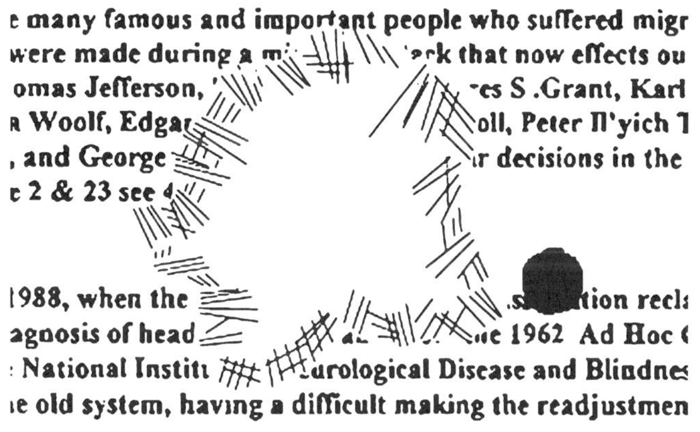

e Greek word "hemikranios", which Galen modified to
" hemicranium" and the Old English translation becam
e many famous and important people who suffered migr
were made during a m
ork that now effects ou
omas Jefferson,
es S .Grant, Karl
a Woolf, Edgar
oll, Peter Il'yich
, and George
r decisions in the
e 2 & 23 see
1988, when the
tion recl
agnosis of head
1962 Ad Hoc
National Instit
urological Disease and Blindne
ie old system, having a difficult making the readjustmen
tem divided vascular headaches into primary and secon
y Vascular Headaches

Blind Spot or negative Scotoma
and ZIGZAG lines or Fortification Spectra

b

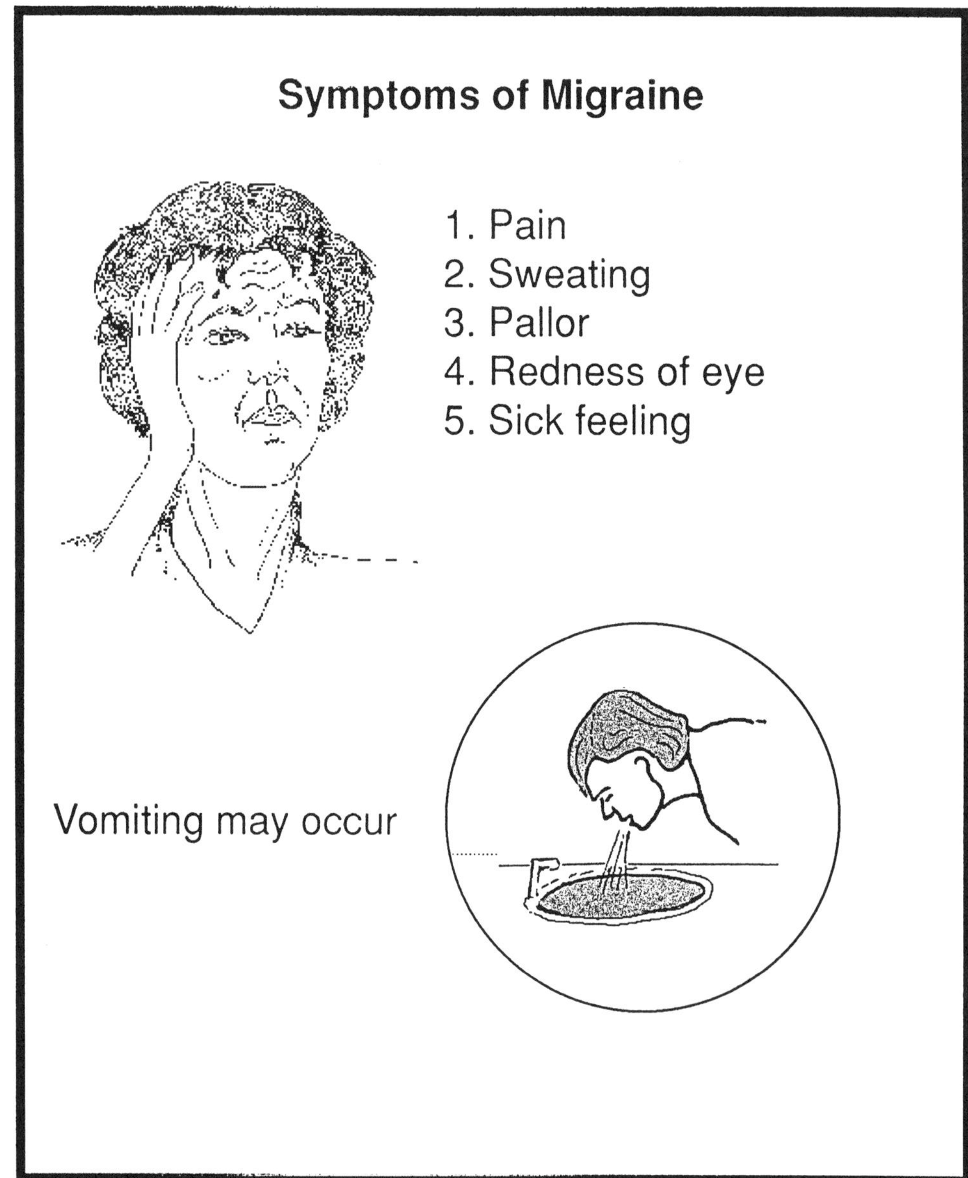

Symptoms of Migraine
1. Pain
2. Sweating
3. Pallor
4. Redness of eye
5. Sick feeling
Vomiting may occur

Figure 6.5 The usual migraine attack is incapacitating. The symptoms are usually unilateral, accompanied by throbbing, pallor, perspiration, and swelling or edema around the eyes. This is almost always accompanied by nausea and sometimes vomiting, and there is photophobia (light sensitivity), sonophobia (noise sensitivity), and sensitivity to odors. The patient will also feel chills. In certain types of migraine, patients will have difficulty with speech, dizziness, confusion, irritability, and visual disturbances. There can be blurred or cloudy vision, with scintillating zigzag lines or fortification spectra, little flashes of light, or blind spots. These patients generally lie down in a quiet, dark room until the attack abates.

TRIGGERING CAUSES OF MIGRAINE

As discussed earlier in this chapter and in Chapter 3, there is now agreement that there seems to be a lowered biological threshold to a variety of external and internal stimuli (see Figure 3.5). Much has been published on these triggering factors. I will only mention some of them. Blows to the head from sports and accidents have been reported to cause migraine. The second part of this book will discuss at length the relationship of head and neck injuries that precipitate or cause migraine-like headaches. Changes in the barometric pressure, for example in airplanes especially in descent, or being in a decompressure chamber, can trigger a migraine. However, Fife and Meyer[19] have reported aborting migraine in their hyperbaric chamber.

Many have reported that weather is responsible for causing their headache. Professor F.G. Sulman[20] has studied the hot, dry wind known as the Sharav in Israel, cool winds like the French Mistral or the Canadian Chinook and others, the Santa Ana of southern California, Arizona desert winds, the Argentine Zonda, the Sirocco of the Mediterrean, the Maltese Xlokk, the Chamsin of the Arab countries, the Foehn of Switzerland, southern Germany and Austria and the North Winds of Melbourne and there appears to be a relationship with these weather changes and reported headaches. Many of my patients tell me that often when the humidity changes, indicating a rain front, they will be able to predict a migraine attack.

Glare and noise can induce migraine. Bright lights, sunlight, flashing lights, and loud blasting noises are frequent triggers in the headache population. Stress, an over-used term, as well as alterations from the daily routine (weekends, holidays, vacations, etc.) are also responsible for the onset of "the pain." Oversleeping is often the culprit, as well as missing meals. Foods and beverages containing nitrite, glutamate, salt, aspartame, tyramine and drugs that contain nitroglycerin, histamine, reserpine, hydralazine, estrogen and others have been reported to trigger migraine.

Excessive amounts of vitamin A, cold foods, fluorescent lighting, allergic reactions, pungent odors such as paint, solvents, smoke, perfumes are all responsible for a possible migraine attack.

IS THERE A MIGRAINE PERSONALITY?

In 1948 Harold Wolff published his research and findings in a masterful collection of his work in "Headache and Other Head Pain." Since then the continuation of his work has been republished and updated and there is a fourth edition printed in 1980.[21]

At that time a great deal of emphasis was placed on psychoanalytical thinking. Fromm-Reichman in 1937 on the basis of eight patients concluded that "they could not be aware of their hostility against beloved persons; therefore, they unconsciously tried to keep their hostility repressed, and finally expressed it by physical symptoms of migraine." She wrote her patients repressed hostility, fearing they would be deprived of the protection of their families. Their envious desire to destroy their rivals' brilliance was turned inward, resulting in symptoms within the patients' heads.

Wolff sustained his studies with this theme and put together characteristics of the migraine personality. As children they were delicate, shy and withdrawn and usually extremely obedient to the desires of their parents. Because these children were sensitive, trustworthy and energetic, they were given responsibility at an early age. When these children reached adult age, they were seen with the following personalities: ambitious and preoccupied with achievement and success, perfection and efficiency, orderliness, doubts and repetitions, resentments, disregarding limits to their body except when they had a migraine attack. They seemed to be cautious with their money, and were socially cautious and prevented intimacy in their social relationships. There was a great deal of sexual dissatisfaction in more than four fifths of the women. Many more symptoms are listed in the fifteen pages describing these personality traits.

As time went on more and more studies were done to evaluate the consistency and accuracy of this hypothesis. As the studies continued, more of the researchers concluded that there was only minimal support for the view that migraine sufferers were more neurotic than age-matched normal subjects.

More recent studies reflect the following: Kudrow and Sutkus[22] reported in 1979 that after evaluating categories of headache — cluster, migraine, scalp muscle contraction, mixed headache sufferers, post trauma and conversion patients — using the MMPI (Minnosota Multiphasic Personality Inventory), cluster and migraine subjects were least neurotic. Neurotic traits were more common among the other categories of headache patients, in the order listed.

In 1982, a study by Andrasic et al.[23] failed to replicate Kudrow's study, but did agree that patients with scalp muscle contraction headache exhibited the greatest psychological distress.

Sternbach et al. in 1890 conducted an empirical statistical study analyzing diagnoses, age, and sex utilizing the MMPI.[24] They felt that the differences in scores may be related to the "pain densities," that is, that the higher scores on the scalp muscle contraction and mixed patients may be due to the fact these individuals experience far fewer pain-free intervals than do the pure vascular headache patients.

Williams et al. in 1986 came to the conclusion, in an article reviewing headache and the MMPI,[25] that headache patients appear to be more disturbed than non-headache patients and the least disturbed are the cluster and migraine patients. The problems increase in the order scalp muscle – mixed – post trauma – conversion, but these disturbances of psychopathology may not be related to the diagnoses.

In 1988, Dieter and Swerdlow did a study that showed that there did not appear to be evidence that chronic headache patients exhibit predictable profile responses to the MMPI, which provides predictable profiles.[26] What we observed was that how patients perceive themselves as headache sufferers was important. We pointed out that many responses to questions on the MMPI may be incorrectly interpreted as far as the psychopathology of the patient is concerned.

In my observations in over 32 years of practice, 16 years of psychiatric practice and 16 years of treating the medical and neurological aspects of headache, I was never able to differentiate any more neurosis between migraine and non-migraine patients. However, this does not mean that I have not seen a number of neurotic migraine patients. My question is, if the amount of pain was reduced, and the fear of impending crippling attacks coming without warning was eliminated, would our test results be the same? What we have to test is, what does chronic pain do to our personality? How many of us really enjoy incapacitating pain as a means of gaining attention or pleasure?

My recollection is that the patient who suffers attacks once a month and is able to abort them with a simple treatment has a different approach to life than the patient who is never able to make any commitments because of ten to twenty attacks a month, for which few treatments are successful. Unfortunately, the medical and the lay public have been inundated with the early concepts that there are unquestionable psychoanalytic dynamics that explain the mechanism of migraine. Hopefully, with all of the physiological research and the education that is being promoted by the National Headache Foundation and The American Association for the Study of Headache, these myths will come to an end.

Case histories have been included after the References. With this introduction to migraine and the case histories, you should be able to understand migraine and the discussions of post traumatic (whiplash) migraine-like headaches.

REFERENCES

1. Saper, J.R., *Headache Disorder*, John Wright-PSG, 1983.
2. Saper, J.R., Magee, K.R., *Freedom From Headaches*, Simon & Schuster, New York, 1978.
3. Swerdlow, B., *The Headache Handbook*, Mayfield Press, 1985.
4. Lance, J.W., *Mechanism and Management of Headaches*, 4th ed., Butterworths, London.
5. International Headache Society, Classification and diagnostic criteria for headache disorders, cranial neuralgias and facial pain, *Cephalalgia*, 8 (Suppl. 7), 1988.
6. Stewart, W.F., Lipton, R.B., Celentano, D.D., Prevalence of migraine headache in the United States: relation to age, income, race, and other sociodemographic factors, *JAMA*, 267, 64–69, 1992.
7. Lipton, R.B., Stewart, W.F., Celentano, D.D., Reed, M.L., Undiagnosed migraine headache: a comparison of symptom based and reported physician diagnosis, *Arch. Intern. Med.*, 152, 1273–1278, 1992.
8. Celentano, D.D., Stewart, W.F., Lipton, R.B., Reed, M.L., Medication use and disability among migraineurs: a national probability sample survey, *Headache*, 32, 223–228, 1992.
9. Raskin, N.H., *Headache*, 2nd ed, Churchill Livingstone, New York, 1988.
10. Swerdlow, B., Dieter, J.N., The persistent migraine "cold patch" and the fixed facial thermogram, *Thermology*, 2, 16–20, 1986.
11. Swerdlow, B., Dieter, J.N., The validity of the vascular "cold patch" in the diagnosis of chronic headache, *Headache*, 26, 22–26, 1986.
12. Swerdlow, B., Dieter, J.N., The vascular "cold patch" is not a prognostic index for headache, *Headache*, 29(9), 562–568, 1989.
13. Swerdlow, B., Dieter, J.N., The thermographically observed effects of hyperoxia on vascular headache patients and non-headache individuals, *Headache*, 27(10), 533–539, 1987.
14. Swerdlow, B., Dieter, J.N., The value of medical thermography for the diagnosis of chronic headache, *Headache Quarterly*, 2, 96–104, 1991.
15. Edmeads, J., Is thermography a marker for vascular headaches? Editorial, *Headache*, 26(1), 47, 1986.
16. Edmeads, J., On negative results. Editorial, *Headache*, 27(1), 1987.
17. Swerdlow, B., Dieter, J.N., Letters to the Editor. Cold spot question heats up, *Headache*, 122–123, Feb. 1989.
18. Diamond, S., Dalessio, D.J., *The Practicing Physician's Approach to Headache*, Williams & Wilkins, Baltimore, 1986.
19. Fife, C.E., Meyer, J.S., Hyperbaric oxygen treatment of acute migraine headache, *Headache Quarterly*, 2(4), 301–306, 1991.
20. Sulman, F.G., unpublished observations.
21. Dalessio, D.J., *Wolff's Headache and Other Head Pain*, 4th ed., Oxford University Press, New York, 1980.
22. Kudrow, L., Sutkus, B.J., MMPI specificity in primary headache disorders, *Headache*, 19, 18–24, 1979.
23. Andrasic, F., Blanchard, E.B., Arena, J.G., Teders, S.J., Rodichok, L.D., Cross validation of The Kudrow-Sutkus MMPI classification system for diagnosing headache type, *Headache*, 22, 2–5, 1982.
24. Sternbach, R.A., Dalessio, D.J., Kunzel, M., Bowman, G.E., MMPI patterns in common headache disorder, *Headache*, 20, 311–315, 1980.
25. Williams, D.E., Thompson, J.K., Haber, J.D., Raczynski, J.M., MMPI and headaches: a special focus on differential diagnosis, prediction of treatment outcome, and patient treatment, *Pain*, 24, 143–158, 1986.
26. Dieter, J.N., Swerdlow, B., A replicative investigation of the reliability of the MMPI in the classification of chronic headaches, *Headache*, 28(3), 212–222, 1988.

CASE HISTORIES*

DEBORAH
Category: Migraine

This is a very interesting case in which a 36-year-old woman came in with complaints of having three different types of headache: incapacitating, interfering and irritating, with different symptoms. Her #1 irritating and #2 interfering headaches started 15 years ago, while the #3 incapacitating headaches started a year and a half ago. There were typical symptoms of migraine with the incapacitating headaches in that the character of her pain was throbbing, and she had nausea, vomiting, sensitivity to light (photophobia), sensitivity to noise (sonophobia), sensitivity to odors, and she would have to go to bed.

She also states that when she was placed on progesterone for premenstrual syndrom (PMS) she began to see zigzag lines (fortification spectra) and blind spots (negative scotomata) and these would last 30 minutes before the headaches started. She had seen an ophthalmologist who had diagnosed her as having an ocular migraine, and at that time, in 1986, had a CT scan which was normal. She also complained of numbness and tingling in both arms, fingers and knees, and has complained of increasing fatigue, with increased sleeping.

Because of the many different symptoms, an MRI was done, which came back negative. Multiple laboratory tests were done to make sure that she was not suffering from any metabolic problems or viral infections that could cause her tiredness. The numbness in her hands turned out to be carpal tunnel syndrome, and the patient's final diagnosis was by the old classification "Classic Migraine," meaning that she has an aura. She was also given a diagnosis not in the classification called "Hormonal Migraine" because it would come monthly with her menstrual periods.

With the treatment that she was getting, her headaches, by the headache log she kept, were reduced by 85%, both in intensity and frequency.

This is a case that seems to start off with a simple headache intake, and turns into being a rather interesting case to rule out the possibility of multiple problems. In the care of a headache specialist, this patient will do very well.

* On the headache assessment forms that accompany these case histories, incapacitating headaches are indicated with solid black lines, interfering headaches with dotted lines, and irritating headaches with gray shading.

MEDICAL HEADACHE HISTORY

Name: Deborah **Age:** 36 **Sex** F **Date:** 1/8/91

Date of Birth: 0/00/54 **Birthplace:** D.C. **Race:** C **Education:** High school

Occupation: Credit Union Branch Manager **Accident:** N/A

Armed Services & Type of Discharge: N/A

PAST HISTORY:

1.	Did you have a normal birth?		Yes	No
	a) forceps used?		Yes	No
	b) cesarean section?		Yes	No
2.	Did you have problems with bedwetting?		Yes	No
	a) If yes, age bedwetting stopped			
3.	Were you car sick as a child (motion)?		Yes	No
	a) If yes, how severe?	Slight	Moderate	Severe
4.	Did you have unexplained abdominal cramps as a child?		Yes	No
5.	Did you have any of the following illnesses in childhood?			
	a) meningitis		Yes	No
	b) encephalitis		Yes	No
	c) scarlet fever		Yes	No
	d) rheumatic fever		Yes	No
6.	Did you have any head injuries as a child?		Yes	No
	a) If yes, please explain:			
7.	Were you treated for emotional illness as a child?		Yes	No

HABITS:

8.	Do you drink alcohol?	Yes	No
	a) If yes, what kind and how much? Maybe 1 or 2 times a year (special occasion)		
	b) Does alcohol bring on or aggravate a headache?	Yes	No
9.	Do you smoke?	Yes	No
	a) If yes, how much? 1½ packs a day		
	b) Does smoking or smoke-filled rooms cause or aggravate headaches?	Yes	No
10.	Do you drink caffeinated beverages?	Yes	No
	a) If yes, how much? Coffee, 3 – 4 cups in a.m.		

MENSTRUAL HISTORY:

At what age did menses begin? 12 Were they regular or irregular? WNL
How were they related to your headache? Increased headaches
Are you or were you ever on Birth Control Pills? No Did they affect your headache? N/A
Have you had a hysterectomy, partial or total, and why? No
Are you in menopause, and if yes, how long? No
Are you on hormones, and if yes, which ones? Progesterone 200 mg SL, Day 12 twice a day for PMS

HEADACHE ASSESSMENT FORM

HA PROFILE	INCAPACITATING #3	INTERFERING #2	IRRITATING #1
ONSET (Years ago and frequency)	1½ years ago, 1 per month	15 years ago, occasionally	15 years ago, occasionally
CURRENT FREQUENCY	One per month	2 to 3 per month	1 per week
TIME OF ONSET	Awaken with	Anytime	Anytime
DURATION	1½ days	1 to 1½ days	1 hour with OTC medications
CHARACTER	Throbbing	Less intense throbbing	Dull ache
PRODROME OR AURA	See zigzag lines, blind spots, blurred vision for 30 minutes	N/A	N/A
ASSOCIATING FEATURES	Nausea; Vomiting; Sensitivity to Light? Noise? Odors? Do you get pale or flush? Do your eyes or nose run? Does your nose get stuffy? Do the whites of your eyes get red? Does your eyelid droop? Do you pace, or go to bed?	Nausea; Vomiting; Sensitivity to Light? Noise? Odors? Do you get pale or flush? Do your eyes or nose run? Does your nose get stuffy? Do the whites of your eyes get red? Does your eyelid droop? Do you pace, or go to bed?	Nausea; Vomiting; Sensitivity to Light? Noise? Odors? Do you get pale or flush? Do your eyes or nose run? Does your nose get stuffy? Do the whites of your eyes get red? Does your eyelid droop? Do you pace, or go to bed?
PRECIPITATING OR AGGRAVATING FEATURES	Movement	Activity	N/A

LOCATION: Mark the location for each type of headache with a different color pen.
Incapacitating #3 is _____ Interfering #2 is -------- Irritating #1 is ▬

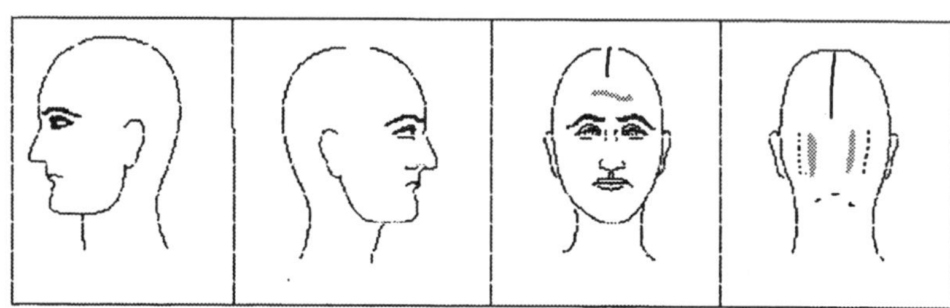

MEDICAL HISTORY:

Have you ever been or are you currently being treated for any of the following?

a) high blood pressure	Yes	No
b) stomach ulcers	Yes	No
c) asthma	Yes	No
d) allergies	Yes	No
e) pneumonia	Yes	No
f) kidney problems	Yes	No
g) low blood sugar	Yes	No
h) glaucoma	Yes	No
i) diabetes	Yes	No
j) heart problems	Yes	No

If you answered yes to any of the above, please describe: Asthmatic bronchitis. Environmental allergies.

List all other medical problems you have had in the past. Include date diagnosed and treatment.
DO NOT LIST OPERATIONS

Food and environmental allergies, 1987. Weekly allergy injections. PMS, 1990 (Progesterone (sublingual) 200 mg 2 x day or more day 12 to start of menses. Migraines, 1984. Started treatment (Cafergot, Fiorinol) in 1984, but moved to Florida in 1985.

SURGICAL HISTORY (List operations and dates performed)

Tonsillectomy, 1976.

PSYCHIATRIC HISTORY (List visits with counselors, psychologists, etc., and type of treatment)

1984 – 3 visits to psychiatrist. (Mother's death. Had a difficult time dealing with it and stepfather problems.)

ACCIDENTS IN ADULT LIFE (Briefly describe any accident that caused any blow to the head or that you feel is related to your headache)

None.A

FAMILY HISTORY:

1. Is your father living? Yes No
   - Age________
   - Cause of death Alcoholic/pneumonia & liver, 51
   - Was there a headache history? Unk Yes No
2. Is your mother living? Yes No
   - Age________
   - Cause of death Cancer (bladder/lung), 63
   - Was there a headache history? Yes No

3. Ages of brothers---Circle the ones with headache
   (47) (44) 32
4. Ages of sisters---Circle the ones with headache
   (41) (33) 33
5. List any other blood relatives with a history of severe headaches.
   Unk

MARITAL HISTORY:
List marriages:

1st marriage age 19 to Present	Did spouse have headaches?	Yes	No
2nd marriage age _____ to _____	Did spouse have headaches?	Yes	No
3rd marriage age _____ to _____	Did spouse have headaches?	Yes	No

Age of current spouse: 38

List ages and sex of all children:

Age _____	Sex _____	Headaches?	Yes	No
Age _____	Sex _____	Headaches?	Yes	No
Age _____	Sex _____	Headaches?	Yes	No

STRESS FACTORS:

List any factors that may be affecting your headaches (money, loneliness, sexual problems, work, etc.)
98% appears to be menstrual-related and the balance allergy and sometimes a tension headache after a long day.

VEGETATIVE SIGNS:

1.	Do you have trouble falling asleep?	Yes	No
2.	Do you have trouble staying asleep?	Yes	No
3.	Has your appetite decreased?	Yes	No
4.	Have you gained or lost weight in the past year?	Yes	No
5.	Have you felt tearful or depressed lately?	Yes	No
6.	Have you had any thoughts of wanting to die?	Yes	No
7.	Have you been forgetful lately?	Yes	No
8.	Any other changes in your normal day-to-day living?		

Please list any medications you are allergic or sensitive to: None that I know of.

Please list any medications you are currently taking (including dosages and frequency per day):
Progesterone 200 mg tab. 2 timesa day begin Day 12 up to menses. Tylox capsules, only if absolultely Cannot tolerate headache pain. Antigen-Prog-1 for headache, but doesn't help and don't take.

PREVIOUS CARE:

1. List doctors who have treated you for headaches: Dr. G., Dr. B., Dr. S., Dr. L., Hospital

2. List any tests you have had for your headache (e.g., EEG, CT scan, MRI, X-Ray, etc.):
CAT scan by Hospital, approx 1986 (with and without contrast) – normal.

3. List any other treatment you have had for your headache (e.g., biofeedback, acupuncture, chiropractic, or any other treatment you had):
None.

TOM
Category: Migraine with aura

This 41-year-old man started getting irritating headaches as a young adult, and he was able to treat those with over-the-counter medication. It was a dull, aching headache. About a year prior to seeing me, the headaches began to increase in intensity and went from an interfering (moderate to severe) headache to incapacitating one month ago, every day. He complained of having "blind spots and zigzag patterns," or fortification spectra, about 20 minutes before the headache, and had all the other typical symptoms of severe migraine, such as nausea, sensitivity to light, having to go to bed, his nose would run, etc. The diagnosis was migraine with aura and also status migraine, which means that the headache would not resolve itself. A work-up was done because his incapacitating headaches had just started a month ago, and there was no indication of an intracranial lesion by the MRI. Because his headaches were intractable and incapacitating and he was incapable of doing any work, the patient was started on the procedure that we used in our clinic in which a catheter was placed in his arm and he was given medicine via a computer that is attached to his belt. He could work all day with this medicine without having to go into the hospital. After four days, the headache broke and the intravenous line was taken out and medication was continued to prevent any future attacks.

The diagnosis was migraine with aura (classical migraine), and status migraine, in remission after treatment.

MEDICAL HEADACHE HISTORY

Name: Tom **Age:** 41 **Sex** M **Date:** 5/22/92

Date of Birth: 00/00/50 **Birthplace:** GA **Race:** W **Education:** 1 yr. college

Occupation: Computer Operations Supervisor **Accident:** N/A

Armed Services & Type of Discharge: 1969-1970 – Marines.

PAST HISTORY:

1.	Did you have a normal birth?	**Yes**	No
	a) forceps used?	Yes	No
	b) cesarean section?	Yes	No
2.	Did you have problems with bedwetting?	Yes	**No**
	a) If yes, age bedwetting stopped	________	
3.	Were you car sick as a child (motion)?	Yes	**No**
	a) If yes, how severe? Slight	Moderate	Severe
4.	Did you have unexplained abdominal cramps as a child?	Yes	**No**
5.	Did you have any of the following illnesses in childhood?		
	a) meningitis	Yes	**No**
	b) encephalitis	Yes	**No**
	c) scarlet fever	Yes	**No**
	d) rheumatic fever	Yes	**No**
6.	Did you have any head injuries as a child?	Yes	**No**
	a) If yes, please explain: ________		
7.	Were you treated for emotional illness as a child?	Yes	**No**

HABITS:

8.	Do you drink alcohol?	**Yes**	No
	a) If yes, what kind and how much? Maybe 6 beers in a month		
	b) Does alcohol bring on or aggravate a headache?	Yes	**No**
9.	Do you smoke?	Yes	**No**
	a) If yes, how much? ________		
	b) Does smoking or smoke-filled rooms cause or aggravate headaches?	Yes	**No**
10.	Do you drink caffeinated beverages?	**Yes**	No
	a) If yes, how much? 2 liters a day (sometimes)		

MENSTRUAL HISTORY:

At what age did menses begin?________ Were they regular or irregular?________
How were they related to your headache?________
Are you or were you ever on Birth Control Pills?________ Did they affect your headache? ________
Have you had a hysterectomy, partial or total, and why?________
Are you in menopause, and if yes, how long?________
Are you on hormones, and if yes, which ones? ________

HEADACHE ASSESSMENT FORM

HA PROFILE	INCAPACITATING #3	INTERFERING #2	IRRITATING #1
ONSET (Years ago and frequency)	A month ago	Nov. 1991 – 1 per week	As a young adult, rare
CURRENT FREQUENCY	Only 2	Every day for a week	Not now, rare before
TIME OF ONSET	Anytime	Anytime	Anytime
DURATION	1 day	Constant	1 hour with OTC medication
CHARACTER	Throbbing	Same, but less intense	Dull ache
PRODROME OR AURA	Had blind spots and zigzag pattern. Headache began 20 minutes later.	N/A	N/A
ASSOCIATING FEATURES	Nausea; Vomiting; Sensitivity to Light? Noise? Odors? Do you get pale or flush? Do your eyes or nose run? Does your nose get stuffy? Do the whites of your eyes get red? Does your eyelid droop? Do you pace, or go to bed?	Nausea; Vomiting; Sensitivity to Light? Noise? Odors? Do you get pale or flush? Do your eyes or nose run? Does your nose get stuffy? Do the whites of your eyes get red? Does your eyelid droop? Do you pace, or go to bed?	Nausea; Vomiting; Sensitivity to Light? Noise? Odors? Do you get pale or flush? Do your eyes or nose run? Does your nose get stuffy? Do the whites of your eyes get red? Does your eyelid droop? Do you pace, or go to bed?
PRECIPITATING OR AGGRAVATING FEATURES	Reflecting lights	Reflecting lights	N/A

LOCATION: Mark the location for each type of headache with a different color pen.

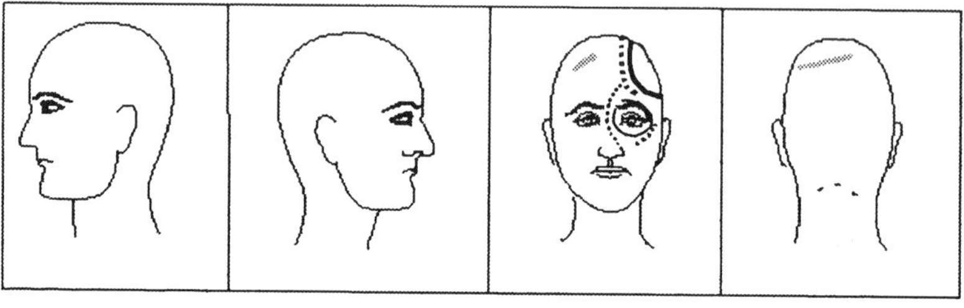

MEDICAL HISTORY:

Have you ever been or are you currently being treated for any of the following?

a) high blood pressure	Yes	No
b) stomach ulcers	Yes	No
c) asthma	Yes	No
d) allergies	Yes	No
e) pneumonia	Yes	No
f) kidney problems	Yes	No
g) low blood sugar	Yes	No
h) glaucoma	Yes	No
i) diabetes	Yes	No
j) heart problems	Yes	No

If you answered yes to any of the above, please describe:. High blood pressure diagnosed 5 years ago. Zestril p.r.n. Environmental allergies. Right Bundle Branch Block (no symptoms).

List all other medical problems you have had in the past. Include date diagnosed and treatment. DO NOT LIST OPERATIONS

SURGICAL HISTORY (List operations and dates performed)

Hernia - 1970. Knee Surgery - 1979.
RK Right Eye - 1985. RK Left Eye - 1986.
Deviated Septum - 1989. Anal Fissure - 1990.

PSYCHIATRIC HISTORY (List visits with counselors, psychologists, etc., and type of treatment)

None.

ACCIDENTS IN ADULT LIFE (Briefly describe any accident that caused any blow to the head or that you feel is related to your headache)

None.

FAMILY HISTORY:

1. Is your father living? Unknown (adopted) Yes No
   Age________
   Cause of death_____?_____
   Was there a headache history? Yes No
2. Is your mother living? Yes No
   Age________
   Cause of death_____?_____
   Was there a headache history? Don't know Yes No

3. Ages of brothers---Circle the ones with headache
   43
4. Ages of sisters---Circle the ones with headache
   ______
5. List any other blood relatives with a history of severe headaches.
   ______

MARITAL HISTORY:
List marriages:

1st marriage age 20 to 29	Did spouse have headaches?	Yes	No (underlined)
2nd marriage age 34 to 35	Did spouse have headaches?	Yes	No (underlined)
3rd marriage age 35 to Present	Did spouse have headaches?	Yes	No (underlined)
4th marriage age ___ to ___	Did spouse have headaches?	Yes	No

Age of current spouse: 38

List ages and sex of all children:

Age 17 Sex F Headaches?	Yes	No (underlined)
Age 15 Sex M Headaches?	Yes (underlined)	No
Age 6 Sex F Headaches?	Yes	No
Age 4 Sex M Headaches?	Yes	No

STRESS FACTORS:

List any factors that may be affecting your headaches (money, loneliness, sexual problems, work, etc.)
Work, Wife's illness, Money, Fear of loss of wife.

VEGETATIVE SIGNS:

1.	Do you have trouble falling asleep?		Yes	No (underlined)
2.	Do you have trouble staying asleep?	?	Yes	No
3.	Has your appetite decreased?		Yes	No (underlined)
4.	Have you gained or lost weight in the past year?		Yes	No (underlined)
5.	Have you felt tearful or depressed lately?		Yes (underlined)	No
6.	Have you had any thoughts of wanting to die?		Yes	No (underlined)
7.	Have you been forgetful lately?		Yes	No (underlined)
8.	Any other changes in your normal day-to-day living?			

Please list any medications you are allergic or sensitive to: Darvocet (increases headaches), Codeine (causes nausea)

Please list any medications you are currently taking (including dosages and frequency per day):
Midrin, maximum of 6 per day; Elavil 75 mg at bedtime; Lorcet Plus.

PREVIOUS CARE:

1. List doctors who have treated you for headaches: Dr. T. Dr. H. Dr. K. Dr. R.

2. List any tests you have had for your headache (e.g., EEG, CT scan, MRI, X-Ray, etc.):
CT scan 2 months ago.

3. List any other treatment you have had for your headache (e.g., biofeedback, acupuncture, chiropractic, or any other treatment you had):
None.

RENEE
Category: Migraine

This 25-year-old woman developed migraine headaches with typical symptoms of throbbing, nausea, vomiting, sensitivity to light, noise and odors, starting at age 9, and increasing as she got older. Eventually, these headaches fell into the categories of also interfering and irritating headaches, a type of combined headache. The patient had to be hospitalized when I saw her because she was having a status migraine and was totally incapacitated. In the hospital she received intravenous medication to abort her headache, which was a success. However, her headaches were rather labile and she would often get attacks. Her medical workup did not show any intracranial lesion or any major medical problem that was causing these continued migraine attacks. She was also taught self-hypnosis to reduce some of the pain that she was having, which was successful about 30% of the time. She continued on an abortive medication whenever she got an attack. From the time that she started treatment until the last I saw her, her headaches had improved about 60%; but she still suffered headaches on a regular basis. I feel this is a patient who would have to be followed carefully and monitored with proper medications and treatment. Diagnosis: Migraine without aura, or non-classical migraine.

MEDICAL HEADACHE HISTORY

Name: Renée **Age:** 25 **Sex** F **Date:** 8/22/85

Date of Birth: 00/00/59 **Birthplace:** FL **Race:** C **Education:** High school

Occupation: Homemaker **Accident:** N/A

Armed Services & Type of Discharge: N/A

PAST HISTORY:

1.	Did you have a normal birth?		Yes (underlined)	No
	a) forceps used?		Yes	No (underlined)
	b) cesarean section?		Yes	No (underlined)
2.	Did you have problems with bedwetting?		Yes	No (underlined)
	a) If yes, age bedwetting stopped		______	
3.	Were you car sick as a child (motion)?		Yes	No (underlined)
	a) If yes, how severe?	Slight	Moderate	Severe
4.	Did you have unexplained abdominal cramps as a child?		Yes	No (underlined)
5.	Did you have any of the following illnesses in childhood?			
	a) meningitis		Yes	No (underlined)
	b) encephalitis		Yes	No (underlined)
	c) scarlet fever		Yes	No (underlined)
	d) rheumatic fever		Yes	No (underlined)
6.	Did you have any head injuries as a child?		Yes	No (underlined)
	a) If yes, please explain: ______			
7.	Were you treated for emotional illness as a child?		Yes	No (underlined)

HABITS:

8.	Do you drink alcohol?	Yes	No (underlined)
	a) If yes, what kind and how much? ______		
	b) Does alcohol bring on or aggravate a headache?	Yes (underlined)	No
9.	Do you smoke?	Yes	No (underlined)
	a) If yes, how much? ______		
	b) Does smoking or smoke-filled rooms cause or aggravate headaches?	Yes	No
10.	Do you drink caffeinated beverages?	Yes	No
	a) If yes, how much? ______		

MENSTRUAL HISTORY:

At what age did menses begin? 12 Were they regular or irregular? WNL

How were they related to your headache? Had headaches 2 to 3 days before period

Are you or were you ever on Birth Control Pills? Yes Did they affect your headache? Worsened

Have you had a hysterectomy, partial or total, and why? No

Are you in menopause, and if yes, how long? No

Are you on hormones, and if yes, which ones? No

HEADACHE ASSESSMENT FORM

HA PROFILE	INCAPACITATING #3	INTERFERING #2	IRRITATING #1
ONSET (Years ago and frequency)	9 years old, came in cycles of every couple months	Teens, 2 a week	Teens, frequently
CURRENT FREQUENCY	Since March, almost every day	Several a week	Couple a month
TIME OF ONSET	N/A	N/A	Afternoon
DURATION	1 day to 5 days	8 to 10 hours	Several hours
CHARACTER	Pressure, throbbing Splitting sensation	Throbbing, tightness	Dull ache
PRODROME OR AURA	N/A	N/A	N/A
ASSOCIATING FEATURES	Nausea; Vomiting; Sensitivity to Light? Noise? Odors? Do you get pale or flush? Do your eyes or nose run? Does your nose get stuffy? Do the whites of your eyes get red? Does your eyelid droop? Do you pace, or go to bed?	Nausea; Vomiting; Sensitivity to Light? Noise? Odors? Do you get pale or flush? Do your eyes or nose run? Does your nose get stuffy? Do the whites of your eyes get red? Does your eyelid droop? Do you pace, or go to bed?	Nausea; Vomiting; Sensitivity to Light? Noise? Odors? Do you get pale or flush? Do your eyes or nose run? Does your nose get stuffy? Do the whites of your eyes get red? Does your eyelid droop? Do you pace, or go to bed?
PRECIPITATING OR AGGRAVATING FEATURES	Red wine, exertion	Red wine, exertion, stress	#1 can become #2

LOCATION: Mark the location for each type of headache with a different color pen.

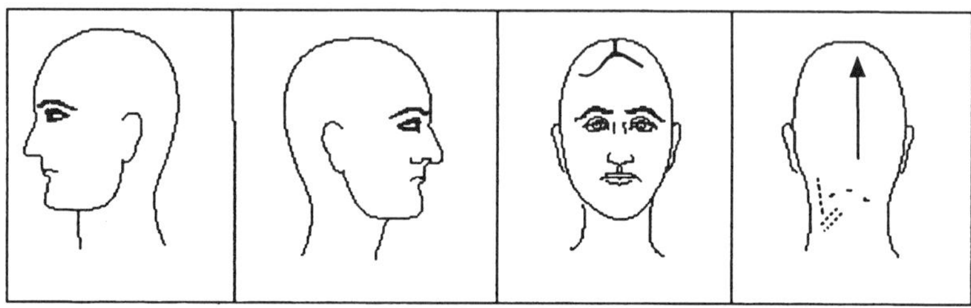

MEDICAL HISTORY:

Have you ever been or are you currently being treated for any of the following?

a) high blood pressure	<u>Yes</u>	No
b) stomach ulcers	Yes	<u>No</u>
c) asthma	Yes	<u>No</u>
d) allergies	Yes	<u>No</u>
e) pneumonia	<u>Yes</u>	No
f) kidney problems	Yes	<u>No</u>
g) low blood sugar	Yes	<u>No</u>
h) glaucoma	Yes	<u>No</u>
i) diabetes	Yes	<u>No</u>
j) heart problems	Yes	<u>No</u>

If you answered yes to any of the above, please describe: High blood pressure during first pregnancy.

List all other medical problems you have had in the past. Include date diagnosed and treatment.
DO NOT LIST OPERATIONS

Hypothyroidism (Hashimoto's disease) diagnosed early 1984. Sinusitis.

SURGICAL HISTORY (List operations and dates performed)

Tonsillectomy, 1974. Lipectomy (right shoulder), 1985.

PSYCHIATRIC HISTORY (List visits with counselors, psychologists, etc., and type of treatment)

No.

ACCIDENTS IN ADULT LIFE (Briefly describe any accident that caused any blow to the head or that you feel is related to your headache)

FAMILY HISTORY:

1. Is your father living? <u>Yes</u> No
   - Age 47
   - Cause of death ______
   - Was there a headache history? Yes <u>No</u>
2. Is your mother living? <u>Yes</u> No
   - Age 46
   - Cause of death ______
   - Was there a headache history? <u>Yes</u> No

3. Ages of brothers---Circle the ones with headache
   22
4. Ages of sisters---Circle the ones with headache
   (28)
5. List any other blood relatives with a history of severe headaches.
   ?

MARITAL HISTORY:
List marriages:

1st marriage age _19_ to Present	Did spouse have headaches?	Yes	No
2nd marriage age ____ to ____	Did spouse have headaches?	Yes	No
3rd marriage age ____ to ____	Did spouse have headaches?	Yes	No

Age of current spouse: 27

List ages and sex of all children:

Age 5	Sex M	Headaches?	Yes	No
Age 2	Sex F	Headaches?	Yes	No
Age ____	Sex ____	Headaches?	Yes	No

STRESS FACTORS:

List any factors that may be affecting your headaches (money, loneliness, sexual problems, work, etc.)

VEGETATIVE SIGNS:

1.	Do you have trouble falling asleep?	Yes	No
2.	Do you have trouble staying asleep?	Yes	No
3.	Has your appetite decreased?	Yes	No
4.	Have you gained or lost weight in the past year?	Yes	No
5.	Have you felt tearful or depressed lately?	Yes	No
6.	Have you had any thoughts of wanting to die?	Yes	No
7.	Have you been forgetful lately?	Yes	No
8.	Any other changes in your normal day-to-day living?		

Please list any medications you are allergic or sensitive to:

Please list any medications you are currently taking (including dosages and frequency per day):
Synthroid 0.175 mg. Fiorinol, Afrin, Tylenol, aspirin

PREVIOUS CARE:

1. List doctors who have treated you for headaches: Dr. G

2. List any tests you have had for your headache (e.g., EEG, CT scan, MRI, X-Ray, etc.):

EEG, CAT scan, 1974.

3. List any other treatment you have had for your headache (e.g., biofeedback, acupuncture, chiropractic, or any other treatment you had):

Chiropractic 1976-77.

WALTER
Category: Migraine headaches

This case shows an interesting variation of migraine. Walter is a 59-year-old man whose headaches started three years ago. He complained of interfering headaches (moderate to severe), which started three years ago. They were occasional. Currently he is getting them every other day. He describes them as lasting one or two hours, if he takes some pain medication. He describes the character of the pain as an ice pick on top of his head, radiating down to the occipital portion of his head. There is no aura, and no associated features. There are no other problems as far as headaches are concerned.

He has been previously worked up by an internist and neurologist, and had a CT scan. He has also seen an ear, nose and throat specialist, and all of this testing has been normal.

Diagnosis: Ice pick headache. This is an interesting headache that has been reported under the group of migraine headaches and has been described as a variant migraine. When treated with certain anti-inflammatories, responses have been very good.

MEDICAL HEADACHE HISTORY

Name: Walter **Age:** 59 **Sex** M **Date:** 1/8/92

Date of Birth: 00/00/32 **Birthplace:** OH **Race:** C **Education:** 2 yrs. College

Occupation: President of Supply Company **Accident:** N/A

Armed Services & Type of Discharge: 1953-1956 - Army

PAST HISTORY:

1.	Did you have a normal birth?		**Yes**	No
	a) forceps used?		Yes	No
	b) cesarean section?		Yes	No
2.	Did you have problems with bedwetting?		Yes	**No**
	a) If yes, age bedwetting stopped		______	
3.	Were you car sick as a child (motion)?		Yes	**No**
	a) If yes, how severe?	Slight	Moderate	Severe
4.	Did you have unexplained abdominal cramps as a child?		Yes	**No**
5.	Did you have any of the following illnesses in childhood?			
	a) meningitis		Yes	**No**
	b) encephalitis		Yes	**No**
	c) scarlet fever		Yes	**No**
	d) rheumatic fever		Yes	**No**
6.	Did you have any head injuries as a child?		Yes	**No**
	a) If yes, please explain:			
7.	Were you treated for emotional illness as a child?		Yes	**No**

HABITS:

8.	Do you drink alcohol?	**Yes**	No
	a) If yes, what kind and how much? 2 times per week		
	b) Does alcohol bring on or aggravate a headache?	Yes	**No**
9.	Do you smoke?	Yes	**No**
	a) If yes, how much?		
	b) Does smoking or smoke-filled rooms cause or aggravate headaches?	Yes	**No**
10.	Do you drink caffeinated beverages?	**Yes**	No
	a) If yes, how much? 4 times per week		

MENSTRUAL HISTORY:

At what age did menses begin?_______ Were they regular or irregular?_______

How were they related to your headache?_______

Are you or were you ever on Birth Control Pills?_______ Did they affect your headache? _______

Have you had a hysterectomy, partial or total, and why?_______

Are you in menopause, and if yes, how long?_______

Are you on hormones, and if yes, which ones?_______

HEADACHE ASSESSMENT FORM

HA PROFILE	INCAPACITATING #3	INTERFERING #2	IRRITATING #1
ONSET (Years ago and frequency)	N/A	3 years ago Occasionally	N/A
CURRENT FREQUENCY	N/A	Every day or Every other day	N/A
TIME OF ONSET	N/A	Anytime	N/A
DURATION	N/A	1 to 2 hours with Fiorinal	N/A
CHARACTER	N/A	Ice pick top of head	N/A
PRODROME OR AURA	N/A	N/A	N/A
ASSOCIATING FEATURES	Nausea; Vomiting; Sensitivity to Light? Noise? Odors? Do you get pale or flush? Do your eyes or nose run? Does your nose get stuffy? Do the whites of your eyes get red? Does your eyelid droop? Do you pace, or go to bed?	Nausea; Vomiting; Sensitivity to Light? Noise? Odors? Do you get pale or flush? Do your eyes or nose run? Does your nose get stuffy? Do the whites of your eyes get red? Does your eyelid droop? Do you pace, or go to bed? Ice pack	Nausea; Vomiting; Sensitivity to Light? Noise? Odors? Do you get pale or flush? Do your eyes or nose run? Does your nose get stuffy? Do the whites of your eyes get red? Does your eyelid droop? Do you pace, or go to bed?
PRECIPITATING OR AGGRAVATING FEATURES	N/A	Heat	N/A

LOCATION: Mark the location for each type of headache with a different color pen.

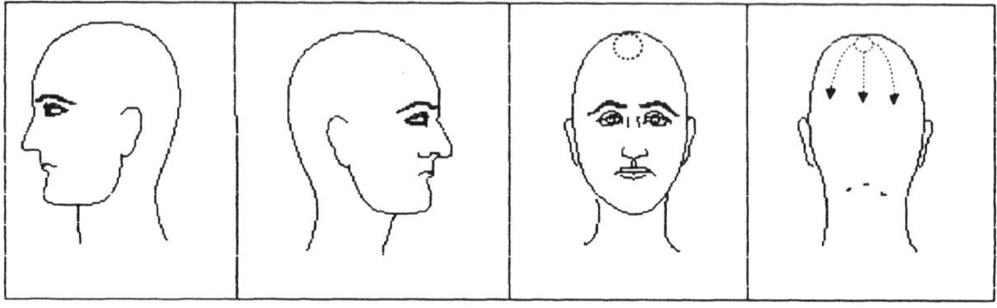

MEDICAL HISTORY:

Have you ever been or are you currently being treated for any of the following?

a) high blood pressure	Yes	No
b) stomach ulcers	Yes	No
c) asthma	Yes	No
d) allergies	Yes	No
e) pneumonia	Yes	No
f) kidney problems	Yes	No
g) low blood sugar	Yes	No
h) glaucoma	Yes	No
i) diabetes	Yes	No
j) heart problems	Yes	No

If you answered yes to any of the above, please describe:____________________

List all other medical problems you have had in the past. Include date diagnosed and treatment.
DO NOT LIST OPERATIONS

None

SURGICAL HISTORY (List operations and dates performed)

Right inguinal hernia – 1965; Left arm radial deviation – 1949; Appendectomy – 1953.

PSYCHIATRIC HISTORY (List visits with counselors, psychologists, etc., and type of treatment)

None

ACCIDENTS IN ADULT LIFE (Briefly describe any accident that caused any blow to the head or that you feel is related to your headache)

None

FAMILY HISTORY:

1. Is your father living? Yes No
   Age________
   Cause of death age 72; hardening of arteries
   Was there a headache history? Yes No
2. Is your mother living? Yes No
   Age 85
   Cause of death________
   Was there a headache history? Yes No
3. Ages of brothers---Circle the ones with headache
   62

4. Ages of sisters---Circle the ones with headache
   ______None______________________________
5. List any other blood relatives with a history of severe headaches.
   ______None______________________________

MARITAL HISTORY:
List marriages:

1st marriage age 26 to 59	Did spouse have headaches?	Yes	No
2nd marriage age ______to______	Did spouse have headaches?	Yes	No
3rd marriage age ______to______	Did spouse have headaches?	Yes	No

Age of current spouse:____________

List ages and sex of all children:

Age 33 Sex M Headaches?	Yes	No
Age 30 Sex M Headaches?	Yes	No
Age 28 Sex F Headaches?	Yes	No

STRESS FACTORS:

List any factors that may be affecting your headaches (money, loneliness, sexual problems, work, etc.)
Ringing in ears; pressure on ears.
____

VEGETATIVE SIGNS:

1.	Do you have trouble falling asleep?	Yes	No
2.	Do you have trouble staying asleep?	Yes	No
3.	Has your appetite decreased?	Yes	No
4.	Have you gained or lost weight in the past year?	Yes	No
5.	Have you felt tearful or depressed lately?	Yes	No
6.	Have you had any thoughts of wanting to die?	Yes	No
7.	Have you been forgetful lately?	Yes	No
8.	Any other changes in your normal day-to-day living?____________		

Please list any medications you are allergic or sensitive to: None
____
____

Please list any medications you are currently taking (including dosages and frequency per day):
Fiorinal
____

PREVIOUS CARE:

1. List doctors who have treated you for headaches: Dr. G; Dr. M; Dr. H.

2. List any tests you have had for your headache (e.g., EEG, CT scan, MRI, X-Ray, etc.):
CT scan in 1991, with and without contrast (normal).
X-rays of head and neck – 1991.

3. List any other treatment you have had for your headache (e.g., biofeedback, acupuncture, chiropractic, or any other treatment you had):
None

RICK
Category: Migraine headaches

This is an interesting type of migraine that is not seen very often. Rick is a 21-year-old aerospace engineering student. His incapacitating headaches started at age 11. They were rare. He had none for two years, and then they started about three weeks ago. They can come on any time and last one day. It is severe pressure, always in the right lateral orbital (around the eye) and temporal region, and goes into his leg 30 minutes before the headache. Associated features are nausea, vomiting, photophobia (sensitivity to light), sonophobia (sensitivity to sound), nasal stuffiness, and he goes to bed. He has loss of equilibrium, and this continues even after the headache. He also has dysarthria, or difficulty in speaking, with these headaches.

He has interfering headaches (moderate to severe), which also started at age 11. They are very similar to the incapacitating headaches, with slightly less intensity.

Irritating headaches (annoying) started as a child. They are occasional. He gets two a month. They come on at any time and last an hour, and he can abort these with over-the-counter medication.

In his family history, his mother also has headaches, but the patient did not recall whether they were similar to his. His neurological examination was normal, and he was diagnosed with vertebral basilar migraine, in which there is loss of equilibrium and difficulty in talking, sometimes double vision; and also hemiplegic migraine, because of the numbness in his leg. The third diagnosis was rule out intracranial lesion, which was done.

Whenever someone has a migraine headache and there are neurological features such as just described, a complete neurological examination and a workup to rule out any type of intracranial lesion such as tumor, aneurysm, etc., must be done.

MEDICAL HEADACHE HISTORY

Name: Rick **Age:** 21 **Sex** M **Date:** 11/4/91

Date of Birth: 00/00/69 **Birthplace:** FL **Race:** W **Education:** Sr. in college

Occupation: College student **Accident:** N/A

Armed Services & Type of Discharge: N/A

PAST HISTORY:

1.	Did you have a normal birth?		Yes	No
	a) forceps used?		Yes	No
	b) cesarean section?		Yes	No
2.	Did you have problems with bedwetting?		Yes	No
	a) If yes, age bedwetting stopped			
3.	Were you car sick as a child (motion)?		Yes	No
	a) If yes, how severe?	Slight	Moderate	Severe
4.	Did you have unexplained abdominal cramps as a child?		Yes	No
5.	Did you have any of the following illnesses in childhood?			
	a) meningitis		Yes	No
	b) encephalitis		Yes	No
	c) scarlet fever		Yes	No
	d) rheumatic fever		Yes	No
6.	Did you have any head injuries as a child?		Yes	No
	a) If yes, please explain: Fell off stool, stitches, age 8 or 9.			
7.	Were you treated for emotional illness as a child?		Yes	No

HABITS:

8.	Do you drink alcohol?	Yes	No
	a) If yes, what kind and how much? Occasional, once a month		
	b) Does alcohol bring on or aggravate a headache?	Yes	No
9.	Do you smoke?	Yes	No
	a) If yes, how much?		
	b) Does smoking or smoke-filled rooms cause or aggravate headaches?	Yes	No
10.	Do you drink caffeinated beverages?	Yes	No
	a) If yes, how much? One a day		

MENSTRUAL HISTORY:

At what age did menses begin?_______ Were they regular or irregular?____________________
How were they related to your headache?____
Are you or were you ever on Birth Control Pills?______ Did they affect your headache? ________
Have you had a hysterectomy, partial or total, and why?_______________________________
Are you in menopause, and if yes, how long?_______________________________________
Are you on hormones, and if yes, which ones?______________________________________

HEADACHE ASSESSMENT FORM

HA PROFILE	INCAPACITATING #3	INTERFERING #2	IRRITATING #1
ONSET (Years ago and frequency)	Age 11, rare	Age 11 Occasionally	As a child Occasionally
CURRENT FREQUENCY	None for 2 years	Had none in 1 year; Started 2 weeks ago	2 per month
TIME OF ONSET	Anytime	Anytime	Anytime
DURATION	1 day	1 to 2 day	1 hour with OTC medications
CHARACTER	Severe pressure	Pressure	Dull ache
PRODROME OR AURA	Same as #2	Blurred vision and flickering, and numbness in hands and leg. Headache starts 30 minutes later.	N/A
ASSOCIATING FEATURES	Nausea; Vomiting; Sensitivity to Light? Noise? Odors? Do you get pale or flush? Do your eyes or nose run? Does your nose get stuffy? Do the whites of your eyes get red? Does your eyelid droop? Do you pace, or go to bed?	Nausea; Vomiting; Sensitivity to Light? Noise? Odors? Do you get pale or flush? Do your eyes or nose run? Does your nose get stuffy? Do the whites of your eyes get red? Does your eyelid droop? Do you pace, or go to bed?	Nausea; Vomiting; Sensitivity to Light? Noise? Odors? Do you get pale or flush? Do your eyes or nose run? Does your nose get stuffy? Do the whites of your eyes get red? Does your eyelid droop? Do you pace, or go to bed?
PRECIPITATING OR AGGRAVATING FEATURES	Loss of equilibrium hangs on after headache	Feels loss of equilibrium a few days after headache	Overtired

LOCATION: Mark the location for each type of headache with a different color pen.

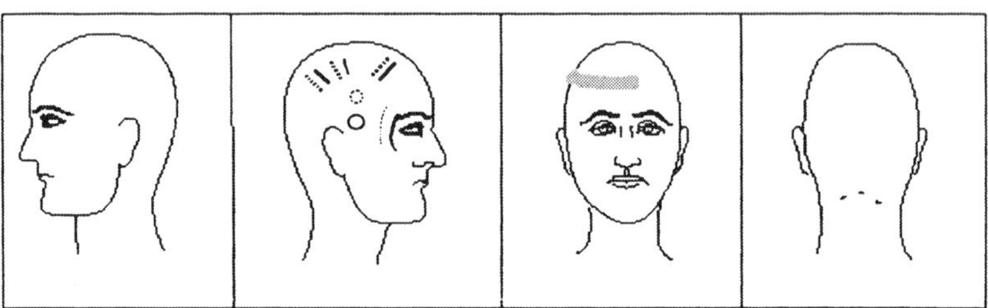

MEDICAL HISTORY:

Have you ever been or are you currently being treated for any of the following?

a) high blood pressure	Yes	No
b) stomach ulcers	Yes	No
c) asthma	Yes	No
d) allergies	Yes	No
e) pneumonia	Yes	No
f) kidney problems	Yes	No
g) low blood sugar	Yes	No
h) glaucoma	Yes	No
i) diabetes	Yes	No
j) heart problems	Yes	No

If you answered yes to any of the above, please describe: Kidney infection 1-1/2 years ago.

List all other medical problems you have had in the past. Include date diagnosed and treatment.
DO NOT LIST OPERATIONS
None

SURGICAL HISTORY (List operations and dates performed)
Possible tonsillectomy and adenoidectomy

PSYCHIATRIC HISTORY (List visits with counselors, psychologists, etc., and type of treatment)
None

ACCIDENTS IN ADULT LIFE (Briefly describe any accident that caused any blow to the head or that you feel is related to your headache)
None

FAMILY HISTORY:

1. Is your father living? Yes No
   Age 50
   Cause of death
   Was there a headache history? Yes No
2. Is your mother living? Yes No
   Age 47
   Cause of death
   Was there a headache history? Yes No
3. Ages of brothers---Circle the ones with headache
   25

4. Ages of sisters---Circle the ones with headache
   None
5. List any other blood relatives with a history of severe headaches.
   My mother's brother died of an aneurysm.

MARITAL HISTORY:
List marriages:

1st marriage age ______ to ______	Did spouse have headaches?	Yes	No
2nd marriage age ______ to ______	Did spouse have headaches?	Yes	No
3rd marriage age ______ to ______	Did spouse have headaches?	Yes	No

Age of current spouse: ____________

List ages and sex of all children:

Age ______ Sex ______	Headaches?	Yes	No
Age ______ Sex ______	Headaches?	Yes	No
Age ______ Sex ______	Headaches?	Yes	No

STRESS FACTORS:

List any factors that may be affecting your headaches (money, loneliness, sexual problems, work, etc.)
School

VEGETATIVE SIGNS:

1.	Do you have trouble falling asleep?	Yes	No
2.	Do you have trouble staying asleep?	Yes	No
3.	Has your appetite decreased?	Yes	No
4.	Have you gained or lost weight in the past year?	Yes	No
5.	Have you felt tearful or depressed lately?	Yes	No
6.	Have you had any thoughts of wanting to die?	Yes	No
7.	Have you been forgetful lately?	Yes	No
8.	Any other changes in your normal day-to-day living? ____________		

Please list any medications you are allergic or sensitive to: No known allergies

Please list any medications you are currently taking (including dosages and frequency per day):
None

PREVIOUS CARE:

1. List doctors who have treated you for headaches: Dr. B.

2. List any tests you have had for your headache (e.g., EEG, CT scan, MRI, X-Ray, etc.):
None.

3. List any other treatment you have had for your headache (e.g., biofeedback, acupuncture, chiropractic, or any other treatment you had):
None.

DOROTHY
Category: Migraine

This 51-year-old woman is a very good example of a typical migraine patient. Her headaches started when she was 12. She was getting them once a week, then once a year. She now seems to get them about once a month. They last one to three days, with typical symptoms of migraine-like throbbing, nausea, vomiting, sensitivity to light, noise, etc. There is also an interfering headache, which is moderate to severe, that precedes this by a day or two before it becomes an incapacitating migraine. This would be a very good example of a non-classical migraine, or, according to the International Headache Society, migraine without aura.

MEDICAL HEADACHE HISTORY

Name: Dorothy **Age:** 51 **Sex** F **Date:** 12/20/89

Date of Birth: 00/00/38 **Birthplace:** TN **Race:** C **Education:** High school

Occupation: Project Control Specialist **Accident:** N/A

Armed Services & Type of Discharge: N/A

PAST HISTORY:

1.	Did you have a normal birth?		Yes	No
	a) forceps used?		Yes	No
	b) cesarean section?		Yes	No
2.	Did you have problems with bedwetting?		Yes	No
	a) If yes, age bedwetting stopped		12	
3.	Were you car sick as a child (motion)?		Yes	No
	a) If yes, how severe?	Slight	Moderate	Severe
4.	Did you have unexplained abdominal cramps as a child?		Yes	No
5.	Did you have any of the following illnesses in childhood?			
	a) meningitis		Yes	No
	b) encephalitis		Yes	No
	c) scarlet fever		Yes	No
	d) rheumatic fever		Yes	No
6.	Did you have any head injuries as a child?		Yes	No
	a) If yes, please explain: Several head blows in high school playing basketball. No headaches.			
7.	Were you treated for emotional illness as a child?		Yes	No

HABITS:

8.	Do you drink alcohol?	Yes	No
	a) If yes, what kind and how much?		
	b) Does alcohol bring on or aggravate a headache?	Yes	No
9.	Do you smoke?	Yes	No
	a) If yes, how much?		
	b) Does smoking or smoke-filled rooms cause or aggravate headaches?	Yes	No
10.	Do you drink caffeinated beverages?	Yes	No
	a) If yes, how much? Approx. 32 oz. day		

MENSTRUAL HISTORY:

At what age did menses begin? 13 Were they regular or irregular? WNL

How were they related to your headache? Increased headaches.

Are you or were you ever on Birth Control Pills? Yes Did they affect your headache? No

Have you had a hysterectomy, partial or total, and why? Partial (Fibroid tumors)

Are you in menopause, and if yes, how long? No

Are you on hormones, and if yes, which ones? Premarin 0.625 mg every day

HEADACHE ASSESSMENT FORM

HA PROFILE	INCAPACITATING #3	INTERFERING #2	IRRITATING #1
ONSET (Years ago and frequency)	Age 12, one a week, then one a year	As a child, rare	N/A
CURRENT FREQUENCY	1 a month	1 a month - #3 starts as a #2	N/A
TIME OF ONSET	Anytime	Anytime	N/A
DURATION	1 to 3 days	1 day before increasing to #3	N/A
CHARACTER	Throbbing	Throbbing	N/A
PRODROME OR AURA	N/A	N/A	N/A
ASSOCIATING FEATURES	Nausea: Vomiting: Sensitivity to Light? Noise? Odors? Do you get pale or flush? Do your eyes or nose run? Does your nose get stuffy? Do the whites of your eyes get red? Does your eyelid droop? Do you pace, or go to bed?	Nausea; Vomiting; Sensitivity to Light? Noise? Odors? Do you get pale or flush? Do your eyes or nose run? Does your nose get stuffy? Do the whites of your eyes get red? Does your eyelid droop? Do you pace, or go to bed?	Nausea; Vomiting; Sensitivity to Light? Noise? Odors? Do you get pale or flush? Do your eyes or nose run? Does your nose get stuffy? Do the whites of your eyes get red? Does your eyelid droop? Do you pace, or go to bed?
PRECIPITATING OR AGGRAVATING FEATURES	Coughing, sneezing, exercise	Exercise	N/A

LOCATION: Mark the location for each type of headache with a different color pen.

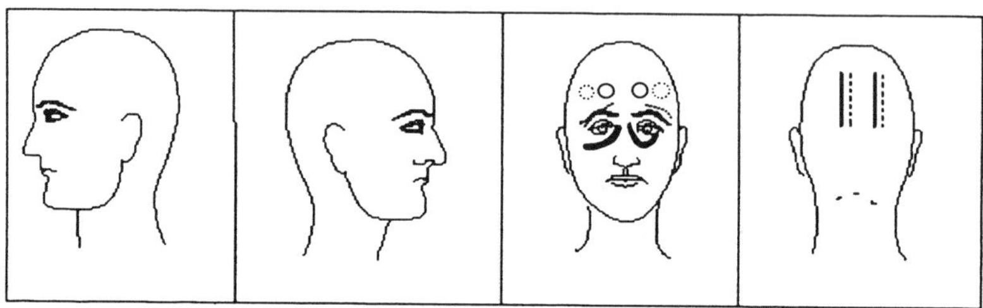

MEDICAL HISTORY:

Have you ever been or are you currently being treated for any of the following?

a) high blood pressure	Yes	No
b) stomach ulcers	Yes	No
c) asthma	Yes	No
d) allergies	Yes	No
e) pneumonia	Yes	No
f) kidney problems	Yes	No
g) low blood sugar	Yes	No
h) glaucoma	Yes	No
i) diabetes	Yes	No
j) heart problems	Yes	No

If you answered yes to any of the above, please describe: Several minor infections.

List all other medical problems you have had in the past. Include date diagnosed and treatment.
DO NOT LIST OPERATIONS

Choroidoiritis since 1963.

SURGICAL HISTORY (List operations and dates performed)

Hysterectomy, 1975. Cosmetic surgery, 1985. Bladder tuck, 1987.

PSYCHIATRIC HISTORY (List visits with counselors, psychologists, etc., and type of treatment)

None.

ACCIDENTS IN ADULT LIFE (Briefly describe any accident that caused any blow to the head or that you feel is related to your headache)

Car accident. Hit head on windshield and received scalp laceration, age 18. Unconscious for over an hour.

FAMILY HISTORY:

1.	Is your father living?	Yes	No
	Age		
	Cause of death Heart attack, age 59		
	Was there a headache history?	Yes	No
2.	Is your mother living?	Yes	No
	Age 46		
	Cause of death Heart attack, age 73		
	Was there a headache history?	Yes	No

3. Ages of brothers---Circle the ones with headache
   54, 49, 48, 47, 41
4. Ages of sisters---Circle the ones with headache
   44
5. List any other blood relatives with a history of severe headaches.
   Paternal cousin

MARITAL HISTORY:
List marriages:

1st marriage age 20 to 24	Did spouse have headaches?	Yes	No
2nd marriage age 26 to 32	Did spouse have headaches?	Yes	No
3rd marriage age ______ to ______	Did spouse have headaches?	Yes	No

Age of current spouse:__________

List ages and sex of all children:

Age 29	Sex M	Headaches? Yes	No
Age 28	Sex F	Headaches? Yes	No
Age 27	Sex M	Headaches? Yes	No

STRESS FACTORS:

List any factors that may be affecting your headaches (money, loneliness, sexual problems, work, etc.)
Work, food, hormones.

VEGETATIVE SIGNS:

1.	Do you have trouble falling asleep?	Yes	No
2.	Do you have trouble staying asleep?	Yes	No
3.	Has your appetite decreased?	Yes	No
4.	Have you gained or lost weight in the past year?	Yes	No
5.	Have you felt tearful or depressed lately?	Yes	No
6.	Have you had any thoughts of wanting to die?	Yes	No
7.	Have you been forgetful lately?	Yes	No
8.	Any other changes in your normal day-to-day living?__________		

Please list any medications you are allergic or sensitive to:__________

Please list any medications you are currently taking (including dosages and frequency per day):
Premarin, 0.625 mg. every day

PREVIOUS CARE:

1. List doctors who have treated you for headaches: None.

2. List any tests you have had for your headache (e.g., EEG, CT scan, MRI, X-Ray, etc.):

3. List any other treatment you have had for your headache (e.g., biofeedback, acupuncture, chiropractic, or any other treatment you had):
Chiropractic.

FRED
Category: Migraine

This 50-year-old man had irritating or tension-type headaches occasionally, and six or seven months ago began to have symptoms that were almost consistent with migraine, except for the character of the pain. Because these started just months ago, it was very important to make sure the patient does not have any intracranial lesion or space-occupying lesion or any tumor or any other medical problem that may have precipitated this headache condition. These conditions were ruled out, and he was treated as a migraine sufferer.

MEDICAL HEADACHE HISTORY

Name: Fred **Age:** 50 **Sex** M **Date:** 10/7/91

Date of Birth: 00/00/41 **Birthplace:** NJ **Race:** W **Education:** 2 yrs. college

Occupation: Insurance Investigator **Accident:** N/A

Armed Services & Type of Discharge: 1958-1962 – Army. Honorable Discharge.

PAST HISTORY:

1.	Did you have a normal birth?		Yes (underlined)	No
	a) forceps used?		Yes	No
	b) cesarean section?		Yes	No
2.	Did you have problems with bedwetting?		Yes	No (underlined)
	a) If yes, age bedwetting stopped		______	
3.	Were you car sick as a child (motion)?		Yes	No (underlined)
	a) If yes, how severe?	Slight	Moderate	Severe
4.	Did you have unexplained abdominal cramps as a child?		Yes	No (underlined)
5.	Did you have any of the following illnesses in childhood?			
	a) meningitis		Yes	No (underlined)
	b) encephalitis		Yes	No (underlined)
	c) scarlet fever		Yes	No (underlined)
	d) rheumatic fever		Yes	No (underlined)
6.	Did you have any head injuries as a child?		Yes	No (underlined)
	a) If yes, please explain: ______			
7.	Were you treated for emotional illness as a child?		Yes	No (underlined)

HABITS:

8.	Do you drink alcohol?	Yes (underlined)	No
	a) If yes, what kind and how much? Moderate		
	b) Does alcohol bring on or aggravate a headache?	Yes (underlined)	No
9.	Do you smoke?	Yes	No (underlined)
	a) If yes, how much? ______		
	b) Does smoking or smoke-filled rooms cause or aggravate headaches?	Yes	No (underlined)
10.	Do you drink caffeinated beverages?	Yes (underlined)	No
	a) If yes, how much? 2 – 3 cups daily		

MENSTRUAL HISTORY:

At what age did menses begin?________ Were they regular or irregular?____________________

How were they related to your headache?____________________

Are you or were you ever on Birth Control Pills?________ Did they affect your headache? ________

Have you had a hysterectomy, partial or total, and why?____________________

Are you in menopause, and if yes, how long?____________________

Are you on hormones, and if yes, which ones? ____________________

HEADACHE ASSESSMENT FORM

HA PROFILE	INCAPACITATING #3	INTERFERING #2	IRRITATING #1
ONSET (Years ago and frequency)	6 – 7 months ago 1/month	6 0 7 months ago 2 – 3/wk	Age 25, occasionally
CURRENT FREQUENCY	1/month	2 – 3 /wk	Not now, occas before these HA
TIME OF ONSET	Awaken with	Awaken with	Anytime
DURATION	12 – 14 hours	4 – 6 hours	1 hour with OTC medication
CHARACTER	Constant sharp pain	Constant ache	Dull ache
PRODROME OR AURA	N/A	N/A	N/A
ASSOCIATING FEATURES	Nausea; Vomiting; Sensitivity to Light? Noise? Odors? Do you get pale or flush? Do your eyes or nose run? Does your nose get stuffy? Do the whites of your eyes get red? Does your eyelid droop? Do you pace, or go to bed?	Nausea; Vomiting; Sensitivity to Light? Noise? Odors? Do you get pale or flush? Do your eyes or nose run? Does your nose get stuffy? Do the whites of your eyes get red? Does your eyelid droop? Do you pace, or go to bed?	Nausea; Vomiting; Sensitivity to Light? Noise? Odors? Do you get pale or flush? Do your eyes or nose run? Does your nose get stuffy? Do the whites of your eyes get red? Does your eyelid droop? Do you pace, or go to bed?
PRECIPITATING OR AGGRAVATING FEATURES	Lying down, bending	N/A	N/A

LOCATION: Mark the location for each type of headache with a different color pen.

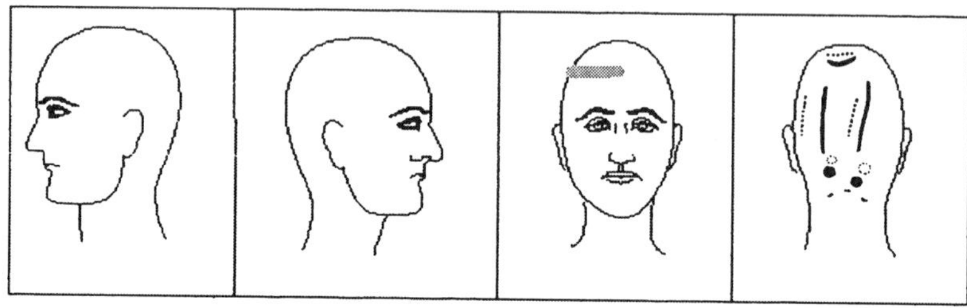

MEDICAL HISTORY:

Have you ever been or are you currently being treated for any of the following?

a) high blood pressure	Yes	No
b) stomach ulcers	Yes	No
c) asthma	Yes	No
d) allergies	Yes	No
e) pneumonia	Yes	No
f) kidney problems	Yes	No
g) low blood sugar	Yes	No
h) glaucoma	Yes	No
i) diabetes	Yes	No
j) heart problems	Yes	No

If you answered yes to any of the above, please describe: Diagnosed with high blood pressure in 1981, with arrhythmia (not now). Arrhythmia, tachycardia one time with reaction to myelogram.

List all other medical problems you have had in the past. Include date diagnosed and treatment.
DO NOT LIST OPERATIONS

Back injury 1981, and reinjury 1987. Physical therapy with chiropractor.

SURGICAL HISTORY (List operations and dates performed)

Tonsillectomy – 1945. Variocelectomy – 1972. Back surgery – 1982.

PSYCHIATRIC HISTORY (List visits with counselors, psychologists, etc., and type of treatment)

Therapy to regain ability to drive after car accident in 1979. Treated for depression and anxiety.

ACCIDENTS IN ADULT LIFE (Briefly describe any accident that caused any blow to the head or that you feel is related to your headache)

None.

FAMILY HISTORY:

1. Is your father living? Yes No
   - Age________
   - Cause of death Killed in WWII
   - Was there a headache history? Yes No
2. Is your mother living? Yes No
   - Age 71
   - Cause of death________
   - Was there a headache history? Yes No

3. Ages of brothers---Circle the ones with headache
   None
4. Ages of sisters---Circle the ones with headache
   None
5. List any other blood relatives with a history of severe headaches.
   None

MARITAL HISTORY:
List marriages:

1st marriage age 22 to Present	Did spouse have headaches?	Yes	No
2nd marriage age ____ to ______	Did spouse have headaches?	Yes	No
3rd marriage age ____ to ______	Did spouse have headaches?	Yes	No
4th marriage age ____ to ______	Did spouse have headaches?	Yes	No

Age of current spouse:__________

List ages and sex of all children:

Age 27 Sex M Headaches?	Yes	No
Age 15 Sex M Headaches?	Yes	No
Age _____ Sex _____ Headaches?	Yes	No
Age _____ Sex _____ Headaches?	Yes	No

STRESS FACTORS:

List any factors that may be affecting your headaches (money, loneliness, sexual problems, work, etc.)
Company being bought out by employees, future uncertain.

VEGETATIVE SIGNS:

1.	Do you have trouble falling asleep?	Yes	No
2.	Do you have trouble staying asleep?	Yes	No
3.	Has your appetite decreased?	Yes	No
4.	Have you gained or lost weight in the past year?	Yes	No
5.	Have you felt tearful or depressed lately?	Yes	No
6.	Have you had any thoughts of wanting to die?	Yes	No
7.	Have you been forgetful lately?	Yes	No
8.	Any other changes in your normal day-to-day living?__________		

Please list any medications you are allergic or sensitive to: Iodine, as the dye used in myelograms, (Anaphylactic shock 1981).

Please list any medications you are currently taking (including dosages and frequency per day):
OTC analgesics – Tylenol, ibuprofen and aspirin. Double doses every 3 to 4 hours when headache present.

PREVIOUS CARE:

1. List doctors who have treated you for headaches: None

2. List any tests you have had for your headache (e.g., EEG, CT scan, MRI, X-Ray, etc.):
None

3. List any other treatment you have had for your headache (e.g., biofeedback, acupuncture, chiropractic, or any other treatment you had):
None.

ROGER
Category: Migraine

This is an interesting type of migraine in which the headache started when this patient was a late teenager. They were occasional. He had the typical symptom of migraine, with the character being throbbing, with nausea and vomiting. He also had a second type of headache that appeared to be both a combination of migraine and perhaps what was called muscle tension headache. They were not frequent and, prior to the patient's coming into our clinic, he was headache-free for 6 to 7 years.

When he came in, he was having the interfering headache (moderate to severe) every day for the past four and a half weeks, which was treated with medication to abort this headache.

There are also irritating headaches that he would get during the week, which were dull and aching, and would be considered muscle tension headaches.

After the patient had his treatment and the headaches were aborted, he telephoned to say that the headaches seemed to be coming back once again. Unfortunately, sometimes migraine sufferers will go into states of remission and then when the headaches come back, they will come back on a more frequent basis. These patients should be treated with both preventative and abortive therapy, with the aim of creating another state of remission that prevents the headaches from returning.

The diagnosis in this case would be status (continuous) nonclassical migraine, or migraine without aura, and muscle contraction headache.

MEDICAL HEADACHE HISTORY

Name: Roger **Age:** 51 **Sex** M **Date:** 8/20/90

Date of Birth: 00/00/39 **Birthplace:** D.C. **Race:** W **Education:** B.S.

Occupation: Estimator **Accident:** N/A

Armed Services & Type of Discharge: N/A

PAST HISTORY:

1.	Did you have a normal birth?		Yes	No
	a) forceps used?		Yes	No
	b) cesarean section?		Yes	No
2.	Did you have problems with bedwetting?		Yes	No
	a) If yes, age bedwetting stopped		10	
3.	Were you car sick as a child (motion)?		Yes	No
	a) If yes, how severe?	Slight	Moderate	Severe
4.	Did you have unexplained abdominal cramps as a child?		Yes	No
5.	Did you have any of the following illnesses in childhood?			
	a) meningitis		Yes	No
	b) encephalitis		Yes	No
	c) scarlet fever		Yes	No
	d) rheumatic fever		Yes	No
6.	Did you have any head injuries as a child?		Yes	No
	a) If yes, please explain:			
7.	Were you treated for emotional illness as a child?		Yes	No

HABITS:

8.	Do you drink alcohol?	Yes	No
	a) If yes, what kind and how much?		
	b) Does alcohol bring on or aggravate a headache?	Yes	No
9.	Do you smoke?	Yes	No
	a) If yes, how much?		
	b) Does smoking or smoke-filled rooms cause or aggravate headaches?	Yes	No
10.	Do you drink caffeinated beverages?	Yes	No
	a) If yes, how much?		

MENSTRUAL HISTORY:

At what age did menses begin?_______ Were they regular or irregular?__________
How were they related to your headache?__________
Are you or were you ever on Birth Control Pills?______ Did they affect your headache? ________
Have you had a hysterectomy, partial or total, and why?__________
Are you in menopause, and if yes, how long?__________
Are you on hormones, and if yes, which ones?__________

HEADACHE ASSESSMENT FORM

HA PROFILE	INCAPACITATING #3	INTERFERING #2	IRRITATING #1
ONSET (Years ago and frequency)	1956, rare	1956, occasionally	1956, occasionally
CURRENT FREQUENCY	Last one was 6 to 7 years ago	Every day for 1-1/2 weeks Last one was 6 months ago	2 per week
TIME OF ONSET	Can awaken with	Wakes up with, increases as day progresses	Anytime
DURATION	4 to 6 hours with ER meds	All day	1 to 4 hours with OTC medication
CHARACTER	Throbbing	Throbbing and pressure	Dull ache
PRODROME OR AURA	N/A	N/A	N/A
ASSOCIATING FEATURES	Nausea; Vomiting; Sensitivity to Light? Noise? Odors? Do you get pale or flush? Do your eyes or nose run? Does your nose get stuffy? Do the whites of your eyes get red? Does your eyelid droop? Do you pace, or go to bed?	Nausea; Vomiting; Sensitivity to Light? Noise? Odors? Do you get pale or flush? Do your eyes or nose run? Does your nose get stuffy? Do the whites of your eyes get red? Does your eyelid droop? Do you pace, or go to bed?	Nausea; Vomiting; Sensitivity to Light? Noise? Odors? Do you get pale or flush? Do your eyes or nose run? Does your nose get stuffy? Do the whites of your eyes get red? Does your eyelid droop? Do you pace, or go to bed?
PRECIPITATING OR AGGRAVATING FEATURES	Lying down, changing position, coughing, sneezing	Temperature changes, bending, physical activity	N/A

LOCATION: Mark the location for each type of headache with a different color pen.

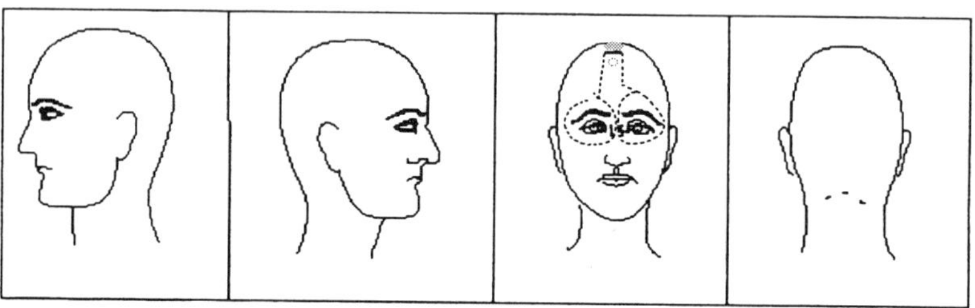

MEDICAL HISTORY:

Have you ever been or are you currently being treated for any of the following?

a) high blood pressure	Yes	**No**
b) stomach ulcers	**Yes**	No
c) asthma	Yes	**No**
d) allergies	**Yes**	No
e) pneumonia	**Yes**	No
f) kidney problems	Yes	**No**
g) low blood sugar	Yes	**No**
h) glaucoma	Yes	**No**
i) diabetes	Yes	**No**
j) heart problems	Yes	**No**

If you answered yes to any of the above, please describe: Ulcers treated 1976 (in remission). Environmental allergies. Pneumonia in 1940 and 1945.

List all other medical problems you have had in the past. Include date diagnosed and treatment.
DO NOT LIST OPERATIONS

Perforated right eardrum. Headaches 1956 to present. Hepatitis 1960.

SURGICAL HISTORY (List operations and dates performed)

Tonsils and adenoids removed – 1943. Pilonidal cyst – 1963. Right inguinal hernia – 1965.
Submucous removal of nose – 1973. Tympanic bone replacement and eardrum graft – 1976.
Left shoulder repair ligaments, calcium removal – 1983. Tympanic bone replacement – 1989.

PSYCHIATRIC HISTORY (List visits with counselors, psychologists, etc., and type of treatment)

Biofeedback 1979.

ACCIDENTS IN ADULT LIFE (Briefly describe any accident that caused any blow to the head or that you feel is related to your headache)

None

FAMILY HISTORY:

1. Is your father living? Yes **No**
   Age_________
   Cause of death Heart attack, age 54
   Was there a headache history? Yes **No**

2. Is your mother living? Yes No
Age________
Cause of death__Old age, 85__________________________
Was there a headache history? Yes No
3. Ages of brothers---Circle the ones with headache
56
4. Ages of sisters---Circle the ones with headache
53
5. List any other blood relatives with a history of severe headaches.
Niece

MARITAL HISTORY:
List marriages:

1st marriage age _23_ to _Present_ Did spouse have headaches?	Yes	No
2nd marriage age ____ to ____ Did spouse have headaches?	Yes	No
3rd marriage age ____ to ____ Did spouse have headaches?	Yes	No

Age of current spouse:__52____

List ages and sex of all children:

Age _28_ Sex _F_ Headaches?	Yes	No
Age _26_ Sex _F_ Headaches?	Yes	No
Age _24_ Sex _F_ Headaches?	Yes	No

STRESS FACTORS:

List any factors that may be affecting your headaches (money, loneliness, sexual problems, work, etc.)
Work sometimes, but stress does not seem to be consistent with all headaches.

VEGETATIVE SIGNS:

1.	Do you have trouble falling asleep?	Yes	No
2.	Do you have trouble staying asleep?	Yes	No
3.	Has your appetite decreased?	Yes	No
4.	Have you gained or lost weight in the past year?	Yes	No
5.	Have you felt tearful or depressed lately?	Yes	No
6.	Have you had any thoughts of wanting to die?	Yes	No
7.	Have you been forgetful lately?	Yes	No
8.	Any other changes in your normal day-to-day living?________		

Please list any medications you are allergic or sensitive to: Gamma globulin

Please list any medications you are currently taking (including dosages and frequency per day):
None

PREVIOUS CARE:

1. List doctors who have treated you for headaches: Dr. H.; Dr. L.; Pain Clinic;
Dr. B., Dr. L., Dr. G

2. List any tests you have had for your headache (e.g., EEG, CT scan, MRI, X-Ray, etc.):
EEG and CT scan in 1990 – both normal.

3. List any other treatment you have had for your headache (e.g., biofeedback, acupuncture, chiropractic, or any other treatment you had):
Biofeedback in 1979. Injections in neck – TP's.

LAURIE
Category: Migraine

This is a case that represents a good example of a hormonal migraine diagnosis. The patient gets these headaches once a month during her menstrual period. She had come to see me because this headache lasted longer than most others. The headache was aborted with proper medication and a plan was made to try to reduce the headaches when they did come. She had all of the symptoms of migraine with the throbbing, nausea, vomiting, sensitivity to light, noise and odors, etc., and the diagnosis here would be migraine without aura (hormonal migraine).

MEDICAL HEADACHE HISTORY

Name: Laurie **Age:** 32 **Sex** F **Date:** 1/28/91

Date of Birth: 00/00/58 **Birthplace:** NY **Race:** W **Education:** 2 yrs college

Occupation: Proof Operator **Accident:** N/A

Armed Services & Type of Discharge: N/A

PAST HISTORY:

1.	Did you have a normal birth?		Yes	No
	a) forceps used?		Yes	No
	b) cesarean section?		Yes	No
2.	Did you have problems with bedwetting?		Yes	No
	a) If yes, age bedwetting stopped			
3.	Were you car sick as a child (motion)?		Yes	No
	a) If yes, how severe?	Slight	Moderate	Severe
4.	Did you have unexplained abdominal cramps as a child?		Yes	No
5.	Did you have any of the following illnesses in childhood?			
	a) meningitis		Yes	No
	b) encephalitis		Yes	No
	c) scarlet fever		Yes	No
	d) rheumatic fever		Yes	No
6.	Did you have any head injuries as a child?		Yes	No
	a) If yes, please explain:			
7.	Were you treated for emotional illness as a child?		Yes	No

HABITS:

8.	Do you drink alcohol?	Yes	No
	a) If yes, what kind and how much? 2 or 3 during holidays		
	b) Does alcohol bring on or aggravate a headache?	Yes	No
9.	Do you smoke?	Yes	No
	a) If yes, how much?		
	b) Does smoking or smoke-filled rooms cause or aggravate headaches?	Yes	No
10.	Do you drink caffeinated beverages?	Yes	No
	a) If yes, how much? 2 cups of coffee, and occasionally a coke		

MENSTRUAL HISTORY:

At what age did menses begin? 13 Were they regular or irregular? WNL

How were they related to your headache? Increase headaches

Are you or were you ever on Birth Control Pills? Yes Did they affect your headache?

Have you had a hysterectomy, partial or total, and why? No

Are you in menopause, and if yes, how long? No

Are you on hormones, and if yes, which ones? No

HEADACHE ASSESSMENT FORM

HA PROFILE	INCAPACITATING #3	INTERFERING #2	IRRITATING #1
ONSET (Years ago and frequency)	Age 30 One a month	N/A	N/A
CURRENT FREQUENCY	One a month	N/A	N/A
TIME OF ONSET	Awaken with	N/A	N/A
DURATION	1 day	This headache has been every day for 2 weeks at #2 level	N/A
CHARACTER	Throbbing and pressure	N/A	N/A
PRODROME OR AURA	N/A	N/A	N/A
ASSOCIATING FEATURES	Nausea: Vomiting: Sensitivity to Light? Noise? Odors? Do you get pale or flush? Do your eyes or nose run? Does your nose get stuffy? Do the whites of your eyes get red? Does your eyelid droop? Do you pace, or go to bed?	Nausea: Vomiting: Sensitivity to Light? Noise? Odors? Do you get pale or flush? Do your eyes or nose run? Does your nose get stuffy? Do the whites of your eyes get red? Does your eyelid droop? Do you pace, or go to bed?	Nausea: Vomiting: Sensitivity to Light? Noise? Odors? Do you get pale or flush? Do your eyes or nose run? Does your nose get stuffy? Do the whites of your eyes get red? Does your eyelid droop? Do you pace, or go to bed?
PRECIPITATING OR AGGRAVATING FEATURES	N/A	N/A	N/A

LOCATION: Mark the location for each type of headache with a different color pen.

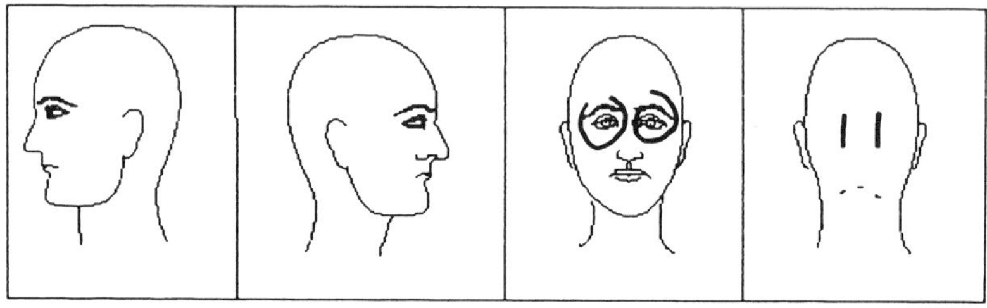

MEDICAL HISTORY:

Have you ever been or are you currently being treated for any of the following?

a) high blood pressure	Yes	No
b) stomach ulcers	Yes	No
c) asthma	Yes	No
d) allergies	Yes	No
e) pneumonia	Yes	No
f) kidney problems	Yes	No
g) low blood sugar	Yes	No
h) glaucoma	Yes	No
i) diabetes	Yes	No
j) heart problems	Yes	No

If you answered yes to any of the above, please describe:.____________________

____

List all other medical problems you have had in the past. Include date diagnosed and treatment.
DO NOT LIST OPERATIONS
None

SURGICAL HISTORY (List operations and dates performed)
None

PSYCHIATRIC HISTORY (List visits with counselors, psychologists, etc., and type of treatment)
None

ACCIDENTS IN ADULT LIFE (Briefly describe any accident that caused any blow to the head or that you feel is related to your headache)
None

FAMILY HISTORY:

1.	Is your father living?	Yes	No
	Age 56		
	Cause of death____________		
	Was there a headache history?	Yes	No
2.	Is your mother living?	Yes	No
	Age 49		
	Cause of death____________		
	Was there a headache history?	Yes	No
3.	Ages of brothers---Circle the ones with headache		
	28		

4. Ages of sisters---Circle the ones with headache
31, 29, 29
5. List any other blood relatives with a history of severe headaches.
None

MARITAL HISTORY:
List marriages:

1st marriage age 25 to 27	Did spouse have headaches?	Yes	No
2nd marriage age ____ to ____	Did spouse have headaches?	Yes	No
3rd marriage age ____ to ____	Did spouse have headaches?	Yes	No

Age of current spouse:________

List ages and sex of all children:

Age 6 Sex M	Headaches?	Yes	No
Age 9 mo. Sex M	Headaches?	Yes	No
Age ____ Sex ____	Headaches?	Yes	No

STRESS FACTORS:

List any factors that may be affecting your headaches (money, loneliness, sexual problems, work, etc.)
Money, future mother-in-law.

VEGETATIVE SIGNS:

1.	Do you have trouble falling asleep?	Yes	No
2.	Do you have trouble staying asleep?	Yes	No
3.	Has your appetite decreased?	Yes	No
4.	Have you gained or lost weight in the past year?	Yes	No
5.	Have you felt tearful or depressed lately?	Yes	No
6.	Have you had any thoughts of wanting to die?	Yes	No
7.	Have you been forgetful lately?	Yes	No
8.	Any other changes in your normal day-to-day living?________		

Please list any medications you are allergic or sensitive to: None

Please list any medications you are currently taking (including dosages and frequency per day):
Phrenilin, one tablet every 6 hours; Pamelor, one at bedtime; Birth control pills daily.

PREVIOUS CARE:

1. List doctors who have treated you for headaches: Dr. K. Dr. M.

2. List any tests you have had for your headache (e.g., EEG, CT scan, MRI, X-Ray, etc.):
CT scan, 4 months ago (normal).

3. List any other treatment you have had for your headache (e.g., biofeedback, acupuncture, chiropractic, or any other treatment you had):
None.

MAXINE
Category: Migraine without aura

I was called to see this 45-year-old woman while she was a patient in the hospital following hip surgery. She had a history of hip surgeries over the years and, following her surgery, she was complaining of severe headaches. The orthopedic surgeon asked if I could help reduce this pain. The patient had typical migraine attacks starting in her twenties, getting attacks once a month, with symptoms of nausea, vomiting, sensitivity to light, noise, etc. While she was in the hospital, she was placed on acute medication therapy for her headaches, receiving Prednisone and other anti-migraine medications and injections, which immediately aborted her pain. She was pain-free from her migraines in the hospital during her recovery from hip surgery. This is a case in which migraine can complicate other medical problems and, if treated properly, can add to the improvement of the general health of the patient.

MEDICAL HEADACHE HISTORY

Name: Maxine **Age:** 45 **Sex** F **Date:** 10/9/90

Date of Birth: 00/00/45 **Birthplace:** PR **Race:** H **Education:** 3 years college

Occupation: Inspector **Accident:** N/A

Armed Services & Type of Discharge: N/A

PAST HISTORY:

1.	Did you have a normal birth?		<u>Yes</u>	No
	a) forceps used?		Yes	No
	b) cesarean section?		Yes	No
2.	Did you have problems with bedwetting?		Yes	<u>No</u>
	a) If yes, age bedwetting stopped			
3.	Were you car sick as a child (motion)?		Yes	<u>No</u>
	a) If yes, how severe?	Slight	Moderate	Severe
4.	Did you have unexplained abdominal cramps as a child?		Yes	<u>No</u>
5.	Did you have any of the following illnesses in childhood?			
	a) meningitis		Yes	<u>No</u>
	b) encephalitis		Yes	<u>No</u>
	c) scarlet fever		Yes	<u>No</u>
	d) rheumatic fever		Yes	<u>No</u>
6.	Did you have any head injuries as a child?		Yes	<u>No</u>
	a) If yes, please explain:			
7.	Were you treated for emotional illness as a child?		Yes	<u>No</u>

HABITS:

8.	Do you drink alcohol?	Yes	<u>No</u>
	a) If yes, what kind and how much?		
	b) Does alcohol bring on or aggravate a headache?	<u>Yes</u>	No
9.	Do you smoke?	Yes	<u>No</u>
	a) If yes, how much?		
	b) Does smoking or smoke-filled rooms cause or aggravate headaches?	<u>Yes</u>	No
10.	Do you drink caffeinated beverages?	Yes	No
	a) If yes, how much?		

MENSTRUAL HISTORY:

At what age did menses begin? 13 Were they regular or irregular? WNL

How were they related to your headache? Increase headaches

Are you or were you ever on Birth Control Pills? No Did they affect your headache?

Have you had a hysterectomy, partial or total, and why? Yes, 8 years ago. Fibroid tumors.

Are you in menopause, and if yes, how long? No

Are you on hormones, and if yes, which ones? Estraderm 0.05 patch

HEADACHE ASSESSMENT FORM

HA PROFILE	INCAPACITATING #3	INTERFERING #2	IRRITATING #1
ONSET (Years ago and frequency)	20's, 1 a month	20's	Occasional
CURRENT FREQUENCY	2 to 3 a month	Headaches start as #2, then go on to #3	N/A
TIME OF ONSET	Anytime	Anytime	Anytime
DURATION	Hours to a week	Same	1 hour with OTC medication
CHARACTER	Tightening	Same	N/A
PRODROME OR AURA	Burning sensation in neck	N/A	N/A
ASSOCIATING FEATURES	Nausea; Vomiting; Sensitivity to Light? Noise? Odors? Do you get pale or flush? Do your eyes or nose run? Does your nose get stuffy? Does the white of your eyes get red? Does your eyelid droop? Do you pace, or go to bed?	Nausea; Vomiting; Sensitivity to Light? Noise? Odors? Do you get pale or flush? Do your eyes or nose run? Does your nose get stuffy? Does the white of your eyes get red? Does your eyelid droop? Do you pace, or go to bed?	Nausea; Vomiting; Sensitivity to Light? Noise? Odors? Do you get pale or flush? Do your eyes or nose run? Does your nose get stuffy? Does the white of your eyes get red? Does your eyelid droop? Do you pace, or go to bed?
PRECIPITATING OR AGGRAVATING FEATURES	Chemicals like paint, perfume, etc.	N/A	N/A

LOCATION: Mark the location for each type of headache with a different color pen.

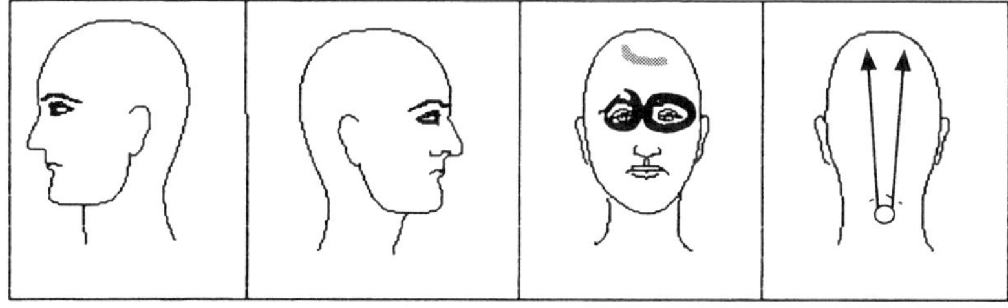

MEDICAL HISTORY:

Have you ever been or are you currently being treated for any of the following?

a) high blood pressure	Yes	No
b) stomach ulcers	Yes	No
c) asthma	Yes	No
d) allergies	Yes	No
e) pneumonia	Yes	No
f) kidney problems	Yes	No
g) low blood sugar	Yes	No
h) glaucoma	Yes	No
i) diabetes	Yes	No
j) heart problems	Yes	No

If you answered yes to any of the above, please describe:____________________

List all other medical problems you have had in the past. Include date diagnosed and treatment.
DO NOT LIST OPERATIONS

N/A

SURGICAL HISTORY (List operations and dates performed)

Hip surgery on right side, age 7, due to birth defects. Four hip implants. Appendectomy age 26. Tubal ligation, age 21. Hysterectomy 8 years ago. Fibroid tumor years ago.

PSYCHIATRIC HISTORY (List visits with counselors, psychologists, etc., and type of treatment)

None

ACCIDENTS IN ADULT LIFE (Briefly describe any accident that caused any blow to the head or that you feel is related to your headache)

None

FAMILY HISTORY:

1. Is your father living? Yes No
   Age__80______
   Cause of death____________________________
   Was there a headache history? Yes No
2. Is your mother living? Yes No
   Age__66______
   Cause of death____________________________
   Was there a headache history? Yes No
3. Ages of brothers---Circle the ones with headache
   ______(46)____________________________
4. Ages of sisters---Circle the ones with headache
   ______43 41 (40) 39________________________
5. List any other blood relatives with a history of severe headaches.
   ______None____________________________

MARITAL HISTORY:

List marriages:

1st marriage age __18__ to __42__ Did spouse have headaches? Yes No
2nd marriage age ______ to ______ Did spouse have headaches? Yes No
3rd marriage age ______ to ______ Did spouse have headaches? Yes No
__________ age ______ to ______ ________________________

Age of current spouse:____________

List ages and sex of all children:

Age __25__ Sex __F__ Headaches? Yes No
Age __24__ Sex __M__ Headaches? Yes No
Age ______ Sex ______ Headaches? Yes No

STRESS FACTORS:

List any factors that may be affecting your headaches (money, loneliness, sexual problems, work, etc.)
____N/A____
____

VEGETATIVE SIGNS:

1. Do you have trouble falling asleep? Yes No
2. Do you have trouble staying asleep? Yes No
3. Has your appetite decreased? Yes No
4. Have you gained or lost weight in the past year? Yes No
5. Have you felt tearful or depressed lately? Yes No
6. Have you had any thoughts of wanting to die? Yes No
7. Have you been forgetful lately? Yes No
8. Any other changes in your normal day-to-day living?____________

Please list any medications you are allergic or sensitive to: Penicillin, Codeine, Darvon

Please list any medications you are currently taking (including dosages and frequency per day):
Cafergot tablets

PREVIOUS CARE:

1. List doctors who have treated you for headaches: None now

2. List any tests you have had for your headache (e.g., EEG, CT scan, MRI, X-Ray, etc.):
Skull x-rays

3. List any other treatment you have had for your headache (e.g., biofeedback, acupuncture, chiropractic, or any other treatment you had):
Chiropractic

CORA
Category: Migraine

This 64-year-old woman reported that, starting in her fifties, she had occasional interfering headaches. Currently, coming into the office, she gets these 3 to 4 times a week. Before that, it was 2 to 3 times a month. She also has "zigzag lines" or fortification spectra.

The interesting part of this patient's headache history is that she never gets the typical incapacitating migraine, although with her interfering headaches, which are moderate to severe, she does have symptoms of classical migraine or migraine with aura, according to the International Headache Society classification. Her headaches were reduced to an occasional irritating headache and she was considered to be doing quite well on treatments.

MEDICAL HEADACHE HISTORY

Name: Cora **Age:** 64 **Sex** F **Date:** 3/5/91

Date of Birth: 00/00/26 **Birthplace:** FL **Race:** W **Education:** High school

Occupation: Part time – 1 day a week **Accident:** N/A

Armed Services & Type of Discharge: N/A

PAST HISTORY:

1.	Did you have a normal birth?		Yes (underlined)	No
	a) forceps used?		Yes	No (underlined)
	b) cesarean section?		Yes	No (underlined)
2.	Did you have problems with bedwetting?		Yes	No (underlined)
	a) If yes, age bedwetting stopped			______
3.	Were you car sick as a child (motion)?		Yes	No (underlined)
	a) If yes, how severe?	Slight	Moderate	Severe
4.	Did you have unexplained abdominal cramps as a child?		Yes	No (underlined)
5.	Did you have any of the following illnesses in childhood?			
	a) meningitis		Yes	No (underlined)
	b) encephalitis		Yes	No (underlined)
	c) scarlet fever		Yes	No (underlined)
	d) rheumatic fever		Yes	No (underlined)
6.	Did you have any head injuries as a child?		Yes	No (underlined)
	a) If yes, please explain: ______			
7.	Were you treated for emotional illness as a child?		Yes	No (underlined)

HABITS:

8.	Do you drink alcohol?	Yes	No (underlined)
	a) If yes, what kind and how much? Not now, did in past		
	b) Does alcohol bring on or aggravate a headache?	Yes	No (underlined)
9.	Do you smoke?	Yes	No (underlined)
	a) If yes, how much? Not now, quit in 1989		
	b) Does smoking or smoke-filled rooms cause or aggravate headaches?	Yes	No (underlined)
10.	Do you drink caffeinated beverages?	Yes (underlined)	No
	a) If yes, how much? Coke occasionally		

MENSTRUAL HISTORY:

At what age did menses begin? 14 Were they regular or irregular? WNL
How were they related to your headache? ______
Are you or were you ever on Birth Control Pills? Yes Did they affect your headache? N/A
Have you had a hysterectomy, partial or total, and why? Total, 1975. Abnormal paps
Are you in menopause, and if yes, how long? ______
Are you on hormones, and if yes, which ones? Premarin 0.625 mg (1-25); Provera 10 mg (½ tab 16-25)

HEADACHE ASSESSMENT FORM

HA PROFILE	INCAPACITATING #3	INTERFERING #2	IRRITATING #1
ONSET (Years ago and frequency)	N/A	In 50's, occasionally	N/A
CURRENT FREQUENCY	N/A	Every day for 3 – 4 days Before that, 2 – 3/month	N/A
TIME OF ONSET	N/A	N/A	N/A
DURATION	N/A	Wax and wane for 1 day	N/A
CHARACTER	N/A	Pressure, throbbing	N/A
PRODROME OR AURA	N/A	Sees zigzag blacklines for 20 minutes, then headache begins	N/A
ASSOCIATING FEATURES	Nausea; Vomiting; Sensitivity to Light? Noise? Odors? Do you get pale or flush? Do your eyes or nose run? Does your nose get stuffy? Do the whites of your eyes get red? Does your eyelid droop? Do you pace, or go to bed?	Nausea; Vomiting; Sensitivity to Light? Noise? Odors? Do you get pale or flush? Do your eyes or nose run? Does your nose get stuffy? Do the whites of your eyes get red? Does your eyelid droop? Do you pace, or go to bed?	Nausea; Vomiting; Sensitivity to Light? Noise? Odors? Do you get pale or flush? Do your eyes or nose run? Does your nose get stuffy? Do the whites of your eyes get red? Does your eyelid droop? Do you pace, or go to bed?
PRECIPITATING OR AGGRAVATING FEATURES	N/A	Coughing	N/A

LOCATION: Mark the location for each type of headache with a different color pen.

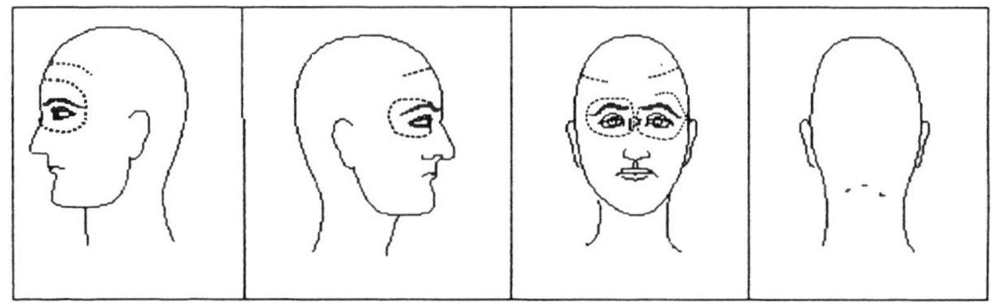

MEDICAL HISTORY:

Have you ever been or are you currently being treated for any of the following?

a) high blood pressure	Yes	No
b) stomach ulcers	Yes	No
c) asthma	Yes	No
d) allergies	Yes	No
e) pneumonia	Yes	No
f) kidney problems	Yes	No
g) low blood sugar	Yes	No
h) glaucoma	Yes	No
i) diabetes	Yes	No
j) heart problems	Yes	No

If you answered yes to any of the above, please describe: High blood pressure diagnosed 2 years ago. Allergies are environmental. Kidney infections on rare occasions.

List all other medical problems you have had in the past. Include date diagnosed and treatment.
DO NOT LIST OPERATIONS

Fibrocystic disease, watched closely by doctor. Emphysema – very early stages. High blood pressure (now taking Lozol daily).

SURGICAL HISTORY (List operations and dates performed)

Hysterectomy, complete – 1975. Gallbladder removed – 1989. Biopsy on breast. Appendix removed during hysterectomy. Tonsils and adenoids removed as a child. Bunion surgery on both feet.

PSYCHIATRIC HISTORY (List visits with counselors, psychologists, etc., and type of treatment)

ACCIDENTS IN ADULT LIFE (Briefly describe any accident that caused any blow to the head or that you feel is related to your headache)

None

FAMILY HISTORY:

1. Is your father living? Yes No
   Age________
   Cause of death 74, accident (surgery, then blood clot)
   Was there a headache history? Yes No
2. Is your mother living? Yes No
   Age________
   Cause of death 42, cancer of the breast
   Was there a headache history? Yes No

3. Ages of brothers---Circle the ones with headache
   None
4. Ages of sisters---Circle the ones with headache
   None
5. List any other blood relatives with a history of severe headaches.
   None

MARITAL HISTORY:
List marriages:

1st marriage age 18 to 21	Did spouse have headaches?	Yes	No
2nd marriage age 27 to 46	Did spouse have headaches?	Yes	No
3rd marriage age 51 to Present	Did spouse have headaches?	Yes	No
3rd marriage age ____ to ____	Did spouse have headaches?	Yes	No

Age of current spouse: 65½

List ages and sex of all children:

Age 37 Sex M Headaches?	Yes	No
Age 32 Sex F Headaches?	Yes	No
Age ____ Sex ____ Headaches?	Yes	No

STRESS FACTORS:

List any factors that may be affecting your headaches (money, loneliness, sexual problems, work, etc.)
Not sure if these problems cause headaches or not, but my son lives here and never calls or comes to see me.

VEGETATIVE SIGNS:

1.	Do you have trouble falling asleep?	Yes	No
2.	Do you have trouble staying asleep?	Yes	No
3.	Has your appetite decreased?	Yes	No
4.	Have you gained or lost weight in the past year?	Yes	No
5.	Have you felt tearful or depressed lately?	Yes	No
6.	Have you had any thoughts of wanting to die?	Yes	No
7.	Have you been forgetful lately?	Yes	No
8.	Any other changes in your normal day-to-day living?		

Please list any medications you are allergic or sensitive to: Penicillin

Please list any medications you are currently taking (including dosages and frequency per day):
Allergy shots twice a week. Lozol – 2.5 mg tablets – 1 daily. Indomethacin for back pain.
Premarin – 0.625 mg taablets – Days 1-25 each month; Provera – 10 mg ½ tablet Days 16-25.
Midrin caps – 1 every 6 hrs. as needed for headache.

PREVIOUS CARE:

1. List doctors who have treated you for headaches: Dr. M·

2. List any tests you have had for your headache (e.g., EEG, CT scan, MRI, X-Ray, etc.):
None

3. List any other treatment you have had for your headache (e.g., biofeedback, acupuncture, chiropractic, or any other treatment you had):
None.

NANCY
Category: Migraine

This 34-year-old woman appeared to have typical symptoms of migraine, starting with her menstrual periods at age 11. She generally had these headaches around her menstrual cycle, with typical symptoms of migraine, such as throbbing, nausea, vomiting, sensitivity to light, noise, odors, and she would have to go to bed.

However, a year ago a new type of headache started, at age 33, and it was constant pressure-type pain. The pain would be primarily in the left parietal side of her head. Because of this new type of headache, a medical workup, including laboratory and CT scan, was done to rule out the possibility of any intracranial lesion or space-occupying lesion, which turned out to be negative.

The patient was treated for migraine headaches, which also reduced this new type of headache, and she did quite well.

MEDICAL HEADACHE HISTORY

Name: Nancy **Age:** 34 **Sex** F **Date:** 12/20/89

Date of Birth: 00/00/53 **Birthplace:** TX **Race:** W **Education:** Some college

Occupation: Homemaker **Accident:** N/A

Armed Services & Type of Discharge: N/A

PAST HISTORY:

1.	Did you have a normal birth?		**Yes**	No
	a) forceps used?		Yes	No
	b) cesarean section?		Yes	**No**
2.	Did you have problems with bedwetting?		Yes	**No**
	a) If yes, age bedwetting stopped			
3.	Were you car sick as a child (motion)?		Yes	**No**
	a) If yes, how severe?	Slight	Moderate	Severe
4.	Did you have unexplained abdominal cramps as a child?		Yes	**No**
5.	Did you have any of the following illnesses in childhood?			
	a) meningitis		Yes	**No**
	b) encephalitis		Yes	**No**
	c) scarlet fever		Yes	**No**
	d) rheumatic fever		Yes	**No**
6.	Did you have any head injuries as a child?		**Yes**	No
	a) If yes, please explain: Hit in the head with a rock and had stitches, age 7			
7.	Were you treated for emotional illness as a child?		Yes	**No**

HABITS:

8.	Do you drink alcohol?	Yes	**No**
	a) If yes, what kind and how much?		
	b) Does alcohol bring on or aggravate a headache?	Yes	No
9.	Do you smoke?	Yes	**No**
	a) If yes, how much?		
	b) Does smoking or smoke-filled rooms cause or aggravate headaches?	Yes	No
10.	Do you drink caffeinated beverages?	**Yes**	No
	a) If yes, how much? 2 to 4 cups of tea a day		

MENSTRUAL HISTORY:

At what age did menses begin? 11 Were they regular or irregular? Severe cramping
How were they related to your headache? Worse
Are you or were you ever on Birth Control Pills? Yes Did they affect your headache? Worse
Have you had a hysterectomy, partial or total, and why?
Are you in menopause, and if yes, how long?
Are you on hormones, and if yes, which ones?

HEADACHE ASSESSMENT FORM

HA PROFILE	INCAPACITATING #3	INTERFERING #2	IRRITATING #1
ONSET (Years ago and frequency)	Age 11 with periods, once a month for 4 to 5 days	Age 33, 3 or 4 weeks at a time	Same
CURRENT FREQUENCY	2 times a month	2 to 3 week cycle	Same
TIME OF ONSET	1 week before period	Anytime	Same
DURATION	Wax and wane, 4 to 5 days	Wax and wane, 3 or 4 weeks	Same
CHARACTER	Throbbing	Constant pressure	Same
PRODROME OR AURA	Sleepy, yawning	N/A	N/A
ASSOCIATING FEATURES	Nausea; Vomiting; Sensitivity to Light? Noise? Odors? Do you get pale or flush? Do your eyes or nose run? Does your nose get stuffy? Do the whites of your eyes get red? Does your eyelid droop? Do you pace, or go to bed?	Nausea; Vomiting; Sensitivity to Light? Noise? Odors? Do you get pale or flush? Do your eyes or nose run? Does your nose get stuffy? Do the whites of your eyes get red? Does your eyelid droop? Do you pace, or go to bed?	Nausea; Vomiting; Sensitivity to Light? Noise? Odors? Do you get pale or flush? Do your eyes or nose run? Does your nose get stuffy? Do the whites of your eyes get red? Does your eyelid droop? Do you pace, or go to bed?
PRECIPITATING OR AGGRAVATING FEATURES	Menstruation, sweets, movement	N/A	N/A

LOCATION: Mark the location for each type of headache with a different color pen.

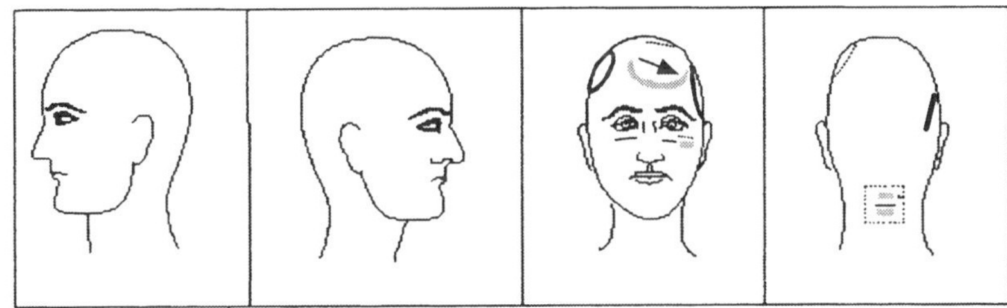

MEDICAL HISTORY:

Have you ever been or are you currently being treated for any of the following?

a) high blood pressure	Yes	No
b) stomach ulcers	Yes	No
c) asthma	Yes	No
d) allergies	Yes	No
e) pneumonia	Yes	No
f) kidney problems	Yes	No
g) low blood sugar	Yes	No
h) glaucoma	Yes	No
i) diabetes	Yes	No
j) heart problems	Yes	No

If you answered yes to any of the above, please describe:____________________

List all other medical problems you have had in the past. Include date diagnosed and treatment.
DO NOT LIST OPERATIONS

Hypoglycemia, 1976. Migraine, sinusitis, polyps in sinus, 1976. Gilbert's Syndrom, 1976.

SURGICAL HISTORY (List operations and dates performed)

Tonsillectomy, 1969. 3rd Nipple removed, 1970. D&C after miscarriage, 1977. Liver biopsy, 1977.

PSYCHIATRIC HISTORY (List visits with counselors, psychologists, etc., and type of treatment)

None

ACCIDENTS IN ADULT LIFE (Briefly describe any accident that caused any blow to the head or that you feel is related to your headache)

FAMILY HISTORY:

1. Is your father living? Yes No
   - Age 66
   - Cause of death__________
   - Was there a headache history? Yes No
2. Is your mother living? Yes No
   - Age 65
   - Cause of death__________
   - Was there a headache history? Yes No
3. Ages of brothers---Circle the ones with headache
   (43) 39

4. Ages of sisters---Circle the ones with headache
   32
5. List any other blood relatives with a history of severe headaches.
   Unknown

MARITAL HISTORY:
List marriages:

1st marriage age 22 to Present	Did spouse have headaches?	<u>Yes</u>	No
2nd marriage age ____ to ____	Did spouse have headaches?	Yes	No
3rd marriage age ____ to ____	Did spouse have headaches?	Yes	No

Age of current spouse: 38

List ages and sex of all children:

Age 9	Sex M	Headaches?	<u>Yes</u>	No
Age 6	Sex M	Headaches?	Yes	<u>No</u>
Age 3	Sex F	Headaches?	Yes	<u>No</u>

STRESS FACTORS:

List any factors that may be affecting your headaches (money, loneliness, sexual problems, work, etc.)

VEGETATIVE SIGNS:

1.	Do you have trouble falling asleep?	<u>Yes</u>	No
2.	Do you have trouble staying asleep?	<u>Yes</u>	No
3.	Has your appetite decreased?	Yes	<u>No</u>
4.	Have you gained or lost weight in the past year?	Yes	<u>No</u>
5.	Have you felt tearful or depressed lately?	Yes	<u>No</u>
6.	Have you had any thoughts of wanting to die?	Yes	<u>No</u>
7.	Have you been forgetful lately?	Yes	<u>No</u>
8.	Any other changes in your normal day-to-day living?		

Please list any medications you are allergic or sensitive to: Penicillin

Please list any medications you are currently taking (including dosages and frequency per day):
Synthroid, 0.1 mg. ½ tablet daily. Fiorinal, 1 or 2 every 6 hours, no more than 6 per day.
Extra Strength Tylenol, 2 tablets. Sinus medication (Sine-Off, SinuTab).
Naldagen T.D., 1 tab 2 times a day, if needed. Nyquil..

PREVIOUS CARE:

1. List doctors who have treated you for headaches: Dr. M. Dr. B.

2. List any tests you have had for your headache (e.g., EEG, CT scan, MRI, X-Ray, etc.):
CT scan – 1976. X-rays.

3. List any other treatment you have had for your headache (e.g., biofeedback, acupuncture, chiropractic, or any other treatment you had):
None.

GINA
Category: Migraine

This patient shows on her intake that her headaches started 6 years prior to seeing me, and they have become a daily occurrence. The patient shows that she had nausea, photophobia, sonophobia and throbbing-like qualities with her headaches, plus many of the precipitating problems that cause migraines, such as alcohol, smoking, menstrual periods, fatigue, diet, and stress, which were all part of the problems that were increasing her headache problem.

The diagnosis based on the headache intake indicates that she was suffering from the International Headache Society classification of Migraine 1.1, which is migraine without an aura, and there also appeared to be a degree of tension-type headache that was mixed in with her migraines. Unfortunately, this patient also had asthma, which did not permit the use of certain medications, and she was very sensitive to other medications. She was started on biofeedback and she was given various medications to abort or to break the migraine attacks.

Again, as you will see with other histories, headaches do not always fall into one category and it requires someone with a great deal of experience to be able to deal with the separate entities of the different types of headaches.

MEDICAL HEADACHE HISTORY

Name: Gina **Age:** 32 **Sex** F **Date:** 4/23/90

Date of Birth: 00/00/57 **Birthplace:** SC **Race:** C **Education:** Graduate

Occupation: Paralegal **Accident:** N/A

Armed Services & Type of Discharge: N/A

PAST HISTORY:

1.	Did you have a normal birth?		<u>Yes</u>	No
	a) forceps used?		Yes	<u>No</u>
	b) cesarean section?		Yes	<u>No</u>
2.	Did you have problems with bedwetting?		Yes	<u>No</u>
	a) If yes, age bedwetting stopped			
3.	Were you car sick as a child (motion)?		<u>Yes</u>	No
	a) If yes, how severe?	Slight	<u>Moderate</u>	Severe
4.	Did you have unexplained abdominal cramps as a child?		Yes	<u>No</u>
5.	Did you have any of the following illnesses in childhood?			
	a) meningitis		Yes	<u>No</u>
	b) encephalitis		Yes	<u>No</u>
	c) scarlet fever		Yes	<u>No</u>
	d) rheumatic fever		Yes	<u>No</u>
6.	Did you have any head injuries as a child?		Yes	<u>No</u>
	a) If yes, please explain:			
7.	Were you treated for emotional illness as a child?		Yes	<u>No</u>

HABITS:

8.	Do you drink alcohol?	Yes	<u>No</u>
	a) If yes, what kind and how much?		
	b) Does alcohol bring on or aggravate a headache?	<u>Yes</u>	No
9.	Do you smoke?	Yes	<u>No</u>
	a) If yes, how much?		
	b) Does smoking or smoke-filled rooms cause or aggravate headaches?	Yes	<u>No</u>
10.	Do you drink caffeinated beverages?	<u>Yes</u>	No
	a) If yes, how much? Decaf tea and diet cola		

MENSTRUAL HISTORY:

At what age did menses begin? 11 Were they regular or irregular? Heavy normal

How were they related to your headache? N/A

Are you or were you ever on Birth Control Pills? No Did they affect your headache? N/A

Have you had a hysterectomy, partial or total, and why? No

Are you in menopause, and if yes, how long? No

Are you on hormones, and if yes, which ones? No

HEADACHE ASSESSMENT FORM

HA PROFILE	INCAPACITATING #3	INTERFERING #2	IRRITATING #1
ONSET (Years ago and frequency)	6 years ago, daily	6 years ago	6 years ago, daily
CURRENT FREQUENCY	1 time a week	Daily	Daily
TIME OF ONSET	Mid a.m., increases to p.m.	Mid a.m. to p.m.	1 to 2 hours after getting up
DURATION	1 day or until goes to bed	Lasts til goes to bed	Until becomes #2, 1 hour to half a day
CHARACTER	Vice-like	Throbs	Dull, steady ache
PRODROME OR AURA	N/A	N/A	N/A
ASSOCIATING FEATURES	Nausea; Vomiting; Sensitivity to Light? Noise? Odors? Do you get pale or flush? Do your eyes or nose run? Does your nose get stuffy? Do the whites of your eyes get red? Does your eyelid droop? Do you pace, or go to bed?	Nausea; Vomiting; Sensitivity to Light? Noise? Odors? Do you get pale or flush? Do your eyes or nose run? Does your nose get stuffy? Do the whites of your eyes get red? Does your eyelid droop? Do you pace, or go to bed?	Nausea; Vomiting; Sensitivity to Light? Noise? Odors? Do you get pale or flush? Do your eyes or nose run? Does your nose get stuffy? Do the whites of your eyes get red? Does your eyelid droop? Do you pace, or go to bed?
PRECIPITATING OR AGGRAVATING FEATURES	Alcohol, smoke, menses, fatigue, dietary, stress	Alcohol, smoke, menses, fatigue, dietary, stress	Alcohol, smoke, menses, fatigue, dietary, stress

LOCATION: Mark the location for each type of headache with a different color pen.

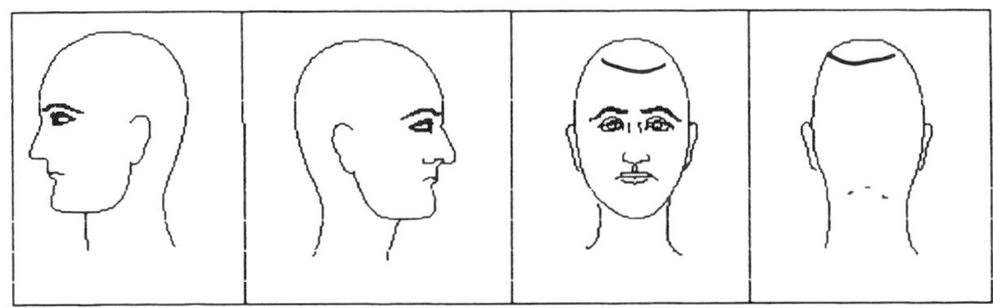

MEDICAL HISTORY:

Have you ever been or are you currently being treated for any of the following?

a) high blood pressure	Yes	No
b) stomach ulcers	Yes	No
c) asthma	Yes	No
d) allergies	Yes	No
e) pneumonia	Yes	No
f) kidney problems	Yes	No
g) low blood sugar	Yes	No
h) glaucoma	Yes	No
i) diabetes	Yes	No
j) heart problems	Yes	No

If you answered yes to any of the above, please describe: Asthma at 3 to 5 years of age. Environmental allergies, and soy.

List all other medical problems you have had in the past. Include date diagnosed and treatment.
DO NOT LIST OPERATIONS

Hyperthyroidism, 1988 or 1989 (take Synthroid). Lifelong allergies, asthma, off and on. Taking allergy shots. Also had allergy shots around 1970 to the mid-1970's.

SURGICAL HISTORY (List operations and dates performed)

Deviated septum, 1974.

PSYCHIATRIC HISTORY (List visits with counselors, psychologists, etc., and type of treatment)

None

ACCIDENTS IN ADULT LIFE (Briefly describe any accident that caused any blow to the head or that you feel is related to your headache)

None

FAMILY HISTORY:

1. Is your father living? Yes No
   Age________
   Cause of death 55, war injury
   Was there a headache history? Yes No
2. Is your mother living? Yes No
   Age 66
   Cause of death________
   Was there a headache history? Yes No

3. Ages of brothers---Circle the ones with headache
   34
4. Ages of sisters---Circle the ones with headache
   None
5. List any other blood relatives with a history of severe headaches.
   None

MARITAL HISTORY:

List marriages:

1st marriage age 32 to Now Did spouse have headaches?	Yes	No
2nd marriage age ____ to ____ Did spouse have headaches?	Yes	No
3rd marriage age ____ to ____ Did spouse have headaches?	Yes	No

Age of current spouse: 32

List ages and sex of all children:

Age ____ Sex ____ Headaches?	Yes	No
Age ____ Sex ____ Headaches?	Yes	No
Age ____ Sex ____ Headaches?	Yes	No

STRESS FACTORS:

List any factors that may be affecting your headaches (money, loneliness, sexual problems, work, etc.)
Traffic, driving, deadlines, stress, caffeine, allergies. Family problems.

VEGETATIVE SIGNS:

1.	Do you have trouble falling asleep?	Yes	No
2.	Do you have trouble staying asleep?	Yes	No
3.	Has your appetite decreased?	Yes	No
4.	Have you gained or lost weight in the past year?	Yes	No
5.	Have you felt tearful or depressed lately?	Yes	No
6.	Have you had any thoughts of wanting to die?	Yes	No
7.	Have you been forgetful lately?	Yes	No
8.	Any other changes in your normal day-to-day living?		

Please list any medications you are allergic or sensitive to: Penicillin

Please list any medications you are currently taking (including dosages and frequency per day):
Synthroid, 0.1 mg. daoily. Triamterene/hctz 50 mg/25/m – every other day.
Aspirin – 2 to 4 per day. Vitamins.

PREVIOUS CARE:

1. List doctors who have treated you for headaches: General Practitioners (2); Neurologist.

2. List any tests you have had for your headache (e.g., EEG, CT scan, MRI, X-Ray, etc.):
CT scan for deviated septum.

3. List any other treatment you have had for your headache (e.g., biofeedback, acupuncture, chiropractic, or any other treatment you had):
None.

DAVID
Category: Migraine

This is another example of migraine without aura, or nonclassical migraine, and tension-type headache. Once again, if one looks at the intake, one sees that there can be variations and that the picture is never clear. This is the reason it is so important to demonstrate the different characteristics of the headaches, to determine what approach must be taken.

It is not uncommon that the headache pattern may start episodically, and eventually, if untreated or by its own course, will become an everyday phenomenon presenting as a different diagnosis.

MEDICAL HEADACHE HISTORY

Name: David **Age:** 29 **Sex** M **Date:** 8/7/91

Date of Birth: 00/00/61 **Birthplace:** IL **Race:** W **Education:** 2 yrs. college

Occupation: Asst. Restaurant Manager **Accident:** N/A

Armed Services & Type of Discharge: N/A

PAST HISTORY:

1.	Did you have a normal birth?		Yes	No
	a) forceps used?		Yes	No
	b) cesarean section?		Yes	No
2.	Did you have problems with bedwetting?		Yes	No
	a) If yes, age bedwetting stopped			
3.	Were you car sick as a child (motion)?		Yes	No
	a) If yes, how severe?	Slight	Moderate	Severe
4.	Did you have unexplained abdominal cramps as a child?		Yes	No
5.	Did you have any of the following illnesses in childhood?			
	a) meningitis		Yes	No
	b) encephalitis		Yes	No
	c) scarlet fever		Yes	No
	d) rheumatic fever		Yes	No
6.	Did you have any head injuries as a child?		Yes	No
	a) If yes, please explain:			
7.	Were you treated for emotional illness as a child?		Yes	No

HABITS:

8.	Do you drink alcohol?	Yes	No
	a) If yes, what kind and how much? Social, 1 to 4, sometimes more		
	b) Does alcohol bring on or aggravate a headache?	Yes	No
9.	Do you smoke?	Yes	No
	a) If yes, how much?		
	b) Does smoking or smoke-filled rooms cause or aggravate headaches?	Yes	No
10.	Do you drink caffeinated beverages?	Yes	No
	a) If yes, how much?		

MENSTRUAL HISTORY:

At what age did menses begin?_______ Were they regular or irregular?____________________

How were they related to your headache?____________________

Are you or were you ever on Birth Control Pills?______ Did they affect your headache? ________

Have you had a hysterectomy, partial or total, and why?____________________

Are you in menopause, and if yes, how long?____________________

Are you on hormones, and if yes, which ones?____________________

HEADACHE ASSESSMENT FORM

HA PROFILE	INCAPACITATING #3	INTERFERING #2	IRRITATING #1
ONSET (Years ago and frequency)	1980 1 to 2 per week	3 weeks ago 1 to 3 per week	In my teens, occasionally
CURRENT FREQUENCY	None since then	1 to 3 per week	Every day
TIME OF ONSET	?	Can awaken with	Can awaken with
DURATION	1 day	1 day	1 hour with OTC medication
CHARACTER	Tight band	Tight band and throbbing	Dull ache
PRODROME OR AURA	N/A	N/A	N/A
ASSOCIATING FEATURES	Nausea; Vomiting; Sensitivity to Light? Noise? Odors? Do you get pale or flush? Do your eyes or nose run? Does your nose get stuffy? Do the whites of your eyes get red? Does your eyelid droop? Do you pace, or go to bed?	Nausea; Vomiting; Sensitivity to Light? Noise? Odors? Do you get pale or flush? Do your eyes or nose run? Does your nose get stuffy? Do the whites of your eyes get red? Does your eyelid droop? Do you pace, or go to bed?	Nausea; Vomiting; Sensitivity to Light? Noise? Odors? Do you get pale or flush? Do your eyes or nose run? Does your nose get stuffy? Do the whites of your eyes get red? Does your eyelid droop? Do you pace, or go to bed?
PRECIPITATING OR AGGRAVATING FEATURES	Movement	Coughing Changing position	N/A

LOCATION: Mark the location for each type of headache with a different color pen.

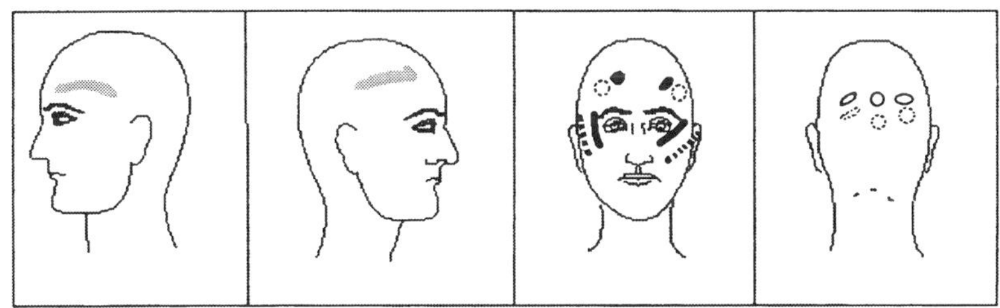

MEDICAL HISTORY:

Have you ever been or are you currently being treated for any of the following?

a) high blood pressure	Yes	No
b) stomach ulcers	Yes	No
c) asthma	Yes	No
d) allergies	Yes	No
e) pneumonia	Yes	No
f) kidney problems	Yes	No
g) low blood sugar	Yes	No
h) glaucoma	Yes	No
i) diabetes	Yes	No
j) heart problems	Yes	No

If you answered yes to any of the above, please describe:____________________

List all other medical problems you have had in the past. Include date diagnosed and treatment.
DO NOT LIST OPERATIONS
N/A

SURGICAL HISTORY (List operations and dates performed)
Dislocated shoulder – 1979. Reconstructive surgery.

PSYCHIATRIC HISTORY (List visits with counselors, psychologists, etc., and type of treatment)
None.

ACCIDENTS IN ADULT LIFE (Briefly describe any accident that caused any blow to the head or that you feel is related to your headache)
N/A

FAMILY HISTORY:

1. Is your father living? Yes No
   Age 48
   Cause of death________________
   Was there a headache history? Yes No
2. Is your mother living? Yes No
   Age 47
   Cause of death________________
   Was there a headache history? Yes No
3. Ages of brothers---Circle the ones with headache
   (28)

4. Ages of sisters---Circle the ones with headache
   None
5. List any other blood relatives with a history of severe headaches.
   Unknown.

MARITAL HISTORY:
List marriages:

1st marriage age _____ to _____	Did spouse have headaches?	Yes	No
2nd marriage age _____ to _____	Did spouse have headaches?	Yes	No
3rd marriage age _____ to _____	Did spouse have headaches?	Yes	No

Age of current spouse: N/A

List ages and sex of all children:

Age _____ Sex _____	Headaches?	Yes	No
Age _____ Sex _____	Headaches?	Yes	No
Age _____ Sex _____	Headaches?	Yes	No

STRESS FACTORS:

List any factors that may be affecting your headaches (money, loneliness, sexual problems, work, etc.)
Money, work.

VEGETATIVE SIGNS:

1.	Do you have trouble falling asleep?	Yes	No
2.	Do you have trouble staying asleep?	Yes	No
3.	Has your appetite decreased?	Yes	No
4.	Have you gained or lost weight in the past year?	Yes	No
5.	Have you felt tearful or depressed lately?	Yes	No
6.	Have you had any thoughts of wanting to die?	Yes	No
7.	Have you been forgetful lately?	Yes	No
8.	Any other changes in your normal day-to-day living?_____		

Please list any medications you are allergic or sensitive to: None

Please list any medications you are currently taking (including dosages and frequency per day):
None

PREVIOUS CARE:

1. List doctors who have treated you for headaches: Dr. R.

2. List any tests you have had for your headache (e.g., EEG, CT scan, MRI, X-Ray, etc.):
EEG and CT scan, X-rays – 1980-81 (all normal).

3. List any other treatment you have had for your headache (e.g., biofeedback, acupuncture, chiropractic, or any other treatment you had):
None

CHAPTER 7

Chronic Daily Headaches

Both for the patient and the physician, treatment of these daily headaches is a most difficult task. The question of how does someone get to the point that a day or almost a day doesn't go by when the patient isn't suffering with pain is quite baffling (Figure 7.1).

These headache sufferers were usually diagnosed as having chronic muscle tension headache or psychogenic headache. The cause of these headaches was generally accepted as ongoing spasms in muscles around the skull. However, studies showed that in evaluating the activity of these muscles using EMG (electromyography) only half of the patients showed increased activity and the other half showed normal or decreased activity. The other interesting finding was that the same results were obtained in subjects without head pain.[1]

Most patients describe their symptoms as being irritating to moderate to occasionally incapacitating pain, on a daily or almost daily basis. Incapacitating pain is experienced weekly, biweekly, or monthly in most cases and when this happens symptoms such as nausea, vomiting, and photophobia and other symptoms of migraine are present. Therefore, it was felt that two different headache types were present, that is, muscle tension and migraine. As more studies are reported, the consensus is that perhaps we are really seeing a continuum of the same type of headache.[2]

Various authors have written excellent studies identifying what may be the process involved in development from occasional to daily headaches. Also reported was that there seems to be a transformation over time from migraine into daily headaches.[3] Another study showed that of 615 patients who presented chronic daily headache, all started with intermittent migraine and 80% had their first episode before age 26. By age 45, 90% of the group had developed daily headaches.[4] Interestingly enough, sometimes the same medication that helps muscle tension headache will help chronic daily headache, just as some migraine medications will do the same. Many of the mechanisms discussed in Chapter 3 on theories of pain have been suggested as the source of pain in the chronic headache problem. At this point serotonin, as a neurotransmitter in the brain, seems to be affected.

Many of the symptoms in chronic daily headache are sleep disturbance, depression, anxiety, and a family history of headache. Kudrow, in a 1982 study, showed that, by decreasing or eliminating analgesic medication there could be a significant improvement in the headache problem.[5] Baumgartner et al.[6] in 1989 found that 80% of patients hospitalized for chronic daily headache and withdrawn from their daily medications were headache-free two weeks after the medications were discontinued. The argument, "Which came first, the chicken or the egg?" is in contention; that is, does the analgesic medication cause the chronic daily headache, or does the headache problem cause the abuse of the medication?

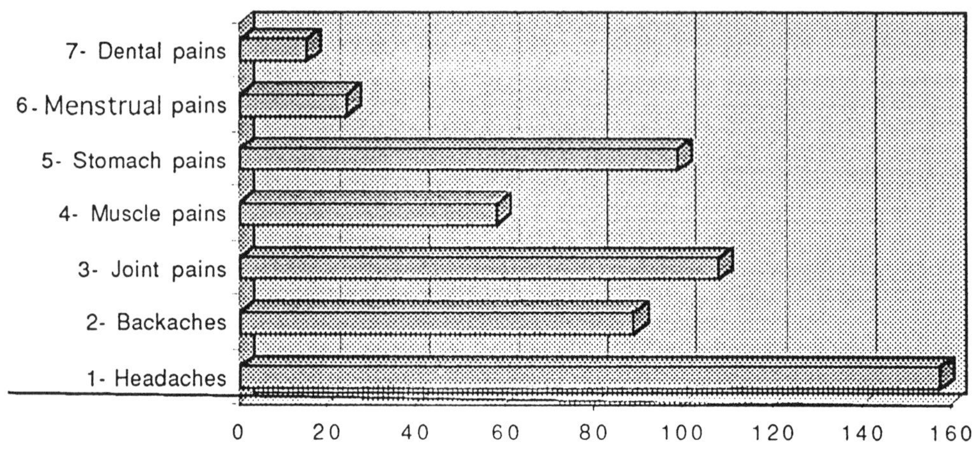

Workdays lost to pain in millions per year

1- Headaches	156.9
2- Backaches	88.8
3- Joint pains	107.8
4- Muscle pains	58.2
5- Stomach pains	98.7
6- Menstrual pains	24.5
7- Dental pains	15.1
Total workdays lost	550.00

Figure 7.1 This figure demonstrates a study that was done in the late 1980s. Of 550 million days lost a year by workers because of pain, the most common cause was headaches, representing approximately 160 million work days lost.

The term "rebound headache" has originated as a result of this medication overuse. Many of the newer books have sections devoted to this problem.[7]

REFERENCES

1. Sheftell, F.D., Chronic daily headache, *Neurology*, 42 (3 Suppl. 2), 32–36, 1992.
2. Raskin, N.H., Appenzeller, O., *Headache*, Churchill Livingstone, New York, 1980.
3. Mathew, N.T., Stubits, E., Nigam, M., Transformation of migraine into daily headaches: analysis of factors, *Headache*, 22, 66–68, 1982.
4. Saper, J.R., Changing perspective on chronic headache, *Clinical Journal of Pain*, 2, 19–28, 1986.
5. Kudrow, L., Paradoxical effects of frequent analgesic use, *Advances in Neurology*, 33, 335–341, 1982.
6. Baumgartner, C.P., Wessely, P., Maly, J., Holzner, F., Long-term prognosis of analgesic withdrawal in patients with drug induced headaches, *Headache*, 29, 510–514, 1989.
7. Rapoport, A.M., Sheftell, F.D., *Headache Relief*, Simon and Schuster, New York, 1991.

CASE HISTORIES*

CHARLES
Category: Daily chronic headaches

A 53-year-old man visited complaining of incapacitating headaches and interfering headaches (moderate to severe). The incapacitating headaches started three years ago. They were occasional. Currently he is getting these every two to three months. They last three hours. There is severe pressure and sometimes throbbing. The pain is located in the periorbital regions (or around the eyes), and the temporal and occipital regions. Associated features are sonophobia, or sensitivity to noise, and he goes to bed. Movement and sneezing will make it worse.

Interfering headaches (moderate to severe) also started three years ago. They were daily and continue to be daily. They are worse in the morning, with constant pain and also severe pressure and throbbing in the areas just described. Again, associated features are sonophobia, and he will go to bed if he can.

There is no headache history in the family. He has seen a neurologist in the past, had a CT scan and been examined, and nothing abnormal was found. The medical examination and neurological examination were basically negative. The diagnosis here would be chronic tension-type headache. This patient was treated with many types of medications, but was having continued problems. Although the incapacitating headaches were reduced in intensity and the interfering headaches were reduced by almost 80%, he continued to have irritating headaches, which are annoying headaches, the rest of the time.

* On the headache assessment forms that accompany these case histories, incapacitating headaches are indicated with solid black lines, interfering headaches with dotted lines, and irritating headaches with gray shading.

MEDICAL HEADACHE HISTORY

Name: Charles **Age:** 53 **Sex** M **Date:** 10/14/91

Date of Birth: 00/00/38 **Birthplace:** FL **Race:** C **Education:** High school

Occupation: Parts Manager for Auto Dealer **Accident:** N/A

Armed Services & Type of Discharge: N/A

PAST HISTORY:

1.	Did you have a normal birth?		Yes	No
	a) forceps used?		Yes	No
	b) cesarean section?		Yes	No
2.	Did you have problems with bedwetting?		Yes	No
	a) If yes, age bedwetting stopped			________
3.	Were you car sick as a child (motion)?		Yes	No
	a) If yes, how severe?	Slight	Moderate	Severe
4.	Did you have unexplained abdominal cramps as a child?		Yes	No
5.	Did you have any of the following illnesses in childhood?			
	a) meningitis		Yes	No
	b) encephalitis		Yes	No
	c) scarlet fever		Yes	No
	d) rheumatic fever		Yes	No
6.	Did you have any head injuries as a child?		Yes	No
	a) If yes, please explain:			
7.	Were you treated for emotional illness as a child?		Yes	No

HABITS:

8.	Do you drink alcohol?	Yes	No
	a) If yes, what kind and how much?		
	b) Does alcohol bring on or aggravate a headache?	Yes	No
9.	Do you smoke?	Yes	No
	a) If yes, how much?		
	b) Does smoking or smoke-filled rooms cause or aggravate headaches?	Yes	No
10.	Do you drink caffeinated beverages?	Yes	No
	a) If yes, how much? Moderate amount of ice tea		

MENSTRUAL HISTORY:

At what age did menses begin?______ Were they regular or irregular?__________________

How were they related to your headache?__________________

Are you or were you ever on Birth Control Pills?______ Did they affect your headache? ________

Have you had a hysterectomy, partial or total, and why?__________________

Are you in menopause, and if yes, how long?__________________

Are you on hormones, and if yes, which ones?__________________

HEADACHE ASSESSMENT FORM

HA PROFILE	INCAPACITATING #3	INTERFERING #2	IRRITATING #1
ONSET (Years ago and frequency)	3 years occasionally	3 years ago, every day	N/A
CURRENT FREQUENCY	1 every 2 to 3 months	Every day	N/A
TIME OF ONSET	Anytime	Worse in morning	N/A
DURATION	2 to 3 hours	Constant	N/A
CHARACTER	Severe pressure, throbbing	Same, less intense	N/A
PRODROME OR AURA	N/A	N/A	N/A
ASSOCIATING FEATURES	Nausea; Vomiting; Sensitivity to Light? Noise? Odors? Do you get pale or flush? Do your eyes or nose run? Does your nose get stuffy? Does the white of your eyes get red? Does your eyelid droop? Do you pace, or go to bed?	Nausea; Vomiting; Sensitivity to Light? Noise? Odors? Do you get pale or flush? Do your eyes or nose run? Does your nose get stuffy? Does the white of your eyes get red? Does your eyelid droop? Do you pace, or go to bed?	Nausea; Vomiting; Sensitivity to Light? Noise? Odors? Do you get pale or flush? Do your eyes or nose run? Does your nose get stuffy? Does the white of your eyes get red? Does your eyelid droop? Do you pace, or go to bed?
PRECIPITATING OR AGGRAVATING FEATURES	N/A	Lying down on left side	N/A

LOCATION: Mark the location for each type of headache with a different color pen.
Incapacitating #3 is ____. Interfering #2 is .... Irritating #1 is ▒▒▒▒

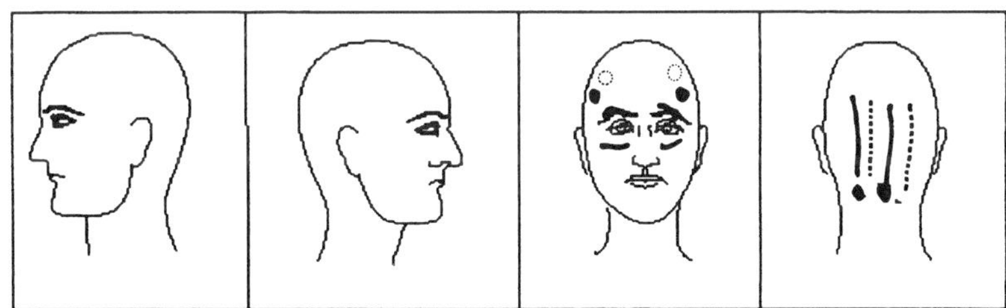

MEDICAL HISTORY:

Have you ever been or are you currently being treated for any of the following?

a) high blood pressure	Yes	No
b) stomach ulcers	Yes	No
c) asthma	Yes	No
d) allergies	Yes	No
e) pneumonia	Yes	No
f) kidney problems	Yes	No
g) low blood sugar	Yes	No
h) glaucoma	Yes	No
i) diabetes	Yes	No
j) heart problems	Yes	No

If you answered yes to any of the above, please describe: High blood pressure diagnosed 3 weeks ago. Ulcers diagnosed in 1981, resolved.

List all other medical problems you have had in the past. Include date diagnosed and treatment.
DO NOT LIST OPERATIONS

None

SURGICAL HISTORY (List operations and dates performed)

Cyst removed from back, 1990.

Gallbladder removed, 1982.

PSYCHIATRIC HISTORY (List visits with counselors, psychologists, etc., and type of treatment)

None

ACCIDENTS IN ADULT LIFE (Briefly describe any accident that caused any blow to the head or that you feel is related to your headache)

None.

FAMILY HISTORY:

1. Is your father living? Yes No
   - Age________
   - Cause of death Heart attack, age 62
   - Was there a headache history? Yes No
2. Is your mother living? Yes No
   - Age________
   - Cause of death Cancer, age 65
   - Was there a headache history? Yes No

3. Ages of brothers---Circle the ones with headache
   36
4. Ages of sisters---Circle the ones with headache
   55 52
5. List any other blood relatives with a history of severe headaches.
   N/A

MARITAL HISTORY:

List marriages:

1st marriage age _20_ to _Present_ Did spouse have headaches? Yes No
2nd marriage age _____ to _______ Did spouse have headaches? Yes No
3rd marriage age _____ to _______ Did spouse have headaches? Yes No

Age of current spouse: _53_

List ages and sex of all children:

Age _31_ Sex _M_ Headaches? Yes No
Age _29_ Sex _F_ Headaches? Yes No
Age _28_ Sex _F_ Headaches? Yes No
Age _27_ Sex _F_ Headaches? Yes No
Age _____ Sex _____ Headaches? Yes No

STRESS FACTORS:

List any factors that may be affecting your headaches (money, loneliness, sexual problems, work, etc.)
Work, normal everyday stress.

VEGETATIVE SIGNS:

1. Do you have trouble falling asleep? Yes No
2. Do you have trouble staying asleep? Yes No
3. Has your appetite decreased? Yes No
4. Have you gained or lost weight in the past year? Yes No
5. Have you felt tearful or depressed lately? Yes No
6. Have you had any thoughts of wanting to die? Yes No
7. Have you been forgetful lately? Yes No
8. Any other changes in your normal day-to-day living?__________

Please list any medications you are allergic or sensitive to: Codeine

Please list any medications you are currently taking (including dosages and frequency per day):
Darvocet, 2 times daily. Halcion, 1 each night.

PREVIOUS CARE:

1. List doctors who have treated you for headaches: Dr. G. Dr. B.

2. List any tests you have had for your headache (e.g., EEG, CT scan, MRI, X-Ray, etc.):
CAT scan – Approximately 2 years ago (normal).

3. List any other treatment you have had for your headache (e.g., biofeedback, acupuncture, chiropractic, or any other treatment you had):
Chiropractic.

JUDY
Category: Daily chronic headache

A 49-year-old woman came in with incapacitating headaches. She said they started when she was 28. At first they occurred infrequently, perhaps two times a month, and over the years they began to occur more frequently and perhaps they have developed for many years, now occurring every day. She said she wakes up with a headache and it is present all day. The majority of the time it is in the right side of her head, either in the temporal area or more recently occurring in the back of the neck area, and then she goes to bed. There are no other associated features. It seems that when she has these headaches, bright lights and noises bother her. She has seen multiple doctors in the past, including family practitioners, neurologists, and is currently under the care of a psychiatrist. She had a CT scan of the brain 15 years before, an MRI of the brain performed 7 years ago, that according to the patient showed a "mild stroke." She has been treated with biofeedback and chiropractic treatment, with no help.

Her medical and neurological examinations were negative. The diagnosis here would be daily chronic headache. The subcategory might be mixed headache (migraine and muscle contraction).

One concern is that with the use of very strong analgesic medication, over the years one has to consider the possibility of rebound headache and attempts would be made to decrease and eliminate those medications to see if the frequency of her headaches and intensity decrease.

MEDICAL HEADACHE HISTORY

Name: Judy **Age:** 49 **Sex** F **Date:** 7/28/92

Date of Birth: 00/00/43 **Birthplace:** FL **Race:** W **Education:** 2 yrs. college

Occupation: Title Company Branch Manager **Accident:** N/A

Armed Services & Type of Discharge: N/A

PAST HISTORY:

1.	Did you have a normal birth?		Yes (underlined)	No
	a) forceps used?		Yes (underlined)	No
	b) cesarean section?		Yes	No (underlined)
2.	Did you have problems with bedwetting?		Yes	No (underlined)
	a) If yes, age bedwetting stopped		______	
3.	Were you car sick as a child (motion)?		Yes (underlined)	No
	a) If yes, how severe?	Slight (underlined)	Moderate	Severe
4.	Did you have unexplained abdominal cramps as a child?		Yes	No (underlined)
5.	Did you have any of the following illnesses in childhood?			
	a) meningitis		Yes	No (underlined)
	b) encephalitis		Yes	No (underlined)
	c) scarlet fever		Yes	No (underlined)
	d) rheumatic fever		Yes	No (underlined)
6.	Did you have any head injuries as a child?		Yes	No (underlined)
	a) If yes, please explain: ______			
7.	Were you treated for emotional illness as a child?		Yes	No (underlined)

HABITS:

8.	Do you drink alcohol?	Yes (underlined)	No
	a) If yes, what kind and how much? Very very rare		
	b) Does alcohol bring on or aggravate a headache?	Yes	No (underlined)
9.	Do you smoke?	Yes (underlined)	No
	a) If yes, how much? 1 pack a day		
	b) Does smoking or smoke-filled rooms cause or aggravate headaches?	Yes	No (underlined)
10.	Do you drink caffeinated beverages?	Yes (underlined)	No
	a) If yes, how much? 3 diet cokes a day		

MENSTRUAL HISTORY:

At what age did menses begin? 15 Were they regular or irregular? WNL
How were they related to your headache? N/A
Are you or were you ever on Birth Control Pills? Yes Did they affect your headache? No
Have you had a hysterectomy, partial or total, and why? '78 – partial; '81 – Oopherectomy (cysts)
Are you in menopause, and if yes, how long? No
Are you on hormones, and if yes, which ones? Premarin 0.625 mg every day

HEADACHE ASSESSMENT FORM

HA PROFILE	INCAPACITATING #3	INTERFERING #2	IRRITATING #1
ONSET (Years ago and frequency)	Age 28 – 2 per month	N/A	N/A
CURRENT FREQUENCY	Every day for 20 years without Vicodin	N/A	N/A
TIME OF ONSET	Awaken with	N/A	N/A
DURATION	All day	N/A	N/A
CHARACTER	Throbbing in temple; pressure in neck	N/A	N/A
PRODROME OR AURA	N/A	N/A	N/A
ASSOCIATING FEATURES	Nausea; Vomiting; Sensitivity to Light? Noise? Odors? Do you get pale or flush? Do your eyes or nose run? Does your nose get stuffy? Do the whites of your eyes get red? Does your eyelid droop? Do you pace, or go to bed?	Nausea; Vomiting; Sensitivity to Light? Noise? Odors? Do you get pale or flush? Do your eyes or nose run? Does your nose get stuffy? Do the whites of your eyes get red? Does your eyelid droop? Do you pace, or go to bed?	Nausea; Vomiting; Sensitivity to Light? Noise? Odors? Do you get pale or flush? Do your eyes or nose run? Does your nose get stuffy? Do the whites of your eyes get red? Does your eyelid droop? Do you pace, or go to bed?
PRECIPITATING OR AGGRAVATING FEATURES	N/A	N/A	N/A

LOCATION: Mark the location for each type of headache with a different color pen.

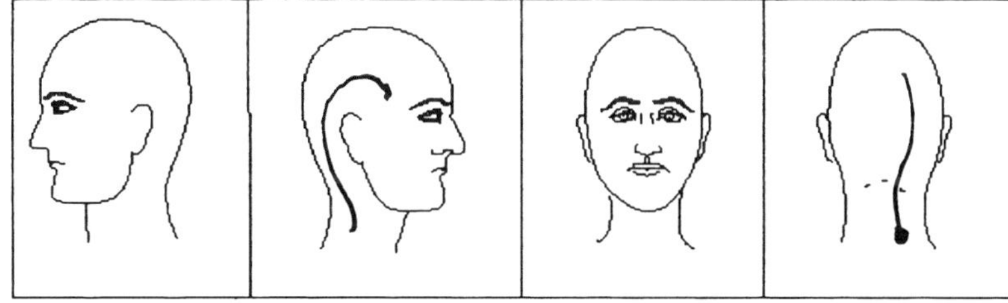

MEDICAL HISTORY:

Have you ever been or are you currently being treated for any of the following?

a) high blood pressure	Yes	No
b) stomach ulcers	Yes	No
c) asthma	Yes	No
d) allergies	Yes	No
e) pneumonia	Yes	No
f) kidney problems	Yes	No
g) low blood sugar	Yes	No
h) glaucoma	Yes	No
i) diabetes	Yes	No
j) heart problems	Yes	No

If you answered yes to any of the above, please describe: Asthma as a child (resolved). Environmental allergies. Pneumonia 5 years ago.

List all other medical problems you have had in the past. Include date diagnosed and treatment. DO NOT LIST OPERATIONS

Slight case of polio on right side 1946. Scarlatina 1948. Have had bronchitis off and on for last 7 years. Shingles 5 years ago right T12.

SURGICAL HISTORY (List operations and dates performed)

Saliva gland removed 1971. Tonsillectomy 1969. Hysterectomy (Partial) 1978; (Total) 1981.

PSYCHIATRIC HISTORY (List visits with counselors, psychologists, etc., and type of treatment)

Dr. B, psychologist, started 3 months ago for headaches.

ACCIDENTS IN ADULT LIFE (Briefly describe any accident that caused any blow to the head or that you feel is related to your headache)

N/A

FAMILY HISTORY:

1. Is your father living? Yes No
   Age 57
   Cause of death Suicide/cancer
   Was there a headache history? Yes No
2. Is your mother living? Yes No
   Age 71
   Cause of death
   Was there a headache history? Yes No

3. Ages of brothers---Circle the ones with headache
   45
4. Ages of sisters---Circle the ones with headache
   N/A
5. List any other blood relatives with a history of severe headaches.
   N/A

MARITAL HISTORY:
List marriages:

1st marriage age 18 to 28	Did spouse have headaches?	Yes	<u>No</u>
2nd marriage age 29 to Present	Did spouse have headaches?	Yes	<u>No</u>
3rd marriage age ____ to ____	Did spouse have headaches?	Yes	No

Age of current spouse: 50

List ages and sex of all children:

Age 27	Sex F	Headaches?	<u>Yes</u>	No
Age ____	Sex ____	Headaches?	Yes	No
Age ____	Sex ____	Headaches?	Yes	No

STRESS FACTORS:

List any factors that may be affecting your headaches (money, loneliness, sexual problems, work, etc.)

VEGETATIVE SIGNS:

1.	Do you have trouble falling asleep?	Yes	<u>No</u>
2.	Do you have trouble staying asleep?	Yes	<u>No</u>
3.	Has your appetite decreased?	Yes	<u>No</u>
4.	Have you gained or lost weight in the past year?	<u>Yes</u>	No
5.	Have you felt tearful or depressed lately?	<u>Yes</u>	No
6.	Have you had any thoughts of wanting to die?	Yes	<u>No</u>
7.	Have you been forgetful lately?	Yes	<u>No</u>
8.	Any other changes in your normal day-to-day living?		

Please list any medications you are allergic or sensitive to: Penicillin, most pain medications

Please list any medications you are currently taking (including dosages and frequency per day):
Premarin – 0.625 gm – 1q a day. Xanax – 0.50 – 2 a day. Sinequan, 150 mg – 1 a day.
Vicodin – 1 or 2 a day.

PREVIOUS CARE:

1. List doctors who have treated you for headaches: Dr. P, Dr. M, Dr. A, Dr. M, Dr. F, Dr. B, Dr. W, Dr. F.

2. List any tests you have had for your headache (e.g., EEG, CT scan, MRI, X-Ray, etc.):
CAT scan (15 years ago – normal); MRI (7 years ago), and x-rays.

3. List any other treatment you have had for your headache (e.g., biofeedback, acupuncture, chiropractic, or any other treatment you had):
Biofeedback (no help), Chiropractic (no help), and massage therapy.

AMY
Category: Daily chronic headache

This is a good example of how a patient develops into a chronic daily headache sufferer. Her headaches started seven years prior to my seeing her. They were occasional, and began to develop into a pattern where they became a daily type headache. What is unusual about this is that most of the muscle contraction headaches generally do not become incapacitating, and this patient claimed that about two times a week the pain is so bad that she has to go to bed. It is interesting that under incapacitating headaches she stated that a precipitating feature is sometimes her menstrual period, which makes one feel that there may be a vascular component. However, this patient does not have any of the typical symptoms of a migraine.

MEDICAL HEADACHE HISTORY

Name: Amy **Age:** 23 **Sex** F **Date:** 3/25/87

Date of Birth: 00/00/64 **Birthplace:** NJ **Race:** C **Education:** High school

Occupation: Catering Coordinator **Accident:** N/A

Armed Services & Type of Discharge: N/A

PAST HISTORY:

1.	Did you have a normal birth?		Yes	No
	a) forceps used?		Yes	No
	b) cesarean section?		Yes	No
2.	Did you have problems with bedwetting?		Yes	No
	a) If yes, age bedwetting stopped			
3.	Were you car sick as a child (motion)?		Yes	No
	a) If yes, how severe?	Slight	Moderate	Severe
4.	Did you have unexplained abdominal cramps as a child?		Yes	No
5.	Did you have any of the following illnesses in childhood?			
	a) meningitis		Yes	No
	b) encephalitis		Yes	No
	c) scarlet fever		Yes	No
	d) rheumatic fever		Yes	No
6.	Did you have any head injuries as a child?		Yes	No
	a) If yes, please explain:			
7.	Were you treated for emotional illness as a child?		Yes	No

HABITS:

8.	Do you drink alcohol?	Yes	No
	a) If yes, what kind and how much? Occasionally		
	b) Does alcohol bring on or aggravate a headache?	Yes	No
9.	Do you smoke?	Yes	No
	a) If yes, how much?		
	b) Does smoking or smoke-filled rooms cause or aggravate headaches?	Yes	No
10.	Do you drink caffeinated beverages?	Yes	No
	a) If yes, how much? One can coke daily		

MENSTRUAL HISTORY:

At what age did menses begin? 13 Were they regular or irregular? WNL

How were they related to your headache? #3 before menses

Are you or were you ever on Birth Control Pills? No Did they affect your headache? N/A

Have you had a hysterectomy, partial or total, and why? No

Are you in menopause, and if yes, how long? No

Are you on hormones, and if yes, which ones? No

HEADACHE ASSESSMENT FORM

HA PROFILE	INCAPACITATING #3	INTERFERING #2	IRRITATING #1
ONSET (Years ago and frequency)	7 years ago	7 years ago Every day	N/A
CURRENT FREQUENCY	2 times a week	Every day	N/A
TIME OF ONSET	Anytime	Anytime	N/A
DURATION	Hours	All day	N/A
CHARACTER	Sharp, dull ache	Sharp, dull ache	N/A
PRODROME OR AURA	N/A	N/A	N/A
ASSOCIATING FEATURES	Nausea; Vomiting; Sensitivity to Light? Noise? Odors? Do you get pale or flush? Do your eyes or nose run? Does your nose get stuffy? Does the white of your eyes get red? Does your eyelid droop? Do you pace, or go to bed?	Nausea; Vomiting; Sensitivity to Light? Noise? Odors? Do you get pale or flush? Do your eyes or nose run? Does your nose get stuffy? Does the white of your eyes get red? Does your eyelid droop? Do you pace, or go to bed?	Nausea; Vomiting; Sensitivity to Light? Noise? Odors? Do you get pale or flush? Do your eyes or nose run? Does your nose get stuffy? Does the white of your eyes get red? Does your eyelid droop? Do you pace, or go to bed?
PRECIPITATING OR AGGRAVATING FEATURES	Menses Left side of neck always knotted	N/A	N/A

LOCATION: Mark the location for each type of headache with a different color pen.

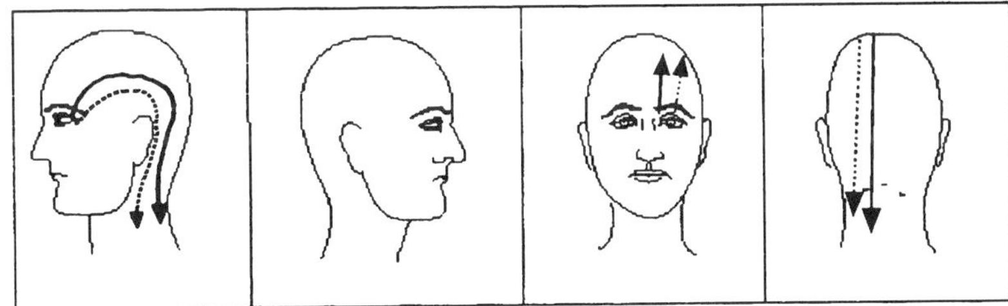

MEDICAL HISTORY:

Have you ever been or are you currently being treated for any of the following?

a) high blood pressure	Yes	No
b) stomach ulcers	Yes	No
c) asthma	Yes	No
d) allergies	Yes	No
e) pneumonia	Yes	No
f) kidney problems	Yes	No
g) low blood sugar	Yes	No
h) glaucoma	Yes	No
i) diabetes	Yes	No
j) heart problems	Yes	No

If you answered yes to any of the above, please describe:____________________

List all other medical problems you have had in the past. Include date diagnosed and treatment.
DO NOT LIST OPERATIONS

None.

SURGICAL HISTORY (List operations and dates performed)

None.

PSYCHIATRIC HISTORY (List visits with counselors, psychologists, etc., and type of treatment)

None.

ACCIDENTS IN ADULT LIFE (Briefly describe any accident that caused any blow to the head or that you feel is related to your headache)

Basketball injury – Hit head into bleachers. Not unconscious. No headache pattern.

FAMILY HISTORY:

1.	Is your father living?	Yes	No
	Age 51		
	Cause of death________________		
	Was there a headache history?	Yes	No
2.	Is your mother living?	Yes	No
	Age 51		
	Cause of death________________		
	Was there a headache history?	Yes	No
3.	Ages of brothers---Circle the ones with headache		

____

4. Ages of sisters---Circle the ones with headache
   ______27 25______
5. List any other blood relatives with a history of severe headaches.
   ______Maternal grandmother______

MARITAL HISTORY:

List marriages:

1st marriage age _____ to _______	Did spouse have headaches?	Yes	No
2nd marriage age _____ to _______	Did spouse have headaches?	Yes	No
3rd marriage age _____ to _______	Did spouse have headaches?	Yes	No

Age of current spouse:___________

List ages and sex of all children:

Age _____ Sex ______	Headaches?	Yes	No
Age _____ Sex ______	Headaches?	Yes	No
Age _____ Sex ______	Headaches?	Yes	No

STRESS FACTORS:

List any factors that may be affecting your headaches (money, loneliness, sexual problems, work, etc.)

____

____

VEGETATIVE SIGNS:

1.	Do you have trouble falling asleep?	Yes	No
2.	Do you have trouble staying asleep?	Yes	No
3.	Has your appetite decreased?	Yes	No
4.	Have you gained or lost weight in the past year?	Yes	No
5.	Have you felt tearful or depressed lately?	Yes	No
6.	Have you had any thoughts of wanting to die?	Yes	No
7.	Have you been forgetful lately?	Yes	No
8.	Any other changes in your normal day-to-day living?___________		

Please list any medications you are allergic or sensitive to: No known allergies

____

____

Please list any medications you are currently taking (including dosages and frequency per day):

____

____

PREVIOUS CARE:

1. List doctors who have treated you for headaches: Neurologist. Optometrist.

2. List any tests you have had for your headache (e.g., EEG, CT scan, MRI, X-Ray, etc.):
CAT scan – 1982. X-rays. Eye exam. Blood test.

3. List any other treatment you have had for your headache (e.g., biofeedback, acupuncture, chiropractic, or any other treatment you had):
Chiropractic.

KAREN
Category: Daily chronic headache

This 26-year-old woman came in with interfering (moderate to severe) and irritating (annoying) headaches. Her interfering headaches started two years ago. She was having two a week, and for the past three months she was having them daily. She awakens with them. They get worse as the day goes on. It is a constant pressure and squeezing sensation in the occipital portion of her head and the cervical region. There is no aura, and sometimes she will have sensitivity to light and noise, and will go to bed if possible.

She had irritating headaches (annoying as a child). They were rare. She was getting them twice a week before two years ago, and she would be able to abort them with over-the-counter medication. Now that she is having the interfering headaches, she no longer can identify the irritating headache.

She was hit on the head about two and a half years ago, but she does not feel this was related to her headache. Her physical examination and neurological examination were essentially negative. She is listed as a daily chronic headache patient. However, one would have to consider there might be some vascular features here and she will be treated with both a course for the muscle tension headache and also for the vascular headache.

MEDICAL HEADACHE HISTORY

Name: Karen **Age:** 26 **Sex** F **Date:** 8/12/92

Date of Birth: 00/00/66 **Birthplace:** D.C. **Race:** C **Education:** Dental Assist.

Occupation: Dental Assistant **Accident:** N/A

Armed Services & Type of Discharge: N/A

PAST HISTORY:

1.	Did you have a normal birth?		Yes	<u>No</u>
	a) forceps used?		Yes	<u>No</u>
	b) cesarean section?		Yes	<u>No</u>
2.	Did you have problems with bedwetting?		Yes	<u>No</u>
	a) If yes, age bedwetting stopped			
3.	Were you car sick as a child (motion)?		<u>Yes</u>	No
	a) If yes, how severe?	<u>Slight</u>	Moderate	Severe
4.	Did you have unexplained abdominal cramps as a child?		Yes	<u>No</u>
5.	Did you have any of the following illnesses in childhood?			
	a) meningitis		Yes	<u>No</u>
	b) encephalitis		Yes	<u>No</u>
	c) scarlet fever		Yes	<u>No</u>
	d) rheumatic fever		Yes	<u>No</u>
6.	Did you have any head injuries as a child?		Yes	<u>No</u>
	a) If yes, please explain:			
7.	Were you treated for emotional illness as a child?		<u>Yes</u>	No

HABITS:

8.	Do you drink alcohol?	<u>Yes</u>	No
	a) If yes, what kind and how much? Maybe 2 drinks a week		
	b) Does alcohol bring on or aggravate a headache?	Yes	<u>No</u>
9.	Do you smoke?	Yes	<u>No</u>
	a) If yes, how much?		
	b) Does smoking or smoke-filled rooms cause or aggravate headaches?	Yes	No
10.	Do you drink caffeinated beverages?	<u>Yes</u>	No
	a) If yes, how much? About 2 cups of coffee a day		

MENSTRUAL HISTORY:

At what age did menses begin? 11 Were they regular or irregular? WNL
How were they related to your headache? Increase headaches
Are you or were you ever on Birth Control Pills? Yes Did they affect your headache? N/A
Have you had a hysterectomy, partial or total, and why? No
Are you in menopause, and if yes, how long? No
Are you on hormones, and if yes, which ones? Yes, Estrogen & Progesterone (not taking now)

HA PROFILE	INCAPACITATING #3	INTERFERING #2	IRRITATING #1
ONSET (Years ago and frequency)	N/A	2 years ago, 2 per week	As a child, rare
CURRENT FREQUENCY	N/A	1-2/wk 'til 2 months ago, every day last 2 months	2/wk until 2 years ago
TIME OF ONSET	N/A	Awaken with, increases as day progresses	Anytime
DURATION	N/A	Constant	1 hour with OTC medication
CHARACTER	N/A	Constant pressure and squeezing	Dull ache
PRODROME OR AURA	N/A	N/A	N/A
ASSOCIATING FEATURES	Nausea; Vomiting; Sensitivity to Light? Noise? Odors? Do you get pale or flush? Do your eyes or nose run? Does your nose get stuffy? Does the white of your eyes get red? Does your eyelid droop? Do you pace, or go to bed?	Nausea; Vomiting; Sensitivity to Light? Noise? Odors? Do you get pale or flush? Do your eyes or nose run? Does your nose get stuffy? Does the white of your eyes get red? Does your eyelid droop? Do you pace, or go to bed?	Nausea; Vomiting; Sensitivity to Light? Noise? Odors? Do you get pale or flush? Do your eyes or nose run? Does your nose get stuffy? Does the white of your eyes get red? Does your eyelid droop? Do you pace, or go to bed?
PRECIPITATING OR AGGRAVATING FEATURES	N/A	Bending over	N/A

LOCATION: Mark the location for each type of headache with a different color pen.

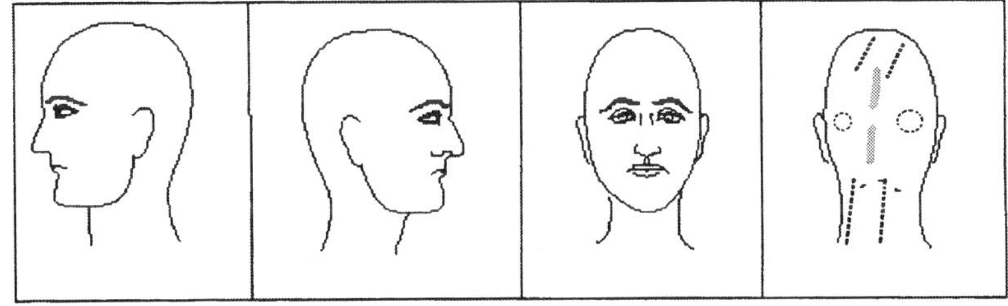

MEDICAL HISTORY:

Have you ever been or are you currently being treated for any of the following?

a) high blood pressure	Yes	No
b) stomach ulcers	Yes	No
c) asthma	Yes	No
d) allergies	Yes	No
e) pneumonia	Yes	No
f) kidney problems	Yes	No
g) low blood sugar	Yes	No
h) glaucoma	Yes	No
i) diabetes	Yes	No
j) heart problems	Yes	No

If you answered yes to any of the above, please describe:____________________

List all other medical problems you have had in the past. Include date diagnosed and treatment. DO NOT LIST OPERATIONS

Hormonal difficulties – treated about 2-1/2 years ago. Stress – currently being treated.

SURGICAL HISTORY (List operations and dates performed)

Surgery on wrist about 14 years ago.

PSYCHIATRIC HISTORY (List visits with counselors, psychologists, etc., and type of treatment)

Saw a psychologist when I was about 16.

ACCIDENTS IN ADULT LIFE (Briefly describe any accident that caused any blow to the head or that you feel is related to your headache)

I've gotten hit in the head and nose, 2-1/2 years ago. Not related to headache.

FAMILY HISTORY:

1.	Is your father living? I was adopted.	Yes	No
	Age________		
	Cause of death________________		
	Was there a headache history?	Yes	No
2.	Is your mother living?	Yes	No
	Age________		
	Cause of death________________		
	Was there a headache history?	Yes	No

3. Ages of brothers---Circle the ones with headache

____

4. Ages of sisters---Circle the ones with headache

____

5. List any other blood relatives with a history of severe headaches.

____

MARITAL HISTORY:

List marriages:

1st marriage age ______ to ______	Did spouse have headaches?	Yes	No
2nd marriage age ______ to ______	Did spouse have headaches?	Yes	No
3rd marriage age ______ to ______	Did spouse have headaches?	Yes	No

Age of current spouse:___________

List ages and sex of all children:

Age _____ Sex ______ Headaches?	Yes	No
Age _____ Sex ______ Headaches?	Yes	No
Age _____ Sex ______ Headaches?	Yes	No

STRESS FACTORS:

List any factors that may be affecting your headaches (money, loneliness, sexual problems, work, etc.)

Work

____

VEGETATIVE SIGNS:

1.	Do you have trouble falling asleep?		Yes	No (underlined)
2.	Do you have trouble staying asleep?	Sometimes	Yes	No
3.	Has your appetite decreased?		Yes (underlined)	No
4.	Have you gained or lost weight in the past year?		Yes (underlined)	No
5.	Have you felt tearful or depressed lately?	Sometimes	Yes	No
6.	Have you had any thoughts of wanting to die?		Yes	No (underlined)
7.	Have you been forgetful lately?		Yes	No (underlined)
8.	Any other changes in your normal day-to-day living?__________			

Please list any medications you are allergic or sensitive to: None

____

____

Please list any medications you are currently taking (including dosages and frequency per day):

BuSpar 5 mg 3 times a day. Erycette topical solution. Advil when needed. Sudafed, one to two times a day for congestion. Actifed for the same.

____

PREVIOUS CARE:

1. List doctors who have treated you for headaches: Dr. R

2. List any tests you have had for your headache (e.g., EEG, CT scan, MRI, X-Ray, etc.):
None.

3. List any other treatment you have had for your headache (e.g., biofeedback, acupuncture, chiropractic, or any other treatment you had):
None.

PATRICK
Category: Daily chronic headache

This is a 29-year-old man who came in suffering daily incapacitating headaches. He said they started at age 12, and then he had nothing until a year after he had some surgery for a hiatal hernia. He said he "felt something pop in his head" and from that point on he has been having these headache attacks. That was five years before he came into the clinic and one year after the surgery. He has these daily. He said these headaches last from three hours to all day. There is sharp, throbbing, ice pick-type pain. It is always in the left temporal region. There is no aura, and associated features are nausea, photophobia, sometimes flushing, redness of his conjunctivae, and he will go to bed.

His father has headaches, and so does a paternal aunt. He is taking Bancap HC every 6 hours and Zantac three times a day. Previous workup indicates that he has been on many of the anti-migraine and headache medications. He has had biofeedback, acupuncture, and chiropractic work, all of no help; CT scan, MRI, an EEG. These were all normal. The psychological test MMPI (Minnesota Multiphasic Personality Inventory) was given in the office and there were significantly increased scales in the area of psychophysiologic distress patterns. We were looking for a specific type of nerve block to see if we could break the pain and also see if we can stop some of the medications he is taking. In this case it is a question of whether this is a chronic daily headache secondary to all the medications he is taking, or whether there is a psychological factor here. At this point, the exact origin of these headaches is difficult to determine. After that visit, for some reason, the patient did not return; but, this is a demonstration of some of the difficulties in treating these daily chronic headaches.

MEDICAL HEADACHE HISTORY

Name: Patrick **Age:** 29 **Sex** M **Date:** 6/26/90

Date of Birth: 00/00/61 **Birthplace:** NYC **Race:** W **Education:** Comm. College

Occupation: Student **Accident:** N/A

Armed Services & Type of Discharge: 1979-82 – Navy. 1983-86 – Army.

PAST HISTORY:

1.	Did you have a normal birth?		Yes	No
	a) forceps used?		Yes	No
	b) cesarean section?		Yes	No
2.	Did you have problems with bedwetting?		Yes	No
	a) If yes, age bedwetting stopped			
3.	Were you car sick as a child (motion)?		Yes	No
	a) If yes, how severe?	Slight	Moderate	Severe
4.	Did you have unexplained abdominal cramps as a child?		Yes	No
5.	Did you have any of the following illnesses in childhood?			
	a) meningitis		Yes	No
	b) encephalitis		Yes	No
	c) scarlet fever		Yes	No
	d) rheumatic fever		Yes	No
6.	Did you have any head injuries as a child?		Yes	No
	a) If yes, please explain:			
7.	Were you treated for emotional illness as a child?		Yes	No

HABITS:

8.	Do you drink alcohol?	Yes	No
	a) If yes, what kind and how much?		
	b) Does alcohol bring on or aggravate a headache?	Yes	No
9.	Do you smoke?	Yes	No
	a) If yes, how much? 1 pack a day		
	b) Does smoking or smoke-filled rooms cause or aggravate headaches?	Yes	No
10.	Do you drink caffeinated beverages?	Yes	No
	a) If yes, how much? 2 liters per day		

MENSTRUAL HISTORY:

At what age did menses begin?_______ Were they regular or irregular?____________________

How were they related to your headache?____________________

Are you or were you ever on Birth Control Pills?______ Did they affect your headache? _______

Have you had a hysterectomy, partial or total, and why?____________________

Are you in menopause, and if yes, how long?____________________

Are you on hormones, and if yes, which ones?____________________

HEADACHE ASSESSMENT FORM

HA PROFILE	INCAPACITATING #3	INTERFERING #2	IRRITATING #1
ONSET (Years ago and frequency)	Age 12, then none until 1 year after surgery	N/A	N/A
CURRENT FREQUENCY	Every day	N/A	N/A
TIME OF ONSET	Awaken with	N/A	N/A
DURATION	3 hours to all day	N/A	N/A
CHARACTER	Sharp, throbbing, Ice pick	N/A	N/A
PRODROME OR AURA	N/A	N/A	N/A
ASSOCIATING FEATURES	Nausea; Vomiting; Sensitivity to Light? Noise? Odors? Do you get pale or flush? Do your eyes or nose run? Does your nose get stuffy? Does the white of your eyes get red? Does your eyelid droop? Do you pace, or go to bed?	Nausea; Vomiting; Sensitivity to Light? Noise? Odors? Do you get pale or flush? Do your eyes or nose run? Does your nose get stuffy? Does the white of your eyes get red? Does your eyelid droop? Do you pace, or go to bed?	Nausea; Vomiting; Sensitivity to Light? Noise? Odors? Do you get pale or flush? Do your eyes or nose run? Does your nose get stuffy? Does the white of your eyes get red? Does your eyelid droop? Do you pace, or go to bed?
PRECIPITATING OR AGGRAVATING FEATURES	Take Bencap every day for headache	N/A	N/A

LOCATION: Mark the location for each type of headache with a different color pen.

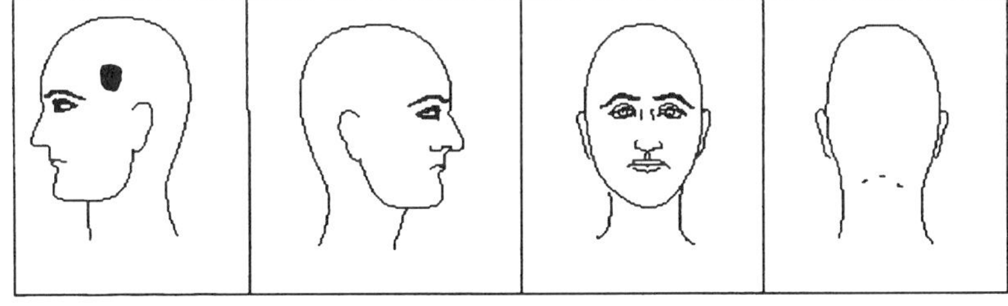

MEDICAL HISTORY:

Have you ever been or are you currently being treated for any of the following?

a) high blood pressure	Yes	No
b) stomach ulcers	Yes	No
c) asthma	Yes	No
d) allergies	Yes	No
e) pneumonia	Yes	No
f) kidney problems	Yes	No
g) low blood sugar	Yes	No
h) glaucoma	Yes	No
i) diabetes	Yes	No
j) heart problems	Yes	No

If you answered yes to any of the above, please describe: Ulcers diagnosed 8 months ago, on Zantac.

List all other medical problems you have had in the past. Include date diagnosed and treatment. DO NOT LIST OPERATIONS

Hiatal hernia w/reflux. Ulcer.

SURGICAL HISTORY (List operations and dates performed)

Hiatal hernia, April 1985.

PSYCHIATRIC HISTORY (List visits with counselors, psychologists, etc., and type of treatment)

Psychologist – Biofeedback for stress and medicine reduction.

ACCIDENTS IN ADULT LIFE (Briefly describe any accident that caused any blow to the head or that you feel is related to your headache)

FAMILY HISTORY:

1. Is your father living? Yes No
   Age 67
   Cause of death
   Was there a headache history? Yes No
2. Is your mother living? Yes No
   Age 58
   Cause of death
   Was there a headache history? Yes No

3. Ages of brothers---Circle the ones with headache
____
4. Ages of sisters---Circle the ones with headache
27
5. List any other blood relatives with a history of severe headaches.
Paternal aunt

MARITAL HISTORY:
List marriages:

1st marriage age 22 to 23	Did spouse have headaches?	Yes	No (underlined)
2nd marriage age 28 to Present	Did spouse have headaches?	Yes	No (underlined)
3rd marriage age ______ to ______	Did spouse have headaches?	Yes	No

Age of current spouse: 23

List ages and sex of all children:

Age _____ Sex ______ Headaches?	Yes	No
Age _____ Sex ______ Headaches?	Yes	No
Age _____ Sex ______ Headaches?	Yes	No
Age _____ Sex ______ Headaches?	Yes	No

STRESS FACTORS:

List any factors that may be affecting your headaches (money, loneliness, sexual problems, work, etc.)
____
____

VEGETATIVE SIGNS:

1.	Do you have trouble falling asleep?	Yes (underlined)	No
2.	Do you have trouble staying asleep?	Yes (underlined)	No
3.	Has your appetite decreased?	Yes	No (underlined)
4.	Have you gained or lost weight in the past year?	Yes	No (underlined)
5.	Have you felt tearful or depressed lately?	Yes	No (underlined)
6.	Have you had any thoughts of wanting to die?	Yes	No (underlined)
7.	Have you been forgetful lately?	Yes	No (underlined)
8.	Any other changes in your normal day-to-day living?______________		

Please list any medications you are allergic or sensitive to: None.
____
____

Please list any medications you are currently taking (including dosages and frequency per day):
Bencap H.C., 1 every 6 hours. Zantac, 1 three times a day.
____

PREVIOUS CARE:

1. List doctors who have treated you for headaches: Dr. G, Dr. M, VA doctors.

2. List any tests you have had for your headache (e.g., EEG, CT scan, MRI, X-Ray, etc.):

CAT scan 3 years ago (with and without contrast) – normal.

MRI 1 year ago – normal.

EEG 3 years ago – normal.

3. List any other treatment you have had for your headache (e.g., biofeedback, acupuncture, chiropractic, or any other treatment you had):

Biofeedback. Acupuncture. Chiropractor.

EDITH
Category: Daily chronic headaches

This is a good example of how a patient starts with periodic headaches and then these become a chronic headache problem.

Edith is a 40-year-old woman whose headaches started at age 20. They were occasional and the symptoms of her headache were similar to migraine and muscle tension type headache, which also appeared to be muscle contraction headaches, on occasion. Now 20 years later, her migraine attacks were about twice a year but she was having the daily interfering headaches. There was no success in her treatment.

This is a good reason why one should begin treatment early, when headaches start increasing, to prevent this chronic problem.

MEDICAL HEADACHE HISTORY

Name: Edith **Age:** 40 **Sex** F **Date:** 7/28/92

Date of Birth: 00/00/52 **Birthplace:** KY **Race:** C **Education:** High school

Occupation: Realtor **Accident:** N/A

Armed Services & Type of Discharge: N/A

PAST HISTORY:

1.	Did you have a normal birth?		<u>Yes</u>	No
	a) forceps used?		Yes	No
	b) cesarean section?		Yes	No
2.	Did you have problems with bedwetting?		Yes	<u>No</u>
	a) If yes, age bedwetting stopped		______	
3.	Were you car sick as a child (motion)?		<u>Yes</u>	No
	a) If yes, how severe?	Slight	<u>Moderate</u>	Severe
4.	Did you have unexplained abdominal cramps as a child?		<u>Yes</u>	No
5.	Did you have any of the following illnesses in childhood?			
	a) meningitis		Yes	<u>No</u>
	b) encephalitis		Yes	<u>No</u>
	c) scarlet fever		Yes	<u>No</u>
	d) rheumatic fever		Yes	<u>No</u>
6.	Did you have any head injuries as a child?		Yes	<u>No</u>
	a) If yes, please explain: ______			
7.	Were you treated for emotional illness as a child?		Yes	<u>No</u>

HABITS:

8.	Do you drink alcohol?	Yes	<u>No</u>
	a) If yes, what kind and how much? ______		
	b) Does alcohol bring on or aggravate a headache?	<u>Yes</u>	No
9.	Do you smoke?	Yes	<u>No</u>
	a) If yes, how much? ______		
	b) Does smoking or smoke-filled rooms cause or aggravate headaches?	Yes	<u>No</u>
10.	Do you drink caffeinated beverages?	<u>Yes</u>	No
	a) If yes, how much? One cup per daily		

MENSTRUAL HISTORY:

At what age did menses begin? 13 Were they regular or irregular? WNL

How were they related to your headache? ______

Are you or were you ever on Birth Control Pills? Yes Did they affect your headache? N/A

Have you had a hysterectomy, partial or total, and why? No

Are you in menopause, and if yes, how long? No

Are you on hormones, and if yes, which ones? No

HEADACHE ASSESSMENT FORM

HA PROFILE	INCAPACITATING #3	INTERFERING #2	IRRITATING #1
ONSET (Years ago and frequency)	Age 25, rare	Age 20 Occasionally	N/A
CURRENT FREQUENCY	2 times a year	Every day for years	N/A
TIME OF ONSET	Anytime	Awaken with	N/A
DURATION	1 day	Constant	N/A
CHARACTER	Severe sharp pressure	Pressure, throbs if bends over	N/A
PRODROME OR AURA	N/A	N/A	N/A
ASSOCIATING FEATURES	Nausea; Vomiting; Sensitivity to Light? Noise? Odors? Do you get pale or flush? Do your eyes or nose run? Does your nose get stuffy? Does the white of your eyes get red? Does your eyelid droop? Do you pace, or go to bed?	Nausea; Vomiting; Sensitivity to Light? Noise? Odors? Do you get pale or flush? Do your eyes or nose run? Does your nose get stuffy? Does the white of your eyes get red? Does your eyelid droop? Do you pace, or go to bed?	Nausea; Vomiting; Sensitivity to Light? Noise? Odors? Do you get pale or flush? Do your eyes or nose run? Does your nose get stuffy? Does the white of your eyes get red? Does your eyelid droop? Do you pace, or go to bed?
PRECIPITATING OR AGGRAVATING FEATURES	N/A	Bending over, clearing throat, sneezing, coughing	N/A

LOCATION: Mark the location for each type of headache with a different color pen.

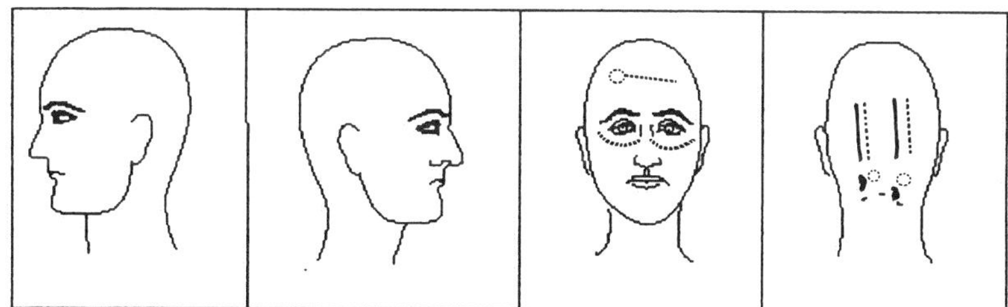

MEDICAL HISTORY:

Have you ever been or are you currently being treated for any of the following?

a) high blood pressure	Yes	No
b) stomach ulcers	Yes	No
c) asthma	Yes	No
d) allergies	Yes	No
e) pneumonia	Yes	No
f) kidney problems	Yes	No
g) low blood sugar	Yes	No
h) glaucoma	Yes	No
i) diabetes	Yes	No
j) heart problems	Yes	No

If you answered yes to any of the above, please describe:____________________

List all other medical problems you have had in the past. Include date diagnosed and treatment.
DO NOT LIST OPERATIONS

N/A

SURGICAL HISTORY (List operations and dates performed)

N/A

PSYCHIATRIC HISTORY (List visits with counselors, psychologists, etc., and type of treatment)

N/A

ACCIDENTS IN ADULT LIFE (Briefly describe any accident that caused any blow to the head or that you feel is related to your headache)

Car accident in 1969.

FAMILY HISTORY:

1. Is your father living? Yes No
   Age 69
   Cause of death____________________
   Was there a headache history? Yes No
2. Is your mother living? Yes No
   Age 61
   Cause of death____________________
   Was there a headache history? Yes No
3. Ages of brothers---Circle the ones with headache
   35 (45)

4. Ages of sisters---Circle the ones with headache
   N/A
5. List any other blood relatives with a history of severe headaches.
   Mother's sister

MARITAL HISTORY:

List marriages:

1st marriage age 17 to 25	Did spouse have headaches?	Yes	No
2nd marriage age 30 to Present	Did spouse have headaches?	Yes	No
3rd marriage age ______ to ______	Did spouse have headaches?	Yes	No

Age of current spouse: 35

List ages and sex of all children:

Age 23 Sex F	Headaches?	Yes	No
Age _____ Sex ______	Headaches?	Yes	No
Age _____ Sex ______	Headaches?	Yes	No

STRESS FACTORS:

List any factors that may be affecting your headaches (money, loneliness, sexual problems, work, etc.)
Mother living with me – terminal illness.

VEGETATIVE SIGNS:

1.	Do you have trouble falling asleep?	Yes	No
2.	Do you have trouble staying asleep?	Yes	No
3.	Has your appetite decreased?	Yes	No
4.	Have you gained or lost weight in the past year?	Yes	No
5.	Have you felt tearful or depressed lately?	Yes	No
6.	Have you had any thoughts of wanting to die?	Yes	No
7.	Have you been forgetful lately?	Yes	No
8.	Any other changes in your normal day-to-day living?________________		

Please list any medications you are allergic or sensitive to: No known allergies

Please list any medications you are currently taking (including dosages and frequency per day):
Fiorinal #3 when needed for pain (maybe one every other day).

PREVIOUS CARE:

1. List doctors who have treated you for headaches: Dr. C., Dr. J.

2. List any tests you have had for your headache (e.g., EEG, CT scan, MRI, X-Ray, etc.):
EEG, CAT scan (with and without contrast) – 1984 (normal). Head X-rays.

3. List any other treatment you have had for your headache (e.g., biofeedback, acupuncture, chiropractic, or any other treatment you had):
Chiropractic.

THELMA
Category: Daily chronic headache

This is a 70-year-old retired nurse, with interfering headaches (moderate to severe). These started at age 21. They were occasional until age 40 when they began to increase. In the last year she has been getting them on a daily basis. It can last anywhere from 2 hours to all day. It is a vice-like pain in the frontal region and posterocervical region. Again, this is another example where headaches begin periodically and develop as time goes on, and also someone in an older age group in which headaches become a daily symptom.

MEDICAL HEADACHE HISTORY

Name: Thelma **Age:** 70 **Sex** F **Date:** 10/28/91

Date of Birth: 00/00/20 **Birthplace:** NC **Race:** C **Education:** High school

Occupation: Retired **Accident:** N/A

Armed Services & Type of Discharge: N/A

PAST HISTORY:

1.	Did you have a normal birth?	?	Yes	No
	a) forceps used?		Yes	No
	b) cesarean section?		Yes	No
2.	Did you have problems with bedwetting?		Yes	No
	a) If yes, age bedwetting stopped			
3.	Were you car sick as a child (motion)?		Yes	No
	a) If yes, how severe?	Slight	Moderate	Severe
4.	Did you have unexplained abdominal cramps as a child?		Yes	No
5.	Did you have any of the following illnesses in childhood?			
	a) meningitis		Yes	No
	b) encephalitis		Yes	No
	c) scarlet fever		Yes	No
	d) rheumatic fever		Yes	No
6.	Did you have any head injuries as a child?		Yes	No
	a) If yes, please explain:			
7.	Were you treated for emotional illness as a child?		Yes	No

HABITS:

8.	Do you drink alcohol?	Yes	No
	a) If yes, what kind and how much?		
	b) Does alcohol bring on or aggravate a headache?	Yes	No
9.	Do you smoke?	Yes	No
	a) If yes, how much?		
	b) Does smoking or smoke-filled rooms cause or aggravate headaches?	Yes	No
10.	Do you drink caffeinated beverages?	Yes	No
	a) If yes, how much?		

MENSTRUAL HISTORY:

At what age did menses begin? 11 Were they regular or irregular? WNL
How were they related to your headache? N/A
Are you or were you ever on Birth Control Pills? No Did they affect your headache?
Have you had a hysterectomy, partial or total, and why? Yes, 1975, total. Hemorrhaging.
Are you in menopause, and if yes, how long? Age 51
Are you on hormones, and if yes, which ones? No

HEADACHE ASSESSMENT FORM

HA PROFILE	INCAPACITATING #3	INTERFERING #2	IRRITATING #1
ONSET (Years ago and frequency)	N/A	Age 21, occasionally until age 40. Increased in last year.	N/A
CURRENT FREQUENCY	N/A	Every day	N/A
TIME OF ONSET	N/A	Anytime	N/A
DURATION	N/A	2 hours to all day	N/A
CHARACTER	N/A	Vicelike	N/A
PRODROME OR AURA	N/A	N/A	N/A
ASSOCIATING FEATURES	Nausea; Vomiting; Sensitivity to Light? Noise? Odors? Do you get pale or flush? Do your eyes or nose run? Does your nose get stuffy? Does the white of your eyes get red? Does your eyelid droop? Do you pace, or go to bed?	Nausea; Vomiting; Sensitivity to Light? Noise? Odors? Do you get pale or flush? Do your eyes or nose run? Does your nose get stuffy? Does the white of your eyes get red? Does your eyelid droop? Do you pace, or go to bed?	Nausea; Vomiting; Sensitivity to Light? Noise? Odors? Do you get pale or flush? Do your eyes or nose run? Does your nose get stuffy? Does the white of your eyes get red? Does your eyelid droop? Do you pace, or go to bed?
PRECIPITATING OR AGGRAVATING FEATURES	N/A	Stress	N/A

LOCATION: Mark the location for each type of headache with a different color pen.

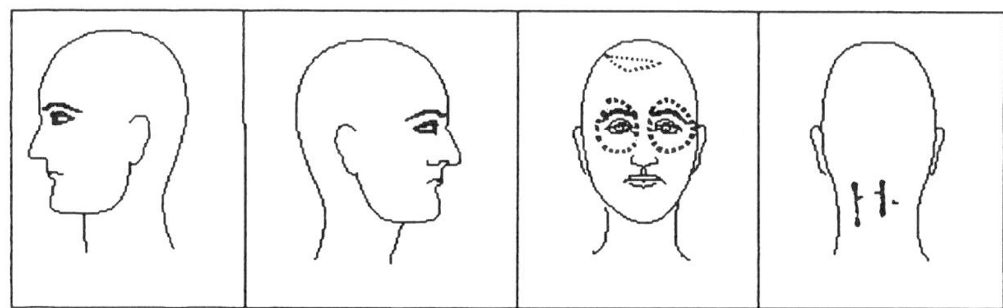

MEDICAL HISTORY:

Have you ever been or are you currently being treated for any of the following?

a) high blood pressure	Yes	No
b) stomach ulcers	Yes	No
c) asthma	Yes	No
d) allergies	Yes	No
e) pneumonia	Yes	No
f) kidney problems	Yes	No
g) low blood sugar	Yes	No
h) glaucoma	Yes	No
i) diabetes	Yes	No
j) heart problems	Yes	No

If you answered yes to any of the above, please describe: High blood pressure diagnosed 15 years ago, on medication. Pneumonia 3 years ago. Borderline diabetes, controlled with diet.

List all other medical problems you have had in the past. Include date diagnosed and treatment. DO NOT LIST OPERATIONS

SURGICAL HISTORY (List operations and dates performed)

Tonsils – 1930. Appendix – 1949. Cesarean – 1951. Hysterectomy – 1975. Gallbladder – 1977. Bladder suspension and repair – 1979.

PSYCHIATRIC HISTORY (List visits with counselors, psychologists, etc., and type of treatment)

Dr. T. Dr. G (depression). Electroshock therapy and analysis. Also Dr. S.

ACCIDENTS IN ADULT LIFE (Briefly describe any accident that caused any blow to the head or that you feel is related to your headache)

None

FAMILY HISTORY:

1. Is your father living? Yes No
   Age________
   Cause of death___Age 54, Heart___________________
   Was there a headache history? Yes No
2. Is your mother living? Yes No
   Age________
   Cause of death___Age 77, Parkinsons_______________
   Was there a headache history? Yes No
3. Ages of brothers---Circle the ones with headache
   ____64 (Deceased, no headaches)_________________
4. Ages of sisters---Circle the ones with headache
   ____None_______________________________________
5. List any other blood relatives with a history of severe headaches.
   ______Grandmother (maternal – Deceased at age 83)_________

MARITAL HISTORY:
List marriages:

1st marriage age _19_ to _22_	Did spouse have headaches?	Yes	No
2nd marriage age _24_ to _35_	Did spouse have headaches?	Yes	No
3rd marriage age _44_ to _Present_	Did spouse have headaches?	Yes	No
_________ age _____ to _______	______________________		

Age of current spouse:___63_________

List ages and sex of all children:

Age _49_ Sex _F_	Headaches?	Yes	No
Age _44_ Sex _F_	Headaches?	Yes	No
Age _39_ Sex _M_	Headaches?	Yes	No

STRESS FACTORS:

List any factors that may be affecting your headaches (money, loneliness, sexual problems, work, etc.)
___Money____
____

VEGETATIVE SIGNS:

1. Do you have trouble falling asleep? Yes No
2. Do you have trouble staying asleep? Yes No
3. Has your appetite decreased? Yes No
4. Have you gained or lost weight in the past year? Yes No
5. Have you felt tearful or depressed lately? Yes No
6. Have you had any thoughts of wanting to die? Yes No
7. Have you been forgetful lately? Yes No
8. Any other changes in your normal day-to-day living?________________________

Please list any medications you are allergic or sensitive to: Sulfa drugs (get hives and shortness of breath)

Please list any medications you are currently taking (including dosages and frequency per day):
Blood pressure medication, Pamelor, Ibuprofen, Restoril and Thorazine (small doses)

PREVIOUS CARE:

1. List doctors who have treated you for headaches: None

2. List any tests you have had for your headache (e.g., EEG, CT scan, MRI, X-Ray, etc.):
CAT scan – January 1990 (normal)

3. List any other treatment you have had for your headache (e.g., biofeedback, acupuncture, chiropractic, or any other treatment you had):
None

LEROY
Category: Daily chronic headaches

This is a 53-year-old man with interfering headaches (moderate to severe). These started in his twenties and he has had them daily since that time. It is a constant headache. He described it as a "vice-like pain" in the frontal part of his head and the superior nasal side, and also the occipital part of his head. He will go to bed if possible. He says that cold drinks or iced drinks make it worse.

Significant medical history is that he was diagnosed as having high blood pressure 20 years ago, and he is on medication for that problem. There is no headache history in his family. There is a daughter who has significant headaches. His neurological examination was normal, and he was diagnosed as

1. chronic muscle contraction headache,
2. rule out muscle contraction headache with atypical vascular features, and
3. rule out headaches caused by chronic hypertension.

He was treated with some medications for his headache, and also placed on biofeedback. Several months later he reported that there was a reduction in the intensity of his headaches, and the patient was referred to a blood pressure specialist in order to help him with that problem.

MEDICAL HEADACHE HISTORY

Name: Leroy **Age:** 53 **Sex** M **Date:** 2/20/92

Date of Birth: 00/00/38 **Birthplace:** SC **Race:** C **Education:** ____

Occupation: Retired **Accident:** N/A

Armed Services & Type of Discharge: 1956-1958 – Army.

PAST HISTORY:

1.	Did you have a normal birth?		Yes	No
	a) forceps used?		Yes	No
	b) cesarean section?		Yes	No
2.	Did you have problems with bedwetting?		Yes	No
	a) If yes, age bedwetting stopped		____	
3.	Were you car sick as a child (motion)?		Yes	No
	a) If yes, how severe?	Slight	Moderate	Severe
4.	Did you have unexplained abdominal cramps as a child?		Yes	No
5.	Did you have any of the following illnesses in childhood?			
	a) meningitis		Yes	No
	b) encephalitis		Yes	No
	c) scarlet fever		Yes	No
	d) rheumatic fever		Yes	No
6.	Did you have any head injuries as a child?		Yes	No
	a) If yes, please explain: ____			
7.	Were you treated for emotional illness as a child?		Yes	No

HABITS:

8.	Do you drink alcohol?	Yes	No
	a) If yes, what kind and how much? ____		
	b) Does alcohol bring on or aggravate a headache?	Yes	No
9.	Do you smoke?	Yes	No
	a) If yes, how much? ____		
	b) Does smoking or smoke-filled rooms cause or aggravate headaches?	Yes	No
10.	Do you drink caffeinated beverages?	Yes	No
	a) If yes, how much? 3 cups of coffee daily		

MENSTRUAL HISTORY:

At what age did menses begin? ____ Were they regular or irregular? ____

How were they related to your headache? ____

Are you or were you ever on Birth Control Pills? ____ Did they affect your headache? ____

Have you had a hysterectomy, partial or total, and why? ____

Are you in menopause, and if yes, how long? ____

Are you on hormones, and if yes, which ones? ____

HEADACHE ASSESSMENT FORM

HA PROFILE	INCAPACITATING #3	INTERFERING #2	IRRITATING #1
ONSET (Years ago and frequency)	N/A	In my 20's Daily	N/A
CURRENT FREQUENCY	N/A	Every day	N/A
TIME OF ONSET	N/A	Anytime	N/A
DURATION	N/A	Constant	N/A
CHARACTER	N/A	Vice-like	N/A
PRODROME OR AURA	N/A	N/A	N/A
ASSOCIATING FEATURES	Nausea; Vomiting; Sensitivity to Light? Noise? Odors? Do you get pale or flush? Do your eyes or nose run? Does your nose get stuffy? Do the whites of your eyes get red? Does your eyelid droop? Do you pace, or go to bed?	Nausea; Vomiting; Sensitivity to Light? Noise? Odors? Do you get pale or flush? Do your eyes or nose run? Does your nose get stuffy? Do the whites of your eyes get red? Does your eyelid droop? Do you pace, or go to bed?	Nausea; Vomiting; Sensitivity to Light? Noise? Odors? Do you get pale or flush? Do your eyes or nose run? Does your nose get stuffy? Do the whites of your eyes get red? Does your eyelid droop? Do you pace, or go to bed?
PRECIPITATING OR AGGRAVATING FEATURES	N/A	Cold drinks or ice cream	N/A

LOCATION: Mark the location for each type of headache with a different color pen.

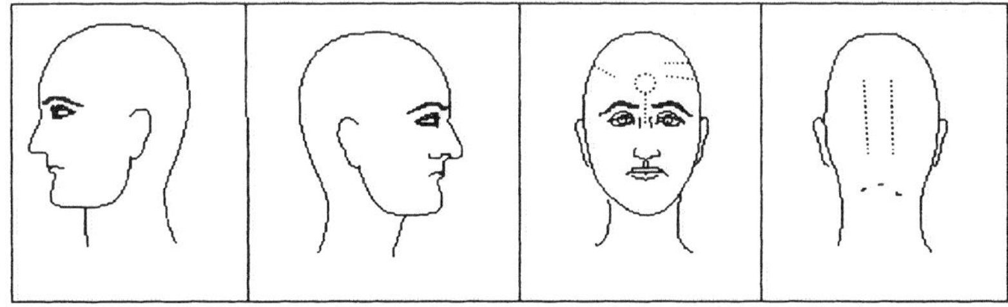

MEDICAL HISTORY:

Have you ever been or are you currently being treated for any of the following?

a) high blood pressure	Yes	No
b) stomach ulcers	Yes	No
c) asthma	Yes	No
d) allergies	Yes	No
e) pneumonia	Yes	No
f) kidney problems	Yes	No
g) low blood sugar	Yes	No
h) glaucoma	Yes	No
i) diabetes	Yes	No
j) heart problems	Yes	No

If you answered yes to any of the above, please describe: Diagnosed 20 years ago. On medication.

List all other medical problems you have had in the past. Include date diagnosed and treatment. DO NOT LIST OPERATIONS

Gout. Urinary infection.

SURGICAL HISTORY (List operations and dates performed)

Surgery for varicose veins, don't remember date. Hemorrhoids – 1989.

PSYCHIATRIC HISTORY (List visits with counselors, psychologists, etc., and type of treatment)

None

ACCIDENTS IN ADULT LIFE (Briefly describe any accident that caused any blow to the head or that you feel is related to your headache)

None

FAMILY HISTORY:

1.	Is your father living?	Yes	No
	Age		
	Cause of death Heart attack, age 38		
	Was there a headache history?	Yes	No
2.	Is your mother living?	Yes	No
	Age 73		
	Cause of death		
	Was there a headache history?	Yes	No

3. Ages of brothers---Circle the ones with headache
   56 55
4. Ages of sisters---Circle the ones with headache
   48
5. List any other blood relatives with a history of severe headaches.
   None

MARITAL HISTORY:
List marriages:

1st marriage age 23 to 37	Did spouse have headaches?	Yes	No
2nd marriage age 40 to Present	Did spouse have headaches?	Yes	No
3rd marriage age ____ to ____	Did spouse have headaches?	Yes	No

(Underlined answers: 1st marriage — Yes; 2nd marriage — No.)

Age of current spouse: 45

List ages and sex of all children:

Age 29 Sex F	Headaches?	Yes	No
Age ____ Sex ____	Headaches?	Yes	No
Age ____ Sex ____	Headaches?	Yes	No

(Underlined answer: first child — Yes.)

STRESS FACTORS:

List any factors that may be affecting your headaches (money, loneliness, sexual problems, work, etc.)
None

VEGETATIVE SIGNS:

1.	Do you have trouble falling asleep?	Yes	No
2.	Do you have trouble staying asleep?	Yes	No
3.	Has your appetite decreased?	Yes	No
4.	Have you gained or lost weight in the past year?	Yes	No
5.	Have you felt tearful or depressed lately?	Yes	No
6.	Have you had any thoughts of wanting to die?	Yes	No
7.	Have you been forgetful lately?	Yes	No
8.	Any other changes in your normal day-to-day living?____		

(Underlined answers: 1 — Yes; 2–7 — No.)

Please list any medications you are allergic or sensitive to:____

Please list any medications you are currently taking (including dosages and frequency per day):
Cardene, 30 mg 3 times a day. Hytran, 5 mg. 1 time a day. Limbitrol 12.5 mg 4 times per day.

PREVIOUS CARE:

1. List doctors who have treated you for headaches: Dr. S

2. List any tests you have had for your headache (e.g., EEG, CT scan, MRI, X-Ray, etc.):
CT scans – 2. Both normal.

3. List any other treatment you have had for your headache (e.g., biofeedback, acupuncture, chiropractic, or any other treatment you had):
None.

LEWIS
Category: Daily chronic headache

This is an 83-year-old man who was headache-free until eight months before seeing me. Interfering headaches (moderate to severe) started eight months before he saw me, and he found that he had them only when he was coughing, bending over, or straining. The pain lasted 30 minutes. It was a sharp and steady pain in the frontal and temporal regions. There is no aura, and no other associated features.

His medical history was essentially unrelated to his headaches and he stated that he had already had a CT scan, which was normal, and his neurological exam was normal. These headaches in elderly people that start all of a sudden are not uncommon in my practice. It is difficult to specify whether this is a muscle contraction headache or a nontypical vascular headache. Increased pressure seems to be a triggering mechanism for his headaches.

He did not respond to medications within a two-month period, and was sent for further testing to a neurological center to see if anything was missed that might have been precipitating intracranial pressure types of headaches.

MEDICAL HEADACHE HISTORY

Name: Lewis **Age:** 83 **Sex** M **Date:** 4/16/91

Date of Birth: 00/00/07 **Birthplace:** AZ **Race:** C **Education:**

Occupation: Retired **Accident:** N/A

Armed Services & Type of Discharge: 1941-1945 – Army; Army Reserves for 20 years

PAST HISTORY:

1.	Did you have a normal birth?		Yes	No
	a) forceps used?		Yes	No
	b) cesarean section?		Yes	No
2.	Did you have problems with bedwetting?		Yes	No
	a) If yes, age bedwetting stopped			
3.	Were you car sick as a child (motion)?		Yes	No
	a) If yes, how severe?	Slight	Moderate	Severe
4.	Did you have unexplained abdominal cramps as a child?		Yes	No
5.	Did you have any of the following illnesses in childhood?			
	a) meningitis		Yes	No
	b) encephalitis		Yes	No
	c) scarlet fever		Yes	No
	d) rheumatic fever		Yes	No
6.	Did you have any head injuries as a child?		Yes	No
	a) If yes, please explain:			
7.	Were you treated for emotional illness as a child?		Yes	No

HABITS:

8.	Do you drink alcohol?	Yes	No
	a) If yes, what kind and how much? 2 oz. per month on average		
	b) Does alcohol bring on or aggravate a headache?	Yes	No
9.	Do you smoke?	Yes	No
	a) If yes, how much?		
	b) Does smoking or smoke-filled rooms cause or aggravate headaches?	Yes	No
10.	Do you drink caffeinated beverages?	Yes	No
	a) If yes, how much? 1 glass of tea 5 times a week		

MENSTRUAL HISTORY:

At what age did menses begin?________ Were they regular or irregular?________
How were they related to your headache?________
Are you or were you ever on Birth Control Pills?______ Did they affect your headache? ________
Have you had a hysterectomy, partial or total, and why?________
Are you in menopause, and if yes, how long?________
Are you on hormones, and if yes, which ones?________

HEADACHE ASSESSMENT FORM

HA PROFILE	INCAPACITATING #3	INTERFERING #2	IRRITATING #1
ONSET (Years ago and frequency)	N/A	Nov. 1990, only when coughing, bending or straining	N/A
CURRENT FREQUENCY	N/A		N/A
TIME OF ONSET	N/A	Anytime	N/A
DURATION	N/A	10 to 30 minutes	N/A
CHARACTER	N/A	Sharp, steady intense pain	N/A
PRODROME OR AURA	N/A	N/A	N/A
ASSOCIATING FEATURES	Nausea; Vomiting; Sensitivity to Light? Noise? Odors? Do you get pale or flush? Do your eyes or nose run? Does your nose get stuffy? Do the whites of your eyes get red? Does your eyelid droop? Do you pace, or go to bed?	Nausea; Vomiting; Sensitivity to Light? Noise? Odors? Do you get pale or flush? Do your eyes or nose run? Does your nose get stuffy? Do the whites of your eyes get red? Does your eyelid droop? Do you pace, or go to bed?	Nausea; Vomiting; Sensitivity to Light? Noise? Odors? Do you get pale or flush? Do your eyes or nose run? Does your nose get stuffy? Do the whites of your eyes get red? Does your eyelid droop? Do you pace, or go to bed?
PRECIPITATING OR AGGRAVATING FEATURES	N/A	Coughing Bending Straining	N/A

LOCATION: Mark the location for each type of headache with a different color pen.

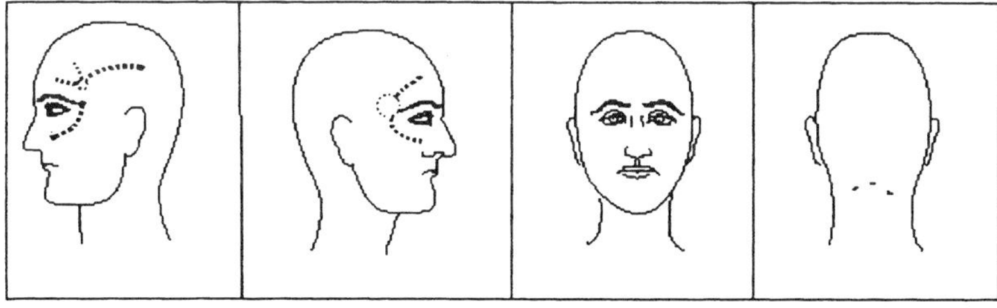

MEDICAL HISTORY:

Have you ever been or are you currently being treated for any of the following?

a) high blood pressure	Yes	No
b) stomach ulcers	Yes	No
c) asthma	Yes	No
d) allergies	Yes	No
e) pneumonia	Yes	No
f) kidney problems	Yes	No
g) low blood sugar	Yes	No
h) glaucoma	Yes	No
i) diabetes	Yes	No
j) heart problems	Yes	No

If you answered yes to any of the above, please describe: Ulcers diagnosed at age 30, but no problems in last 10 years. Arrhythmia 8 years ago. Thrombophlebitis in 1989.

List all other medical problems you have had in the past. Include date diagnosed and treatment. DO NOT LIST OPERATIONS

Possible Parkinsonism in right arm and hand.

SURGICAL HISTORY (List operations and dates performed)

Tonsillectomy in 1925. Appendectomy in 1939.

PSYCHIATRIC HISTORY (List visits with counselors, psychologists, etc., and type of treatment)

None

ACCIDENTS IN ADULT LIFE (Briefly describe any accident that caused any blow to the head or that you feel is related to your headache)

None

FAMILY HISTORY:

1. Is your father living? Yes No
   - Age________
   - Cause of death Leukemia
   - Was there a headache history? Yes No
2. Is your mother living? Yes No
   - Age________
   - Cause of death Tuberculosis, age 23
   - Was there a headache history? Yes No

3. Ages of brothers---Circle the ones with headache
   None
4. Ages of sisters---Circle the ones with headache
   None
5. List any other blood relatives with a history of severe headaches.
   Paternal grandfather

MARITAL HISTORY:
List marriages:

1st marriage age 28 to Present	Did spouse have headaches?	Yes	No
2nd marriage age ______to______	Did spouse have headaches?	Yes	No
3rd marriage age ______to______	Did spouse have headaches?	Yes	No

Age of current spouse: 84

List ages and sex of all children:

Age 53 Sex M	Headaches?	Yes	No
Age 50 Sex M	Headaches?	Yes	No
Age ______ Sex ______	Headaches?	Yes	No

STRESS FACTORS:

List any factors that may be affecting your headaches (money, loneliness, sexual problems, work, etc.)
None

VEGETATIVE SIGNS:

1.	Do you have trouble falling asleep?	Yes	No
2.	Do you have trouble staying asleep?	Yes	No
3.	Has your appetite decreased?	Yes	No
4.	Have you gained or lost weight in the past year?	Yes	No
5.	Have you felt tearful or depressed lately?	Yes	No
6.	Have you had any thoughts of wanting to die?	Yes	No
7.	Have you been forgetful lately?	Yes	No
8.	Any other changes in your normal day-to-day living?______		

Please list any medications you are allergic or sensitive to: Penicillin

Please list any medications you are currently taking (including dosages and frequency per day):
Lanoxin – 0.125 mg. 1 time per day; Phenobartital 30 mg. 3 times per day;
One enteric-coated aspirin per day Sometimes take Mylanta.

PREVIOUS CARE:

1. List doctors who have treated you for headaches: None

2. List any tests you have had for your headache (e.g., EEG, CT scan, MRI, X-Ray, etc.):
CT scan with contrast – normal.

3. List any other treatment you have had for your headache (e.g., biofeedback, acupuncture, chiropractic, or any other treatment you had):
None.

FRED
Category: Daily chronic headache

This patient provides an example of a headache that starts periodically and develops into a daily headache. Fred is a 48-year-old man who is self-employed and drives his own truck and is relatively healthy.

Interfering headaches (moderate to severe) started two years ago. He had them once a week. Currently, for the past year they have become daily. He awakens with them. The headache gets worse as the day goes on. The pain lasts all day. The pressure-type pain starts in the frontal temporal regions and works its way back to the occipital and cervical regions (back of the neck). He sometimes will go to bed because of the pain. This man is an example of a chronic muscle-tension headache, but could also be secondary to problems associated with the cervical facet joints. (See Chapter 14 on cervicogenic headaches.)

MEDICAL HEADACHE HISTORY

Name: Fred **Age:** 48 **Sex** M **Date:** 5/23/91

Date of Birth: 00/00/42 **Birthplace:** FL **Race:** C **Education:** High school

Occupation: Self employed truck driver **Accident:** N/A

Armed Services & Type of Discharge: 1960-1961 – Air Force – Medical Discharge

PAST HISTORY:

1.	Did you have a normal birth?		**Yes**	No
	a) forceps used?		Yes	**No**
	b) cesarean section?		Yes	**No**
2.	Did you have problems with bedwetting?		Yes	**No**
	a) If yes, age bedwetting stopped		______	
3.	Were you car sick as a child (motion)?		Yes	**No**
	a) If yes, how severe?	Slight	Moderate	Severe
4.	Did you have unexplained abdominal cramps as a child?		Yes	**No**
5.	Did you have any of the following illnesses in childhood?			
	a) meningitis		Yes	**No**
	b) encephalitis		Yes	**No**
	c) scarlet fever		Yes	**No**
	d) rheumatic fever		**Yes**	No
6.	Did you have any head injuries as a child?		Yes	**No**
	a) If yes, please explain: Rheumatic fever at age 5			
7.	Were you treated for emotional illness as a child?		Yes	**No**

HABITS:

8.	Do you drink alcohol?	Yes	**No**
	a) If yes, what kind and how much? ______		
	b) Does alcohol bring on or aggravate a headache?	Yes	**No**
9.	Do you smoke?	**Yes**	No
	a) If yes, how much? 2 packs a day		
	b) Does smoking or smoke-filled rooms cause or aggravate headaches?	Yes	**No**
10.	Do you drink caffeinated beverages?	**Yes**	No
	a) If yes, how much? Coke, tea, coffee – 1 quart a day		

MENSTRUAL HISTORY:

At what age did menses begin?______ Were they regular or irregular?______
How were they related to your headache?______
Are you or were you ever on Birth Control Pills?______ Did they affect your headache? ______
Have you had a hysterectomy, partial or total, and why?______
Are you in menopause, and if yes, how long?______
Are you on hormones, and if yes, which ones?______

HEADACHE ASSESSMENT FORM

HA PROFILE	INCAPACITATING #3	INTERFERING #2	IRRITATING #1
ONSET (Years ago and frequency)	N/A	2 years ago 1 per week	N/A
CURRENT FREQUENCY	N/A	Every day for 1 year	N/A
TIME OF ONSET	N/A	Awaken with	N/A
DURATION	N/A	All day	N/A
CHARACTER	N/A	Pressure	N/A
PRODROME OR AURA	N/A	N/A	N/A
ASSOCIATING FEATURES	Nausea; Vomiting; Sensitivity to Light? Noise? Odors? Do you get pale or flush? Do your eyes or nose run? Does your nose get stuffy? Does the white of your eyes get red? Does your eyelid droop? Do you pace, or go to bed?	Nausea; Vomiting; Sensitivity to Light? Noise? Odors? Do you get pale or flush? Do your eyes or nose run? Does your nose get stuffy? Does the white of your eyes get red? Does your eyelid droop? Do you pace, or <u>go to bed?</u>	Nausea; Vomiting; Sensitivity to Light? Noise? Odors? Do you get pale or flush? Do your eyes or nose run? Does your nose get stuffy? Does the white of your eyes get red? Does your eyelid droop? Do you pace, or go to bed?
PRECIPITATING OR AGGRAVATING FEATURES	N/A	N/A	N/A

LOCATION: Mark the location for each type of headache with a different color pen.

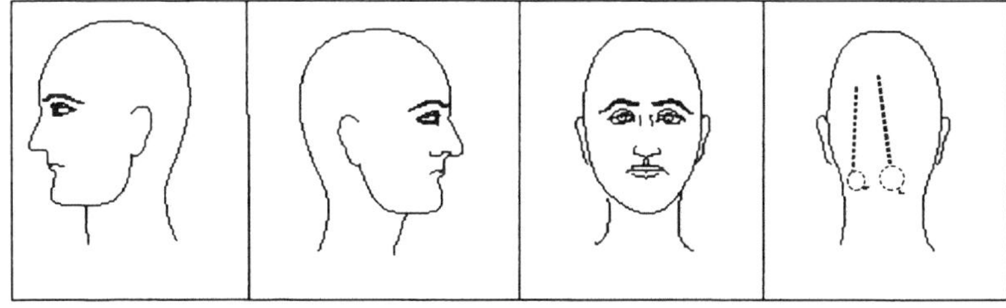

MEDICAL HISTORY:

Have you ever been or are you currently being treated for any of the following?

a) high blood pressure	Yes	No
b) stomach ulcers	Yes	No
c) asthma	Yes	No
d) allergies	Yes	No
e) pneumonia	Yes	No
f) kidney problems	Yes	No
g) low blood sugar	Yes	No
h) glaucoma	Yes	No
i) diabetes	Yes	No
j) heart problems	Yes	No

If you answered yes to any of the above, please describe:____________________________

List all other medical problems you have had in the past. Include date diagnosed and treatment.
DO NOT LIST OPERATIONS

None

SURGICAL HISTORY (List operations and dates performed)

None

PSYCHIATRIC HISTORY (List visits with counselors, psychologists, etc., and type of treatment)

None.

ACCIDENTS IN ADULT LIFE (Briefly describe any accident that caused any blow to the head or that you feel is related to your headache)

None.

FAMILY HISTORY:

1. Is your father living? Yes No
   Age________
   Cause of death Heart attack, age 72
   Was there a headache history? Yes No

2. Is your mother living? Yes No
   Age 77
   Cause of death ______
   Was there a headache history? Yes No
3. Ages of brothers---Circle the ones with headache
   None
4. Ages of sisters---Circle the ones with headache
   None
5. List any other blood relatives with a history of severe headaches.
   Paternal aunt

MARITAL HISTORY:

List marriages:

1st marriage age 25 to Present Did spouse have headaches? Yes No
2nd marriage age ______ to ______ Did spouse have headaches? Yes No
3rd marriage age ______ to ______ Did spouse have headaches? Yes No

Age of current spouse: 44

List ages and sex of all children:

Age 15 Sex F Headaches? Yes No
Age ______ Sex ______ Headaches? Yes No

STRESS FACTORS:

List any factors that may be affecting your headaches (money, loneliness, sexual problems, work, etc.)
None that I know of.

VEGETATIVE SIGNS:

1. Do you have trouble falling asleep? Yes No
2. Do you have trouble staying asleep? Yes No
3. Has your appetite decreased? Yes No
4. Have you gained or lost weight in the past year? Yes No
5. Have you felt tearful or depressed lately? Yes No
6. Have you had any thoughts of wanting to die? Yes No
7. Have you been forgetful lately? Yes No
8. Any other changes in your normal day-to-day living? ______

Please list any medications you are allergic or sensitive to: No known allergies

Please list any medications you are currently taking (including dosages and frequency per day):
Parafon Forte, as needed

PREVIOUS CARE:

1. List doctors who have treated you for headaches: Dr. C.

2. List any tests you have had for your headache (e.g., EEG, CT scan, MRI, X-Ray, etc.):
None

3. List any other treatment you have had for your headache (e.g., biofeedback, acupuncture, chiropractic, or any other treatment you had):
None

HOWARD
Category: Daily chronic headache

Howard is an 82-year-old man, and is an example of a senior citizen who appeared to be headache-free most of his life and then later on headaches seemed to start for some particular reason and become a chronic, daily problem.

Interfering headaches (moderate to severe) started three to four years ago, and the patient would get them several times a week. For the last year he has been experiencing them on a daily basis. The time of onset is one hour after arising, and the duration can be anywhere from two hours to all day. The character of the pain is a tight band which is located around the frontal portion of his head. There is no nausea, vomiting, photophobia, sonophobia, which are features of migraine.

Several months after treatment, the patient told me that he had had a CT scan which was normal. I recommended that he have an MRI of the brain to make sure there was no lesion that was causing this daily headache.

There is a question as to whether endorphins, our own antipain analgesics, may be reduced as we age and perhaps a latent headache problem will now arise because there is no mechanism to fight the pain. However, this is speculation as to why these headaches come on with elderly people, and it is not something that is uncommon.

Diagnosis: Chronic tension headache.

MEDICAL HEADACHE HISTORY

Name: Howard **Age:** 82 **Sex** M **Date:** 5/3/89

Date of Birth: 00/00/06 **Birthplace:** IN **Race:** C **Education:** High school

Occupation: Retired **Accident:** N/A

Armed Services & Type of Discharge: 1944-1945 – Navy – Honorable Discharge

PAST HISTORY:

1.	Did you have a normal birth?		Yes	No
	a) forceps used?		Yes	No
	b) cesarean section?		Yes	No
2.	Did you have problems with bedwetting?		Yes	No
	a) If yes, age bedwetting stopped		______	
3.	Were you car sick as a child (motion)?		Yes	No
	a) If yes, how severe?	Slight	Moderate	Severe
4.	Did you have unexplained abdominal cramps as a child?		Yes	No
5.	Did you have any of the following illnesses in childhood?			
	a) meningitis		Yes	No
	b) encephalitis		Yes	No
	c) scarlet fever		Yes	No
	d) rheumatic fever		Yes	No
6.	Did you have any head injuries as a child?		Yes	No
	a) If yes, please explain:______			
7.	Were you treated for emotional illness as a child?		Yes	No

HABITS:

8.	Do you drink alcohol?	Yes	No
	a) If yes, what kind and how much? 2 or 3 highballs each week		
	b) Does alcohol bring on or aggravate a headache?	Yes	No
9.	Do you smoke?	Yes	No
	a) If yes, how much?______		
	b) Does smoking or smoke-filled rooms cause or aggravate headaches?	Yes	No
10.	Do you drink caffeinated beverages?	Yes	No
	a) If yes, how much?______		

MENSTRUAL HISTORY:

At what age did menses begin?______ Were they regular or irregular?______
How were they related to your headache?______
Are you or were you ever on Birth Control Pills?______ Did they affect your headache? ______
Have you had a hysterectomy, partial or total, and why?______
Are you in menopause, and if yes, how long?______
Are you on hormones, and if yes, which ones?______

HEADACHE ASSESSMENT FORM

HA PROFILE	INCAPACITATING #3	INTERFERING #2	IRRITATING #1
ONSET (Years ago and frequency)	N/A	3 to 4 years ago 2 to 3 per week	N/A
CURRENT FREQUENCY	N/A	Every day for the last year	N/A
TIME OF ONSET	N/A	1 hour after arising	N/A
DURATION	N/A	2 hours to all day	N/A
CHARACTER	N/A	Tight band	N/A
PRODROME OR AURA	N/A	N/A	N/A
ASSOCIATING FEATURES	Nausea: Vomiting: Sensitivity to Light? Noise? Odors? Do you get pale or flush? Do your eyes or nose run? Does your nose get stuffy? Does the white of your eyes get red? Does your eyelid droop? Do you pace, or go to bed?	Nausea; Vomiting; Sensitivity to Light? Noise? Odors? Do you get pale or flush? Do your eyes or nose run? Does your nose get stuffy? Does the white of your eyes get red? Does your eyelid droop? Do you pace, or go to bed?	Nausea: Vomiting; Sensitivity to Light? Noise? Odors? Do you get pale or flush? Do your eyes or nose run? Does your nose get stuffy? Does the white of your eyes get red? Does your eyelid droop? Do you pace, or go to bed?
PRECIPITATING OR AGGRAVATING FEATURES	N/A	N/A	N/A

LOCATION: Mark the location for each type of headache with a different color pen.

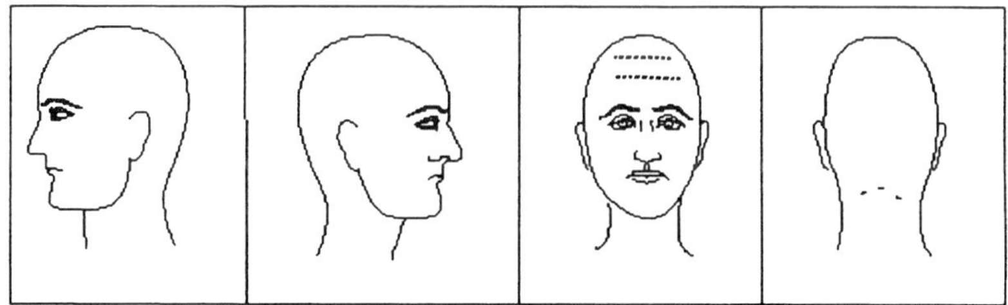

MEDICAL HISTORY:

Have you ever been or are you currently being treated for any of the following?

a) high blood pressure	<u>Yes</u>	No
b) stomach ulcers	<u>Yes</u>	No
c) asthma	Yes	<u>No</u>
d) allergies	<u>Yes</u>	No
e) pneumonia	Yes	<u>No</u>
f) kidney problems	Yes	<u>No</u>
g) low blood sugar	Yes	<u>No</u>
h) glaucoma	Yes	<u>No</u>
i) diabetes	Yes	<u>No</u>
j) heart problems	Yes	<u>No</u>

If you answered yes to any of the above, please describe: High blood pressure diagnosed in 1986, Take medication. Bleeding ulcers in 1963 and 1972; resolved. Environmental allergies.

List all other medical problems you have had in the past. Include date diagnosed and treatment. DO NOT LIST OPERATIONS

Duodenal ulcer, Nov. 1963, and Oct. 1982 (resolved). Heart valve dysfunction.

SURGICAL HISTORY (List operations and dates performed)

Appendectomy, Dec. 1947.
Large intestine removed, Dec. 1987 (diverticulosis).
Tonsillectomy & Adenoidectomy, 1930.
Cataract removal, right eye, Aug. 1987.

PSYCHIATRIC HISTORY (List visits with counselors, psychologists, etc., and type of treatment)

None.

ACCIDENTS IN ADULT LIFE (Briefly describe any accident that caused any blow to the head or that you feel is related to your headache)

None.

FAMILY HISTORY:

1. Is your father living? Yes No
   Age________
   Cause of death____Heart failure, age 70____________
   Was there a headache history? Yes No
2. Is your mother living? Yes No
   Age________
   Cause of death____Complications, age 82____________
   Was there a headache history? Yes No
3. Ages of brothers---Circle the ones with headache
   ______84______________________________
4. Ages of sisters---Circle the ones with headache
   ______84 (died)______________________________
5. List any other blood relatives with a history of severe headaches.
   ______None______________________________

MARITAL HISTORY:

List marriages:

1st marriage age __25__ to __30__	Did spouse have headaches?	Yes	No
2nd marriage age __31__ to Present	Did spouse have headaches?	Yes	No
3rd marriage age ______ to ______	Did spouse have headaches?	Yes	No

Age of current spouse:___76_______

List ages and sex of all children:

Age __49__ Sex __M__	Headaches?	Yes	No
Age ______ Sex ______	Headaches?	Yes	No

STRESS FACTORS:

List any factors that may be affecting your headaches (money, loneliness, sexual problems, work, etc.)

____

____

VEGETATIVE SIGNS:

1.	Do you have trouble falling asleep?	Yes	No
2.	Do you have trouble staying asleep?	Yes	No
3.	Has your appetite decreased?	Yes	No
4.	Have you gained or lost weight in the past year?	Yes	No
5.	Have you felt tearful or depressed lately?	Yes	No
6.	Have you had any thoughts of wanting to die?	Yes	No
7.	Have you been forgetful lately?	Yes	No
8.	Any other changes in your normal day-to-day living?______________		

Please list any medications you are allergic or sensitive to:___Sulfa______________

____

Please list any medications you are currently taking (including dosages and frequency per day):

Benadryl, 50 mg. Isocom. Capoten, 25 mg. every day. Zantac, 150 mg. Vitamin C.
Potassium. Lukinate, 550 mg. Nyacinamid, 100 mg. Organic zinc. Chelated iron.

PREVIOUS CARE:

1. List doctors who have treated you for headaches:

2. List any tests you have had for your headache (e.g., EEG, CT scan, MRI, X-Ray, etc.):

CT scan, without contrast (normal), 1982.

3. List any other treatment you have had for your headache (e.g., biofeedback, acupuncture, chiropractic, or any other treatment you had):

None

LUTHER
Category: Daily chronic headache

This is a 73-year-old man who has daily headaches. These are interfering headaches, which are moderate to severe. The pain is constant, and it is in the area around the eyes, the periorbital region, and the posterior occipital and cervical regions. The character of the pain is a dull ache. There are no other associated features.

He states that his headaches seemed to start after he was given medication for hypertension six months previous to coming into the office. Other significant history is that he had a stroke on the right side of his brain in 1989 and it left him with some minor disabilities on the left side of his body, but he did not have a headache as a result of this.

When I saw him, he was taking multiple medications for his medical problems and had been taking eight Tylenol a day for the past six months.

The diagnosis is a daily chronic headache, and this may be aggravated by taking too much pain medication, which may result in rebound headache. This could add to the headache problem. There are certain medications that are used to reduce blood pressure that can aggravate a headache; but, generally, when they are eliminated the headache will go in remission. As discussed with other cases, headaches starting in elderly people for some reason take on daily characteristics and they seem to be most difficult to treat because they don't seem to be very responsive to the usual medications that are often successful.

MEDICAL HEADACHE HISTORY

Name: Luther **Age:** 73 **Sex** M **Date:** 5/14/91

Date of Birth: 00/00/17 **Birthplace:** SC **Race:** C **Education:**________

Occupation: Retired **Accident:** N/A

Armed Services & Type of Discharge: 1942-1945 – Air Force – Honorable Discharge

PAST HISTORY:

1.	Did you have a normal birth?		Yes (underlined)	No
	a) forceps used?		Yes	No (underlined)
	b) cesarean section?		Yes	No (underlined)
2.	Did you have problems with bedwetting?		Yes	No (underlined)
	a) If yes, age bedwetting stopped		________	
3.	Were you car sick as a child (motion)?		Yes	No (underlined)
	a) If yes, how severe?	Slight	Moderate	Severe
4.	Did you have unexplained abdominal cramps as a child?		Yes	No (underlined)
5.	Did you have any of the following illnesses in childhood?			
	a) meningitis		Yes	No (underlined)
	b) encephalitis		Yes	No (underlined)
	c) scarlet fever		Yes	No (underlined)
	d) rheumatic fever		Yes	No (underlined)
6.	Did you have any head injuries as a child?		Yes	No (underlined)
	a) If yes, please explain: Rheumatic fever at age 5			
7.	Were you treated for emotional illness as a child?		Yes	No (underlined)

HABITS:

8.	Do you drink alcohol?		Yes	No (underlined)
	a) If yes, what kind and how much?________			
	b) Does alcohol bring on or aggravate a headache?		Yes	No (underlined)
9.	Do you smoke?		Yes	No (underlined)
	a) If yes, how much?________			
	b) Does smoking or smoke-filled rooms cause or aggravate headaches?		Yes	No (underlined)
10.	Do you drink caffeinated beverages?		Yes (underlined)	No
	a) If yes, how much? 1 coffee, 1 tea			

MENSTRUAL HISTORY:

At what age did menses begin?_______ Were they regular or irregular?________
How were they related to your headache?________
Are you or were you ever on Birth Control Pills?______ Did they affect your headache? _______
Have you had a hysterectomy, partial or total, and why?________
Are you in menopause, and if yes, how long?________
Are you on hormones, and if yes, which ones?________

HEADACHE ASSESSMENT FORM

HA PROFILE	INCAPACITATING #3	INTERFERING #2	IRRITATING #1
ONSET (Years ago and frequency)	N/A	1 day after taking meds for hypertension 6 months ago	N/A
CURRENT FREQUENCY	N/A	Every day	N/A
TIME OF ONSET	N/A	Awaken with, and increasing during day	N/A
DURATION	N/A	Constant	N/A
CHARACTER	N/A	Dull ache	N/A
PRODROME OR AURA	N/A	N/A	N/A
ASSOCIATING FEATURES	Nausea; Vomiting; Sensitivity to Light? Noise? Odors? Do you get pale or flush? Do your eyes or nose run? Does your nose get stuffy? Does the white of your eyes get red? Does your eyelid droop? Do you pace, or go to bed?	Nausea; Vomiting; Sensitivity to Light? Noise? Odors? Do you get pale or flush? Do your eyes or nose run? Does your nose get stuffy? Does the white of your eyes get red? Does your eyelid droop? Do you pace, or go to bed?	Nausea; Vomiting; Sensitivity to Light? Noise? Odors? Do you get pale or flush? Do your eyes or nose run? Does your nose get stuffy? Does the white of your eyes get red? Does your eyelid droop? Do you pace, or go to bed?
PRECIPITATING OR AGGRAVATING FEATURES	N/A	Stress	N/A

LOCATION: Mark the location for each type of headache with a different color pen.

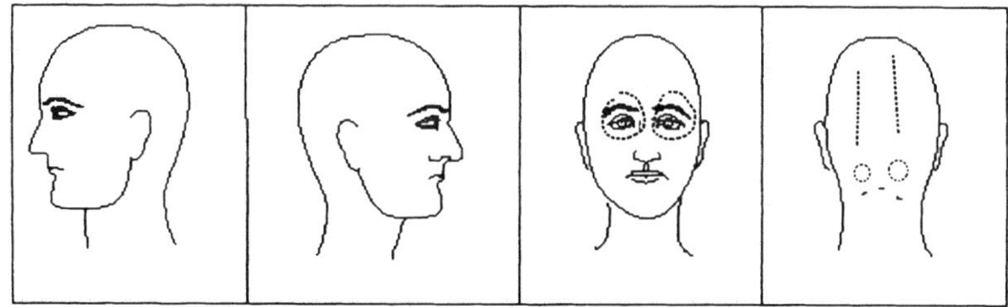

MEDICAL HISTORY:

Have you ever been or are you currently being treated for any of the following?

a) high blood pressure	**Yes**	No
b) stomach ulcers	Yes	**No**
c) asthma	Yes	**No**
d) allergies	Yes	**No**
e) pneumonia	Yes	**No**
f) kidney problems	Yes	**No**
g) low blood sugar	Yes	**No**
h) glaucoma	Yes	**No**
i) diabetes	Yes	**No**
j) heart problems	Yes	**No**

If you answered yes to any of the above, please describe: High blood pressure diagnosed 6 months ago, on medication.

List all other medical problems you have had in the past. Include date diagnosed and treatment. DO NOT LIST OPERATIONS

Stroke, left side of body (right side of brain) – 1989.

SURGICAL HISTORY (List operations and dates performed)

Stomach operation, 1960. Hernia operation, 1960. Prostate operation, 1982.

PSYCHIATRIC HISTORY (List visits with counselors, psychologists, etc., and type of treatment)

Psychiatrist, 1965. Biofeedback training, 1990.

ACCIDENTS IN ADULT LIFE (Briefly describe any accident that caused any blow to the head or that you feel is related to your headache)

Car ran into back of my car, 1985.

FAMILY HISTORY:

1.	Is your father living?	Yes	**No**
	Age______		
	Cause of death 75		
	Was there a headache history?	Yes	**No**
2.	Is your mother living?	Yes	**No**
	Age______		
	Cause of death 86, diabetes complications		
	Was there a headache history?	Yes	**No**

3. Ages of brothers---Circle the ones with headache
   None
4. Ages of sisters---Circle the ones with headache
   1 sister, died of brain tumor at age 28
5. List any other blood relatives with a history of severe headaches.
   None

MARITAL HISTORY:
List marriages:

1st marriage age 23 to Present	Did spouse have headaches?	Yes	No
2nd marriage age ______ to ______	Did spouse have headaches?	Yes	No
3rd marriage age ______ to ______	Did spouse have headaches?	Yes	No

Age of current spouse: 71

List ages and sex of all children:

Age 49 Sex F	Headaches?	Yes	No
Age 30 Sex F	Headaches?	Yes	No

STRESS FACTORS:

List any factors that may be affecting your headaches (money, loneliness, sexual problems, work, etc.)
Shin splints. Frustration over results of stroke. Inability to play tennis and to maintain yard and garden.

VEGETATIVE SIGNS:

1.	Do you have trouble falling asleep?	Yes	No
2.	Do you have trouble staying asleep?	Yes	No
3.	Has your appetite decreased?	Yes	No
4.	Have you gained or lost weight in the past year?	Yes	No
5.	Have you felt tearful or depressed lately?	Yes	No
6.	Have you had any thoughts of wanting to die?	Yes	No
7.	Have you been forgetful lately?	Yes	No
8.	Any other changes in your normal day-to-day living? ______		

Please list any medications you are allergic or sensitive to: Voltarin

Please list any medications you are currently taking (including dosages and frequency per day):
Desyrel, 50 mg. at bedtime. Lopressor, 50 mg. 1 a day. Feldene, 20 mg. 1 a day.
Tranxene, 3.75 mg., as needed. Tylenol, 6 to 8 per day.

PREVIOUS CARE:

1. List doctors who have treated you for headaches: Dr. T., Dr. P.

2. List any tests you have had for your headache (e.g., EEG, CT scan, MRI, X-Ray, etc.):
X-rays

3. List any other treatment you have had for your headache (e.g., biofeedback, acupuncture, chiropractic, or any other treatment you had):
Biofeedback.

THERESA
Category: Daily chronic headache

This 54-year-old woman came into the office with a rather interesting history. She was relatively headache-free all of her life until 6 months ago, and then she began getting headaches every day. They were constant with sharp, pressure-type pain, occasional throbbing, but mostly a dull and steady ache. It was moderate to severe every single day. The patient had had extensive workup by multiple physicians to rule out any medical or neurological problem, which was not found. After several attempts to help her as an outpatient, she was placed in the hospital and given intraveneous medication to treat what might have been an atypical vascular or migraine-type headache, which was only partially successful. She was discharged from the hospital with minimal relief. She was diagnosed with daily chronic tension headache.

Unfortunately, we sometimes see patients who will develop daily headaches later in life and they become extremely difficult to treat, primarily because the etiology of the headache is really not known. Sometimes they will go into their own remission, and sometimes will improve with medication or other types of therapy, but they are not predictable, and unfortunately for the patient, this turned out to be a very unpleasant course.

MEDICAL HEADACHE HISTORY

Name: Theresa **Age:** 54 **Sex** F **Date:** 8/6/91

Date of Birth: 00/00/37 **Birthplace:** FL **Race:** W **Education:** 11th grade

Occupation: Accounting **Accident:** N/A

Armed Services & Type of Discharge: N/A

PAST HISTORY:

1.	Did you have a normal birth?		Yes (underlined)	No
	a) forceps used?		Yes	No
	b) cesarean section?		Yes	No
2.	Did you have problems with bedwetting?		Yes	No (underlined)
	a) If yes, age bedwetting stopped			
3.	Were you car sick as a child (motion)?		Yes	No (underlined)
	a) If yes, how severe?	Slight	Moderate	Severe
4.	Did you have unexplained abdominal cramps as a child?		Yes	No (underlined)
5.	Did you have any of the following illnesses in childhood?			
	a) meningitis		Yes	No (underlined)
	b) encephalitis		Yes	No (underlined)
	c) scarlet fever		Yes	No (underlined)
	d) rheumatic fever		Yes	No (underlined)
6.	Did you have any head injuries as a child?		Yes	No (underlined)
	a) If yes, please explain:			
7.	Were you treated for emotional illness as a child?		Yes	No (underlined)

HABITS:

8.	Do you drink alcohol?		Yes (underlined)	No
	a) If yes, what kind and how much? 5 to 7 glasses of wine a week, but not since headaches			
	b) Does alcohol bring on or aggravate a headache?		Yes	No (underlined)
9.	Do you smoke?		Yes	No (underlined)
	a) If yes, how much?			
	b) Does smoking or smoke-filled rooms cause or aggravate headaches?		Yes ?	No
10.	Do you drink caffeinated beverages?		Yes (underlined)	No
	a) If yes, how much? 1 to 3 cups in morn			

MENSTRUAL HISTORY:

At what age did menses begin? 12 Were they regular or irregular? WNL
How were they related to your headache? N/A
Are you or were you ever on Birth Control Pills? No Did they affect your headache? N/A
Have you had a hysterectomy, partial or total, and why? '65, Partial. Fibroids
Are you in menopause, and if yes, how long?
Are you on hormones, and if yes, which ones? Premarin 0.9 mg every day

HEADACHE ASSESSMENT FORM

HA PROFILE	INCAPACITATING #3	INTERFERING #2	IRRITATING #1
ONSET (Years ago and frequency)	N/A	6 months ago Every day	N/A
CURRENT FREQUENCY	N/A	Every day	N/A
TIME OF ONSET	N/A	Constant	N/A
DURATION	N/A	Constant	N/A
CHARACTER	N/A	Pressure – sharp; occas. throb – dull steady ache	N/A
PRODROME OR AURA	N/A	N/A	N/A
ASSOCIATING FEATURES	Nausea; Vomiting; Sensitivity to Light? Noise? Odors? Do you get pale or flush? Do your eyes or nose run? Does your nose get stuffy? Do the whites of your eyes get red? Does your eyelid droop? Do you pace, or go to bed?	Nausea; Vomiting; Sensitivity to Light? Noise? Odors? Do you get pale or flush? Do your eyes or nose run? Does your nose get stuffy? Do the whites of your eyes get red? Does your eyelid droop? Do you pace, or go to bed?	Nausea; Vomiting; Sensitivity to Light? Noise? Odors? Do you get pale or flush? Do your eyes or nose run? Does your nose get stuffy? Do the whites of your eyes get red? Does your eyelid droop? Do you pace, or go to bed?
PRECIPITATING OR AGGRAVATING FEATURES	N/A	Laughing, sneezing	N/A

LOCATION: Mark the location for each type of headache with a different color pen.

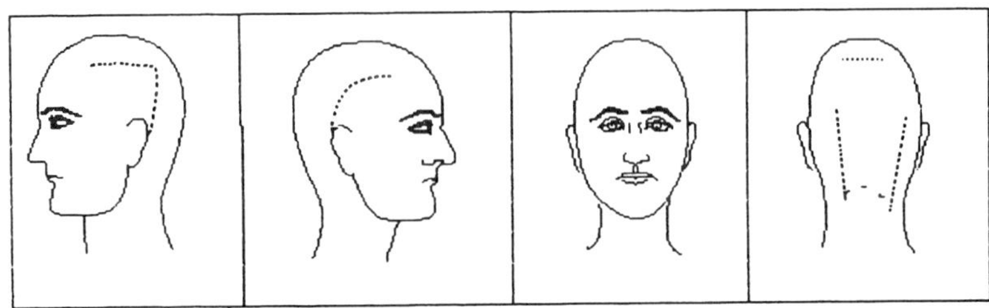

MEDICAL HISTORY:

Have you ever been or are you currently being treated for any of the following?

a) high blood pressure	Yes	No
b) stomach ulcers	Yes	No
c) asthma	Yes	No
d) allergies	Yes	No
e) pneumonia	Yes	No
f) kidney problems	Yes	No
g) low blood sugar	Yes	No
h) glaucoma	Yes	No
i) diabetes	Yes	No
j) heart problems	Yes	No

If you answered yes to any of the above, please describe:____________________

____

List all other medical problems you have had in the past. Include date diagnosed and treatment.
DO NOT LIST OPERATIONS

Back problems about last 20 years.

____

SURGICAL HISTORY (List operations and dates performed)

Hysterectomy – June 1965 (Fibroids). Gallbladder – 1983. Cystocele – 1986.

Laser surgery (eyes) – 1990.

____

PSYCHIATRIC HISTORY (List visits with counselors, psychologists, etc., and type of treatment)

1 time after father's death.

____

ACCIDENTS IN ADULT LIFE (Briefly describe any accident that caused any blow to the head or that you feel is related to your headache)

None that I recall.

____

FAMILY HISTORY:

1.	Is your father living?	Yes	No
	Age________		
	Cause of death Heart – 75		
	Was there a headache history?	Yes	No
2.	Is your mother living?	Yes	No
	Age 72		
	Cause of death________		
	Was there a headache history?	Yes	No

3. Ages of brothers---Circle the ones with headache
56 51 48 40
4. Ages of sisters---Circle the ones with headache
None
5. List any other blood relatives with a history of severe headaches.
None

MARITAL HISTORY:
List marriages:

1st marriage age 16 to 21	Did spouse have headaches?	Yes (underlined)	No
2nd marriage age 22 to 36	Did spouse have headaches?	Yes	No (underlined)
3rd marriage age ____ to ____	Did spouse have headaches?	Yes	No

Age of current spouse:__________

List ages and sex of all children:

Age 34 Sex F Headaches?	Yes	No (underlined)
Age 37 Sex F Headaches?	Yes (underlined)	No
Age ____ Sex ____ Headaches?	Yes	No

STRESS FACTORS:

List any factors that may be affecting your headaches (money, loneliness, sexual problems, work, etc.)
Money, work problems

VEGETATIVE SIGNS:

1.	Do you have trouble falling asleep?	Yes	No (underlined)
2.	Do you have trouble staying asleep?	Yes	No (underlined)
3.	Has your appetite decreased?	Yes	No (underlined)
4.	Have you gained or lost weight in the past year?	Yes	No (underlined)
5.	Have you felt tearful or depressed lately?	Yes	No (underlined)
6.	Have you had any thoughts of wanting to die?	Yes	No (underlined)
7.	Have you been forgetful lately?	Yes	No (underlined)
8.	Any other changes in your normal day-to-day living?__________		

Please list any medications you are allergic or sensitive to: Penicillin - rash

Please list any medications you are currently taking (including dosages and frequency per day):
Premarin, 0.9 mg 1 time a day. Timoptic, 0.05% 2 times a day. Anexsia 7.5, 2-3 times a day.

PREVIOUS CARE:

1. List doctors who have treated you for headaches: Dr. M. Dr. O.

2. List any tests you have had for your headache (e.g., EEG, CT scan, MRI, X-Ray, etc.):
CAT scan 2 weeks ago (with and without contrast) – normal.

3. List any other treatment you have had for your headache (e.g., biofeedback, acupuncture, chiropractic, or any other treatment you had):
None.

NETTIE
Category: Daily chronic headache

This 36-year-old woman came in with what appears to have started as a migraine headache as a teenager, and increased both in frequency and intensity over the years. Then in her twenties the interfering headaches, or more severe headaches, started. They were occasional and have now become a daily occurrence. The migraine headache has the typical symptoms of being a throbbing-type headache with nausea, sensitivity to light and noise, etc., and she would have to go to bed; however, the daily headaches got to the point where the patient had become disabled.

In further history taking, information came that she had a past history of being abused significantly, and that a psychological component added now to this chronic headache problem. This patient would need treatment of both medications for migraine and biofeedback to help relax her, and also psychological treatment to help her cope with her past history that was adding to the continued daily headache problem.

After a year of treatment, her headaches were reduced significantly and she went back to community college and was attempting to become a productive individual, and seemed to be responding significantly to treatment.

MEDICAL HEADACHE HISTORY

Name: Nettie **Age:** 36 **Sex** F **Date:** 3/25/91

Date of Birth: 00/00/54 **Birthplace:** NY **Race:** H **Education:** High school

Occupation: Unemployed **Accident:** N/A

Armed Services & Type of Discharge: N/A

PAST HISTORY:

1.	Did you have a normal birth?		Yes	No
	a) forceps used?		Yes	No
	b) cesarean section?		Yes	No
2.	Did you have problems with bedwetting?		Yes	No
	a) If yes, age bedwetting stopped			
3.	Were you car sick as a child (motion)?		Yes	No
	a) If yes, how severe?	Slight	Moderate	Severe
4.	Did you have unexplained abdominal cramps as a child?		Yes	No
5.	Did you have any of the following illnesses in childhood?			
	a) meningitis		Yes	No
	b) encephalitis		Yes	No
	c) scarlet fever		Yes	No
	d) rheumatic fever		Yes	No
6.	Did you have any head injuries as a child?		Yes	No
	a) If yes, please explain:			
7.	Were you treated for emotional illness as a child?		Yes	No

HABITS:

8.	Do you drink alcohol?	Yes	No
	a) If yes, what kind and how much?		
	b) Does alcohol bring on or aggravate a headache?	Yes	No
9.	Do you smoke?	Yes	No
	a) If yes, how much? ½ pack a day		
	b) Does smoking or smoke-filled rooms cause or aggravate headaches?	Yes	No
10.	Do you drink caffeinated beverages?	Yes	No
	a) If yes, how much? Coffee, 4 or 5 cups		

MENSTRUAL HISTORY:

At what age did menses begin? 11 Were they regular or irregular? Severe cramps, edema
How were they related to your headache? Increase headaches
Are you or were you ever on Birth Control Pills? No Did they affect your headache? N/A
Have you had a hysterectomy, partial or total, and why? No
Are you in menopause, and if yes, how long? No
Are you on hormones, and if yes, which ones? No

HEADACHE ASSESSMENT FORM

HA PROFILE	INCAPACITATING #3	INTERFERING #2	IRRITATING #1
ONSET (Years ago and frequency)	Teenager, occasionally	In 20's, occasionally	N/A
CURRENT FREQUENCY	Increased 2 yrs. ago 1 to 2 wk now	Every day in the last few months	N/A
TIME OF ONSET	Anytime	Anytime	N/A
DURATION	1 day	All day	N/A
CHARACTER	Throbbing at temples "twisted feeling inside head"	Throbbing	N/A
PRODROME OR AURA	Scintillating scotomata blurred vision	N/A	N/A
ASSOCIATING FEATURES	Nausea; Vomiting; Sensitivity to Light? Noise? Odors? Do you get pale or flush? Do your eyes or nose run? Does your nose get stuffy? Does the white of your eyes get red? Does your eyelid droop? Do you pace, or go to bed?	Nausea; Vomiting; Sensitivity to Light? Noise? Odors? Do you get pale or flush? Do your eyes or nose run? Does your nose get stuffy? Does the white of your eyes get red? Does your eyelid droop? Do you pace, or go to bed?	Nausea; Vomiting; Sensitivity to Light? Noise? Odors? Do you get pale or flush? Do your eyes or nose run? Does your nose get stuffy? Does the white of your eyes get red? Does your eyelid droop? Do you pace, or go to bed?
PRECIPITATING OR AGGRAVATING FEATURES	Any movement	Coughing	N/A

LOCATION: Mark the location for each type of headache with a different color pen.

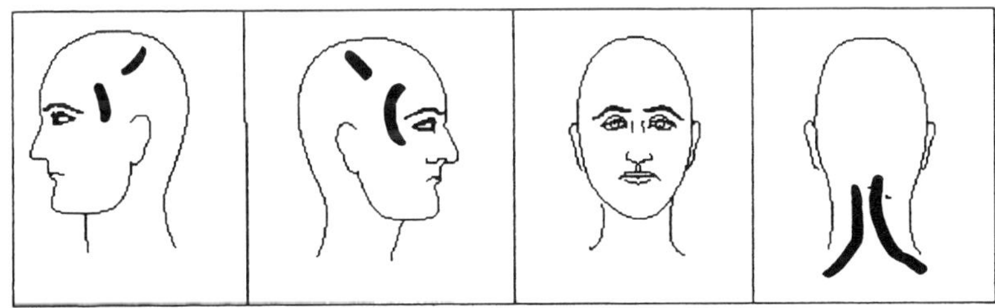

MEDICAL HISTORY:

Have you ever been or are you currently being treated for any of the following?

a) high blood pressure	Yes	No
b) stomach ulcers	Yes	No
c) asthma	Yes	No
d) allergies	Yes	No
e) pneumonia	Yes	No
f) kidney problems	Yes	No
g) low blood sugar	Yes	No
h) glaucoma	Yes	No
i) diabetes	Yes	No
j) heart problems	Yes	No

If you answered yes to any of the above, please describe: Asthma diagnosed as teenager. Allergies are environmental. Pneumonia as a child. Last kidney infection 1½ years ago.

List all other medical problems you have had in the past. Include date diagnosed and treatment. DO NOT LIST OPERATIONS

PMS a few years ago.

SURGICAL HISTORY (List operations and dates performed)

Cesarean sections – 1978, 1982. Cyst removed from right breast 16 years ago.
Tonsillectomy & Adenoidectomy – age 5.

PSYCHIATRIC HISTORY (List visits with counselors, psychologists, etc., and type of treatment)

Counselor for vocational.

ACCIDENTS IN ADULT LIFE (Briefly describe any accident that caused any blow to the head or that you feel is related to your headache)

Head injuries as a child, not related to headache.

FAMILY HISTORY:

1. Is your father living? I do not know my father — Yes No
   - Age________
   - Cause of death________
   - Was there a headache history? — Yes No
2. Is your mother living? — Yes No
   - Age 53
   - Cause of death________
   - Was there a headache history? Don't know — Yes No

3. Ages of brothers---Circle the ones with headache
   31
4. Ages of sisters---Circle the ones with headache
   29 20
5. List any other blood relatives with a history of severe headaches.
   None that I know of

MARITAL HISTORY:
List marriages:

1st marriage age 23 to 26	Did spouse have headaches?	Yes	No
2nd marriage age ______ to ______	Did spouse have headaches?	Yes	No
3rd marriage age ______ to ______	Did spouse have headaches?	Yes	No

Age of current spouse:___________

List ages and sex of all children:

Age 12 Sex M	Headaches?	Yes	<u>No</u>
Age 8 Sex M	Headaches?	Yes	<u>No</u>
Age _____ Sex ______	Headaches?	Yes	No

STRESS FACTORS:

List any factors that may be affecting your headaches (money, loneliness, sexual problems, work, etc.)

____

____

VEGETATIVE SIGNS:

1.	Do you have trouble falling asleep?	<u>Yes</u>	No
2.	Do you have trouble staying asleep?	<u>Yes</u>	No
3.	Has your appetite decreased?	Yes	<u>No</u>
4.	Have you gained or lost weight in the past year?	<u>Yes</u>	No
5.	Have you felt tearful or depressed lately?	Yes	<u>No</u>
6.	Have you had any thoughts of wanting to die?	Yes	<u>No</u>
7.	Have you been forgetful lately?	<u>Yes</u>	No
8.	Any other changes in your normal day-to-day living?________________		

Please list any medications you are allergic or sensitive to: None

____

Please list any medications you are currently taking (including dosages and frequency per day):
Motrin only when headaches appear.

____

PREVIOUS CARE:

1. List doctors who have treated you for headaches: Dr. C. Hospital emergency room.

2. List any tests you have had for your headache (e.g., EEG, CT scan, MRI, X-Ray, etc.):

CT scan – with and without contrast (normal).

3. List any other treatment you have had for your headache (e.g., biofeedback, acupuncture, chiropractic, or any other treatment you had):

None.

ANITA
Category: Daily chronic headache

This patient, a 50-year-old woman, started having moderate headaches at age 14, and they developed into daily headaches. Five years prior to seeing me, she began getting incapacitating headaches that seemed to have similar symptoms to migraine, but somewhat variant. The patient had taken medication, especially over-the-counter medication, for many years in an attempt to relieve her pain and this made a case in which the patient had developed rebound headaches, which is a result of taking too much pain medication.

Her diagnosis would be tension headache, possibly migraine without aura, or rebound headache secondary to too much medication.

MEDICAL HEADACHE HISTORY

Name: Anita **Age:** 50 **Sex** F **Date:** 11/16/89

Date of Birth: 00/00/39 **Birthplace:** MN **Race:** W **Education:** 1 yr. college

Occupation: Unemployed **Accident:** N/A

Armed Services & Type of Discharge: N/A

PAST HISTORY:

1.	Did you have a normal birth?		Yes (underlined)	No
	a) forceps used?		Yes	No (underlined)
	b) cesarean section?		Yes	No (underlined)
2.	Did you have problems with bedwetting?		Yes	No (underlined)
	a) If yes, age bedwetting stopped		______	
3.	Were you car sick as a child (motion)?		Yes (underlined)	No
	a) If yes, how severe?	Slight (underlined)	Moderate	Severe
4.	Did you have unexplained abdominal cramps as a child?		Yes	No (underlined)
5.	Did you have any of the following illnesses in childhood?			
	a) meningitis		Yes	No (underlined)
	b) encephalitis		Yes	No (underlined)
	c) scarlet fever		Yes	No (underlined)
	d) rheumatic fever		Yes	No (underlined)
6.	Did you have any head injuries as a child?		Yes	No (underlined)
	a) If yes, please explain: ______			
7.	Were you treated for emotional illness as a child?		Yes	No (underlined)

HABITS:

8.	Do you drink alcohol?	Yes	No (underlined)
	a) If yes, what kind and how much? ______		
	b) Does alcohol bring on or aggravate a headache?	Yes	No (underlined)
9.	Do you smoke?	Yes	No (underlined)
	a) If yes, how much? ______		
	b) Does smoking or smoke-filled rooms cause or aggravate headaches?	Yes (underlined)	No
10.	Do you drink caffeinated beverages?	Yes	No
	a) If yes, how much? ______		

MENSTRUAL HISTORY:

At what age did menses begin? 13 Were they regular or irregular? WNL

How were they related to your headache? N/A

Are you or were you ever on Birth Control Pills? Yes Did they affect your headache? No

Have you had a hysterectomy, partial or total, and why? '78 – Partial (Endometriosis)

Are you in menopause, and if yes, how long? No

Are you on hormones, and if yes, which ones? Premarin 0.625 mg Day 1-28 for osteoporosis

HEADACHE ASSESSMENT FORM

HA PROFILE	INCAPACITATING #3	INTERFERING #2	IRRITATING #1
ONSET (Years ago and frequency)	5 years ago 1per month	Age 14 3 per week	N/A
CURRENT FREQUENCY	None now since Inderal and Elavil	Every day	N/A
TIME OF ONSET	Anytime	Late p.m. or early evening	N/A
DURATION	3 days	1 hour with Fiorinal #3	N/A
CHARACTER	Steady vicelike	Same, less intense	N/A
PRODROME OR AURA	N/A	N/A	N/A
ASSOCIATING FEATURES	Nausea; Vomiting; Sensitivity to Light? Noise? Odors? Do you get pale or flush? Do your eyes or nose run? Does your nose get stuffy? Do the whites of your eyes get red? Does your eyelid droop? Do you pace, or go to bed?	Nausea; Vomiting; Sensitivity to Light? Noise? Odors? Do you get pale or flush? Do your eyes or nose run? Does your nose get stuffy? Do the whites of your eyes get red? Does your eyelid droop? Do you pace, or go to bed?	Nausea; Vomiting; Sensitivity to Light? Noise? Odors? Do you get pale or flush? Do your eyes or nose run? Does your nose get stuffy? Do the whites of your eyes get red? Does your eyelid droop? Do you pace, or go to bed?
PRECIPITATING OR AGGRAVATING FEATURES	Movement	Not eating Stress	N/A

LOCATION: Mark the location for each type of headache with a different color pen.

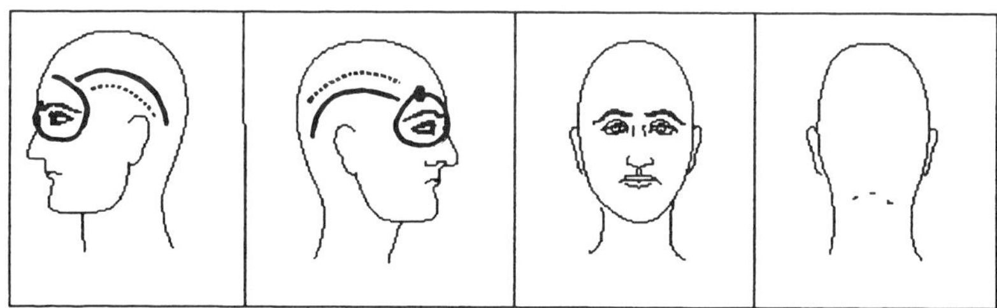

MEDICAL HISTORY:

Have you ever been or are you currently being treated for any of the following?

a) high blood pressure	Yes	<u>No</u>
b) stomach ulcers	Yes	<u>No</u>
c) asthma	Yes	<u>No</u>
d) allergies	<u>Yes</u>	No
e) pneumonia	Yes	<u>No</u>
f) kidney problems	Yes	<u>No</u>
g) low blood sugar	<u>Yes</u>	No
h) glaucoma	Yes	<u>No</u>
i) diabetes	Yes	<u>No</u>
j) heart problems	Yes	<u>No</u>

If you answered yes to any of the above, please describe: Environmental allergies. Low blood sugar diagnosed 10 years ago, controlled with diet.

List all other medical problems you have had in the past. Include date diagnosed and treatment.
DO NOT LIST OPERATIONS

Hypoglycemia diagnosed 10½ years ago, diet control.
Environmental illness and immune system – 3 years ago.

SURGICAL HISTORY (List operations and dates performed)

Sinus surgery 4 years ago. Partial hysterectomy 11 years ago. Cysts on ovaries and appendix removed 13 years ago. Benign lumps removed from breasts 18 years ago. Tonsillectomy 46 years ago.

PSYCHIATRIC HISTORY (List visits with counselors, psychologists, etc., and type of treatment)

None.

ACCIDENTS IN ADULT LIFE (Briefly describe any accident that caused any blow to the head or that you feel is related to your headache)

Slight whiplash 3 years ago.

FAMILY HISTORY:

1.	Is your father living?	Yes	<u>No</u>
	Age________		
	Cause of death Alzheimers, 75		
	Was there a headache history?	<u>Yes</u>	No
2.	Is your mother living?	<u>Yes</u>	No
	Age 77		
	Cause of death Has Parkinsons Disease		
	Was there a headache history?	<u>Yes</u>	No

3. Ages of brothers---Circle the ones with headache
   46 (44)
4. Ages of sisters---Circle the ones with headache
   N/A
5. List any other blood relatives with a history of severe headaches.
   N/A

MARITAL HISTORY:

List marriages:

1st marriage age 18 to 48	Did spouse have headaches?	Yes	No
2nd marriage age ____ to ____	Did spouse have headaches?	Yes	No
3rd marriage age ____ to ____	Did spouse have headaches?	Yes	No

Age of current spouse:__________

List ages and sex of all children:

Age 30	Sex M	Headaches?	Yes	No
Age 29	Sex M	Headaches?	Yes	No
Age 22	Sex M	Headaches?	Yes	No
Age 18	Sex M	Headaches?	Yes	No
Age ____	Sex ____	Headaches?	Yes	No

STRESS FACTORS:

List any factors that may be affecting your headaches (money, loneliness, sexual problems, work, etc.)

VEGETATIVE SIGNS:

1.	Do you have trouble falling asleep?	Yes	No
2.	Do you have trouble staying asleep?	Yes	No
3.	Has your appetite decreased?	Yes	No
4.	Have you gained or lost weight in the past year?	Yes	No
5.	Have you felt tearful or depressed lately?	Yes	No
6.	Have you had any thoughts of wanting to die?	Yes	No
7.	Have you been forgetful lately?	Yes	No
8.	Any other changes in your normal day-to-day living?__________		

Please list any medications you are allergic or sensitive to: Nystatin, Nyzerol

Please list any medications you are currently taking (including dosages and frequency per day):

Premarin – 0.625 mg - 28 days on, 5 days off. Amitriptyline 75 mg – 2 at bedtime.
Fiorinal #3 – 1 each 4 hours as needed. Inderal – 60 mg – 1 in afternoon; 120 mg – 1 each morning.
Prozac – 20 mg – 1 each a.m. Synthroid – 0.175 mg – 1 each a.m. Wigraine – 2 at onset of headache followed by 1 each half hour to 6 a day.

PREVIOUS CARE:

1. List doctors who have treated you for headaches: D.O., Arthritis Specialist, Osteopath, Neurologist, Nasal Surgeon, Environmental Illness Specialist.

2. List any tests you have had for your headache (e.g., EEG, CT scan, MRI, X-Ray, etc.):
CAT scan (2 years ago – "blocked sinuses").

3. List any other treatment you have had for your headache (e.g., biofeedback, acupuncture, chiropractic, or any other treatment you had):
Chiropractic (no help). Acupuncture (no help).

LYNN
Category: Daily chronic headache

This is a very good example of "rebound" headaches. This 33-year-old woman came in with the following history.

Incapacitating headaches: she states that she rarely had a migraine type of headache in the past. When she did, it was severe throbbing pain, and she had nausea, and was bothered by bright lights and loud noises. She had not had any for many years.

Interfering headaches (moderate to severe): These began approximately 5 to 6 years ago and occurred occasionally. Over the last six months, however, they have been present on a daily basis. They can awaken her. She has constant pain and has pressure and throbbing with it. It characteristically starts out both posteriorly, that is, in the back of her head, and then radiates to the front. There is nausea, and bright lights and loud noises bother her. She knows, however, that lying down makes the pain worse. It is not worsened by coughing or sneezing, and there is no visual loss, numbness or weakness.

Irritating headaches (annoying): These began in high school and occurred occasionally. They were occurring three times a week until six months ago, when the other headaches were so severe that she does not feel these headaches anymore. She said that she takes various over-the-counter analgesics to abort these headaches.

In taking the history, I found that she used 10 or 12 different types of over-the-counter medication, and she has been doing this for the last six months, and taking many pills that she does not recall each day. It appears that she is taking over 100 pain pills a week. This patient's neurological workup was negative and this type of problem is seen quite frequently when patients begin to take too much medication, and just the opposite happens — that is, the headaches get worse, instead of better. We diagnosed analgesic rebound headache, and under that would be chronic muscular contraction headache.

MEDICAL HEADACHE HISTORY

Name: Lynn **Age:** 33 **Sex** F **Date:** 7/28/92

Date of Birth: 00/00/58 **Birthplace:** WI **Race:** W **Education:** B.A.

Occupation: Homemaker **Accident:** N/A

Armed Services & Type of Discharge: N/A

PAST HISTORY:

1.	Did you have a normal birth?		Yes (underlined)	No
	a) forceps used?		Yes	No (underlined)
	b) cesarean section?		Yes	No (underlined)
2.	Did you have problems with bedwetting?		Yes	No (underlined)
	a) If yes, age bedwetting stopped		______	
3.	Were you car sick as a child (motion)?		Yes (underlined)	No
	a) If yes, how severe?	Slight	Moderate (underlined)	Severe
4.	Did you have unexplained abdominal cramps as a child?		Yes	No (underlined)
5.	Did you have any of the following illnesses in childhood?			
	a) meningitis		Yes	No (underlined)
	b) encephalitis		Yes	No (underlined)
	c) scarlet fever		Yes	No (underlined)
	d) rheumatic fever		Yes	No (underlined)
6.	Did you have any head injuries as a child?		Yes	No (underlined)
	a) If yes, please explain: ______			
7.	Were you treated for emotional illness as a child?		Yes	No (underlined)

HABITS:

8.	Do you drink alcohol?	Yes (underlined)	No
	a) If yes, what kind and how much? 1 drink every 2 to 4 weeks		
	b) Does alcohol bring on or aggravate a headache?	Yes	No (underlined)
9.	Do you smoke?	Yes	No (underlined)
	a) If yes, how much? ______		
	b) Does smoking or smoke-filled rooms cause or aggravate headaches?	Yes (underlined)	No
10.	Do you drink caffeinated beverages?	Yes (underlined)	No
	a) If yes, how much? One a day		

MENSTRUAL HISTORY:

At what age did menses begin? 16 Were they regular or irregular? WNL

How were they related to your headache? N/A

Are you or were you ever on Birth Control Pills? Yes Did they affect your headache? No

Have you had a hysterectomy, partial or total, and why? No

Are you in menopause, and if yes, how long? No

Are you on hormones, and if yes, which ones? No

HEADACHE ASSESSMENT FORM

HA PROFILE	INCAPACITATING #3	INTERFERING #2	IRRITATING #1
ONSET (Years ago and frequency)	N/A	5 to 6 years ago Occasionally	High school, occasionally
CURRENT FREQUENCY	N/A	Every day for 6 months	2 to 3 per week until 6 months ago
TIME OF ONSET	N/A	Awaken with	Anytime
DURATION	N/A	Constant	1 to 2 hours with OTC
CHARACTER	N/A	Pressure and throbbing	Same, but less intense
PRODROME OR AURA	N/A	N/A	N/A
ASSOCIATING FEATURES	Nausea; Vomiting; Sensitivity to Light? Noise? Odors? Do you get pale or flush? Do your eyes or nose run? Does your nose get stuffy? Does the white of your eyes get red? Does your eyelid droop? Do you pace, or go to bed?	Nausea; Vomiting; Sensitivity to Light? Noise? Odors? Do you get pale or flush? Do your eyes or nose run? Does your nose get stuffy? Does the white of your eyes get red? Does your eyelid droop? Do you pace, or go to bed?	Nausea; Vomiting; Sensitivity to Light? Noise? Odors? Do you get pale or flush? Do your eyes or nose run? Does your nose get stuffy? Does the white of your eyes get red? Does your eyelid droop? Do you pace, or go to bed?
PRECIPITATING OR AGGRAVATING FEATURES	N/A	Lying down	N/A

LOCATION: Mark the location for each type of headache with a different color pen.

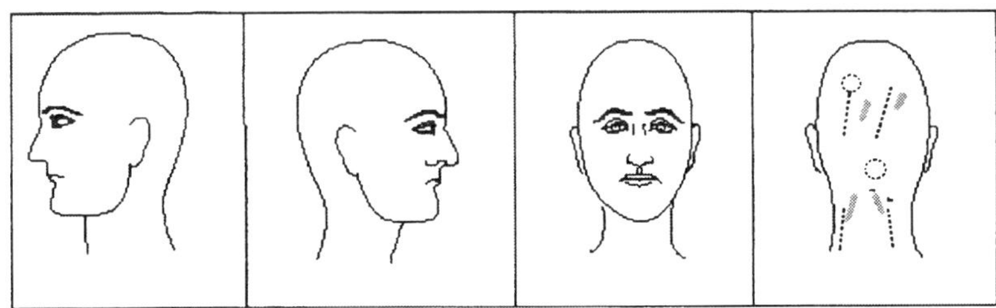

MEDICAL HISTORY:

Have you ever been or are you currently being treated for any of the following?

a) high blood pressure	Yes	<u>No</u>
b) stomach ulcers	Yes	<u>No</u>
c) asthma	<u>Yes</u>	No
d) allergies	<u>Yes</u>	No
e) pneumonia	Yes	<u>No</u>
f) kidney problems	Yes	<u>No</u>
g) low blood sugar	<u>Yes</u>	No
h) glaucoma	Yes	<u>No</u>
i) diabetes	Yes	<u>No</u>
j) heart problems	Yes	<u>No</u>

If you answered yes to any of the above, please describe: Asthma diagnosed a year ago. Environmental allergies. Low blood sugar diagnosed 1980, controlled with diet.

List all other medical problems you have had in the past. Include date diagnosed and treatment.
DO NOT LIST OPERATIONS

None.

SURGICAL HISTORY (List operations and dates performed)

Tonsillectomy, 1980. Cesarean, 1988.

PSYCHIATRIC HISTORY (List visits with counselors, psychologists, etc., and type of treatment)

None.

ACCIDENTS IN ADULT LIFE (Briefly describe any accident that caused any blow to the head or that you feel is related to your headache)

None.

FAMILY HISTORY:

1.	Is your father living?	Yes	<u>No</u>
	Age________		
	Cause of death Cancer		
	Was there a headache history?	Yes	<u>No</u>
2.	Is your mother living?	<u>Yes</u>	No
	Age 60		
	Cause of death________		
	Was there a headache history?	<u>Yes</u>	No
3.	Ages of brothers---Circle the ones with headache		
	35		

4. Ages of sisters---Circle the ones with headache
   (25)
5. List any other blood relatives with a history of severe headaches.
   None

MARITAL HISTORY:
List marriages:

1st marriage age 21 to Present	Did spouse have headaches?	Yes	No
2nd marriage age ____ to ____	Did spouse have headaches?	Yes	No
3rd marriage age ____ to ____	Did spouse have headaches?	Yes	No

Age of current spouse: 34

List ages and sex of all children:

Age 8	Sex F	Headaches?	Yes	No
Age 4	Sex F	Headaches?	Yes	No
Age 2	Sex F	Headaches?	Yes	No

STRESS FACTORS:

List any factors that may be affecting your headaches (money, loneliness, sexual problems, work, etc.)
Stress?

VEGETATIVE SIGNS:

1.	Do you have trouble falling asleep?	Yes	No
2.	Do you have trouble staying asleep?	Yes	No
3.	Has your appetite decreased?	Yes	No
4.	Have you gained or lost weight in the past year?	Yes	No
5.	Have you felt tearful or depressed lately?	Yes	No
6.	Have you had any thoughts of wanting to die?	Yes	No
7.	Have you been forgetful lately?	Yes	No
8.	Any other changes in your normal day-to-day living?		

Please list any medications you are allergic or sensitive to: Penicillin

Please list any medications you are currently taking (including dosages and frequency per day):
Allergy injections, 3 times a week. Over the counter medications – 10 to 12 a day.

PREVIOUS CARE:

1. List doctors who have treated you for headaches: None.

2. List any tests you have had for your headache (e.g., EEG, CT scan, MRI, X-Ray, etc.):
None.

3. List any other treatment you have had for your headache (e.g., biofeedback, acupuncture, chiropractic, or any other treatment you had):
None.

Chapter 8

Cluster Headache

In 1979 I was privileged to meet Dr. Lee Kudrow, who is internationally known for his work and writings on cluster headache. He was completing his book, *Cluster Headaches*, published by Oxford University Press, 1980, and he handed me an article he had just published in the journal *Headache*.[1,2] In that article he presents a description of a cluster attack he has experienced. I think that anyone who has suffered this type of attack will relate to his description of his own attack and how accurate a clinical picture is presented.

> Following a period of perhaps several hours, during which time I feel quite elated and energetic, I experience a fullness in my ears, somewhat more on the right than the left, having a character not unlike that which occurs during rapid descent in an airplane or elevator. I next become aware of a dull discomfort, an extension of ear fullness at the base of my skull — further extending over the entire head, on both sides, although more on the right. At this point two or three minutes have elapsed; seemingly short but long enough for me to know that indeed a 'cluster' has begun and will ultimately get worse. Such anticipation causes me considerable consternation regarding any decision to my activities or cancel plans and find a place to be alone; giving way to a slowly increasing anxiety, fear, panic, and withdrawal. I become aware of myself, 'listening' for changes in my head. Is the cluster prematurely aborting itself, progressing further, or unchanging? A sudden stab, only fleeting, strikes my temple, then again — somewhere near the apex of my skull and upper molars in my face — always on the right side. It strikes me again, deep into the skull base and as quickly, changes location to a small area above my eyebrow. My nose is stuffed yet runs simultaneously. If I could sneeze I feel the attack would end. But in spite of all the tricks I find myself unable to induce sneezing.
>
> While sharp stabs continue in this fashion, a slow crescendo of dull pain presents itself in an area of a hand's length and breadth over the eye and temporal region. The area of pain narrows into a smaller area but as if magnified, enlarges in intensity. I find my self bending my neck downward, though slightly, as if my head is being pushed from behind. My neck up to the base of my skull is tight and feels as if I were wearing a neck collar. I am compelled to remove my tie and loosen my shirt collar even though I know that it will not offer me even a modicum of relief.
>
> In an attempt to alter this persistent discomfort, I drop my head between my legs, while seated. My face and eyes seem to fill with fluid but the pain remains unchanged. In spite of my suntan, as I look into the mirror, a gaunt, sickly pale face appears back. My right lid is only slightly drooping and the white of my eye is charted with many red vessels, giving it an overall color of pink.
>
> Having difficulty standing in one place too long, I leave the mirror to continue my alternating pacing and sitting.

As usual, I am struck with the additional fear that the pain will never end, but dismiss it as impossible, since even if it were the case, I would surely kill myself.

The pain, now located somewhere behind my eye and slightly above, worsens. The pain is best described as a 'force' pushing with such incredible power through my eye that my head appears to be moving backward, yielding its resistance. The 'force' wanes and waxes, but the duration of successive exacerbations seems to increase. The cluster is at its peak, which is celebrated by an outpouring of tears from my right eye only. I have now been in cluster for 35 minutes — 10 minutes at its peak.

My wife peeks in the room in which I hold forth. I look up and see her expression of pity, frustration and helplessness. She sees my tortured face as I have seen it in the mirror at this stage before; a drooling mouth, agape, gray face wet on one side, an almost closed eyelid, and smelling of pain and anguish. She closes the door and leaves, feeling hurt for me, anger for the stupidity of medical science, and guilt — since deep within her mind is the suspicion that she is the cause of my suffering.

I cry for her, but more for myself. The pain is so incredible. Suddenly I am overwhelmed by a fury. I lift a chair high above my head and crash it to the floor. With doubled fist I strike the wall. The pain persists.

Waning periods soon become longer in duration and I allow myself to suspect that the peak is behind me — but cautiously, since I have been too often disappointed.

Indeed, the pain is ending. The descent from the mountain of pain is rapid. The 'force' is gone. Only the severe pain remains. My nose and eyes continue to run. The road back, as with all travels, covers the same territory — but faster. Stabbing, easily tolerated pain is felt. Then gone. Dull, aching fullness, neck stiffness — all disappear in turn, to be replaced by a welcome sensation of pins and needles over the right scalp area — not unlike after one's leg has been 'asleep.' Thus my head has awakened after a nightmare of torment.

Eye and nose dry, I let out a sigh. I collect my pile of wet tissues strewn all over the floor and deposit them in a wastepaper basket. The innocent chair now uprighted, I rub my slightly bruised fist. Thus, having ended the battle and cleaned up its field, I open the door and enter my pain-free world — until tomorrow.

Cluster headache was often under-diagnosed and misdiagnosed, although it is one of the most severe forms of head pain known to man. Fortunately, they are not a common problem following a flexion/extension type of injury and if they appear may resemble a cluster-like headache.

Cluster headache has been referred to by many other names: red migraine, erythroprosopalgia, erythromelalgia, sphenopalatine neuralgia, vidian neuralgia, ciliary neuralgia, periodic migrainous neuralgia, histaminic cephalgia, and Horton's disease.[3]

Although migraine is seen three to four times more often in women, cluster is seen five to eight times more often in men. It generally is seen beginning about age 20 and reduces or goes into its own remission in the fifth or sixth decade. However, it can certainly begin at any age and no one can predict that there is a certain age at which it will disappear. Mathew states in his article[3] that there have been reports of infants at age one who have had symptoms that appeared as cluster-like headaches.

Prior to the International Headache Society's classification in 1988, the classification of cluster headaches was as shown in Table 8.1. Table 8.2 shows the IHS classification.

Table 8.1 Early Classification

1. Episodic or periodic
2. Chronic
   - A. Primary
   - B. Secondary
   - C. Chronic paroxysmal hemicrania (CPH)
3. Atypical variant
   - A. Cluster–migraine
   - B. Cluster–vertigo

Table 8.2 International Headache Society Classification of Cluster Headache

3.1	Cluster headache		
	3.1.1	Cluster headache, periodicity undetermined	
	3.1.2	Episodic cluster headache	
	3.1.3	Chronic cluster headache	
		3.1.3.1	Chronic cluster headache unremitting from onset
		3.1.3.2	Chronic cluster headache evolved from episodic
3.2	Chronic paroxysmal hemicrania		
3.3	Cluster-like headache disorder not fulfilling above criteria		
	A.	Cluster tic syndrome	
	B.	Cluster-vertigo	
	C.	Cluster-migraine	
	D.	Following head trauma	
	E.	Following infection	
	F.	Associated with intracranial vascular and space-taking lesions	

CLINICAL FEATURES

Usually cluster patients will have their attacks once or twice a year. The periods of attack last about 2 to 3 months. The attacks usually occur during the night after the patient goes to sleep. However, as in most cases in medicine, nothing is fixed and attacks may occur at any time. The attacks seem more prevalent in the autumn or the spring. This changes if the pattern becomes chronic.

There is a great difference between cluster and migraine. There is no aura with cluster and there are no gastrointestinal symptoms like nausea and vomiting. The pain is not felt as throbbing and the cluster patient does not retire to a dark, quiet room in a prone position. The pain usually does not last longer than 2 to 3 hours.

The reason the term cluster is used is that these headaches come in groups several times a year and attacks may be from one to three attacks a day. The pain is usually from 45 minutes to $1^1/_2$ to 2 hours. The pain can be anywhere in the face or head but usually behind the eye, the cheek bone, or the temporal region, and is almost always one-sided (unilateral).

During the attack one can often see or feel the superficial temporal artery on the side of the head. Other features seen during the attack are a drooping of the eyelid (ptosis), running of the eye (lacrimation), redness of the eye (injection of the conjunctiva), nasal stuffiness or running (rhinorrhea). Often there is sweating on the side of the face that is in pain. A consistent complaint of the cluster patient is that he describes the pain as a stabbing pain, often as a hot poker going through his eye or his scalp.

Dr. John Graham described certain features of the cluster patient.[4] He found that they were men who tended to have a "lionine facial appearance," ruddy complexion, deep furrows on the face, vertical forehead creases, and orange-peel facial skin. Many of them are tall and rugged looking, with a broad deep chin and skull. Many of these patients are cigarette smokers and alcohol and coffee drinkers. During the cluster period even a bar rag can precipitate an attack and these men will stop drinking during that period! What is most interesting is that even though this is a most debilitating pain, these men always seem to continue working. It is only when the condition becomes chronic and daily that work becomes unbearable (Figure 8.1).

Often attacks are associated with reduction of oxygen intake, such as obstruction of the airways, and high altitude may precipitate an attack. There seems to be a significant number of patients who have cluster headaches who also show symptoms of peptic ulcer.

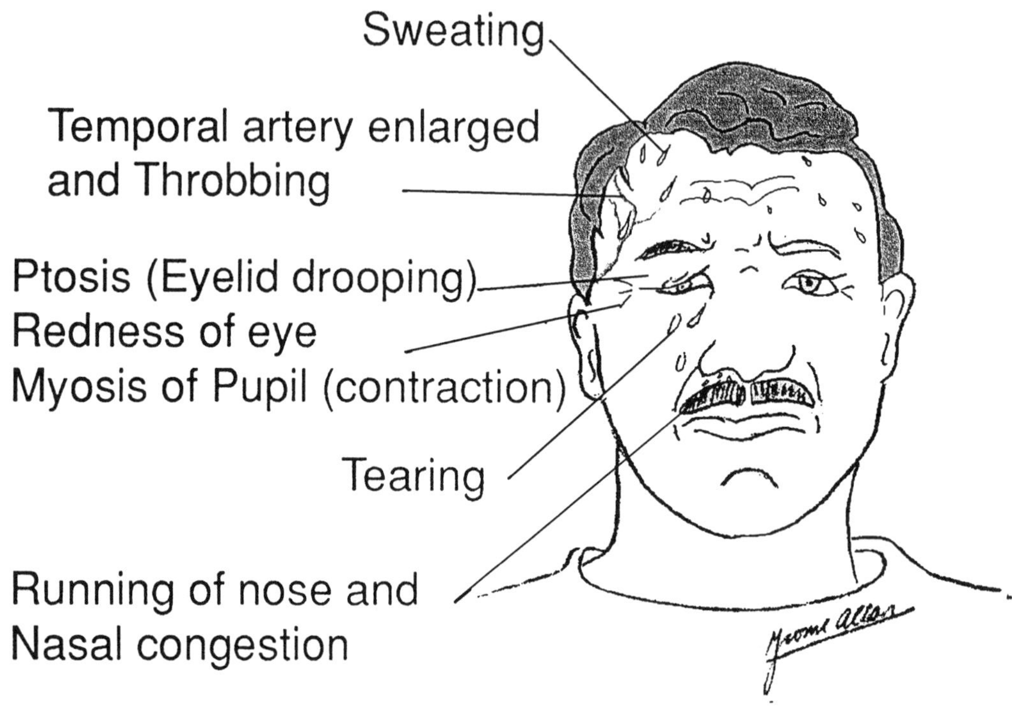

Figure 8.1 The typical symptoms of cluster headache. The temporal artery enlarges and is pulsating. The pain is usually poker-like behind the eye on the side of the headache. There is unilateral ptosis (closing of the eyelid) and swelling and redness of that eyelid. Pinpoint pupils (myosis) and redness of the conjunctivae, tearing, flushing of the side of the face, sweating, nasal congestion, and rhinorrhea (running of the nose) are typical symptoms of cluster headache.

Chronic Cluster Headache

There seem to be two ways that chronic daily cluster headache takes place. One is that the headache starts as an episodic cluster and eventually becomes chronic. The other is that they start immediately as a chronic daily phenomenon, and it has been reported that a small percentage may become episodic. Fortunately, today there are newer treatments that may be very helpful; some are discussed in Part two of this book. Prior to these treatments these headaches were called the "suicide headache" because there seemed to be no other way out of this constant debilitating pain.

Chronic Paroxysmal Hemicrania or CPH

This headache seems to be the woman's answer to cluster headache. Almost as many women get this type of cluster as men get episodic cluster. The attacks are short, from a few minutes to 20 minutes, and they may get up to thirty attacks a day. Many of the symptoms seen in cluster headache are also seen in CPH. Fortunately, almost all of these headaches can be helped and prevented with a drug called indomethocin or Indocin.

CLUSTER-LIKE HEADACHE DISORDERS

Cluster–tic syndrome: These patients present with a tic-like syndrome and cluster headache. There seems to be a relationship between cluster headache and trigeminal neuralgia.

Cluster–vertigo: There has been a report of a patient with a cluster headache attack and severe vertigo.

Cluster–migraine: I have seen a good number of these patients. Often they present with mixed features. That is, they may come in with episodic attacks but have similar features of migraine such as nausea and vomiting, or have features of migraine with symptoms of cluster as described.

Cluster-like headache following head and facial injury: Lance[5] describes 8 out of 60 patients who he observed had cluster headache after facial surgery following an automobile accident. He also described some patients who had cluster headaches they seemed to have gotten years after the accident. Mathew also found some patients who had cluster-like headaches after injury close to the trigeminal nerve.[6] However, Lance points out that in Kudrow's large study, he has not been able to validate this type of headache secondary to head trauma.

The treatment of cluster headaches that may be concomitant to a post traumatic syndrome is discussed in Chapter 25.

After reading the case histories that follows the References, you should have a better understanding of the cluster headache and any similar type of headache that may be related to post traumatic head injury or whiplash.

REFERENCES

1. Kudrow, L., *Cluster Headache*, Oxford University Press, New York, 1980.
2. Kudrow, L., Cluster headache: diagnosis and management, *Headache*, 142–150, April 1979.
3. Mathew, N.T., Cluster headache, *Neurology*, 42 (Suppl. 2), 22–31, 1992.
4. Graham, J.R., Cluster headaches, *Headache*, 11, 175–185, 1972.
5. Lance, J.W., *Mechanism and Management of Headaches*, 4th ed., Buttersworth, London, 1982.
6. Mathew, N.T., Rueveni, U., Cluster-like headache following head trauma, *Headache*, 28 (Abstr.), 307, 1988.

CASE HISTORIES*

KEN
Category: Episode cluster headache

This is a 36-year-old man with a typical history of cluster headaches starting 6 years previously. He gets these attacks that last one to two hours. The character of the pain is sharp, knifelike, and throbbing. They awaken him in the middle of the night with excruciating pain, and this patient was diagnosed with episodic cluster. He was treated with some steroids and oxygen, and his headaches were aborted. A plan was set up that, for any future attacks he would call immediately during that particular episode. He also had a CT scan to make sure there was no intracranial lesion, which was negative. This is a very good example of being able to treat an excruciating headache problem with a simple procedure. Diagnosis: Episodic cluster headache.

* On the headache assessment forms that accompany these case histories, incapacitating headaches are indicated with solid black lines, interfering headaches with dotted lines, and irritating headaches with gray shading.

MEDICAL HEADACHE HISTORY

Name: <u>Ken</u> **Age:** <u>36</u> **Sex** <u>M</u> **Date:** <u>10/10/90</u>

Date of Birth: <u>00/00/54</u> **Birthplace:** <u>RI</u> **Race:** <u>C</u> **Education:** <u>11th Grade</u>

Occupation: <u>Sales Director</u> **Accident:** <u>N/A</u>

Armed Services & Type of Discharge: <u>1972-1975 – Army, Bad Conduct Discharge</u>

PAST HISTORY:

1.	Did you have a normal birth?		<u>Yes</u>	No
	a) forceps used?		Yes	<u>No</u>
	b) cesarean section?		Yes	<u>No</u>
2.	Did you have problems with bedwetting?		Yes	<u>No</u>
	a) If yes, age bedwetting stopped		______	
3.	Were you car sick as a child (motion)?		Yes	<u>No</u>
	a) If yes, how severe?	Slight	Moderate	Severe
4.	Did you have unexplained abdominal cramps as a child?		Yes	<u>No</u>
5.	Did you have any of the following illnesses in childhood?			
	a) meningitis		Yes	<u>No</u>
	b) encephalitis		Yes	<u>No</u>
	c) scarlet fever		Yes	<u>No</u>
	d) rheumatic fever		Yes	<u>No</u>
6.	Did you have any head injuries as a child?		Yes	<u>No</u>
	a) If yes, please explain:______			
7.	Were you treated for emotional illness as a child?		Yes	<u>No</u>

HABITS:

8.	Do you drink alcohol?	<u>Yes</u>	No
	a) If yes, what kind and how much?______		
	b) Does alcohol bring on or aggravate a headache?	Yes	<u>No</u>
9.	Do you smoke?	<u>Yes</u>	No
	a) If yes, how much? <u>2 packs a day</u>		
	b) Does smoking or smoke-filled rooms cause or aggravate headaches?	Yes	<u>No</u>
10.	Do you drink caffeinated beverages?	<u>Yes</u>	No
	a) If yes, how much? <u>5 cups coffee + coke daily</u>		

MENSTRUAL HISTORY:

At what age did menses begin?______ Were they regular or irregular?______
How were they related to your headache?______
Are you or were you ever on Birth Control Pills?______ Did they affect your headache?______
Have you had a hysterectomy, partial or total, and why?______
Are you in menopause, and if yes, how long?______
Are you on hormones, and if yes, which ones?______

HEADACHE ASSESSMENT FORM

HA PROFILE	INCAPACITATING #3	INTERFERING #2	IRRITATING #1
ONSET (Years ago and frequency)	6 years ago 4 to 6 weeks, every day	N/A	N/A
CURRENT FREQUENCY	4 weeks ago, every day last cycle May 1990	N/A	N/A
TIME OF ONSET	Awakens with	N/A	N/A
DURATION	1 to 2 hours	N/A	N/A
CHARACTER	Sharp knifelike and throbbing	N/A	N/A
PRODROME OR AURA	N/A	N/A	N/A
ASSOCIATING FEATURES	Nausea; Vomiting; Sensitivity to Light? Noise? Odors? Do you get pale or flush? Do your eyes or nose run? Does your nose get stuffy? Does the white of your eyes get red? Does your eyelid droop? Do you pace, or go to bed? Sits quietly	Nausea; Vomiting; Sensitivity to Light? Noise? Odors? Do you get pale or flush? Do your eyes or nose run? Does your nose get stuffy? Does the white of your eyes get red? Does your eyelid droop? Do you pace, or go to bed?	Nausea; Vomiting; Sensitivity to Light? Noise? Odors? Do you get pale or flush? Do your eyes or nose run? Does your nose get stuffy? Does the white of your eyes get red? Does your eyelid droop? Do you pace, or go to bed?
PRECIPITATING OR AGGRAVATING FEATURES	Bending over Movement	N/A	N/A

LOCATION: Mark the location for each type of headache with a different color pen.

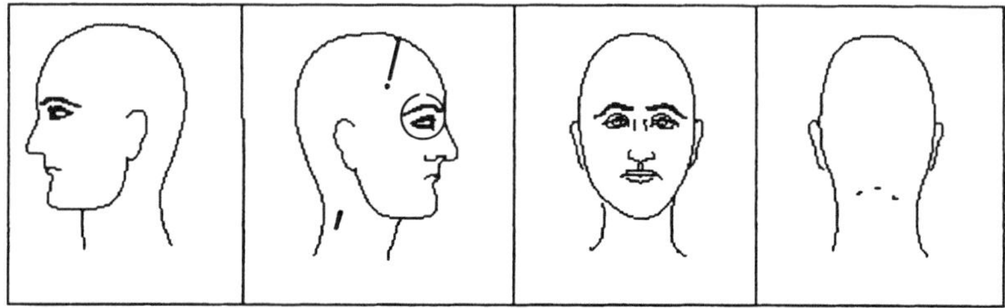

MEDICAL HISTORY:

Have you ever been or are you currently being treated for any of the following?

a) high blood pressure	Yes	No
b) stomach ulcers	Yes	No
c) asthma	Yes	No
d) allergies	Yes	No
e) pneumonia	Yes	No
f) kidney problems	Yes	No
g) low blood sugar	Yes	No
h) glaucoma	Yes	No
i) diabetes	Yes	No
j) heart problems	Yes	No

If you answered yes to any of the above, please describe).

List all other medical problems you have had in the past. Include date diagnosed and treatment.
DO NOT LIST OPERATIONS

None.

SURGICAL HISTORY (List operations and dates performed)

None.

PSYCHIATRIC HISTORY (List visits with counselors, psychologists, etc., and type of treatment)

None.

ACCIDENTS IN ADULT LIFE (Briefly describe any accident that caused any blow to the head or that you feel is related to your headache)

FAMILY HISTORY:

1.	Is your father living?	Yes	No
	Age 59		
	Cause of death		
	Was there a headache history?	Yes	No
2.	Is your mother living?	Yes	No
	Age 59		
	Cause of death		
	Was there a headache history?	Yes	No

3. Ages of brothers---Circle the ones with headache
   22
4. Ages of sisters---Circle the ones with headache
   37 34 32 26 24
5. List any other blood relatives with a history of severe headaches.
   None

MARITAL HISTORY:
List marriages:

1st marriage age 23 to 35 Did spouse have headaches? Yes No
2nd marriage age _____ to ______ Did spouse have headaches? Yes No
3rd marriage age ______to ______ Did spouse have headaches? Yes No
Age of current spouse: 42

List ages and sex of all children:

Age 10 Sex M Headaches? Yes No
Age 5 Sex M Headaches? Yes No
Age ______ Sex ______ Headaches? Yes No
Age ______ Sex ______ Headaches? Yes No

STRESS FACTORS:

List any factors that may be affecting your headaches (money, loneliness, sexual problems, work, etc.)
None.

VEGETATIVE SIGNS:

1. Do you have trouble falling asleep? Yes No
2. Do you have trouble staying asleep? Yes No
3. Has your appetite decreased? Yes No
4. Have you gained or lost weight in the past year? Yes No
5. Have you felt tearful or depressed lately? Yes No
6. Have you had any thoughts of wanting to die? Yes No
7. Have you been forgetful lately? Yes No
8. Any other changes in your normal day-to-day living?________________

Please list any medications you are allergic or sensitive to: No known allergies.

Please list any medications you are currently taking (including dosages and frequency per day):
None.

PREVIOUS CARE:

1. List doctors who have treated you for headaches:____________________

____

____

____

2. List any tests you have had for your headache (e.g., EEG, CT scan, MRI, X-Ray, etc.):

CAT scan – 1985 (normal).

____

____

____

3. List any other treatment you have had for your headache (e.g., biofeedback, acupuncture, chiropractic, or any other treatment you had):

____

____

____

DAVID
Category: Episodic cluster headache

This patient is 37 years old, with headaches that started at age 32. He has typical symptoms of cluster headache with the sharp pain and some throbbing. He feels there is a slight muscle spasm in his neck before the headache. He states that he had had acupuncture a year ago, and the headaches went away for six months but then came back. The patient was worked up to make sure there were no other medical problems, and he was treated with medications and did very well. He was also told that if the headaches become continuous and will not break, there is a surgical procedure that may be able to help him in the future; but, for the present, we would work on the basis of how frequently he gets his attacks. His diagnosis was episodic cluster headache.

MEDICAL HEADACHE HISTORY

Name: David **Age:** 37 **Sex** M **Date:** 10/7/91

Date of Birth: 00/00/54 **Birthplace:** NY **Race:** C **Education:** 3 yrs. college

Occupation: Hair Stylist **Accident:** 5/89

Armed Services & Type of Discharge: N/A

PAST HISTORY:

1.	Did you have a normal birth?		<u>Yes</u>	No
	a) forceps used?		Yes	No
	b) cesarean section?		Yes	No
2.	Did you have problems with bedwetting?		Yes	<u>No</u>
	a) If yes, age bedwetting stopped			
3.	Were you car sick as a child (motion)?		Yes	<u>No</u>
	a) If yes, how severe?	Slight	Moderate	Severe
4.	Did you have unexplained abdominal cramps as a child?		Yes	<u>No</u>
5.	Did you have any of the following illnesses in childhood?			
	a) meningitis		Yes	<u>No</u>
	b) encephalitis		Yes	<u>No</u>
	c) scarlet fever		Yes	<u>No</u>
	d) rheumatic fever		Yes	<u>No</u>
6.	Did you have any head injuries as a child?		Yes	<u>No</u>
	a) If yes, please explain:			
7.	Were you treated for emotional illness as a child?		Yes	<u>No</u>

HABITS:

8.	Do you drink alcohol?	<u>Yes</u>	No
	a) If yes, what kind and how much? On occasion, a few beers		
	b) Does alcohol bring on or aggravate a headache?	<u>Yes</u>	No
9.	Do you smoke?	<u>Yes</u>	No
	a) If yes, how much? A pack a day		
	b) Does smoking or smoke-filled rooms cause or aggravate headaches?	<u>Yes</u>	No
10.	Do you drink caffeinated beverages?	<u>Yes</u>	No
	a) If yes, how much? 6 cups		

MENSTRUAL HISTORY:

At what age did menses begin?______ Were they regular or irregular?______

How were they related to your headache?______

Are you or were you ever on Birth Control Pills?______ Did they affect your headache? ______

Have you had a hysterectomy, partial or total, and why?______

Are you in menopause, and if yes, how long?______

Are you on hormones, and if yes, which ones?______

HEADACHE ASSESSMENT FORM

HA PROFILE	INCAPACITATING #3	INTERFERING #2	IRRITATING #1
ONSET (Years ago and frequency)	Age 32 Every day	N/A	N/A
CURRENT FREQUENCY	Every day	N/A	N/A
TIME OF ONSET	Usually at night	N/A	N/A
DURATION	1 to 18 hours	N/A	N/A
CHARACTER	Ice pick left temple and severe throbbing	N/A	N/A
PRODROME OR AURA	Always has muscle contraction in neck minutes before headache	N/A	N/A
ASSOCIATING FEATURES	Nausea; Vomiting; Sensitivity to Light? Noise? Odors? Do you get pale or flush? Do your eyes or nose run? Does your nose get stuffy? Does the white of your eyes get red? Does your eyelid droop? Do you pace, or go to bed?	Nausea; Vomiting; Sensitivity to Light? Noise? Odors? Do you get pale or flush? Do your eyes or nose run? Does your nose get stuffy? Does the white of your eyes get red? Does your eyelid droop? Do you pace, or go to bed?	Nausea; Vomiting; Sensitivity to Light? Noise? Odors? Do you get pale or flush? Do your eyes or nose run? Does your nose get stuffy? Does the white of your eyes get red? Does your eyelid droop? Do you pace, or go to bed?
PRECIPITATING OR AGGRAVATING FEATURES	Alcohol	N/A	N/A

LOCATION: Mark the location for each type of headache with a different color pen.

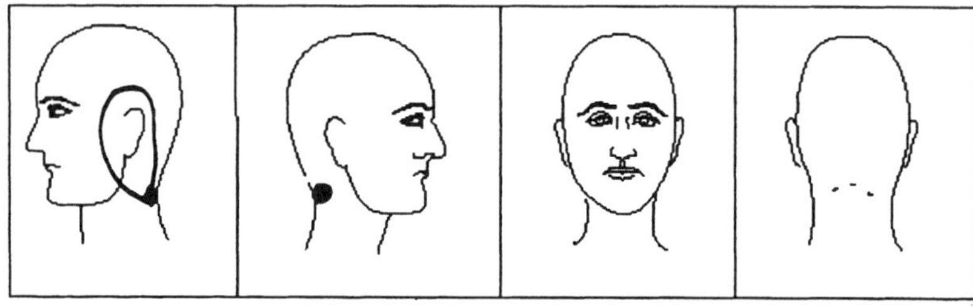

MEDICAL HISTORY:

Have you ever been or are you currently being treated for any of the following?

a) high blood pressure	Yes	No
b) stomach ulcers	Yes	No
c) asthma	Yes	No
d) allergies	Yes	No
e) pneumonia	Yes	No
f) kidney problems	Yes	No
g) low blood sugar	Yes	No
h) glaucoma	Yes	No
i) diabetes	Yes	No
j) heart problems	Yes	No

If you answered yes to any of the above, please describe:____________________

List all other medical problems you have had in the past. Include date diagnosed and treatment.
DO NOT LIST OPERATIONS

Optic neuritis. Chronic cluster headache.

SURGICAL HISTORY (List operations and dates performed)

N/A.

PSYCHIATRIC HISTORY (List visits with counselors, psychologists, etc., and type of treatment)

N/A.

ACCIDENTS IN ADULT LIFE (Briefly describe any accident that caused any blow to the head or that you feel is related to your headache)

Auto – head through windshield 1979.

FAMILY HISTORY:

1. Is your father living? Yes No
   Age 70
   Cause of death____________________
   Was there a headache history? Yes No
2. Is your mother living? Yes No
   Age 68
   Cause of death____________________
   Was there a headache history? Yes No
3. Ages of brothers---Circle the ones with headache
   41

4. Ages of sisters---Circle the ones with headache
   None
5. List any other blood relatives with a history of severe headaches.
   None

MARITAL HISTORY:
List marriages:

1st marriage age _____ to _______	Did spouse have headaches?	Yes	No
2nd marriage age _____ to _______	Did spouse have headaches?	Yes	No
3rd marriage age _____ to _______	Did spouse have headaches?	Yes	No

Age of current spouse:___________

List ages and sex of all children:

Age _____ Sex _____	Headaches?	Yes	No
Age _____ Sex _____	Headaches?	Yes	No
Age _____ Sex _____	Headaches?	Yes	No
Age _____ Sex _____	Headaches?	Yes	No

STRESS FACTORS:

List any factors that may be affecting your headaches (money, loneliness, sexual problems, work, etc.)

VEGETATIVE SIGNS:

1.	Do you have trouble falling asleep?	Yes	No
2.	Do you have trouble staying asleep?	Yes	No
3.	Has your appetite decreased?	Yes	No
4.	Have you gained or lost weight in the past year?	Yes	No
5.	Have you felt tearful or depressed lately?	Yes	No
6.	Have you had any thoughts of wanting to die?	Yes	No
7.	Have you been forgetful lately?	Yes	No
8.	Any other changes in your normal day-to-day living?__________		

Please list any medications you are allergic or sensitive to: None

Please list any medications you are currently taking (including dosages and frequency per day):
None.

PREVIOUS CARE:

1. List doctors who have treated you for headaches: Dr. H,

2. List any tests you have had for your headache (e.g., EEG, CT scan, MRI, X-Ray, etc.):
EEG, CAT scan, MRI (all normal).

3. List any other treatment you have had for your headache (e.g., biofeedback, acupuncture, chiropractic, or any other treatment you had):
Biofeedback (helps). Acupuncture (helps). Chiropractic.

ALVIN
Category: Chronic cluster headache

This is a history of an unfortunate patient who began having cluster headaches as a teenager, and they developed from an episodic cluster attack until they became chronic and continuous. Because they were so severe, the patient was unable to work and became disabled. This is the headache that previously was called the "suicide headache" because it was so painful and, because there was no treatment, many men would give up on the excruciating pain that they had.

At the time of his visit, he had been getting these attacks every day for the past one and a half years. He had the typical intralateral symptoms, on the side of the headache, with tearing, or lacrimation; ptosis, or drooping of the eyelid; and diaphoresis, or sweating, on the left side of the head. The patient had a great deal of workup in many particular areas, and fortunately there is a surgical procedure that seems to be effective with a certain group of people that can give almost total relief. That operation is called radiofrequency trigeminal gangliorhizolysis, and the patient was sent to Houston where the operation was done. Unfortunately, I have not had a follow up as to the success of the procedure, but this is an example of a chronic cluster headache that started as an episodic cluster headache.

MEDICAL HEADACHE HISTORY

Name: Alvin **Age:** 43 **Sex** M **Date:** 5/24/90

Date of Birth: 00/00/47 **Birthplace:** TN **Race:** W **Education:** 10th Grade

Occupation: Disability **Accident:** N/A

Armed Services & Type of Discharge: N/A

PAST HISTORY:

1.	Did you have a normal birth?		Yes (underlined)	No
	a) forceps used?		Yes	No
	b) cesarean section?		Yes	No
2.	Did you have problems with bedwetting?		Yes	No (underlined)
	a) If yes, age bedwetting stopped			______
3.	Were you car sick as a child (motion)?		Yes	No (underlined)
	a) If yes, how severe?	Slight	Moderate	Severe
4.	Did you have unexplained abdominal cramps as a child?		Yes	No (underlined)
5.	Did you have any of the following illnesses in childhood?			
	a) meningitis		Yes	No
	b) encephalitis		Yes	No
	c) scarlet fever		Yes	No
	d) rheumatic fever		Yes	No
6.	Did you have any head injuries as a child?		Yes	No (underlined)
	a) If yes, please explain: ______			
7.	Were you treated for emotional illness as a child?		Yes	No (underlined)

HABITS:

8.	Do you drink alcohol?	Yes (underlined)	No
	a) If yes, what kind and how much? Occasionally		
	b) Does alcohol bring on or aggravate a headache?	Yes	No (underlined)
9.	Do you smoke?	Yes (underlined)	No
	a) If yes, how much? 1 pack a day		
	b) Does smoking or smoke-filled rooms cause or aggravate headaches?	Yes	No (underlined)
10.	Do you drink caffeinated beverages?	Yes (underlined)	No
	a) If yes, how much? 2 coffee 1 coke		

MENSTRUAL HISTORY:

At what age did menses begin?______ Were they regular or irregular?______
How were they related to your headache?______
Are you or were you ever on Birth Control Pills?______ Did they affect your headache? ______
Have you had a hysterectomy, partial or total, and why?______
Are you in menopause, and if yes, how long?______
Are you on hormones, and if yes, which ones?______

HEADACHE ASSESSMENT FORM

HA PROFILE	INCAPACITATING #3	INTERFERING #2	IRRITATING #1
ONSET (Years ago and frequency)	30 yrs. ago 1 to 2 a week	N/A	N/A
CURRENT FREQUENCY	1 to 7 a day for 1½ years	N/A	N/A
TIME OF ONSET	Anytime	N/A	N/A
DURATION	30 minutes to 4 hours	N/A	N/A
CHARACTER	Burning, ice pick pain	N/A	N/A
PRODROME OR AURA	N/A	N/A	N/A
ASSOCIATING FEATURES	Nausea; Vomiting; Sensitivity to Light? Noise? Odors? Do you get pale or flush? Do your eyes or nose run? Does your nose get stuffy? Does the white of your eyes get red? Does your eyelid droop? Do you pace, or go to bed?	Nausea; Vomiting; Sensitivity to Light? Noise? Odors? Do you get pale or flush? Do your eyes or nose run? Does your nose get stuffy? Does the white of your eyes get red? Does your eyelid droop? Do you pace, or go to bed?	Nausea; Vomiting; Sensitivity to Light? Noise? Odors? Do you get pale or flush? Do your eyes or nose run? Does your nose get stuffy? Does the white of your eyes get red? Does your eyelid droop? Do you pace, or go to bed?
PRECIPITATING OR AGGRAVATING FEATURES	N/A	N/A	N/A

LOCATION: Mark the location for each type of headache with a different color pen.

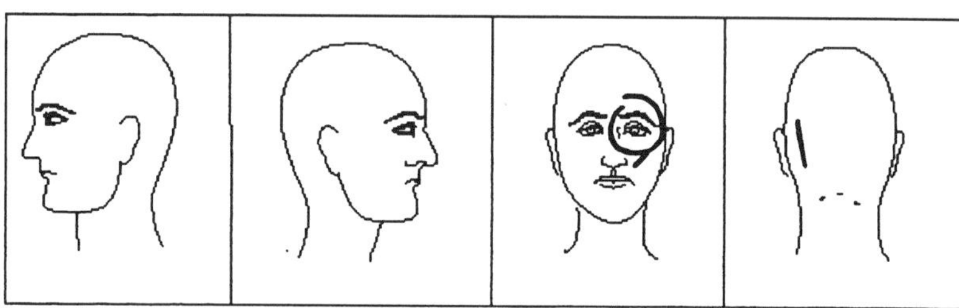

MEDICAL HISTORY:

Have you ever been or are you currently being treated for any of the following?

a) high blood pressure	<u>Yes</u>	No
b) stomach ulcers	<u>Yes</u>	No
c) asthma	Yes	<u>No</u>
d) allergies	<u>Yes</u>	No
e) pneumonia	<u>Yes</u>	No
f) kidney problems	Yes	<u>No</u>
g) low blood sugar	Yes	<u>No</u>
h) glaucoma	Yes	<u>No</u>
i) diabetes	Yes	<u>No</u>
j) heart problems	<u>Yes</u>	No

If you answered yes to any of the above, please describe: High blood pressure diagnosed 1 yr. ago. Ulcers diagnosed 1 yr. ago (take Tagamet twice a day). Environmental allergies. Pneumonia 2 yrs. ago. Arrhythmia.

List all other medical problems you have had in the past. Include date diagnosed and treatment. DO NOT LIST OPERATIONS

Crohn's Disease, diagnosed 1 year ago. Lung problems (collapsed lung 15 years ago).

SURGICAL HISTORY (List operations and dates performed)

Tumor removed from neck, 1989. Tumor removed from hand, 1988. Sinus surgery, 1988.

PSYCHIATRIC HISTORY (List visits with counselors, psychologists, etc., and type of treatment)

Dr. P., Dr. W., Dr. H., Dr. H.

ACCIDENTS IN ADULT LIFE (Briefly describe any accident that caused any blow to the head or that you feel is related to your headache)

FAMILY HISTORY:

1.	Is your father living?	<u>Yes</u>	No
	Age 78		
	Cause of death		
	Was there a headache history?	Yes	<u>No</u>
2.	Is your mother living?	<u>Yes</u>	No
	Age 68		
	Cause of death		
	Was there a headache history?	Yes	<u>No</u>

3. Ages of brothers---Circle the ones with headache
____

4. Ages of sisters---Circle the ones with headache
45 48

5. List any other blood relatives with a history of severe headaches.
None

MARITAL HISTORY:
List marriages:

1st marriage age 20 to 39	Did spouse have headaches?	Yes	No
2nd marriage age 43 to Present	Did spouse have headaches?	Yes	No
3rd marriage age ______ to ______	Did spouse have headaches?	Yes	No

Age of current spouse: 42

List ages and sex of all children:

Age 22 Sex M Headaches?	Yes	No
Age 18 Sex M Headaches?	Yes	No
Age 15 Sex M Headaches?	Yes	No
Age 10 Sex M Headaches?	Yes	No

STRESS FACTORS:

List any factors that may be affecting your headaches (money, loneliness, sexual problems, work, etc.)
None.

VEGETATIVE SIGNS:

1.	Do you have trouble falling asleep?	Yes	No
2.	Do you have trouble staying asleep?	Yes	No
3.	Has your appetite decreased?	Yes	No
4.	Have you gained or lost weight in the past year?	Yes	No
5.	Have you felt tearful or depressed lately?	Yes	No
6.	Have you had any thoughts of wanting to die?	Yes	No
7.	Have you been forgetful lately?	Yes	No
8.	Any other changes in your normal day-to-day living?______		

Please list any medications you are allergic or sensitive to: Bee stings

Please list any medications you are currently taking (including dosages and frequency per day):
Cafergot PB; Tagamet, 2 every day; Azulfidine, four every day; Darvocet, at bedtime.

PREVIOUS CARE:

1. List doctors who have treated you for headaches: Dr. H, Dr. P, Dr. S, Dr. H.

2. List any tests you have had for your headache (e.g., EEG, CT scan, MRI, X-Ray, etc.):
CAT scan, EEG, X-ray.

3. List any other treatment you have had for your headache (e.g., biofeedback, acupuncture, chiropractic, or any other treatment you had):
None.

SKIP
Category: Cluster headache

This is a good example of a typical episodic cluster headache patient. The patient is a 50-year-old man, who started getting headaches 4 years ago. They generally come on in the spring of the year; however, this time they started in the fall, which is not unusual. He gets these attacks daily, lasting 20 minutes to 3 hours, with a jabbing and burning pain. There are no features that we see in migraine. Lots of the features were on the side of the headache, such as the eye running, or lacrimation; the nose running, or rhinorrhea. The patient's eye on the side of the headache seems to droop, which is called ptosis, and he must pace. These are all very typical symptoms of cluster headache. He was diagnosed with episodic cluster headache, was treated, and his headache attacks were aborted. He was instructed to return the next time an attack started.

MEDICAL HEADACHE HISTORY

Name: Skip **Age:** 50 **Sex** M **Date:** 10/10/88

Date of Birth: 00/00/38 **Birthplace:** FL **Race:** W **Education:** High school

Occupation: Truck Driver **Accident:** N/A

Armed Services & Type of Discharge: N/A

PAST HISTORY:

1.	Did you have a normal birth?		Yes	No
	a) forceps used?		Yes	No
	b) cesarean section?		Yes	No
2.	Did you have problems with bedwetting?		Yes	No
	a) If yes, age bedwetting stopped		______	
3.	Were you car sick as a child (motion)?		Yes	No
	a) If yes, how severe?	Slight	Moderate	Severe
4.	Did you have unexplained abdominal cramps as a child?		Yes	No
5.	Did you have any of the following illnesses in childhood?			
	a) meningitis		Yes	No
	b) encephalitis		Yes	No
	c) scarlet fever		Yes	No
	d) rheumatic fever		Yes	No
6.	Did you have any head injuries as a child?		Yes	No
	a) If yes, please explain:______			
7.	Were you treated for emotional illness as a child?		Yes	No

HABITS:

8.	Do you drink alcohol?	Yes	No
	a) If yes, what kind and how much? Moderate		
	b) Does alcohol bring on or aggravate a headache?	Yes	No
9.	Do you smoke?	Yes	No
	a) If yes, how much? Pipe		
	b) Does smoking or smoke-filled rooms cause or aggravate headaches?	Yes	No
10.	Do you drink caffeinated beverages?	Yes	No
	a) If yes, how much? 4 – 5 cups coffee		

MENSTRUAL HISTORY:

At what age did menses begin?______ Were they regular or irregular?______
How were they related to your headache?______
Are you or were you ever on Birth Control Pills?______ Did they affect your headache? ______
Have you had a hysterectomy, partial or total, and why?______
Are you in menopause, and if yes, how long?______
Are you on hormones, and if yes, which ones?______

HEADACHE ASSESSMENT FORM

HA PROFILE	INCAPACITATING #3	INTERFERING #2	IRRITATING #1
ONSET (Years ago and frequency)	4 yrs. ago spring only	N/A	Has had #1 headaches twice a month. Able to abort with food or apirin.
CURRENT FREQUENCY	This cycle began 3 weeks ago. Every other day	N/A	
TIME OF ONSET	Anytime. 1 to 3 a day	N/A	
DURATION	20 minutes to 3 hours	N/A	1 hour with aspirin
CHARACTER	Constant pain, jabbing and burning.	N/A	Dull ache
PRODROME OR AURA	N/A	N/A	N/A
ASSOCIATING FEATURES	Nausea; Vomiting; Sensitivity to Light? Noise? Odors? Do you get pale or flush? Do your eyes or nose run? Does your nose get stuffy? Does the white of your eyes get red? Does your eyelid droop? Do you pace, or go to bed?	Nausea; Vomiting; Sensitivity to Light? Noise? Odors? Do you get pale or flush? Do your eyes or nose run? Does your nose get stuffy? Does the white of your eyes get red? Does your eyelid droop? Do you pace, or go to bed?	Nausea; Vomiting; Sensitivity to Light? Noise? Odors? Do you get pale or flush? Do your eyes or nose run? Does your nose get stuffy? Does the white of your eyes get red? Does your eyelid droop? Do you pace, or go to bed?
PRECIPITATING OR AGGRAVATING FEATURES	N/A	N/A	N/A

LOCATION: Mark the location for each type of headache with a different color pen.

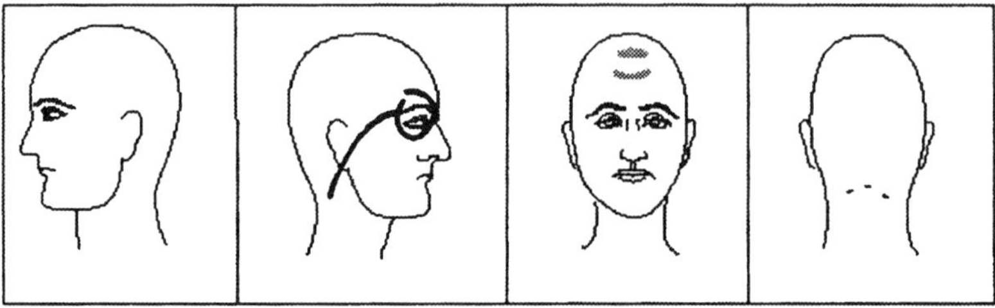

MEDICAL HISTORY:

Have you ever been or are you currently being treated for any of the following?

a) high blood pressure	Yes	No
b) stomach ulcers	Yes	No
c) asthma	Yes	No
d) allergies	Yes	No
e) pneumonia	Yes	No
f) kidney problems	Yes	No
g) low blood sugar	Yes	No
h) glaucoma	Yes	No
i) diabetes	Yes	No
j) heart problems	Yes	No

If you answered yes to any of the above, please describe:____________________

List all other medical problems you have had in the past. Include date diagnosed and treatment. DO NOT LIST OPERATIONS

None.

SURGICAL HISTORY (List operations and dates performed)

Vasectomy – 20 years ago. Tonsillectomy – as a child.

PSYCHIATRIC HISTORY (List visits with counselors, psychologists, etc., and type of treatment)

None.

ACCIDENTS IN ADULT LIFE (Briefly describe any accident that caused any blow to the head or that you feel is related to your headache)

None.

FAMILY HISTORY:

1.	Is your father living?	Yes	No
	Age________		
	Cause of death________________		
	Was there a headache history?	Yes	No
2.	Is your mother living?	Yes	No
	Age 70		
	Cause of death________________		
	Was there a headache history?	Yes	No
3.	Ages of brothers---Circle the ones with headache		
	44		

4. Ages of sisters---Circle the ones with headache
   None
5. List any other blood relatives with a history of severe headaches.
   None .

MARITAL HISTORY:
List marriages:

1st marriage age 18 to 34 Did spouse have headaches?	Yes	No
2nd marriage age 35 to Present Did spouse have headaches?	Yes	No
3rd marriage age ______ to ______ Did spouse have headaches?	Yes	No

Age of current spouse:__________

List ages and sex of all children:

Age 31 Sex M Headaches?	Yes	No
Age 29 Sex F Headaches?	Yes	No
Age _____ Sex ______ Headaches?	Yes	No
Age _____ Sex ______ Headaches?	Yes	No

STRESS FACTORS:

List any factors that may be affecting your headaches (money, loneliness, sexual problems, work, etc.)
None.

VEGETATIVE SIGNS:

1.	Do you have trouble falling asleep?	Yes	No
2.	Do you have trouble staying asleep?	Yes	No
3.	Has your appetite decreased?	Yes	No
4.	Have you gained or lost weight in the past year?	Yes	No
5.	Have you felt tearful or depressed lately?	Yes	No
6.	Have you had any thoughts of wanting to die?	Yes	No
7.	Have you been forgetful lately?	Yes	No
8.	Any other changes in your normal day-to-day living?__________		

Please list any medications you are allergic or sensitive to: None

Please list any medications you are currently taking (including dosages and frequency per day):
Ergostat.

PREVIOUS CARE:

1. List doctors who have treated you for headaches: Dr. P,

2. List any tests you have had for your headache (e.g., EEG, CT scan, MRI, X-Ray, etc.):
None.

3. List any other treatment you have had for your headache (e.g., biofeedback, acupuncture, chiropractic, or any other treatment you had):
None.

PEGGY
Category: Cluster headache

This is a 55-year-old woman who came in with excruciating headaches, lasting over half a day, totally incapacitating and disabling the patient. It is interesting that this cluster patient was a woman, inasmuch as men generally have cluster headache eight times more than women. However, she also had some of the symptoms seen with migraine, and this frequently could be confused as an atypical migraine diagnosis. The patient was treated as a status cluster, meaning that the cluster headache would not break, and also was given a diagnosis of cluster headache with migraine features.

The patient was hospitalized and treated intravenously with specific medication that broke the headache totally, and the patient became headache-free. Records show that she did not have another attack until three years later, when she was treated once again for the same condition.

MEDICAL HEADACHE HISTORY

Name: Peggy **Age:** 55 **Sex** F **Date:** 10/20/86

Date of Birth: 00/00/31 **Birthplace:** SC **Race:** W **Education:** High school

Occupation: Cashier **Accident:** N/A

Armed Services & Type of Discharge: N/A

PAST HISTORY:

1.	Did you have a normal birth?		<u>Yes</u>	No
	a) forceps used?		Yes	<u>No</u>
	b) cesarean section?		Yes	<u>No</u>
2.	Did you have problems with bedwetting?		Yes	<u>No</u>
	a) If yes, age bedwetting stopped		______	
3.	Were you car sick as a child (motion)?		Yes	<u>No</u>
	a) If yes, how severe?	Slight	Moderate	Severe
4.	Did you have unexplained abdominal cramps as a child?		Yes	<u>No</u>
5.	Did you have any of the following illnesses in childhood?			
	a) meningitis		Yes	<u>No</u>
	b) encephalitis		Yes	<u>No</u>
	c) scarlet fever		Yes	<u>No</u>
	d) rheumatic fever		Yes	<u>No</u>
6.	Did you have any head injuries as a child?		Yes	<u>No</u>
	a) If yes, please explain: ______			
7.	Were you treated for emotional illness as a child?		Yes	<u>No</u>

HABITS:

8.	Do you drink alcohol?	Yes	<u>No</u>
	a) If yes, what kind and how much? ______		
	b) Does alcohol bring on or aggravate a headache?	<u>Yes</u>	No
9.	Do you smoke?	<u>Yes</u>	No
	a) If yes, how much? ½ a pack a day		
	b) Does smoking or smoke-filled rooms cause or aggravate headaches?	Yes	<u>No</u>
10.	Do you drink caffeinated beverages?	Yes	No
	a) If yes, how much? ______		

MENSTRUAL HISTORY:

At what age did menses begin? 16 Were they regular or irregular? WNL

How were they related to your headache? N/A

Are you or were you ever on Birth Control Pills? No Did they affect your headache? No

Have you had a hysterectomy, partial or total, and why? Partial, 1971. Uterine cancer.

Are you in menopause, and if yes, how long? No

Are you on hormones, and if yes, which ones? Estrace, 1 mg. Metandrin 5 mg.

HEADACHE ASSESSMENT FORM

HA PROFILE	INCAPACITATING #3	INTERFERING #2	IRRITATING #1
ONSET (Years ago and frequency)	Dec. 1983 – every day, 3 month cycles	N/A	N/A
CURRENT FREQUENCY	Every day – Cycle started in Sept.	N/A	N/A
TIME OF ONSET	3 – 4 p.m.	N/A	N/A
DURATION	8 – 10 hours	N/A	N/A
CHARACTER	Severe pressure	N/A	N/A
PRODROME OR AURA	N/A	N/A	N/A
ASSOCIATING FEATURES	Nausea; Vomiting; Sensitivity to Light? Noise? Odors? Do you get pale or flush? Do your eyes or nose run? Does your nose get stuffy? Does the white of your eyes get red? Does your eyelid droop? Do you pace, or go to bed? Sits in chair	Nausea; Vomiting; Sensitivity to Light? Noise? Odors? Do you get pale or flush? Do your eyes or nose run? Does your nose get stuffy? Does the white of your eyes get red? Does your eyelid droop? Do you pace, or go to bed?	Nausea; Vomiting; Sensitivity to Light? Noise? Odors? Do you get pale or flush? Do your eyes or nose run? Does your nose get stuffy? Does the white of your eyes get red? Does your eyelid droop? Do you pace, or go to bed?
PRECIPITATING OR AGGRAVATING FEATURES	Lying down	N/A	N/A

LOCATION: Mark the location for each type of headache with a different color pen.

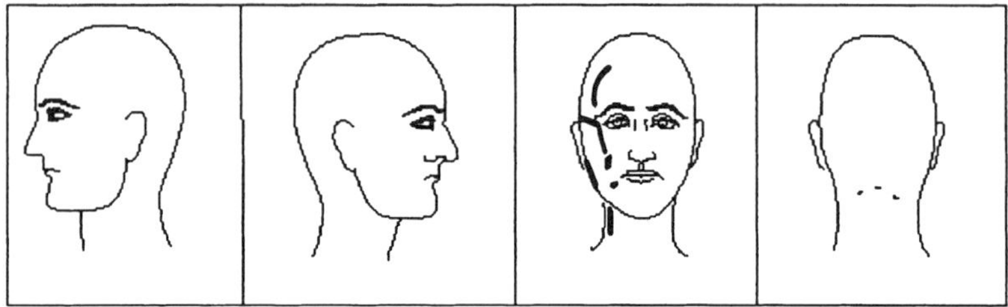

MEDICAL HISTORY:

Have you ever been or are you currently being treated for any of the following?

a) high blood pressure	Yes	No
b) stomach ulcers	Yes	No
c) asthma	Yes	No
d) allergies	Yes	No
e) pneumonia	Yes	No
f) kidney problems	Yes	No
g) low blood sugar	Yes	No
h) glaucoma	Yes	No
i) diabetes	Yes	No
j) heart problems	Yes	No

If you answered yes to any of the above, please describe: Pinpoint ulcer, dissolved 1956. Kidney infections 3 times. Was taking Timolol for headaches, caused bradycardia.

List all other medical problems you have had in the past. Include date diagnosed and treatment.
DO NOT LIST OPERATIONS

Pinpoint ulcer 1956, dissolved. Cancer of uterus, partial hysterectomy 1971. Bursitis in both shoulders. Tumor on right ovary, 1962. Kidney infections.

SURGICAL HISTORY (List operations and dates performed)

Partial hysterectomy, 1971. Tumor in left upper arm, 1979. Exploratory, excessive uterine bleeding, 1962.

PSYCHIATRIC HISTORY (List visits with counselors, psychologists, etc., and type of treatment)

Paralysis after hysterectomy (H. Hospital)

ACCIDENTS IN ADULT LIFE (Briefly describe any accident that caused any blow to the head or that you feel is related to your headache)

Tripped while watering plants. Landed on ground. Stunned, unconscious for a few minutes. Not examined. 1983.

FAMILY HISTORY:

1.	Is your father living?	Yes	No
	Age 83		
	Cause of death ______		
	Was there a headache history?	Yes	No
2.	Is your mother living?	Yes	No
	Age 83		
	Cause of death ______		
	Was there a headache history?	Yes	No

3. Ages of brothers---Circle the ones with headache
____

4. Ages of sisters---Circle the ones with headache
(57)

5. List any other blood relatives with a history of severe headaches.
____

MARITAL HISTORY:
List marriages:

1st marriage age 24 to 28	Did spouse have headaches?	Yes (underlined)	No
2nd marriage age 38 to 41	Did spouse have headaches?	Yes	No (underlined)
3rd marriage age 44 to Present	Did spouse have headaches?	Yes	No (underlined)

Age of current spouse: 57

List ages and sex of all children:

Age 29 Sex M	Headaches?	Yes (underlined)	No
Age ____ Sex ____	Headaches?	Yes	No
Age ____ Sex ____	Headaches?	Yes	No

STRESS FACTORS:

List any factors that may be affecting your headaches (money, loneliness, sexual problems, work, etc.)
A little of each.

VEGETATIVE SIGNS:

1.	Do you have trouble falling asleep?	Yes (underlined)	No
2.	Do you have trouble staying asleep?	Yes (underlined)	No
3.	Has your appetite decreased?	Yes (underlined)	No
4.	Have you gained or lost weight in the past year?	Yes (underlined)	No
5.	Have you felt tearful or depressed lately?	Yes (underlined)	No
6.	Have you had any thoughts of wanting to die?	Yes (underlined)	No
7.	Have you been forgetful lately?	Yes (underlined)	No
8.	Any other changes in your normal day-to-day living?______		

Please list any medications you are allergic or sensitive to: Timolol

Please list any medications you are currently taking (including dosages and frequency per day):
Fiorinal #3 – 2 twice a day as needed. Phenaphen #3 as needed. Estrace 1 mg at night.
Metandren 5 mg. every other night.

PREVIOUS CARE:

1. List doctors who have treated you for headaches: Dr. F., Dr. R., Dr. R., Dr. G., Dr. E., Dr. N.

2. List any tests you have had for your headache (e.g., EEG, CT scan, MRI, X-Ray, etc.): EEG, CAT scan of head. X-rays of head. (negative)

3. List any other treatment you have had for your headache (e.g., biofeedback, acupuncture, chiropractic, or any other treatment you had):

CARLA
Category: Cluster headache

This is a 41-year-old woman who demonstrated typical symptoms of cluster headache. Again, this is unusual for women, but this is a typical cluster-type patient and her attacks would last 20 minutes to 2 hours, several times a day. She had not had an attack for the past 5 years and she described the character of pain as a "boring, ice-pick." She was treated with the appropriate medications, and the headaches were aborted. She was discharged to be seen again as needed, if the headaches started again. Her diagnosis was episodic cluster headache.

MEDICAL HEADACHE HISTORY

Name: Carla **Age:** 41 **Sex** F **Date:** 12/9/91

Date of Birth: 00/00/50 **Birthplace:** IL **Race:** C **Education:** Some college

Occupation: Computer Programmer **Accident:** N/A

Armed Services & Type of Discharge: N/A

PAST HISTORY:

1.	Did you have a normal birth?		Yes (underlined)	No
	a) forceps used?		Yes	No
	b) cesarean section?		Yes	No (underlined)
2.	Did you have problems with bedwetting?		Yes	No (underlined)
	a) If yes, age bedwetting stopped		______	
3.	Were you car sick as a child (motion)?		Yes	No (underlined)
	a) If yes, how severe?	Slight	Moderate	Severe
4.	Did you have unexplained abdominal cramps as a child?		Yes (underlined)	No
5.	Did you have any of the following illnesses in childhood?			
	a) meningitis		Yes	No (underlined)
	b) encephalitis		Yes	No (underlined)
	c) scarlet fever		Yes	No (underlined)
	d) rheumatic fever		Yes	No (underlined)
6.	Did you have any head injuries as a child?		Yes	No (underlined)
	a) If yes, please explain: ______			
7.	Were you treated for emotional illness as a child?		Yes	No (underlined)

HABITS:

8.	Do you drink alcohol?	Yes	No (underlined)
	a) If yes, what kind and how much? ______		
	b) Does alcohol bring on or aggravate a headache?	Yes	No
9.	Do you smoke?	Yes (underlined)	No
	a) If yes, how much? Smoke one day per week		
	b) Does smoking or smoke-filled rooms cause or aggravate headaches?	Yes	No (underlined)
10.	Do you drink caffeinated beverages?	Yes (underlined)	No
	a) If yes, how much? 2 per day		

MENSTRUAL HISTORY:

At what age did menses begin? 13 Were they regular or irregular? WNL
How were they related to your headache? N/A
Are you or were you ever on Birth Control Pills? Yes Did they affect your headache? No
Have you had a hysterectomy, partial or total, and why? No
Are you in menopause, and if yes, how long? No
Are you on hormones, and if yes, which ones? No

HEADACHE ASSESSMENT FORM

HA PROFILE	INCAPACITATING #3	INTERFERING #2	IRRITATING #1
ONSET (Years ago and frequency)	Age 17, 2 to 4 every day for 6 to 7 weeks	N/A	As a teenager, occasionally
CURRENT FREQUENCY	None for last 5 years had headache yesterday	N/A	2 to 3 a week
TIME OF ONSET	All day, usually 2 to 4 every day	N/A	Mid-morning
DURATION	20 minutes to 2 hours	N/A	1 hour with OTC medication
CHARACTER	Boring, ice-pick	N/A	Tightness
PRODROME OR AURA	N/A	N/A	N/A
ASSOCIATING FEATURES	Nausea; Vomiting; Sensitivity to Light? Noise? Odors? Do you get pale or flush? Do your eyes or nose run? Does your nose get stuffy? Does the white of your eyes get red? Does your eyelid droop? Do you pace, or go to bed?	Nausea; Vomiting; Sensitivity to Light? Noise? Odors? Do you get pale or flush? Do your eyes or nose run? Does your nose get stuffy? Does the white of your eyes get red? Does your eyelid droop? Do you pace, or go to bed?	Nausea; Vomiting; Sensitivity to Light? Noise? Odors? Do you get pale or flush? Do your eyes or nose run? Does your nose get stuffy? Does the white of your eyes get red? Does your eyelid droop? Do you pace, or go to bed?
PRECIPITATING OR AGGRAVATING FEATURES	Coughing	N/A	N/A

LOCATION: Mark the location for each type of headache with a different color pen.

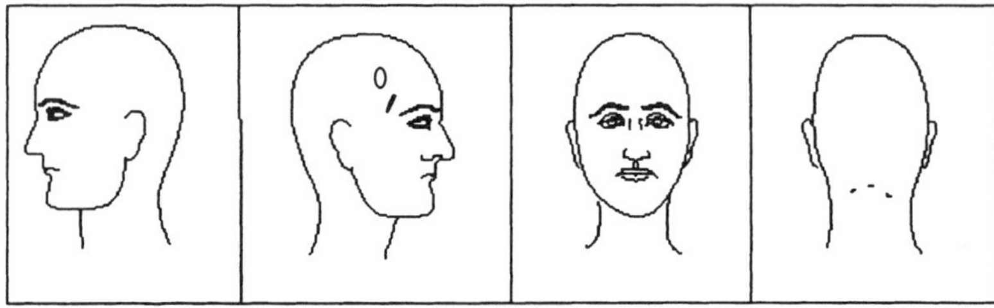

MEDICAL HISTORY:

Have you ever been or are you currently being treated for any of the following?

a) high blood pressure	Yes	No
b) stomach ulcers	Yes	No
c) asthma	Yes	No
d) allergies	Yes	No
e) pneumonia	Yes	No
f) kidney problems	Yes	No
g) low blood sugar	Yes	No
h) glaucoma	Yes	No
i) diabetes	Yes	No
j) heart problems	Yes	No

If you answered yes to any of the above, please describe:__________

List all other medical problems you have had in the past. Include date diagnosed and treatment.
DO NOT LIST OPERATIONS

1988 – Inpatient treatment for alcoholism and drug addiction.

SURGICAL HISTORY (List operations and dates performed)

1973 – Breast augmentation. 1955 – Tonsillectomy. 1990 – D&C after miscarriage.

PSYCHIATRIC HISTORY (List visits with counselors, psychologists, etc., and type of treatment)

Treatment in recovery (see above).

ACCIDENTS IN ADULT LIFE (Briefly describe any accident that caused any blow to the head or that you feel is related to your headache)

None.

FAMILY HISTORY:

1. Is your father living? Yes No
   - Age 64
   - Cause of death__________
   - Was there a headache history? Yes No
2. Is your mother living? Yes No
   - Age 61
   - Cause of death__________
   - Was there a headache history? Yes No

3. Ages of brothers---Circle the ones with headache
   39 36 30
4. Ages of sisters---Circle the ones with headache
   None. .
5. List any other blood relatives with a history of severe headaches.
   None.

MARITAL HISTORY:
List marriages:

1st marriage age 19 to 20	Did spouse have headaches?	Yes	No
2nd marriage age 31 to 32	Did spouse have headaches?	Yes	No
3rd marriage age 35 to 38	Did spouse have headaches?	Yes	No

Age of current spouse: N/A

List ages and sex of all children:

Age ______	Sex ______	Headaches?	Yes	No
Age ______	Sex ______	Headaches?	Yes	No
Age ______	Sex ______	Headaches?	Yes	No

STRESS FACTORS:

List any factors that may be affecting your headaches (money, loneliness, sexual problems, work, etc.)
Money, loneliness, work problems.

VEGETATIVE SIGNS:

1.	Do you have trouble falling asleep?		Yes	No
2.	Do you have trouble staying asleep?		Yes	No
3.	Has your appetite decreased?		Yes	No
4.	Have you gained or lost weight in the past year?	?	Yes	No
5.	Have you felt tearful or depressed lately?		Yes	No
6.	Have you had any thoughts of wanting to die?		Yes	No
7.	Have you been forgetful lately?		Yes	No
8.	Any other changes in your normal day-to-day living?______			

Please list any medications you are allergic or sensitive to: Darvon

Please list any medications you are currently taking (including dosages and frequency per day):
None

PREVIOUS CARE:

1. List doctors who have treated you for headaches: Dr. C., Dr. D.

2. List any tests you have had for your headache (e.g., EEG, CT scan, MRI, X-Ray, etc.):

EEG 5 years ago (abnormal).

CT scan of head without contrast 5 years ago (normal)

3. List any other treatment you have had for your headache (e.g., biofeedback, acupuncture, chiropractic, or any other treatment you had):

Chiropractic (no help).

GARY
Category: Cluster headaches

This 37-year-old man came in having headache attacks three to four times a day. The pain was described as both "ice pick" and "throbbing" and he also gives unusual symptoms for a cluster headache, such as having nausea, vomiting, and sensitivity to light, noise, and odors.

Alcohol will precipitate an attack, which is almost always seen when someone is in a cluster period. The patient has to pace when he gets a headache and, again, this is fairly normal with a cluster headache patient. Another interesting feature of many cluster patients is they smoke a great deal. He smokes at least two packs of cigarettes a day, and drinks 15 cups of coffee a day. He is a large man, 6 ft, 2 in., 212 pounds, and looks like a very tough man, except when he gets a headache attack. As Dr. John Graham says, they become extremely passive.

The patient was treated with the appropriate course to abort these headaches. After his cluster attacks were aborted, the patient did not return for further treatment. His diagnosis would be episodic cluster headache.

MEDICAL HEADACHE HISTORY

Name: Gary **Age:** 37 **Sex** M **Date:** 5/23/89

Date of Birth: 00/00/52 **Birthplace:** D.C. **Race:** C **Education:** 11th Grade

Occupation: Drywall Contractor **Accident:** N/A

Armed Services & Type of Discharge: Army 1970-1971, Undesirable

PAST HISTORY:

1.	Did you have a normal birth?		<u>Yes</u>	No
	a) forceps used?		Yes	<u>No</u>
	b) cesarean section?		Yes	<u>No</u>
2.	Did you have problems with bedwetting?		Yes	<u>No</u>
	a) If yes, age bedwetting stopped		______	
3.	Were you car sick as a child (motion)?		Yes	<u>No</u>
	a) If yes, how severe?	Slight	Moderate	Severe
4.	Did you have unexplained abdominal cramps as a child?		Yes	<u>No</u>
5.	Did you have any of the following illnesses in childhood?			
	a) meningitis		Yes	<u>No</u>
	b) encephalitis		Yes	<u>No</u>
	c) scarlet fever		Yes	<u>No</u>
	d) rheumatic fever		Yes	<u>No</u>
6.	Did you have any head injuries as a child?		Yes	<u>No</u>
	a) If yes, please explain:______			
7.	Were you treated for emotional illness as a child?		Yes	<u>No</u>

HABITS:

8.	Do you drink alcohol?	<u>Yes</u>	No
	a) If yes, what kind and how much? Case of beer per week		
	b) Does alcohol bring on or aggravate a headache?	<u>Yes</u>	No
9.	Do you smoke?	<u>Yes</u>	No
	a) If yes, how much? Two packs a day		
	b) Does smoking or smoke-filled rooms cause or aggravate headaches?	Yes	<u>No</u>
10.	Do you drink caffeinated beverages?	<u>Yes</u>	No
	a) If yes, how much? 15 cups coffee per day		

MENSTRUAL HISTORY:

At what age did menses begin?______ Were they regular or irregular?______
How were they related to your headache?______
Are you or were you ever on Birth Control Pills?______ Did they affect your headache? ______
Have you had a hysterectomy, partial or total, and why?______
Are you in menopause, and if yes, how long?______
Are you on hormones, and if yes, which ones?______

HEADACHE ASSESSMENT FORM

HA PROFILE	INCAPACITATING #3	INTERFERING #2	IRRITATING #1
ONSET (Years ago and frequency)	16 years ago – 1 a year 3 – 4 a day	N/A	N/A
CURRENT FREQUENCY	Started 1 wk ago. Had none for 3 years	N/A	N/A
TIME OF ONSET	Anytime, usually at night	N/A	N/A
DURATION	1 to 3 hours	N/A	N/A
CHARACTER	Ice pick pain, throbbing	N/A	N/A
PRODROME OR AURA	N/A	N/A	N/A
ASSOCIATING FEATURES	Nausea; Vomiting; Sensitivity to Light? Noise? Odors? Do you get pale or flush? Do your eyes or nose run? Does your nose get stuffy? Does the white of your eyes get red? Does your eyelid droop? Do you pace, or go to bed?	Nausea; Vomiting; Sensitivity to Light? Noise? Odors? Do you get pale or flush? Do your eyes or nose run? Does your nose get stuffy? Does the white of your eyes get red? Does your eyelid droop? Do you pace, or go to bed?	Nausea; Vomiting; Sensitivity to Light? Noise? Odors? Do you get pale or flush? Do your eyes or nose run? Does your nose get stuffy? Does the white of your eyes get red? Does your eyelid droop? Do you pace, or go to bed?
PRECIPITATING OR AGGRAVATING FEATURES	Alcohol Vomiting eases pain momentarily	N/A	N/A

LOCATION: Mark the location for each type of headache with a different color pen.

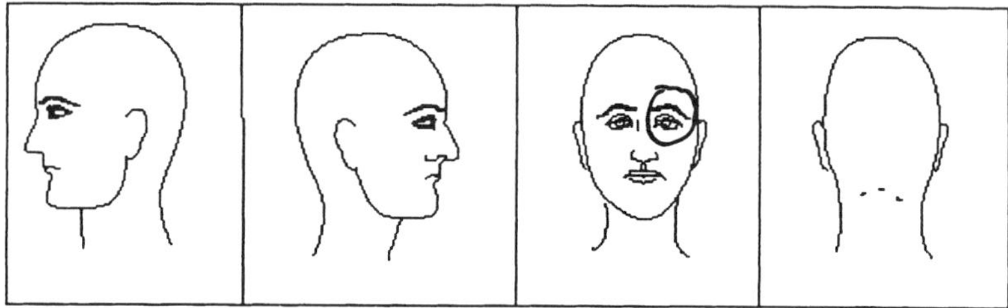

MEDICAL HISTORY:

Have you ever been or are you currently being treated for any of the following?

a) high blood pressure	Yes	No
b) stomach ulcers	Yes	No
c) asthma	Yes	No
d) allergies	Yes	No
e) pneumonia	Yes	No
f) kidney problems	Yes	No
g) low blood sugar	Yes	No
h) glaucoma	Yes	No
i) diabetes	Yes	No
j) heart problems	Yes	No

If you answered yes to any of the above, please describe:____________________

List all other medical problems you have had in the past. Include date diagnosed and treatment. DO NOT LIST OPERATIONS

Car accident, age 11. Broken left femur. Dislocated and broken right shoulder. Broken left ankle.

SURGICAL HISTORY (List operations and dates performed)

Pin put in left femur, removed 1 year later. Shoulder muscle operated on 1 year after accident.

Tonsillectomy & Adenoidectomy, age 6.

PSYCHIATRIC HISTORY (List visits with counselors, psychologists, etc., and type of treatment)

N/A.

ACCIDENTS IN ADULT LIFE (Briefly describe any accident that caused any blow to the head or that you feel is related to your headache)

N/A.

FAMILY HISTORY:

1. Is your father living? Yes No
   - Age 63
   - Cause of death________________
   - Was there a headache history? Yes No
2. Is your mother living? Yes No
   - Age________
   - Cause of death Car accident, age 31
   - Was there a headache history? Yes No
3. Ages of brothers---Circle the ones with headache
   - None

4. Ages of sisters---Circle the ones with headache
   None
5. List any other blood relatives with a history of severe headaches.
   None

MARITAL HISTORY:
List marriages:

1st marriage age 21 to Now Did spouse have headaches?	Yes	No
2nd marriage age ___ to ___ Did spouse have headaches?	Yes	No
3rd marriage age ___ to ___ Did spouse have headaches?	Yes	No

Age of current spouse:___________

List ages and sex of all children:

Age 14 Sex M Headaches?	Yes	No
Age 9 Sex M Headaches?	Yes	No
Age 3 Sex F Headaches?	Yes	No
Age ___ Sex ___ Headaches?	Yes	No

STRESS FACTORS:

List any factors that may be affecting your headaches (money, loneliness, sexual problems, work, etc.)
Money

VEGETATIVE SIGNS:

1.	Do you have trouble falling asleep?	Yes	No
2.	Do you have trouble staying asleep?	Yes	No
3.	Has your appetite decreased?	Yes	No
4.	Have you gained or lost weight in the past year?	Yes	No
5.	Have you felt tearful or depressed lately?	Yes	No
6.	Have you had any thoughts of wanting to die?	Yes	No
7.	Have you been forgetful lately?	Yes	No
8.	Any other changes in your normal day-to-day living?___		

Please list any medications you are allergic or sensitive to: Codeine

Please list any medications you are currently taking (including dosages and frequency per day):
Methadone, every day.

PREVIOUS CARE:

1. List doctors who have treated you for headaches: Dr. C., Dr. D.

2. List any tests you have had for your headache (e.g., EEG, CT scan, MRI, X-Ray, etc.):

CAT scan, 1984 (normal).

Spinal tap, 15 years ago (normal).

3. List any other treatment you have had for your headache (e.g., biofeedback, acupuncture, chiropractic, or any other treatment you had):

N/A.

JANE
Category: Cluster headache

This is a rather interesting case of a 33-year-old woman who started having headaches several years before I saw her. When she came into the office three years later, the headaches had started to become a daily problem, for the past six months. The Headache Intake Form shows she was getting them daily. She awakens with them, and she can abort them in one hour after she takes medication. She does not have the typical symptoms of migraine, with nausea and vomiting, although there is throbbing and the pain is localized in the right back side of her head.

There is a diagnosis called chronic paroxysmal hemicrania, which is the female counterpart to cluster headache, although in this particular headache syndrome, the attacks are generally shorter and multiple. This particular woman has a variation of that type of headache, and was treated as a patient with CPH, or chronic paroxysmal hemicrania.

The value of this report shows that headache phenomena do not fall into easy-to-find categories, and sometimes one has to stretch the imagination in order to reduce the suffering of the patient.

She was placed on the appropriate medication for this, and did experience significant reduction of her pain. She was told that she would have to be on guard for further attacks of this type of headache.

MEDICAL HEADACHE HISTORY

Name: Jane **Age:** 33 **Sex** F **Date:** 4/23/90

Date of Birth: 00/00/57 **Birthplace:** D.C. **Race:** C **Education:** B.S.

Occupation: Homemaker **Accident:** N/A

Armed Services & Type of Discharge: N/A

PAST HISTORY:

1.	Did you have a normal birth?		Yes	No
	a) forceps used?		Yes	No
	b) cesarean section?		Yes	No
2.	Did you have problems with bedwetting?		Yes	No
	a) If yes, age bedwetting stopped			
3.	Were you car sick as a child (motion)?		Yes	No
	a) If yes, how severe?	Slight	Moderate	Severe
4.	Did you have unexplained abdominal cramps as a child?		Yes	No
5.	Did you have any of the following illnesses in childhood?			
	a) meningitis		Yes	No
	b) encephalitis		Yes	No
	c) scarlet fever		Yes	No
	d) rheumatic fever		Yes	No
6.	Did you have any head injuries as a child?		Yes	No
	a) If yes, please explain:			
7.	Were you treated for emotional illness as a child?		Yes	No

HABITS:

8.	Do you drink alcohol?	Yes	No
	a) If yes, what kind and how much?		
	b) Does alcohol bring on or aggravate a headache?	Yes	No
9.	Do you smoke?	Yes	No
	a) If yes, how much?		
	b) Does smoking or smoke-filled rooms cause or aggravate headaches?	Yes	No
10.	Do you drink caffeinated beverages?	Yes	No
	a) If yes, how much?		

MENSTRUAL HISTORY:

At what age did menses begin? 13 Were they regular or irregular? WNL

How were they related to your headache? N/A

Are you or were you ever on Birth Control Pills? Yes Did they affect your headache? No

Have you had a hysterectomy, partial or total, and why? No

Are you in menopause, and if yes, how long? No

Are you on hormones, and if yes, which ones? No

HEADACHE ASSESSMENT FORM

HA PROFILE	INCAPACITATING #3	INTERFERING #2	IRRITATING #1
ONSET (Years ago and frequency)	N/A	4/87 4 p.m. 11/89 to present	N/A
CURRENT FREQUENCY	N/A	Daily	N/A
TIME OF ONSET	N/A	Sometimes awaken with Usually a.m.	N/A
DURATION	N/A	½ to 1 hour with medication	N/A
CHARACTER	N/A	Throbbing	N/A
PRODROME OR AURA	N/A	N/A	N/A
ASSOCIATING FEATURES	Nausea; Vomiting; Sensitivity to Light? Noise? Odors? Do you get pale or flush? Do your eyes or nose run? Does your nose get stuffy? Does the white of your eyes get red? Does your eyelid droop? Do you pace, or go to bed?	Nausea; Vomiting; Sensitivity to Light? Noise? Odors? Do you get pale or flush? Do your eyes or nose run? Does your nose get stuffy? Does the white of your eyes get red? Does your eyelid droop? Do you pace, or go to bed?	Nausea; Vomiting; Sensitivity to Light? Noise? Odors? Do you get pale or flush? Do your eyes or nose run? Does your nose get stuffy? Does the white of your eyes get red? Does your eyelid droop? Do you pace, or go to bed?
PRECIPITATING OR AGGRAVATING FEATURES	N/A	N/A	N/A

LOCATION: Mark the location for each type of headache with a different color pen.

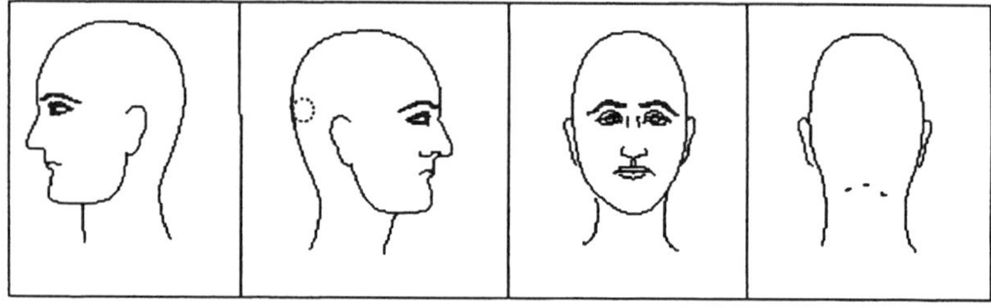

MEDICAL HISTORY:

Have you ever been or are you currently being treated for any of the following?

a) high blood pressure	Yes	No
b) stomach ulcers	Yes	No
c) asthma	Yes	No
d) allergies	Yes	No
e) pneumonia	Yes	No
f) kidney problems	Yes	No
g) low blood sugar	Yes	No
h) glaucoma	Yes	No
i) diabetes	Yes	No
j) heart problems	Yes	No

If you answered yes to any of the above, please describe: Pneumonia in 1970.

List all other medical problems you have had in the past. Include date diagnosed and treatment.
DO NOT LIST OPERATIONS

1987 – Onset of headaches, lasted approximately 4 months. Had eye examination, sinus exam, CAT scan, blood workup. Nothing conclusive reported. Ongoing problem with heel.

SURGICAL HISTORY (List operations and dates performed)

Hernia – 1958. Appendectomy – 1974. Tonsillectoy – 1975. Cesarean section – 1988.

PSYCHIATRIC HISTORY (List visits with counselors, psychologists, etc., and type of treatment)

N/A.

ACCIDENTS IN ADULT LIFE (Briefly describe any accident that caused any blow to the head or that you feel is related to your headache)

N/A.

FAMILY HISTORY:

1. Is your father living? Yes No
   - Age 70
   - Cause of death
   - Was there a headache history? Yes No
2. Is your mother living? Yes No
   - Age 63
   - Cause of death
   - Was there a headache history? Yes No

3. Ages of brothers---Circle the ones with headache
   42 4.1 36 34 21
4. Ages of sisters---Circle the ones with headache
   32 31 (25)
5. List any other blood relatives with a history of severe headaches.
   None.

MARITAL HISTORY:
List marriages:

1st marriage age __26__ to __Present__ Did spouse have headaches? Yes __No__
2nd marriage age _____ to _______ Did spouse have headaches? Yes No
3rd marriage age _____ to _______ Did spouse have headaches? Yes No
Age of current spouse: __33__

List ages and sex of all children:
Age __21 mo.__ Sex __M__ Headaches? Yes __No__
Age _____ Sex _____ Headaches? Yes No
Age _____ Sex _____ Headaches? Yes No

STRESS FACTORS:

List any factors that may be affecting your headaches (money, loneliness, sexual problems, work, etc.)
None.

VEGETATIVE SIGNS:

1. Do you have trouble falling asleep? Yes __No__
2. Do you have trouble staying asleep? Yes __No__
3. Has your appetite decreased? __Yes__ No
4. Have you gained or lost weight in the past year? Yes __No__
5. Have you felt tearful or depressed lately? Yes __No__
6. Have you had any thoughts of wanting to die? Yes __No__
7. Have you been forgetful lately? __Yes__ No
8. Any other changes in your normal day-to-day living? ______

Please list any medications you are allergic or sensitive to: None.

Please list any medications you are currently taking (including dosages and frequency per day):
Motrin IB as needed for headache (approximately 2 to 3 a day).

PREVIOUS CARE:

1. List doctors who have treated you for headaches: Dr. S.

2. List any tests you have had for your headache (e.g., EEG, CT scan, MRI, X-Ray, etc.):
CAT scan, sinus x-ray, sed rate test, eye exam.

3. List any other treatment you have had for your headache (e.g., biofeedback, acupuncture, chiropractic, or any other treatment you had):

Chapter 9

Sinus Headache

During the years of my practice, a day wouldn't go by without at least one of my new patients telling me one of their headaches was a sinus headache. While looking at television, advertisements in newspapers or magazines, or listening to the radio, one cannot go through the day without being told of some special medicine to cure "sinus headache." When walking through the supermarket or drugstore, one's eye is drawn to shelves of medications to treat sinus headaches. The amount of money spent to alleviate this problem is astronomical and yet it has been demonstrated that less than 2% of headaches are probably "sinus headaches."

The reason a chapter is devoted to this problem is that an attempt will be made to clarify this over-used term.

Sinusitis, or vasomotor rhinitis, is a very common disorder, but it is questionable how many people with this problem actually get a headache from it. Most studies indicate that if a headache is related to congestion of the sinuses, it is generally in the acute phase and rarely in the chronic phase of the condition. Most headache specialists are in agreement that most patients who complain of ongoing or recurrent sinus headache are probably suffering from one of the variants of migraine (Figure 9.1).

Sinuses are air pockets within bony structures in the nose, cheeks, and the frontal skull. These bony structures are covered with membranes that secrete mucus, which eventually flows down through the nose. During an acute infection or some type of inflammation, a severe allergic episode causes the sinuses to become congested. There is no opportunity for the flow of air through these sinuses, and pressure from this and the increased fluids will build and this will cause pain. As long as there is complete obstruction there will be pain. The pain is usually in the frontal part of the face and forehead (Figure 9.2) and generally mild to moderate and dull or aching. It is constant and nonthrobbing. The headache is relieved when there is a significant reduction of the fluids and a restoration of the air flow.

When the membranes lining the sinuses are inflamed, there is production of this fluid. However, during a vascular headache such as migraine, or cluster or migraine-like headaches, there is also dilatation of the blood vessels in these linings and this also causes secretion of fluids and similar sensations, mimicking the symptoms of a sinus headache. Another confusing element is that some medications that help sinus headache also help migraine. In many of the over-the-counter medications for sinus headache are decongestants and analgesics (aspirin or acetaminophen) and caffeine which often will help reduce the pain of migraine. Hence, the confusion over which type of headache was helped by this so-called sinus medication.

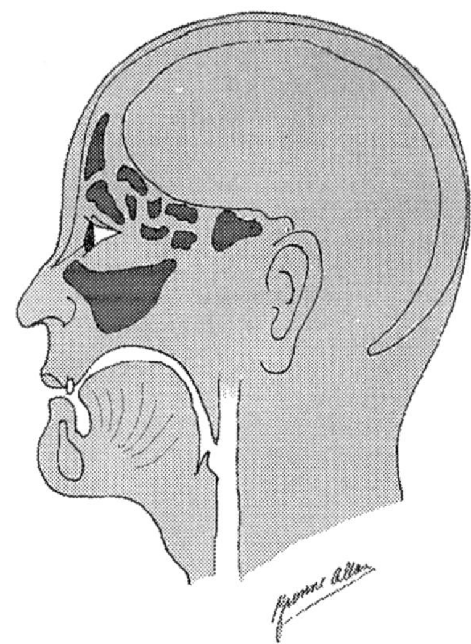

Figure 9.1 This illustration shows the various sinuses. Sinus headache is generally related to an acute sinusitis where there is total blockage. This may cause headache in the frontal, temporal, or occipital regions of the head. Often people who have migraine or muscle tension headache think they are having sinus headache. Sinus headaches are less frequent than advertisements lead us to believe.

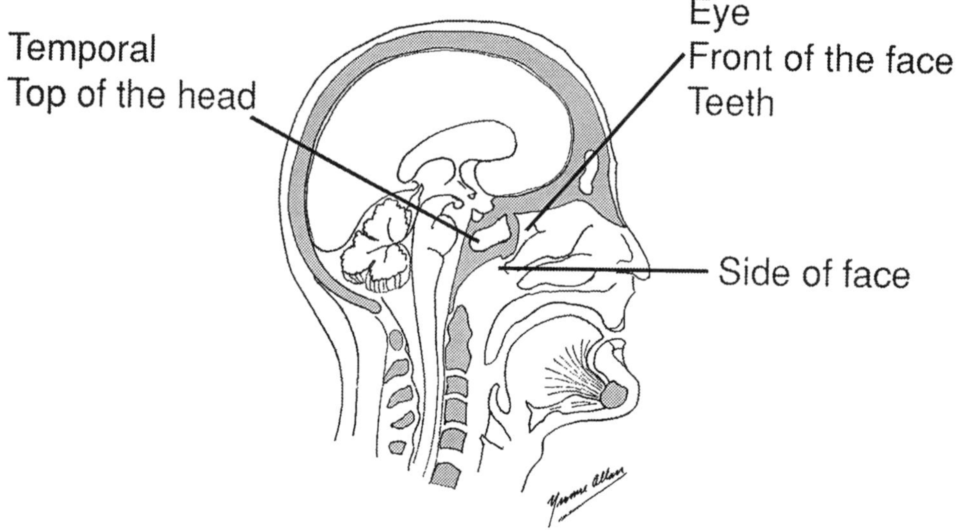

Figure 9.2 Shows pain from sinus obstruction referred to other regions of the head.

Other studies have shown that if a person has a chronic sinus condition there is usually enough of a passage between the sinuses and therefore not a complete obstruction and the severe pressure that causes the headache. Again, if someone has a chronic sinus condition and constant headaches, then the probability of a migraine variant is the more likely culprit.

If there is continued pain and discharge of fluids from the nasal passages, then an investigation of more serious diseases should be pursued. Mucous cysts called mucoceles could develop and this might cause obstruction of the sinus or cause erosion of the bone, which is very painful. Although sinus headache is exaggerated, infection of the sinuses can be extremely dangerous. If there is a collection of pus there is a possibility that this could lead to a cerebral abscess or spread an infection to the blood stream. Although rare, continued pain and discharge should be evaluated by an ear, nose and throat specialist (otolaryngologist) to rule out the possibility of a malignant disease.

Once the patient understands, taking unnecessary medications that may mask serious situations and the likelihood of delaying proper treatment for vascular headaches may be avoided.

The following case history should provide you with a better understanding of the sinus headache and any similar type of headache that may be related to post traumatic head injury or whiplash.

CASE HISTORY*

ROBIN
Category: Sinus headache

Although this is not a true sinus headache condition, this history is placed in this chapter because it appears that the headache followed some nasal reconstructive surgery and appeared to be a vascular type of headache. Symptoms were throbbing, photophobia, sonophobia, and the patient has to go to bed. Quick movements and lifting any weight seemed to increase the headache.

This patient stated that seven years before seeing me she had some nasal surgery for reconstruction of her sinuses and the headaches seemed to start almost at that point. She did report, though, that there were some occasional headaches prior to the surgery. However, since the surgery, she had been having these attacks four to five times a week. Her initial diagnosis was

1. atypical vascular headaches,
2. atypical muscle contraction headaches,
3. rule out reconstructive sinus condition.

An x-ray series of the sinuses was done and was reported back as normal. Most likely these headaches are a vascular type of headache that were precipitated or triggered by the sinus surgery. That is something that happens with migraine-type headaches, in that there are various triggering mechanisms that precipitate this kind of headache. So, in fact, this is a migraine-type headache.

* On the headache assessment form that accompanies this case history, the patient's interfering headaches are shown with dotted lines.

MEDICAL HEADACHE HISTORY

Name: Robin **Age:** 30 **Sex** F **Date:** 1/7/91

Date of Birth: 00/00/60 **Birthplace:** IL **Race:** C **Education:** High school

Occupation: Receptionist **Accident:** N/A

Armed Services & Type of Discharge: N/A

PAST HISTORY:

1.	Did you have a normal birth?		Yes	No
	a) forceps used?		Yes	No
	b) cesarean section?		Yes	No
2.	Did you have problems with bedwetting?		Yes	No
	a) If yes, age bedwetting stopped			
3.	Were you car sick as a child (motion)?		Yes	No
	a) If yes, how severe?	Slight	Moderate	Severe
4.	Did you have unexplained abdominal cramps as a child?		Yes	No
5.	Did you have any of the following illnesses in childhood?			
	a) meningitis		Yes	No
	b) encephalitis		Yes	No
	c) scarlet fever		Yes	No
	d) rheumatic fever		Yes	No
6.	Did you have any head injuries as a child?		Yes	No
	a) If yes, please explain:			
7.	Were you treated for emotional illness as a child?		Yes	No

HABITS:

8.	Do you drink alcohol?	Yes	No
	a) If yes, what kind and how much? Occasional		
	b) Does alcohol bring on or aggravate a headache?	Yes	No
9.	Do you smoke?	Yes	No
	a) If yes, how much?		
	b) Does smoking or smoke-filled rooms cause or aggravate headaches?	Yes	No
10.	Do you drink caffeinated beverages?	Yes	No
	a) If yes, how much?		

MENSTRUAL HISTORY:

At what age did menses begin? 12 Were they regular or irregular? WNL

How were they related to your headache? N/A

Are you or were you ever on Birth Control Pills? Yes Did they affect your headache? No

Have you had a hysterectomy, partial or total, and why? No

Are you in menopause, and if yes, how long? No

Are you on hormones, and if yes, which ones? No

HEADACHE ASSESSMENT FORM

HA PROFILE	INCAPACITATING #3	INTERFERING #2	IRRITATING #1
ONSET (Years ago and frequency)	N/A	8 years ago Occasional	N/A
CURRENT FREQUENCY	N/A	3 to 4 times a week; headaches have increased since nose surgery	N/A
TIME OF ONSET	N/A	Anytime	N/A
DURATION	N/A	All day	N/A
CHARACTER	N/A	Throbbing	N/A
PRODROME OR AURA	N/A	N/A	N/A
ASSOCIATING FEATURES	Nausea; Vomiting; Sensitivity to Light? Noise? Odors? Do you get pale or flush? Do your eyes or nose run? Does your nose get stuffy? Do the whites of your eyes get red? Does your eyelid droop? Do you pace, or go to bed?	Nausea; Vomiting; Sensitivity to Light? Noise? Odors? Do you get pale or flush? Do your eyes or nose run? Does your nose get stuffy? Do the whites of your eyes get red? Does your eyelid droop? Do you pace, or go to bed?	Nausea; Vomiting; Sensitivity to Light? Noise? Odors? Do you get pale or flush? Do your eyes or nose run? Does your nose get stuffy? Do the whites of your eyes get red? Does your eyelid droop? Do you pace, or go to bed?
PRECIPITATING OR AGGRAVATING FEATURES	N/A	Lifting weights Quick movement	N/A

LOCATION: Mark the location for each type of headache with a different color pen.

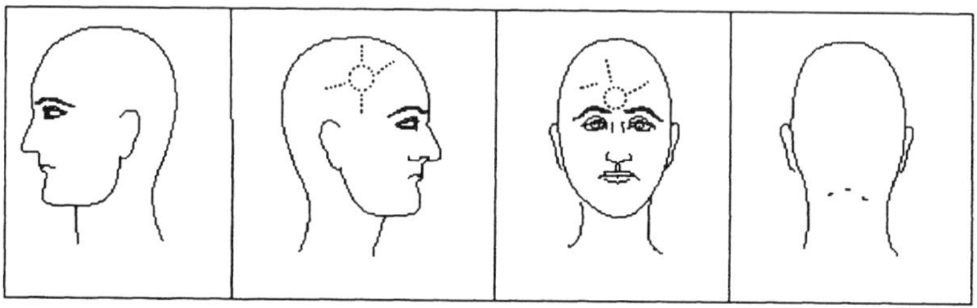

MEDICAL HISTORY:

Have you ever been or are you currently being treated for any of the following?

a) high blood pressure	Yes	No
b) stomach ulcers	Yes	No
c) asthma	Yes	No
d) allergies	Yes	No
e) pneumonia	Yes	No
f) kidney problems	Yes	No
g) low blood sugar	Yes	No
h) glaucoma	Yes	No
i) diabetes	Yes	No
j) heart problems	Yes	No

If you answered yes to any of the above, please describe:____________________

List all other medical problems you have had in the past. Include date diagnosed and treatment.
DO NOT LIST OPERATIONS

Mammogram – refrain from caffeine.

SURGICAL HISTORY (List operations and dates performed)

Nose reconstructive surgery – 1994. Tonsillectomy & Adenoidectomy – age 10.

PSYCHIATRIC HISTORY (List visits with counselors, psychologists, etc., and type of treatment)

None

ACCIDENTS IN ADULT LIFE (Briefly describe any accident that caused any blow to the head or that you feel is related to your headache)

Pulled a muscle in right shoulder 6 months ago.

FAMILY HISTORY:

1.	Is your father living?	Yes	No
	Age________		
	Cause of death Unknown		
	Was there a headache history?	Yes	No
2.	Is your mother living?	Yes	No
	Age 60		
	Cause of death________		
	Was there a headache history?	Yes	No

3. Ages of brothers---Circle the ones with headache
   24, 27, 36, 40
4. Ages of sisters---Circle the ones with headache
   38
5. List any other blood relatives with a history of severe headaches.
   N/A

MARITAL HISTORY:
List marriages:

1st marriage age 19 to 21	Did spouse have headaches?	Yes	No
2nd marriage age 22 to 30	Did spouse have headaches?	Yes	No
3rd marriage age ______ to ______	Did spouse have headaches?	Yes	No

Age of current spouse: N/A

List ages and sex of all children:

Age _____ Sex ______	Headaches?	Yes	No
Age _____ Sex ______	Headaches?	Yes	No
Age _____ Sex ______	Headaches?	Yes	No

STRESS FACTORS:

List any factors that may be affecting your headaches (money, loneliness, sexual problems, work, etc.)
Fast paced, stressful job.

VEGETATIVE SIGNS:

1.	Do you have trouble falling asleep?	Yes	No
2.	Do you have trouble staying asleep?	Yes	No
3.	Has your appetite decreased?	Yes	No
4.	Have you gained or lost weight in the past year?	Yes	No
5.	Have you felt tearful or depressed lately?	Yes	No
6.	Have you had any thoughts of wanting to die?	Yes	No
7.	Have you been forgetful lately?	Yes	No
8.	Any other changes in your normal day-to-day living?______		

Please list any medications you are allergic or sensitive to: None

Please list any medications you are currently taking (including dosages and frequency per day):
Birth control pills – TriPhasil.

PREVIOUS CARE:

1. List doctors who have treated you for headaches: None

2. List any tests you have had for your headache (e.g., EEG, CT scan, MRI, X-Ray, etc.):
None

3. List any other treatment you have had for your headache (e.g., biofeedback, acupuncture, chiropractic, or any other treatment you had):
None.

Chapter 10

Other Causes of Headache

There are hundreds of reasons why patients suffer the pain of headache. In this chapter I will list the International Headache Society's Classification of Headaches that can be associated with causes from inside or outside of the body. These headaches may be a primary or secondary symptom of this precipitating event. An attempt will be made to explain some of these events.[1]

Ice pick headache (idiopathic stabbing headache) — These headaches have been described as transient stabs of pain that do not have any physical cause. The pain is usually in the upper part of the head, around the eyes, the temples, and the side of the head (parietal). The pain lasts only a fraction of a second and occurs as a single stab or a series of stabs. The frequency is irregular and commonly is seen more often with migraine patients, and often the pain is at the site of that headache. Indomethacin 25 mg three times a day is the treatment of choice.

Swim-goggle headache (external compression headache) — This headache results from the application of pressure around the head causing a stimulation of the nerves around that part of the head. It is a constant pain and is corrected by removing the stimulus. If the stimulus is prolonged, it might lead to a migraine attack.

Cold stimulus headache — This is a headache from an external source such as being exposed to sub-zero weather or diving into very cold water. Eliminating the source is all that is necessary to relieve this problem.

Internal stimulus headache — Also called ice cream headache. This is caused by the passage of very cold material over the palate and the posterior pharyngeal wall. Again the people most subject to this pain are the migraine population. The pain is usually felt in the middle forehead. Eating or drinking this food slowly will often eliminate this problem.

Benign cough headache — This is a bilateral headache precipitated by coughing and is not related to any lesion in the cranium, and lasts less than one minute.

Weight-lifters headache or benign exertional headache — This headache is brought on by exercise. My experience has been that exercise where there is significant neck movement will cause this headache and exercises such as swimming or stationary cycling often avoid this problem. The headache is usually throbbing and may develop migrainous features and will last minutes to an entire day.

Orgasmic cephalgia or headache associated with sexual activity — There appears to be three types of headache secondary to sexual activity. One type of headache may be related to excessive contraction of head and neck muscles. This is often seen in men who have muscular necks and the pain is dull and increases during the evolution of sexual excitement. The pain subsides

Table 10.1

4. Miscellaneous headaches not associated with structural lesion
   - 4.1 Idiopathic stabbing headache, previously called ice pick pains
   - 4.2 External compression headache
   - 4.3 Cold stimulus headache
     - 4.3.1 External application of a cold stimulus
     - 4.3.2 Ingestion of a cold stimulus
   - 4.4 Benign cough headache
   - 4.5 Benign exertional headache
   - 4.6 Headache associated with sexual activity
     - 4.6.1 Dull type
     - 4.6.2 Explosive type
     - 4.6.3 Postural type

5. Headache associated with head trauma
   - 5.1 Acute post traumatic headache
     - 5.1.1 With significant head trauma and/or confirmatory signs
     - 5.1.2 With minor head trauma and no confirmatory signs
   - 5.2 Chronic post traumatic headache
     - 5.2.1 With significant head trauma and/or confirmatory signs
     - 5.2.2 With minor head trauma and no confirmatory signs

6. Headache associated with vascular disorders
   - 6.1 Acute ischemic cerebrovascular disease
     - 6.1.1 Transient ischemic attack (TIA)
     - 6.1.2 Thromboembolic stroke
   - 6.2 Intracranial hematoma
     - 6.2.1 Intracerebral hematoma
     - 6.2.2 Subdural hematoma
     - 6.2.3 Epidural hematoma
   - 6.3 Subarachnoid hemorrhage
   - 6.4 Unruptured vascular malformation
     - 6.4.1 Arteriovenous malformation
     - 6.4.2 Saccular aneurysm
   - 6.5 Arteritis
     - 6.5.1 Giant cell arteritis
     - 6.5.2 Other systemic arteritides
     - 6.5.3 Primary intracranial arterites
   - 6.6 Carotid or vertebral artery pain
     - 6.6.1 Carotid or vertebral dissection
     - 6.6.2 Carotidynia (idiopathic)
     - 6.6.3 Postendarterectomy headache
   - 6.7 Venous thrombosis
   - 6.8 Arterial hypertension
     - 6.8.1 Acute pressor response to exogenous agent
     - 6.8.2 Pheochromocytoma
     - 6.8.3 Malignant (accelerated) hypertension
     - 6.8.4 Preeclampsia and eclampsia
   - 6.9 Headache associated with other vascular disorder

7. Headache associated with nonvascular intracranial disorder
   - 7.1 High cerebrospinal fluid pressure
     - 7.1.1 Benign intracranial hypertension
     - 7.1.2 High pressure hydrocephalus
   - 7.2 Low cerebrospinal fluid pressure
     - 7.2.1 Postlumbar puncture headache
     - 7.2.2 Cerebrospinal fluid fistula headache
   - 7.3 Intracranial infection
   - 7.4 Intracranial sarcoidosis and other noninfectious inflammatory diseases
   - 7.5 Headache related to intrathecal injections

Table 10.1 (continued)

7.5.1 Direct effect
7.5.2 Due to chemical meningitis
7.6 Intracranial neoplasm
7.7 Headache associated with other intracranial disorder

8. Headache associated with substance or with withdrawal
8.1 Headache induced by acute substance use or exposure
8.1.1 Nitrate/nitrite-induced headache
8.1.2 Monosodium glutamate-induced headache
8.1.3 Carbon monoxide-induced headache
8.1.4 Alcohol-induced headache
8.1.5 Other substances
8.2 Headache induced by chronic substance use or exposure
8.2.1 Ergotamine and related compounds (methysergide [Sansert])-induced headache
8.2.2 Analgesics abuse headache
8.2.3 Other substances
8.3 Headache from substance withdrawal (acute use)
8.3.1 Alcohol withdrawal headache (hangover)
8.3.2 Other substances
8.4 Headache from substance withdrawal (chronic use)
8.4.1 Ergotomine withdrawal headache
8.4.2 Caffeine withdrawal headache
8.4.3 Narcotics abstinence headache
8.4.4 Other substances
8.5 Headache associated with substances but with uncertain mechanism
8.5.1 Birth control pills or estrogens
8.5.2 Other substances

9. Headache associated with noncephalic infection
9.1 Viral infection
9.1.1 Focal noncephalic
9.1.2 Systemic
9.2 Bacterial infection
9.2.1 Focal noncephalic
9.2.2 Systemic (septicemia)
9.3 Headache related to other infection

10. Headache associated with metabolic disorder
10.1 Hypoxia
10.1.1 High altitude headache
10.1.2 Hypoxic headache
10.1.3 Sleep apnea headache
10.2 Hypercapnia
10.3 Mixed hypoxia and hypercapnia
10.4 Hypoglycemia
10.5 Dialysis
10.6 Headache related to other metabolic abnormality

11. Headache or facial pain associated with disorder of cranium, neck, eyes, nose, sinuses, teeth, mouth, or other facial or cranial structures
11.1 Cranial bone
11.2 Neck
11.2.1 Cervical spine
11.2.2 Retropharyngeal tendinitis
11.3 Eyes
11.3.1 Acute glaucoma
11.3.2 Refractive errors
11.3.3 Heterophoria or heterotropia
11.4 Ears

Table 10.1 (continued)

	11.5	Nose and sinuses		
		11.5.1	Acute sinus headache	
		11.5.2	Other diseases of nose and sinuses	
	11.6	Teeth, jaws, and related structures		
	11.7	Temporomandibular joint disease		
12.	Cranial neuralgias, nerve trunk pain and deafferentation pain			
	12.1	Persistent (in contrast to tic-like) pain of cranial nerve origin		
		12.1.1	Compression or distortion of cranial nerves and second or third cervical roots	
		12.1.2	Demyelination of cranial nerves	
			12.1.2.1	Optic neuritis (retrobulbar neuritis)
		12.1.3	Infarction of cranial nerves	
			12.1.3.1	Diabetic neuritis
		12.1.4	Inflammation of cranial nerves	
			12.1.4.1	Herpes zoster
			12.1.4.2	Chronic post-herpetic neuralgia
		12.1.5	Tolosa-Hunt syndrome	
		12.1.6	Neck tongue syndrome	
		12.1.7	Other causes of persistent pain of cranial nerve origin	
	12.2	Trigeminal neuralgia		
		12.2.1	Idiopathic trigeminal neuralgia	
		12.2.2	Symptomatic trigeminal neuralgia	
			12.2.2.1	Compression of trigeminal root or ganglion
			12.2.2.2	Central lesions
	12.3	Glossopharyngeal neuralgia		
		12.3.1	Idiopathic glossopharyngeal neuralgia	
		12.3.2	Symptomatic glossopharyngeal neuralgia	
	12.4	Nervus intermedia neuralgia		
	12.5	Superior laryngeal neuralgia		
	12.6	Occipital neuralgia		
	12.7	Central causes of head and facial pain other than tic douloureux		
		12.7.1	Anesthesia dolorosa	
		12.7.2	Thalamic pain	
	12.8	Facial pain not fulfilling criteria in groups 11 or 12		
13.	Headaches not classifiable			

with relaxation. A second type of headache is characterized by an intense, explosive pain generally during orgasm. This pain may be due to a rapid increase in blood pressure and dilatation of the arterial blood vessels. A third type is seen when a standing position is attempted and is relieved when a reclining position is taken. This headache may be due to a change in the pressure of the cerebrospinal fluid, suggesting a tear in the covering of the brain (arachnoid membrane). This is a benign condition. These headaches are seen more in men than women and are considered benign. However, abnormalities in the brain may also cause these headaches with increased pressure. If this problem arises, a neurological examination is recommended as soon as these symptoms display themselves. Some anti-migraine medications taken before intercourse may relieve benign sexual activity headaches.

Headache associated with head trauma — These headaches are discussed in Part two of this book.

Headache associated with vascular disorders — Alterations of the pressure in the brain generally cause headache. Therefore, in any condition in which there is bleeding or an abnormal increase in the size of the blood vessel that causes an increase of intracranial pressure, a headache will ensue.

Transient ischemic attack or TIA — About 40% of people who have this attack will get a headache. In this attack there is not an increase of pressure in the brain. Also, these attacks resolve themselves within 24 hours. The symptoms are similar to the symptoms of a stroke and then go into a remission. The headache can last from minutes to days. The headache can be steady or throbbing. The mechanism of the headache is not clear and probably there is an alteration of the chemistry affecting serotonin that sets off other headaches like migraine.

Temporal arteritis or giant cell arteritis or Horton disease — This disease is found in women three to four times more frequently than men and generally is seen in people over the age of 50. This is an inflammatory disorder of the arteries. Symptoms of this disease are headache, pain in jaw muscles, double vision or blindness, weight loss, fever, night sweats, and some anemia. This is often associated with pain and stiffness of the joints (polymyalgia rheumatica). The headache is generally one-sided, often located in the temporal region, and is generally boring and burning. The pain is often worse at night and in cold weather. The area around the superficial temporal artery is often tender and reddened. It is important to have the diagnosis made as soon as possible, because blindness is a realistic possibility, and because there is compromise of the ophthalmic artery to the optic nerve. Laboratory blood work, especially the sedimentation rate and a biopsy of the artery, will help in making the diagnosis. Prednisone is often started as soon as the diagnosis is suspected, to prevent blindness (Figure 10.1).

Carotidynia — There is a relationship between this disease and migraine about 50% of the time. Along with the headache is throbbing discomfort in the neck. It is found in people of all ages and the attacks last from minutes to hours and occur over several days. Medications for migraine plus prednisone are often effective. There are many different arterial diseases that have to be considered.

Hypertension and headache — Although for many years it was thought that there was a direct relationship between high blood pressure and headache, the evidence to support this concept has been subject to controversy. Chronic high blood pressure that does not fluctuate does not seem to be responsible for headache. However, a sudden rise in pressure secondary to exertion or a pathological condition can cause headache. A tumor of the adrenal gland called pheochromocytoma. which causes excessive production of chemicals that produce a rapid increase of blood pressure will cause a significant headache. Other symptoms of this tumor are rapid heart beat (tachycardia), sweating, pallor, and sometimes a loss of consciousness. The symptoms of the headache are throbbing and sometimes nausea and vomiting and the headache is often experienced for less than an hour. Laboratory and radiological methods are used to make the diagnosis. Other causes of rapid increase of blood pressure, such as sneezing, laughing, yawning, coughing, or sexual exertion, can also precipitate a headache that has throbbing, stabbing, or lancinating pain. These symptoms are generally seen more frequently with people who have a preexisting problem with headaches.

Dialysis and headache — Both patients with migraine and many without will experience a severe migraine like headache within hours of having dialysis. The headache is throbbing, often accompanied with nausea and vomiting, and is bilateral.

Pseudotumor cerebri — This disease acts as though there is a tumor in the brain, but in fact there is no mass or tumor. There is an increase of intracranial hypertension and this causes headache and gradually diminishing vision. There are many other diseases that are associated with pseudotumor cerebri that may be responsible for increasing intracranial pressure. This problem is seen more often in obese women. The headache of pseudotumor cerebri is nonspecific and diagnosing this condition is mostly done by excluding space-occupying lesions and other conditions that cause increased intracranial pressure.

Hypoglycemia — Missing meals or fasting for more than 5 to 6 hours reduces the glucose or sugar levels in the blood. Persons with migraine will often develop severe headache. Persons who were never diagnosed with migraine may also get headache and my suspicion is that these people, if they never experienced a migraine attack, are latent migraine sufferers. Although the exact mechanism of what causes the headache is unknown, the alteration of the metabolism may create excitement in the brain and this may trigger the headache pattern that was discussed in Chapter 3.

Vitamins and headache — It has been shown that high doses of vitamin A may aggravate headache disorders. Large doses of vitamin A may also cause other unpleasant symptoms. This

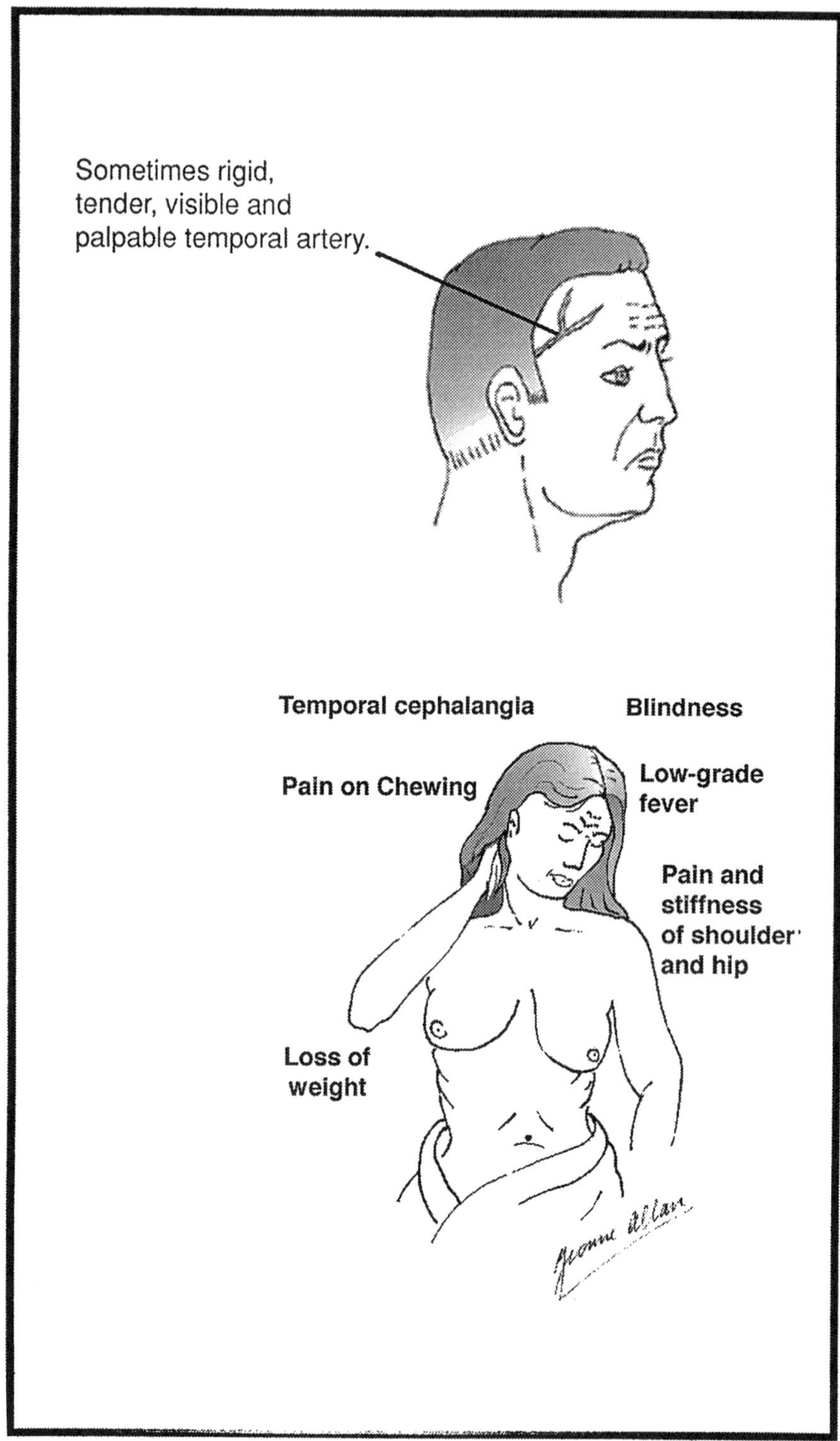

Figure 10.1 Temporal arteritis, seen twice as often in women, may be demonstrated by a rigid, tender, nonpulsating temporal artery which may be visible or palpable. Other symptoms are pain on chewing, loss of weight, weakness of muscles, symmetrical pain in the shoulders and hips, and low grade fever. Blindness may develop.

was originally discovered when arctic explorers ate large amounts of polar bear liver and became ill and had headaches. The headache is nonspecific and can be throbbing or nonthrobbing. Other symptoms of vitamin A overdosage are gastrointestinal distress, vertigo, pseudotumor cerebri, especially in children, blurred vision, double vision (diplopia), enlarged liver (hepatomegaly), joint pain, loss of hair (alopecia), textural skin changes, and fissures of the lips.

Alcohol and headache — Persons with migraine and cluster are well aware of the headaches that are experienced after the ingestion of alcohol. Aged alcohol in liquors and wines usually will precipitate a headache in migraine sufferers and very small amounts of alcohol can initiate an incapacitating attack with cluster patients who are in the cluster cycle. The hangover headache has all the features of a migraine headache. Migraineurs seem to be very sensitive to the histamines or tyramines in the beverages.

Altitude and headache — High altitudes can precipitate a migraine attack. Mountain sickness includes throbbing headache, nausea, shortness of breath, visual disturbance, palpitations, fluid in the lungs and the brain. I have treated some skiers with migraine by having them take antimigraine medications before ascending the ski run.

Constipation and headache — The problem of headache from constipation has been reported in many people. Whether the headaches are related to the effects of overuse of medications or from the absorption of toxins produced by the stool or psychological factors is not known.

Drug abuse and headache — This area was discussed in Chapter 7 on chronic daily headache. It is well known that overuse of medication to eliminate headache can actually cause worse headaches — "rebound headaches" — and in order to improve the headache problem it is necessary to eliminate or greatly reduce the amount of medication. Not only does the candidate create more headaches but runs the risk of causing other problems in the body. Overuse of many of these medications can cause kidney problems leading to chronic kidney disorder, as well as disorders of the stomach, such as ulcer, bleeding, and gastritis, plus disorders of the blood, such as bleeding disorders and anemia. Too much medication can also cause unexplained neurologic symptoms and may also cause personality changes.

There are many other causes of headaches. It is beyond the scope of this book to present the conditions of intracranial lesions. However, other books are available that provide more complete information (see References 2 to 5).

The case histories after the References will give you information about other causes of headaches.

REFERENCES

1. *Cephalgia Journal*, 1988, Norwegian Press.
2. Saper, J.R., *Headache Disorder*, John Wright-PSG, 1983.
3. Raskin, N.H., *Headache*, 2nd ed., Churchill Livingstone, New York, 1988.
4. Lance, J.W., *Mechanism and Management of Headaches*, 4th ed., Butterworths, London, 1982.
5. Diamond, S., Dalessio, D.J., *The Practicing Physician's Approach to Headache*, Williams & Wilkins, Baltimore, 1986.

CASE HISTORIES*

JOHN
Category: Other conditions causing headaches

The patient is a 49-year-old man who was seen as an emergency patient. He complained of incapacitating headaches which started in his early twenties. They were occasional, and he states that he had an occasional migraine attack, but had no headaches for many years until almost four weeks before he came to the clinic. He states his mother died and he came from out of town for the funeral and about a week later, he started having these headaches on a daily basis. He also complains about being lethargic and has difficulty in balance. His headaches last all day. It is a throbbing headache in the frontal part of his head. There is no aura, and associated features are none except for tiredness, and he must stay in bed.

Although his neurological examination was normal, it was diagnosed as headaches of unknown etiology, and to rule out the possibility of intracranial lesion. The patient states that he had a cold or the flu before this, and he says that since that time his problems of balance and the rapidity of his thinking processes have been altered. I explained to the patient that it would be extremely important to do a total medical examination and an MRI or a CT scan to make sure that there wasn't an intracranial lesion or some disease that was causing these headaches. Although it would be easy to consider that the trauma of his mother's death might have precipitated this response, one has to make sure that there isn't something going on that's organic at the same time. Unfortunately, the patient lived out of town and did not want to be worked up in this area. He went back to his residence and I lost contact with him.

* On the headache assessment forms that accompany these case histories, incapacitating headaches are indicated with solid black lines, interfering headaches with dotted lines, and irritating headaches with gray shading.

MEDICAL HEADACHE HISTORY

Name: John **Age:** 49 **Sex** M **Date:** 1/9/91

Date of Birth: 00/00/41 **Birthplace:** FL **Race:** W **Education:** B.A.

Occupation: Retired **Accident:** N/A

Armed Services & Type of Discharge: N/A

PAST HISTORY:

1.	Did you have a normal birth?		Yes	No
	a) forceps used?		Yes	No
	b) cesarean section?		Yes	No
2.	Did you have problems with bedwetting?		Yes	No
	a) If yes, age bedwetting stopped		______	
3.	Were you car sick as a child (motion)?		Yes	No
	a) If yes, how severe?	Slight	Moderate	Severe
4.	Did you have unexplained abdominal cramps as a child?		Yes	No
5.	Did you have any of the following illnesses in childhood?			
	a) meningitis		Yes	No
	b) encephalitis		Yes	No
	c) scarlet fever		Yes	No
	d) rheumatic fever		Yes	No
6.	Did you have any head injuries as a child?		Yes	No
	a) If yes, please explain: ______			
7.	Were you treated for emotional illness as a child?		Yes	No

HABITS:

8.	Do you drink alcohol?	Yes	No
	a) If yes, what kind and how much? Moderately		
	b) Does alcohol bring on or aggravate a headache?	Yes	No
9.	Do you smoke?	Yes	No
	a) If yes, how much? ______		
	b) Does smoking or smoke-filled rooms cause or aggravate headaches?	Yes	No
10.	Do you drink caffeinated beverages?	Yes	No
	a) If yes, how much? 3 cups of coffee per day		

MENSTRUAL HISTORY:

At what age did menses begin? ______ Were they regular or irregular? ______

How were they related to your headache? ______

Are you or were you ever on Birth Control Pills? ______ Did they affect your headache? ______

Have you had a hysterectomy, partial or total, and why? ______

Are you in menopause, and if yes, how long? ______

Are you on hormones, and if yes, which ones? ______

HEADACHE ASSESSMENT FORM

HA PROFILE	INCAPACITATING #3	INTERFERING #2	IRRITATING #1
ONSET (Years ago and frequency)	Early 20's, occasionally	N/A	N/A
CURRENT FREQUENCY	No HA for 4 months until mother died Dec. 1990	N/A	N/A
TIME OF ONSET	Every day since 12/90 Awaken with	N/A	N/A
DURATION	All day	N/A	N/A
CHARACTER	Throbbing	N/A	N/A
PRODROME OR AURA	N/A	N/A	N/A
ASSOCIATING FEATURES	Nausea; Vomiting; Sensitivity to Light? Noise? Odors? Do you get pale or flush? Do your eyes or nose run? Does your nose get stuffy? Does the white of your eyes get red? Does your eyelid droop? Do you pace, or go to bed? tired	Nausea; Vomiting; Sensitivity to Light? Noise? Odors? Do you get pale or flush? Do your eyes or nose run? Does your nose get stuffy? Does the white of your eyes get red? Does your eyelid droop? Do you pace, or go to bed?	Nausea; Vomiting; Sensitivity to Light? Noise? Odors? Do you get pale or flush? Do your eyes or nose run? Does your nose get stuffy? Does the white of your eyes get red? Does your eyelid droop? Do you pace, or go to bed?
PRECIPITATING OR AGGRAVATING FEATURES	Physical activity	N/A	N/A

LOCATION: Mark the location for each type of headache with a different color pen.

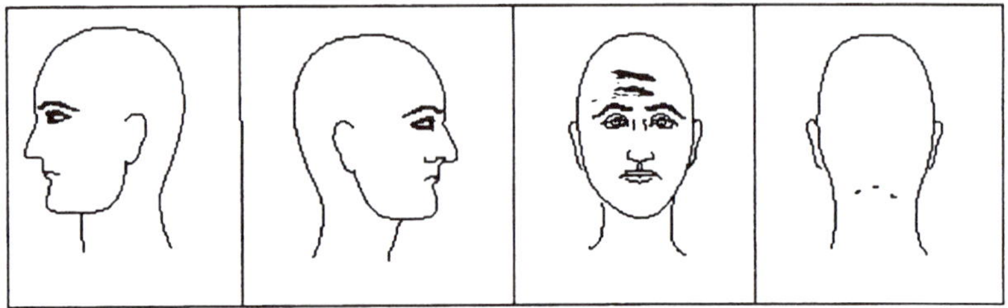

MEDICAL HISTORY:

Have you ever been or are you currently being treated for any of the following?

a) high blood pressure	Yes (underlined)	No
b) stomach ulcers	Yes	No (underlined)
c) asthma	Yes	No (underlined)
d) allergies	Yes	No (underlined)
e) pneumonia	Yes (underlined)	No
f) kidney problems	Yes	No (underlined)
g) low blood sugar	Yes	No (underlined)
h) glaucoma	Yes	No (underlined)
i) diabetes	Yes	No (underlined)
j) heart problems	Yes	No (underlined)

If you answered yes to any of the above, please describe: Pneumonia 3 years ago.

List all other medical problems you have had in the past. Include date diagnosed and treatment.
DO NOT LIST OPERATIONS

None.

SURGICAL HISTORY (List operations and dates performed)

Tonsillectomy & Adenoidectomy, age 10.

Appendectomy, age 14.

PSYCHIATRIC HISTORY (List visits with counselors, psychologists, etc., and type of treatment)

None.

ACCIDENTS IN ADULT LIFE (Briefly describe any accident that caused any blow to the head or that you feel is related to your headache)

None.

FAMILY HISTORY:

1. Is your father living?	Yes	No (underlined)
Age ________		
Cause of death Suicide, age 55		
Was there a headache history?	Yes	No (underlined)
2. Is your mother living?	Yes	No (underlined)
Age ________		
Cause of death Lung cancer, age 80		
Was there a headache history?	Yes	No (underlined)

3. Ages of brothers---Circle the ones with headache
   53
4. Ages of sisters---Circle the ones with headache
   None
5. List any other blood relatives with a history of severe headaches.
   None

MARITAL HISTORY:
List marriages:

1st marriage age 20 to 27 Did spouse have headaches?	Yes	No
2nd marriage age 31 to 49 Did spouse have headaches?	Yes	No
3rd marriage age ______ to ______ Did spouse have headaches?	Yes	No

Age of current spouse:__________

List ages and sex of all children:

Age 27 Sex M Headaches?	Yes	No
Age 24 Sex M Headaches?	Yes	No
Age 21 Sex F Headaches?	Yes	No
Age ______ Sex ______ Headaches?	Yes	No

STRESS FACTORS:

List any factors that may be affecting your headaches (money, loneliness, sexual problems, work, etc.)
Death of mother.

VEGETATIVE SIGNS:

1.	Do you have trouble falling asleep?	Yes	No
2.	Do you have trouble staying asleep?	Yes	No
3.	Has your appetite decreased?	Yes	No
4.	Have you gained or lost weight in the past year?	Yes	No
5.	Have you felt tearful or depressed lately?	Yes	No
6.	Have you had any thoughts of wanting to die?	Yes	No
7.	Have you been forgetful lately?	Yes	No
8.	Any other changes in your normal day-to-day living?__________		

Please list any medications you are allergic or sensitive to: None.

Please list any medications you are currently taking (including dosages and frequency per day):
Tylenol, 2 tablets 5 times a day.

PREVIOUS CARE:

1. List doctors who have treated you for headaches: None.

2. List any tests you have had for your headache (e.g., EEG, CT scan, MRI, X-Ray, etc.):

None

3. List any other treatment you have had for your headache (e.g., biofeedback, acupuncture, chiropractic, or any other treatment you had):

None

PATRICK
Category: Other conditions causing headaches

The patient is a 76-year-old man who complained of interfering headaches (moderate to severe). He stated that these headaches started two years ago and mentioned that he had angioplasty at that time, but is not sure if they were related. He said after that the pain became daily and persistent. He describes the pain as being in the back of his head, the front of his head, and involving the whole head. There was constant pain that occasionally has sharp features, and feels at times there might be some throbbing. He said he also experienced some zigzag lines in front of his vision, and he has also had these without headache. When the pain is severe, there is nausea and he needs to go to bed. He does not know of anything that precipitates or aggravates the headache.

He has had a significant medical history with angioplasty and cardiac surgery and surgery on the carotid artery. The patient takes three Darvocet a day and other medications. Although his diagnosis is chronic daily headache, he was placed in the category of Other Conditions because I had seen at times that surgical interventions affecting the arteries may sometimes be a precipitating factor, but the cause is unknown. Whether this is just a chronic tension headache or caused by another problem at this point is unknown.

MEDICAL HEADACHE HISTORY

Name: Patrick **Age:** 76 **Sex** M **Date:** 6/11/92

Date of Birth: 00/00/15 **Birthplace:** PA **Race:** C **Education:** ______

Occupation: Retired **Accident:** N/A

Armed Services & Type of Discharge: 1941-42 – Army.

PAST HISTORY:

1.	Did you have a normal birth?		<u>Yes</u>	No
	a) forceps used?		Yes	No
	b) cesarean section?		Yes	No
2.	Did you have problems with bedwetting?		Yes	<u>No</u>
	a) If yes, age bedwetting stopped		______	
3.	Were you car sick as a child (motion)?		Yes	<u>No</u>
	a) If yes, how severe?	Slight	Moderate	Severe
4.	Did you have unexplained abdominal cramps as a child?		Yes	<u>No</u>
5.	Did you have any of the following illnesses in childhood?			
	a) meningitis		Yes	<u>No</u>
	b) encephalitis		Yes	<u>No</u>
	c) scarlet fever		Yes	<u>No</u>
	d) rheumatic fever		Yes	<u>No</u>
6.	Did you have any head injuries as a child?		Yes	<u>No</u>
	a) If yes, please explain: ______			
7.	Were you treated for emotional illness as a child?		Yes	<u>No</u>

HABITS:

8.	Do you drink alcohol?	Yes	<u>No</u>
	a) If yes, what kind and how much? ______		
	b) Does alcohol bring on or aggravate a headache?	Yes	<u>No</u>
9.	Do you smoke?	Yes	<u>No</u>
	a) If yes, how much? ______		
	b) Does smoking or smoke-filled rooms cause or aggravate headaches?	Yes	<u>No</u>
10.	Do you drink caffeinated beverages?	Yes	<u>No</u>
	a) If yes, how much? ______		

MENSTRUAL HISTORY:

At what age did menses begin? ______ Were they regular or irregular? ______
How were they related to your headache? ______
Are you or were you ever on Birth Control Pills? ______ Did they affect your headache? ______
Have you had a hysterectomy, partial or total, and why? ______
Are you in menopause, and if yes, how long? ______
Are you on hormones, and if yes, which ones? ______

HEADACHE ASSESSMENT FORM

HA PROFILE	INCAPACITATING #3	INTERFERING #2	IRRITATING #1
ONSET (Years ago and frequency)	N/A	2 years ago, every day after angioplasty	N/A
CURRENT FREQUENCY	N/A	Every day	N/A
TIME OF ONSET	N/A	Constant	N/A
DURATION	N/A	Constant	N/A
CHARACTER	N/A	Very sharp, throbbing	N/A
PRODROME OR AURA	N/A	Ringing in ears	N/A
ASSOCIATING FEATURES	Nausea; Vomiting; Sensitivity to Light? Noise? Odors? Do you get pale or flush? Do your eyes or nose run? Does your nose get stuffy? Does the white of your eyes get red? Does your eyelid droop? Do you pace, or go to bed?	Nausea; Vomiting; Sensitivity to Light? Noise? Odors? Do you get pale or flush? Do your eyes or nose run? Does your nose get stuffy? Does the white of your eyes get red? Does your eyelid droop? Do you pace, or go to bed?	Nausea; Vomiting; Sensitivity to Light? Noise? Odors? Do you get pale or flush? Do your eyes or nose run? Does your nose get stuffy? Does the white of your eyes get red? Does your eyelid droop? Do you pace, or go to bed?
PRECIPITATING OR AGGRAVATING FEATURES	N/A	N/A	N/A

LOCATION: Mark the location for each type of headache with a different color pen.

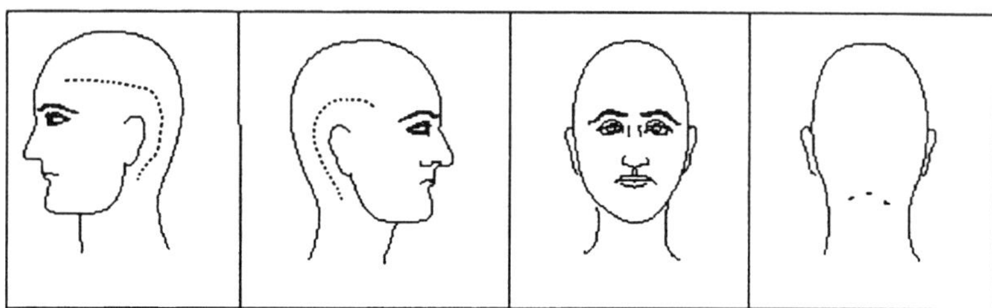

MEDICAL HISTORY:

Have you ever been or are you currently being treated for any of the following?

a) high blood pressure	Yes	<u>No</u>
b) stomach ulcers	<u>Yes</u>	No
c) asthma	Yes	<u>No</u>
d) allergies	Yes	<u>No</u>
e) pneumonia	<u>Yes</u>	No
f) kidney problems	Yes	<u>No</u>
g) low blood sugar	Yes	<u>No</u>
h) glaucoma	Yes	<u>No</u>
i) diabetes	Yes	<u>No</u>
j) heart problems	<u>Yes</u>	No

If you answered yes to any of the above, please describe: Ulcers diagnosed 25 years ago, resolved. Pneumonia 5 years ago. Angioplasty 2 years ago. Bypass surgery 1975.

List all other medical problems you have had in the past. Include date diagnosed and treatment. DO NOT LIST OPERATIONS

SURGICAL HISTORY (List operations and dates performed)

Bypass Heart Surgery, 1975. Carotid Artery, 1976. Gallbladder, ? Angioplasty 2 years ago. Tonsillectomy & Adenoidectomy. Appendectomy. Temporal artery biopsy, 1991.

PSYCHIATRIC HISTORY (List visits with counselors, psychologists, etc., and type of treatment)

1991, 5 EST's - treatment for depression.

ACCIDENTS IN ADULT LIFE (Briefly describe any accident that caused any blow to the head or that you feel is related to your headache)

None.

FAMILY HISTORY:

1. Is your father living? Yes <u>No</u>

   Age________

   Cause of death Flu, age 46

   Was there a headache history? Yes <u>No</u>

2. Is your mother living? Yes <u>No</u>
   Age________
   Cause of death___Heart attack, age 65_______________
   Was there a headache history? Yes <u>No</u>
3. Ages of brothers---Circle the ones with headache
   ___3 brothers, died of coronary___________________
4. Ages of sisters---Circle the ones with headache
   ___5 sisters, 4 deceased. 1 age 74________________
5. List any other blood relatives with a history of severe headaches.
   ___None___________________________________

MARITAL HISTORY:

List marriages:

1st marriage age _24_ to _Present_ Did spouse have headaches? <u>Yes</u> No
2nd marriage age _____ to _______ Did spouse have headaches? Yes No
3rd marriage age _____ to _______ Did spouse have headaches? Yes No
Age of current spouse:__74_______

List ages and sex of all children:
Age _____ Sex ______ Headaches? Yes No
Age _____ Sex ______ Headaches? Yes No
Age _____ Sex ______ Headaches? Yes No
Age _____ Sex ______ Headaches? Yes No

STRESS FACTORS:

List any factors that may be affecting your headaches (money, loneliness, sexual problems, work, etc.)
____
____

VEGETATIVE SIGNS:

1. Do you have trouble falling asleep? <u>Yes</u> No
2. Do you have trouble staying asleep? <u>Yes</u> No
3. Has your appetite decreased? Yes <u>No</u>
4. Have you gained or lost weight in the past year? Yes <u>No</u>
5. Have you felt tearful or depressed lately? <u>Yes</u> No
6. Have you had any thoughts of wanting to die? Yes <u>No</u>
7. Have you been forgetful lately? Yes <u>No</u>
8. Any other changes in your normal day-to-day living?_______________

Please list any medications you are allergic or sensitive to:__None.__________________
____

Please list any medications you are currently taking (including dosages and frequency per day):
___Procardia. Nitroglycerin. Darvocet as needed. Valium.____________
____

PREVIOUS CARE:

1. List doctors who have treated you for headaches: Dr. L, Dr. M.

2. List any tests you have had for your headache (e.g., EEG, CT scan, MRI, X-Ray, etc.):

CT scan 1 year ago (normal).

EEG 1 year ago (normal).

Carotid ultrasound.

3. List any other treatment you have had for your headache (e.g., biofeedback, acupuncture, chiropractic, or any other treatment you had):

None.

NICK
Category: Other conditions causing headaches

Nick is a 37-year-old man who complained of interfering headaches (moderate to severe). These started two weeks ago and occur daily. He wakes up with them, and they get worse as the day progresses. It is a constant headache and a burning headache. The pain seems to start in the top of his head and works itself downward or inferiorly to the posterior cervical region. There is no aura and no other associated features. He must sit quietly. In the beginning, he said lying down would make it worse.

Cervical and neurological examinations are normal. His diagnosis was acute headache of unknown etiology (origin) and rule out intracranial lesion. A workup was done in order to rule out any intracranial lesion and his CT scan was normal. His laboratory workup was also normal, and he was placed on an anti-inflammatory medication to see whether this would decrease what may now be just an extremely severe tension headache.

MEDICAL HEADACHE HISTORY

Name: Nick **Age:** 37 **Sex** M **Date:** 10/3/90

Date of Birth: 00/00/53 **Birthplace:** FL **Race:** B **Education:** 2 years college

Occupation: Electrician **Accident:** N/A

Armed Services & Type of Discharge: N/A

PAST HISTORY:

1.	Did you have a normal birth?		Yes (underlined)	No
	a) forceps used?		Yes	No
	b) cesarean section?		Yes	No
2.	Did you have problems with bedwetting?		Yes	No (underlined)
	a) If yes, age bedwetting stopped		______	
3.	Were you car sick as a child (motion)?		Yes	No (underlined)
	a) If yes, how severe?	Slight	Moderate	Severe
4.	Did you have unexplained abdominal cramps as a child?		Yes	No (underlined)
5.	Did you have any of the following illnesses in childhood?			
	a) meningitis		Yes	No
	b) encephalitis		Yes	No
	c) scarlet fever		Yes	No
	d) rheumatic fever		Yes	No
6.	Did you have any head injuries as a child?		Yes	No (underlined)
	a) If yes, please explain: ______			
7.	Were you treated for emotional illness as a child?		Yes	No (underlined)

HABITS:

8.	Do you drink alcohol?	Yes	No (underlined)
	a) If yes, what kind and how much? ______		
	b) Does alcohol bring on or aggravate a headache?	Yes	No (underlined)
9.	Do you smoke?	Yes	No (underlined)
	a) If yes, how much? ______		
	b) Does smoking or smoke-filled rooms cause or aggravate headaches?	Yes	No (underlined)
10.	Do you drink caffeinated beverages?	Yes	No (underlined)
	a) If yes, how much? ______		

MENSTRUAL HISTORY:

At what age did menses begin? ______ Were they regular or irregular? ______

How were they related to your headache? ______

Are you or were you ever on Birth Control Pills? ______ Did they affect your headache? ______

Have you had a hysterectomy, partial or total, and why? ______

Are you in menopause, and if yes, how long? ______

Are you on hormones, and if yes, which ones? ______

HEADACHE ASSESSMENT FORM

HA PROFILE	INCAPACITATING #3	INTERFERING #2	IRRITATING #1
ONSET (Years ago and frequency)	N/A	2 weeks ago, every day	N/A
CURRENT FREQUENCY	N/A	Every day, Increases at night	N/A
TIME OF ONSET	N/A	Wake up with, gets worse during day	N/A
DURATION	N/A	Constant	N/A
CHARACTER	N/A	Burning	N/A
PRODROME OR AURA	N/A	Ringing in ears	N/A
ASSOCIATING FEATURES	Nausea; Vomiting; Sensitivity to Light? Noise? Odors? Do you get pale or flush? Do your eyes or nose run? Does your nose get stuffy? Does the white of your eyes get red? Does your eyelid droop? Do you pace, or go to bed?	Nausea; Vomiting; Sensitivity to Light? Noise? Odors? Do you get pale or flush? Do your eyes or nose run? Does your nose get stuffy? Does the white of your eyes get red? Does your eyelid droop? Do you pace, or go to bed? Sits quietly	Nausea; Vomiting; Sensitivity to Light? Noise? Odors? Do you get pale or flush? Do your eyes or nose run? Does your nose get stuffy? Does the white of your eyes get red? Does your eyelid droop? Do you pace, or go to bed?
PRECIPITATING OR AGGRAVATING FEATURES	N/A	Lying down on left side	N/A

LOCATION: Mark the location for each type of headache with a different color pen.

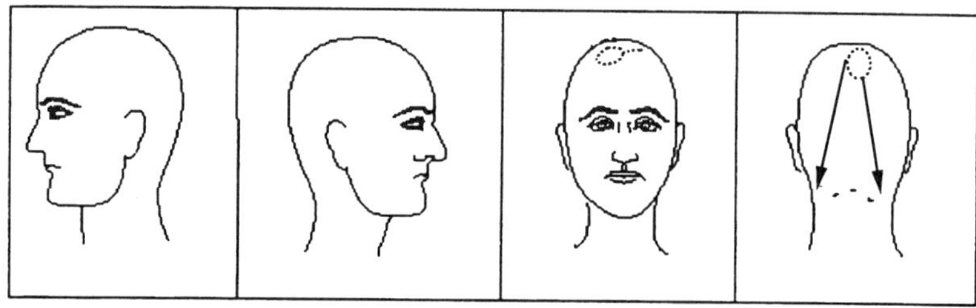

MEDICAL HISTORY:

Have you ever been or are you currently being treated for any of the following?

a) high blood pressure	Yes	No
b) stomach ulcers	Yes	No
c) asthma	Yes	No
d) allergies	Yes	No
e) pneumonia	Yes	No
f) kidney problems	Yes	No
g) low blood sugar	Yes	No
h) glaucoma	Yes	No
i) diabetes	Yes	No
j) heart problems	Yes	No

If you answered yes to any of the above, please describe: Environmental allergies.

List all other medical problems you have had in the past. Include date diagnosed and treatment.
DO NOT LIST OPERATIONS

None

SURGICAL HISTORY (List operations and dates performed)

None

PSYCHIATRIC HISTORY (List visits with counselors, psychologists, etc., and type of treatment)

None

ACCIDENTS IN ADULT LIFE (Briefly describe any accident that caused any blow to the head or that you feel is related to your headache)

None.

FAMILY HISTORY:

1. Is your father living? Yes No
   Age____
   Cause of death 54, CVA
   Was there a headache history? Yes No

2. Is your mother living? Yes No
   Age 64
   Cause of death____
   Was there a headache history? Yes No

3. Ages of brothers---Circle the ones with headache
   42 31
4. Ages of sisters---Circle the ones with headache
   44 38 34 32
5. List any other blood relatives with a history of severe headaches.
   None

MARITAL HISTORY:
List marriages:

1st marriage age 22 to Present	Did spouse have headaches?	Yes	No
2nd marriage age _____ to _______	Did spouse have headaches?	Yes	No
3rd marriage age _____ to _______	Did spouse have headaches?	Yes	No

Age of current spouse: 36

List ages and sex of all children:

Age 13 Sex F Headaches?	Yes	No
Age 7 Sex F Headaches?	Yes	No
Age _____ Sex ______ Headaches?	Yes	No
Age _____ Sex ______ Headaches?	Yes	No

STRESS FACTORS:

List any factors that may be affecting your headaches (money, loneliness, sexual problems, work, etc.)

____

____

VEGETATIVE SIGNS:

1.	Do you have trouble falling asleep?	Yes	No
2.	Do you have trouble staying asleep?	Yes	No
3.	Has your appetite decreased?	Yes	No
4.	Have you gained or lost weight in the past year?	Yes	No
5.	Have you felt tearful or depressed lately?	Yes	No
6.	Have you had any thoughts of wanting to die?	Yes	No
7.	Have you been forgetful lately?	Yes	No
8.	Any other changes in your normal day-to-day living?__________		

Please list any medications you are allergic or sensitive to: No known allergies.

____

____

Please list any medications you are currently taking (including dosages and frequency per day):
None.

____

PREVIOUS CARE:

1. List doctors who have treated you for headaches: None

2. List any tests you have had for your headache (e.g., EEG, CT scan, MRI, X-Ray, etc.):
None.

3. List any other treatment you have had for your headache (e.g., biofeedback, acupuncture, chiropractic, or any other treatment you had):
None.

ALFRED
Category: Other conditions causing headaches

This is an interesting case of an 80-year-old man who is currently retired. He experiences irritating headaches (annoying) which started two years after he states he was straining having a bowel movement and he had them daily for three months. Then they went into their own remission. The current headaches started several months before he came to see me and he was now having them daily. They seem to come on after dinner in the evening, but they come on only when he coughs. They last 30 minutes to an hour and he takes Anacin. The character of the pain is dull pressure and burning on the top of his head. The pain is in the orbital, frontal and crown of his head. There is no prodrome, that is a warning that he is going to get a headache, and there are no associated features, such as seen with vascular and migraine headaches. Coughing and bending over will make his headaches worse.

His neurological workup was normal, and the diagnosis at that time was

1. daily headache, etiology unknown, and
2. rule out an intracranial lesion.

A CT scan was done, which was essentially normal. He was treated with minimum medication and improved, but months later he called and said he feels his headaches are better but he still gets them when he coughs. Although his condition was benign and there was no intracranial lesion, evidently the triggering mechanism of increased pressure from the cough was one of the mechanisms that started his headache. The best that he was able to get was a reduction, but not an elimination, of that problem.

MEDICAL HEADACHE HISTORY

Name: Alfred **Age:** 80 **Sex** M **Date:** 6/22/92

Date of Birth: 00/00/12 **Birthplace:** CN **Race:** C **Education:** College

Occupation: Retired **Accident:** N/A

Armed Services & Type of Discharge: Army – 1944; National Guard – 10 years.

PAST HISTORY:

1.	Did you have a normal birth?		<u>Yes</u>	No
	a) forceps used?		Yes	No
	b) cesarean section?		Yes	No
2.	Did you have problems with bedwetting?		Yes	<u>No</u>
	a) If yes, age bedwetting stopped		______	
3.	Were you car sick as a child (motion)?		Yes	<u>No</u>
	a) If yes, how severe?	Slight	Moderate	Severe
4.	Did you have unexplained abdominal cramps as a child?		Yes	<u>No</u>
5.	Did you have any of the following illnesses in childhood?			
	a) meningitis		Yes	<u>No</u>
	b) encephalitis		Yes	<u>No</u>
	c) scarlet fever		<u>Yes</u>	No
	d) rheumatic fever		Yes	<u>No</u>
6.	Did you have any head injuries as a child?		Yes	<u>No</u>
	a) If yes, please explain: ______			
7.	Were you treated for emotional illness as a child?		Yes	<u>No</u>

HABITS:

8.	Do you drink alcohol?	Yes	<u>No</u>
	a) If yes, what kind and how much? ______		
	b) Does alcohol bring on or aggravate a headache?	Yes	<u>No</u>
9.	Do you smoke?	Yes	<u>No</u>
	a) If yes, how much? ______		
	b) Does smoking or smoke-filled rooms cause or aggravate headaches?	Yes	<u>No</u>
10.	Do you drink caffeinated beverages?	Yes	<u>No</u>
	a) If yes, how much? ______		

MENSTRUAL HISTORY:

At what age did menses begin? ______ Were they regular or irregular? ______
How were they related to your headache? ______
Are you or were you ever on Birth Control Pills? ______ Did they affect your headache? ______
Have you had a hysterectomy, partial or total, and why? ______
Are you in menopause, and if yes, how long? ______
Are you on hormones, and if yes, which ones? ______

HEADACHE ASSESSMENT FORM

HA PROFILE	INCAPACITATING #3	INTERFERING #2	IRRITATING #1
ONSET (Years ago and frequency)	N/A	N/A	2 years ago Every day for 3 months
CURRENT FREQUENCY	N/A	N/A	Started again 4/92 Every day
TIME OF ONSET	N/A	N/A	6:00 – 7:00 p.m., only when cough
DURATION	N/A	N/A	30 min. to 1 hour with Anacin
CHARACTER	N/A	N/A	Dull pressure
PRODROME OR AURA	N/A	N/A	N/A
ASSOCIATING FEATURES	Nausea: Vomiting: Sensitivity to Light? Noise? Odors? Do you get pale or flush? Do your eyes or nose run? Does your nose get stuffy? Do the whites of your eyes get red? Does your eyelid droop? Do you pace, or go to bed?	Nausea: Vomiting: Sensitivity to Light? Noise? Odors? Do you get pale or flush? Do your eyes or nose run? Does your nose get stuffy? Do the whites of your eyes get red? Does your eyelid droop? Do you pace, or go to bed?	Nausea: Vomiting: Sensitivity to Light? Noise? Odors? Do you get pale or flush? Do your eyes or nose run? Does your nose get stuffy? Do the whites of your eyes get red? Does your eyelid droop? Do you pace, or go to bed?
PRECIPITATING OR AGGRAVATING FEATURES	N/A	N/A	Coughing Bending over

LOCATION: Mark the location for each type of headache with a different color pen.

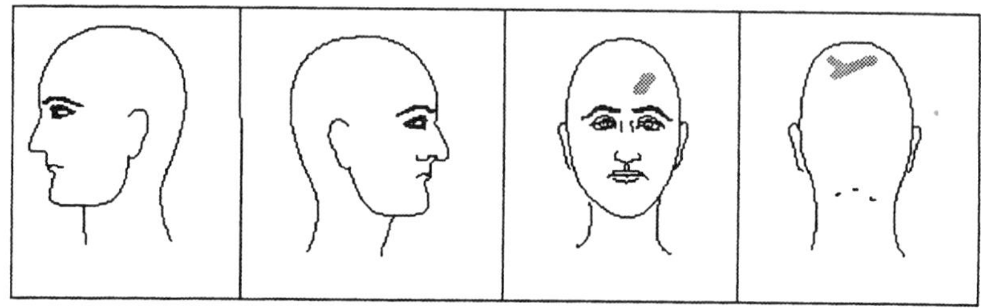

MEDICAL HISTORY:

Have you ever been or are you currently being treated for any of the following?

a) high blood pressure	Yes	No
b) stomach ulcers	Yes	No
c) asthma	Yes	No
d) allergies	Yes	No
e) pneumonia	Yes	No
f) kidney problems	Yes	No
g) low blood sugar	Yes	No
h) glaucoma	Yes	No
i) diabetes	Yes	No
j) heart problems	Yes	No

If you answered yes to any of the above, please describe:____________________

List all other medical problems you have had in the past. Include date diagnosed and treatment.
DO NOT LIST OPERATIONS
None.

SURGICAL HISTORY (List operations and dates performed)
Hernias – 1969 and 1972. Tonsillectomy & Adenoidectomy as a child.

PSYCHIATRIC HISTORY (List visits with counselors, psychologists, etc., and type of treatment)
None

ACCIDENTS IN ADULT LIFE (Briefly describe any accident that caused any blow to the head or that you feel is related to your headache)
None

FAMILY HISTORY:

1.	Is your father living?	Yes	No
	Age________		
	Cause of death Leukemia, age 81		
	Was there a headache history?	Yes	No
2.	Is your mother living?	Yes	No
	Age________		
	Cause of death A fall, age 87		
	Was there a headache history?	Yes	No
3.	Ages of brothers---Circle the ones with headache		
	Three brothers		

4. Ages of sisters—Circle the ones with headache
   Four sisters
5. List any other blood relatives with a history of severe headaches.
   None

MARITAL HISTORY:

List marriages:

1st marriage age 23 to Now	Did spouse have headaches?	Yes	No
2nd marriage age ____ to ____	Did spouse have headaches?	Yes	No
3rd marriage age ____ to ____	Did spouse have headaches?	Yes	No

Age of current spouse: 72

List ages and sex of all children:

Age 49	Sex F	Headaches?	Yes	No
Age 47	Sex F	Headaches?	Yes	No
Age 42	Sex M	Headaches?	Yes	No

STRESS FACTORS:

List any factors that may be affecting your headaches (money, loneliness, sexual problems, work, etc.)
None

VEGETATIVE SIGNS:

1.	Do you have trouble falling asleep?	Yes	No
2.	Do you have trouble staying asleep?	Yes	No
3.	Has your appetite decreased?	Yes	No
4.	Have you gained or lost weight in the past year?	Yes	No
5.	Have you felt tearful or depressed lately?	Yes	No
6.	Have you had any thoughts of wanting to die?	Yes	No
7.	Have you been forgetful lately?	Yes	No
8.	Any other changes in your normal day-to-day living?		

Please list any medications you are allergic or sensitive to: None that I'm aware of.

Please list any medications you are currently taking (including dosages and frequency per day):
Anacin, 2 tablets twice a day.

PREVIOUS CARE:

1. List doctors who have treated you for headaches: Dr. D

2. List any tests you have had for your headache (e.g., EEG, CT scan, MRI, X-Ray, etc.):
None.

3. List any other treatment you have had for your headache (e.g., biofeedback, acupuncture, chiropractic, or any other treatment you had):
None.

GERALD
Category: Other conditions causing headaches

This is an example of triggering mechanisms that may start the headache process for reasons that we are unaware of. This patient was seen about a year after he had spinal anesthesia for some surgery, and from that point on he continued to get irritating headaches on a daily basis. It is not uncommon that patients will get headaches following spinal anesthesia, but generally they go into their own remission within the first 10 days, and rarely continue as a chronic problem. However, this is an example of how certain situations can trigger the headache mechanism.

MEDICAL HEADACHE HISTORY

Name: Gerald **Age:** 71 **Sex** M **Date:** 1/11/90

Date of Birth: 00/00/18 **Birthplace:** ________ **Race:** C **Education:** 2-1/2 yrs college

Occupation: Retired **Accident:** N/A

Armed Services & Type of Discharge: Army – World War II

PAST HISTORY:

1.	Did you have a normal birth?		<u>Yes</u>	No
	a) forceps used?		<u>Yes</u>	No
	b) cesarean section?		Yes	<u>No</u>
2.	Did you have problems with bedwetting?		Yes	<u>No</u>
	a) If yes, age bedwetting stopped		________	
3.	Were you car sick as a child (motion)?		<u>Yes</u>	No
	a) If yes, how severe?	Slight	<u>Moderate</u>	Severe
4.	Did you have unexplained abdominal cramps as a child?		Yes	<u>No</u>
5.	Did you have any of the following illnesses in childhood?			
	a) meningitis		Yes	<u>No</u>
	b) encephalitis		Yes	<u>No</u>
	c) scarlet fever		Yes	<u>No</u>
	d) rheumatic fever		Yes	<u>No</u>
6.	Did you have any head injuries as a child?		Yes	<u>No</u>
	a) If yes, please explain: ________			
7.	Were you treated for emotional illness as a child?		Yes	<u>No</u>

HABITS:

8.	Do you drink alcohol?	<u>Yes</u>	No
	a) If yes, what kind and how much? Very moderately		
	b) Does alcohol bring on or aggravate a headache?	Yes	<u>No</u>
9.	Do you smoke?	Yes	<u>No</u>
	a) If yes, how much? ________		
	b) Does smoking or smoke-filled rooms cause or aggravate headaches?	Yes	<u>No</u>
10.	Do you drink caffeinated beverages?	Yes	<u>No</u>
	a) If yes, how much? ________		

MENSTRUAL HISTORY:

At what age did menses begin?_______ Were they regular or irregular?________
How were they related to your headache?________
Are you or were you ever on Birth Control Pills?______ Did they affect your headache? ________
Have you had a hysterectomy, partial or total, and why?________
Are you in menopause, and if yes, how long?________
Are you on hormones, and if yes, which ones?________

HEADACHE ASSESSMENT FORM

HA PROFILE	INCAPACITATING #3	INTERFERING #2	IRRITATING #1
ONSET (Years ago and frequency)	N/A	N/A	Dec. 4, after surgery with a spinal
CURRENT FREQUENCY	N/A	N/A	Constantly awaken with
TIME OF ONSET	N/A	N/A	Continuous
DURATION	N/A	N/A	Continuous
CHARACTER	N/A	N/A	Dull achy
PRODROME OR AURA	N/A	N/A	N/A
ASSOCIATING FEATURES	Nausea; Vomiting; Sensitivity to Light? Noise? Odors? Do you get pale or flush? Do your eyes or nose run? Does your nose get stuffy? Do the whites of your eyes get red? Does your eyelid droop? Do you pace, or go to bed?	Nausea; Vomiting; Sensitivity to Light? Noise? Odors? Do you get pale or flush? Do your eyes or nose run? Does your nose get stuffy? Do the whites of your eyes get red? Does your eyelid droop? Do you pace, or go to bed?	Nausea; Vomiting; Sensitivity to Light? Noise? Odors? Do you get pale or flush? Do your eyes or nose run? Does your nose get stuffy? Do the whites of your eyes get red? Does your eyelid droop? Do you pace, or go to bed?
PRECIPITATING OR AGGRAVATING FEATURES	N/A	N/A	Reading Going to movies

LOCATION: Mark the location for each type of headache with a different color pen.

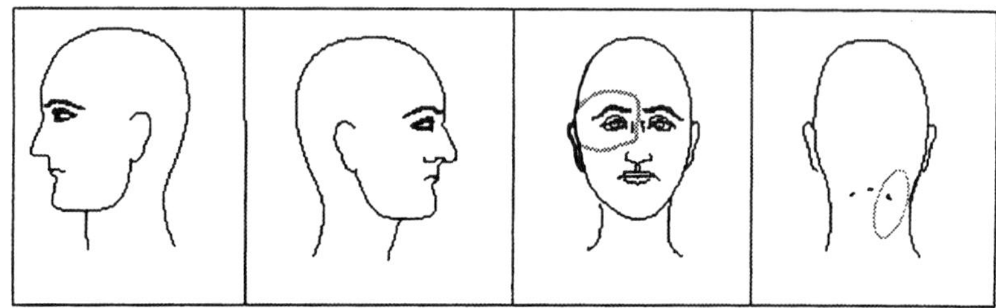

MEDICAL HISTORY:

Have you ever been or are you currently being treated for any of the following?

a) high blood pressure	<u>Yes</u>	No
b) stomach ulcers	Yes	<u>No</u>
c) asthma	Yes	<u>No</u>
d) allergies	Yes	<u>No</u>
e) pneumonia	Yes	<u>No</u>
f) kidney problems	Yes	<u>No</u>
g) low blood sugar	Yes	<u>No</u>
h) glaucoma	Yes	<u>No</u>
i) diabetes	Yes	<u>No</u>
j) heart problems	Yes	<u>No</u>

If you answered yes to any of the above, please describe:______________________________

List all other medical problems you have had in the past. Include date diagnosed and treatment.
DO NOT LIST OPERATIONS

Hypertension.

SURGICAL HISTORY (List operations and dates performed)

Appendectomy – 1934. Melanoma – 1976. Zenkers Diverticulosis – 1986. Prostate reaming – 1986.
Hernia – 1986. Double hernia – 1989.

PSYCHIATRIC HISTORY (List visits with counselors, psychologists, etc., and type of treatment)

None

ACCIDENTS IN ADULT LIFE (Briefly describe any accident that caused any blow to the head or that you feel is related to your headache)

None

FAMILY HISTORY:

1. Is your father living?	Yes	<u>No</u>
Age________		
Cause of death Don't know		
Was there a headache history?	Yes	No
2. Is your mother living?	Yes	<u>No</u>
Age________		
Cause of death Stroke, age 82		
Was there a headache history?	Yes	<u>No</u>

3. Ages of brothers---Circle the ones with headache
   None
4. Ages of sisters---Circle the ones with headache
   None
5. List any other blood relatives with a history of severe headaches.
   None

MARITAL HISTORY:

List marriages:

1st marriage age 25 to Present	Did spouse have headaches?	Yes	No
2nd marriage age _____ to _____	Did spouse have headaches?	Yes	No
3rd marriage age _____ to _____	Did spouse have headaches?	Yes	No

Age of current spouse: 68

List ages and sex of all children:

Age 40 Sex F	Headaches?	Yes	No
Age 36 Sex M	Headaches?	Yes	No
Age _____ Sex _____	Headaches?	Yes	No

STRESS FACTORS:

List any factors that may be affecting your headaches (money, loneliness, sexual problems, work, etc.)
None

VEGETATIVE SIGNS:

1.	Do you have trouble falling asleep?	Yes	No
2.	Do you have trouble staying asleep?	Yes	No
3.	Has your appetite decreased?	Yes	No
4.	Have you gained or lost weight in the past year?	Yes	No
5.	Have you felt tearful or depressed lately?	Yes	No
6.	Have you had any thoughts of wanting to die?	Yes	No
7.	Have you been forgetful lately?	Yes	No
8.	Any other changes in your normal day-to-day living?_____		

Please list any medications you are allergic or sensitive to: Demerol

Please list any medications you are currently taking (including dosages and frequency per day):
Cardizem, twice daily.

PREVIOUS CARE:

1. List doctors who have treated you for headaches: Dr. N; Dr. H; Dr. M

2. List any tests you have had for your headache (e.g., EEG, CT scan, MRI, X-Ray, etc.):
X-rays.

3. List any other treatment you have had for your headache (e.g., biofeedback, acupuncture, chiropractic, or any other treatment you had):
Neck therapy. Physical therapy, which gave temporary relief.

LENORA
Category: Other conditions causing headaches

This 41-year-old woman came into the office approximately five months after she began getting headaches following the flu. She was having interfering headaches (moderate to severe). After the flu, she found that she awakened with them. They last all day. It is a throbbing headache, 95% of the time on the right side of her periorbital or eye region and also on the right posterior cervical region. There is no aura. Associated features are nausea, sonophobia (sensitivity to noise), pallor, and she will go to bed if possible.

There was a history of slight car sickness as a child, and there is also a history of a mother who suffered severe headaches.

This patient did not have any headache history until she got the flu about five months before I saw her. At that time there was a great deal of literature on headaches secondary to the Epstein-Barr virus, and the thought was that this may be responsible for causing these atypical vascular headaches. A blood virus panel was ordered to rule out this particular cause of the headache problem.

She was diagnosed with:

1. atypical migraine,
2. daily vascular headaches, and
3. rule out headaches secondary to the Epstein-Barr virus.

She was treated as a migraine patient and her headaches decreased from 100% to 8% over a period of four months. She was doing well a year after I had seen her, until she called to say that the headaches had started once again after she was exposed to her house being sprayed for flea control. This makes me feel that this was an atypical migraine and it was caused by these various triggering mechanisms that are discussed in Chapter 3.

MEDICAL HEADACHE HISTORY

Name: Lenora **Age:** 41 **Sex** F **Date:** 5/6/91

Date of Birth: 00/00/49 **Birthplace:** FL **Race:** C **Education:** 1 yr. college

Occupation: Day Care **Accident:** N/A

Armed Services & Type of Discharge: N/A

PAST HISTORY:

1.	Did you have a normal birth?		Yes	No
	a) forceps used?		Yes	No
	b) cesarean section?		Yes	No
2.	Did you have problems with bedwetting?		Yes	No
	a) If yes, age bedwetting stopped		______	
3.	Were you car sick as a child (motion)?		Yes	No
	a) If yes, how severe?	Slight	Moderate	Severe
4.	Did you have unexplained abdominal cramps as a child?		Yes	No
5.	Did you have any of the following illnesses in childhood?			
	a) meningitis		Yes	No
	b) encephalitis		Yes	No
	c) scarlet fever		Yes	No
	d) rheumatic fever		Yes	No
6.	Did you have any head injuries as a child?		Yes	No
	a) If yes, please explain: ______			
7.	Were you treated for emotional illness as a child?		Yes	No

HABITS:

8.	Do you drink alcohol?	Yes	No
	a) If yes, what kind and how much? ______		
	b) Does alcohol bring on or aggravate a headache?	Yes	No
9.	Do you smoke?	Yes	No
	a) If yes, how much? ______		
	b) Does smoking or smoke-filled rooms cause or aggravate headaches?	Yes	No
10.	Do you drink caffeinated beverages?	Yes	No
	a) If yes, how much? ______		

MENSTRUAL HISTORY:

At what age did menses begin? 9 Were they regular or irregular? WNL

How were they related to your headache? N/A

Are you or were you ever on Birth Control Pills? Yes Did they affect your headache? No

Have you had a hysterectomy, partial or total, and why? No

Are you in menopause, and if yes, how long? No

Are you on hormones, and if yes, which ones? No

HEADACHE ASSESSMENT FORM

HA PROFILE	INCAPACITATING #3	INTERFERING #2	IRRITATING #1
ONSET (Years ago and frequency)	N/A	1/91 after the flu Every day	N/A
CURRENT FREQUENCY	N/A	Every day	N/A
TIME OF ONSET	N/A	Can awaken with	N/A
DURATION	N/A	All day	N/A
CHARACTER	N/A	Throbbing	N/A
PRODROME OR AURA	N/A	N/A	N/A
ASSOCIATING FEATURES	Nausea; Vomiting; Sensitivity to Light? Noise? Odors? Do you get pale or flush? Do your eyes or nose run? Does your nose get stuffy? Do the whites of your eyes get red? Does your eyelid droop? Do you pace, or go to bed?	Nausea; Vomiting; Sensitivity to Light? Noise? Odors? Do you get pale or flush? Do your eyes or nose run? Does your nose get stuffy? Do the whites of your eyes get red? Does your eyelid droop? Do you pace, or go to bed?	Nausea; Vomiting; Sensitivity to Light? Noise? Odors? Do you get pale or flush? Do your eyes or nose run? Does your nose get stuffy? Do the whites of your eyes get red? Does your eyelid droop? Do you pace, or go to bed?
PRECIPITATING OR AGGRAVATING FEATURES	N/A	N/A	N/A

LOCATION: Mark the location for each type of headache with a different color pen.

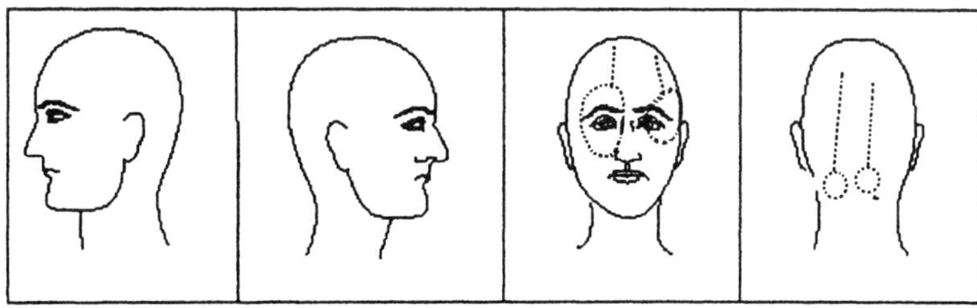

MEDICAL HISTORY:

Have you ever been or are you currently being treated for any of the following?

a) high blood pressure	Yes	No
b) stomach ulcers	Yes	No
c) asthma	Yes	No
d) allergies	Yes	No
e) pneumonia	Yes	No
f) kidney problems	Yes	No
g) low blood sugar	Yes	No
h) glaucoma	Yes	No
i) diabetes	Yes	No
j) heart problems	Yes	No

If you answered yes to any of the above, please describe:________________

List all other medical problems you have had in the past. Include date diagnosed and treatment.
DO NOT LIST OPERATIONS
Asthma as a small child. Scoliosis, age 20. Hepatitis, age 36.

SURGICAL HISTORY (List operations and dates performed)
None.

PSYCHIATRIC HISTORY (List visits with counselors, psychologists, etc., and type of treatment)
None

ACCIDENTS IN ADULT LIFE (Briefly describe any accident that caused any blow to the head or that you feel is related to your headache)
None

FAMILY HISTORY:

1. Is your father living? Yes No
   Age________
   Cause of death Liver cancer, age 77
   Was there a headache history? Yes No
2. Is your mother living? Yes No
   Age________
   Cause of death Lupus, age 78
   Was there a headache history? Yes No
3. Ages of brothers---Circle the ones with headache
   47

4. Ages of sisters---Circle the ones with headache
None
5. List any other blood relatives with a history of severe headaches.
None

MARITAL HISTORY:
List marriages:

1st marriage age 23 to Now	Did spouse have headaches?	Yes	No
2nd marriage age ___ to ___	Did spouse have headaches?	Yes	No
3rd marriage age ___ to ___	Did spouse have headaches?	Yes	No

Age of current spouse: 49

List ages and sex of all children:

Age 15 Sex F	Headaches?	Yes	No
Age 9 Sex F	Headaches?	Yes	No
Age 5 Sex F	Headaches?	Yes	No

STRESS FACTORS:

List any factors that may be affecting your headaches (money, loneliness, sexual problems, work, etc.)
Money, work, teenager has boyfriend 5 years older. I don't get a day off.

VEGETATIVE SIGNS:

1.	Do you have trouble falling asleep?	Yes	No
2.	Do you have trouble staying asleep?	Yes	No
3.	Has your appetite decreased?	Yes	No
4.	Have you gained or lost weight in the past year?	Yes	No
5.	Have you felt tearful or depressed lately?	Yes	No
6.	Have you had any thoughts of wanting to die?	Yes	No
7.	Have you been forgetful lately?	Yes	No
8.	Any other changes in your normal day-to-day living?		

Please list any medications you are allergic or sensitive to: Penicillin

Please list any medications you are currently taking (including dosages and frequency per day):
Valium, 5 mg. at night only. Halcion (haven't been taking). Fiorinal 1 to 2 times a day.

PREVIOUS CARE:

1. List doctors who have treated you for headaches: Dr. S

2. List any tests you have had for your headache (e.g., EEG, CT scan, MRI, X-Ray, etc.):
None.

3. List any other treatment you have had for your headache (e.g., biofeedback, acupuncture, chiropractic, or any other treatment you had):
None.

WALTER
Category: Other conditions causing headaches

This patient stated that his headaches started two years before we saw him in our office. Several months prior to that he had an emergency neurosurgical procedure done because of a spontaneous subdural hematoma.

Incapacitating headaches: These began several months after the above-mentioned surgical intervention. He says he gets them on a daily basis. They begin upon awakening as soon as he gets out of bed, and they last until he lies down. He said his headache is always relieved by his lying down. He describes the pain as a tight cap sitting over his head. There is no pressure-type feeling in the back, but it stays in the bifrontal, bitemporal and biparietal regions. There are no warning signs and no symptoms of migraine.

Interfering headaches (moderate to severe): These have the same features and quality as the incapacitating headaches, but they are not incapacitating. Again, he states that these headaches are relieved by lying down. The patient's neurological examination was essentially negative, and there was a shunt in the left temporal area proceeding down to his neck that was placed in him in the original operation. His diagnoses were

1. low pressure headache, and
2. history of subdural hematoma, spontaneous.

An MRI did not disclose any significant findings. After testing, the patient was referred to another neurosurgeon who saw him and a clip ligation was placed on the original shunt to prevent leakage of cerebrospinal fluid. The report back from the neurosurgeon two months after the patient came into our office was that his low pressure headaches have resolved and he was doing quite well.

It is interesting to note in reviewing all the records of the patient how many times he was told by various clinicians that these headaches were secondary to depression, and were most likely psychological. Perhaps we should consider the other side of the circle, that is, that depression and any psychological symptoms came as a result of the incapacitating chronic pain.

MEDICAL HEADACHE HISTORY

Name: Walter **Age:** 70 **Sex** M **Date:** 9/22/92

Date of Birth: 00/00/22 **Birthplace:** AL **Race:** C **Education:** 3 yrs. college

Occupation: Retired **Accident:** N/A

Armed Services & Type of Discharge: 1939-1945 – Army.

PAST HISTORY:

1.	Did you have a normal birth?		Yes	No
	a) forceps used?		Yes	No
	b) cesarean section?		Yes	No
2.	Did you have problems with bedwetting?		Yes	No
	a) If yes, age bedwetting stopped		______	
3.	Were you car sick as a child (motion)?		Yes	No
	a) If yes, how severe?	Slight	Moderate	Severe
4.	Did you have unexplained abdominal cramps as a child?		Yes	No
5.	Did you have any of the following illnesses in childhood?			
	a) meningitis		Yes	No
	b) encephalitis		Yes	No
	c) scarlet fever		Yes	No
	d) rheumatic fever		Yes	No
6.	Did you have any head injuries as a child?		Yes	No
	a) If yes, please explain: ______			
7.	Were you treated for emotional illness as a child?		Yes	No

HABITS:

8.	Do you drink alcohol?	Yes	No
	a) If yes, what kind and how much?______		
	b) Does alcohol bring on or aggravate a headache?	Yes	No
9.	Do you smoke?	Yes	No
	a) If yes, how much?______		
	b) Does smoking or smoke-filled rooms cause or aggravate headaches?	Yes	No
10.	Do you drink caffeinated beverages?	Yes	No
	a) If yes, how much?______		

MENSTRUAL HISTORY:

At what age did menses begin?______ Were they regular or irregular?______
How were they related to your headache?______
Are you or were you ever on Birth Control Pills?______ Did they affect your headache? ______
Have you had a hysterectomy, partial or total, and why?______
Are you in menopause, and if yes, how long?______
Are you on hormones, and if yes, which ones?______

HEADACHE ASSESSMENT FORM

HA PROFILE	INCAPACITATING #3	INTERFERING #2	IRRITATING #1
ONSET (Years ago and frequency)	October 27, 1990 Daily	October 27, 1990 Daily	N/A
CURRENT FREQUENCY	Daily	Daily	N/A
TIME OF ONSET	Comes on 5 to 10 minutes after awakening	Comes on 5 to 10 minutes after awakening	N/A
DURATION	Lasts until I go to bed	Lasts until I go to bed	N/A
CHARACTER	Pressure	Inside pressure	N/A
PRODROME OR AURA	N/A	N/A	N/A
ASSOCIATING FEATURES	Nausea: Vomiting: Sensitivity to Light? Noise? Odors? Do you get pale or flush? Do your eyes or nose run? Does your nose get stuffy? Do the whites of your eyes get red? Does your eyelid droop? Do you pace, or go to bed?	Nausea: Vomiting: Sensitivity to Light? Noise? Odors? Do you get pale or flush? Do your eyes or nose run? Does your nose get stuffy? Do the whites of your eyes get red? Does your eyelid droop? Do you pace, or go to bed?	Nausea: Vomiting: Sensitivity to Light? Noise? Odors? Do you get pale or flush? Do your eyes or nose run? Does your nose get stuffy? Do the whites of your eyes get red? Does your eyelid droop? Do you pace, or go to bed?
PRECIPITATING OR AGGRAVATING FEATURES	N/A	N/A	N/A

LOCATION: Mark the location for each type of headache with a different color pen.

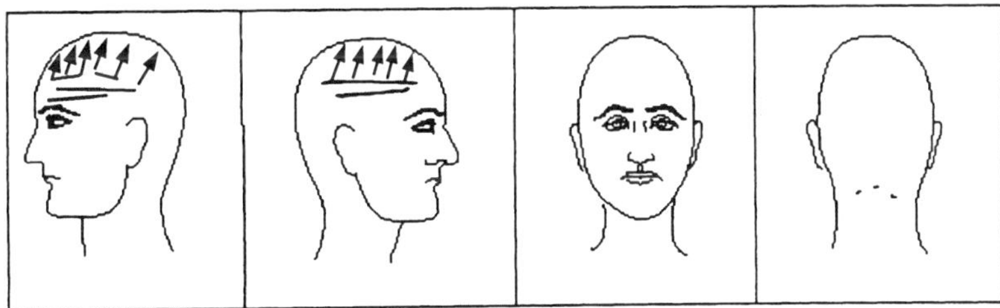

MEDICAL HISTORY:

Have you ever been or are you currently being treated for any of the following?

a) high blood pressure	Yes	No
b) stomach ulcers	Yes	No
c) asthma	Yes	No
d) allergies	Yes	No
e) pneumonia	Yes	No
f) kidney problems	Yes	No
g) low blood sugar	Yes	No
h) glaucoma	Yes	No
i) diabetes	Yes	No
j) heart problems	Yes	No

If you answered yes to any of the above, please describe: Pneumonia 5 to 10 years ago.
Prostate.

List all other medical problems you have had in the past. Include date diagnosed and treatment.
DO NOT LIST OPERATIONS
1976 – Problem with stomach and hiatal hernia.

SURGICAL HISTORY (List operations and dates performed)
1935 – Appendectomy. 1973 – Hiatal hernia. 1973 – Spleen removed with adhesions.
1985 – Subdural hematoma; drained (no plate).

PSYCHIATRIC HISTORY (List visits with counselors, psychologists, etc., and type of treatment)
None

ACCIDENTS IN ADULT LIFE (Briefly describe any accident that caused any blow to the head o that you feel is related to your headache)
None

FAMILY HISTORY:

1.	Is your father living?	Yes	No
	Age________		
	Cause of death Kidney cancer, age 67		
	Was there a headache history?	Yes	No
2.	Is your mother living?	Yes	No
	Age________		
	Cause of death Colon cancer, age 55		
	Was there a headache history?	Yes	No

3. Ages of brothers---Circle the ones with headache
   72
4. Ages of sisters---Circle the ones with headache
   66
5. List any other blood relatives with a history of severe headaches.
   None

MARITAL HISTORY:

List marriages:

1st marriage age 25 to 50	Did spouse have headaches?	Yes	No (underlined)
2nd marriage age 50 to 71	Did spouse have headaches?	Yes (underlined)	No
3rd marriage age ____ to ____	Did spouse have headaches?	Yes	No

Age of current spouse: 62

List ages and sex of all children:

Age 34 Sex M	Headaches?	Yes	No (underlined)
Age 42 Sex F	Headaches?	Yes	No (underlined)
Age ____ Sex ____	Headaches?	Yes	No

STRESS FACTORS:

List any factors that may be affecting your headaches (money, loneliness, sexual problems, work, etc.)
None

VEGETATIVE SIGNS:

1.	Do you have trouble falling asleep?	Yes	No (underlined)
2.	Do you have trouble staying asleep?	Yes	No (underlined)
3.	Has your appetite decreased?	Yes	No (underlined)
4.	Have you gained or lost weight in the past year?	Yes	No (underlined)
5.	Have you felt tearful or depressed lately?	Yes	No (underlined)
6.	Have you had any thoughts of wanting to die?	Yes	No (underlined)
7.	Have you been forgetful lately?	Yes	No (underlined)
8.	Any other changes in your normal day-to-day living?		

Please list any medications you are allergic or sensitive to: Morphine

Please list any medications you are currently taking (including dosages and frequency per day):
Prilosec – 20 mg. 1 per day; Creon and Fiorinal, as needed.

PREVIOUS CARE:

1. List doctors who have treated you for headaches: Dr. H.; Dr. B.

2. List any tests you have had for your headache (e.g., EEG, CT scan, MRI, X-Ray, etc.):
CT and MRI in 1990.

3. List any other treatment you have had for your headache (e.g., biofeedback, acupuncture, chiropractic, or any other treatment you had):
Chiropractic in 1991. Helped for a short time.

LISA
Category: Other conditions causing headaches

This is a 31-year-old nurse who came in with daily incapacitating headaches. She gives an interesting history that she was headache-free until she went on a trip to Peru approximately a year before I saw her. She became ill there, had severe diarrhea and other types of symptoms related to food poisoning, and also came back with 35 to 40 insect bites, even though she wore insect repellant. There had been a gradual downhill course for the patient in terms of her having multiple symptoms such as lethargy, etc., and incapacitating headaches. She has been worked up by multiple physicians. She has seen infectious disease experts. She has seen neurologists, and was seen at the Mayo Clinic in Jacksonville, Florida. At this point, I feel that she had some type of virus that affected her neurological system.

She has daily incapacitating headaches. They are constant, stabbing and boring in the medial orbital range by the eyes and radiate posteriorly to the back of the head. There is no aura. Associated features are nausea, vomiting, photophobia, sonophobia, sensitivity to odors, and she must go to bed.

Diagnosis here is

1. headaches of unknown etiology (source),
2. daily incapacitating intractable vascular headaches (migraine) secondary to viral disease.

Unfortunately, the prognosis for this patient is not very good.

MEDICAL HEADACHE HISTORY

Name: Lisa **Age:** 31 **Sex** F **Date:** 10/28/91

Date of Birth: 00/00/60 **Birthplace:** CN **Race:** W **Education:** A.S.

Occupation: Unemployed **Accident:** N/A

Armed Services & Type of Discharge: N/A

PAST HISTORY:

1.	Did you have a normal birth?		<u>Yes</u>	No
	a) forceps used?		Yes	<u>No</u>
	b) cesarean section?		Yes	<u>No</u>
2.	Did you have problems with bedwetting?		Yes	<u>No</u>
	a) If yes, age bedwetting stopped		______	
3.	Were you car sick as a child (motion)?		<u>Yes</u>	No
	a) If yes, how severe?	Slight	<u>Moderate</u>	Severe
4.	Did you have unexplained abdominal cramps as a child?		Yes	<u>No</u>
5.	Did you have any of the following illnesses in childhood?			
	a) meningitis		Yes	<u>No</u>
	b) encephalitis		Yes	<u>No</u>
	c) scarlet fever		<u>Yes</u>	No
	d) rheumatic fever		Yes	<u>No</u>
6.	Did you have any head injuries as a child?		Yes	<u>No</u>
	a) If yes, please explain: ______			
7.	Were you treated for emotional illness as a child?		Yes	<u>No</u>

HABITS:

8.	Do you drink alcohol?	<u>Yes</u>	No
	a) If yes, what kind and how much? Prior to illness, 1 to 2 oz. per week		
	b) Does alcohol bring on or aggravate a headache?	Yes	<u>No</u>
9.	Do you smoke?	Yes	<u>No</u>
	a) If yes, how much? ______		
	b) Does smoking or smoke-filled rooms cause or aggravate headaches?	<u>Yes</u>	No
10.	Do you drink caffeinated beverages?	<u>Yes</u>	No
	a) If yes, how much? One coffee and one Pepsi per day		

MENSTRUAL HISTORY:

At what age did menses begin? 12 Were they regular or irregular? WNL
How were they related to your headache? N/A
Are you or were you ever on Birth Control Pills? No Did they affect your headache? ______
Have you had a hysterectomy, partial or total, and why? No
Are you in menopause, and if yes, how long? No
Are you on hormones, and if yes, which ones? No

HEADACHE ASSESSMENT FORM

HA PROFILE	INCAPACITATING #3	INTERFERING #2	IRRITATING #1
ONSET (Years ago and frequency)	Oct. 1990, every day for 2 weeks after returning from Peru	N/A	As a child, occasionally
CURRENT FREQUENCY	Every day	N/A	None since 10/90, occasionally before that
TIME OF ONSET	Awaken with	N/A	Anytime
DURATION	Constant	N/A	1 hour with OTC medications
CHARACTER	Stabbing, boring	N/A	Dull ache
PRODROME OR AURA	N/A	N/A	N/A
ASSOCIATING FEATURES	Nausea; Vomiting; Sensitivity to Light? Noise? Odors? Do you get pale or flush? Do your eyes or nose run? Does your nose get stuffy? Does the white of your eyes get red? Does your eyelid droop? Do you pace, or go to bed?	Nausea; Vomiting; Sensitivity to Light? Noise? Odors? Do you get pale or flush? Do your eyes or nose run? Does your nose get stuffy? Does the white of your eyes get red? Does your eyelid droop? Do you pace, or go to bed?	Nausea; Vomiting; Sensitivity to Light? Noise? Odors? Do you get pale or flush? Do your eyes or nose run? Does your nose get stuffy? Does the white of your eyes get red? Does your eyelid droop? Do you pace, or go to bed?
PRECIPITATING OR AGGRAVATING FEATURES	Movement	N/A	Hunger

LOCATION: Mark the location for each type of headache with a different color pen.

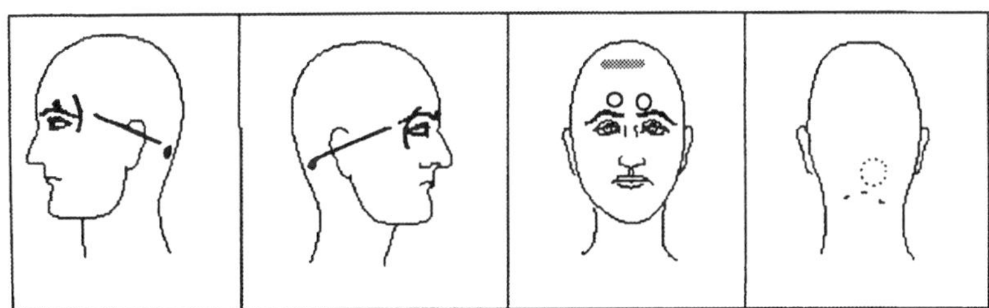

MEDICAL HISTORY:

Have you ever been or are you currently being treated for any of the following?

a) high blood pressure	Yes	No
b) stomach ulcers	Yes	No
c) asthma	Yes	No
d) allergies	Yes	No
e) pneumonia	Yes	No
f) kidney problems	Yes	No
g) low blood sugar	Yes	No
h) glaucoma	Yes	No
i) diabetes	Yes	No
j) heart problems	Yes	No

If you answered yes to any of the above, please describe:____________________

List all other medical problems you have had in the past. Include date diagnosed and treatment. DO NOT LIST OPERATIONS

After a trip to Peru in Sept. 1990, had severe diarrhea, food poisoning, insect bites, and gradually declining health. Have seen numerous doctors. Possibly some type of encephalo virus. Have been unemployed as a result.

SURGICAL HISTORY (List operations and dates performed)

Jan. 1990 – Maxillary down graft and mandibular osteotomy with screws and fixation and cadaver bone implants due to congenital law malformation. Sept. 1989, excision of two benign lumps in breasts.

PSYCHIATRIC HISTORY (List visits with counselors, psychologists, etc., and type of treatment)

Dr. G, therapist, for problems associated with prolonged illness.

ACCIDENTS IN ADULT LIFE (Briefly describe any accident that caused any blow to the head or that you feel is related to your headache)

N/A

FAMILY HISTORY:

1. Is your father living? Yes No
   - Age 69
   - Cause of death____________________
   - Was there a headache history? Yes No
2. Is your mother living? Yes No
   - Age 62
   - Cause of death____________________
   - Was there a headache history? Yes No

3. Ages of brothers---Circle the ones with headache
   30
4. Ages of sisters---Circle the ones with headache
   (37) 36 35 29 22
5. List any other blood relatives with a history of severe headaches.
   ______

MARITAL HISTORY:

List marriages:

1st marriage age ______ to ______ Did spouse have headaches?	Yes	No
2nd marriage age ______ to ______ Did spouse have headaches?	Yes	No
3rd marriage age ______ to ______ Did spouse have headaches?	Yes	No

Age of current spouse:______

List ages and sex of all children:

Age ______ Sex ______ Headaches?	Yes	No
Age ______ Sex ______ Headaches?	Yes	No
Age ______ Sex ______ Headaches?	Yes	No

STRESS FACTORS:

List any factors that may be affecting your headaches (money, loneliness, sexual problems, work, etc.)

______

______

VEGETATIVE SIGNS:

1.	Do you have trouble falling asleep?	Yes	No
2.	Do you have trouble staying asleep?	Yes	No
3.	Has your appetite decreased?	Yes	No
4.	Have you gained or lost weight in the past year?	Yes	No
5.	Have you felt tearful or depressed lately?	Yes	No
6.	Have you had any thoughts of wanting to die?	Yes	No
7.	Have you been forgetful lately?	Yes	No
8.	Any other changes in your normal day-to-day living?______		

Please list any medications you are allergic or sensitive to: No known allergies

______

______

Please list any medications you are currently taking (including dosages and frequency per day):

Phenergan, 50 mg., twice a day; Lopressor, 100 mg., twice a day

Dolobid, 500 mg. twice a day; Elevil, 75 mg., twice a day.

______

______

PREVIOUS CARE:

1. List doctors who have treated you for headaches: Dr. C., Dr. D., Dr. B.

2. List any tests you have had for your headache (e.g., EEG, CT scan, MRI, X-Ray, etc.):

CT brain

MRI – Jan. 1991 (normal)

EEG (normal)

3. List any other treatment you have had for your headache (e.g., biofeedback, acupuncture, chiropractic, or any other treatment you had):

EMILY
Category: Other conditions causing headache

This is an interesting case in which a 39-year-old woman came in who was disabled and on workers compensation as a result of an accident that happened five years before I saw her. According to the patient, she was working at an agricultural chemical shipping company as an administrative secretary working with these chemicals in a building which she said had no ventilation and no protective gear. The chemical was shipped to the office one month after she began to work there and it was stored near her office. She says her headaches began immediately and states that she had no headaches prior to the incident. She also said that she did not suffer asthma before this. The name of the chemical was proprionic acid.

Incapacitating headaches: The patient states that since the day of exposure she began to get these headaches. They come any time she is exposed to a strong odor. They last one to two days and it is a severe pressure in the paranasal area and the supraorbital regions above the eyes. There is no prodrome or aura, and associated features are sensitivity to odors, and she will go to bed.

Interfering headaches (moderate to severe): These also started the day of exposure and she had these daily and still has them daily. They are very similar to the incapacitating headaches, with slightly less pain. She says that blowing her nose will make her headaches worse. She says that she can be in bed for three days at a time with her incapacitating headaches. At the present time she states that if she is not exposed to any volatile fumes, she can be relatively headache-free.

She has had multiple surgeries in her sinus areas, and she currently has to see the ENT specialist for a weekly cleaning of her sinuses. She has chronic drainage whenever there is accumulated nasal discharge. She has seen multiple physicians, and has been seen at both the University of Pennsylvania and the University of Florida for help with her problems.

This is an example of headaches secondary to chemical exposure by her history.

MEDICAL HEADACHE HISTORY

Name: Emily **Age:** 39 **Sex** F **Date:** 9/24/92

Date of Birth: 00/00/52 **Birthplace:** VA **Race:** W **Education:** 2 yrs. college

Occupation: W.C. **Accident:** 1987

Armed Services & Type of Discharge: N/A

PAST HISTORY:

1.	Did you have a normal birth?		**Yes**	No
	a) forceps used?		Yes	**No**
	b) cesarean section?		Yes	**No**
2.	Did you have problems with bedwetting?		Yes	**No**
	a) If yes, age bedwetting stopped		________	
3.	Were you car sick as a child (motion)?		Yes	**No**
	a) If yes, how severe?	Slight	Moderate	Severe
4.	Did you have unexplained abdominal cramps as a child?		Yes	**No**
5.	Did you have any of the following illnesses in childhood?			
	a) meningitis		Yes	**No**
	b) encephalitis		Yes	**No**
	c) scarlet fever		Yes	**No**
	d) rheumatic fever		Yes	**No**
6.	Did you have any head injuries as a child?		Yes	**No**
	a) If yes, please explain: ________			
7.	Were you treated for emotional illness as a child?		Yes	**No**

HABITS:

8.	Do you drink alcohol?	**Yes**	No
	a) If yes, what kind and how much? Only occasionally		
	b) Does alcohol bring on or aggravate a headache?	Yes	**No**
9.	Do you smoke?	Yes	**No**
	a) If yes, how much? ________		
	b) Does smoking or smoke-filled rooms cause or aggravate headaches?	**Yes**	No
10.	Do you drink caffeinated beverages?	**Yes**	No
	a) If yes, how much? One coffee daily		

MENSTRUAL HISTORY:

At what age did menses begin? 9 Were they regular or irregular? WNL

How were they related to your headache? N/A

Are you or were you ever on Birth Control Pills? Yes Did they affect your headache? No

Have you had a hysterectomy, partial or total, and why? Partial, 1975. Increased bleeding.

Are you in menopause, and if yes, how long? No

Are you on hormones, and if yes, which ones? No

HEADACHE ASSESSMENT FORM

HA PROFILE	INCAPACITATING #3	INTERFERING #2	IRRITATING #1
ONSET (Years ago and frequency)	Day of exposure 1 per week	Day of exposure Every day	N/A
CURRENT FREQUENCY	Anytime exposed to a strong odor	Still every day	N/A
TIME OF ONSET	Anytime	Anytime	N/A
DURATION	1 to 2 days	All day	N/A
CHARACTER	Severe pressure	Same, but less intense	N/A
PRODROME OR AURA	N/A	N/A	N/A
ASSOCIATING FEATURES	Nausea; Vomiting; Sensitivity to Light? Noise? Odors? Do you get pale or flush? Do your eyes or nose run? Does your nose get stuffy? Does the white of your eyes get red? Does your eyelid droop? Do you pace, or go to bed?	Nausea; Vomiting; Sensitivity to Light? Noise? Odors? Do you get pale or flush? Do your eyes or nose run? Does your nose get stuffy? Does the white of your eyes get red? Does your eyelid droop? Do you pace, or go to bed?	Nausea; Vomiting; Sensitivity to Light? Noise? Odors? Do you get pale or flush? Do your eyes or nose run? Does your nose get stuffy? Does the white of your eyes get red? Does your eyelid droop? Do you pace, or go to bed?
PRECIPITATING OR AGGRAVATING FEATURES	N/A	Blowing nose, sniffing	N/A

LOCATION: Mark the location for each type of headache with a different color pen.

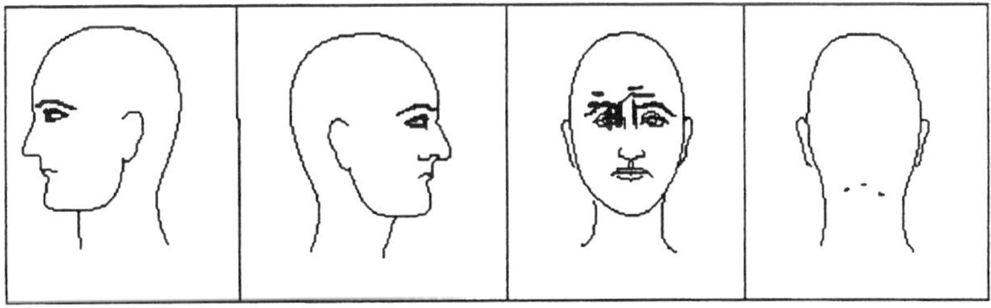

MEDICAL HISTORY:

Have you ever been or are you currently being treated for any of the following?

a) high blood pressure	Yes	No
b) stomach ulcers	Yes	No
c) asthma	Yes	No
d) allergies	Yes	No
e) pneumonia	Yes	No
f) kidney problems	Yes	No
g) low blood sugar	Yes	No
h) glaucoma	Yes	No
i) diabetes	Yes	No
j) heart problems	Yes	No

If you answered yes to any of the above, please describe:______________________

List all other medical problems you have had in the past. Include date diagnosed and treatment.
DO NOT LIST OPERATIONS

Mitral valve prolapse; gastric ulcers; asthma; have had pneumonia and kidney problems; hypocholesterolemia.
Chemical inhalation at work.

SURGICAL HISTORY (List operations and dates performed)

Partial hysterectomy, 1975. Tonsillectomy, 1965. Septoplasty; bilateral maxillary antrostomies; bilateral submucous rseections of inferior turbinates; endoscopic ethmoidectomy; revision of endoscopic ethmoidectomy; lysis of nasal adhesions; chronic ozena treatments.

PSYCHIATRIC HISTORY (List visits with counselors, psychologists, etc., and type of treatment)

C. Counseling Center, depression due to my illness and work accident.

ACCIDENTS IN ADULT LIFE (Briefly describe any accident that caused any blow to the head or that you feel is related to your headache)

Exposure to toxic fumes at work (proprionic acid) and other chemicals – 18 months.

FAMILY HISTORY:

1.	Is your father living?	Yes	No
	Age 64		
	Cause of death______________		
	Was there a headache history?	Yes	No
2.	Is your mother living?	Yes	No
	Age 58		
	Cause of death______________		
	Was there a headache history?	Yes	No

3. Ages of brothers---Circle the ones with headache
 34
4. Ages of sisters---Circle the ones with headache
 None
5. List any other blood relatives with a history of severe headaches.
 None

MARITAL HISTORY:
List marriages:

1st marriage age 18 to 25	Did spouse have headaches?	Yes	No
2nd marriage age 29 to Present	Did spouse have headaches?	Yes	No
3rd marriage age ____ to ____	Did spouse have headaches?	Yes	No

Age of current spouse: 42

List ages and sex of all children:

Age 19 Sex F Headaches?	Yes	No
Age 18 Sex F Headaches?	Yes	No
Age ____ Sex ____ Headaches?	Yes	No

STRESS FACTORS:

List any factors that may be affecting your headaches (money, loneliness, sexual problems, work, etc.)
 None

VEGETATIVE SIGNS:

1.	Do you have trouble falling asleep?	Yes	No
2.	Do you have trouble staying asleep?	Yes	No
3.	Has your appetite decreased?	Yes	No
4.	Have you gained or lost weight in the past year?	Yes	No
5.	Have you felt tearful or depressed lately?	Yes	No
6.	Have you had any thoughts of wanting to die?	Yes	No
7.	Have you been forgetful lately?	Yes	No
8.	Any other changes in your normal day-to-day living?		

Please list any medications you are allergic or sensitive to: Tagamet

Please list any medications you are currently taking (including dosages and frequency per day):
Chalydyl, twice a day. Ventolin inhaler, 2 puffs 4 x per day. Atrovent, 2 puffs per day.
Intal, 2 puffs 4 x per day. Reglan, 20 mg 4 x per day. Prozac, 1 daily. Zantac, 300 mg at bedtime.
Fioricet, 2 tablets every 6 hours. Tylenol #3, 1 o 2 x per day. Beconase, 3 x per day.

PREVIOUS CARE:

1. List doctors who have treated you for headaches: Dr. C., Dr. S., Dr. K.

2. List any tests you have had for your headache (e.g., EEG, CT scan, MRI, X-Ray, etc.):

CAT scan last one 1 month ago (without contrast)

X-rays

3. List any other treatment you have had for your headache (e.g., biofeedback, acupuncture, chiropractic, or any other treatment you had):

Nerve blockers (no help).

CHAPTER 11

Headaches in Children

Children are not spared headaches. The number of headache attacks in children and the young age at which they occur are far more prevalent than one expects. In young children not yet able to talk, the flu or other gastrointestinal disease is often the diagnosis, while in fact they may be suffering from a migraine attack.

Unfortunately, headache studies in children are both difficult and few as to the frequency of this problem. Some studies indicate by age 15 years about 20% of children have migraine or nonvascular headaches. The fortunate aspect is that the vast majority of headaches are not caused by dangerous conditions such as brain tumors or severe disease. This is not to say that if a child presents with a severe headache problem one should not do a complete headache workup. It just says that fortunately any major disease that may be causing a headache is a rarity.

A Swedish study in 1962 showed that by age seven, 2.5% of 9000 school children had frequent nonmigrainous headaches, 1.4% had true migraine, and 35% had infrequent headaches of various types.

By age 15, 16% had frequent nonmigrainous headache, 5.3% had migraine, and 54% had infrequent headaches. Other studies have shown that before puberty boys and girls have migraine almost equally and after puberty girls show a ratio 3 to 4 times higher. It also has been shown that by age 15, 5% of adolescents have experienced a migraine attack. In 50% of all individuals who have migraine attacks, the attacks start before age 20. There seems to be a positive relationship with family history for similar types of headaches in anywhere from 50% to 90% of the cases.

With children losing more than one million school days a year, it is important to review the types of headaches they have.[1]

Sinus headaches — As stated in Chapter 9, sinus headaches are over-diagnosed and this is as true for children as it is for adults. Only about 13% of children with sinusitis actually get a headache from this problem. These children usually have other symptoms, such as coughing, nasal congestion, runny nose, postnasal drip, ear infections and other similar symptoms. X-rays of the sinuses will generally show thickening of the membranes and also mucus filling the spaces of some of the sinuses. Generally treatment of these symptoms not only clears the sinus problems but also the headache.

Vision headaches — Rarely are frequent headaches associated with severe diseases of the eye and most of the time they are usually related to overstrain of the muscles that control eye movements. Proper glasses and better reading habits, especially in this era of the computer, are important. A visit to the ophthalmologist to rule out any serious medical disease should be done first, in the case of any major problem, in order not to permit a disease to continue to progress.

Dental headaches — Infections can sometimes irritate the nerve that sends pain messages to the front of the face and head (trigeminal nerve). Anatomical abnormalities that cause chewing dysfunction, such as temporomandibular joint dysfunction (TMJ) or abnormal bites can create "trigger points" in the muscles of mastication, which in turn can cause headaches. Trigger points are discussed in more detail in Part two of this book in Chapter 18. However, I have seen many patients who have had extensive treatments to correct their dental problems and even when the correction was made the headaches continued. This may be due to the fact that we were dealing with two different problems, one a dental disease, and two a migraine or migraine variant. I was fortunate to have been able to refer to dental specialists who also were knowledgeable in the area of headaches and who had an ongoing dialog with me about the patients. This also helped relieve the anxiety and expectations of the parents of these children.

Ice cream headache — Eating ice cream rapidly may cause a severe sharp pain to the forehead or temple. Several major nerves of the head seem to be responsible for the different locations of these pains (trigeminal, glossopharyngeal, and vagus). A study by Raskin and Knittle[2] has found that over 90% of these patients were in the population of migraine sufferers. If the child complains frequently of these episodes, the parent should be aware that there may be a migraine condition lurking in the future.

Headache from fever — Whenever a child has a high fever and complains of a headache, the important area to be concerned about is the fever. The headache may be the body's way of warning that something serious is going on. A bacterial infection of the brain causing meningitis or a viral infection causing encephalitis may be lurking and the headache may be a blessing in disguise to warn the parent to find immediate attention. Often headache is associated with infections in other parts of the body. Although the exact mechanism of why people get headaches with generalized infections is not exactly known, it may be that in children who already have a potential for headache problems the infection acts as a triggering factor to set into motion that particular headache. At any rate, look for symptoms other than headache that are also part of the infectious process.

Migraine in children — The symptoms of migraine in children are similar to adults (see Chapter 6), and unfortunately they are often misdiagnosed as tension headaches. It is important for the family to realize that 70% to 90% of children who have migraine have a close relative who also has migraine. The adults must realize that often their headaches are not diagnosed correctly.

When a child gets a headache attack he or she looks sick, hence the term "sick headache." Children become pale, with reddened eyes and sometimes experience sweating, nausea, vomiting, often abdominal pain, and they retreat to a dark quiet area. Our studies indicate that 65% of the time children who have or are going to eventually have migraine, will have one or a combination of the following symptoms: bed wetting (enuresis), motion sickness, or abdominal cramps before puberty. In tracing 2000 adult migraine patients, almost 65% had one or more of these symptoms.

The same mechanisms that trigger a migraine attack in adults trigger migraines in children. Before starting any treatment, it is best to take the child to a headache specialist or someone who has an interest in headache and children. A detailed history of the child and family is essential, followed by a thorough physical and neurological examination. Then all the proper tests should be done. This is far more important than a "speedy diagnosis" and a fast approach to relieve the pain. The encouraging news is that more often than not children have a better response to conservative treatment than adults do.

After a neurological evaluation, a medical examination of the child's metabolism, infectious problems, review of all his or her internal systems, allergies, sensitivity to foods, and living habits should be taken into account. The last step is to evaluate "stress problems." If one starts off with the assumption that stress is the primary problem, then medical diseases can be missed and the condition may get worse. There is no child or adult who does not have to deal with some discomfort, but I have seen too many parents who have been told to alter the child's life only to find that the frequency of the headaches has not changed.

It is important to keep in mind that many very young children do not have the ability or language developed to communicate the fact that they are having headaches.

Often, just changing diets or meal times and sleep habits may help reduce attacks. Relaxation treatments like biofeedback, proper exercise, and correcting vision and posture may be of benefit. Correcting dental and orthopedic abnormalities may also be of help. What is very important to understand is that before a medication program is devised, look for non-medication therapy. Medication should not be ruled out, and fortunately children respond to minimal amounts of medication.

Other types of migraine that were discussed in Chapter 6 also have neurological symptoms accompanying them. These same types can also appear in children and always should be evaluated by a neurologist.

Vertebrobasilar migraine involves the lower part of the brain, called the brainstem. It was always believed that constriction of the basilar artery reduces the supply of blood to the brainstem. This reduction of blood was supposed to cause the following symptoms: loss of equilibrium, disturbed balance, double vision, trouble pronouncing words, slurred speech, confusion, and sometimes coma. Newer thinking on the migraine mechanism is that the blood vessel constriction may be the result of a neurochemical mechanism alteration in the nervous system of the brain that starts a whole series of events in the neurophysiology that causes this type of migraine. Fortunately, this disease by itself is benign and does not lead to permanent damage. The other positive news is that there are many ways to treat this condition.

Ophthalmoplegic migraine is another type of migraine that should be evaluated by a neurologist to make sure there is no other neurological illness. The headaches are acute and repetitive and are associated with double vision (diplopia), due to a partial paralysis (paresis) of the muscles directing the eyeball (extraocular muscles). The pupil is often dilated.

Hemiplegic migraine is accompanied by paralysis on one half or one side of the body. Often this paralysis comes one half to one hour before the headache. This headache can start as early as one to two years of age and now is shown to be an inherited disease by chromosome identification. Newer studies have isolated the chromosome that may be responsible for this condition.

Retinal migraine is described as repeated attacks of headache, generally preceded by visual impairment or blindness involving one eye. The visual impairment lasts about an hour. This condition is often benign or does not progress into a worse disease, but any other neurological condition causing this problem must be ruled out.

There are also **migraine variants or equivalents**, in which, although there are no headaches there are symptoms that are similar to migraine and often respond to the same treatments of migraine. Some of these symptoms are vertigo, motion sickness, periodic fainting, flashing lights, rapid heart beat, mood alterations, sleep disturbances, and sometimes distortions of smell, vision, and body images. Other symptoms are confusion, bedwetting, night terrors, sometimes sleepwalking, but there are almost always gastrointestinal symptoms. There always seem to be abdominal cramps and vomiting with no other disease being found. Many times these gastrointestinal symptoms are relieved by antimigraine treatments. Later on after childhood about 75% of these children get typical migraine attacks.

Cluster headache — This type of headache is rarely seen in children; less than 2% in children under 10. The symptoms are similar to adults in that the pain is intense on one side of the head and it is a boring type of pain. There is a ptosis (drooping of the eyelid), a redness and tearing of the eye, stuffed nose and a running nostril on the same side of the pain. This is a diagnosis that could easily be missed by anyone who is not well trained in headache diagnosis.

Tension-type headache — This headache has been discussed fully in Chapter 5. There is no difference in symptoms whether this headache is in children or adults. The symptoms are usually band-like, aching, pressing, tightening or dull. The pain is generally mild or irritating to moderate, which I describe as interfering. Often they are described as getting worse or starting after the person wakes up, and often become more painful as the day goes on. There are no signs of nausea, vomiting or throbbing-like pain, but when these signs become apparent we suspect that this is progressing into a migraine-like headache.

There are multiple approaches to the treatment of tension-like headaches, which are discussed in many of the books that are published today on the subject. Most of these treatments are behavioral approaches to reduce stress caused by the environment surrounding the child, which may be precipitating the headaches. Other treatments include diet changes, exercise programs, sleep pattern alterations, counseling, biofeedback training, and very conservative medication therapy.

One area that rarely is talked about is the influence that headache suffering parents have on promoting a "headache child." I have had many of my patients bring their children to me and the analysis of the problem is often that the child is mimicking the behavior of the parent. If a parent expects the child to observe and carry out the positive messages that are being conveyed, why not the negative ones? If a child sees that the parent doesn't have to go to work, do household chores, or go to church, and can avoid any unpleasant event by lying down in a dark room complaining of head pain, while everyone else in the family gives special care to the headache sufferer, why not do the same thing?

When treating the child with a headache complaint it is often wise to investigate the parents and work with the whole family, if this is the situation in the home setting. It is important to correct this problem in childhood before another "headache parent" is developed.

REFERENCES

1. Rapoport, A.M., Sheftel, F.D., *Headache Relief*, Simon and Schuster, New York, 1990.
2. Raskin, N.H., *Headache*, 2nd ed., Churchill Livingstone. New York, 1988.

CASE HISTORIES*

HELEN
Category: Headache in children

This is another case in which headaches started as a child and, although I saw the patient when she was 42, certainly this would be someone who should have been treated as a child to perhaps prevent further increase of headaches, or at least to have them under more control.

These headaches started when the patient was 6 and she would get several a week, and then the pattern stopped at age 16. Then the pattern began to take place during the menstrual periods and also the ovulation cycles.

The diagnosis of this patient would be nonclassical migraine or migraine without aura according to the classification of the International Headache Society, and she also would be considered to have hormonal migraine and be treated during the hormonal and ovulation periods.

* On the headache assessment forms that accompany these case hisories, incapacitating headaches are indicated with solid black lines, interfering headaches with dotted lines, and irritating headaches with gray shading.

MEDICAL HEADACHE HISTORY

Name: Helen **Age:** 42 **Sex** F **Date:** 12/10/86

Date of Birth: 00/00/44 **Birthplace:** NY **Race:** W **Education:** 1 year college

Occupation: Accountant **Accident:** N/A

Armed Services & Type of Discharge: N/A

PAST HISTORY:

1.	Did you have a normal birth?		Yes	No
	a) forceps used?		Yes	No
	b) cesarean section?		Yes	No
2.	Did you have problems with bedwetting?		Yes	No
	a) If yes, age bedwetting stopped		______	
3.	Were you car sick as a child (motion)?		Yes	No
	a) If yes, how severe?	Slight	Moderate	Severe
4.	Did you have unexplained abdominal cramps as a child?		Yes	No
5.	Did you have any of the following illnesses in childhood?			
	a) meningitis		Yes	No
	b) encephalitis		Yes	No
	c) scarlet fever		Yes	No
	d) rheumatic fever		Yes	No
6.	Did you have any head injuries as a child?		Yes	No
	a) If yes, please explain: ______			
7.	Were you treated for emotional illness as a child?		Yes	No

HABITS:

8.	Do you drink alcohol?	Yes	No
	a) If yes, what kind and how much? ______		
	b) Does alcohol bring on or aggravate a headache?	Yes	No
9.	Do you smoke?	Yes	No
	a) If yes, how much? ______		
	b) Does smoking or smoke-filled rooms cause or aggravate headaches?	Yes	No
10.	Do you drink caffeinated beverages?	Yes	No
	a) If yes, how much? ______		

MENSTRUAL HISTORY:

At what age did menses begin? 13-14 Were they regular or irregular? WNL
How were they related to your headache? Has headaches around periods
Are you or were you ever on Birth Control Pills? Yes Did they affect your headache? ______
Have you had a hysterectomy, partial or total, and why? No
Are you in menopause, and if yes, how long? No
Are you on hormones, and if yes, which ones? Medroxy, Progesterone

HEADACHE ASSESSMENT FORM

HA PROFILE	INCAPACITATING #3	INTERFERING #2	IRRITATING #1
ONSET (Years ago and frequency)	Age 6-16 couple times a week; Age 16-now, couple times a month	N/A	Age 39, 4 times a year
CURRENT FREQUENCY	Several times a month	N/A	4 times a year
TIME OF ONSET	Usually before period; can be during or after	N/A	Change of seasons, wakes up with
DURATION	Wakes up with; 24 to 48 hours	N/A	20 minutes, if taking medications
CHARACTER	Throbbing	Slight throbbing, pressure	N/A
PRODROME OR AURA	N/A	N/A	N/A
ASSOCIATING FEATURES	Nausea; Vomiting; Sensitivity to Light? Noise? Odors? Do you get pale or flush? Do your eyes or nose run? Does your nose get stuffy? Do the whites of your eyes get red? Does your eyelid droop? Do you pace, or go to bed?	Nausea; Vomiting; Sensitivity to Light? Noise? Odors? Do you get pale or flush? Do your eyes or nose run? Does your nose get stuffy? Do the whites of your eyes get red? Does your eyelid droop? Do you pace, or go to bed?	Nausea; Vomiting; Sensitivity to Light? Noise? Odors? Do you get pale or flush? Do your eyes or nose run? Does your nose get stuffy? Do the whites of your eyes get red? Does your eyelid droop? Do you pace, or go to bed?
PRECIPITATING OR AGGRAVATING FEATURES	Lying down Menstruation Alcohol Walking	N/A	Change of seasons

LOCATION: Mark the location for each type of headache with a different color pen.

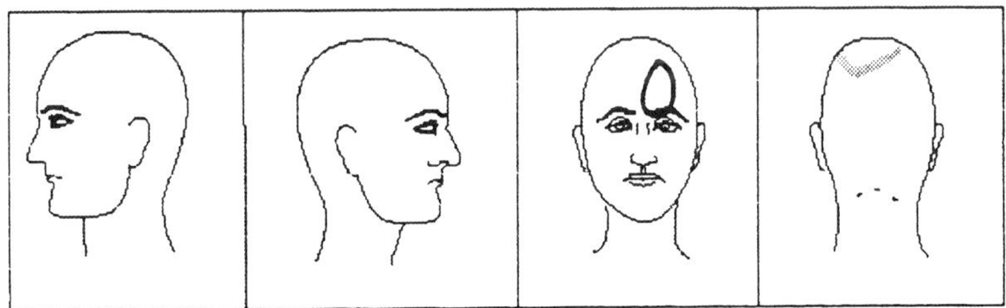

MEDICAL HISTORY:

Have you ever been or are you currently being treated for any of the following?

a) high blood pressure	Yes	<u>No</u>
b) stomach ulcers	Yes	<u>No</u>
c) asthma	Yes	<u>No</u>
d) allergies	Yes	<u>No</u>
e) pneumonia	Yes	<u>No</u>
f) kidney problems	Yes	<u>No</u>
g) low blood sugar	Yes	<u>No</u>
h) glaucoma	Yes	<u>No</u>
i) diabetes	Yes	<u>No</u>
j) heart problems	Yes	<u>No</u>

If you answered yes to any of the above, please describe:____________________

List all other medical problems you have had in the past. Include date diagnosed and treatment.
DO NOT LIST OPERATIONS

1986 – Pinched nerve in neck/shoulder area. Treated with acupuncture.
1984 – Degenerative disk in neck. Traction and anti-inflammatory drugs.

SURGICAL HISTORY (List operations and dates performed)

Appendectomy 1954. Tonsillectomy 1964. Ectopic pregnancy 1968.

PSYCHIATRIC HISTORY (List visits with counselors, psychologists, etc., and type of treatment)

None

ACCIDENTS IN ADULT LIFE (Briefly describe any accident that caused any blow to the head or that you feel is related to your headache)

None

FAMILY HISTORY:

1. Is your father living? <u>Yes</u> No
   - Age 86
   - Cause of death____________________
   - Was there a headache history? Yes <u>No</u>
2. Is your mother living? <u>Yes</u> No
   - Age 67
   - Cause of death____________________
   - Was there a headache history? Yes <u>No</u>

3. Ages of brothers---Circle the ones with headache
   40
4. Ages of sisters---Circle the ones with headache
   44 38
5. List any other blood relatives with a history of severe headaches.
   None

MARITAL HISTORY:

List marriages:

1st marriage age 1966 to Present	Did spouse have headaches?	Yes	<u>No</u>
2nd marriage age _____ to _______	Did spouse have headaches?	Yes	No
3rd marriage age _____ to _______	Did spouse have headaches?	Yes	No

Age of current spouse: 41

List ages and sex of all children:

Age 16 Sex F	Headaches?	Yes	<u>No</u>
Age 14 Sex M	Headaches?	<u>Yes</u>	No
Age _____ Sex _____	Headaches?	Yes	No

STRESS FACTORS:

List any factors that may be affecting your headaches (money, loneliness, sexual problems, work, etc.)
None

VEGETATIVE SIGNS:

1.	Do you have trouble falling asleep?	Yes	<u>No</u>
2.	Do you have trouble staying asleep?	Yes	<u>No</u>
3.	Has your appetite decreased?	Yes	<u>No</u>
4.	Have you gained or lost weight in the past year?	Yes	<u>No</u>
5.	Have you felt tearful or depressed lately?	Yes	<u>No</u>
6.	Have you had any thoughts of wanting to die?	Yes	<u>No</u>
7.	Have you been forgetful lately?	<u>Yes</u>	<u>No</u>
8.	Any other changes in your normal day-to-day living?		

Please list any medications you are allergic or sensitive to: None. Aspirin upsets stomach.

Please list any medications you are currently taking (including dosages and frequency per day):
Medroxy, Progesterone, 1 tablet daily 14 days before menstrual cycle.

PREVIOUS CARE:

1. List doctors who have treated you for headaches: Dr. R, Dr. W.

2. List any tests you have had for your headache (e.g., EEG, CT scan, MRI, X-Ray, etc.):
None.

3. List any other treatment you have had for your headache (e.g., biofeedback, acupuncture, chiropractic, or any other treatment you had):
Acupuncture.

DANIEL
Category: Headaches in children

This young boy of 11 had been having headaches that were identified since age 4. The intake indicates that he has typical symptoms of migraine, with the throbbing qualities, nausea, vomiting, and sensitivity to light, noise, and odors. Unfortunately, they were interfering with his ability to do his school work properly. There was no indication that there was any neurological problem, and he was treated conservatively with aspirin and an antihistamine twice a day, and also given a short course in biofeedback, which tends to work well with children.

MEDICAL HEADACHE HISTORY

Name: Daniel **Age:** 11 **Sex** M **Date:** 3/19/91

Date of Birth: 00/00/79 **Birthplace:** FL **Race:** W **Education:** 6th Grade

Occupation: Student **Accident:** N/A

Armed Services & Type of Discharge: N/A

PAST HISTORY:

1.	Did you have a normal birth?		<u>Yes</u>	No
	a) forceps used?		<u>Yes</u>	No
	b) cesarean section?		Yes	No
2.	Did you have problems with bedwetting?		Yes	<u>No</u>
	a) If yes, age bedwetting stopped			______
3.	Were you car sick as a child (motion)?		Yes	<u>No</u>
	a) If yes, how severe?	Slight	Moderate	Severe
4.	Did you have unexplained abdominal cramps as a child?		Yes	<u>No</u>
5.	Did you have any of the following illnesses in childhood?			
	a) meningitis		Yes	<u>No</u>
	b) encephalitis		Yes	<u>No</u>
	c) scarlet fever		Yes	<u>No</u>
	d) rheumatic fever		Yes	<u>No</u>
6.	Did you have any head injuries as a child?		Yes	<u>No</u>
	a) If yes, please explain:______			
7.	Were you treated for emotional illness as a child?		Yes	<u>No</u>

HABITS:

8.	Do you drink alcohol?	Yes	<u>No</u>
	a) If yes, what kind and how much?______		
	b) Does alcohol bring on or aggravate a headache?	Yes	No
9.	Do you smoke?	Yes	<u>No</u>
	a) If yes, how much?______		
	b) Does smoking or smoke-filled rooms cause or aggravate headaches?	Yes	<u>No</u>
10.	Do you drink caffeinated beverages?	<u>Yes</u>	No
	a) If yes, how much? Pepsi		

MENSTRUAL HISTORY:

At what age did menses begin?______ Were they regular or irregular?______

How were they related to your headache?______

Are you or were you ever on Birth Control Pills?______ Did they affect your headache? ______

Have you had a hysterectomy, partial or total, and why?______

Are you in menopause, and if yes, how long?______

Are you on hormones, and if yes, which ones?______

HEADACHE ASSESSMENT FORM

HA PROFILE	INCAPACITATING #3	INTERFERING #2	IRRITATING #1
ONSET (Years ago and frequency)	Age 6 – 2/month	Age 4 – 5, Occasionally	Age 4 – 5, Occasionally
CURRENT FREQUENCY	1/wk	1 – 2 mo.	3 – 4/wk
TIME OF ONSET	Anytime	Anytime	Anytime
DURATION	2 – 3 days	1 day	1 hour with OTC medications
CHARACTER	Throbbing	Same, less intense	Dull ache
PRODROME OR AURA	N/A	N/A	N/A
ASSOCIATING FEATURES	Nausea; Vomiting; Sensitivity to Light? Noise? Odors? Do you get pale or flush? Do your eyes or nose run? Does your nose get stuffy? Does the white of your eyes get red? Does your eyelid droop? Do you pace, or go to bed?	Nausea; Vomiting; Sensitivity to Light? Noise? Odors? Do you get pale or flush? Do your eyes or nose run? Does your nose get stuffy? Does the white of your eyes get red? Does your eyelid droop? Do you pace, or go to bed?	Nausea; Vomiting; Sensitivity to Light? Noise? Odors? Do you get pale or flush? Do your eyes or nose run? Does your nose get stuffy? Does the white of your eyes get red? Does your eyelid droop? Do you pace, or go to bed?
PRECIPITATING OR AGGRAVATING FEATURES	Activity, coughing	Coughing	N/A

LOCATION: Mark the location for each type of headache with a different color pen.

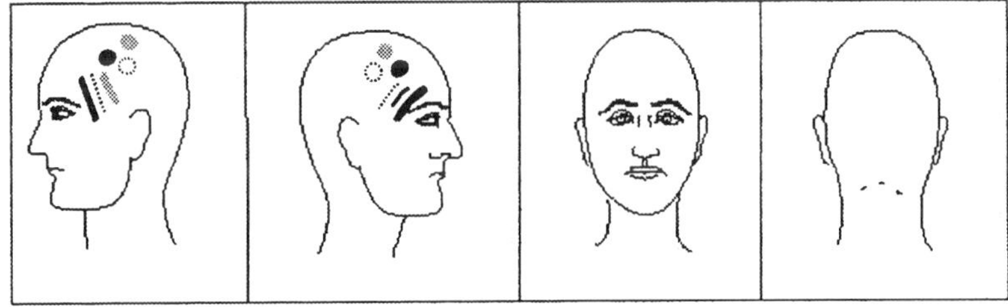

MEDICAL HISTORY:

Have you ever been or are you currently being treated for any of the following?

a) high blood pressure	Yes	No
b) stomach ulcers	Yes	No
c) asthma	Yes	No
d) allergies	Yes	No
e) pneumonia	Yes	No
f) kidney problems	Yes	No
g) low blood sugar	Yes	No
h) glaucoma	Yes	No
i) diabetes	Yes	No
j) heart problems	Yes	No

If you answered yes to any of the above, please describe:____________________

List all other medical problems you have had in the past. Include date diagnosed and treatment.
DO NOT LIST OPERATIONS

Hospitalized in 1988 or 1989 for low blood sugar.

Surgical History (List operations and date performed).

None

PSYCHIATRIC HISTORY (List visits with counselors, psychologists, etc., and type of treatment)

None

ACCIDENTS IN ADULT LIFE (Briefly describe any accident that caused any blow to the head or that you feel is related to your headache)

None.

FAMILY HISTORY:

1.	Is your father living?	Yes	No
	Age 43		
	Cause of death__________		
	Was there a headache history?	Yes	No
2.	Is your mother living?	Yes	No
	Age 39		
	Cause of death__________		
	Was there a headache history?	Yes	No
3.	Ages of brothers---Circle the ones with headache		
	(14) has "grown out" of them		

4. Ages of sisters---Circle the ones with headache
   ___7____
5. List any other blood relatives with a history of severe headaches.
   ___Great aunt, paternal cousin___________________

MARITAL HISTORY:
List marriages:

1st marriage age	to	Did spouse have headaches?	Yes	No
2nd marriage age _____	to _______	Did spouse have headaches?	Yes	No
3rd marriage age _____	to _______	Did spouse have headaches?	Yes	No

Age of current spouse:___________

List ages and sex of all children:

Age _____	Sex ______	Headaches?	Yes	No
Age _____	Sex ______	Headaches?	Yes	No
Age _____	Sex ______	Headaches?	Yes	No

STRESS FACTORS:

List any factors that may be affecting your headaches (money, loneliness, sexual problems, work, etc.)
___Baseball, school_____________________________________
____

VEGETATIVE SIGNS:

1.	Do you have trouble falling asleep?	Yes	No
2.	Do you have trouble staying asleep?	Yes	No
3.	Has your appetite decreased?	Yes	No
4.	Have you gained or lost weight in the past year?	Yes	No
5.	Have you felt tearful or depressed lately?	Yes	No
6.	Have you had any thoughts of wanting to die?	Yes	No
7.	Have you been forgetful lately?	Yes	No
8.	Any other changes in your normal day-to-day living?____________		

Please list any medications you are allergic or sensitive to:____________________
____

Please list any medications you are currently taking (including dosages and frequency per day):
___Tylenol #3 and Ventolin_______________________________
____

PREVIOUS CARE:

1. List doctors who have treated you for headaches:____________________
____
____
____

2. List any tests you have had for your headache (e.g., EEG, CT scan, MRI, X-Ray, etc.):
___CT scan 1990 (normal).________________________________
____
____
____

3. List any other treatment you have had for your headache (e.g., biofeedback, acupuncture, chiropractic, or any other treatment you had):
___None.____
____
____

SHIRLEY
Category: Headaches in children

Although this is a history on a 45-year-old adult, these headaches started when the patient was a child, approximately age 5, and therefore we place the case history in this chapter to show that this is an important problem that must be treated early to prevent the continuous increase of headaches that will become disabling in adult life.

This patient appears to have started having migraines at age 7, and they would have been considered to be classical migraine or migraine with aura under the International Headache Society classification because of the "squiggly lines" that preceded the headache, starting way back. These headaches had developed from migraine into daily intractable headache, which means that it is constantly interfering and preventing her from functioning in a progressive way during her life. You will notice early on in the medical history that high elevations or airplane flights would increase her headaches.

Although these headaches most likely started as migraine with aura, that is with the so-called "squiggly lines", she also reported that she would sometimes have these auras without a headache. Eventually, she began to have the less severe interfering headaches and they began to come on a daily basis. One year before she came to our office, she was having them every day.

A neurological examination and an MRI did not indicate any tumor or intracranial lesion, and the last time the patient was seen it appeared that she was having a very difficult time because of being hypersensitive to all medications.

MEDICAL HEADACHE HISTORY

Name: Shirley **Age:** 45 **Sex** F **Date:** 8/24/92

Date of Birth: 00/00/47 **Birthplace:** WI **Race:** W **Education:** High school

Occupation: Data Processing **Accident:** N/A

Armed Services & Type of Discharge: N/A

PAST HISTORY:

1.	Did you have a normal birth?		Yes	No
	a) forceps used?		Yes	No
	b) cesarean section?		Yes	No
2.	Did you have problems with bedwetting?		Yes	No
	a) If yes, age bedwetting stopped			
3.	Were you car sick as a child (motion)?		Yes	No
	a) If yes, how severe?	Slight	Moderate	Severe
4.	Did you have unexplained abdominal cramps as a child?		Yes	No
5.	Did you have any of the following illnesses in childhood?			
	a) meningitis		Yes	No
	b) encephalitis		Yes	No
	c) scarlet fever		Yes	No
	d) rheumatic fever		Yes	No
6.	Did you have any head injuries as a child?		Yes	No
	a) If yes, please explain:			
7.	Were you treated for emotional illness as a child?		Yes	No

HABITS:

8.	Do you drink alcohol?		Yes	No
	a) If yes, what kind and how much?			
	b) Does alcohol bring on or aggravate a headache?		Yes	No
9.	Do you smoke?		Yes	No
	a) If yes, how much? 1 pack a day			
	b) Does smoking or smoke-filled rooms cause or aggravate headaches?		Yes	No
10.	Do you drink caffeinated beverages?		Yes	No
	a) If yes, how much? 2 cups coffee 1 coke a day			

MENSTRUAL HISTORY:

At what age did menses begin? 15 Were they regular or irregular? WNL
How were they related to your headache? N/A
Are you or were you ever on Birth Control Pills? Yes Did they affect your headache? Increased HA
Have you had a hysterectomy, partial or total, and why? Partial 1983, Total 1985. Cysts
Are you in menopause, and if yes, how long? No
Are you on hormones, and if yes, which ones? Premarin 1.25 mg 5/wk

HEADACHE ASSESSMENT FORM

HA PROFILE	INCAPACITATING #3	INTERFERING #2	IRRITATING #1
ONSET (Years ago and frequency)	Age 7, occasionally	As a child, occasionally	N/A
CURRENT FREQUENCY	1 to 2 in 6 months	Every day for more than a year	N/A
TIME OF ONSET	Anytime	Anytime	N/A
DURATION	1 day	2 hours to all day	N/A
CHARACTER	Throbbing	Slight throbbing, pressure	N/A
PRODROME OR AURA	Sees "squiggly lines" – Headache 20 to 30 min. later.	N/A	N/A
ASSOCIATING FEATURES	Nausea; Vomiting; Sensitivity to Light? Noise? Odors? Do you get pale or flush? Do your eyes or nose run? Does your nose get stuffy? Do the whites of your eyes get red? Does your eyelid droop? Do you pace, or go to bed?	Nausea; Vomiting; Sensitivity to Light? Noise? Odors? Do you get pale or flush? Do your eyes or nose run? Does your nose get stuffy? Do the whites of your eyes get red? Does your eyelid droop? Do you pace, or go to bed?	Nausea; Vomiting; Sensitivity to Light? Noise? Odors? Do you get pale or flush? Do your eyes or nose run? Does your nose get stuffy? Do the whites of your eyes get red? Does your eyelid droop? Do you pace, or go to bed?
PRECIPITATING OR AGGRAVATING FEATURES	Movement. Has aura 2 to 3 times a week without headache for a month	Airplane flight Higher elevation	N/A

LOCATION: Mark the location for each type of headache with a different color pen.

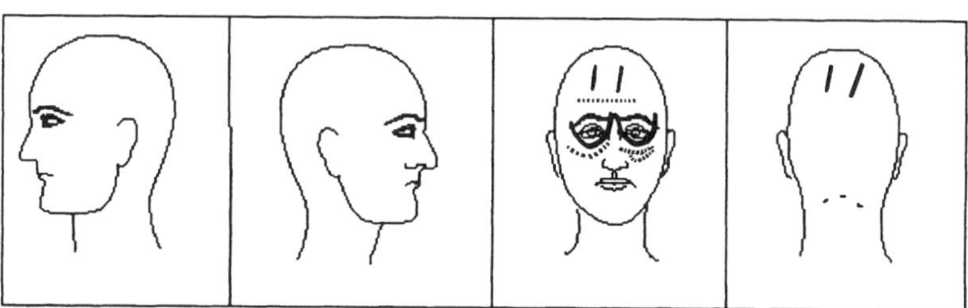

MEDICAL HISTORY:

Have you ever been or are you currently being treated for any of the following?

a) high blood pressure	Yes	No
b) stomach ulcers	Yes	No
c) asthma	Yes	No
d) allergies	Yes	No
e) pneumonia	Yes	No
f) kidney problems	Yes	No
g) low blood sugar	Yes	No
h) glaucoma	Yes	No
i) diabetes	Yes	No
j) heart problems	Yes	No

If you answered yes to any of the above, please describe:____________________

List all other medical problems you have had in the past. Include date diagnosed and treatment.
DO NOT LIST OPERATIONS

Sinusitis.

SURGICAL HISTORY (List operations and dates performed)

Tonsillectomy 1967. Hysterectomy (partial) 1983, (total) 1985. Breast reduction 1980.

PSYCHIATRIC HISTORY (List visits with counselors, psychologists, etc., and type of treatment)

None

ACCIDENTS IN ADULT LIFE (Briefly describe any accident that caused any blow to the head or that you feel is related to your headache)

Car accident. Hit in the back of the head with a tennis racket (16 years ago).

FAMILY HISTORY:

1. Is your father living? Yes No
   Age 72
   Cause of death________________
   Was there a headache history? Yes No
2. Is your mother living? Yes No
   Age 70
   Cause of death________________
   Was there a headache history? Yes No

3. Ages of brothers---Circle the ones with headache
____

4. Ages of sisters---Circle the ones with headache
(49) 47 42 40

5. List any other blood relatives with a history of severe headaches.
None

MARITAL HISTORY:
List marriages:

1st marriage age 17 to 21	Did spouse have headaches?	Yes	No
2nd marriage age 34 to 34	Did spouse have headaches?	Yes	No
3rd marriage age 36 to Present	Did spouse have headaches?	Yes	No

Age of current spouse: 40

List ages and sex of all children:

Age 28 Sex F	Headaches?	Yes	No
Age ______ Sex ______	Headaches?	Yes	No
Age ______ Sex ______	Headaches?	Yes	No

STRESS FACTORS:

List any factors that may be affecting your headaches (money, loneliness, sexual problems, work, etc.)
____
____

VEGETATIVE SIGNS:

1.	Do you have trouble falling asleep?	Yes	No
2.	Do you have trouble staying asleep?	Yes	No
3.	Has your appetite decreased?	Yes	No
4.	Have you gained or lost weight in the past year?	Yes	No
5.	Have you felt tearful or depressed lately?	Yes	No
6.	Have you had any thoughts of wanting to die?	Yes	No
7.	Have you been forgetful lately?	Yes	No
8.	Any other changes in your normal day-to-day living?______		

Please list any medications you are allergic or sensitive to: Sulfa

Please list any medications you are currently taking (including dosages and frequency per day):
Premarin 1.25 mg. 5 days a week. Tylenol 2 to 4 a day.
____

PREVIOUS CARE:

1. List doctors who have treated you for headaches:____________________

2. List any tests you have had for your headache (e.g., EEG, CT scan, MRI, X-Ray, etc.):
CAT scan on sinus 2 weeks ago.

3. List any other treatment you have had for your headache (e.g., biofeedback, acupuncture, chiropractic, or any other treatment you had):
None.

CHAPTER 12

How to Diagnose Headaches

THE HISTORY

In Chapter 4, "The Headache Intake Form," the emphasis was on how important the initial history is in making the diagnosis. At this point the reader has to recognize that headache is not a simple problem, and unless an accurate diagnosis is made the ability to help manage the problem will not improve but could become worse. What might become a tolerable situation, under poor management could become a disability. Whoever the patient goes to for a headache workup should be someone who has an excellent grasp of diagnosis and treatment. That person should also know when the problem has become more complex than he or she is trained to manage, and to whom to refer the patient.

Fortunately, most headache patients do not present a life-threatening disease but it is extremely important that any underlying medical, neurological, or dental disease be eliminated as a cause of the headache symptom. That is why a headache specialist or a physician who has an interest in headaches should be utilized in the evaluation of an ongoing or chronic headache problem. In my own practice over the years I have been able to recognize many of the above problems, and if I could not treat them I had other specialists resolve the disorder.

The history is the most important phase in establishing the diagnosis of any headache condition.[1] As discussed in Chapter 4, the onset, frequency, duration, intensity, character of the pain, prodromes or auras, associating features, aggravating factors, and the location are essential to know.

Other variables that have to be known are: age, gender, occupation; if it applies, menstrual history; birth information; bed wetting problems, motion or car sickness, or abdominal cramps before puberty; any history of meningitis, encephalitis, scarlet fever, or rheumatic fever; sensitivity to alcohol, smoke filled rooms, or caffeine; any and all previous medical conditions; any surgical procedures; any psychiatric or psychological treatments; any family history of headaches; any stress factors that are currently happening; any signs of depression, i.e., appetite decrease, difficulty with sleep, loss of libido, loss of concentration; any previous medications that were used to treat the headache problem and which ones helped; what current medications are being taken, and how much. Any medications that cause adverse effects, any factors that may provoke a headache, any hormonal changes, contraceptives, menstrual periods, menopause, hormone replacement, exertion, weather, bright lights, altitude, paints or solvents, any physical alterations that cause headache, must be noted.

Foods that may cause a headache include:

Aged cheeses: cheddar, Gruyere, Stilton, Brie, Camembert, etc.
Alcohol: wine, beer, aged liquor
Caffeine: coffee, tea, cola, various medications that have caffeine in them
Chocolate
Sugar products
Dairy products: milk, ice cream, yogurt, cream
Fermented, pickled foods: herring, sour cream, vinegar, marinated meats
Fruits: bananas, avocado, figs, raisins, oranges and other citrus foods
Monosodium glutamate (MSG): Chinese foods, seasoned salt products, instant foods, TV dinners, processed meats, roasted nuts, potato chips
Meats with nitrites: bologna, hot dogs, pepperoni, salami, pastrami, bacon, sausages, canned ham, corned beef, smoked fish
Sugar substitutes: diet drinks, or diet foods
Sulfites: salad bars, shrimp, soft drinks, certain wines
Vegetables: onions, broad beans, pea pods, nuts, peanuts
Yeast products: yeast extract, fresh breads, raised coffee cakes, doughnuts

Headache sufferers should be prepared to list any foods that they are aware of that have caused a headache, and to give a history of anyone who has treated them for a headache including his or her professional title. They should be able to list all tests and treatments that were done.

THE PHYSICAL EXAMINATION

After the history is taken, the physical examination is the next step. It is also important that the physical examination be as complete as the history intake. Based on the information gathered from all this, the examiner will determine what other tests are necessary. The rationale for laboratory tests, any neurodiagnostic studies, electrocardiography, x-rays, dental studies, psychological studies, and any other investigations should be based on the information derived from the history and physical examination. Even the information that a patient does *not* give may be a clue to the examiner that further testing is necessary. Often I have heard patients say, "I know this may seem silly, doctor…" when, in fact, that information leads the examiner to consider medical diseases that the patient was unaware existed.

Dr. Joel Saper has said, "Patients have illnesses and symptoms long before doctors understand them or have the means to diagnose or treat them."

The physical examination includes two parts, examination of the body as a whole, and a neurological examination.

Examination of the body should include: temperature, respiration, pulse, blood pressure on both arms, height, and weight. The rest of the examination includes the face, scalp, eyes, nose, ears, mouth, teeth, gums, tongue, temporomandibular joint, sinuses, neck (lymph nodes, carotid arteries, thyroid and the muscles of the neck and shoulders), lungs, heart, abdomen, and extremities. Normally a rectal and genital examination are not done, but if infection or cancer is suspected then this should be evaluated. I have always placed a great deal of emphasis on the muscles and tendons of the neck and shoulders and will discuss trigger points in greater detail in Part two of this book.

The neurological examination includes evaluation of the cranial nerves, especially II through XII, the cerebellar, the motor and sensory systems, the pulses in the legs and feet, and the major reflexes.

Finally, as part of the initial examination the mental status is done to make sure there are no organic psychiatric diseases.

Once the initial examination is complete the physician must now decide what types of tests should be done to rule out any organic disease. This decision is based on the medical knowledge and the experience of the clinician. Ordering a great many tests has several drawbacks: one, they are very expensive, and two, random testing can often lead the examiner in the wrong direction and perhaps even give a false sense of security.

LABORATORY TESTING

Because there are several hundred causes that may produce headaches, laboratory testing is essential for helping to rule out medical disease. It also establishes baseline results that may be used later on to follow any changes that occur if a disease gets worse and then begins to demonstrate abnormal findings. It is also helpful in determining any abnormalities that may come as a result of changes due to medication that is used in treating the headache problem.

Because many patients underestimate or deliberately do not report the amount of prescribed or over-the-counter medications they use drug evaluations using blood or urine can detect toxic levels of drugs. As discussed in Chapter 7 overuse or abuse of medications may cause "rebound headaches," and reducing or eliminating the drugs may significantly diminish or even eliminate the headaches.

The tests that are suggested to start with are a complete chemistry profile, a complete blood count, and urinalysis. Further testing may include drug screening, thyroid testing, estrogen studies for women, and bleeding time for patients who present with hematomas or black and blue marks from taking too much aspirin.

Because there are so many diseases that may have headache as a secondary symptom, laboratory testing is the best way to zero in on these disorders. Abnormalities in the chemistry profile, the blood count, and urinalysis may give clues to the following:

1. Diseases of the gastrointestinal system
2. Diseases of the cardiovascular system
3. Diseases of the respiratory system
4. Diseases of the nervous system
5. Diseases of muscle
6. Diseases of the immune system
7. Diseases of calcium metabolism and bone
8. Diseases of the kidney
9. Diseases of metabolism
10. Diseases of the endocrine system
11. Diseases of the skin
12. Diseases due to physical agents
13. Disorders of water and electrolyte metabolism and of acid/base balance
14. Disorders resulting from vitamin deficiencies
15. Disorders of the blood
16. Infectious diseases
17. Tropical diseases
18. Worms
19. Venereal diseases
20. Abnormal reactions to drugs
21. Poisons

Neurodiagnostic Testing

The following tests are necessary under certain indications: computerized tomography (CT) scan, magnetic resonance imaging (MRI), lumbar puncture (LP), electroencephalography (EEG), electrocardiography (EKG), routine x-rays, arteriography, ultrasound testing, evoked response testing.[1]

Computerized Tomographic (CT) Scan

Benign headaches such as migraine, cluster, and muscle tension headache may be masking another organic illness that has not yet shown its own individual symptoms. Sometimes medications, by relieving pain, may also mask a hidden disorder. Discovering this hidden illness early enough may prevent a disabling or even a fatal outcome. The CT scan may show tumor, abscess, hydrocephalus, stroke, subdural hematomas, obstructive hydrocephephalus, hemorrhage, and arteriovenous (AV) malformation. The CT scan views calcification and bony structure problems with clarity.

Magnetic Resonance Imaging (MRI)

The cost of the MRI is significantly more than the CT scan. The MRI has much better resonance or intensification and visualization of certain areas of the head and neck. It can demonstrate regions of the brain without the use of the contrast material that is used so often with the CT scan. However, a different type of signal intensity enhancer is used with the MRI called gadolinium and is considered safe. Another addition to the MRI is the MRA, magnetic resonance angiography, which allows better visualization of the vascular anatomy without the risk or pain of angiography. At this point the MRA is not considered a total replacement for the invasive angiography.

The MRI is felt to be superior to the CT scan in identifying various lesions in the brainstem, cervical disc disease, and spondylosis (an abnormal immobility and fixation of a joint). It is also superior to the CT scan in visualizing the pituitary region, and demyelinating (destruction of a fatty sheath around the nerve), ischemic (obstruction of the circulation of a part), and inflammatory disease. It is also considered a better way to evaluate the soft tissue of the neck, the carotid artery circulation, and the facial and retropharyngeal regions.

CT scans are the procedure of choice with patients in the emergency room because CT is much quicker than MRI and is better suited for that kind of patient. The CT scan has the ability to view any acute type of intracranial bleeding. The procedure is considered safe except with pregnant women, because the effects of magnetic fields and radio waves on the unborn fetus are not known. Patients with pacemakers are also not exposed to this procedure.

The decision as to whether to use the CT vs. the MRI (and MRA) must be left in the hands of the experts (neurologists, neurosurgeons, and radiologists), who have the responsibility and expertise in making these critical decisions, and should not be based on cost or economics.

Lumbar Puncture

The lumbar puncture is done to measure the cerebral spinal fluid (CSF) pressure. It also is used to determine if there is any bleeding, infection, inflammation or abnormal cells from tumors in the central nervous system.

The indications for a lumbar puncture are the following:

Abrupt or sudden onset of a headache;
Headache accompanied by signs or symptoms of infection (fever, stiff neck, etc.);
Suspicion of bleeding;

Suspicion of elevated or reduced pressure;
Headache attacks associated with cranial nerve deficits that may result from infiltrative tumor, or infectious involvement of the brainstem.

The LP should not be performed until a CT scan or an MRI has ruled out the presence of any intracranial disease that might increase the risk of this procedure. If a scanner or an MRI is not available, the neurologist or neurosurgeon must use his or her judgment as to the importance of or need for the information.

Electroencephalography (EEG)

By measuring the electrical activity of the brain, several types of information can be established. Bursts or alterations of electrical activity may indicate a predisposition to seizure activity or disturbances resulting from drug or metabolic illness and primary neurological disease. Some drugs or medications may increase the possibility of seizures or mental confusion, memory impairment, amnesia, and personality changes, while other medications may lower the seizure threshold. This may be an indication for a baseline EEG with follow up studies.

Electrocardiography (ECG)

Although primary cardiac disease is rarely responsible for headache, some of the headache medications may alter the rhythm of the heart. Again, baseline examination may be prudent.

Routine X-rays

Cervical spine and skull x-rays are indicated when fracture or bone disease is suspected.

Arteriography

This test is indicated when there is a strong suspicion of aneurysm, vasculitis or stroke or any disease that evaluation of cerebral circulation will help to determine.[1]

Ultrasound

This is a noninvasive way to examine the carotid vascular system and heart if the dynamics of artery flow produce neurological symptoms with the headache syndrome.

Evoked Response Testing

Evoked response testing is used where various neurological conditions are associated with headache. There are auditory evoked response, visual evoked response, and somatosensory evoked response tests.

Tests for Suspected Stroke or Vasculitis

Patients with headache and periodic neurological symptoms are sometimes evaluated for the risk of stroke. There are many laboratory tests that can be done and specialists such as neurologists, hematologists, etc., are aware of these tests.

Dental Evaluations

Dental abnormalities may be responsible for primary headache symptoms or exacerbation of preexisting headache conditions. Abcesses, infections, various tumors, malocclusions and other conditions may contribute to the headache problem. These conditions are discussed in Chapter 18.

Fortunately, most headache conditions are primary and not secondary to neurological, medical, or dental disease. However, as part of a complete headache evaluation any of these above conditions must be considered. A headache specialist often is able to discriminate the various possibilities of these causes with a comprehensive history and physical examination and then choose the proper tests or referral to a particular specialist without redundancy or excessive testing that is costly and unnecessary.

REFERENCES

1. Saper, J.R., Silbertstein, S.D., Gordon, C.D., Hamel, R.I., *Handbook of Headache Management*, Williams and Wilkins, Baltimore, 1993.

PART TWO

Chapter 13

Post Traumatic Headache Syndrome

This diagnosis has several classifications: post traumatic headache syndrome, post concussion headache syndrome, subjective post traumatic headache syndrome, headache associated with head trauma, acute post traumatic headache, chronic post traumatic headache and the post head trauma syndrome.

Regardless of the classification, the problem is enormous. Head injury in the past 12 years caused more deaths than all the deaths from all the wars this country has been in since its founding. Headaches of all types cause more lost work days (over 160 million days a year) than any other pain disease. The number of people involved in head and neck injuries is staggering. Various studies estimate ranges anywhere between four to twelve million a year. About 10% to 15% of these injured people will end up with ongoing headaches. These patients require many different specialists as part of the total *treatment team*. The lost work days, medical costs, and legal expenses are estimated to be about $25 to $30 billion a year.

Who are the members of this team? Let us start with a family of four going for a ride on a Sunday afternoon. The father is driving, the mother is in the passenger seat, and their teenage daughter and her six year old brother are in the back seat. The car stops for a red light. A pick-up truck (with two young men who have consumed several cans of beer and are not paying attention) plows into their car at 20 plus miles per hour.

After the accident all six are taken to the emergency room. The family complains to the ER staff they all have headaches and are "sore all over." The mother and father remember hitting their heads on part of the front and side windows of their car. After they are examined and have CT scans, they are given prescriptions for pain medication and some advice for when they get home. They are all reassured that there was no brain damage or fractures of their skulls or neck bones.

The next day they continue to have headaches and severe soreness in their heads, necks, backs, and muscles around the body. *Now the team begins to build.* They see their family practice doctor and he prescribes different medications and tells them to rest for a few days. After a few days the father calls and says his head and neck hurt so much he cannot function, and this is true for the other members of the family. The family doctor refers them all to an orthopedic specialist. The orthopedic specialist tells them after examinations and cervical x-rays that they have cervical sprains, orders new medication, and sends them to a physical therapist.

After several months of physical therapy the family returns to the orthopedist and lists the following complaints. (Incidentally, the young men in the pickup truck are fine.) The father says his headaches are incapacitating three to four days of the week. The mother complains that whenever she tries to do housework her headaches get so bad she vomits. The teenage daughter and the six year old brother have the same complaints and the orthopedic specialist sends them off to the neurologist.

After a thorough examination, MRIs, blood tests and even one spinal tap, the neurologist alters the medication and again reassures the family there is no brain damage and tells them to reduce any stress in their life.

After one month, they return to the neurologist. Beside the headaches they have the following complaints: the father is irritable, can't sleep, is depressed, and has lost his libido. The mother's headaches are so bad she stays in a dark room and is sick to her stomach. The teenage daughter's periods are irregular, she is very irritable, does not socialize anymore, and can't concentrate. The six year old brother holds his head all the time and is doing poorly in school. The neurologist sends the mother and father to a psychiatrist and the younger two to a psychologist or counselor.

The psychiatrist changes the medication and has them all evaluated by the neuropsychologist to see if there is brain damage that cannot be seen on the MRI or CT scan. All start psychotherapy.

Though the family is not attending church regularly anymore, they now begin to see the minister to straighten out this problem. The minister tells the family that he has had some parishioners with the same problems who have done well with acupuncture and biofeedback. The family's friends are also concerned and know people with the same problem who have done well with homeopathy, chiropractors, alternative medicine, spiritual therapy, and massages. The more people the family meet, the more recommendations for different types of help are suggested.

Now, after a year of no progress, the insurance company begins to deny payments for these treatments. The family is angry about their situation; after all, they were innocent people on a Sunday afternoon excursion and were whiplashed by "intoxicated, irresponsible young men." Now the family gets their lawyer and their lawyer engages the lawyers of the insurance company. From there begins the search to investigate all the people involved in the various treatments, and then everyone goes to court. Now the jury and the judge become part of "the team." Is it any wonder that the cost of this minor accident becomes staggering?

This book attempts to bridge the gap by transforming the complex medical terminology into terminology that all members of the "team" will understand.

Having been involved in so many of these cases and having testified many times on either side of the fence, I have come to realize how all of these people involved interpret headache differently. There does not seem to be a similar concept or language on the problem of chronic post traumatic headache. It doesn't seem to matter, whether it is the patients, the doctors, the ancillary therapists, the insurance examiners, the lawyers, the jury, the judge, the clergy, or all the people who participate in recommendations, everyone seems to march to his own drummer, and everyone is certain he is correct.

Perhaps so many concepts exist because headache as a medical symptom has never had significant scientific evidence to justify objective findings and has always been interpreted by subjective anecdotes. The last ten years have produced significant science in the area of headache and the future looks promising for much more investigation and explanation in the scientific arena.

In 1979, Dr. Russell Packard[1] published a study that is considered to be a landmark in significant information for the medical community. In his study, he questioned both doctors and patients. He found that the *doctors* felt the patients' foremost concern was pain relief and medications. He then found that the *patients'* major concern was the explanation of their pain. Hopefully, this book will meet the criteria to explain this very great, gray area.

If we consider the number of readers who comprise "the team" we are reaching out to millions of people. My observations of thousands of victims have been that they are far more interested in understanding why they are suffering and what options they have to get better, than in the outcome of the litigation.

The enormous number of medical therapists in all areas of treatment need a source of information that gives a global perspective of cause and effect that makes sense in their efforts to help the victim. Third party carriers, insurance companies, etc., plus all the lawyers on both sides of the courtroom, need the same information. When we think of all the people involved in accidents during the last year and multiply this by the last five years, we are easily considering millions of people.

Why is it that when a patient walks into a doctor's office and says, "I have headaches; I can't sleep; I can't tolerate noise; I lose my temper easily; I can't concentrate; I forget things all the time; I feel depressed; I have nightmares; I have lost sexual enjoyment," the doctor is ready to take on this complex problem. Then when the doctor says, "When did these symptoms start?" and the patient says, "Right after the accident, nine months ago," the doctor's zeal plunges to the bottom of the canyon. Why does this doctor begin to question the validity of these symptoms he was so ready to cure only seconds ago? Why does the doctor so quickly challenge the motives of the patient and question whether these symptoms are real or contrived?

How and when did all this start? It seems that the railroads were the origin of this problem going back over 150 years ago.[2] In the mid-1800s, as the railroad companies were rapidly laying tracks and more passengers were traveling, injuries were also increasing. Many of these injuries came as a result of the sudden starting and stopping of the trains. Physicians become more involved and the question of identifying the relationship between the injury and the clinical symptoms began to evolve as a problem.

Dr. Michael R. Trimble in the early 1860s wrote his book, *Post Traumatic Neurosis — From Railway Spine to the Whiplash*, which began many debates and lectures on this enigma.

At that time Dr. John Erichsen of the University College Hospital in London lectured on "certain obscure injuries of the nervous system commonly met with as a result of shocks to the body received in collisions on railways." He proposed that the post traumatic disorder resulted from mechanical damage to brain and spinal cord. Eventually he wrote a book in 1882, *Concussion of the Spine: Nervous Shock and other Obscure Injuries of the Nervous System and Their Clinical and Medical/Legal Aspects*. He observed that if the train was struck from behind and the passengers were sitting with their backs toward the end of the train, or if they were sitting with their backs to the front of the train and the train was struck from the front, these injuries seemed to be the more important ones. He further suggested that the injury to the spinal cord was due to an inflammatory reaction similar to the inflammation of an infection.

He brought attention to the fact of how frequently medical persons had to give evidence in a court for damages against the railway companies for injuries to the nervous system in which there were so many discrepancies and the possibilities for so much mischief. It has been written that Dr. Erichsen's book was often quoted in court.

In 1893, Dr. Herbert Page, who was employed by the Northwest Railway, wrote *Injuries of the Spine and the Spinal Cord Without Apparent Mechanical Lesion*. Page pointed out that in the absence of specific injury to the spine, the concept of "railway spine" should be discounted. He felt that these complaints were a series of exaggerations.

In 1883, the *Boston Medical Surgical Journal* also wrote an editorial disputing Dr. Erichsen's work as having no scientific merit.

While all of this was going on, another major change in medicine was taking place. The era of psychiatry was in a state of upheaval and psychoanalysis was born. Charcot, Gowers, Janet, Freud, Adler and many more began to focus on the contribution of illnesses that were a product of the mind. Words like hysteria, functional, and psychosomatic were now being used to explain illnesses that were not demonstrated by organic evidence. And soon after, even illnesses that had organic lesions were thought to have a psychological origin. All of these terms became fodder for the physicians who disagreed with the concept of Erichsen.

Page took it one step further and used these hysterical disorders to describe that there was a relationship between these post-accident symptoms to malingering. The fact that there was compensation and no measured disability was enough to justify that the patient was using these "contrived symptoms" for monetary gain.

As a result of all this activity, workman's compensation laws were introduced, and in 1880 the Employers Liability Act (ELA) was passed giving compensation to workmen as long as the injury was not a direct result of the worker's negligence. Then in 1906 that criterion was eliminated and the Workman's Compensation Act was passed. It was found that although the number of workers remained the same in the following six years, the number of accidents rose by 44%. The law also would only pay compensation if the worker was out for two or more weeks and would not pay if the worker returned before the fourteen days were up. But if the worker was out more than fourteen days then he would be compensated for the first two weeks he was out. These laws encouraged abuse, and unexplainable railway injuries became widespread and malingering was common. It is easy to understand why the medical community became suspicious and nonempathetic to the worker with many symptoms and no physical injury to back these claims.

Over the next century opinions and studies were done to support each side of the controversy. In 1917 Collie wrote that the longer the injured person was off, the more difficult it was for him to return to work. Other studies pointed out that work habits were related to the worker's culture and depending on that individual's culture would determine the degree of malingering.

More and more studies were concerned with damage to the brain that was not identifiable with the technology that was available.

In 1941, Denny-Brown and Russell did experiments creating head trauma in animals, and they were convinced that there was interference with highly organized nervous system mechanisms.

In 1945 and 1946, Holburn and then Pudenz and Sheldon suggested that acceleration forces that were responsible for damage were rotational rather than linear.

In 1950, Groat and Simmons reported that a simple concussion could be responsible for considerable loss of neurons in the brainstem. More and more studies supported the idea that there was microscopic destructive lesions even after minor head injuries.

While tissue damage was one of the areas explored, the other was the result of psychological testing. Researchers like Wechsler, Reusch, Gronwall, Wrightson, Courville, Merskey, Woodforde and many more began to show the effects of head injury, both major and minor, to children as well as adults. Their results indicated that "hysteria" may be the result of the accident rather than a preexisting personality. They also found a change in intellectual and visual judgment even in minor injuries. Courville found headache, psychic symptoms, dizziness, and emotional disturbances in children in significant percentages. He found these symptoms irrespective of compensation and suggested that the neurosis theories were being kept alive by the physicians who worked for the insurance companies.

Bella and Moraitis demonstrated that two years after settlement these symptoms were persistent and they did not find that early settlement meant an early return to work.

A landmark paper written by Miller in 1961 in the *British Medical Journal* reported that in a study of fifty of his own patients only two were disabled two years after their settlement. He found that forty-five patients made a complete recovery and he concluded that the symptoms were not due to the accident but rather compensation and financial gain. Much of Miller's work is supported today even though there is growing evidence to the contrary.

Miller's concepts state:

1. No one suffering from post traumatic syndrome recovers and returns to work before settlement.
2. Post traumatic syndrome never occurs in patients when there is no possibility of obtaining compensation.
3. The syndrome never follows severe head injury.
4. The post traumatic syndrome never occurs in professional or managerial people.
5. These patients always return to work, free of symptoms, once they have received compensation.

After Miller's paper a slew of presentations were made to dispute his results. Kelly in 1972 and 1975 wrote two papers, "The Post-Traumatic Syndrome" and "The Post Traumatic Syndrome

— An Iatrogenic Disease," that strongly disagreed with Miller's findings. In the two papers Kelly found that (1) 84 out of 110 patients returned to work before settlement and were completely recovered; (2) 24 out of 34 patients who were not involved in claim or pension developed post traumatic syndrome; (3) 49 out of 62 patients who developed post traumatic syndrome were from professional or managerial classes; (4) 26 out of 56 patients who had severe head injuries developed post traumatic syndrome.

As studies continued, reports now included in these post traumatic syndromes not only head injuries but also flexion/extension or acceleration/deceleration or "whiplash" injuries that did not have actual trauma to the skull. Studies indicate that the force is so great in these injuries that there is injury to the upper brain as well as the brainstem.

McNab in 1974 found, in a study of 266 patients, that following flexion/extension injury 121 of 145 patients still were without relief two or more years after legal settlement.

The fact that today we recognize we cannot separate the mind from the body, and that significant symptoms are not necessarily related to a significant destruction of tissue, continues the battle as to what is real and what is contrived. Although all agree that there is a small number of malingerers, the two sides continue to battle on and those with the syndrome continue to suffer.

POST TRAUMATIC HEADACHE SECONDARY TO HEAD TRAUMA

The distinction will be made between a headache syndrome that is caused by injury to the skull and, in the next chapter, a headache syndrome that is caused by an injury to the neck. Each injury can cause the same type of headaches. It is beyond the scope of this book to go into great detail concerning head trauma that causes obvious damage to the brain, its blood vessels, and the structures that make up the contents within the cranium.

The International Headache Society uses the classification shown in Table 13.1.

Another system of classification was presented by the Mild Traumatic Brain Injury (MTBI) Committee of the Head Injury Interdisciplinary Special Interest Group to the American Congress of Rehabilitation Medicine in 1991.[3]

A person with MTBI is a person who has had a traumatically induced physiological disruption of brain function, as manifested by at least one of the following:

1. Any period of loss of consciousness
2. Any loss of memory for events immediately before or after the accident
3. Any alteration in mental state at the time of the accident (e.g., feeling dazed, disoriented or confused)
4. Focal neurological deficit(s) that may or may not be transient but where the severity of the injury does not exceed the following:
    a. Loss of consciousness of approximately 30 minutes or less
    b. After 30 minutes, a Glascow Coma Scale of 13–15
    c. Post traumatic amnesia (PTA), not greater than 24 hours

One of the major problems with these classifications is that the diagnosis of post traumatic headache syndrome is based on a period of unconsciousness and/or amnesia. In clinical practice, when patients are interviewed some time after the accident, many of them are not sure if they lost consciousness, and unless there were observers who recorded the event these facts are not reliable. Even professional boxers who are "knocked out" during a fight cannot accurately tell the exact amount of time they were unconscious or do not know the time of their confusion.

The syndrome with its symptoms appears to be consistent regardless of the degree of trauma or presence of fracture, or loss of consciousness, presence or absence of retrograde amnesia, blood in the cerebrospinal fluid, or other identifiable abnormalities.

Table 13.1

5.1 Acute post traumatic headache

5.1.1 *With significant head trauma and/or confirmatory signs*

Diagnostic criteria:

A. Significance of head trauma documented by at least one of the following:
1. Loss of consciousness
2. Post traumatic amnesia lasting more than 10 minutes
3. At least two of the following exhibit relevant abnormality: clinical neurological examination, x-ray of the skull, neuroimaging, evoked potentials, spinal fluid examination, vestibular function test, neuropsychological testing

B. Headache occurs less than 14 days after regaining consciousness (or after trauma, if there has been no loss of consciousness)

5.1.2 *With minor head trauma and no confirmatory signs*

Diagnostic criteria:

A. Head trauma that does not satisfy 5.1.1 A.

B. Headache occurs less than 14 days after injury

C. Headache disappears within 8 weeks after injury

5.2 Chronic post traumatic headache

5.2.1 *With significant head trauma and/or confirmatory signs*

Diagnostic criteria:

A. Significance of head trauma documented by at least one of the following:
1. Loss of consciousness
2. Post traumatic amnesia lasting more than 10 minutes
3. At least two of the following exhibit relevant abnormality: clinical neurological examination, x-ray of the skull, neuroimaging, evoked potentials, spinal fluid examination, vestibular function test, and neuropsychological testing

B. Headache occurs less than 14 days after regaining consciousness (or after trauma, if there is no loss of consciousness)

C. Headache continues more than 8 weeks after regaining consciousness (or after trauma, if there has been no loss of consciousness)

5.2.2 *With minor head trauma and no confirmatory signs*

Diagnostic criteria:

A. Head trauma that does not satisfy 5.2.1 A

B. Headache occurs less than 14 days after injury

C. Headache continues more than 8 weeks after injury

There are many causes of head injury, some intentional and some unintentional, and they can affect infants to elderly people. These injuries may occur at home, work, or on the road. Children are often injured by falls or miscalculations in their activities. Older people can fall as a result of their becoming unstable. Young adults are often careless, and men younger than 25 pose the greatest risk as drivers (Figure 13.1). Automobile accidents are responsible for most of the head injuries, and poor judgment, alcohol, social drugs, prescription medications, medical illnesses that interfere with eyesight, hearing, or cause epilepsy, dizziness, or even problems that restrict movements of the head all contribute to this epidemic.

Intentional injuries, such as abuse against the young (shaken baby syndrome), women, the elderly, and persons of all ages from beatings, muggings, rape, and gunshot wounds are frequent causes of traumatic brain injury.

There are many different types of injury to the brain and some can be revealed with clinical testing, medical procedures, and neuroimaging, while others are based on clinical experience and, unfortunately, autopsy.

Head injuries often include brain injury, but not necessarily so. Head injuries without obvious brain injury may produce the post trauma headache or the post head trauma syndrome. Damage to the neck, jaw, eyes, nose, lacerations to the scalp with poor healing, blows to the head from sporting events or fights may cause head damage but not obvious brain injury. With the diagnosis of post trauma headache, this distinction must be made (Figure 13.2).

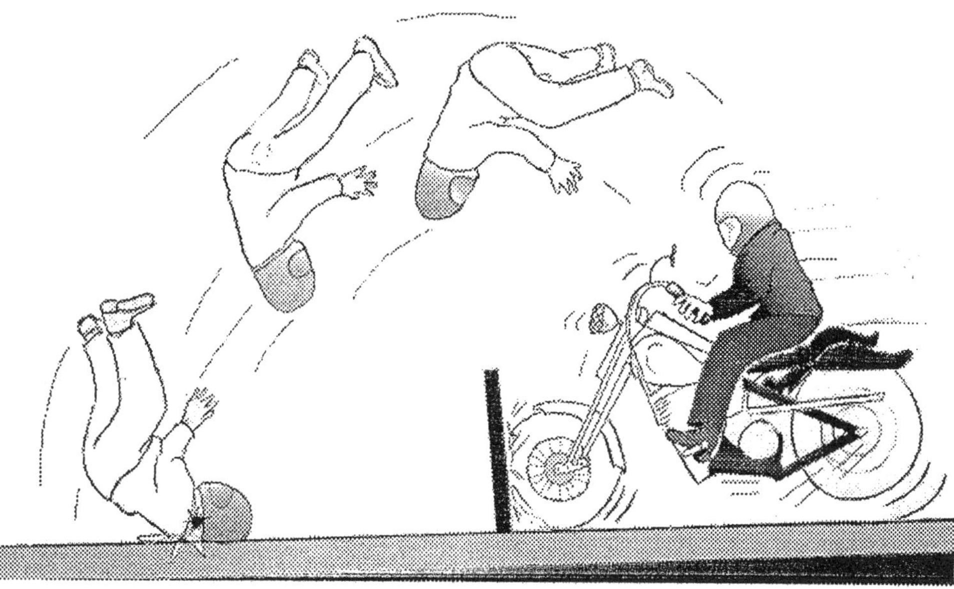

Figure 13.1 A great many head injuries come as a result of motorcycles, motorbikes, or bicycles in which the driver hits a solitary object and then is thrown from the seat of the cycle to the solitary object or the ground, causing a post traumatic head injury. It is obvious that the lack of a helmet, even with bicycles, will increase the chances for significant head and possibly brain trauma.

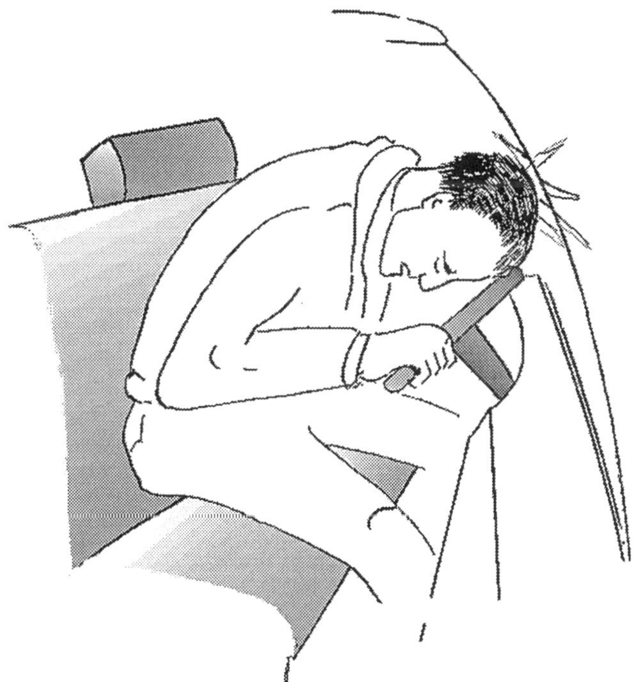

Figure 13.2 Person striking head from automobile accident. Many auto accidents, whether they are rear-end collisions or others, will cause not only flexion-extension or whiplash injuries, but also most people will strike their heads on the windshield, the side of the car, the side glass pane, or even have their heads rotated and hit the ceiling of the car. As a result of this, there is head injury, and following this are often the symptoms associated with post traumatic headache syndrome.

The various types of brain injury may cause the following damage:

1. *Concussion* is a jar, jolt, or blow to the head that creates several symptoms, such as loss or clouding of memory of events leading to or following the injury (antegrade or retrograde amnesia), plus headache, neck pain, dizziness, mood changes, insomnia, lassitude, etc. Most of these symptoms will resolve in days to months.
2. *Contusion* is a bruise or bruises to the brain. With these bruises are swellings and bleeding. These bruises can be caused by strikes to the skull or penetration of the skull. The damage to the brain can be produced by an object penetrating the skull or the brain striking the inner surfaces of the skull.
3. *Edema* is swelling caused by minor or major injuries. When edema is diffuse there is an elevation of intracranial pressure which can cause herniation of the brain. This is compounded when there is associated hemorrhage within the brain. When the edema is diffuse the patient will be critically ill or obtunded. Because there is loss of cortical surface and the boundaries become lost, the CT or MRI will demonstrate this loss.
4. *Hemorrhage* may result from head trauma. Contusion and axonal injury may be associated with small amounts of bleeding. Penetrating injuries may cause a great amount of bleeding. When there is fracture of the temporal bone and a tearing of the medial meningeal artery or there is tearing of the large venous sinuses (dural), the end result can be an epidural hematoma and this is a life-threatening situation. Subdural and subarachnoid hemorrhage are often associated with blows to the head. Infants may develop this disorder when violently shaken. This condition may also be seen in older persons with minimal head trauma.
5. *Axonal injury* may be focal or diffuse. When nerve filaments are stretched or separated by rotational or translational forces, fracture of the brain tissue ensues. These forces can stretch or snap nerve cell filaments between the different structures of the brain. The brain within the skull can act like a bowl of "Jello" and form fracture lines when shaken. This can take place in acceleration/deceleration (whiplash) accidents or a blunt force to the head. There can be bleeding with axonal injury. This type of injury has also been described in the explanation of "soft neurological symptoms." Diffuse axonal injury is life threatening.
6. *Coup-contrecoup injury* is generally seen in whiplash or acceleration/deceleration injuries or a fall of several feet. The coup injury occurs on the side of the primary impact and is generally more serious than the contrecoup on the opposite side of the brain. Sometimes after a fall in which the back of the head (occiput) is struck, the contrecoup on the frontal brain is worse. This may be due to the shape of the skull in the front of the head which is rougher than the back.
7. *Head injury* is where there is an open fracture and damage to the cranial vault, there may be exposure to the outside environment and a CSF (cerebral spinal fluid) leak, with the possibility of infection, which could lead to meningitis.
8. *Herniation* is a serious or death dealing situation. When the brain swells or there is bleeding, the brain pushes through the closed compartments of the skull. There are different types of herniation which lead to compression of the cerebral arteries and eventually the collapse of the brain.

Therefore, traumatic brain injury can be caused by both open and closed head injuries. Open head injuries are usually caused by penetration of the skull by knives, ice picks, bullets, large blunt objects, or striking one's head against a fixed object. Continuous beatings of the skull in boxing and other similar events may also cause brain injury, most likely because of axonal injury which will lead to the postconcussive syndrome. It is interesting that there seems to be an inverse ratio between the extent of the injury and the intensity of the headache syndrome; that is, the worse the injury to the brain the less the extent of the headaches in duration, intensity, and frequency. However, I have treated some patients who had invasive neurosurgery and had continued headaches for years after their surgery.

The causes of post traumatic headaches have been listed by Barnat as:[4]

Blunt head contact, 57.3%
Whiplash, 43.6%
Object hit head, 13.7%
Other, 13.7%
Body shaken, 9.4%

The types of headaches that follow head trauma are similar to the headaches described in the earlier chapters. In other words, head pain that is not created by scalp injuries, nerve entrapments, bone fractures or pain that is specific to the area of injury are headaches that are like tension, migraine, cluster, mixed (migraine and tension), and a specific headache called dysautonomic cephalgia. Another type of headache, called "cervicogenic headache," is discussed in Chapter 19.

As you can see from the case histories presented, it is difficult to distinguish the differences between the symptoms of non-trauma headaches from injury or trauma headaches. This is why I call them muscle tension-like, migraine-like, cluster-like, etc.

Post trauma tension-like headaches are generally mild to moderate, with dull, aching, pressing, tightening feelings, and are nonpulsating. They are generally bilateral and band-like. There is no nausea or vomiting and they are not aggravated by bright lights, noise, or odors. The eyes do not get red and the person does not get flushed or pale. There is no eyelid droop and the eyes do not tear. There is no nasal running or stuffiness and the muscles are often tender to touch. These headaches can be caused by the trauma or aggravated in intensity, frequency, and duration if they existed before the trauma or accident.

Post trauma migraine-like headaches are similar to migraine headaches and can been caused by the accident or trauma, or they can be aggravated if they preexisted. These headaches are generally moderate to severe to incapacitating. They can be unilateral or bilateral, are generally pulsating, throbbing, or pounding. There is nausea and sometimes vomiting, and bright lights, noise, and various types of odors will make them worse. There can be warning signs (prodromes or auras) that will precede the headache. Exercise, walking, climbing stairs, and various movements of the neck will start an attack or make the headache worse.

Post trauma cluster-like headaches are similar to cluster headaches. It is extremely rare that cluster headache is caused by an accident, and some experts dispute that this can happen. However, a person who is a cluster sufferer may precipitate an already existing condition during a quiet period of the cluster cycle, although this is not common.

These attacks can take place once to several times a day and are almost always so severe that they are incapacitating and disabling. The attacks last one half to two hours and the pain is stabbing, often described as a hot poker being driven into the eye or head. There is no aura, no nausea or vomiting, no throbbing, and lights, noise, and odors do not intensify the headache. On the side of the headache there is sweating, both the eye and nose run, and often the eyelid droops (ptosis).

Post traumatic dysautonomic cephalgia, described by Vijayn and Dreyful[5] as a result of neck injury, is similar to migraine with several other features. The pain is unilateral, throbbing, and has pupillary dilatation and excessive sweating on the side of the headache during the headache phase. Between headaches there is a partial lid droop (ptosis) and a smaller pupil (miosis). Otherwise the other symptoms are similar to migraine. This was documented by Swerdlow using electronic telethermography.[6]

Once the post traumatic headaches become a syndrome, other symptoms become part of this complex problem. Barnat classifies these symptoms, from most frequent complaints to least.[4]

Headache, 82.9%
Irritability, 66.7%
Insomnia, 63.2%
Anxiety, 58.1%
Memory problems, 57.3%
Other pain, 56.4%
Concentration problems, 52.1%
Depression, 52.1%
Dizziness, 41.1%
Confusion, 36.8%
No control of emotions, 36.8%
Loss of libido, 35.0%

Tinnitus, 29.1%
Cannot carry out plans, 29.1%
Cannot plan, 28.4%
Flashbacks, 28.2%
Do not enjoy sex, 26.5%
Nightmares, 26.5%
Arithmetic problems, 17.9%

If one compares the symptoms of the post traumatic headache syndrome to the post concussive syndrome, then one has to question how important is the distinction and how important is diagnosis based on unconsciousness and amnesia.[3] Common symptoms of post concussive syndrome are:

Lightheadedness
Vertigo/dizziness
Neck pain
Headache
Photophobia
Phonophobia
Tinnitus
Impaired memory
Easy distractibility
Impaired comprehension
Forgetfulness
Impaired logical thought
Difficulty with new or abstract concepts
Insomnia
Irritability
Easy fatigability
Apathy
Outbursts of anger
Mood swings
Depression
Loss of libido
Personality change
Intolerance to alcohol

Another study by Lees-Healey and Brown listed neuropsychological complaints on 170 personal injury claimants:[7]

Anxiety or nervousness, 93%
Sleeping problems, 92%
Depression, 89%
Headaches, 88%
Back pain, 80%
Fatigue (mental or physical), 79%
Concentration problems, 78%
Worries about health, 77%
Irritability, 77%
Neck pain, 74%
Impatience, 65%
Restlessness, 62%
Feeling disorganized, 61%
Loss of interest, 60%
Confusion, 59%
Loss of efficiency in carrying out everyday tasks, 56%
Shoulder pain, 55%
Memory problems, 53%
Dizziness, 44%
Sexual problems, 41%
Numbness, 39%
Nausea, 38%
"Not finding the word you want or using the wrong word", 34%
"Visual problems, blurring, or seeing double", 32%
Trembling or tremors, 30%
Hearing problems, 29%

Constipation, 29%
Foot pain, 24%
Trouble reading, 24%
Bumping into things, 21%
Elbow pain, 21%
Speech problems, 18%
Impotence, 15%

In the other chapters on whiplash (acceleration/deceleration) and on cervicogenic headaches the reader will notice the consistency of the complaints of these patients and will take notice why clinicians who treat these patients are comfortable with the diagnosis without having to have objective evidence of brain tissue destruction.

An attempt to explain the mechanisms for the above symptoms unfortunately is difficult because at the moment minute destruction of brain tissue can only be observed microscopically and examination is only done at autopsy. There have been controlled studies on animals approximating minor head injuries in humans, and observations of tissue change in the animals are similar to what have been observed in the brains of humans at autopsy.

What has been seen microscopically is that there is alteration and some nerve cell loss. Also observed are blood vessel (vascular) alterations in all the levels of the brain, cortical, subcortical, and in the brainstem. There is also degeneration of the material that connects the nerve cells (microglia) and also the body of the nerve (axones).

The exact cause of the pain of these headaches may be due to the disturbance of the pain modulating system in the brainstem that passes that information to the upper brain for interpretation of the pain mechanism. An attempt to explain this mechanism can be read in Chapter 3.

The other pain as described before could come from injury to the muscles, tendons, blood vessels, and nerves surrounding the skull, as well as damage to the cervical area, cervical roots, spinal cord, the joints, temporomandibular joint, and other areas of the face and neck. Besides pain from these places, the pain itself could be a triggering mechanism to start the headache process. Trigger points in the muscles around the neck and shoulders can refer pain to the head; this is discussed in Chapter 17.

Another area to consider is whether there was a predisposition either biologically or psychologically, that renders that accident victim a candidate for a chronic headache condition. This does not mean that these symptoms are not real, but rather attempts to explain why some recover from these accidents or injuries and others do not.

After the trauma takes place the patient will generally complain of headache almost immediately or within the first 24 to 48 hours. Sometimes these symptoms may not present for weeks or months. If there are more severe pains in the neck or shoulders, or other parts of the body that were injured, then this particular pain may mask the headache. I have often seen patients who did not report headache in the emergency room for this reason and later were told they were contriving this symptom, when in fact they were so distressed by their other injuries that headache was not their priority at that moment. There are situations where headache does not appear at all for days or weeks. When headaches appear months later it is much more difficult to make the connection between the headache and the accident, and all the symptoms of the syndrome must now be evaluated.

However, it is not uncommon for neurological symptoms or other conditions to take months to develop or be recognized. As an example, in rare cases there is a condition known as post traumatic epilepsy, which is a delayed condition. Conditions that impair memory, or the ability to process information, or reduced concentration, or cognitive deficits (awareness or perception), and neuropsychiatric symptoms, such as personality change, depression, rage attacks (see the above lists) develop over a period of time. Other symptoms such as dizziness and vertigo or sleep disturbance may start immediately or develop over time.

Other conditions that may be precipitated by the trauma are blackouts or fainting (syncope), true seizures or pseudoseizures (staring spells, dizziness, amnesia or confusion, episodic disorientation and fugue states, personality dissociation and impulsive behavior with loss of memory for that event). All these conditions are rare and an attempt must be made to differentiate in the absence of physiological documentation, the difference between a "spell' or a factitious or malingering set of symptoms. Not having objective physical evidence does not rule out a condition caused by a trauma.

After head and brain injury there may be a disruption in the area of the brain that controls physiological balance, or homeostasis. These areas of the brain are the hypothalamus and the master gland, the pituitary, which in turn controls the adrenal gland. As a result of this disruption the following alterations may take place: weight loss or gain, changes in appetite, increased thirst, alcohol intolerance, menstrual irregularities, amenorrhea, sexual dysfunction, and others.[8]

As the syndrome develops and the patient continues with chronic pain and the other accompanying problems over a long period of time, those who are in close relationship with the patient also begin to pay a price. Family members who start out with total support of the patient begin to become frustrated with the lack of improvement and resent the dependency of the victim and the time that is consumed in caring for him or her. Also, because of the lack of physical evidence to support the disability, the other members of the family become suspicious of how real this illness is, and soon empathy turns to rejection, anger, and frustration. If this continues and no hope for improvement is apparent, relationships begin to crumble and breakups become inevitable. What started out as a relatively minor accident can become a devastating experience in a psychosocial setting.

The essential elements in establishing the diagnosis of the post traumatic headache syndrome is to rule out any other condition that might account for these symptoms. As discussed earlier in this chapter, head injury can cause organic disorders that could mimic this syndrome. Cerebral hemorrhage, blood clots under the coverings of the brain (subdural/epidural hematoma), low pressure in the brain (CSF hypotension), blood clots in the large cerebral veins or in the sinuses of the brain (cavernous), aneurysms, increased pressure in the brain because of accumulation of cerebral spinal fluid (post traumatic hydrocephalus), true seizures, damage to the vertebrae, cervical nerves, jaw, temporomandibular joint, styloid ligament, face, and muscles are some of the conditions that must be ruled out.

KEY TO DIAGNOSIS

The most important start is a comprehensive history of the patient which attempts to compare the pre-traumatic status: medical, social, performance at work, school or home, sexual, intellectual (cognitive), and personality. Beside taking the history from the patient, it is also important to get as much information as possible from the closest member of the family who can objectively differentiate the pre- to the post trauma changes.

After the history, a comprehensive physical and neurological examination is next. When this information is evaluated, the proper testing can be done to rule out any physical and psychological abnormalities. The value of a good history and physical is to help prevent the overuse and over-expense of unnecessary testing.

Laboratory testing will help to rule out medical and metabolic disease. Brain abnormalities may be distinguished with the use of visual, auditory, and somatosensory evoked potentials, electroencephalography (EEG), CT and MRI scans, and recently the positron emission tomography (PET) scan is being considered in post traumatic behavioral changes.[9] Otolaryngological (ENT) testing for dizziness and vertigo using vestibular evaluations and electronystagmography evaluations, and dental specialists for TMJ and jaw and face problems, are also part of a necessary evaluation (see Chapter 18).

Sometimes nerve blocks in the neck and face not only can be valuable as treatment, but may also serve as a diagnostic aid.

Because many of the complaints of the post traumatic headache patient are difficulty in concentration, memory, cognitive difficulties, personality changes, etc., a neuropsychological battery is critical in evaluating "soft" neurological and psychological disturbances.

Treatments of these conditions will be discussed in the chapter on treatments and treatment plans.

The major issue of convincing the legal profession and the insurance companies on the legitimacy of this syndrome is convincing them of the consistency of these symptoms in so many of the studies that have been done and the clinical experience of the specialist examining the patient.

Cynicism of the medical profession has been based on a small percentage of persons who have had preexisting personality disorders and who psychologically need the attention and illness as a means of dealing with their unconscious unresolved conflicts. The other group of people with personality disorders, who are willing to feign illness and be deceptive for the purpose of financial gain, revenge, avoidance of responsibilities, and to control others, also are responsible for compromising the legitimacy of those who are the real sufferers. Weeding out the malingerers, the factitious disorders and those who are only interested in secondary gain falls upon the professionals who will be able to construct examinations and testing that will identify this group.

However, it must be realized that not being able to identify this disorder by objective biological markers does not mean the disease is absent, but rather that we have not yet developed the diagnostic sophistication to identify this microscopic and molecular disruption. Since World War II advances in medicine have been short of a miracle, and in the last 25 years it appears that advances have come in geometric proportions. Since I have been in medicine, starting in 1957, so many diseases that were based only on clinical observation and so many diseases that were identified as "psychosomatic" have now been objectified in the laboratory, in radiology, with other imaging techniques, biochemically, and genetically that it makes me realize that we are getting closer to identifying this disorder.

It wasn't long ago that migraine was considered a disorder of an angry perfectionist, and today through research, while attempting to understand how a certain medication helps a migraine attack, an entire neurochemical explanation of migraine has been developed. The identification of genetic material in hemiplegic migraine is pushing us that much closer to the genetics of migraine in general. Unfortunately, there are still some clinicians who stick with the angry perfectionist model and cloud scientific progress.

The brain is very intricate and complicated and has an extraordinary network of transmitters, both neurological and chemical, that are very sensitive and vulnerable to even minor changes. The fact that people react differently when exposed to many different types of negative stimuli should not change when exposed to head trauma. That is, as Symonds said in 1937, "It's not so much what happens to the head, but whose head it happens to." Symonds would be that much more proud of his statement had he realized the advances in science in the past 60 years.[8] The more we are aware that emotional illness is predicated on a neurochemical system that may be out of balance the more it would be obvious that another insult to this system would only disrupt it further. Someone who suffers from severe anxiety or depression and now is presented with new distress signals will react with a greater excess of physiological responsiveness that will continue to add to these already preexisting symptoms. This is not to say that the symptoms of post traumatic headache syndrome are only found in those who had preexisting emotional illness. It is the experience of all headache specialists that the majority of persons with this syndrome were considered quite stable before the accident.

As long as the physician maintains objectivity and recognizes that early and proper intervention is the key to minimize suffering, the long haul of overutilization of testing and unnecessary and costly treatments could reduce the enormous burden of expense to society. All involved with these patients must realize there is physiological legitimacy for the existence of the post-traumatic headache syndrome.

REFERENCES

1. Packard, R.C., What does the headache patient want?, *Headache*, 19, 370–374, 1979.
2. Saper, J.R., Post Head Trauma Syndrome, History and Definition, Lecture Note from the American Association for the Study of Headache, New York, 1985.
3. Foreman, S.F., Croft, A.C., *Whiplash Injuries, The Cervical Acceleration/Deceleration Syndrome*, 2nd ed., Williams & Wilkins, Baltimore, 1995.
4. Barnat, M.R., Post traumatic headache patient 1: demographics, injuries, headaches, and health status, *Headache*, 26, 271–277, 1986.
5. Vijayn, N., Dreyful, P.M., Post traumatic dysautonomic celphalgia, *Archives of Neurology*, 32, 649–652, 1975.
6. Swerdlow, B., Thermographic documentation in a case of post-traumatic dysautonomic cephalgia, *Thermology*, 1, 102–105, 1985.
7. Lees-Healy, P.R., Brown, R.S., Neuropsychological complaint base rates in 170 personal injury claimants, *Archives of Clinical Neuropsychology*, 8, 203–209, 1993.
8. Symonds, C.P., Mental disorders following head injury, *Proceedings of the Royal Society of Medicine*, 30, 1081, 1937.
9. Sharkstein, C.P., Mayberg, H.S, Bertweir, M.L., et al., Mania after brain injury: neuroradiological and metabolic findings, *Annals of Neurology*, 27, 652–659, 1990.

CASE HISTORIES*

The following are case histories and summaries that will help identify post traumatic headaches. There are also actual medical reports that help you understand how the physician comes to the diagnosis. Identifying details have been left out to protect the privacy of the individuals.

* On the headache assessment forms that accompany these case histories, incapacitating headaches are indicated with solid black lines, interfering headaches with dotted lines, and irritating headaches with gray shading.

MEDICAL HEADACHE HISTORY

Name: Leslie **Age:** 30 **Sex** F **Date:** 10/24/94

Date of Birth: 00/00/64 **Birthplace:** PA **Race:** ____ **Education:** MBA

Occupation: Accounting **Accident:** 1991

Armed Services & Type of Discharge: N/A

PAST HISTORY:

1.	Did you have a normal birth? Unknown		Yes	No
	a) forceps used?		Yes	No
	b) cesarean section?		Yes	No
2.	Did you have problems with bedwetting?		**Yes**	No
	a) If yes, age bedwetting stopped		5	
3.	Were you car sick as a child (motion)?		**Yes**	No
	a) If yes, how severe?	Slight	**Moderate**	Severe
4.	Did you have unexplained abdominal cramps as a child?		Yes	**No**
5.	Did you have any of the following illnesses in childhood?			
	a) meningitis		Yes	**No**
	b) encephalitis		Yes	**No**
	c) scarlet fever		Yes	**No**
	d) rheumatic fever		Yes	**No**
6.	Did you have any head injuries as a child?		**Yes**	No
	a) If yes, please explain: Concussions x 2			
7.	Were you treated for emotional illness as a child?		Yes	**No**

HABITS:

8.	Do you drink alcohol?	**Yes**	No
	a) If yes, what kind and how much? Occasionally (3 times/wk)		
	b) Does alcohol bring on or aggravate a headache?	Yes	**No**
9.	Do you smoke?	**Yes**	No
	a) If yes, how much? 2 pks a week		
	b) Does smoking or smoke-filled rooms cause or aggravate headaches?	Yes	**No**
10.	Do you drink caffeinated beverages?	Yes	**No**
	a) If yes, how much? ____		

MENSTRUAL HISTORY:

At what age did menses begin? 14 Were they regular or irregular? WNL

How were they related to your headache? N/A

Are you or were you ever on Birth Control Pills? N/A Did they affect your headache? N/A

Have you had a hysterectomy, partial or total, and why? No

Are you in menopause, and if yes, how long? No

Are you on hormones, and if yes, which ones? No

HEADACHE ASSESSMENT FORM

HA PROFILE	INCAPACITATING #3	INTERFERING #2	IRRITATING #1
ONSET (Years ago and frequency)	N/A	3 months ago Daily	Since teens; one a week
CURRENT FREQUENCY	N/A	Neck pain daily, with 3-4 per week	2 to 3/week
TIME OF ONSET	N/A	Wake with it, go to bed with it	At end of day
DURATION	N/A	All day	Till she goes home and has a few beers
CHARACTER	N/A	Sharp, constant jabbing pain	Dull ache
PRODROME OR AURA	N/A	N/A	N/A
ASSOCIATING FEATURES	Nausea; Vomiting; Sensitivity to Light? Noise? Odors? Do you get pale or flush? Do your eyes or nose run? Does your nose get stuffy? Do the whites of your eyes get red? Does your eyelid droop? Do you pace, or go to bed?	Nausea; Vomiting; <u>Sensitivity to Light</u>? Noise? Odors? Do you get pale or flush? Do your eyes or nose run? Does your nose get stuffy? Do the whites of your eyes get red? Does your eyelid droop? Do you pace, or go to bed?	Nausea; Vomiting; Sensitivity to Light? Noise? Odors? Do you get pale or flush? Do your eyes or nose run? Does your nose get stuffy? Do the whites of your eyes get red? Does your eyelid droop? Do you pace, or go to bed?
PRECIPITATING OR AGGRAVATING FEATURES	N/A	N/A	Stress

LOCATION: Mark the location for each type of headache with a different color pen.

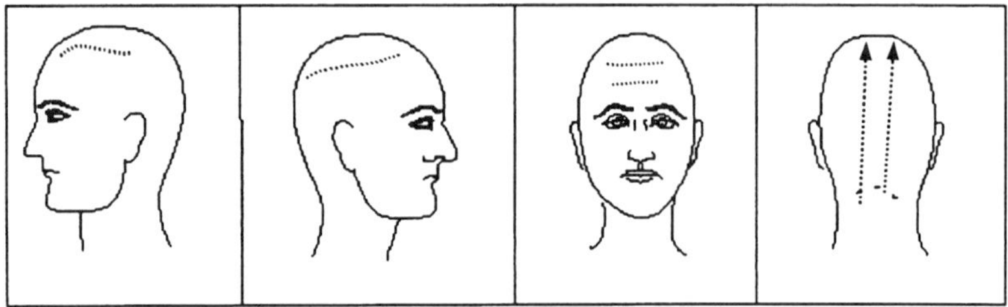

MEDICAL HISTORY:

Have you ever been or are you currently being treated for any of the following?

a) high blood pressure	Yes	No (underlined)
b) stomach ulcers	Yes (underlined)	No
c) asthma	Yes	No (underlined)
d) allergies	Yes (underlined)	No
e) pneumonia	Yes (underlined)	No
f) kidney problems	Yes (underlined)	No
g) low blood sugar	Yes	No (underlined)
h) glaucoma	Yes	No (underlined)
i) diabetes	Yes	No (underlined)
j) heart problems	Yes	No (underlined)

If you answered yes to any of the above, please describe: Ulcers diagnosed 5 years ago. Environmental allergies. Pneumonia 3 times; hospitalized twice. Kidney problems since childhood.

List all other medical problems you have had in the past. Include date diagnosed and treatment.
DO NOT LIST OPERATIONS

TMJ – caused shift in jaw after removal of wisdom teeth.

SURGICAL HISTORY (List operations and dates performed)

Wisdom teeth removed 1981.

PSYCHIATRIC HISTORY (List visits with counselors, psychologists, etc., and type of treatment)

Depression, 1989 to 1992. Medication and psychotherapy.

ACCIDENTS IN ADULT LIFE (Briefly describe any accident that caused any blow to the head or that you feel is related to your headache)

Auto accident, 1991. Hit on driver's side door, without seatbelt. Was driving and at a complete stop. Thrown to other side of car and hit head (left posterior). Conscious, but had amnesia for 14 hours. Hospitalized for 2 days. Concussion found on x-rays and CT scan.

FAMILY HISTORY:

1. Is your father living? Yes (underlined) No
   - Age 60
   - Cause of death ______
   - Was there a headache history? Yes No
2. Is your mother living? Yes (underlined) No
   - Age 57
   - Cause of death ______
   - Was there a headache history? Yes No

3. Ages of brothers---Circle the ones with headache
   34 23
4. Ages of sisters---Circle the ones with headache
   29
5. List any other blood relatives with a history of severe headaches.
   None.

MARITAL HISTORY:
List marriages:

1st marriage age 20 to 29	Did spouse have headaches?	Yes	No
2nd marriage age ___ to ___	Did spouse have headaches?	Yes	No
3rd marriage age ___ to ___	Did spouse have headaches?	Yes	No

Age of current spouse: N/A

List ages and sex of all children:

Age ___	Sex ___	Headaches?	Yes	No
Age ___	Sex ___	Headaches?	Yes	No
Age ___	Sex ___	Headaches?	Yes	No

STRESS FACTORS:

List any factors that may be affecting your headaches (money, loneliness, sexual problems, work, etc.)
Daily living activities.

VEGETATIVE SIGNS:

1.	Do you have trouble falling asleep?	Yes	No
2.	Do you have trouble staying asleep?	Yes	No
3.	Has your appetite decreased?	Yes	No
4.	Have you gained or lost weight in the past year?	Yes	No
5.	Have you felt tearful or depressed lately?	Yes	No
6.	Have you had any thoughts of wanting to die?	Yes	No
7.	Have you been forgetful lately?	Yes	No
8.	Any other changes in your normal day-to-day living? ___		

Please list any medications you are allergic or sensitive to: No known allergies

Please list any medications you are currently taking (including dosages and frequency per day):
Tylenol #3, 2 to 3 a day. Motrin 800 mg p.r.n. (1 tablet q.h.s.)

PREVIOUS CARE:

1. List doctors who have treated you for headaches: Dr. R.

2. List any tests you have had for your headache (e.g., EEG, CT scan, MRI, X-Ray, etc.):
CT scan

3. List any other treatment you have had for your headache (e.g., biofeedback, acupuncture, chiropractic, or any other treatment you had):
Chiropractic (not helpful). Physical therapy (helpful).

The following is an example of an actual medical report demonstrating the diagnosis:

Dear Dr. :

Thank you for the kind referral of Ms. Leslie for headache evaluation and treatment.

Leslie is a 30-year-old white female born 00/00/64 in Pennsylvania. She has completed a graduate level MA degree and has lived in Florida for the last 12 years where she is employed in accounting.

HEADACHE PROFILE:

The patient had only a mild headache history prior to a motor vehicle accident on 00/00/94. At that time the patient was an unrestrained driver of a motor vehicle when she was sitting stationary at an intersection and a pickup truck hit her car on the driver's side. The patient was thrown to the other side of the car, striking the left posterior portion of her head. There was no loss of consciousness, but the patient did have amnesia for approximately 14 hours after the accident. Amnesia of those 14 hours persists to this time. The patient remained hospitalized at the County Hospital for 2 days for the diagnosis of concussion. A CT scan was performed at that time. It should also be noted that the patient did have a significant laceration of the scalp from the accident.

Incapacitating Headaches: None.

Interfering Headaches (moderate to severe): The patient developed these headaches approximately one month after her motor vehicle accident. Immediately after the accident the patient was seen by a chiropractor who did chiropractic manipulations to her cervical region. This treatment provided transient, i.e., one hour, of relief and then the patient noted that the cervical pain would develop into headache pain. This has resolved greatly with the discontinuing of chiropractic medicine. The patient states that she then transferred to physical therapy and has found relief with her muscle pain; however, the cervical or neck pain is persistent and remains on a daily basis. The patient will awake with the pain and it will progress throughout the day. The patient describes the pain as a sharp constant jabbing pain in the midline of the cervical region. There is no prodrome with this pain or associated features.

Irritating Headaches (annoying): The patient noted the onset of these headaches when she was in her teens and they occurred approximately on a weekly basis at that time. These headaches have increased in frequency to 2 to 3 times per week. The patient will note these headaches at the end of the day and they will persist until she is able to relax and have a "few beers." The pain is described as a dull aching pain in a band-like distribution around the head. There is no prodrome or associated features with these headaches. They are, however, precipitated by stress.

Menstrual History: Began at age 14 and is reported to be normal with no increase in headache symptoms with menstrual cycle.

PAST HISTORY: The patient's birth history is unknown. There is a history of enuresis until age 5. There is no history of unexplained abdominal cramps pre-puberty. There is a history of mild car sickness as a child. There is no history of meningitis, encephalitis, scarlet fever or rheumatic fever. The patient had a concussion at age 5. No treatment for emotional illness.

Habits: The patient drinks approximately 3 alcoholic beverages per week and smokes 2 packs of cigarettes per week. She does not consume caffeinated beverages.

Medical History:

1. History of Peptic Ulcer Disease – bleeding ulcer. The patient is not under treatment at this time.
2. Environmental allergies since childhood, especially smoke.
3. Pneumonia x 3, requiring hospitalization.
4. Renal calculi – frequent problem since childhood.
5. TMJ disease. After removal of wisdom teeth, the patient does have some crepitus in the TMJ with some increase in headache symptoms from this area.

Surgical History: Removal of wisdom teeth in 1981.

Psychiatric History: Depression from 1989 to 1992 treated with medication and psychotherapy.

Head Injuries in Adult Life: As described in history of present illness.

Family History: Her father is living, age 60, with no headache history. Her mother is living, age 57, with no headache history. The patient has 2 brothers and 1 sister, with no headache history. The patient is currently single and does not have any children.

Stress Factors: The patient states that daily living activities provide stress that increases her headache symptoms.

Vegetative Signs: The patient does not complain of trouble both falling and staying asleep. No depression, suicidal ideation or memory defect noted.

Allergies to Medications: None.

Current Medications: The patient is currently taking Tylenol #3 two to three per day, and Motrin p.r.n.

Doctors Seen in the Past for Headaches: The patient has been evaluated by Dr. for her headache problems, including CT scan of the brain done on 00/00/94 and that was negative for intracranial pathology.

Physical Examination: Height 5'4", weight 143 pounds, pulse 76, respirations 18, left BP 102/74, right BP 110/80. The patient is awake, alert, oriented and cooperative to history and physical examination. The face did not show any asymmetry. The temporomandibular joint area was grossly normal. The patient had her vision checked two months ago. The nose appeared normal. The auditory canals were clear and the tympanic membranes appeared intact. The mouth and throat appeared normal. Gums, tongue, buccal mucosa and teeth were grossly normal. The patient has pain on palpation at the midline at the spinous process of C7 and T1. The normal lordosis is well preserved at that area. Good range of motion cervically. Carotid bruits could not be heard. Cervical nodes were not enlarged. The lungs were clear to auscultation and percussion. The heart had a regular sinus rhythm with no murmurs. The abdomen was soft and nontender. The patient had a GYN examination two years ago and she was advised to follow up with this.

Neurological Examination: Cranial nerve II: Visual fields were grossly normal. III, IV and VI: No strabismus, nystagmus or ptosis. V: Normal sensation and corneal reflex. VII: Normal facial movements (wrinkle, frown, smile and strength of eyelids). VIII: Normal Weber and Rinne. IX and X: Good gag reflex. XI: Normal sternocleidomastoid and trapezius. XII: Normal protrusion and strength of tongue. Cerebellar: Negative Rhomberg. Normal finger-to-nose, diadochokinesis, heel-shin, tandem and heel and toes walking. Motor System: No atrophy, fasciculations, wasting or tremors. Good muscle strength in arms, wrists, fingers and legs. Sensory System: Superficial tactile, pain and vibrations (wrists, elbows, knees and ankles) were normal. Normal motion and positions of fingers and toes. Normal 2-point discrimination. Reflexes: Normal 2+ reflexes of triceps, biceps, knee jerk, ankle jerk, etc. Normal pulses in dorsalis pedis, posterior tibial and popliteal.

DIAGNOSES:

1. Post-traumatic headache.
2. Rule out post-traumatic cervicogenic headache. The patient may have underlying cervical spine sprain/strain and myofascial pain contributing to her headache syndrome. Certainly the pain on palpation would be indicative of this.
3. History of pre-existing, prior to motor vehicle accident, episodic tension-type headaches.

RECOMMENDED TESTS:

1. Headache profile to rule out any metabolic causes of the patient's complaints. The patient has had a CT scan in the recent past which was negative.
2. I would also like to obtain cervical spine x-rays, AP, lateral, flexion and extension views.

The patient does not have any clinical indication at this time that would warrant a CT or an MRI of the cervical spine.

INITIAL THERAPY: I would initially suggest for medication management:

1. Amitriptyline 10 mg q.h.s.

2. I would suggest trial of non-steroidal anti-inflammatory medication. However, the patient did have non-steroidal anti-inflammatory medication after the accident and did have symptom improvement, but she was unable to tolerate it. We will try Orudis as an alternative.
3. Cervical plexus regional block given the area of pain on palpation.
4. The possibility of cervical facet blocks with fluoroscopic guidance will be considered.
5. We will also add deep neuromuscular mobilization and kinetic activity at our office. This will allow us to supervise the patient from both a medical management point of view and from her physical medicine point of view.

Dr. , thank you again for the kind referral of this most pleasant patient. If you have any questions or if there is anything further I can do, please feel free to contact me.

Sincerely,

R. , M.D.

TO THE READER: As you can see, this patient could fall in the category of Chapter 13 (Post Traumatic Headache), Chapter 14 (Whiplash Headache), or under Chapter 19 (Cervicogenic Headache). I chose this particular chapter because the patient did strike her head.

March 22, 1993

[Doctor's name and address omitted].

RE: SAMANTHA

Dear Dr. [...]:

Thank you for the referral of Samantha.

This is a 17-year-old female born [...] in [...] and living in [...] for [...] years. She is in the twelfth grade at [...] school.

On [...] she was in a significant accident in which she was a passenger without a seat belt. Another car pulled out in front of her and hit the passenger side of their car. Her head hit the windshield and she was taken to the emergency room. X-rays were taken of the neck and knee and she states she had some glass embedded in her forehead. Her headaches began immediately but she had taken Tylenol for two days and states that there was no headache problem prior to the accident.

HEADACHE PROFILE

Incapacitating headaches: These started the day of the accident. She had them daily for about a week and she still has them daily. They last two to three hours. It is a throbbing headache upon wakening and then it is a steady ache. The pain is in the temporal areas, either side, the lateral orbital regions and the cervical regions. There is no aura. There is some nausea, photophobia, phonophobia, and she goes to bed if possible. Movement will make it worse.

Interfering headaches (moderate to severe): Patient had two episodes in which she fainted and does complain of being lightheaded.

Irritating headaches (annoying): N/A.

Menstrual history: Began at age twelve. She was on birth control pills to regulate her menses at age twelve for six months with no adverse effects.

Past history: She was a cesarean section delivery. There is no history of enuresis or unexplained abdominal cramps pre-puberty. There is no history of car sickness as a child. There is no history of meningitis, encephalitis, scarlet fever, or rheumatic fever. There were no head injuries as a child.

Habits: She does not smoke or drink.

Review of systems: Pulmonary negative, cardiovascular negative, gastrointestinal negative, urogenital negative.

The patient denies fever, rash, chest pain, palpitations, nausea, vomiting, change in bowel habits, blood in stool, indigestion, change in urination, jaw claudication, arthralgias, myalgias, change in weight, mental changes, seizures, visual obscuration, blurred vision, blindness, diplopia, tinnitus, weakness, paralysis, sensory changes, incontinence, depression, or suicidal ideation.

Medical history: The patient has no history of high blood pressure, stomach ulcers, asthma, allergies, pneumonia, kidney problems, low blood sugar, glaucoma, diabetes, or heart problems.

Surgical history: She had a T&A at age seven.

Psychiatric history: Negative.

Head injuries in adult life: Negative.

Family history: Her father is living, age 48, with no headaches. Her mother is living, age 49, with no headaches. There is a brother and two sisters with no headaches.

Allergies to medications: NKA.

Current medications: She is on Tetracycline 250 mg b.i.d. for some dermatological problems. She has had no imaging tests.

Doctors seen in the past for headaches: None.

Physical examination: Height 5' 5$^1/_2$", weight 135 pounds, pulse 80, left BP 102/68, right BP 108/70. The face did not show any asymmetry. The temporomandibular joint area was grossly normal. The eyes appeared normal. Conjunctivae were clear and the pupils reacted equally to light and accommodation. Retinal fundus examination revealed no papilledema and no abnormalities with the arteries and veins. There were no bruits over the supraorbital region. The nose appeared normal. The auditory canals were clear and the tympanic membranes appeared intact. The mouth and throat appeared normal. Gums, tongue, buccal mucosa and teeth were grossly normal. There were several myofascial trigger points in the upper trapezius muscle bilaterally. There were no masses felt in the thyroid gland. Carotid bruits could not be heard. Cervical nodes were not enlarged. The lungs were clear to auscultation and percussion. The heart had a regular sinus rhythm with no murmurs. The abdomen was soft and nontender. A rectal or vaginal exam was not done.

Neurological examination: Cranial nerve II: Visual fields were grossly normal. III, IV and VI: No strabismus, nystagmus or ptosis. V: Normal sensation and corneal reflex. VII: Normal facial movements (wrinkle, frown, smile, and strength of eyelids). VIII: Normal Weber and Rinne. IX and X: Good gag reflex. XI: Normal sternocleidomastoid and trapezius. XII: Normal protrusion and strength of tongue. Cerebellar: Negative Rhomberg. Normal finger-to-nose, diadochokinesis, heel-shin, tandem, and heel and toes walking. Motor System: No atrophy, fasciculations, wasting, or tremors. Good muscle strength in arms, wrists, fingers, and legs. Sensory System: Superficial tactile, pain and vibrations (wrists, elbows, knees, and ankles) were normal. Normal motion and positions of fingers and toes. Normal 2-point discrimination. Reflexes: Normal 2+ reflexes of triceps, biceps, knee jerk, ankle jerk, etc. Normal pulses in dorsalis pedis, posterior tibial and popliteal.

Diagnoses:

1. Post traumatic daily headache.
2. Rule out post traumatic structural lesion.
3. Post traumatic vascular headache.
4. Post traumatic muscle contraction with myofascial trigger points.

Impression: This pleasant 17-year-old young woman was in a significant accident in 1993. Along with her headaches, which appear to be vascular, there are also some myofascial trigger points. The patient also complains of some dizziness and has fainted twice. I feel that one has to rule out the possibility of any intracranial structural lesion.

I will do an EEG and MRI of the patient. In order to help her with the trigger points, I will do trigger points with deep neuromuscular mobilization and kinetic activity, and she will be placed on Amitriptyline 10 mg h.s., Bellergal-S h.s., and Midrin to help abort her headaches.

She will maintain a monthly headache log and we will have another consultation in one month.

Again, thank you for the referral of this very pleasant patient. If there are any questions, please do not hesitate to call or write.

Sincerely,

BERNARD SWERDLOW, M.D.

These notes were dictated with the patient present.

MEDICAL HEADACHE HISTORY

Name: Samantha **Age:** 17 **Sex** F **Date:** 3/22/93

Date of Birth: 00/00/75 **Birthplace:** OH **Race:** W **Education:** High School

Occupation: Student **Accident:** 1993

Armed Services & Type of Discharge: N/A

PAST HISTORY:

1.	Did you have a normal birth?		Yes	No
	a) forceps used?		Yes	No
	b) cesarean section?		Yes	No
2.	Did you have problems with bedwetting?		Yes	No
	a) If yes, age bedwetting stopped		______	
3.	Were you car sick as a child (motion)?		Yes	No
	a) If yes, how severe?	Slight	Moderate	Severe
4.	Did you have unexplained abdominal cramps as a child?		Yes	No
5.	Did you have any of the following illnesses in childhood?			
	a) meningitis		Yes	No
	b) encephalitis		Yes	No
	c) scarlet fever		Yes	No
	d) rheumatic fever		Yes	No
6.	Did you have any head injuries as a child?		Yes	No
	a) If yes, please explain: ______			
7.	Were you treated for emotional illness as a child?		Yes	No

HABITS:

8.	Do you drink alcohol?	Yes	No
	a) If yes, what kind and how much? ______		
	b) Does alcohol bring on or aggravate a headache?	Yes	No
9.	Do you smoke?	Yes	No
	a) If yes, how much? ______		
	b) Does smoking or smoke-filled rooms cause or aggravate headaches?	Yes	No
10.	Do you drink caffeinated beverages?	Yes	No
	a) If yes, how much? ______		

MENSTRUAL HISTORY:

At what age did menses begin? 12 Were they regular or irregular? WNL

How were they related to your headache? N/A

Are you or were you ever on Birth Control Pills? Yes Did they affect your headache? N/A

Have you had a hysterectomy, partial or total, and why? No

Are you in menopause, and if yes, how long? No

Are you on hormones, and if yes, which ones? No

HEADACHE ASSESSMENT FORM

HA PROFILE	INCAPACITATING #3	INTERFERING #2	IRRITATING #1
ONSET (Years ago and frequency)	N/A	Day of accident Every day for 1 week	N/A
CURRENT FREQUENCY	N/A	Every day	N/A
TIME OF ONSET	N/A	Awakens with	N/A
DURATION	N/A	2 to 3 hours	N/A
CHARACTER	N/A	Throbbing upon awakening, then steady ache	N/A
PRODROME OR AURA	N/A	N/A	N/A
ASSOCIATING FEATURES	Nausea; Vomiting; Sensitivity to Light? Noise? Odors? Do you get pale or flush? Do your eyes or nose run? Does your nose get stuffy? Do the whites of your eyes get red? Does your eyelid droop? Do you pace, or go to bed?	Nausea; Vomiting; Sensitivity to Light? Noise? Odors? Do you get pale or flush? Do your eyes or nose run? Does your nose get stuffy? Do the whites of your eyes get red? Does your eyelid droop? Do you pace, or go to bed?	Nausea; Vomiting; Sensitivity to Light? Noise? Odors? Do you get pale or flush? Do your eyes or nose run? Does your nose get stuffy? Do the whites of your eyes get red? Does your eyelid droop? Do you pace, or go to bed?
PRECIPITATING OR AGGRAVATING FEATURES	N/A	Movement	N/A

LOCATION: Mark the location for each type of headache with a different color pen.

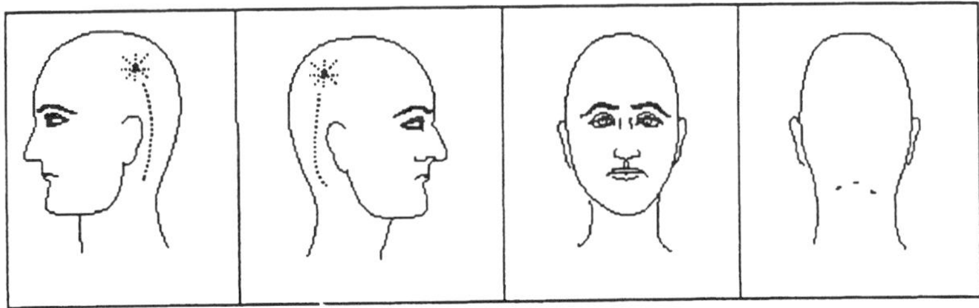

MEDICAL HISTORY:

Have you ever been or are you currently being treated for any of the following?

a) high blood pressure	Yes	No
b) stomach ulcers	Yes	No
c) asthma	Yes	No
d) allergies	Yes	No
e) pneumonia	Yes	No
f) kidney problems	Yes	No
g) low blood sugar	Yes	No
h) glaucoma	Yes	No
i) diabetes	Yes	No
j) heart problems	Yes	No

If you answered yes to any of the above, please describe:________________

List all other medical problems you have had in the past. Include date diagnosed and treatment.
DO NOT LIST OPERATIONS

SURGICAL HISTORY (List operations and dates performed)

Tonsillectomy, age 7

PSYCHIATRIC HISTORY (List visits with counselors, psychologists, etc., and type of treatment)

Currently in treatment w/Dr. P for personal problems.

ACCIDENTS IN ADULT LIFE (Briefly describe any accident that caused any blow to the head or that you feel is related to your headache)

Auto accident, 1993. Passenger without seat belt. Another car pulled out of the lot and hit passenger side of car. Head hit windshield. Taken to emergency room, x-rayed neck and knee. Had glass embedded in forehead. Headaches began immediately, but had Tylenol #3 x 2 days. No headaches prior to the accident.

FAMILY HISTORY:

1. Is your father living? Yes No
   Age 48
   Cause of death________________
   Was there a headache history? Yes No
2. Is your mother living? Yes No
   Age 49
   Cause of death________________
   Was there a headache history? Yes No

3. Ages of brothers---Circle the ones with headache
One brother
4. Ages of sisters---Circle the ones with headache
Two sisters
5. List any other blood relatives with a history of severe headaches.
None

MARITAL HISTORY:
List marriages:

1st marriage age _____ to _______	Did spouse have headaches?	Yes	No
2nd marriage age _____ to _______	Did spouse have headaches?	Yes	No
3rd marriage age ______to _______	Did spouse have headaches?	Yes	No

Age of current spouse:________

List ages and sex of all children:

Age _____ Sex ______	Headaches?	Yes	No
Age _____ Sex ______	Headaches?	Yes	No
Age _____ Sex ______	Headaches?	Yes	No

STRESS FACTORS:

List any factors that may be affecting your headaches (money, loneliness, sexual problems, work, etc.)

____

____

VEGETATIVE SIGNS:

1.	Do you have trouble falling asleep?	Yes	No (underlined)
2.	Do you have trouble staying asleep?	Yes	No (underlined)
3.	Has your appetite decreased?	Yes	No (underlined)
4.	Have you gained or lost weight in the past year?	Yes (underlined)	No
5.	Have you felt tearful or depressed lately?	Yes	No (underlined)
6.	Have you had any thoughts of wanting to die?	Yes	No (underlined)
7.	Have you been forgetful lately?	Yes	No (underlined)

8. Any other changes in your normal day-to-day living?________________

Please list any medications you are allergic or sensitive to: No known allergies

Please list any medications you are currently taking (including dosages and frequency per day):
Tetracycline, 250 mg twice a day for skin..

____

____

PREVIOUS CARE:

1. List doctors who have treated you for headaches: None.

2. List any tests you have had for your headache (e.g., EEG, CT scan, MRI, X-Ray, etc.):
None.

3. List any other treatment you have had for your headache (e.g., biofeedback, acupuncture, chiropractic, or any other treatment you had):
None.

TAMI
Category: Post traumatic headache

The headache intake form indicates that this 28-year-old woman was in an accident four months prior to my seeing her. She states that "a driver pulled out in front of me, causing me to hit him." There was immediate impact. She says that there was no locking of the seatbelts and she hit her head against the windshield. Although the window didn't break, it could be seen where she hit her head. She was dazed, but not unconscious. She was taken to a hospital, x-rayed and released.

Incapacitating headaches: The first one of these occurred approximately three weeks after the accident. She had three of them. They began in mid-morning and lasted all day, and she described it as a hot, searing pain with pressure. It always involves the right eye area. With the headache, she has nausea, vomiting, light sensitivity or photophobia, sonophobia or noise sensitivity, and she has to go to bed. Any movement makes it worse. There is no aura or warning sign that she is going to get the headache.

Interfering headaches (moderate to severe): She does recall having these occasionally from age 15. When they occur, they occur once a week. Since the accident, they have increased in frequency and have been on a daily basis.

A history of headaches in her family reveals that the maternal side of her family has headaches, and her sister has headaches.

This is another case in which the patient had what appeared to have been some vascular headaches prior to the accident that now are increased in both intensity and frequency. She would be diagnosed as having a chronic, post-traumatic headache with migraine features. This is a pleasant story, in that three months after coming to the office and being placed on a migraine diet and some medications, she became headache-free. The medications were discontinued and the patient was told to come back if she had any further problems.

MEDICAL HEADACHE HISTORY

Name: Tami **Age:** 28 **Sex** F **Date:** 10/15/92

Date of Birth: 00/00/64 **Birthplace:** FL **Race:** C **Education:** A.A.

Occupation: Office Administrator **Accident:** June 1992

Armed Services & Type of Discharge: N/A

PAST HISTORY:

1.	Did you have a normal birth?		Yes (underlined)	No
	a) forceps used?		Yes	No (underlined)
	b) cesarean section?		Yes	No (underlined)
2.	Did you have problems with bedwetting?		Yes	No (underlined)
	a) If yes, age bedwetting stopped		______	
3.	Were you car sick as a child (motion)?		Yes	No (underlined)
	a) If yes, how severe?	Slight (underlined)	Moderate	Severe
4.	Did you have unexplained abdominal cramps as a child?		Yes	No (underlined)
5.	Did you have any of the following illnesses in childhood?			
	a) meningitis		Yes	No (underlined)
	b) encephalitis		Yes	No (underlined)
	c) scarlet fever		Yes	No (underlined)
	d) rheumatic fever		Yes	No (underlined)
6.	Did you have any head injuries as a child?		Yes	No (underlined)
	a) If yes, please explain: ______			
7.	Were you treated for emotional illness as a child?		Yes	No (underlined)

HABITS:

8.	Do you drink alcohol?	Yes (underlined)	No
	a) If yes, what kind and how much? 1 – 2 per week		
	b) Does alcohol bring on or aggravate a headache?	Yes	No (underlined)
9.	Do you smoke?	Yes	No (underlined)
	a) If yes, how much? ______		
	b) Does smoking or smoke-filled rooms cause or aggravate headaches?	Yes	No (underlined)
10.	Do you drink caffeinated beverages?	Yes (underlined)	No
	a) If yes, how much? 1 – 2 daily		

MENSTRUAL HISTORY:

At what age did menses begin? 12 Were they regular or irregular? WNL
How were they related to your headache? N/A
Are you or were you ever on Birth Control Pills? Yes Did they affect your headache? ______
Have you had a hysterectomy, partial or total, and why? No
Are you in menopause, and if yes, how long? No
Are you on hormones, and if yes, which ones? No

HEADACHE ASSESSMENT FORM

HA PROFILE	INCAPACITATING #3	INTERFERING #2	IRRITATING #1
ONSET (Years ago and frequency)	3 weeks after accident, have had only 3 last one Oct. 12	Age 15 – Occasionally, then 1 week after accident 2/week	N/A
CURRENT FREQUENCY	Last one 10/12	1/wk. Every day since 10/12	N/A
TIME OF ONSET	Mid-morning	Mid-morning	N/A
DURATION	1 day	All day	N/A
CHARACTER	"hot searing pain" and pressure	Same, but less intense	Dull ache
PRODROME OR AURA	N/A	N/A	N/A
ASSOCIATING FEATURES	Nausea; Vomiting; Sensitivity to Light? Noise? Odors? Do you get pale or flush? Do your eyes or nose run? Does your nose get stuffy? Do the whites of your eyes get red? Does your eyelid droop? Do you pace, or go to bed? dizzy	Nausea; Vomiting; Sensitivity to Light? Noise? Odors? Do you get pale or flush? Do your eyes or nose run? Does your nose get stuffy? Do the whites of your eyes get red? Does your eyelid droop? Do you pace, or go to bed?	Nausea; Vomiting; Sensitivity to Light? Noise? Odors? Do you get pale or flush? Do your eyes or nose run? Does your nose get stuffy? Do the whites of your eyes get red? Does your eyelid droop? Do you pace, or go to bed?
PRECIPITATING OR AGGRAVATING FEATURES	Sudden movement	N/A	N/A

LOCATION: Mark the location for each type of headache with a different color pen.

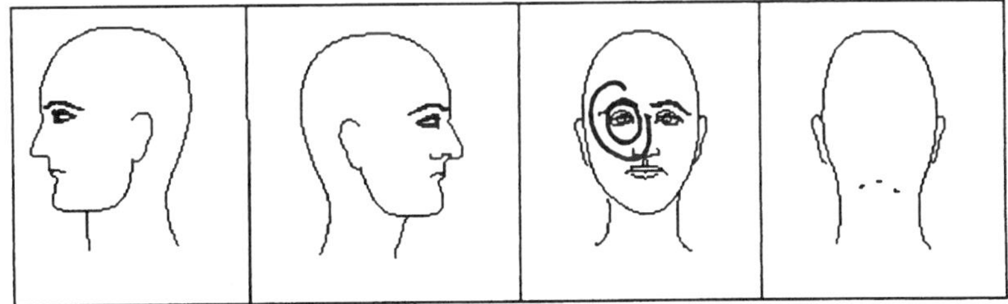

MEDICAL HISTORY:

Have you ever been or are you currently being treated for any of the following?

a) high blood pressure	Yes	No
b) stomach ulcers	Yes	No
c) asthma	Yes	No
d) allergies	Yes	No
e) pneumonia	Yes	No
f) kidney problems	Yes	No
g) low blood sugar	Yes	No
h) glaucoma	Yes	No
i) diabetes	Yes	No
j) heart problems	Yes	No

If you answered yes to any of the above, please describe:____________________

List all other medical problems you have had in the past. Include date diagnosed and treatment.
DO NOT LIST OPERATIONS

Knee problem, spastic colon, low blood pressure.

SURGICAL HISTORY (List operations and dates performed)

Ear surgery, 1983.

PSYCHIATRIC HISTORY (List visits with counselors, psychologists, etc., and type of treatment)

Currently in treatment w/Dr. P for personal problems.

ACCIDENTS IN ADULT LIFE (Briefly describe any accident that caused any blow to the head or that you feel is related to your headache)

June, 1992 – Driver pulled out in front of me causing me to hit him. Immediate impact, no locking of seatbelts. Hit head against windshield. Dazed, but not unconscious. Taken to hospital, x-rayed and released. Headaches began one week after.

FAMILY HISTORY:

1.	Is your father living?	Yes	No
	Age______		
	Cause of death 52, murdered		
	Was there a headache history?	Yes	No
2.	Is your mother living?	Yes	No
	Age 52		
	Cause of death______		
	Was there a headache history?	Yes	No

3. Ages of brothers---Circle the ones with headache
   31 and 16
4. Ages of sisters---Circle the ones with headache
   (28)
5. List any other blood relatives with a history of severe headaches.
   Maternal grandmother

MARITAL HISTORY:

List marriages:

1st marriage age ______ to ______	Did spouse have headaches?	Yes	No
2nd marriage age ______ to ______	Did spouse have headaches?	Yes	No
3rd marriage age ______ to ______	Did spouse have headaches?	Yes	No

Age of current spouse:________

List ages and sex of all children:

Age _____ Sex ______	Headaches?	Yes	No
Age _____ Sex ______	Headaches?	Yes	No
Age _____ Sex ______	Headaches?	Yes	No

STRESS FACTORS:

List any factors that may be affecting your headaches (money, loneliness, sexual problems, work, etc.)
Loneliness.

VEGETATIVE SIGNS:

1.	Do you have trouble falling asleep?	Yes	No
2.	Do you have trouble staying asleep?	Yes	No
3.	Has your appetite decreased?	Yes	No
4.	Have you gained or lost weight in the past year?	Yes	No
5.	Have you felt tearful or depressed lately?	Yes	No
6.	Have you had any thoughts of wanting to die?	Yes	No
7.	Have you been forgetful lately?	Yes	No
8.	Any other changes in your normal day-to-day living?________		

Please list any medications you are allergic or sensitive to: None.

Please list any medications you are currently taking (including dosages and frequency per day):
None.

PREVIOUS CARE:

1. List doctors who have treated you for headaches: None.

2. List any tests you have had for your headache (e.g., EEG, CT scan, MRI, X-Ray, etc.):
MRI – brain (normal).

3. List any other treatment you have had for your headache (e.g., biofeedback, acupuncture, chiropractic, or any other treatment you had):
Chiropractic (helped temporarily).

JOHN
Category: Post traumatic headache

This is a 33-year-old man who was working as a maintenance mechanic for a large commercial airline. Four months before I saw him, he had walked into a small aircraft with a low overhead. He stated that he "jammed my head onto my neck." He was not unconscious. He went to the emergency room 24 hours later with severe headache and states he had an occasional headache prior to the accident.

Incapacitating headaches started in his twenties, and he had them occasionally. Since the accident, he gets them two or three times a week. It is a throbbing headache around both his eyes and the back of his neck. With these headaches, he has nausea, light sensitivity or photophobia, noise sensitivity or sonophobia, and must go to bed. Movement will make his headache worse.

Interfering headaches also started in his twenties, and he also now gets them two to three times a week since the accident. He said that if he doesn't take pain medication, they will become incapacitating and the pain is similar to the incapacitating headaches.

He was given a psychological test which showed some depression and some tension.

This is a case in which there probably were some preexisting migraine attacks, and the trauma caused the increased frequency of these headaches. The patient continued to work and is a very dedicated person; however, the increased frequency of his already preexisting condition is going to be very difficult to control. Often medication that will work on non-traumatic headaches will not be effective with traumatic headaches. The prognosis here is guarded.

MEDICAL HEADACHE HISTORY

Name: John **Age:** 33 **Sex** M **Date:** 7/11/90

Date of Birth: 00/00/56 **Birthplace:** MI **Race:** C **Education:** High school

Occupation: Aircraft maintenance **Accident:** 3/90

Armed Services & Type of Discharge: None

PAST HISTORY:

1.	Did you have a normal birth?		Yes	No
	a) forceps used?		Yes	No
	b) cesarean section?		Yes	No
2.	Did you have problems with bedwetting?		Yes	No
	a) If yes, age bedwetting stopped		______	
3.	Were you car sick as a child (motion)?		Yes	No
	a) If yes, how severe?	Slight	Moderate	Severe
4.	Did you have unexplained abdominal cramps as a child?		Yes	No
5.	Did you have any of the following illnesses in childhood?			
	a) meningitis		Yes	No
	b) encephalitis		Yes	No
	c) scarlet fever		Yes	No
	d) rheumatic fever		Yes	No
6.	Did you have any head injuries as a child?		Yes	No
	a) If yes, please explain:______			
7.	Were you treated for emotional illness as a child?		Yes	No

HABITS:

8.	Do you drink alcohol?	Yes	No
	a) If yes, what kind and how much? Has never had alcohol		
	b) Does alcohol bring on or aggravate a headache?	Yes	No
9.	Do you smoke?	Yes	No
	a) If yes, how much?______		
	b) Does smoking or smoke-filled rooms cause or aggravate headaches?	Yes	No
10.	Do you drink caffeinated beverages?	Yes	No
	a) If yes, how much? 16 or 32 oz. a week		

MENSTRUAL HISTORY:

At what age did menses begin?______ Were they regular or irregular?______
How were they related to your headache?______
Are you or were you ever on Birth Control Pills?______ Did they affect your headache? ______
Have you had a hysterectomy, partial or total, and why?______
Are you in menopause, and if yes, how long?______
Are you on hormones, and if yes, which ones?______

HEADACHE ASSESSMENT FORM

HA PROFILE	INCAPACITATING #3	INTERFERING #2	IRRITATING #1
ONSET (Years ago and frequency)	In 20's, occasionally	In 20's, 1 a month before accident	N/A
CURRENT FREQUENCY		2 to 3 a week, which can increase to #3 if pain medication not taken	N/A
TIME OF ONSET	Anytime	Anytime	N/A
DURATION	4 – 8 hours	2 – 4 hours with pain medication	N/A
CHARACTER	Throbbing	Same, less severe	N/A
PRODROME OR AURA	N/A	N/A	N/A
ASSOCIATING FEATURES	Nausea; Vomiting; Sensitivity to Light? Noise? Odors? Do you get pale or flush? Do your eyes or nose run? Does your nose get stuffy? Does the white of your eyes get red? Does your eyelid droop? Do you pace, or go to bed?	Nausea; Vomiting; Sensitivity to Light? Noise? Odors? Do you get pale or flush? Do your eyes or nose run? Does your nose get stuffy? Does the white of your eyes get red? Does your eyelid droop? Do you pace, or go to bed?	Nausea; Vomiting; Sensitivity to Light? Noise? Odors? Do you get pale or flush? Do your eyes or nose run? Does your nose get stuffy? Does the white of your eyes get red? Does your eyelid droop? Do you pace, or go to bed?
PRECIPITATING OR AGGRAVATING FEATURES	Movement	Not taking pain medication	N/A

LOCATION: Mark the location for each type of headache with a different color pen.

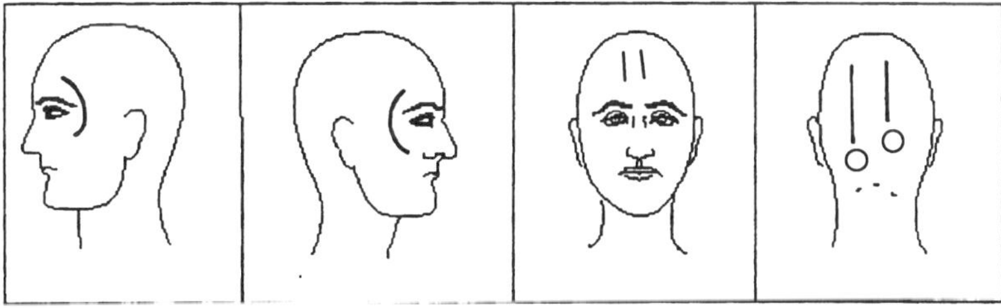

MEDICAL HISTORY:

Have you ever been or are you currently being treated for any of the following?

a) high blood pressure	Yes	No
b) stomach ulcers	Yes	No
c) asthma	Yes	No
d) allergies	Yes	No
e) pneumonia	Yes	No
f) kidney problems	Yes	No
g) low blood sugar	Yes	No
h) glaucoma	Yes	No
i) diabetes	Yes	No
j) heart problems	Yes	No

If you answered yes to any of the above, please describe:____________________

List all other medical problems you have had in the past. Include date diagnosed and treatment.
DO NOT LIST OPERATIONS

SURGICAL HISTORY (List operations and dates performed)

Foot (operated on for burn) – 1978. Upper lip (sutures) – 1979. Left shoulder (dislocation) – 1985.
Right elbow (loose body) – 1983.

PSYCHIATRIC HISTORY (List visits with counselors, psychologists, etc., and type of treatment)

None.

ACCIDENTS IN ADULT LIFE (Briefly describe any accident that caused any blow to the head or that you feel is related to your headache)

In March, 1990, I was walking into an aircraft wiyth low overhead. I jammed my head into my Neck. Not unconscious. Went to ER 24 hours later for severe headahe. Had occasional Headaches before accident.

FAMILY HISTORY:

1. Is your father living? Yes No
   Age 69
   Cause of death____________________
   Was there a headache history? Yes No
2. Is your mother living? Yes No
   Age 62
   Cause of death____________________
   Was there a headache history? Yes No

3. Ages of brothers---Circle the ones with headache
   27 30 35 37 40
4. Ages of sisters---Circle the ones with headache
   None
5. List any other blood relatives with a history of severe headaches.
   ?

MARITAL HISTORY:
List marriages:

1st marriage age 27 to Now	Did spouse have headaches?	Yes	No
2nd marriage age ___ to ___	Did spouse have headaches?	Yes	No
3rd marriage age ___ to ___	Did spouse have headaches?	Yes	No

Age of current spouse: 26

List ages and sex of all children:

Age 2	Sex F	Headaches? Yes	No
Age ___	Sex ___	Headaches? Yes	No
Age ___	Sex ___	Headaches? Yes	No
Age ___	Sex ___	Headaches? Yes	No

STRESS FACTORS:

List any factors that may be affecting your headaches (money, loneliness, sexual problems, work, etc.)
None

VEGETATIVE SIGNS:

1.	Do you have trouble falling asleep?	Yes	No
2.	Do you have trouble staying asleep?	Yes	No
3.	Has your appetite decreased?	Yes	No
4.	Have you gained or lost weight in the past year?	Yes	No
5.	Have you felt tearful or depressed lately?	Yes	No
6.	Have you had any thoughts of wanting to die?	Yes	No
7.	Have you been forgetful lately?	Yes	No
8.	Any other changes in your normal day-to-day living?		

Please list any medications you are allergic or sensitive to: Sulfa

Please list any medications you are currently taking (including dosages and frequency per day):
Just pain med. When I start to get headache.

PREVIOUS CARE:

1. List doctors who have treated you for headaches: Dr. N.,

2. List any tests you have had for your headache (e.g., EEG, CT scan, MRI, X-Ray, etc.):
CAT scan and x-rays

3. List any other treatment you have had for your headache (e.g., biofeedback, acupuncture, chiropractic, or any other treatment you had):
Physical Therapy (no help).

CONSULTATION

PATIENT: DANA

DATE: November 30, 1994

Ms. Dana [...] is a 19-year-old female born [...] in Florida who presented herself for headache evaluation and treatment.

The patient has lived in [...] her entire life and is currently a full-time college student.

HEADACHE PROFILE

The patient was involved in a motor vehicle accident on [...], when the car she was driving was struck by another automobile. Although she was wearing a seatbelt, it "came undone." The other driver allegedly ran a stop sign, hitting the patient's automobile head-on. The patient estimates she was traveling at approximately 45 mph and did not see the other car and therefore was unable to brake. The other driver died in the car accident. The patient did strike her head, although it is unsure exactly where, and she also received a laceration on her forehead on the right side. The patient was transported to City Hospital, evaluated but not hospitalized, and was told that she sustained "swelling of the brain." The patient is not sure if x-rays were performed of her head and neck. The patient did experience loss of consciousness of unknown duration. The next day the patient saw [Dr. P] for follow-up and was told that the headache symptoms she suffered immediately after the accident were due to stress. He did not perform x-rays at that time. She was given medication — prescription type unknown — which did not improve her symptoms.

Prior to this motor vehicle accident, the patient never had a #3 or incapacitating headache. The patient states that prior to the accident she had only rare mild headaches that responded to over-the-counter medication. These headaches were very mild and never interfered with any of her activities.

Incapacitating headaches: This headache occurred the day of the accident and lasted for the next week. The patient currently suffers one of these headaches every 7 to 14 days. This headache will occur at any time of the day and will last 48 hours. The pain is characterized as a throbbing pressure sensation localized in the temporal area and radiating to the cervical region bilaterally. There is no prodrome with these headaches; however, they are associated with nausea but not vomiting, photophobia, pallor, and the patient will seek bed rest if possible. The patient does note that movement will increase the symptoms.

Interfering headaches (moderate to severe): These headaches developed approximately one month after the accident and the first one lasted approximately 2 weeks. The patient currently suffers one of these headaches every 7 to 14 days. This headache can occur at any time of the day and will generally last 24 hours. The pain location and characterization is the same as with the #3 or incapacitating headaches, except less intense. There is no prodrome with these headaches; however, they are associated with some nausea — no vomiting, photophobia, sensitivity to odors, and the patient will seek bed rest if possible.

Irritating headaches (annoying): None.

Menstrual history: Began at age 11 and is reported to be normal. The patient is currently taking oral contraceptives and has been since age 18. No other hormone supplementation.

Past history: The patient was most probably a normal delivery. There is no history of enuresis or unexplained abdominal cramps pre-puberty. There is no history of car sickness as a child. There is no history of meningitis, encephalitis, scarlet fever, or rheumatic fever. There were no head injuries as a child.

Habits: The patient does not drink alcohol and does not smoke; however, she does note that secondary smoke will increase her headaches. The patient does drink approximately four caffeinated beverages per day.

Medical history: TMJ. The patient is scheduled for dental implant and TMJ evaluation following that.

The patient has no history of high blood pressure, stomach ulcers, asthma, allergies, pneumonia, kidney problems, low blood sugar, glaucoma, diabetes, or heart problems.

Review of systems: Pulmonary negative, cardiovascular negative, gastrointestinal negative, urogenital negative.

Surgical history: In 1990, orthodontic surgery with excision of 9 teeth.

Psychiatric history: The patient has seen [...] for one year and Dr. [...] for six months for psychotherapy and Prozac, and [...] for six months. These treatments were for dealing with the accident and depression.

Family history: Her father is living, age 42, with no headache history. Her mother is living, age 41, with no headache history. The patient has no brothers and one sister with a history of #2 or interfering headaches. The patient has a great uncle who died of a brain tumor. The patient is single and does not have children.

Stress factors: The patient lists stress factors of sleep and sister returning back home.

Vegetative signs: The patient reports difficulty both in falling and staying asleep. Depression without suicidal ideation. No memory difficulty.

Allergies to medications: None.

Current medications: The patient is currently taking Excedrin and Advil p.r.n. and oral contraceptives.

Doctors seen in the past for headaches: The patient has been evaluated by [Dr. P] who stated that her headaches were stress-related. The patient has not had any other evaluation or treatment for her headaches.

Physical examination: Height 5'½", weight 113 pounds, pulse 76, left BP 100/74, right BP 96/78. The face did not show any asymmetry. The temporomandibular joint area was grossly normal. The eyes appeared normal. Conjunctivae were clear and the pupils reacted equally to light and accommodation. Retinal fundus examination revealed no papilledema and no abnormalities with the arteries and veins. There were no bruits over the supraorbital region. The nose appeared normal. The auditory canals were clear and the tympanic membranes appeared intact. The mouth and throat appeared normal. Gums, tongue, buccal mucosa and teeth were grossly normal. Neck: The patient has approximately 4 to 6 myofascial trigger points in the trapezius muscle group. Carotid bruits could not be heard. Cervical nodes were not enlarged. The lungs were clear to auscultation and percussion. The heart had a regular sinus rhythm with no murmurs. The abdomen was soft and nontender. Rectal and vaginal exams were deferred to her regular physician.

Neurological examination: Cranial nerve II: Visual fields were grossly normal. III, IV and VI: No strabismus, nystagmus or ptosis. V: Normal sensation and corneal reflex. VII: Normal facial movements (wrinkle, frown, smile and strength of eyelids). VIII: Normal Weber and Rinne. IX and X: Good gag reflex. XI: Normal sternocleidomastoid and trapezius. XII: Normal protrusion and strength of tongue. Cerebellar: Negative Rhomberg. Normal finger-to-nose, diadochokinesis, heel-shin, tandem and heel and toes walking. Motor system: No atrophy, fasciculations, wasting or tremors. Good muscle strength in arms, wrists, fingers and legs. Sensory system: Superficial tactile, pain and vibrations (wrists, elbows, knees and ankles) were normal. Normal motion and positions of fingers and toes. Normal 2-point discrimination. Reflexes: Normal 2+ reflexes of triceps, biceps, knee jerk, ankle jerk, etc. Normal pulses in dorsalis pedis, posterior tibial and popliteal.

DIAGNOSES

1. Post traumatic headache — vascular. International Headache Society classification 5.2.
2. Chronic post traumatic myofascial syndrome. The patient has not had any problem with myofascial symptoms prior to motor vehicle accident and the symptoms occurred immediately after.

Fortunately, the patient is not suffering any problems with memory per her history; however, she is having problems with depression which could be a component of the post traumatic headache syndrome; and also problems with sleep disturbance which, again, could be problems from the post traumatic headache syndrome. The throbbing nature of the pain, associated with gastrointestinal and sensory changes, indicates a vascular nature to this headache.

I would recommend:

1. MRI of the brain with and without contrast to rule out any structural lesions in this patient with persistent headache symptoms.
2. Headache profile to rule out any metabolic etiologies that could be contributing to the headache.

Relative to therapy, we will start the patient on:

1. Amitriptyline 10 mg q.h.s. approximately 2 hours before bedtime. This will also help associated sleep disturbance.
2. Inderal 20 mg t.i.d. to be used in combination with Elavil as a prophylactic measure.
3. The patient reports one headache every 1 to 2 weeks and we will start with a combination of Midrin and Fioricet for an abortive measure. If this is not successful, then will start Ergopak with Promethazine for second line of defense of abortive medication.
4. Physical therapy and trigger point injections for myofascial component.

The patient will also be given a headache log and a headache diet to observe, and will return to the office in approximately 4 weeks for reevaluation and further medical management.

MEDICAL HEADACHE HISTORY

Name: Dana **Age:** 19 **Sex** F **Date:** 11/30/94

Date of Birth: 00/00/75 **Birthplace:** FL **Race:** C **Education:** In College

Occupation: Student. **Accident:** 1992

Armed Services & Type of Discharge: N/A

PAST HISTORY:

1.	Did you have a normal birth?		Yes (underlined)	No
	a) forceps used?		Yes	No (underlined)
	b) cesarean section?		Yes	No (underlined)
2.	Did you have problems with bedwetting?		Yes	No (underlined)
	a) If yes, age bedwetting stopped		______	
3.	Were you car sick as a child (motion)?		Yes	No (underlined)
	a) If yes, how severe?	Slight	Moderate	Severe
4.	Did you have unexplained abdominal cramps as a child?		Yes	No (underlined)
5.	Did you have any of the following illnesses in childhood?			
	a) meningitis		Yes	No (underlined)
	b) encephalitis		Yes	No (underlined)
	c) scarlet fever		Yes	No (underlined)
	d) rheumatic fever		Yes	No (underlined)
6.	Did you have any head injuries as a child?		Yes	No (underlined)
	a) If yes, please explain: ______			
7.	Were you treated for emotional illness as a child?		Yes	No (underlined)

HABITS:

8.	Do you drink alcohol?	Yes	No (underlined)
	a) If yes, what kind and how much? ______		
	b) Does alcohol bring on or aggravate a headache?	Yes	No (underlined)
9.	Do you smoke?	Yes	No (underlined)
	a) If yes, how much? ______		
	b) Does smoking or smoke-filled rooms cause or aggravate headaches?	Yes (underlined)	No
10.	Do you drink caffeinated beverages?	Yes (underlined)	No
	a) If yes, how much? Many during the day, 4 glasses		

MENSTRUAL HISTORY:

At what age did menses begin? 11 Were they regular or irregular? WNL
How were they related to your headache? N/A
Are you or were you ever on Birth Control Pills? Yes Did they affect your headache? N/A
Have you had a hysterectomy, partial or total, and why? No
Are you in menopause, and if yes, how long? No
Are you on hormones, and if yes, which ones? No

HEADACHE ASSESSMENT FORM

HA PROFILE	INCAPACITATING #3	INTERFERING #2	IRRITATING #1
ONSET (Years ago and frequency)	Day of accident 1 a week	One month after accident 1 every 2 weeks	N/A
CURRENT FREQUENCY	1 every 7 to 14 days	1 every 7 to 14 days	N/A
TIME OF ONSET	Anytime	Anytime	N/A
DURATION	48 hours	1 day	N/A
CHARACTER	Throbbing, pressure	Same, less intense	N/A
PRODROME OR AURA	N/A	N/A	N/A
ASSOCIATING FEATURES	Nausea; Vomiting; Sensitivity to Light? Noise? Odors? Do you get pale or flush? Do your eyes or nose run? Does your nose get stuffy? Do the whites of your eyes get red? Does your eyelid droop? Do you pace, or go to bed?	Nausea; Vomiting; Sensitivity to Light? Noise? Odors? Do you get pale or flush? Do your eyes or nose run? Does your nose get stuffy? Do the whites of your eyes get red? Does your eyelid droop? Do you pace, or go to bed?	Nausea; Vomiting; Sensitivity to Light? Noise? Odors? Do you get pale or flush? Do your eyes or nose run? Does your nose get stuffy? Do the whites of your eyes get red? Does your eyelid droop? Do you pace, or go to bed?
PRECIPITATING OR AGGRAVATING FEATURES	Movement	N/A	N/A

LOCATION: Mark the location for each type of headache with a different color pen.

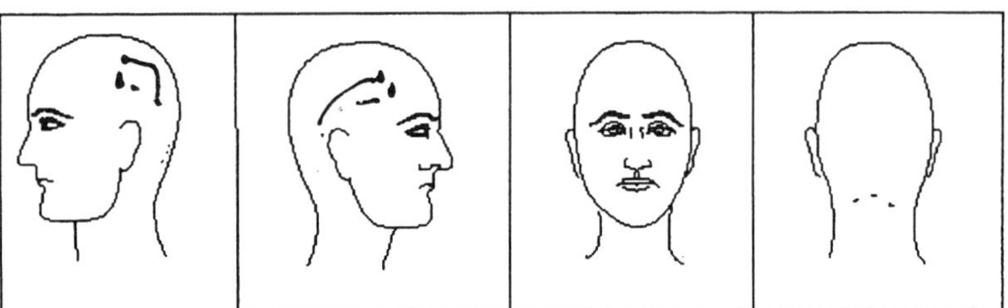

MEDICAL HISTORY:

Have you ever been or are you currently being treated for any of the following?

a) high blood pressure	Yes	No
b) stomach ulcers	Yes	No
c) asthma	Yes	No
d) allergies	Yes	No
e) pneumonia	Yes	No
f) kidney problems	Yes	No
g) low blood sugar	Yes	No
h) glaucoma	Yes	No
i) diabetes	Yes	No
j) heart problems	Yes	No

If you answered yes to any of the above, please describe:________________

List all other medical problems you have had in the past. Include date diagnosed and treatment.
DO NOT LIST OPERATIONS

TMJ – no treatment so far, scheduled for implants.

SURGICAL HISTORY (List operations and dates performed)

Orthodontia – 1990. Had 9 teeth removed.

PSYCHIATRIC HISTORY (List visits with counselors, psychologists, etc., and type of treatment)

Ms. W, Dr. M, Ms. T.

ACCIDENTS IN ADULT LIFE (Briefly describe any accident that caused any blow to the head or that you feel is related to your headache)

Car accident, 1992. Driver, wearing seat belt, which "came undone." Another driver ran stop sign and hit me head-on. I was traveling about 45 mph. Did not see other car and did not brake. Other driver died in accident. Hit head (don't know where), lacerated right forehead. Told of swelling of brain, but was not hospitalized. Treated and released from emergency room. X-rays taken of head or neck. Was unconscious, but don't know how long; came to in passenger seat. Did not have severe headaches prior to accident. Had #3 headache the day after the accident.

FAMILY HISTORY:

1. Is your father living? Yes No
   Age 42
   Cause of death________________
   Was there a headache history? Yes No

2. Is your mother living? Yes No
    Age 41
    Cause of death________________
    Was there a headache history? Yes No

3. Ages of brothers---Circle the ones with headache
    ____

4. Ages of sisters---Circle the ones with headache
    (22)

5. List any other blood relatives with a history of severe headaches.
    Great uncle died of brain tumor.

MARITAL HISTORY:
List marriages:

1st marriage age _____ to _______	Did spouse have headaches?	Yes	No
2nd marriage age _____ to _______	Did spouse have headaches?	Yes	No
3rd marriage age _____ to _______	Did spouse have headaches?	Yes	No

Age of current spouse:________

List ages and sex of all children:

Age _____ Sex _____	Headaches?	Yes	No
Age _____ Sex _____	Headaches?	Yes	No
Age _____ Sex _____	Headaches?	Yes	No

STRESS FACTORS:

List any factors that may be affecting your headaches (money, loneliness, sexual problems, work, etc.)
Sleep and sister moving back home.
____

VEGETATIVE SIGNS:

1.	Do you have trouble falling asleep?	Yes	No
2.	Do you have trouble staying asleep?	Yes	No
3.	Has your appetite decreased?	Yes	No
4.	Have you gained or lost weight in the past year?	Yes	No
5.	Have you felt tearful or depressed lately?	Yes	No
6.	Have you had any thoughts of wanting to die?	Yes	No
7.	Have you been forgetful lately?	Yes	No
8.	Any other changes in your normal day-to-day living?________________		

Please list any medications you are allergic or sensitive to: No known allergies

Please list any medications you are currently taking (including dosages and frequency per day):
Excedrin, Advil, BCP.

PREVIOUS CARE:

1. List doctors who have treated you for headaches: Dr. P.

2. List any tests you have had for your headache (e.g., EEG, CT scan, MRI, X-Ray, etc.):
TMJ test.

3. List any other treatment you have had for your headache (e.g., biofeedback, acupuncture, chiropractic, or any other treatment you had):
None.

ROBERT
Category: Post traumatic headache

This is a 31-year-old man who approximately seven months before he saw me was driving with his seatbelt on when a semi-tractor-trailer rear-ended him, knocking him into the median and causing him to be hit again by the same truck. The trailer ran over the back of his car. He hit his head on the sunroof several times, causing him to be unconscious briefly. He went to the emergency room where he was treated and released. He said his headaches began immediately, and states there was no headache history prior to the accident.

Incapacitating headaches: These started about a month after the accident. They occur approximately several times a month. They can last a full day. The headaches are throbbing in the bilateral periorbital (around the eye sockets), frontal, occipital (rear), and cervical regions of his head. There is no aura. Associated features include nausea, vomiting, sonophobia (sound sensitivity), sensitivity to odors, pallor, and he must go to bed. Driving long distances and movement will make his headache worse.

Interfering headaches: These started the day of the accident, and he has been having these daily. They are mild upon awakening and increase in intensity during the day. It is constant pain and pressure in the frontal, occipital, and posterocervical regions. There are no associated features.

The diagnosis here would be post traumatic/concussion vascular headaches and post traumatic/concussion daily headaches (most likely a muscle tension type).

Prior to seeing me, the patient had multiple treatments including chiropractic, biofeedback, etc. with minimal success. This patient probably will end up also having a cervicogenic-type headache as a result of the injury to the cervical vertebrae; but we will take some time later to identify this.

MEDICAL HEADACHE HISTORY

Name: Robert **Age:** 31 **Sex** M **Date:** 12/14/92

Date of Birth: 00/00/61 **Birthplace:** OH **Race:** C **Education:** Some college

Occupation: Sales **Accident:** 5/89

Armed Services & Type of Discharge: N/A

PAST HISTORY:

1.	Did you have a normal birth?		Yes (underlined)	No
	a) forceps used?		Yes	No (underlined)
	b) cesarean section?		Yes	No (underlined)
2.	Did you have problems with bedwetting?		Yes	No
	a) If yes, age bedwetting stopped		______	
3.	Were you car sick as a child (motion)?		Yes	No (underlined)
	a) If yes, how severe?	Slight	Moderate	Severe
4.	Did you have unexplained abdominal cramps as a child?		Yes	No (underlined)
5.	Did you have any of the following illnesses in childhood?			
	a) meningitis		Yes	No (underlined)
	b) encephalitis		Yes	No (underlined)
	c) scarlet fever		Yes	No (underlined)
	d) rheumatic fever		Yes	No (underlined)
6.	Did you have any head injuries as a child?		Yes	No (underlined)
	a) If yes, please explain:______			
7.	Were you treated for emotional illness as a child?		Yes	No (underlined)

HABITS:

8.	Do you drink alcohol?	Yes (underlined)	No
	a) If yes, what kind and how much? Maybe 1 beer a month		
	b) Does alcohol bring on or aggravate a headache?	Yes	No (underlined)
9.	Do you smoke?	Yes	No (underlined)
	a) If yes, how much?______		
	b) Does smoking or smoke-filled rooms cause or aggravate headaches?	Yes	No (underlined)
10.	Do you drink caffeinated beverages?	Yes	No (underlined)
	a) If yes, how much?______		

MENSTRUAL HISTORY:

At what age did menses begin?______ Were they regular or irregular?______
How were they related to your headache?______
Are you or were you ever on Birth Control Pills?______ Did they affect your headache? ______
Have you had a hysterectomy, partial or total, and why?______
Are you in menopause, and if yes, how long?______
Are you on hormones, and if yes, which ones?______

HEADACHE ASSESSMENT FORM

HA PROFILE	INCAPACITATING #3	INTERFERING #2	IRRITATING #1
ONSET (Years ago and frequency)	1 month after accident occasionally	Day of accident Every day	N/A
CURRENT FREQUENCY	Approximately 1 – 2 month	Every day	N/A
TIME OF ONSET	Anytime	Mild upon awakening, increases during the day	N/A
DURATION	8 to 10 hours	Constant	N/A
CHARACTER	Throbbing	Throbbing	N/A
PRODROME OR AURA	N/A	N/A	N/A
ASSOCIATING FEATURES	Nausea; Vomiting; Sensitivity to Light? Noise? Odors? Do you get pale or flush? Do your eyes or nose run? Does your nose get stuffy? Does the white of your eyes get red? Does your eyelid droop? Do you pace, or go to bed?	Nausea; Vomiting; Sensitivity to Light? Noise? Odors? Do you get pale or flush? Do your eyes or nose run? Does your nose get stuffy? Does the white of your eyes get red? Does your eyelid droop? Do you pace, or go to bed?	Nausea; Vomiting; Sensitivity to Light? Noise? Odors? Do you get pale or flush? Do your eyes or nose run? Does your nose get stuffy? Does the white of your eyes get red? Does your eyelid droop? Do you pace, or go to bed?
PRECIPITATING OR AGGRAVATING FEATURES	Long distance driving Movement	Long distance driving	N/A

LOCATION: Mark the location for each type of headache with a different color pen.

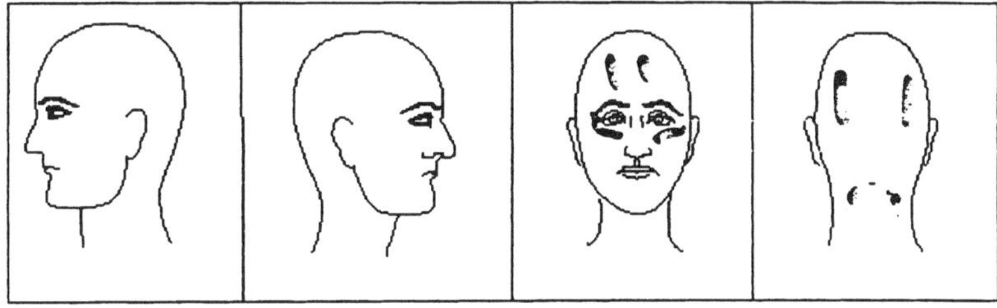

MEDICAL HISTORY:

Have you ever been or are you currently being treated for any of the following?

a) high blood pressure	Yes	No
b) stomach ulcers	Yes	No
c) asthma	Yes	No
d) allergies	Yes	No
e) pneumonia	Yes	No
f) kidney problems	Yes	No
g) low blood sugar	Yes	No
h) glaucoma	Yes	No
i) diabetes	Yes	No
j) heart problems	Yes	No

If you answered yes to any of the above, please describe:____________________

List all other medical problems you have had in the past. Include date diagnosed and treatment.
DO NOT LIST OPERATIONS

Bulging disk, lower back. Neck sprain. Whiplash.

SURGICAL HISTORY (List operations and dates performed)

Tonsillectomy & Adenoidectomy – age 5.

PSYCHIATRIC HISTORY (List visits with counselors, psychologists, etc., and type of treatment)

Dr. T (biofeedback).

ACCIDENTS IN ADULT LIFE (Briefly describe any accident that caused any blow to the head or that you feel is related to your headache)

May 1989 – I was rear-ended by a semi-truck, knocked across the median, hit a second time by same truck in front left fener. Then tractor trailer ran over back of car. Since my head was so close to the roof, I hit my head and jammed my neck. September 1987 – Rear-ended and had back pain, but no headache.

FAMILY HISTORY:

1.	Is your father living?	Yes	No
	Age 53		
	Cause of death____________________		
	Was there a headache history?	Yes	No
2.	Is your mother living?	Yes	No
	Age 51		
	Cause of death____________________		
	Was there a headache history?	Yes	No

3. Ages of brothers---Circle the ones with headache
   29 28
4. Ages of sisters---Circle the ones with headache
   33
5. List any other blood relatives with a history of severe headaches.
   None

MARITAL HISTORY:

List marriages:

1st marriage age 28 to Present	Did spouse have headaches?	Yes	No
2nd marriage age ____ to ____	Did spouse have headaches?	Yes	No
3rd marriage age ____ to ____	Did spouse have headaches?	Yes	No

Age of current spouse: 24

List ages and sex of all children:

Age 2 ½ Sex F	Headaches?	Yes	No
Age 7 mo Sex M	Headaches?	Yes	No
Age ____ Sex ____	Headaches?	Yes	No
Age ____ Sex ____	Headaches?	Yes	No

STRESS FACTORS:

List any factors that may be affecting your headaches (money, loneliness, sexual problems, work, etc.)

____

____

VEGETATIVE SIGNS:

1.	Do you have trouble falling asleep?	Yes	No
2.	Do you have trouble staying asleep?	Yes	No
3.	Has your appetite decreased?	Yes	No
4.	Have you gained or lost weight in the past year?	Yes	No
5.	Have you felt tearful or depressed lately?	Yes	No
6.	Have you had any thoughts of wanting to die?	Yes	No
7.	Have you been forgetful lately?	Yes	No
8.	Any other changes in your normal day-to-day living? ____		

Please list any medications you are allergic or sensitive to: NKA

____

____

Please list any medications you are currently taking (including dosages and frequency per day):

None.

____

PREVIOUS CARE:

1. List doctors who have treated you for headaches: Dr. M, Dr. T, Dr. B

2. List any tests you have had for your headache (e.g., EEG, CT scan, MRI, X-Ray, etc.):
MRI of neck and lower back.

3. List any other treatment you have had for your headache (e.g., biofeedback, acupuncture, chiropractic, or any other treatment you had):
Biofeedback (helps a little). Neuromuscular massage (helps). Chiropractic (helps).

TERRY
Category: Post traumatic headache

This is a 28-year-old man who was in an accident about six months before he came to the clinic. He was driving with his seatbelt on. He was trying to avoid a dog and hit a tree. His seatbelt broke, his head hit the windshield, and he was unconscious briefly. He was taken home by a friend and seen by a doctor three days later. His headaches began the day of the accident. He did not suffer any headaches prior to the accident.

Incapacitating headaches: These started the day of the accident and he was having them daily. He awakens with them. They will last from one hour to all day, and then come back. They will wax and wane. It starts as a sharp pain and then becomes throbbing in the bilateral temporal regions and the occipital portion of his head. There is no aura. Associated features are nausea, vomiting, light sensitivity, and he will have to go to bed. Exertion will make it worse.

This is very typical of a migraine-type headache that follows a head trauma. This is a good example of how these headaches can be precipitated and continue, and why they should be treated soon after the accident.

MEDICAL HEADACHE HISTORY

Name: Terry **Age:** 28 **Sex** M **Date:** 4/8/91

Date of Birth: 00/00/62 **Birthplace:** FL **Race:** B **Education:** 1 yr. college

Occupation: Construction **Accident:** 1990

Armed Services & Type of Discharge: N/A

PAST HISTORY:

1.	Did you have a normal birth?		Yes	No
	a) forceps used?		Yes	No
	b) cesarean section?		Yes	No
2.	Did you have problems with bedwetting?		Yes	No
	a) If yes, age bedwetting stopped			____
3.	Were you car sick as a child (motion)?		Yes	No
	a) If yes, how severe?	Slight	Moderate	Severe
4.	Did you have unexplained abdominal cramps as a child?		Yes	No
5.	Did you have any of the following illnesses in childhood?			
	a) meningitis		Yes	No
	b) encephalitis		Yes	No
	c) scarlet fever		Yes	No
	d) rheumatic fever		Yes	No
6.	Did you have any head injuries as a child?		Yes	No
	a) If yes, please explain:____			
7.	Were you treated for emotional illness as a child?		Yes	No

HABITS:

8.	Do you drink alcohol?	Yes	No
	a) If yes, what kind and how much?____		
	b) Does alcohol bring on or aggravate a headache?	Yes	No
9.	Do you smoke?	Yes	No
	a) If yes, how much?____		
	b) Does smoking or smoke-filled rooms cause or aggravate headaches?	Yes	No
10.	Do you drink caffeinated beverages?	Yes	No
	a) If yes, how much?____		

MENSTRUAL HISTORY:

At what age did menses begin?____ Were they regular or irregular?____
How were they related to your headache?____
Are you or were you ever on Birth Control Pills?____ Did they affect your headache? ____
Have you had a hysterectomy, partial or total, and why?____
Are you in menopause, and if yes, how long?____
Are you on hormones, and if yes, which ones?____

HEADACHE ASSESSMENT FORM

HA PROFILE	INCAPACITATING #3	INTERFERING #2	IRRITATING #1
ONSET (Years ago and frequency)	Day of accident Every day	N/A	N/A
CURRENT FREQUENCY	Every day	N/A	N/A
TIME OF ONSET	Can awaken with	N/A	N/A
DURATION	1 hour to all day, comes and goes	N/A	N/A
CHARACTER	Starts with sharp pain, then throbbing	N/A	N/A
PRODROME OR AURA	N/A	N/A	N/A
ASSOCIATING FEATURES	Nausea; Vomiting; Sensitivity to Light? Noise? Odors? Do you get pale or flush? Do your eyes or nose run? Does your nose get stuffy? Does the white of your eyes get red? Does your eyelid droop? Do you pace, or go to bed?	Nausea; Vomiting; Sensitivity to Light? Noise? Odors? Do you get pale or flush? Do your eyes or nose run? Does your nose get stuffy? Does the white of your eyes get red? Does your eyelid droop? Do you pace, or go to bed?	Nausea; Vomiting; Sensitivity to Light? Noise? Odors? Do you get pale or flush? Do your eyes or nose run? Does your nose get stuffy? Does the white of your eyes get red? Does your eyelid droop? Do you pace, or go to bed?
PRECIPITATING OR AGGRAVATING FEATURES	Movement	N/A	N/A

LOCATION: Mark the location for each type of headache with a different color pen.

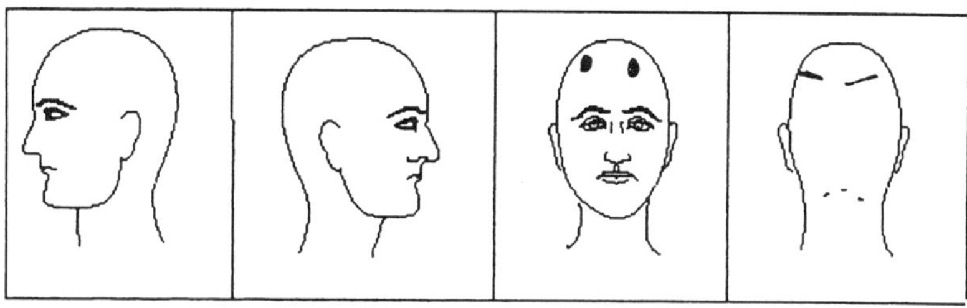

MEDICAL HISTORY:

Have you ever been or are you currently being treated for any of the following?

a) high blood pressure	Yes	No
b) stomach ulcers	Yes	No
c) asthma	Yes	No
d) allergies	Yes	No
e) pneumonia	Yes	No
f) kidney problems	Yes	No
g) low blood sugar	Yes	No
h) glaucoma	Yes	No
i) diabetes	Yes	No
j) heart problems	Yes	No

If you answered yes to any of the above, please describe:____________________

List all other medical problems you have had in the past. Include date diagnosed and treatment.
DO NOT LIST OPERATIONS

None

SURGICAL HISTORY (List operations and dates performed)

None.

PSYCHIATRIC HISTORY (List visits with counselors, psychologists, etc., and type of treatment)

None.

ACCIDENTS IN ADULT LIFE (Briefly describe any accident that caused any blow to the head or that you feel is related to your headache)

Car accident. Driving with seat belt. Trying to avoid a dog and hit a tree. Seatbelt broke and head went into the windshield. Unconscious briefly. Taken home by a friend. Seen by doctor 3 days later. Headaches began day of accident. No headaches before accident.

FAMILY HISTORY:

1. Is your father living? Yes No
   - Age 58
   - Cause of death____________________
   - Was there a headache history? Yes No
2. Is your mother living? Yes No
   - Age 56
   - Cause of death____________________
   - Was there a headache history? Yes No

3. Ages of brothers---Circle the ones with headache
   36 32 23 18
4. Ages of sisters---Circle the ones with headache
   40 37 34 33
5. List any other blood relatives with a history of severe headaches.
   None

MARITAL HISTORY:
List marriages:

1st marriage age _____ to _______ Did spouse have headaches? Yes No
2nd marriage age _____ to _______ Did spouse have headaches? Yes No
3rd marriage age _____ to _______ Did spouse have headaches? Yes No
Age of current spouse:__________

List ages and sex of all children:
Age _____ Sex _____ Headaches? Yes No
Age _____ Sex _____ Headaches? Yes No
Age _____ Sex _____ Headaches? Yes No
Age _____ Sex _____ Headaches? Yes No

STRESS FACTORS:

List any factors that may be affecting your headaches (money, loneliness, sexual problems, work, etc.)
____
____

VEGETATIVE SIGNS:

1. Do you have trouble falling asleep? Yes No
2. Do you have trouble staying asleep? Yes No
3. Has your appetite decreased? Yes No
4. Have you gained or lost weight in the past year? Yes No
5. Have you felt tearful or depressed lately? Yes No
6. Have you had any thoughts of wanting to die? Yes No
7. Have you been forgetful lately? Yes No
8. Any other changes in your normal day-to-day living?__________

Please list any medications you are allergic or sensitive to: None
____
____

Please list any medications you are currently taking (including dosages and frequency per day):
Tylenol 3.
____

PREVIOUS CARE:

1. List doctors who have treated you for headaches: Dr. D

2. List any tests you have had for your headache (e.g., EEG, CT scan, MRI, X-Ray, etc.):

CAT scan 1990 (without contrast) – normal.

X-rays.

3. List any other treatment you have had for your headache (e.g., biofeedback, acupuncture, chiropractic, or any other treatment you had):

May 14, 1992

[Doctor's name and address omitted]

RE: MICHELLE

Dear Dr. [...]

Thank you for your referral. This is a 31-year-old female born [...] in Florida. She has a high school education. She started working last month as a security guard.

The patient states that in 1991 she was in an automobile accident. She was a passenger in the front seat without a seat belt. They were making a U-turn when they were broad-sided on the driver's side. She was thrown into the rearview mirror and hit her left forehead. She was not unconscious. She was taken to the emergency room where she had sutures in the left forehead. She was x-rayed and released. Her headaches began two days later. She states that she had a rare, annoying headache that was controlled with aspirin prior to the accident.

HEADACHE PROFILE

Incapacitating headaches: These started two days after the accident. She had them daily for three weeks. Currently she is getting two to three a week. They come on at any time. They will last all day. It is a sharp, boring, occasional throbbing pain always in the left side in the left periorbital, frontal and occipital and cervical regions. There is no aura. The patient states that she has to go to bed with these headaches. There are no other associated features.

Interfering headaches (moderate to severe): These started three weeks after the accident and she has been having them daily. It is a constant pain. It is also boring and occasional throbbing in the same location just described, always on the left side. She will go to bed, if possible.

Irritating headaches (annoying): These started at age 20. They were very rare. She may get one a month. She can abort them with over-the-counter medication. It is a dull ache in the frontal part of her head.

Menstrual history: Menses began at age 12 and are within normal limits. She used to get an occasional annoying headache with her periods. She was on birth control pills for two days at age 19, but had nausea and vomiting problems and stopped them.

Past history: The patient was a normal delivery. There is no history of enuresis or unexplained abdominal cramps pre-puberty. There is no history of car sickness as a child. There is no history of meningitis, encephalitis, scarlet fever, or rheumatic fever. There were no head injuries as a child.

Habits: She does not drink. She does not smoke.

Medical history: Essentially negative.

Review of systems: Pulmonary negative, cardiovascular negative, gastrointestinal negative, urogenital negative.

Surgical history: She had significant burns as a child when a hot water heater exploded on her. She had a rebuilt knee on the right side and multiple scarring as a result of it. She had skin grafts every year until she was 17 years old.

Psychiatric history: Negative.

Family history: Father living, 56, no headaches. Mother deceased at age 50 of a coronary, with no headache history. There are four brothers, 32, 24, 22, and 16, and a sister, 24, with no headaches. A maternal aunt has headaches.

Marital history: The patient has been married from age 18 to present. There are three children, a girl 9, and two boys, 7 and 4, with no headaches. Her husband is 34 and is a route driver and cabinet maker.

Allergies to medications: She thinks that caffeine might increase her headaches.

Medications: She is currently taking Triavil p.r.n. for sleep, but says this makes her very lethargic and she is not comfortable with it.

Previous work-up: She had some x-rays of her skull, which I assume were negative. She has had some physical therapy which helped her back, but not her headache.

Physical examination: Height 5'3", weight 174 pounds, pulse 82, left arm BP 110/64, right arm BP 104/68. The face did not show any asymmetry. The temporomandibular joint area was grossly normal. The eyes appeared normal. Conjunctivae were clear and the pupils reacted equally to light and accommodation. Retinal fundus examination revealed no papilledema and no abnormalities with the arteries and veins. There were no bruits over the supraorbital region. The nose appeared normal. The auditory canals were clear and the tympanic membranes appeared intact. The mouth and throat appeared normal. Gums, tongue, buccal mucosa and teeth were grossly normal. The neck revealed multiple myofascial trigger points in the upper trapezius and middle trapezius with exquisite tenderness. There were no masses felt in the thyroid gland. Carotid bruits could not be heard. Cervical nodes were not enlarged. The lungs were clear to auscultation and percussion. The heart had a regular sinus rhythm with no murmurs. The abdomen was soft and nontender. A rectal or vaginal examination was not done.

Neurological examination: Cranial nerve II: Visual fields grossly normal. III, IV and VI: No strabismus, nystagmus or ptosis. V: Normal sensation and corneal reflex. VII: Normal facial movements (wrinkle, frown, smile and strength of eyelids). VIII: Normal Weber and Rinne. IX and X: Good gag reflex. XI: Normal strength of sternocleidomastoid and trapezius. XII: Normal protrusion and strength of tongue. Cerebellar: Negative Romberg. Normal finger-to-nose, diadochokinesis, heel-shin, tandem and heel and toes walking. Motor system: No atrophy, fasciculations, wasting or tremors. Good muscle strength in arms, wrists, fingers and legs. Sensory system: Superficial tactile, pain and vibrations (wrists, elbows, knees and ankles) were normal. Normal motion and positions of fingers and toes. Normal 2-point discrimination. Reflexes: Normal 2+ reflexes of triceps, biceps, knee jerk, ankle jerk, etc. Normal pulses in dorsalis pedis, posterior tibial and popliteal.

DIAGNOSES

1. Post traumatic headache.
2. Post traumatic vascular headache daily.
3. Post traumatic daily muscle contraction headache with myofascial trigger points.
4. Preexisting rare, annoying headache, tension-type.

IMPRESSION/RECOMMENDATION

This 31-year-old woman comes in with significant, almost daily, headaches as a result of an accident she had in 1991. Examination reveals myofascial trigger points in the middle and upper trapezius region and what appears to be both a vascular and muscle contraction headache. The patient had a significant injury in which she required 25 sutures in her forehead on the left side. I feel it is necessary that one consider the possibility of any intracranial mechanism that may be causing it as a result of a concussion. The patient will have an MRI of the brain. She will be started on Verapamil 80 mg t.i.d., Prednisone 10 mg q.i.d., reduce by 10 mg daily, and Flexeril 10 mg t.i.d. To abort the headache, she will have Midrin and Fiorinal. The patient will be on this treatment for about a month and will have myofascial trigger points and deep neuromuscular mobilization with kinetic activity. If this is not effective, then she may be a candidate for ambulatory infusion therapy with Dihydroergotamine, which often can abort the headache totally. However, we will wait to see what her response is for one month prior to considering this mode of treatment. The ambulatory infusion therapy is done through a peripherally inserted central catheter.

Thank you once again for the referral of this patient. I will keep you posted as to her progress. If there are any questions, please do not hesitate to call or write.

Sincerely,

Bernard Swerdlow, M.D.

MEDICAL HEADACHE HISTORY

Name: Michelle **Age:** 31 **Sex** F **Date:** 5/14/92

Date of Birth: 00/00/61 **Birthplace:** FL **Race:** C **Education:** High School

Occupation: Security Personnel **Accident:** 1991

Armed Services & Type of Discharge: N/A

PAST HISTORY:

1.	Did you have a normal birth?		Yes (underlined)	No
	a) forceps used?		Yes	No
	b) cesarean section?		Yes	No
2.	Did you have problems with bedwetting?		Yes	No (underlined)
	a) If yes, age bedwetting stopped		______	
3.	Were you car sick as a child (motion)?		Yes	No (underlined)
	a) If yes, how severe?	Slight	Moderate	Severe
4.	Did you have unexplained abdominal cramps as a child?		Yes	No (underlined)
5.	Did you have any of the following illnesses in childhood?			
	a) meningitis		Yes	No (underlined)
	b) encephalitis		Yes	No (underlined)
	c) scarlet fever		Yes	No (underlined)
	d) rheumatic fever		Yes	No (underlined)
6.	Did you have any head injuries as a child?		Yes	No (underlined)
	a) If yes, please explain: ______			
7.	Were you treated for emotional illness as a child?		Yes	No (underlined)

HABITS:

8.	Do you drink alcohol?	Yes	No (underlined)
	a) If yes, what kind and how much? ______		
	b) Does alcohol bring on or aggravate a headache?	Yes	No (underlined)
9.	Do you smoke?	Yes	No (underlined)
	a) If yes, how much? ______		
	b) Does smoking or smoke-filled rooms cause or aggravate headaches?	Yes	No (underlined)
10.	Do you drink caffeinated beverages?	Yes (underlined)	No
	a) If yes, how much? Maybe one coke in a day		

MENSTRUAL HISTORY:

At what age did menses begin? 12 Were they regular or irregular? WNL

How were they related to your headache? Increased #1 headaches

Are you or were you ever on Birth Control Pills? Yes Did they affect your headache? N/A

Have you had a hysterectomy, partial or total, and why? No

Are you in menopause, and if yes, how long? No

Are you on hormones, and if yes, which ones? No

HEADACHE ASSESSMENT FORM

HA PROFILE	INCAPACITATING #3	INTERFERING #2	IRRITATING #1
ONSET (Years ago and frequency)	2 days after accident, Every day x 3 weeks	3 weeks after accident, Every day	Age 20, Rare
CURRENT FREQUENCY	2 – 3/week	Every other day	1 – 2/month
TIME OF ONSET	Anytime	Can awaken with	Anytime
DURATION	All day	Constant	1 hr. with OTC meds
CHARACTER	Sharp, boring, occasional throbbing	Same, but less intense	Dull
PRODROME OR AURA	N/A	N/A	N/A
ASSOCIATING FEATURES	Nausea; Vomiting; Sensitivity to Light? Noise? Odors? Do you get pale or flush? Do your eyes or nose run? Does your nose get stuffy? Do the whites of your eyes get red? Does your eyelid droop? Do you pace, or go to bed?	Nausea; Vomiting; Sensitivity to Light? Noise? Odors? Do you get pale or flush? Do your eyes or nose run? Does your nose get stuffy? Do the whites of your eyes get red? Does your eyelid droop? Do you pace, or go to bed?	Nausea; Vomiting; Sensitivity to Light? Noise? Odors? Do you get pale or flush? Do your eyes or nose run? Does your nose get stuffy? Do the whites of your eyes get red? Does your eyelid droop? Do you pace, or go to bed?
PRECIPITATING OR AGGRAVATING FEATURES	N/A	N/A	N/A

LOCATION: Mark the location for each type of headache with a different color pen.

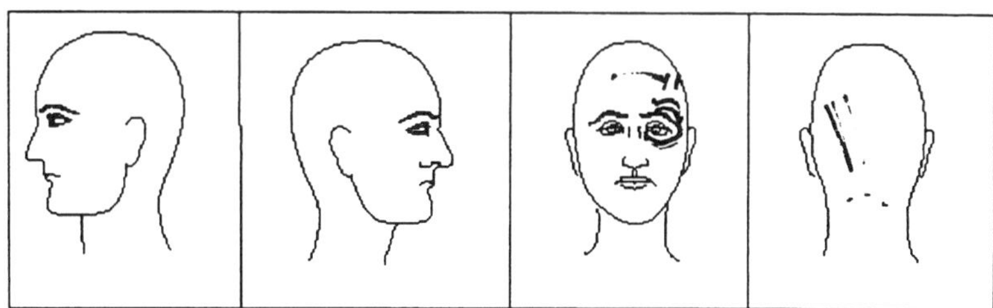

MEDICAL HISTORY:

Have you ever been or are you currently being treated for any of the following?

a) high blood pressure	Yes	No
b) stomach ulcers	Yes	No
c) asthma	Yes	No
d) allergies	Yes	No
e) pneumonia	Yes	No
f) kidney problems	Yes	No
g) low blood sugar	Yes	No
h) glaucoma	Yes	No
i) diabetes	Yes	No
j) heart problems	Yes	No

If you answered yes to any of the above, please describe:________________________

List all other medical problems you have had in the past. Include date diagnosed and treatment.
DO NOT LIST OPERATIONS

Burned as a child. Had two skin grafts every year until I was 17 years old.

SURGICAL HISTORY (List operations and dates performed)

Skin grafts every year until 17.

PSYCHIATRIC HISTORY (List visits with counselors, psychologists, etc., and type of treatment)

None.

ACCIDENTS IN ADULT LIFE (Briefly describe any accident that caused any blow to the head or that you feel is related to your headache)

In 1991 a car hit us. I was a passenger in the front seat with a seat belt. Making a U-turn, we were Broad-sided on the driver's side. Thrown into the rearview mirror and cut my head. Not unconscious. Taken to emergeny room. Received 25 sutures to the left forehead, x-rayed, and released. Headaches began two days later.

FAMILY HISTORY:

1. Is your father living? Yes No
   - Age 56
   - Cause of death________________
   - Was there a headache history? Yes No
2. Is your mother living? Yes No
   - Age________
   - Cause of death Heart attack, age 50
   - Was there a headache history? Yes No

3. Ages of brothers---Circle the ones with headache
   32 24 22 16
4. Ages of sisters---Circle the ones with headache
   24
5. List any other blood relatives with a history of severe headaches.
   Maternal aunt.

MARITAL HISTORY:
List marriages:

1st marriage age 18 to Present	Did spouse have headaches?	Yes	No
2nd marriage age ____ to ____	Did spouse have headaches?	Yes	No
3rd marriage age ____ to ____	Did spouse have headaches?	Yes	No

Age of current spouse: 34

List ages and sex of all children:

Age 9	Sex F	Headaches? Yes	No
Age 7	Sex M	Headaches? Yes	No
Age 4	Sex M	Headaches? Yes	No

STRESS FACTORS:

List any factors that may be affecting your headaches (money, loneliness, sexual problems, work, etc.)
None.

VEGETATIVE SIGNS:

1.	Do you have trouble falling asleep?	Yes	No
2.	Do you have trouble staying asleep?	Yes	No
3.	Has your appetite decreased?	Yes	No
4.	Have you gained or lost weight in the past year?	Yes	No
5.	Have you felt tearful or depressed lately?	Yes	No
6.	Have you had any thoughts of wanting to die?	Yes	No
7.	Have you been forgetful lately?	Yes	No
8.	Any other changes in your normal day-to-day living?		

Please list any medications you are allergic or sensitive to: Caffeine increases headaches

Please list any medications you are currently taking (including dosages and frequency per day):
Triavil p.r.n. (for sleep).

PREVIOUS CARE:

1. List doctors who have treated you for headaches: None.

2. List any tests you have had for your headache (e.g., EEG, CT scan, MRI, X-Ray, etc.):
X-rays.

3. List any other treatment you have had for your headache (e.g., biofeedback, acupuncture, chiropractic, or any other treatment you had):
Physical therapy (helped back, but not headache).

January 20, 1994

[Doctor's name and address omitted]

RE: RANDY

Dear Dr. [...]:

Thank you for the referral of Mr. [...]

This is a 46-year-old male born 00/00/47 in [...], New York, and living in Florida since [...]. The patient was not working at the time of the accident on 00/00/93. In this accident, the patient was driving and was hit in the rear by a car traveling, by the patient's history, at 80 mph. There were witnesses to the speed of that car. The patient hit his head on the steering wheel and there was no loss of consciousness. He was treated at the scene of the accident by paramedics and was taken to [...] Hospital E.R. where he had x-rays and was released with a collar and medications. The patient went back to the hospital in a day or two because he felt he had a fracture and more severe injuries. The hospital took some more x-rays.

HEADACHE PROFILE

Incapacitating headaches: These headaches started within the first week after the accident. The patient gets these headaches daily. They last from one half hour to three or four hours, and he will get multiple attacks during the day. It is a pressure-type headache, primarily in the posterior cervical occipital and the crown of his head and also the parietal temporal regions. There is no aura and there is some photophobia and he will go to bed. There is some dizziness with the headache.

Interfering headaches (moderate to severe): The patient had this type of headache prior to the accident, which then went into remission. The patient had tension headaches back in the area of 1985 to about 1986 and these went into remission. He was in remission with these headaches until the day of the accident of 00/00/93. Since that time, he has been having these headaches daily. It is also similar to the incapacitating headache with somewhat less intensity. The area and location of headaches are the same as before, and the associated features are the same as before.

Irritating headaches (annoying): N/A.

PAST HISTORY: The patient was most probably a normal delivery. There is no history of enuresis or unexplained abdominal cramps pre-puberty. There is no history of car sickness as a child. There is no history of meningitis, encephalitis, scarlet fever, or rheumatic fever. There were no head injuries as a child.

Habits: The patient does not drink. He does smoke a pack of cigarettes a day.

Medical history: The patient's medical history is essentially negative.

Review of systems: Pulmonary negative, cardiovascular negative, gastrointestinal negative, urogenital negative.

Surgical history: The patient had a tonsillectomy at age 8 or 9.

Psychiatric history: The patient has seen a psychiatrist at the Veteran's Hospital for a period of time, and since 1985 has been seeing [...]. He is being treated for panic disorder and is taking Klonopin and Nardil and doing quite well.

Head injuries in adult life: Other than the accident reported, the patient stated he had no head injuries prior to this.

Family history: His father is deceased, at age 57, of liver cancer, with no headache history. His mother is living, age 72, with no headache history. There is a 49-year-old sister with no headache history. The patient was married from 1972 to 1976, and from 1979 to present. There is a 13-year-old son with no headache history.

Allergies to medications: The patient is allergic to Sulfa and Penicillin.

Current medications: The patient is currently taking Nardil 30 mg t.i.d., Klonopin 2 mg a.m. and 2 mg p.m.

Doctors seen in the past for headaches: The patient has been seeing [...] and has used a pain suppressor, with no help.

Tests done in the past: The patient had a CT scan and x-rays in 1993, the results of which were negative.

The patient had the following radiological reports: On 00/00/93 he had a cervical spine series and there are degenerative changes of C6/7. A cervical spine CT revealed: C1/2 negative, C2/3 negative, C3/4 negative, C4/5 small posterior osteophyte is visualized, the neural foramen are open, there is no stenosis. C5/6 reveals large ventral osteophyte indents in the interior dural sac with disk extension. There is loss of the epidural space at this level and minimal cord flattening. C6/7 — large broad-based osteophyte is evident extending eccentrically to the left where there is evidence of neural foramen narrowing. There is no discrete herniation. There is no significant stenosis. C7/T1 negative.

Impression: Degenerative changes at C5/6 and C6/7 with evidence of left neural foramenal narrowing at C6/7 (read by [...], M.D. at [...] Hospital).

The patient also had some x-rays on 00/00/93. They were read by [...] and some cervical spine minimal degenerative changes were described.

Physical examination: Height 5'11", weight 226 pounds, pulse 88, left BP 114/76, right BP 118/90. The face did not show any asymmetry. The temporomandibular joint area was grossly normal. The eyes appeared normal. Conjunctivae were clear and the pupils reacted equally to light and accommodation. Retinal fundus examination revealed no papilledema and no abnormalities with the arteries and veins. There were no bruits over the supraorbital region. The nose appeared normal. The auditory canals were clear and the tympanic membranes appeared intact. The mouth and throat appeared normal. Gums, tongue, buccal mucosa, and teeth were grossly normal. The neck was supple and there were no masses felt in the thyroid gland. Carotid bruits could not be heard. Cervical nodes were not enlarged. The lungs were clear to auscultation and percussion. The heart had a regular sinus rhythm with no murmurs. The abdomen was soft and nontender. A rectal exam was not done.

Neurological examination: Cranial nerve II: Visual fields were grossly normal. III, IV and VI: No strabismus, nystagmus, or ptosis. V: Normal sensation and corneal reflex. VII: Normal facial movements (wrinkle, frown, smile, and strength of eyelids). VIII: Normal Weber and Rinne. IX and X: Good gag reflex. XI: Normal sternocleidomastoid and trapezius. XII: Normal protrusion and strength of tongue. Cerebellar: Negative Rhomberg. Normal finger-to-nose, diadochokinesis, heel-shin, tandem, and heel and toes walking. Motor system: No atrophy, fasciculations, wasting, or tremors. Good muscle strength in arms, wrists, fingers and legs. Sensory system: Superficial tactile, pain, and vibrations (wrists, elbows, knees and ankles) were normal. Normal motion and positions of fingers and toes. Normal 2-point discrimination. Reflexes: Normal 2+ reflexes of triceps, biceps, knee jerk, ankle jerk, etc. Normal pulses in dorsalis pedis, posterior tibial and popliteal.

DIAGNOSES

1. Post traumatic headache.
2. Rule out cervicogenic headache.
3. Rule out post traumatic muscle contraction headache.
4. Preexisting tension headache from 1967-1985 (on an on-and-off basis).

IMPRESSION

This 46-year-old gentleman comes in with headaches which he states started on the day of an accident he had in which he was rear-ended by a car going "80 mph" on 00/00/93. There is also a history that the patient suffered tension headaches prior to that from 1967 to 1985 on an "on and off" basis. Once he started his Nardil for his panic disorder in 1985, most of his headaches disappeared, and now these headaches seem to have either been exacerbated by the accident or may be a new type of headache. There does not seem to be a vascular component to this headache by the patient's history.

Part of the problem with the patient is that there is a tendency to overextend information which is superfluous to the information we are trying to get and history taking becomes somewhat difficult. I explained to the patient that he would have to answer questions as I ask them and stay away from all the other data that he thinks is necessary.

The final analysis is that there appears to be a cervicogenic type headache as the result of a cervicogenic strain, which may cause some headaches with a minor vascular component. For this, I would recommend that he have a posterior regional block of C1, 2 and 3, which we can do here, and see if he gets the response that would give him significant relief for a short period of time, such as a week to ten days. If he gets that kind of response and we can identify the origin of the headache, then we will consider doing an epidural block or facet block in that area. I also explained to the patient that we are also able to do blocks at C5/6 if they are related to his current problem from the accident.

Thank you for the referral of this patient. If there are any questions, please do not hesitate to call or write.

Sincerely,

BERNARD SWERDLOW, M.D.

These notes were dictated with the patient present. Again, this is a situation where this history could be placed in this chapter, or in Chapter 14 (whiplash) and Chapter 19 (cervicogenic headache).

MEDICAL HEADACHE HISTORY

Name: Randy **Age:** 46 **Sex** M **Date:** 1/20/94

Date of Birth: 00/00/47 **Birthplace:** NY **Race:** W **Education:** 3 yrs. college

Occupation: Unable to work **Accident:** 00/93

Armed Services & Type of Discharge: U.S. Army

PAST HISTORY:

1.	Did you have a normal birth?		Yes (underlined)	No
	a) forceps used?		Yes	No (underlined)
	b) cesarean section?		Yes	No (underlined)
2.	Did you have problems with bedwetting?		Yes	No (underlined)
	a) If yes, age bedwetting stopped		______	
3.	Were you car sick as a child (motion)?		Yes	No (underlined)
	a) If yes, how severe?	Slight	Moderate	Severe
4.	Did you have unexplained abdominal cramps as a child?		Yes	No (underlined)
5.	Did you have any of the following illnesses in childhood?			
	a) meningitis		Yes	No (underlined)
	b) encephalitis		Yes	No (underlined)
	c) scarlet fever		Yes	No (underlined)
	d) rheumatic fever		Yes	No (underlined)
6.	Did you have any head injuries as a child?		Yes	No (underlined)
	a) If yes, please explain:______			
7.	Were you treated for emotional illness as a child?		Yes	No (underlined)

HABITS:

8.	Do you drink alcohol?	Yes	No (underlined)
	a) If yes, what kind and how much?______		
	b) Does alcohol bring on or aggravate a headache?	Yes	No
9.	Do you smoke?	Yes (underlined)	No
	a) If yes, how much? 1 pack a day		
	b) Does smoking or smoke-filled rooms cause or aggravate headaches?	Yes	No (underlined)
10.	Do you drink caffeinated beverages?	Yes (underlined)	No
	a) If yes, how much? Coffee, 2 or 3 times a week; cola once in awhile		

MENSTRUAL HISTORY:

At what age did menses begin?______ Were they regular or irregular?______
How were they related to your headache?______
Are you or were you ever on Birth Control Pills?______ Did they affect your headache? ______
Have you had a hysterectomy, partial or total, and why?______
Are you in menopause, and if yes, how long?______
Are you on hormones, and if yes, which ones?______

HEADACHE ASSESSMENT FORM

HA PROFILE	INCAPACITATING #3	INTERFERING #2	IRRITATING #1
ONSET (Years ago and frequency)	Within first week after accident	Day of accident	N/A
CURRENT FREQUENCY	2 a week	Every day if not #3	N/A
TIME OF ONSET	When awaken	When awaken	N/A
DURATION	½ to 3 or 4 hours	Constant	N/A
CHARACTER	Pressure	Pressure, less than #3	N/A
PRODROME OR AURA	N/A	N/A	N/A
ASSOCIATING FEATURES	Nausea; Vomiting; Sensitivity to Light? Noise? Odors? Do you get pale or flush? Do your eyes or nose run? Does your nose get stuffy? Does the white of your eyes get red? Does your eyelid droop? Do you pace, or go to bed? Dizziness	Nausea; Vomiting; Sensitivity to Light? Noise? Odors? Do you get pale or flush? Do your eyes or nose run? Does your nose get stuffy? Does the white of your eyes get red? Does your eyelid droop? Do you pace, or go to bed? Dizziness	Nausea; Vomiting; Sensitivity to Light? Noise? Odors? Do you get pale or flush? Do your eyes or nose run? Does your nose get stuffy? Does the white of your eyes get red? Does your eyelid droop? Do you pace, or go to bed?
PRECIPITATING OR AGGRAVATING FEATURES	N/A	N/A	N/A

LOCATION: Mark the location for each type of headache with a different color pen.

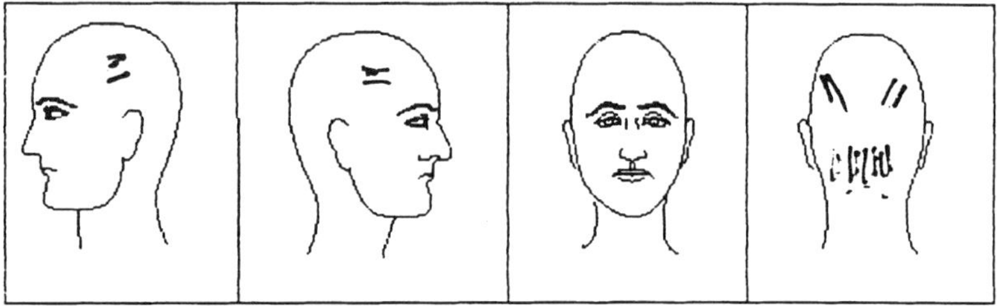

MEDICAL HISTORY:

Have you ever been or are you currently being treated for any of the following?

a) high blood pressure	Yes	No
b) stomach ulcers	Yes	No
c) asthma	Yes	No
d) allergies	Yes	No
e) pneumonia	Yes	No
f) kidney problems	Yes	No
g) low blood sugar	Yes	No
h) glaucoma	Yes	No
i) diabetes	Yes	No
j) heart problems	Yes	No

If you answered yes to any of the above, please describe:____________________

List all other medical problems you have had in the past. Include date diagnosed and treatment.
DO NOT LIST OPERATIONS

After accident, fracture of 6 teeth and C7.

SURGICAL HISTORY (List operations and dates performed)

Tonsillectomy, age 8 or 9.

PSYCHIATRIC HISTORY (List visits with counselors, psychologists, etc., and type of treatment)

Seeing psychiatrist at VA. Since 1985 seeing Dr. G. Panic disorder. Take Klonopin and Nardil.

ACCIDENTS IN ADULT LIFE (Briefly describe any accident that caused any blow to the head or that you feel is related to your headache)

Car accident, 1993. Driving, wearing seatbelt. Hit in rear by car traveling 80 mph. Hit head on steering wheel. Did not lose consciousness. Treated at scene by paramedics and transported to hospital emergency room. Had x-rays, CT scan, released with collar and medications.

FAMILY HISTORY:

1.	Is your father living?	Yes	No
	Age________		
	Cause of death Liver cancer, age 57		
	Was there a headache history?	Yes	No
2.	Is your mother living?	Yes	No
	Age 72		
	Cause of death________		
	Was there a headache history?	Yes	No

3. Ages of brothers---Circle the ones with headache
   None
4. Ages of sisters---Circle the ones with headache
   49
5. List any other blood relatives with a history of severe headaches.
   None

MARITAL HISTORY:

List marriages:

1st marriage age 1972 to 1976	Did spouse have headaches?	Yes	No
2nd marriage age 1979 to Present	Did spouse have headaches?	Yes	No
3rd marriage age _____ to _______	Did spouse have headaches?	Yes	No

Age of current spouse:___________

List ages and sex of all children:

Age 13 Sex M	Headaches?	Yes	No
Age _____ Sex ______	Headaches?	Yes	No
Age _____ Sex ______	Headaches?	Yes	No
Age _____ Sex ______	Headaches?	Yes	No

STRESS FACTORS:

List any factors that may be affecting your headaches (money, loneliness, sexual problems, work, etc.)
This headache started directly after accident, with dizziness.

VEGETATIVE SIGNS:

1.	Do you have trouble falling asleep?	Yes	No
2.	Do you have trouble staying asleep?	Yes	No
3.	Has your appetite decreased?	Yes	No
4.	Have you gained or lost weight in the past year?	Yes	No
5.	Have you felt tearful or depressed lately?	Yes	No
6.	Have you had any thoughts of wanting to die?	Yes	No
7.	Have you been forgetful lately?	Yes	No
8.	Any other changes in your normal day-to-day living?__________		

Please list any medications you are allergic or sensitive to: Sulfa, Penicillin. Many medications and foods that are contraindicated by Nardil (Phenelzine) that I take.

Please list any medications you are currently taking (including dosages and frequency per day):
Nardil (Phenelzine), 30 mg t.i.d.; Klonopin 2 mg. a.m. and 2 mg p.m.

PREVIOUS CARE:

1. List doctors who have treated you for headaches: Dr. D.

2. List any tests you have had for your headache (e.g., EEG, CT scan, MRI, X-Ray, etc.):
CAT scan and x-rays, since 1993 accident.

3. List any other treatment you have had for your headache (e.g., biofeedback, acupuncture, chiropractic, or any other treatment you had):
Pain suppressor (electronic).

February 14, 1984

[Name and address of Attorney deleted]

RE: SUSAN

Dear Mr. [...]:

Susan [...] was seen in this office because of incapacitating headaches and interfering headaches. She is a 35-year-old female, born 00/00/48 in [...], and has been living in [...] for thirty years. She has had a year of college, and presently is an insurance agent.

The patient stated that prior to 1977, she had never suffered any headaches except an occasional mild one, which was so infrequent it was never a problem. She remembers the infrequent headaches sometimes being associated with her periods. In 1977 the patient was in an automobile accident, and for the first time she began to have the incapacitating and interfering headaches. This was in June of 1977, and the patient states that she suffered "a whiplash injury," and did not hit her head. She was hospitalized, and was diagnosed as having cervical strain because of neck pain and headaches. She was readmitted to County Memorial Hospital on 00/00/77 because of her headaches and muscular spasm in her neck, and was diagnosed at that time with torticollis. In the beginning the patient states that she was getting these incapacitating headaches almost every other day, and prior to her accident in 1982 she was getting them about once a month. They would come on at any time, and could last anywhere from 1 to 7 days. These headaches were bifrontal, and actually the patient drew a ring around her entire head covering her eyes, and the occipital portion including the nuchal ridge. The character of this headache was burning and sometimes throbbing. She was feeling "rushed" and her blood pressure would drop. She had nausea, vomiting, photophobia, acousticophobia, and sensitivity to odors. She would become white and have to go to bed. She noticed that alcohol made them worse. She also complained, in 1977, of spasms in the back and shoulders, which was diagnosed as torticollis.

There was also an accompanying, interfering headache, moderate to severe, which started also in 1977. She would have this headache once a week, coming at any time, lasting the same amount of time as the incapacitating headache, and covering the same area, including pain in her neck and back. The character was also burning and throbbing, and all the associated features were the same as the incapacitating headaches, except that it was with less intensity.

Then in 1982 the patient was involved in another accident. She was driving down the street when a police car came out from a side street and hit her on the passenger side. The patient was driving, on her way to a florist to get flowers, and was hit on the way back to the office. She states that her temple hit the mirror, and she blacked out. The patient states that since the 1982 accident, her headache became worse. Incidentally, the patient's litigation for the first accident was settled, and the patient is presently in litigation for the 1982 accident. She described the incapacitating headache from the 1982 accident as coming every other day, or once a week, comes on at any time, and lasts 1 to 7 days. The location of this headache is exactly the same as the other one, except that there are two areas, one on the right temple, and an area on the right side of the upper cervical area that goes into spasms and swells. She also gets muscle spasms all the way down her back. The character of the pain of this headache is also throbbing. There is also blurring of vision in both eyes, and tearing of the right eye during a headache. There is nausea, vomiting, photophobia, acousticophobia, sensitivity to odors, pallor, lacrimation, and the patient goes to bed. She states that she feels like she wants to bang her head against the wall. The patient does not describe any interfering or irritating headaches associated with this second accident.

The patient began menstruating at age 13, and had "painful periods." At age 27 she had a hysterectomy, still has her ovaries, and is not on any hormones. She was on the birth control pill in 1969 for one year, and they were discontinued. The patient did not get these headaches during her menstruation before her hysterectomy.

Past history: The patient's birth was normal, and there is no history of meningitis, encephalitis, or scarlet fever. There is no history of enuresis, motion illness, or abdominal cramps. She denies any head injury as a child.

Habits: Currently the patient drinks on rare occasions, but does not drink during a headache. She states that smoke-filled rooms make her headaches worse.

Medical history: Essentially negative, except five hospitalizations between the period of 1977 through 1979 for headaches, and four hospitalizations for her headaches since her 1982 accident. Her average length of stay was 7 to 9 days, and she was generally placed on narcotics and physical exercise.

Surgical history: The patient had a partial hysterectomy in 1975.

Psychiatric history: The patient saw a psychiatrist in 1968 when her mother and father were divorced, and that depression was resolved.

Family history: Her father is living, is 57 years old, with no headaches. Her mother is also living, is 56 years of age, with no headaches. There are two sisters, 36 and 28, with no headaches. She was married the first time at age 20 through 23, and there is a son age 13 with no headaches. She was married the second time at age 25, and her husband is 36. There is no history of other blood relatives suffering from headaches.

Vegetative signs: The patient states that she has not slept well since her 1977 accident. Her appetite is all right, there is no weight change, and she cries and gets depressed only when her headaches get out of control. There are some thoughts of dying when her headaches are so severe that she has no way of stopping the pain.

Previous care: She has been seen since 1977 by [Dr. ...], who has been treating her for chronic cervical strain. The patient also had a CAT scan and skull x-rays which were normal. Other than medications, the patient has been treated with hot packs, massage, acupuncture, which gave her relief while the needles were in her, and TENS which gave her relief at times. She has seen a chiropractor, which gave her some temporary relief. The patient has been on an assortment of medications such as Fiorinal #3, Demerol, Midrin, Soma, Robaxin, and Flexeril for her back pain. Some of these gave her temporary relief, and some not at all.

Physical examination: While in the office, the patient had a physical examination which revealed a 5'3", 137 pound, white female, with a pulse of 80, blood pressure of 128/84 in the left arm, and 132/86 in the right arm. There was no TMJ tenderness or carotid bruits, and her eyes reacted equally to light and accommodation. Her neck was supple, with no lymph nodes or enlarged thyroid that could be felt. The muscles in the cervical area and upper back felt very tight to palpation. The lungs were clear to auscultation and percussion, and her heart had a regular sinus rhythm with no murmurs. Rectal and vaginal examinations were not done.

Neurological examination: Cranial nerves II-XII were grossly normal. Cerebellar, motor, and sensory systems did not show any pathology. Her reflexes were 1+ and somewhat sluggish. Femoral, dorsalis pedis, posterior tibial, and popliteal pulses were normal and bounding.

The patient also had an MMPI (Minnesota Multiphasic Personality Inventory) showing a mild level of underlying depression secondary to her headaches. Other than that, the patient's profile was essentially normal. The patient also had a directional Doppler analysis which was grossly normal (see attached report), and cerebrovascular/migraine thermography and was having a headache that day; therefore, a vascular cold patch could not be demonstrated. There were also extreme areas of heat on her back and neck, which are typical of muscle contraction spasm (see attached report).

DIAGNOSES

1. Post traumatic headache — muscle contraction type.
2. Post traumatic headache — mixed type.
3. Post traumatic headache — migraine-like.
4. Atypical vascular headache.
5. Rule out cervicogenic headache.

Post traumatic type I headache is typical of a muscle contraction headache syndrome. Type II is the same as type I plus a vascular component distinguished by circumscribed tenderness as a major feature. Type III resembles migraine headache. The atypical vascular headache has features of migraine combined with cluster-like symptoms, such as teary eyes, running nose, pacing and wanting to bang her head against the wall, and the swelling that she complains of. The diagnoses just mentioned are supported through the objective findings of the cerebrovascular thermography.

Recommendations: It was suggested that the patient have biofeedback to reduce the pain that she is having. She was placed on amitriptyline 10 mg at bedtime for her muscle contraction pain. For migraine-type pain, she was placed on Inderal 40 mg twice a day, and was given a prescription for suppositories of Cafergot and Phenergan to abort the attack. For the atypical vascular headache, she was placed on Indocin 25 mg three times a day, and it was recommended for her to take oxygen treatment for 15 minutes four times a day to abort the headache if necessary. On 00/00/84, she had a biofeedback treatment, with minimal success using both temperature and EMG.

The patient will be seen in two weeks for another biofeedback treatment, plus evaluation of her headache log.

Summary: This 35-year-old white female, who had no headache history prior to 1977 when she had a "whiplash" type accident, started getting both severe and incapacitating headaches. The headaches seemed to reduce their frequency and their intensity until the second accident in 1982, in which the patient hit her right temple on the mirror and had a blackout.

Since that time she has been having incapacitating headaches at least once a week, lasting several days, and the intensity and frequency has increased. It would appear that the second accident exacerbated the patient's condition, and that this increase in intensity and frequency is related to this accident. An attempt is being made to reduce the patient's suffering, and to stabilize the patient into having an infrequent headache pattern. According to the patient, she is losing a great deal of time from work, and must reduce her activities to spend at least 25% of her waking time in bed because of these headaches.

If there are any questions, please do not hesitate to call or write.

Sincerely,

Bernard Swerdlow, M.D.

This case demonstrates some of the complexities in getting a history from a patient and deciding which accident may be responsible for her headaches.

MEDICAL HEADACHE HISTORY

Name: Susan **Age:** 35 **Sex** F **Date:** 1/24/84

Date of Birth: 00/00/48 **Birthplace:** MS **Race:** ____ **Education:** 1 Yr. College

Occupation: Insurance **Accident:** 1977/1982

Armed Services & Type of Discharge: N/A

PAST HISTORY:

1.	Did you have a normal birth?		Yes (underlined)	No
	a) forceps used?		Yes	No
	b) cesarean section?		Yes	No
2.	Did you have problems with bedwetting?		Yes	No (underlined)
	a) If yes, age bedwetting stopped		____	
3.	Were you car sick as a child (motion)?		Yes	No (underlined)
	a) If yes, how severe?	Slight	Moderate	Severe
4.	Did you have unexplained abdominal cramps as a child?		Yes	No (underlined)
5.	Did you have any of the following illnesses in childhood?			
	a) meningitis		Yes	No (underlined)
	b) encephalitis		Yes	No (underlined)
	c) scarlet fever		Yes	No (underlined)
	d) rheumatic fever		Yes	No (underlined)
6.	Did you have any head injuries as a child?		Yes	No (underlined)
	a) If yes, please explain: ____			
7.	Were you treated for emotional illness as a child?		Yes	No (underlined)

HABITS:

8.	Do you drink alcohol?	Yes (underlined)	No
	a) If yes, what kind and how much? On occasion		
	b) Does alcohol bring on or aggravate a headache?	Yes	No (underlined)
9.	Do you smoke?	Yes	No (underlined)
	a) If yes, how much? ____		
	b) Does smoking or smoke-filled rooms cause or aggravate headaches?	Yes (underlined)	No
10.	Do you drink caffeinated beverages?	Yes	No
	a) If yes, how much? ____		

MENSTRUAL HISTORY:

At what age did menses begin? 13 Were they regular or irregular? WNL, painful

How were they related to your headache? Increased #1 HAs

Are you or were you ever on Birth Control Pills? Yes Did they affect your headache? N/A

Have you had a hysterectomy, partial or total, and why? Yes, Partial at age 27.

Are you in menopause, and if yes, how long? No

Are you on hormones, and if yes, which ones? No

HEADACHE ASSESSMENT FORM

HA PROFILE	INCAPACITATING #3	INTERFERING #2	IRRITATING #1
ONSET (Years ago and frequency)	Accident in 1977 Constant at first	1977 A lot	N/A
CURRENT FREQUENCY	None for a month, then constantly for several days	1/wk	N/A
TIME OF ONSET	No set time, can wake her up	Anytime	N/A
DURATION	1 day to 7 days	1 day to 1 week	N/A
CHARACTER	Burning, throbbing, pressure, or band around head	Burning, throbbing, pressure, or band around head	N/A
PRODROME OR AURA	Have "rush", draining sensation; turn white; BP drops;	Back spasms	N/A
ASSOCIATING FEATURES	Nausea; Vomiting; Sensitivity to Light? Noise? Odors? Do you get pale or flush? Do your eyes or nose run? Does your nose get stuffy? Do the whites of your eyes get red? Does your eyelid droop? Do you pace, or go to bed? Heat to back	Nausea; Vomiting; Sensitivity to Light? Noise? Odors? Do you get pale or flush? Do your eyes or nose run? Does your nose get stuffy? Do the whites of your eyes get red? Does your eyelid droop? Do you pace, or go to bed?	Nausea; Vomiting; Sensitivity to Light? Noise? Odors? Do you get pale or flush? Do your eyes or nose run? Does your nose get stuffy? Do the whites of your eyes get red? Does your eyelid droop? Do you pace, or go to bed?
PRECIPITATING OR AGGRAVATING FEATURES	Back spasms (shoulder), spasms lower in back	Same as #3, only less severe	Used to get with periods

LOCATION: Mark the location for each type of headache with a different color pen.

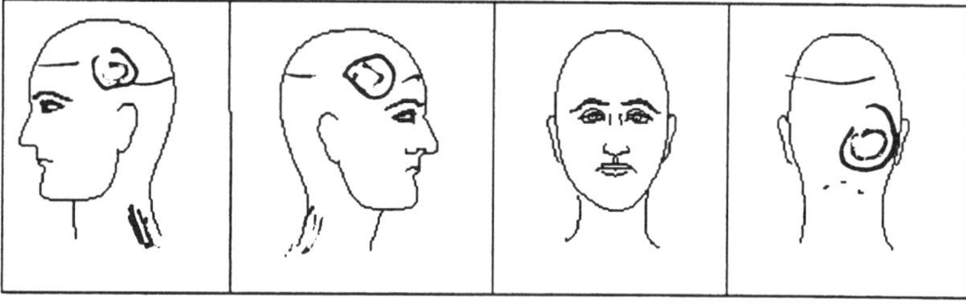

MEDICAL HISTORY:

Have you ever been or are you currently being treated for any of the following?

a) high blood pressure	Yes	No
b) stomach ulcers	Yes	No
c) asthma	Yes	No
d) allergies	Yes	No
e) pneumonia	Yes	No
f) kidney problems	Yes	No
g) low blood sugar	Yes	No
h) glaucoma	Yes	No
i) diabetes	Yes	No
j) heart problems	Yes	No

If you answered yes to any of the above, please describe:____________________________

List all other medical problems you have had in the past. Include date diagnosed and treatment.
DO NOT LIST OPERATIONS

Headaches, hospitalized 2 times in 1983, 2 times in 1982, 5 times from 1977-1979.

SURGICAL HISTORY (List operations and dates performed)

Partial hysterectomy, 1975.

PSYCHIATRIC HISTORY (List visits with counselors, psychologists, etc., and type of treatment)

When mother and father divorced.

ACCIDENTS IN ADULT LIFE (Briefly describe any accident that caused any blow to the head or that you feel is related to your headache)

Auto accident, 1977. Whiplash. Hospitalized. Auto accident, 1982. Hit by police car. Right temple hit mirror. Blacked out. Hit on passenger side.

FAMILY HISTORY:

1. Is your father living? Yes No
   Age 57
   Cause of death____________________
   Was there a headache history? Yes No
2. Is your mother living? Yes No
   Age 56
   Cause of death____________________
   Was there a headache history? Yes No
3. Ages of brothers---Circle the ones with headache

____

4. Ages of sisters---Circle the ones with headache
   28 36
5. List any other blood relatives with a history of severe headaches.
   None.

MARITAL HISTORY:
List marriages:

1st marriage age 20 to 23	Did spouse have headaches?	Yes	No
2nd marriage age 25 to Present	Did spouse have headaches?	Yes	No
3rd marriage age ____ to ____	Did spouse have headaches?	Yes	No

Age of current spouse: 36

List ages and sex of all children:

Age 13 Sex M	Headaches?	Yes	No
Age ____ Sex ____	Headaches?	Yes	No
Age ____ Sex ____	Headaches?	Yes	No

STRESS FACTORS:

List any factors that may be affecting your headaches (money, loneliness, sexual problems, work, etc.)
None.

VEGETATIVE SIGNS:

1.	Do you have trouble falling asleep?	Yes	No
2.	Do you have trouble staying asleep?	Yes	No
3.	Has your appetite decreased?	Yes	No
4.	Have you gained or lost weight in the past year?	Yes	No
5.	Have you felt tearful or depressed lately?	Yes	No
6.	Have you had any thoughts of wanting to die?	Yes	No
7.	Have you been forgetful lately?	Yes	No
8.	Any other changes in your normal day-to-day living? ____		

Please list any medications you are allergic or sensitive to: No known allergies

Please list any medications you are currently taking (including dosages and frequency per day):

PREVIOUS CARE:

1. List doctors who have treated you for headaches: Dr. O.

2. List any tests you have had for your headache (e.g., EEG, CT scan, MRI, X-Ray, etc.):
CT scan
Skull x-rays

3. List any other treatment you have had for your headache (e.g., biofeedback, acupuncture, chiropractic, or any other treatment you had):
Hot packs, massage, chiropractor, acupuncture, TENS

December 24, 1992

[Doctor's name and address omitted)

Dear Dr. [...]:

I saw Keith [...] at [...] on December 24, 1992.

Identifying data: This is a 36-year-old power plant operator.

Chief complaint: Headache.

The patient was in his usual state of health until the first week of [...], 1992, when he was involved in an automobile accident. The patient relates he was the driver of an El Camino that was struck in the rear end by a car going at an unknown speed. He was wearing a seat belt. His body went backwards and his head shattered the back window. He then lost consciousness for seconds to minutes. He was taken to the emergency room where cervical spine x-rays and a CAT scan of the head were performed. He was then treated and released. He had the onset of a dazed feeling, nonspecific confusion, neck pain, entire back pain, and left hand pain.

HEADACHE PROFILE

Incapacitating headaches: He did not have these prior to the accident. He is currently having one per week without any special timing. Once present, it lasts from one to three days. It is a diffuse pain that begins posteriorly and then radiates up into the head symmetrically and bilaterally. There is nausea, light sensitivity, facial flushing, watering of the eyes, and the need to go to bed.

Interfering headaches: These began the day of the accident and have been constant and unrelenting since the accident. It is the same as the #3 headache, but does not incapacitate him.

Irritating headache: These occurred in high school. He has not had these for years. It was a nonspecific pain in the temple that is totally different from the current pain.

There has not been any loss of vision, further loss of consciousness, or other new features associated with the headache.

Childhood history: The patient was most probably a normal delivery. There is no history of enuresis or unexplained abdominal cramps pre-puberty. There is no history of meningitis, encephalitis, scarlet fever, or rheumatic fever. There were no head injuries as a child.

Habits: He drinks socially, but does not smoke or use illicit drugs.

Review of Systems: Positive since the accident for nausea, weight loss, nonspecific dizziness, nonspecific memory problem, blurred vision, ringing in the ears, a subjective sense of weakness, and decreased sensation involving the entire left hand, and a sense of depression. In addition, he has noted some difficulty walking at times.

He denies fever, rash, cough, chest pain, palpitations, vomiting, change in bowel habits, blood in stool, indigestion, urination difficulty, pain on chewing, arthritis, muscle aches, seizures, visual loss, double vision, persistent paralysis, loss of bowel or bladder control. There has been questionably some suicidal thoughts, but we have discussed this and he agrees not to act on any of these thoughts.

Medical history: The patient has no history of high blood pressure, stomach ulcers, asthma, allergies, pneumonia, kidney problems, low blood sugar, glaucoma, diabetes, or heart problems.

Surgical history: Bilateral hernia repair, 1992.

Psychiatric history: Negative.

Family history: Positive for headaches in his mother.

Vegetative signs: There has been sleep difficulty, and the above-mentioned weight loss.

Medical allergies: None.

Current medications: Consist of over-the-counter drugs such as Advil, Motrin, aspirin, and Tylenol without relief.

Doctors seen in the past: Include Dr. [...], a physician who he has seen three times per week for help with his neck and back. He has also seen Dr. [...], a neurologist who did not provide him with relief.

Tests done in the past: Include plain spine films, CT of brain, MRI of the brain, and brain mapping. We do not have the results of any of these.

Other treatments tried: Chiropractic.

Physical examination: Height 5'9", weight 181 pounds, BP left 136/92, BP right 132/92, pulse 76.

Mental status: Patient is alert and oriented with no apparent speech or cognitive dysfunction. There is a slightly depressed affect.

Cranial nerve exam: The optic discs are flat with good venous pulsations. Visual fields are full to confrontation. The pupils are round, regular, and equal, and respond to light and accommodation both directly and consensually. Extraocular muscle movement is intact. There is no nystagmus in any direction. Facial sensation is intact to temperature. Corneal reflexes are intact and equal. There is no facial asymmetry, wrinkling of the forehead, or burying of the eyelashes. Retraction of the corner of the mouth on smiling and showing the teeth are equal. Hearing is intact to whisper. The Weber and Rinne tests are normal. Gag reflex is present. The palate elevates in the midline. Strength of the sternocleidomastoid and trapezius muscles are normal. The tongue protrudes in the midline. There is no tremor or atrophy of the tongue. No dysarthria is noted.

Motor and coordination examination: Normal heel, toe and tandem gait. Negative Rhomberg's. No drift. Finger-nose-finger, rapid alternating movements and heel-knee-shin are intact. Strength on direct testing is normal. Tone is normal. Bulk is normal. There is no tremor, involuntary movements, atrophy or fasciculations. Subjectively, he feels weak in the left forearm and arm "like he had just finished working out."

Reflexes: 2+ and symmetric with clear bilateral plantar flexor response. No pathologic reflexes.

Sensation: Position, vibration and temperature are intact throughout. Stereognosis and graphesthesia are intact.

Vascular: Carotid and temporal artery pulses are present and equal. No bruits are heard over the head or carotids. No tenderness of the carotid or temporal arteries.

Head: Atraumatic, normocephalic. No areas of tenderness on palpation.

TMJ: No pain is elicited on palpation of the temporomandibular joints. No crepitation is heard.

Neck: Supple. Full range of motion. 4+ muscle spasm with decreased range of motion in all planes. Negative Kernig's and Brudzinski's.

IMPRESSION

1. Post traumatic/concussion headache syndrome.
2. Post concussion syndrome (dizziness, memory difficulty, blurred vision, ringing in the ears, depression).
3. Subjective left hand/arm symptoms.
4. Subjective gait difficulty.

DIFFERENTIAL DIAGNOSIS: Headache.

1. Post traumatic migraine.
2. Post traumatic muscle tension type headache.

PLAN

1. I need to obtain the results of all the prior testing, including MRI and CT of brain, spine films, brain mapping, lab work, neurologic and chiropractic exam.
2. If these are unremarkable and if symptoms persist, I would recommend an MRI of the neck, EMG/NCV of the left upper extremity to look for correctable causes of his gait difficulty and left upper extremity difficulty.
3. MMPI to evaluate the depression, as well as other symptoms that might have resulted from the accident.
4. Continuation of chiropractic and massage therapy.
5. Biofeedback.
6. For symptoms, Midrin, Norgesic and Orudis.
7. For prevention and to try to decrease these symptoms, Doxepin and Bellergal.
8. We will follow him up in one month's time. In the meantime, we will obtain the results as above. If there are any side effects or problems or his symptoms change, he will call.
9. Due to the severity of his symptoms, we will give him a four-day pulse of Prednisone to try to stop these symptoms.

Thank you for the referral of this patient. If there are any questions, please do not hesitate to call or write.

Sincerely,

BERNARD SWERDLOW, M.D.

MEDICAL HEADACHE HISTORY

Name: Keith **Age:** 36 **Sex** M **Date:** 12/24/92

Date of Birth: 00/00/56 **Birthplace:** MI **Race:** W **Education:** High school

Occupation: Power Plant Operator **Accident:** 00/92

Armed Services & Type of Discharge: Reserves

PAST HISTORY:

1.	Did you have a normal birth?		Yes	No
	a) forceps used?		Yes	No
	b) cesarean section?		Yes	No
2.	Did you have problems with bedwetting?		Yes	No
	a) If yes, age bedwetting stopped			
3.	Were you car sick as a child (motion)?		Yes	No
	a) If yes, how severe?	Slight	Moderate	Severe
4.	Did you have unexplained abdominal cramps as a child?		Yes	No
5.	Did you have any of the following illnesses in childhood?			
	a) meningitis		Yes	No
	b) encephalitis		Yes	No
	c) scarlet fever		Yes	No
	d) rheumatic fever		Yes	No
6.	Did you have any head injuries as a child?		Yes	No
	a) If yes, please explain:			
7.	Were you treated for emotional illness as a child?		Yes	No

HABITS:

8.	Do you drink alcohol?	Yes	No
	a) If yes, what kind and how much? Little to none at all		
	b) Does alcohol bring on or aggravate a headache?	Yes	No
9.	Do you smoke?	Yes	No
	a) If yes, how much?		
	b) Does smoking or smoke-filled rooms cause or aggravate headaches?	Yes	No
10.	Do you drink caffeinated beverages?	Yes	No
	a) If yes, how much? 2 to 3 cups of coffee		

MENSTRUAL HISTORY:

At what age did menses begin?_______ Were they regular or irregular?____________________
How were they related to your headache?____________________
Are you or were you ever on Birth Control Pills?______ Did they affect your headache? _______
Have you had a hysterectomy, partial or total, and why?____________________
Are you in menopause, and if yes, how long?____________________
Are you on hormones, and if yes, which ones?____________________

HEADACHE ASSESSMENT FORM

HA PROFILE	INCAPACITATING #3	INTERFERING #2	IRRITATING #1
ONSET (Years ago and frequency)	Since accident 00/92, 1 per week	Since accident, Constant	After high school, 1 per month
CURRENT FREQUENCY	1 per week	Unless it increases to #3, Constant	None
TIME OF ONSET	Anytime	Constant	N/A
DURATION	½ to 3 or 4 hours	Constant	N/A
CHARACTER	Pressure	Pressure, but less severe than #3	N/A
PRODROME OR AURA	N/A	N/A	N/A
ASSOCIATING FEATURES	Nausea: Vomiting: Sensitivity to Light? Noise? Odors? Do you get pale or flush? Do your eyes or nose run? Does your nose get stuffy? Does the white of your eyes get red? Does your eyelid droop? Do you pace, or go to bed?	Nausea: Vomiting: Sensitivity to Light? Noise? Odors? Do you get pale or flush? Do your eyes or nose run? Does your nose get stuffy? Does the white of your eyes get red? Does your eyelid droop? Do you pace, or go to bed?	Nausea: Vomiting: Sensitivity to Light? Noise? Odors? Do you get pale or flush? Do your eyes or nose run? Does your nose get stuffy? Does the white of your eyes get red? Does your eyelid droop? Do you pace, or go to bed?
PRECIPITATING OR AGGRAVATING FEATURES	N/A	N/A	N/A

LOCATION: Mark the location for each type of headache with a different color pen.

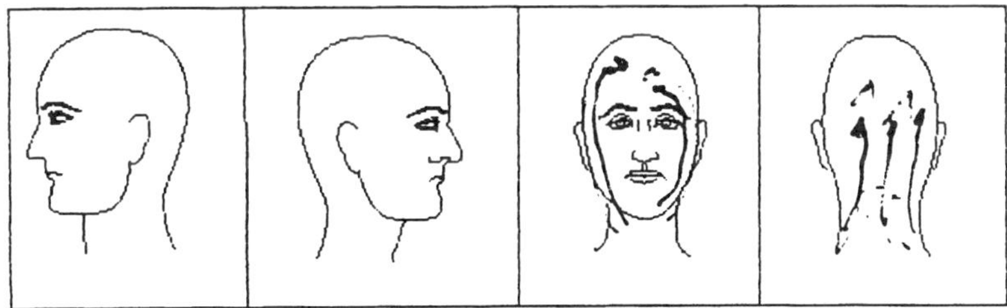

MEDICAL HISTORY:

Have you ever been or are you currently being treated for any of the following?

a) high blood pressure	Yes	No
b) stomach ulcers	Yes	No
c) asthma	Yes	No
d) allergies	Yes	No
e) pneumonia	Yes	No
f) kidney problems	Yes	No
g) low blood sugar	Yes	No
h) glaucoma	Yes	No
i) diabetes	Yes	No
j) heart problems	Yes	No

If you answered yes to any of the above, please describe:____________________

List all other medical problems you have had in the past. Include date diagnosed and treatment.
DO NOT LIST OPERATIONS

None.

SURGICAL HISTORY (List operations and dates performed)

1992, Bilateral hernia

PSYCHIATRIC HISTORY (List visits with counselors, psychologists, etc., and type of treatment)

None.

ACCIDENTS IN ADULT LIFE (Briefly describe any accident that caused any blow to the head or that you feel is related to your headache)

Car accident, 1992. Driving, wearing seatbelt. Stopped at light. Hit in rearend by car going at unknown speed. Body went backwards and head shattered the back window. Lost consciousness. Taken to emergency room, x-rays, CAT scan, treated and released.

FAMILY HISTORY:

1.	Is your father living?	Yes	No
	Age________		
	Cause of death __Stomach cancer__		
	Was there a headache history?	Yes	No
2.	Is your mother living?	Yes	No
	Age __70__		
	Cause of death________		
	Was there a headache history?	Yes	No

3. Ages of brothers---Circle the ones with headache

____

4. Ages of sisters---Circle the ones with headache

____

5. List any other blood relatives with a history of severe headaches.

____

MARITAL HISTORY:

List marriages:

1st marriage age 21 to 23	Did spouse have headaches?	Yes	No
2nd marriage age 26 to 36	Did spouse have headaches?	Yes	No
3rd marriage age ____ to ____	Did spouse have headaches?	Yes	No

Age of current spouse:__________

List ages and sex of all children:

Age 6 Sex M	Headaches?	Yes	No
Age ____ Sex ____	Headaches?	Yes	No
Age ____ Sex ____	Headaches?	Yes	No
Age ____ Sex ____	Headaches?	Yes	No

STRESS FACTORS:

List any factors that may be affecting your headaches (money, loneliness, sexual problems, work, etc.)

____

____

VEGETATIVE SIGNS:

1.	Do you have trouble falling asleep?	Yes	No
2.	Do you have trouble staying asleep?	Yes	No
3.	Has your appetite decreased?	Yes	No
4.	Have you gained or lost weight in the past year?	Yes	No
5.	Have you felt tearful or depressed lately?	Yes	No
6.	Have you had any thoughts of wanting to die?	Yes	No
7.	Have you been forgetful lately?	Yes	No
8.	Any other changes in your normal day-to-day living?__________		

Please list any medications you are allergic or sensitive to: None.

____

Please list any medications you are currently taking (including dosages and frequency per day):

Advil, 3 most days. Tylenol. Motrin. Aspirin.

____

____

PREVIOUS CARE:

1. List doctors who have treated you for headaches: Dr. D.

2. List any tests you have had for your headache (e.g., EEG, CT scan, MRI, X-Ray, etc.):
Spine films, CT of brain, MRI of brain, brain mapping.

3. List any other treatment you have had for your headache (e.g., biofeedback, acupuncture, chiropractic, or any other treatment you had):
None.

KATRINA
Category: Post traumatic headache

This is an example of a post traumatic headache where the patient was not unconscious and was not hospitalized after the accident. Seven months before I had seen her, she was in an auto accident where a car turned in front of the car in which she was a passenger, and the cars hit head-on. She hit her head on the windshield, but she was not unconscious. She was not hospitalized, but was taken to the emergency room, x-rayed, had a CT scan, which was normal, and she was given some pain medication.

Incapacitating headaches: These started four and a half months after the accident and she was getting two or three a month before she saw me, and when she saw me she was getting one a month and it would last two or three days. The pain was both pressure and throbbing, and at times vice-like. The associated features are typical of vascular or migraine-like headaches, with nausea, photophobia (light sensitivity), sonophobia (sound sensitivity), and she would have to go to bed.

Interfering headaches (moderate to severe): These started on the same day of the accident, and she was getting them anywhere from two to four times a week. They would last about three hours, and she would take medication to end the pain. The pain in both the headaches was in the regions around the eyes and the temporal regions of the head, the parietal and the occipital-cervical regions, or the back of the head, and both had similar symptoms.

Irritating headaches: Interestingly enough, five months before the accident she had gotten some irritating headaches in the frontal part of her head and was given some Midrin, which she said she took to abort her headaches. But, after that she did not have a headache like this again until the accident. She also gave a history of having some sinus headaches several times a year while she was in college.

A diagnosis here would have been a post-traumatic headache, and even though she was not unconscious, having hit her head against the windshield, I would consider this also to be a concussion-type headache and these headaches would be a post-trauma/concussion with migraine symptoms.

MEDICAL HEADACHE HISTORY

Name: Katrina **Age:** 33 **Sex** F **Date:** 6/27/91

Date of Birth: 00/00/57 **Birthplace:** IL **Race:** C **Education:** B.A.

Occupation: Contract Specialist **Accident:** September 1990

Armed Services & Type of Discharge: N/A

PAST HISTORY:

1.	Did you have a normal birth?		Yes	No
	a) forceps used?		Yes	No
	b) cesarean section?		Yes	No
2.	Did you have problems with bedwetting?		Yes	No
	a) If yes, age bedwetting stopped			
3.	Were you car sick as a child (motion)?		Yes	No
	a) If yes, how severe?	Slight	Moderate	Severe
4.	Did you have unexplained abdominal cramps as a child?		Yes	No
5.	Did you have any of the following illnesses in childhood?			
	a) meningitis		Yes	No
	b) encephalitis		Yes	No
	c) scarlet fever		Yes	No
	d) rheumatic fever		Yes	No
6.	Did you have any head injuries as a child?		Yes	No
	a) If yes, please explain:			
7.	Were you treated for emotional illness as a child?		Yes	No

HABITS:

8.	Do you drink alcohol?	Yes	No
	a) If yes, what kind and how much?		
	b) Does alcohol bring on or aggravate a headache?	Yes	No
9.	Do you smoke?	Yes	No
	a) If yes, how much?		
	b) Does smoking or smoke-filled rooms cause or aggravate headaches?	Yes	No
10.	Do you drink caffeinated beverages?	Yes	No
	a) If yes, how much?		

MENSTRUAL HISTORY:

At what age did menses begin? 13 Were they regular or irregular? WNL

How were they related to your headache? Increased severity

Are you or were you ever on Birth Control Pills? No Did they affect your headache?

Have you had a hysterectomy, partial or total, and why? No

Are you in menopause, and if yes, how long? No

Are you on hormones, and if yes, which ones? Prior Progesterone prn for PMS (none in 6 months)

HEADACHE ASSESSMENT FORM

HA PROFILE	INCAPACITATING #3	INTERFERING #2	IRRITATING #1
ONSET (Years ago and frequency)	Feb. 1991 – 2 to 3 times a month	Sept. 30 – 3 to 4 times a week	Sept. 30 – always there
CURRENT FREQUENCY	1 time a month	2 to 3 a week	Always there
TIME OF ONSET	Late P.M. Awaken with - rare	P.M. – late evening Awaken with – rare	Always there
DURATION	3 days	2 to 3 hours	Always there
CHARACTER	Throbbing, Pressure	Throbbing	Dull ache
PRODROME OR AURA	Pressure behind eye, right side of neck starts hurting	Pressure behind eyes	N/A
ASSOCIATING FEATURES	Nausea; Vomiting; Sensitivity to Light? Noise? Odors? Do you get pale or flush? Do your eyes or nose run? Does your nose get stuffy? Do the whites of your eyes get red? Does your eyelid droop? Do you pace, or go to bed?	Nausea; Vomiting; Sensitivity to Light? Noise? Odors? Do you get pale or flush? Do your eyes or nose run? Does your nose get stuffy? Do the whites of your eyes get red? Does your eyelid droop? Do you pace, or go to bed?	Nausea; Vomiting; Sensitivity to Light? Noise? Odors? Do you get pale or flush? Do your eyes or nose run? Does your nose get stuffy? Do the whites of your eyes get red? Does your eyelid droop? Do you pace, or go to bed?
PRECIPITATING OR AGGRAVATING FEATURES	N/A	N/A	N/A

LOCATION: Mark the location for each type of headache with a different color pen.

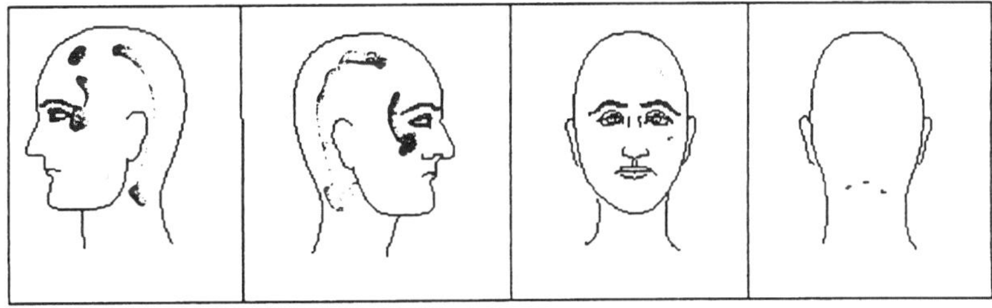

MEDICAL HISTORY:

Have you ever been or are you currently being treated for any of the following?

a) high blood pressure	Yes	No
b) stomach ulcers	Yes	No
c) asthma	Yes	No
d) allergies	Yes	No
e) pneumonia	Yes	No
f) kidney problems	Yes	No
g) low blood sugar	Yes	No
h) glaucoma	Yes	No
i) diabetes	Yes	No
j) heart problems	Yes	No

If you answered yes to any of the above, please describe: Ulcers diagnosed 8/90.

List all other medical problems you have had in the past. Include date diagnosed and treatment.
DO NOT LIST OPERATIONS

Peptic ulcer disease, 8/90. Spastic colon, March 1990.

SURGICAL HISTORY (List operations and dates performed)

Tonsillectomy, 1961.
Hysterectomy 1965. Tonsillectomy & Adenoidectomy age 4.

PSYCHIATRIC HISTORY (List visits with counselors, psychologists, etc., and type of treatment)

N/A

ACCIDENTS IN ADULT LIFE (Briefly describe any accident that caused any blow to the head or that you feel is related to your headache)

Car turned in front of the car in which I was a passenger. Front of our car hit the side of the other car. My head hit the windshield and cracked it. Car was traveling at about 30 mph. Taken to hospital emergency room, x-rayed, had CT scan, given pain pills.

FAMILY HISTORY:

1. Is your father living? Yes No
   Age 53
   Cause of death
   Was there a headache history? Yes No
2. Is your mother living? Yes No
   Age 53
   Cause of death
   Was there a headache history? Yes No

3. Ages of brothers---Circle the ones with headache
   ____None____________________________
4. Ages of sisters---Circle the ones with headache
   ____32 30____________________________
5. List any other blood relatives with a history of severe headaches.
   ____

MARITAL HISTORY:

List marriages:

1st marriage age __25__ to Present	Did spouse have headaches?	Yes	No
2nd marriage age _____ to _______	Did spouse have headaches?	Yes	No
3rd marriage age ______to _______	Did spouse have headaches?	Yes	No

Age of current spouse:___38_____

List ages and sex of all children:

Age __3___	Sex __M__	Headaches?	Yes	No
Age __8___	Sex __M__	Headaches?	Yes	No
Age _____	Sex ______	Headaches?	Yes	No
Age _____	Sex ______	Headaches?	Yes	No

STRESS FACTORS:

List any factors that may be affecting your headaches (money, loneliness, sexual problems, work, etc.)
____Possible work problems.______________________________
____

VEGETATIVE SIGNS:

1.	Do you have trouble falling asleep?	Yes	No
2.	Do you have trouble staying asleep?	Yes	No
3.	Has your appetite decreased?	Yes	No
4.	Have you gained or lost weight in the past year?	Yes	No
5.	Have you felt tearful or depressed lately?	Yes	No
6.	Have you had any thoughts of wanting to die?	Yes	No
7.	Have you been forgetful lately?	Yes	No
8.	Any other changes in your normal day-to-day living?______________		

Please list any medications you are allergic or sensitive to:___Penicillin____________________

Please list any medications you are currently taking (including dosages and frequency per day):
___Tagamet 400 mg 2 times a day.________________________
____
____

PREVIOUS CARE:

1. List doctors who have treated you for headaches: Dr. S. Dr. C.

2. List any tests you have had for your headache (e.g., EEG, CT scan, MRI, X-Ray, etc.):
MRI – Neck.
CAT scan – head and neck.
X-rays – neck.

3. List any other treatment you have had for your headache (e.g., biofeedback, acupuncture, chiropractic, or any other treatment you had):
Physical therapy for 4 months. Trigger points x 3.

Chapter 14

Cervical Acceleration/Deceleration Syndrome (Whiplash)

I remember some time ago testifying in court on a post concussion head injury and an acceleration/deceleration injury. After I explained to the jury the nature of the accident and why this 35-year-old man was suffering, the defense attorney stood between me and the jury while staring at them and said, "You mean, doctor, this is really only a whiplash." In one fell swoop, after a careful scientific presentation of a post head trauma syndrome, all of the credibility of this explanation was to be washed away with the word *whiplash*.

In 1928 H.E. Crowe presented a paper at the meeting of the Western Orthopedic Association in San Francisco and used the word whiplash to explain the biomechanics of a rear ended accident. Unfortunately, the term became synonymous with litigation and the term has lost its meaning and credibility. The term whiplash has been described as "the manna for the plaintiff's attorney, pestilence for the defense attorney, and a paid vacation for the unscrupulous patient."

What then would be a better term to use to describe this condition? Terms often used are flexion/extension or hyperflexion/hyperextension injury. These terms attempt to explain a rear ended injury but would be opposite if it were a front ended accident. These words do not take into account the fact that there is a rotational component to this injury. Therefore, in order to account for all the biomechanics of this injury the term cervical acceleration/deceleration (CAD) will be used[1] Figure 14.1.

Cervical acceleration/deceleration (CAD) or whiplash will be defined as an injury to the neck without a direct strike to the head. Interestingly, many of the symptoms that present themselves in post head trauma syndrome are also seen in CAD syndrome — that is, neck pains, headaches, visual disturbances, dizziness, weakness, parathesias, concentration and memory disturbances, and psychological symptoms. Although most people who are involved in motor vehicle accidents improve to be symptom-free within a few months, there is a small percentage of patients who will continue to have symptoms for years and this small number of injured persons represents an enormous cost to our society. The question of whether litigation promotes ongoing symptoms or how litigation is handled that adds to this problem has to be examined.

Although there are many conditions that are responsible for hyperflexion and hyperextension of the neck (falls from a height, diving accidents, sport injuries, etc.), the greatest percentage of this trauma is caused by motor vehicle accidents (MVA). Most of these accidents follow a rear end impact but may also follow lateral or frontal collisions. The term "whiplash" was actually used to

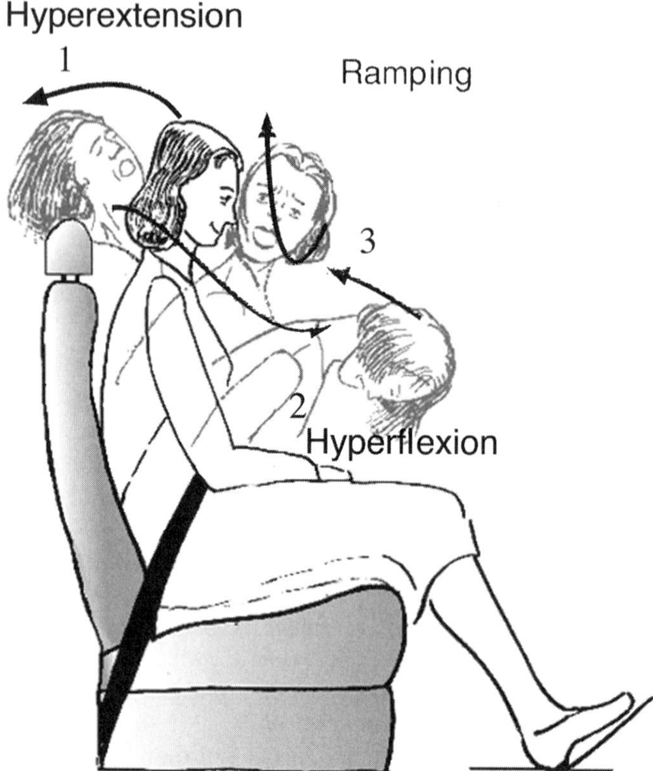

Figure 14.1 Acceleration/deceleration (or whiplash). After a rear-end collision, the occupant is forced backward into the seat back (hyperextension). There may be a vertical motion (called ramping). Following this, the occupant is forced forward or in hyperflexion (see Chapter 15).

describe the mechanism of the accident but since its inception it has also taken on the definition of a syndrome or the disease that follows this mechanism.

Following World War I the Navy instituted the launching of planes from the decks of battleships and cruisers using catapults. Because the pilot was not protected, there was violence to the cervical spine. The force was so great that the pilot blacked out for a few seconds and accidents occurred. This was certainly due to the whiplash effect. The Navy quickly recognized this and provided head rests and shoulder harnesses and corrected the problem. It took another 50 years before it became mandatory for auto makers to use headrests and shoulder harnesses in the production of cars.

Evans[2] reports, "In 1928, in presenting a report (never published) on eight cases of neck injuries resulting from traffic accidents before the Western Orthopedic Association in San Francisco, Crowe used the term 'whiplash'. Later on in 1963, Crowe in a symposium stated, 'I used the unfortunate term whiplash. This expression was intended to be a description of motion, but it has been accepted by physicians, patients, and attorneys as the name of a disease; and the misunderstanding has led to its misapplication by many physicians and others over the years'."

The actual term whiplash was not used in the medical literature until 1945 and became popular in the 1950s. In 1953, Gay and Abbott reported in an article on whiplash that, "Characteristically, these patients were more disabled and remained handicapped for longer periods than was anticipated, considering the mild character of the accident."

In 1955 Severy et al.[3] accomplished a major breakthrough by doing controlled studies using humans and dummies, photographing the sequences of hyperextension followed by flexion, and reversed the incorrect assumptions that were previously reported that flexion was followed by extension. They reported, "The low-speed rear-end collision is one of the more common types of urban automobile accidents and it is probably the most misleading. Unlike most types of collisions, the rear-end collision frequently results in minor car damage with major bodily injury. Also, unlike most injury producing accidents, there is generally no visible sign of injury for the rear-end collision victim."

In article after article that I researched the conclusion of all authors is that the amount of damage to the automobile and the speed of the cars involved in the collision bear little relationship to the injury sustained by the cervical spine. All attempts to correlate clinical outcome with the extent of damage to the involved cars and their speed have been shown to have little or no prognostic value. Even the passenger position in the car, use of seat belts, and the presence of a head restraint showed no significant relationship with the symptoms (Figure 14.2). However, rotated or inclined head

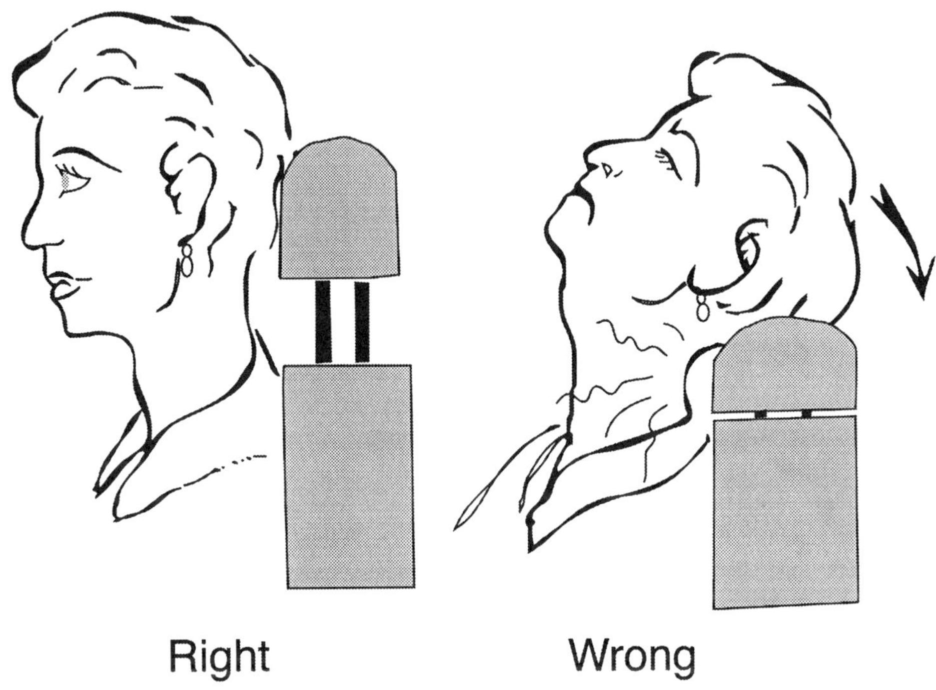

Figure 14.2 Improper use of a cervical restraint that is too low may aggravate the hyperextension phase. The proper height of the restraint should support the occipital region.

position at the moment of impact was associated with a higher frequency of multiple symptoms and with more severe symptoms and signs of musculoligamental cervical strain and of neural, particularly radicular, damage. Unprepared occupants had a higher frequency of multiple symptoms and more severe headaches. Rear-end collision was associated with a higher frequency of multiple, especially of cranial and brainstem dysfunction. Sturzenegger et al.[4] concluded that three features of the accident mechanism were associated with more severe symptoms: (1) an unprepared occupant; (2) rear-end collision, with or without subsequent frontal impact, and (3) rotated or inclined head position at the moment of impact. Another interesting finding of MacNab[5] is that seat belts have significantly reduced injuries in automobile accidents in general, but a belted passenger will suffer more neck pain than an unbelted passenger.

Evans reported that in 1989 the National Safety Council estimated 12,800,000 motor vehicle accidents in the U.S., and of these 3,280,000 were rear-end collisions with an estimated 1,000,000 whiplash injuries. More recent data suggest that there may be as many as 3,000,000 whiplash injuries. Pearce[6] reports that the Motor Accidents Board in Victoria reviewed 2352 cases of whiplash and found 43% rear-end collision, 32% head-on collision, and 35% side impact. Barnsley, Lord, and Bogduk[7] report that in the early 1970s there were 3.8 million rear-end impact MVAs when the population was 200 million. Today we exceed 250 million. They estimate from the 3.8 million approximately 20% will develop symptoms from the neck; therefore the annual incidence of symptoms from whiplash is 3.8 per 1000 population. They point out the results of another study during that time frame which showed that of disabling neck injury of women workers was 14.5 per 1000 defined by medical assessment rather than by insurance claim.

Barnsley et al. point out that in countries where there is only one insurer the incidence is lower:[7] Switzerland, 0.44 per 1000; Norway, 2 per 1000; Australia, 1 per 1000; New Zealand, 0.1 per 1000; all in the period of 1978 to 1981. Unpublished figures in 1992 from New South Wales Motor Accident Authority indicate an annual incidence of 0.8 per 1000. They continue to report that these numbers are derived from insurance and compensation claims and the many variables and barriers to make a claim may skew the data; therefore, it does not give an accurate estimate of the number of whiplash or acceleration/deceleration disabling neck injuries. Their report includes information on the Motor Accident Board in Australia where legislation has created bureaucratic barriers, disincentives, and up-front costs for people intending to file claims. Because there was a fall in insurance claims, statements have been made that legislation will reduce the number of whiplash accidents and whiplash is a behavioral problem and not an injury. Barnsley et al.[7] counter this by saying that if you set up the same barriers in reporting sexually transmitted diseases and less people report, does that mean that the incidence of these diseases are falling? In epidemiological terms, extrapolating these numbers is potentially dangerous.

PERSISTENCE OF SYMPTOMS

It appears that most patients will recover in two to three months and after that recovery slows dramatically. If the symptoms do not remiss in the first several months then they do not seem to change after two years. There have been many studies and the results of chronic neck pain vary.

Taking percentages of most of these studies reported, it appears that anywhere between 14% and 42% of these patients will develop chronic neck pain, and of these about 10% will have constant severe pain indefinitely.

PREVALENCE

Barnsley et al.[7] calculated, allowing for the crudeness of this estimate, that given an incidence of 1 per 1000, and that approximately 25% of patients with whiplash injury progress to chronic symptoms with 10% suffering severe pain, one could expect 0.25% new cases per 1000 population per annum developing chronic pain, and 0.1 cases with severe pain. They go on to say if the average age of the person sustaining a whiplash injury is 30 and the average life span is 70 years, the cumulative effect over 40 years yields a prevalence in the entire population of about 1% with chronic pain and 0.4% with severe pain. Even if this figure is discounted by two, there is still a significant number of 0.5% of chronic pain and 0.4% with severe pain. Interestingly, they compare this figure as being the same as the prevalence of epilepsy.

SYMPTOMS AND SIGNS

Evans lists the sequelae (conditions following and resulting from disease) of whiplash injuries.[2]

Neck and back injuries
  Myofascial (muscles and ligaments)

- Fractures and dislocations
- Disk herniation

Cord compression
- Spondylosis
- Radiculopathy
- Facet joint
- Increased development of spondylosis

Headaches
- Muscle contraction type
- Greater occipital neuralgia
- Temporomandibular joint injury
- Migraine

Dizziness
- Vestibular dysfunction
- Brainstem dysfunction
- Cervical origin
- Barre syndrome
- Hyperventilation syndrome

Paresthesias
- Trigger points
- Thoracic outlet syndrome
- Cervical radiculopathy
- Carpal tunnel syndrome
- Ulnar neuropathy at the elbow

Cognitive, somatic, and psychologic sequelae
- Memory, attention, and concentration impairment
- Nervousness and irritability
- Sleep disturbances
- Fatigability
- Depression
- Personality change
- Compensation neurosis

Rare sequelae
- Torticollis
- Transient global amnesia
- Esophageal perforation and descending mediastinitis

Barnsley et al.[7] include visual disturbances in their list of symptoms and that will be discussed below.

Neck Pain

Evans[2] found that following a motor vehicle accident (MVA) 62% of patients presenting to the emergency room complained of neck pain. Within 6 hours, 65% complain of neck pain; within 24 hours an additional 28%, and within 72 hours the remaining 7%.

The majority of neck pain is associated with cervical sprains, that is injury to the joint, muscles or ligaments. Rarely are there rupture to the muscles, cervical disk herniations, cervical spine fractures or dislocations. The lower cervical area is more at risk than the upper first two cervical vertebrae (atlas and axis) and their associated ligaments.

Between the vertebrae there is a structure called the zygapophyseal joint that may have some significance in the pain in the neck and injections to produce therapeutic blocks may determine if these patients have zygapophyseal disease. Barnsley et al.,[7] in their studies, describe the neck pain as dull and aching and it gets worse with movement and then is sometimes sharp. There is neck stiffness and pain may radiate to the head, shoulder, arm, or inner scapular area. Attempts to localize the source of the pain by using x-rays, CT scans, and MRI are unsuccessful because we do not have a standard for "pain pathology."

In 1988 Bogduk and Marsland developed a technique to anesthetize the cervical zygapophyseal joints. This technique was studied and refined and further information[8] revealed that between 25% and 62% of whiplash patients were suffering from cervical zygapophyseal pain. Barnsley and Bogduk,[9] Barnsley, Lord and Bogduk,[10] and Barnsley, Lord, Wallis and Bogduk[11] have demonstrated that by following this stringent protocol under double-blind, controlled conditions, 54% of the pain in the neck that these patients complained of came from at least one of these zygapophyseal joints. They claim that no other source of pain in the neck has been so clearly defined or found to be so common. This work represents a most meaningful advance in objectifying that the neck pain in whiplash can be identified. Perhaps then what has been classified so frequently in the past as a psychological disorder will now be considered as a chronic physical disease.

Headache

After neck pain, headache is the most frequent complaint after whiplash injury. In a prospective study by Balla and Karnaghan[12] of 180 patients seen within four weeks of the whiplash injury, 82% complained of headaches, which were occipitally located in 46%, generalized in 34%, and in other locations in 20%. More than 50% had headache more than one half the time, and after three months, headache persisted in 73% of these patients and 33% had headache more than one half the time.

Interestingly, the International Headache Society in their heading of "Headache associated with head trauma" mentions acceleration/deceleration, but does not have a specific diagnosis, other than saying it does not satisfy the criteria for post traumatic headache (see Chapter 13).

Most authors refer to the major percentage of headaches as muscle contraction type and feel that this is associated with greater occipital neuralgia. This is explained as coming from a blow to the suboccipital region or by an entrapment of the semispinalis capitis muscle. However, pain may come from any of the muscles around the neck, such as the superior trapezius, semispinalis capitis, semispinalis cervicis, rectus capitis posterior minor and major, obliquus capitis superior and inferior, their tendons and ligaments. The anatomy of these structures is discussed in Chapter 16 (see also Figures 14.3 and 14.4). Headache pain may also come from a traumatized temporomandibular joint (see Chapter 18).

Out of over 10,000 scientific articles published on whiplash there are only a handful that discuss migraine or vascular headaches associated with this type of trauma. However, in my practice I have seen numerous patients that either had a migraine or migraine-like headache *de novo* or as an exacerbation of a previous condition as a result of a whiplash accident. Whenever a patient would come in with an incapacitating headache as just described a regional nerve block in the occipital area would almost always abort that migraine-like headache. Much more of this is discussed in Chapter 19 on cervicogenic headache. At the end of this chapter patient histories will be presented to demonstrate this point. Although there are not many articles published, this observation has been noticed by many of my colleagues who are headache specialists.

Whether the pain is transmitted by irritation or damage to the nerve, muscle, tendon, ligament, or myofascial trigger points, a headache can be precipitated by palpating or irritating this area. The pain will often start in the neck, usually one sided, and travel up over the top of the head (cephalad) to the frontal area and what seems to start as a muscle contraction-like headache ends up as a migraine-like headache. However, there have been many patients whose neck pain is bilateral and the frontal headaches will be unilateral or bilateral.

Why these patients have migraine headaches is certainly an enigma at this time; however, there are some who have attempted to explain the phenomenon. In 1985, Swerdlow[13] reported on thermographic studies using the "cold patch" as a biologic marker in vascular headaches and found the following: (1) "Cold patches" in post traumatic type I (muscle contraction) and headache-free

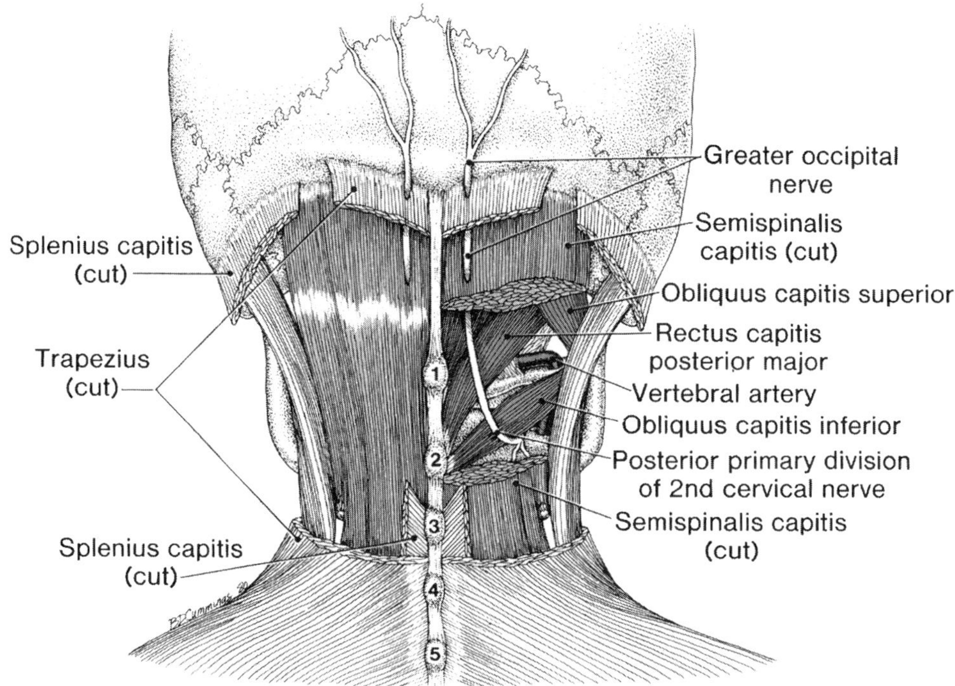

Figure 14.3 This demonstrates a dissection of the muscles of the neck and the anatomy of that area that can be injured as a result of an acceleration/deceleration accident. (From Travell, J.G., Simons, D.G., *Myofascial Pain and Dysfunction, the Trigger Point Manual*, Williams & Wilkins, Baltimore, 1983. With permission.)

and scalp muscle contraction patients were few and statistically insignificant. (2) "Cold patches" in post traumatic types I and II (muscle contraction and vascular) and type III (migraine-like) did show a significantly greater number of "cold patches" than type I or headache-free patients. Our conclusion at that time was that there may be a biologically preset condition for migraine-like headaches that was precipitated by trauma (Figure 14.5).

Bogduk in 1986 (see Barnsley, et al.[7]) provided a neuroanatomical explanation that there is a connection between the cervical nerves (C1–C3) and the cervical portion of the trigeminal nucleus forming the trigemino-cervical nucleus. What this means is that afferents (going in the direction of the brain) from the first three cervical nerves send their messages to the trigeminal nerve which sends the impulses to the front of the face, or the distribution of the trigeminal nerve. Pain from the upper cervical nerves is then referred to the ophthalmic division of the trigeminal nerve and this pain is felt in the orbital, frontal and the temporal regions. Therefore, it is possible to explain how injury in the upper back of the neck (suboccipital headache) through the trigemino-cervical nucleus can also cause pain in the front and side of the face (Figure 14.6).

Foreman and Croft[1] discuss how pain-mediating chemicals may be responsible for triggering a headache. They talk about a chronic local inflammation as a product of a tear or rupture of muscle, myofascia, tendon, or ligament that can release substance P, bradykinin, and other pain-producing peptides, as well as proteolytic enzymes that are released from damaged tissues which cause pain. Ischemia (local anemia) from muscle spasm can also produce pain. The nerve endings stimulated from these chemicals send messages to the spinal cord and then through a reflex increases the contraction. Through an intricate process in the spinal cord via specialized neurons, a feedback loop is created and the cycle is perpetuated and tissue repair is impeded.

As was stated in Chapter 3, the migraine attack is precipitated from a triggering mechanism. If a patient has been suffering migraine before the whiplash accident and the neck pain is extreme,

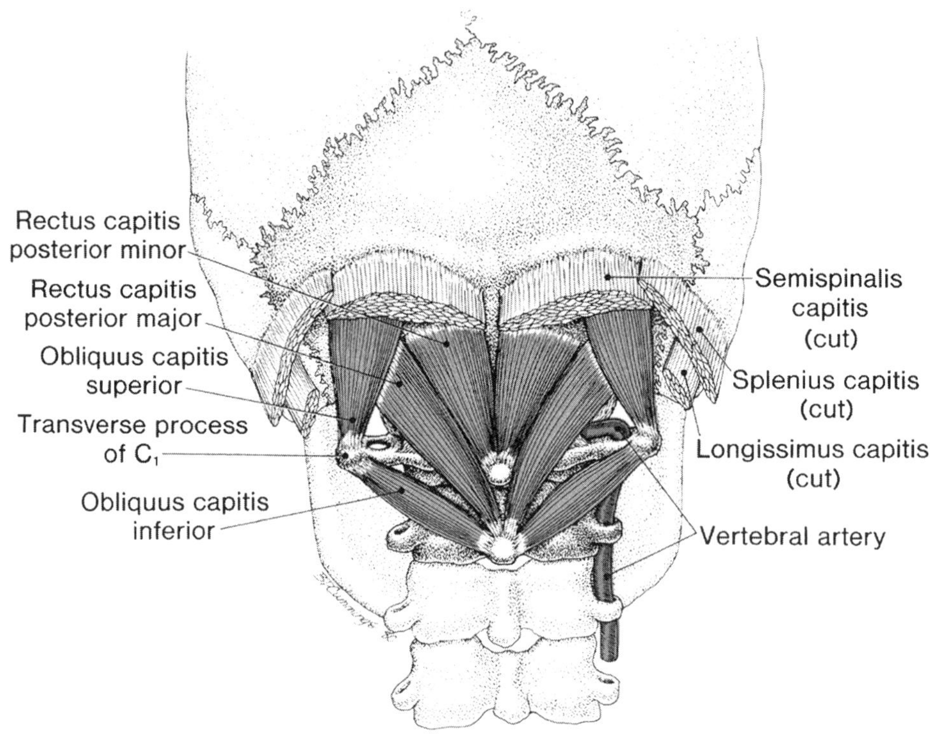

Figure 14.4 Further dissection of the neck muscles reveals the suboccipital muscles. (From Travell, J.G., Simons, D.G., *Myofascial Pain and Dysfunction, the Trigger Point Manual*, Williams & Wilkins, Baltimore, 1983. With permission.)

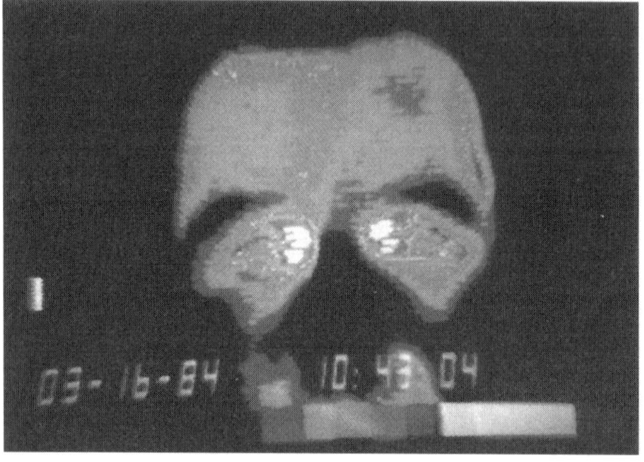

Figure 14.5 A vascular "cold patch" (right frontal region). This cold patch was demonstrated in 82% of migraine patients. (From Swerdlow, B., Dieter, J.N., *Headache*, 26(1), 22–26, 1986. With permission.)

then the stress from pain is enough to create a migraine attack. This will cause the brain, which already has a weakened threshold, to start a neurochemical sequence that provokes the migraine attack. On the other hand, as explained by Bogduk, if the trigeminal nerve is stimulated by the damaged cervical nerves then this may also precipitate a migraine or migraine-like attack. Foreman

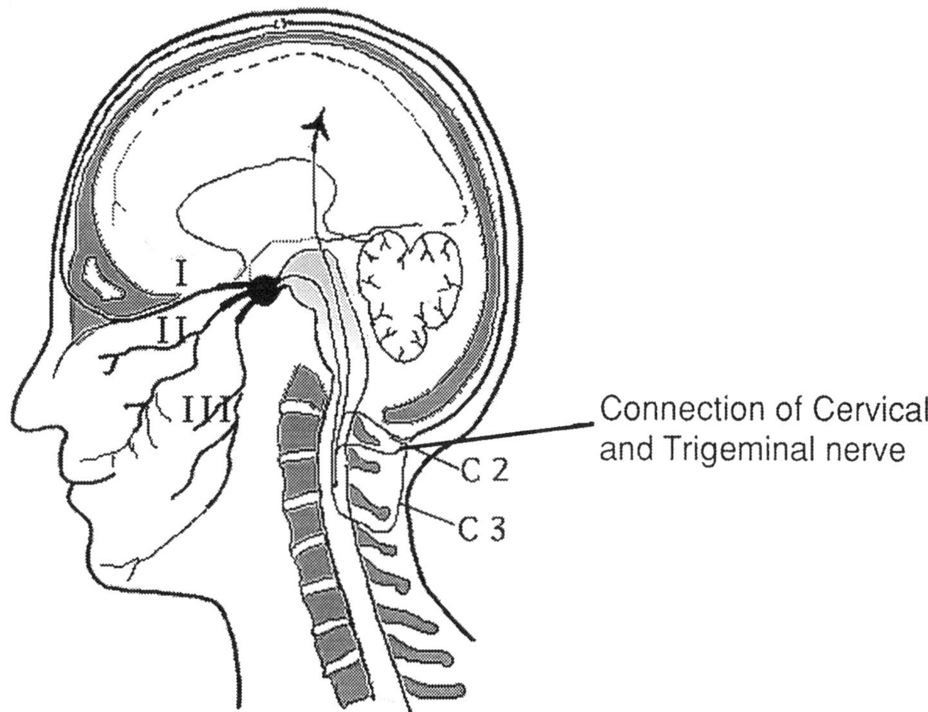

Figure 14.6 This illustration demonstrates that beneath the skin, the fifth cranial nerve (trigeminal) and its divisions I, II or III, plus irritation of the cervical nerves 1, 2 or 3, can send messages to the brain, and the brain in turn will interpret the pain. There is also a connection between the cervical nerves in a lower segment of the trigeminal nerve that comes down to the first and second cervical vertebra, and this connection sends messages from the cervical nerves to the trigeminal nerve and vice versa. Therefore, someone who may be having irritation in the back of the neck may end up with pain in the front of the face as a result of these connections. This is demonstrated in the chapters on whiplash and cervicogenic headache.

and Croft's thoughts on pain-producing peptides are another way of stimulating the trigeminal system to trigger a vascular type of headache.

As the diagram demonstrates, external trigger factors exceed a threshold and activate serotonin and norepinephrine-containing neurons in the brainstem. Once this activation of various neurons, connective tissues, and blood vessels takes place, pain-provoking and neuroinflammatory chemicals are generated within the cerebral cortex and its connective tissues. Once these chemicals are generated, pain receptors in the trigeminovascular system within the coverings of the brain (meninges) will stimulate neurons within the brain to create the awareness of pain.

While this is happening there is activation within the artery of its own pain-provoking chemicals (substance P, neurokinen A, and calcitonin-gene related peptide) which causes a sterile inflammatory process, which sensitizes nerve endings and then causes severe pain, and then this pain is sustained long after the initial trigger has disappeared.

Based on this information it would appear that there is enough justification to consider that whiplash or acceleration/deceleration accidents could precipitate or aggravate a migraine-like headache.

Dizziness

There have been many reports that dizziness and disequilibrium are frequent complaints following whiplash or acceleration/deceleration accidents. Evans[2] reports on several studies with patients who have neck pain and headache who also complain of vertigo (the sensation of moving around in space or objects moving around the person), floating sensations, tinnitus (ringing or tinkling sound in the ear), and hearing impairment, in that order. These symptoms have been attributed to injuries to various structures, such as the vestibular apparatus, the brainstem, the cervical sympathetics, vertebral insufficiency, and the cervical proprioceptive system (awareness of posture, movement, and changes in equilibrium). In anxious patients who are in pain one may often see hyperventilation, which may cause dizziness and paresthesias in their hands or fingers (numbness, prickling, or tingling sensations) which can be unilateral or bilateral.

There have been many studies using various tests to explain these symptoms. ENG (electronystagmograph) studies have shown abnormalities in 54% to 67% of patients complaining of dizziness. These studies were significantly abnormal when comparing whiplash patients to a control group. Barnsley et al.[7] review multiple studies and conclude that these studies indicate vestibular dysfunction either from a central or peripheral injury. In the chronic post cervical acceleration/deceleration population (whiplash) patients have shown both symptoms and abnormal ENG studies well over 12 months.

Evans[2] discusses Tamura's report that 20 patients were found to have disk protrusions at C3/C4 and had cervical diskectomy and fusion and 19 of the 20 were completely relieved of symptoms at an average of 30 months. Nineteen patients who did not have surgery had persistent symptoms after follow up at an average of 24 months.

Once again, one has to extend caution with this group of persistent post cervical acceleration/deceleration (whiplash) syndrome that a specific organic lesion may be responsible for these symptoms and the diagnosis of a post accident neurosis or malingering diagnosis may prevent proper diagnosis and treatment.

Paresthesias

Paresthesias are abnormal sensations, such as tingling, prickling, numbness, or heightened sensations. These are symptoms that are often seen after whiplash in the upper extremities. They are symptoms that are not accompanied by objective findings such as abnormal neurological signs. Evans reports on several studies that find 33% complained of these symptoms acutely and 37% reported paresthesias after a mean follow up of 19.7 months.[2] Of the patients who had a reduced range of cervical movement and evidence of objective neurologic loss, 100% complained of paresthesias and 60% still reported these symptoms 24.7 months later.

Paresthesias can be caused by several factors. Trigger points in the muscles around the neck, shoulders, chest and arms can refer pain and/or paresthesias to the upper extremities. This is explained in more detail in Chapters 16 and 17.

Entrapment neuropathies, such as carpal tunnel syndrome, can also cause paresthesias (Figure 14.7). Some patients complain of hand numbness and tingling after whiplash injury and are documented as having carpal tunnel syndrome. If this problem was not preexisting, this syndrome may come about by a hyperextension injury to the wrist while gripping the steering wheel or bracing the hands on the dashboard during the collision. Carpal tunnel syndrome could also come from any disease of the roots of the spinal cord in the cervical region caused by a crush to this area or a compression to the spinal cord.

Another cause of paresthesias following a whiplash is thoracic outlet syndrome. Thoracic outlet syndrome is seen four times more in women than men and therefore this syndrome is seen much more in women than men following whiplash. Women seem to have more problems with neck injuries than men because of the weaker neck muscles. Thoracic outlet syndrome is most likely caused by compression of the lower cords of the brachial plexus as they pass between the scalenus anterior muscle and the scalenus medius muscle and under the clavicle (Figure 14.8). The condition starts with subjective sensory symptoms followed by pain and paresthesias, and the syndrome then includes headache, neck pain, and paresthesias radiating down the ulnar arm and forearm into the

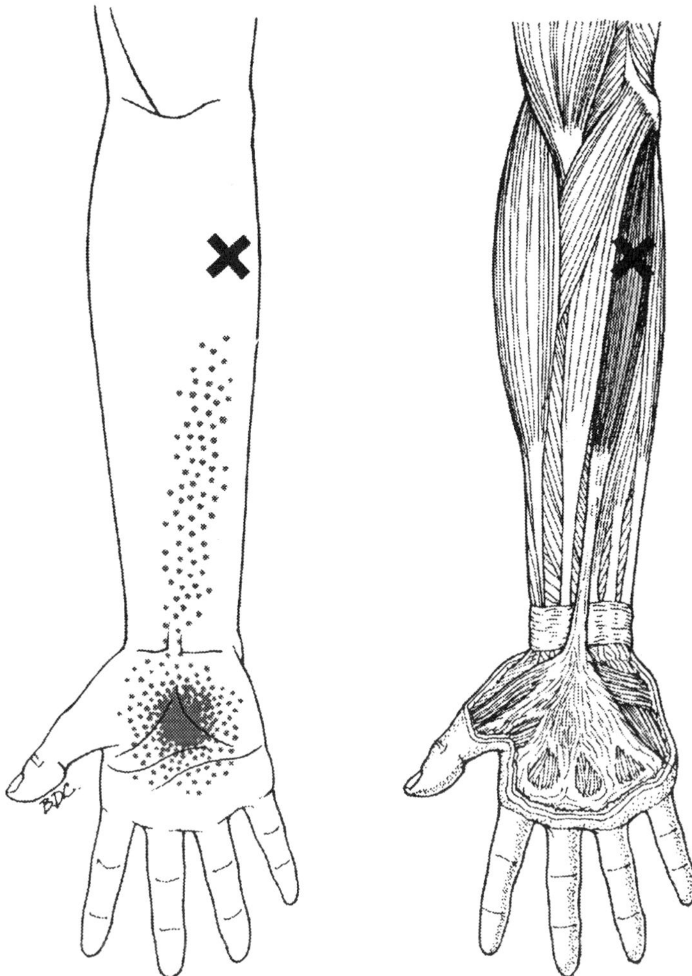

Figure 14.7 Trigger points in the upper arm or forearm can refer paresthesias (tingling sensations) or pain in the hand. (From Travell, J.G., Simons, D.G., *Myofascial Pain and Dysfunction, the Trigger Point Manual*, Williams & Wilkins, Baltimore, 1983. With permission.)

4th and 5th fingers. There are some tests such as Adson's test and others, but they are not specific because there may be a positive test in normal subjects. There has been some objective evidence with some slowed nerve conduction across the thoracic outlet. The fact that a significant number of positive results appeared after whiplash provides reason to support real abnormalities of ulnar nerve conduction in patients with arm symptoms following whiplash injury. The work done in this area provides reason for further research.

Visual Disturbances

Visual disturbances are another of the complaints following whiplash injury. Patients may complain of blurred vision for long periods of time. There are many attempts to explain the very intricate neuroanatomic and neurophysiologic reasons for this symptom. One reason may be that cervical pain alters sympathetic nervous system activity and causes unsuitable accommodation of the eye and produces blurring and difficulty focusing. As studies continue, hopefully, there will be an objective test to locate the specific pathology.

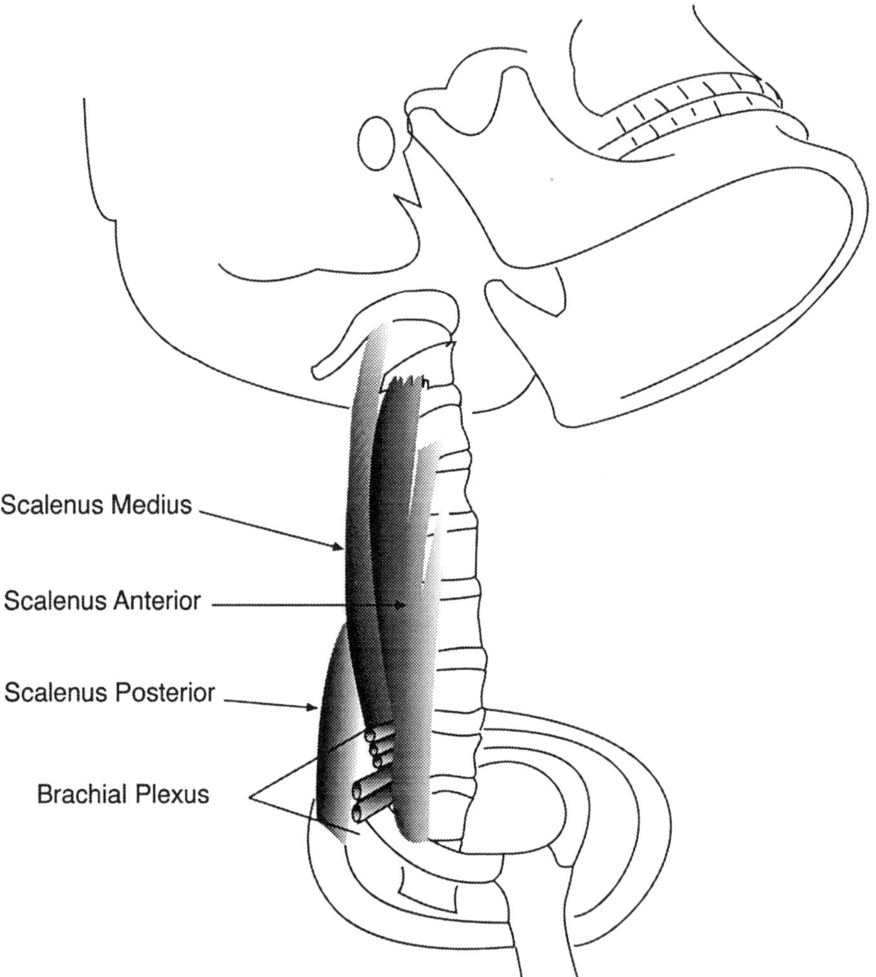

Figure 14.8 The nerves of the brachial plexus, along with the subclavian blood vessels, can be compromised by compression of the muscles concerned with flexion and lateral flexion of the neck. (Adapted from Foreman, S.M., and Croft, A.C., *Whiplash Injuries: The Cervical Acceleration/Deceleration Syndrome*, 2nd ed., Williams & Wilkins, Baltimore, 1995. With permission.)

Neuropsychological Symptoms

Although there is no direct head trauma with whiplash injury, there have been many studies (with monkeys) that indicate that acceleration/deceleration accidents can cause cerebral concussion and cerebral hemorrhages on the surface of the brain and upper cervical spinal cord. Ommaya and Yarnell[14] reported two cases of humans with subdural hematomas after whiplash injuries. There have been other studies of injury to the nerves of the eye muscles suggesting brainstem injury.

Evans[2] reports, on reviewing several studies, that patients with chronic symptoms after a whiplash injury fall into the following percentages: nervousness and irritability 67%; cognitive disturbances 44%; depression 85%; headache 100%; neck pain 72%; vertigo 60%. As discussed earlier, these symptoms are also common in post head trauma syndrome, chronic pain syndromes, and chronic psychiatric disease such as panic disorder, anxiety disorder, and somatization disorder.

This area of neuropsychological symptoms has led to a wide debate and controversy over whether this was a preexisting problem or the result of the accident itself. Radanov et al.,[15] in a very well controlled study, demonstrated that psychological factors, negative affectivity, and personality traits were not significant in predicting the duration of these symptoms. They found other factors that seem to be significant:

1. Older patients
2. If the head was rotated or inclined at the time of impact
3. A higher incidence of pretraumatic headache
4. A higher incidence of intensity of initial neck pain
5. Complained of a greater number of symptoms
6. A higher incidence of radicular deficits (nerve roots)
7. A higher incidence and scores on multiple symptoms analysis
8. Displayed more degenerative signs (i.e., osteoarthrosis) on x-ray

In addition, symptomatic patients scored higher with regard to impaired well being and performed worse on tasks of attentional functioning and showed more concern with regard to long-term suffering and disability. No difference was found between the disabled and the nondisabled symptomatic patients.

It appears then that psychological factors do not predict chronicity of symptoms and that perhaps constant refractory pain, disbelieving doctors, loss of employment, and the stress of the legal battles contribute to the psychological symptoms. If patients have significant psychopathology before the accident, then perhaps we are dealing with two different independent conditions.

Cognition (Perception and Memory)

Some patients will complain of memory and concentration disturbances after whiplash injury (acceleration/deceleration), while others have reported that they do not wish to discuss these symptoms for fear that they will be considered neurotic or malingering. Neuropsychometric testing studies have been conflicting in confirming objective cognitive impairments. In a closer look at these studies it appears that patients with a history of chronic somatic illness not related to trauma have similar problems. This raises the possibility that the cognitive problems are related to the chronic head and neck pain and not to direct injury to the brain.

Objective testing using CT scans, MRI, and electroencephalograms (EEGs) have also not been conclusive and, like with neuropsychometric testing, the reports are conflicting.

Where there seems to be agreement is that impairment of cognitive functioning appears to be consistently related to chronic pain, depression, anxiety, effects of medication, and headache is always present.[4,7,15]

Radiographic Studies

Both for the medical and legal professions objective information is extremely important to document the diagnosis and proof of a lesion or no lesion, depending who is being represented. Therefore using radiographic techniques has always been an important tool. However, with soft tissue injuries this documentation is difficult to assess.

Many times if there are preexisting asymptomatic findings and if this has been seen in examinations prior to the date of the accident, then a relationship may be made with symptoms appearing after the accident.

Cervical spondylosis (the breaking down of a vertebral structure) is generally asymptomatic and increases with age. Between ages 20 to 29, 13% of men and 5% of women will have signs of spondylosis. After age 70, 100% of men and 96% of women are affected.[2] Degenerative disc disease also increases with age and is also asymptomatic. Between ages 30 to 40, changes are seen in 6% of both men and women, and 75% between the ages of 60 to 70. These changes are seen in C5–C6 and C6–C7.

Another anatomical change that alters with age is cervical disc protrusion, which may also be asymptomatic. Studies have shown that disc protrusion may occur in patients ages 45 to 54 20% of the time. This increases to 57% in patients older than 64 years. As a result of these disc protrusions, there can be spinal cord impingement in 16% of patients between the ages of 45 to 64, and this increases to 26% in patients over 64. Also, as a result of disc protrusion there can be spinal cord compression.

Reexamining patients who had disease prior to whiplash and following them after whiplash shows a significant increase in the disease. One study showed that in patients with a mean age of 30 who had no evidence of degenerative disc disease, 39% developed degenerative disc disease where the expectation would be 6%. Other studies showed that where there was degenerative disease at one level there were now degenerative changes at another level in 55% of the patients.

These studies were done originally on patients who did not have symptoms before the whiplash accident and who now were complaining of painful symptoms described in the whiplash syndrome.

PROGNOSIS

Fortunately, most whiplash (cervical acceleration/deceleration) patients do well and are completely returned to feeling normal in two to three months. However, there are a significant number of patients who report that they feel disabled after six months. Many factors have to be taken into consideration that may be responsible for continued symptoms. Neck pain and headache are the two most frequent symptoms, and other symptoms discussed earlier are much less frequent.

Inasmuch as pain is the leading cause of complaint, it is important to find objective reasons for this complaint. If objective evidence is not found, then the consistent symptoms from the data collected from the hundreds of thousands of cases reported in the literature are also relevant. If symptoms are dizziness, vertigo, paresthesias, back pain, etc., objective testing may verify these disorders or these symptoms may fall into the category of consistent complaints.

If the symptoms are related to cerebral complaints such as nervousness, anxiety, depression, memory loss, concentration problems, fatigue, sleep disturbance, etc., these symptoms may be measured by neuropsychological testing or clinical observation or these symptoms may be consistent as part of the syndrome.

Then the gray area of speculation comes into consideration. What has the accident contributed to the pre-accident status of the patient? What was the nature of the accident? Was the accident caused by the patient? Was the accident caused by a negligent individual? Was the accident caused by an intoxicated (alcohol, medications, street drugs) individual? Was the accident caused by careless teenagers on a joy ride? Was the accident caused by a felon being chased by the police? Did the accident occur while the patient was working, and was it a job the patient loved or hated?

It is extremely important to see if the accident altered a happy life or an unhappy life of the patient. Problems that may contribute to a chronic condition, whether there are objective findings or not, are extremely important to help in the treatment of this whiplash syndrome. Finding social, psychological, or economic problems must not make the examiner come to conclusions that the patient is a malingerer or has developed a factitious illness. Having psychological problems as a result of the accident may mean that two types of treatment have to be initiated, one for the physical and one for the psychological symptoms.

Questions that I think are important for the evaluation are the following:

How much education have you had?
What kind of work do you do, and do you like your job?
If you are not working, why not?
Were you ever in the armed service, and if yes, what branch were you in, when? Any action? Any injury? Any medical history? What type of discharge did you have?

Was there any treatment for emotional problems in childhood?
Were there any head injuries as a child?
Do you drink alcohol, and if so, what kind and how much?
Do you use any kind of drugs that are not prescribed, and if so, why?
Any chronic medical problem? (see medical intake for complete medical history)
Any previous psychological or psychiatric therapy or consultation?
List all previous accidents both in childhood and adulthood. It is important to inform the patient that any omission may be held against him if litigation is pursued.
A complete family history (see intake form, Chapter 4).
A complete marital history and any current problems (see Chapter 4).
A history of all your children and any current problems.
Any current stress factor. List all problems (e.g., money, loneliness, sexual problems, work problems, etc.) either before or after the accident.
Are you currently: depressed, having trouble falling asleep, trouble staying asleep?
Has your appetite changed? Is your memory OK? Do you have thoughts about wanting to die?
Are you currently taking any medications?

It is obvious that chronic pain has a secondary psychological effect, just as much as psychological problems may add to the pain problem. If a successful surgeon has a whiplash syndrome and cannot perform, this is certainly going to affect his or her psyche no differently than a long-distance eighteen-wheel hauler. However, if an unhappy, unstable surgeon or truck driver has the same whiplash accident, this may certainly add to the chronicity of the pain and disability of the syndrome.

Although much of the pain in whiplash accidents is related to soft tissue (myofascial) injuries, other types of pathology such as disc disease, bone disease, or radiculopathy should be ruled out using tests such as MRI, computed tomography (CT) scans, myelography and other nerve conduction studies.

Evans,[2] using his own and other studies of neck pain and headaches, reported that 49% were asymptomatic after three months and 57% by six months. After one year 26.3% still reported pain, and after two years one third of the patients still reported pain (neck pain 89%, neck stiffness 40%, shoulder pain 37%, headache 26%, interscapular pain 29%, referred symptoms 40%). Patients who reported pain at two years still reported symptoms at a study 10 years later.

Balla and Karnaghan[12] reported in a study of 100 patients that 90% were seen in six months and three years after the accident and 80% were still having headaches. Half the patients were having headaches daily while the rest were having headaches once a week or more.

Prognostic Variables

The following are variables that appear to be a significant factor in the prognosis of patients who have continued symptoms[2]

1. Older patients; those over 50 have a poorer prognosis
2. Interscapular or upper back pain
3. Occipital headache
4. Multiple symptoms or paresthesias at presentation
5. Reduced range of movement of the cervical spine
6. Objective neurologic deficit
7. Preexisting degenerative osteoarthritic changes
8. Cervical stenosis (for development of myelopathy [spinal cord pathology])
9. Abnormal cervical spine curves (have been reported as and as not a prognostic sign)

Interestingly, in the area of occupations related to poor prognosis it seems that upper middle occupational categories have an increased incidence of symptoms persisting longer than six months as compared to lower and higher occupational categories.

Continued symptoms longer than six months was also seen in rear-end collisions as compared to other types of collisions. The speed or severity of collision and the extent of damage to the vehicle did not seem to affect the prognosis of the patients studied.

In several studies of medicolegal cases, Evans[2] reports that one study showed 79% of patients returned to work by one month, 86% by three months, 91% by six months, and 94% by one year. Another study reported that permanent medical disability occurred in 9.6% of patients involved in rear-end collisions, and 3.8% involved in front-end or side-impact accidents.

Other studies reported that in over 5000 cases of whiplash injury, 26% of the patients were not able to return to normal activities at six months. In another study of 102 patients seen in the emergency room, the group was broken down into two groups, a good prognostic group and a poor prognostic group. The good prognostic group (66% of the total of 102 patients) all returned to work within 16 weeks; one third took no time off at all, and the average time off was two weeks. Of the poor prognostic group of patients, the average time off was six weeks; 20% took no time off work, and 9% did not return to work by two years.

Patients who are involved in whiplash (cervical acceleration/deceleration) injuries have a high rate of litigation. In the United States where we have a system of tort law in which a party is held responsible for the injury, then one would expect a high rate of litigation. As the symptoms increase in severity from mild to severe, the litigation increases twofold.[2]

There have been many papers published that seem to represent one side or the other. That is, some physicians have made it known that they feel this is a syndrome that has developed out of litigation and financial compensation. Other papers published recognize that a small percentage of injured people are attempting to "cash in" on the accident. However, they stress that most of the severely injured who do not recover are so consistent with their symptoms that it would be hard to deny the reality of this syndrome. It appears that the most recent of the papers published, from the late 1970s to the present, justify this syndrome with clinical evidence that lends credibility to this problem. (See the section below, "A Model".)

I have seen hundreds of whiplash patients with chronic headache and have felt only a small percentage of these patients were malingerers and patients who are in need of secondary gain only. Most of the patients I have seen who are involved for secondary gain (money or attention, etc.) seem to be the same type of patient regardless of whether they were involved in an accident or not. Every attempt should be made to identify the severely neurotic, the histrionic personality, the factitious illness sufferer, and the sociopath. It is also imperative that the treating physician does not feel an obligation to support these psychiatric disorders in a litigation situation.

On the other hand, as stated above, patients with psychiatric disease or those people who may be psychologically labile are not immune to injury and their symptoms of pain are no different from those who do not have these problems. As discussed in the preceding chapter, there are many factors that may contribute psychological symptoms as a result of the accident; first, the frustration of what takes place with a patient who has had the insult of an accident that now causes ongoing pain that changes the patient's life and lifestyle. Next, add the insult of what that patient has to endure with unsuccessful medical treatment and victimization by family, friends, employers, insurance companies, and the legal system. Add this kind of stress and frustration to anyone's life and there are enough ingredients to cause "psychological symptoms" plus the pain they have to endure, and it is predictable that any psychological test is going to demonstrate some abnormalities.

It has been shown that many of the papers that have taken the stance that whiplash is solely a litigation syndrome and has no merit as a medical condition have been flawed as a scientific presentation. Often the population used was too small to be representative of significant figures. Control groups were not used and conclusions drawn were often interpreted by a biased interrogator.

A MODEL

Barnsley and coworkers[7] have suggested a model for whiplash based on a review of the literature and their own studies. There appears to be enough evidence, anatomical, biomechanical, and experimental, to support various injuries in the whiplash (cervical acceleration/deceleration) accident. Damage has been demonstrated to the pre-vertebral (in front of) and post-vertebral (in back of) muscles. There can be damage to the zygapophyseal joints (an articular process of a vertebra) and the intervertebral discs. Other damage that is not seen often is damage to the sympathetic nervous system trunk, the brain, the inner ear, and the esophagus.

Pain can be produced from tears in the muscles and ligaments and when these heal the pain should clear in the span of several weeks. Ligament healing may take longer because of a poorer blood supply. Minor fractures with some bleeding also will heal, taking somewhat longer — two to three months. However, damage to the zygapophyseal joints and the intervertebral discs present a different problem and a different prognostic picture.

Because there is little or no blood supply to the discs, tears to this structure (annulus fibrosis) or separation of the disc from the adjacent vertebral body will not heal. This damage will cause interruption of the nerves supplying these structures and are a source of pain. Experimental studies, postmortem studies, and imaging studies support this concept. However, there is no proof that these disc injuries occur only in patients with pain and that these lesions are always painful.

Injury to the zygapophyseal joints has been produced experimentally, found in postmortem examinations, and has been found in clinical studies. When there is injury to the zygapophyseal joint, there is disruption to the joint surface and this can lead to an osteoarthritis of that joint and ongoing pain. Also bleeding into the joint (hemarthrosis) or injury to the intra-articular structure may lead to a chronic, post traumatic synovitis (inflammation of the synovial membrane lining the joint) that will cause ongoing pain and joint damage. With this problem there is little chance of healing or spontaneous healing (Figure 14.9).

Unfortunately, these zygapophyseal joint problems are almost impossible to detect with x-ray, and can be detected only with special techniques or high resolution CT scans. However, enormous work and studies have been done to demonstrate the credibility of these conclusions by using local anesthetic blocks.[8-11] By using large patient population studies plus double-blind, controlled diagnostic blocks, Barnsley and colleagues have been able to show the prevalence of zygapophysial joint pain to be 54%. This certainly gives evidence that there is a physiological reason for pain secondary to injury to this joint.

The model demonstrated discusses two types of injury: (1) acute tears in muscle and sprains, which constitute the majority of the patients and will heal in a relatively short period of time (weeks to six months), and (2) injuries to the discs and zygapophyseal joints, which do not resolve and lead to chronic pain (Figure 14.10). Because zygapophyseal joint problems cannot be detected on current imaging techniques and because there are no neurological signs or demonstrable disease, doctors will often miss the diagnosis or not be aware of this diagnosis and then not believe the patient and soon the patient is labeled a malingerer. From this point on, psychological symptoms that did not exist previously come into play.

An extremely important research paper by Wallis, Lord and Bogduk was published in the journal *Pain* in October 1997.[16] These authors have been quoted many times during the writing of this book for their work with chronic pain after whiplash injury or cervical acceleration-deceleration syndrome using the zygapophyseal joint as one of the major reasons for the chronic pain that follows this injury. As mentioned previously, they have done various nerve blocks in this area and have been able to exhibit complete pain relief for a period of time, demonstrating that the pain arising from this specific area is the major component of the chronic pain that exists after whiplash when this joint is affected.

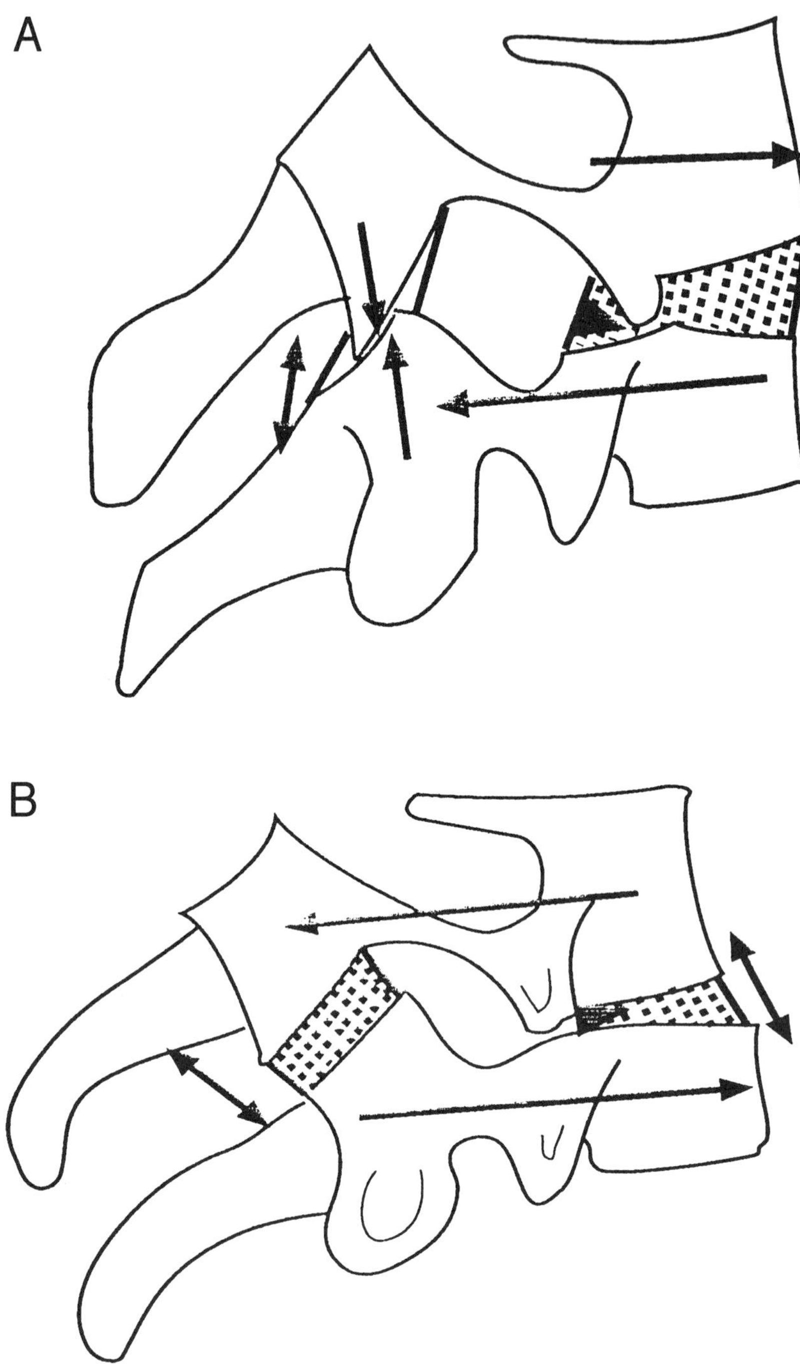

Figure 14.9 The shearing forces that take place in an acceleration/deceleration injury. (A) The smaller arrows demonstrate the resistance of the zygapophyseal joints and tension within the intervertebral discs. (B) The opposite movement. (Adapted from Barnsley, L., Lord, S., Bogduk, N., *Pain*, 58, 283–307, 1994).

Their most recent paper[16] reports that if the pain is relieved by this neurosurgical technique, the psychological symptoms that accompanied this pain also become resolved. What is extremely important about this paper is that it demonstrates that there does not have to be any psychotherapy

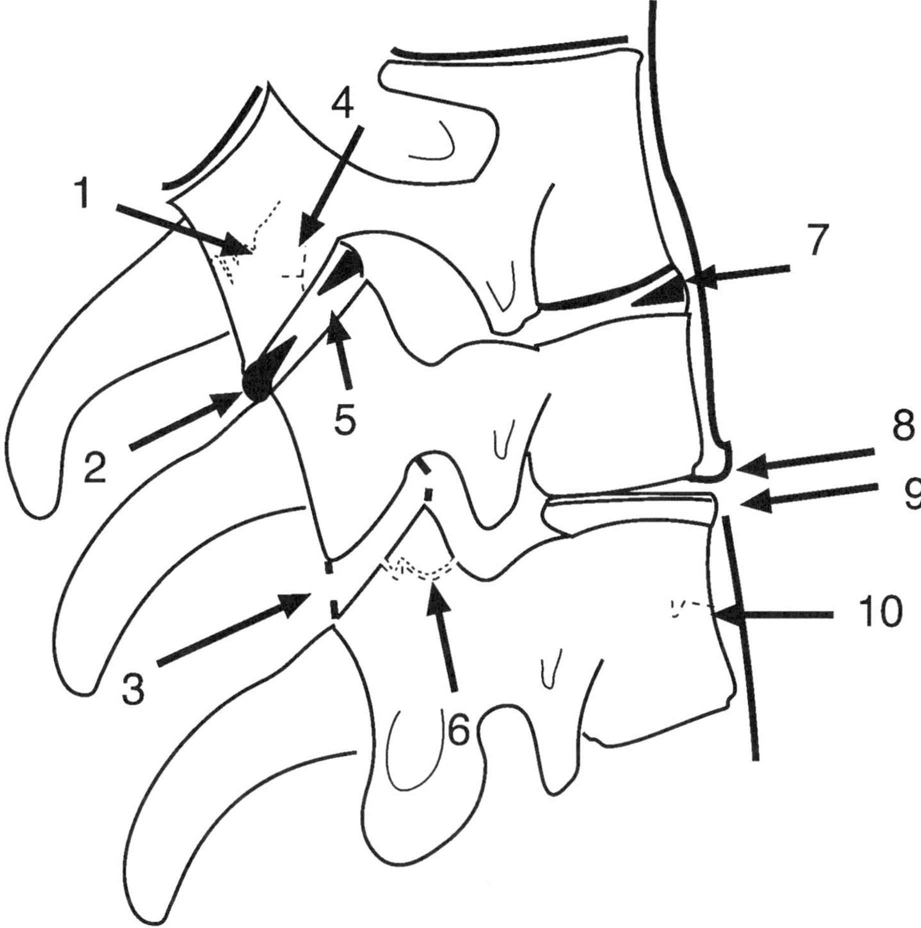

Figure 14.10 Some of the injuries that can take place following an acceleration/deceleration (whiplash injury). (**1**) Fracture of the vertebral lamina (arch); (**2**) bleeding of the zygapophyseal joint; (**3**) tearing of the zygapophyseal joint capsule; (**4**) fracture of the subcartilage plate; (**5**) bruising of intra-articular cartilage; (**6**) fracture of the articular surface; (**7**) tearing of the annulus fibrosus of intervertebral disc; (**8**) tearing of the anterior longitudinal ligament; (**9**) separation or fracture of the endplate; (**10**) vertebral body fracture. (Adapted from Barnsley, L., Lord, S., Bogduk, N., *Pain*, 58, 283–307, 1994.)

involved in treating the patient's depression and psychological complaints if the pain is relieved. This then shows that, in cases where the patient's psychological symptoms did not exist prior to the accident, when the pain is relieved the psychological symptoms are relieved and the patient returns to a normal way of life, or certainly to his or her state prior to the accident. Wallis et al. point out that this radiofrequency neurotomy does not provide a permanent cure but it may give long-term analgesia. The pain relief can last many months or even years, and the psychological symptoms also will abate for that period of time. Interestingly enough, when the symptoms of pain again arise, then the psychological symptoms return and there is a definite relationship between the specific pain and the psychological symptoms. What is so important is that these patients become disabled, both psychologically and from pain, as a result of the inflammatory response of the zygapophyseal joint. There may be both a diagnostic and treatment potential to eliminate this problem and a large and expensive disability problem that coexists with this particular injury. The authors point out that pain and psychological symptoms coming from other sources of chronic pain may well need a different type of treatment and continuing psychotherapeutic counseling.

The chronicity of this neck problem would certainly explain the continued headache symptoms, but there is another headache problem that we see in the headache clinic, and that is, often when the neck pain seems to be healing, the headaches continue. In Chapter 19 we attempt to explain why these headaches continue and why this clinical entity has been neglected until recently. It has been my experience that patients who had migraine previously on a periodic basis now complain of very frequent migraine-like headaches combined with muscle tension-like headaches. My other experience with this entity is that the medications that seemed effective to abort the migraine attack before the accident no longer appear to work. Another interesting observation is that prior to the accident these sufferers would place the location of their headache at the front or side of their head (temporal), but after the accident they complain that the headache starts in the back of their neck . They also found that they were sensitive to an attack with any extra movements of their neck. Another interesting observation is that even though the prior medications did not work, a nerve block to the upper neck and occipital region would almost always abort the headache pain both in the back and the front of the head. These patients would come into the clinic with severe migraine symptoms: nausea, vomiting, an inflamed eye, pallor, sweating, photophobia, and a flu-like appearance, and within five minutes all the symptoms would be gone.

It was also noted that patients who did not improve almost always were those who likely had a personality disorder with secondary gain as their greatest need.

The method of the nerve block is discussed in Chapter 25. Another treatment using intravenous medication is discussed in Chapter 25.

SUMMARY

There are an enormous number of motor vehicle accidents in this country and all over the world, and a large percentage of these are rear-ended, frontal or lateral accidents that cause injuries to the neck without the head striking an immovable object. Cervical acceleration/deceleration or whiplash occurs when the head accelerates relative to the body. These forces cause shear and excessive torque to the structures of the neck. When this happens there is compression and derangement of the tissues in the neck. Studies that have been performed on animals and cadavers and postmortem examinations have shown that there have been injuries to the muscles, ligaments, intervertebral discs and the cervical zygapophyseal joints. The studies have also shown that in spite of these obvious injuries they may not necessarily be demonstrated clinically or with radiological testing.

The majority of these patients or victims will heal spontaneously over a period of one to six months; these are the group of victims who suffered minor injury to the muscles and ligaments. However, there are a group of patients who will not get better and will become chronically sick. Their major complaints are neck pain and headache. Other symptoms may be visual disturbance, dizziness, weakness, paresthesias, cognitive deficits, depression, anxiety, sleep disturbance related to pain and also psychological symptoms related to the litigation process.

Chronicity of symptoms appears to be related to older patients, rotated or inclined head position at the time of the accident, and a higher incidence of pretraumatic headache. These persons displayed more degenerative cervical vertebrae disease, complained of more symptoms than the average victim, and had a higher incidence of radicular symptoms. They also displayed higher scores on tests that demonstrated impaired well-being, performed worse on tasks concerned with attentional functioning, and showed more concern with regard to long-term suffering.

All objective studies find no sound evidence to sustain the belief that psychological factors or a desire for monetary gain affects the eventual outcome of the whiplash patient, barring the malingerer or a pretraumatic severe personality disorder.

See the case histories following the References.

REFERENCES

1. Foreman, S.M., Croft, A.C., *Whiplash Injuries: The Cervical Acceleration/Deceleration Syndrome*, 2nd ed., Williams & Wilkins, Baltimore, 1995.
2. Evans, R.W., Some observations on whiplash injuries, *Neurologic Clinics*, 10(4), 975–997, 1992.
3. Severy, D.M, Mathewson, J.H., Bechtol, Co., Controlled automobile rear end collisions, an investigation of related engineering and medical phenomena. *Canadian Service Medical Journal*, 11, 1955.
4. Sturzenegger, M., Distefano, G., Radanov, B.P., Schnidrig, A., Presenting symptoms and signs after whiplash injury: the influence of accident mechanisms, 44, 688–699, 1994.
5. Macnab, I., The whiplash syndrome, *Orthopedic Clinics of North America*, 2(2), 389–403, 1971.
6. Pearce, J.M.S., Polemics of chronic whiplash injury, 44, 1993–1997, 1994.
7. Barnsley, L., Lord, S., Bogduk, N., Clinical review: whiplash injury, *Pain*, 58, 283–307, 1994.
8. Aprill, C., Bogduk, N., The prevalence of cervical zygapophyseal joint pain: a first approximation. *Spine*, 17(7), 1992.
9. Barnsley, L., Bogduk, N., Medial branch blocks are specific for the diagnosis of cervical zygapophyseal joint pain, *Reg Anesthesia*, 18(6), 1993.
10. Barnsley, L., Lord, S., Bogduk, N., Comparative local anaesthetic blocks in the diagnosis of cervical zygapophyseal joint pain, *Pain*, 55, 99–106, 1993.
11. Barnsley, L., Lord, S., Wallis, B., Bogduk, N., False-positive rates of cervical zygapophyseal joint blocks, *Clinical Journal of Pain*, 9, 124–130, 1993.
12. Balla, J., Karnaghan, J., Whiplash headache, *Clinical and Experimental Neurology*, 23, 179–182, 1987.
13. Swerdlow, B., Thermographic documentation in a case of post-traumatic dysautonomic cephalalgia, *Thermology*, 1, 102–105, 1985.
14. Ommaya, A.K., Yarnell, P., Subdural hematoma after whiplash injury, *Lancet*, 2, 237–239, 1969.
15. Radanov, B.P., Sturzenegger, M., Di Stefano, G., Long-term outcome after whiplash injury, a 2 year follow-up considering features of injury mechanism and somatic, radiologic, and psychosocial findings, *Medicine*, 74, 281–297, 1995.
16. Wallis, B., Lord, S., Bogduk, N., Resolution of psychological distress of whiplash patients following radiofrequency neurotomy: a randomized, double-blind, placebo-controlled trial, *Pain Journal*, October 1997.

CASE HISTORIES*

The following are case histories and summaries that will help you identify cervical acceleration/deceleration syndrome headaches. There are also actual medical reports to help you understand how the physician comes to the diagnosis.

* On the headache assessment forms that accompany these case histories, incapacitating headaches are indicated with solid black lines, interfering headaches with dotted lines, and irritating headaches with gray shading.

June 23, 1993

[Doctor's name and address omitted]

RE: GEORGE

Dear Dr. [...]:

Thank you for the referral of George [...]. This is a 33-year-old male born 00/00/59 in Florida who was in the Army from 1979 to 1987.

He was working for [...] and was in an accident on 00/00/93. He was driving, wearing his seat belt, when his brakes locked and he was rear-ended by another car. He was thrown back over the seat (the seat had no neck support), and then was thrown forward. He had a significant flexion extension injury. He was taken to the hospital emergency room, x-rayed and released. His headaches began on the same day. He states he did not have any headaches prior to the accident.

HEADACHE PROFILE

Incapacitating headaches: On the day of the accident he said they started but about two days after the accident he began to get daily incapacitating headaches. These last twenty to thirty minutes. It is a throbbing headache in the posterior cervical, parietal and temporal region and the lateral orbital regions, left worse than right. There is no aura. Associated features are nausea, vomiting, photophobia, phonophobia, pallor, and he goes to bed. Multiple things will precipitate the headache.

Interfering headaches (moderate to severe): These are identical to the incapacitating headaches with less intensity. When he doesn't have the half-hour to hour incapacitating headache, he has a daily, constant, moderate to severe headache.

Past history: The patient was most probably a normal delivery. There is no history of enuresis or unexplained abdominal cramps pre-puberty. There is no history of car sickness as a child. There is no history of meningitis, encephalitis, scarlet fever, or rheumatic fever. There were no head injuries as a child.

Habits: He does not drink. He smokes about a pack and a half of cigarettes a day at present.

Medical history: The patient has no history of high blood pressure, stomach ulcers, asthma, allergies, pneumonia, kidney problems, low blood sugar, glaucoma, diabetes, or heart problems.

Review of systems: Pulmonary negative, cardiovascular negative, gastrointestinal negative, urogenital negative.

Surgical history: In 1986 he had a kidney infection in the left kidney, and in 1987 he had an accident in which he had cut both arms.

Psychiatric history: Negative.

Family history: His father is living, age 59, with no headache history. His mother is living, age 52, with no headache history. He has two sisters, ages 34 and 37, with no headache history.

Patient was married from age 19 to 21 and from 24 to present. There are two boys, ages 2 and 5, with no headaches.

Stress factors: There are multiple stress factors that are causing depression, insomnia, etc. He was fired from his job because of the accident. He has financial problems, personal problems, and is close to divorce because of his current attitude since the accident. He has been depressed and forgetful since the accident.

Allergies to medications: NKA.

Current medications: He is currently taking Hydrocodone, cyclobenzaprine (Flexeril three times a day), and ibuprofen.

Doctors seen in the past for headaches: He is seeing his family doctor where he got the Hydrocodone. He is currently seeing you. He says that when he has any traction or physical therapy, his headaches increase. He finds the TENS are not helping.

Physical examination: Height 5' 9$^1/_2$", weight 145 pounds, pulse 70, left BP 118/72, right BP 110/70. The face did not show any asymmetry. The temporomandibular joint area was grossly normal. The eyes appeared normal. Conjunctivae were clear and the pupils reacted equally to light and accommodation. Retinal fundus examination revealed no papilledema and no abnormalities with the arteries and veins. There were no bruits over the supraorbital region. The nose appeared normal. The auditory canals were clear, and the tympanic membranes appeared intact. The mouth and throat appeared normal. Gums, tongue, buccal mucosa and teeth were grossly normal. There are multiple latent trigger points in the upper cervical region. Carotid bruits could not be heard. Cervical nodes were not enlarged. The lungs were clear to auscultation and percussion. The heart had a regular sinus rhythm with no murmurs. The abdomen was soft and nontender. In the extremities, he is unable to approximate a right finger, secondary to an old injury. A rectal exam was not done.

Neurological examination: Cranial nerve II: Visual fields were grossly normal. III, IV and VI: No strabismus, nystagmus or ptosis. V: Normal sensation and corneal reflex. VII: Normal facial movements (wrinkle, frown, smile, and strength of eyelids). VIII: Normal Weber and Rinne. IX and X: Good gag reflex. XI: Normal sternocleidomastoid and trapezius. XII: Normal protrusion and strength of tongue. Cerebellar: Negative Rhomberg. Normal finger-to-nose, diadochokinesis, heel-shin, tandem, and heel and toes walking. Motor system: No atrophy, fasciculations, wasting, or tremors. Good muscle strength in arms, wrists, fingers, and legs. Sensory system: Superficial tactile, pain and vibrations (wrists, elbows, knees, and ankles) were normal. Normal motion and positions of fingers and toes. Normal 2-point discrimination. Reflexes: Normal 2+ reflexes of triceps, biceps, knee jerk, ankle jerk, etc. Normal pulses in dorsalis pedis, posterior tibial and popliteal.

DIAGNOSES

1. Post traumatic (flexion/extension-whiplash) daily incapacitating headaches.
2. Post traumatic (flexion/extension-whiplash) daily vascular headaches.
3. Post traumatic (flexion/extension-whiplash) muscle contraction headache with latent myofascial trigger points.
4. Rule out cervicogenic headache.
5. Rule out intracranial structural lesion.
6. Severe depression.

IMPRESSION

This is a 33-year-old gentleman who comes in with constant intractable headache problems since an accident he had on 00/00/93. At the present time, he is involved with chiropractic treatment and it appears that this accident (see initial description of accident) has caused vascular headaches (migraine-like) and also muscle contraction headaches with myofascial trigger points.

As a medication route, I feel that patient should have Amitriptyline 10 mg at h.s., Propranolol 20 mg t.i.d., Bellergal-S b.i.d., Midrin to abort his headaches, and Relafen 500 mg times two, once a day, for his pain problem. I think that the patient needs a regional block of C1, 2, 3, starting with the left side which is worse, in order to break this headache and also to give the ligaments a chance to rest. I would also consider the possibility of doing cervical facet blocks with fluoroscopic guidance if the diagnosis of cervicogenic headache could be established. I would also consider biofeedback as a means of reducing a lot of the muscle tension, depression, anxiety, etc., that he is having. If his depression continues, we will recommend that the patient see a psychiatrist for both psychotherapy and medication therapy.

At the present time, we are waiting for an okay from the insurance company to start the procedures on him and as soon as they give us the okay we will.

Thank you once again for referring this patient to our office. If there are any questions, please do not hesitate to call or write.

Sincerely,

BERNARD SWERDLOW, M.D.

These notes were dictated with the patient present.

MEDICAL HEADACHE HISTORY

Name: George **Age:** 33 **Sex** M **Date:** 6/3/93

Date of Birth: 00/00/59 **Birthplace:** FL **Race:** C **Education:** 14 years

Occupation: Unemployed **Accident:** 1993

Armed Services & Type of Discharge: U.S. Army 1979-1987

PAST HISTORY:

1.	Did you have a normal birth?		Yes	No
	a) forceps used?		Yes	No
	b) cesarean section?		Yes	No
2.	Did you have problems with bedwetting?		Yes	No
	a) If yes, age bedwetting stopped			
3.	Were you car sick as a child (motion)?		Yes	No
	a) If yes, how severe?	Slight	Moderate	Severe
4.	Did you have unexplained abdominal cramps as a child?		Yes	No
5.	Did you have any of the following illnesses in childhood?			
	a) meningitis		Yes	No
	b) encephalitis		Yes	No
	c) scarlet fever		Yes	No
	d) rheumatic fever		Yes	No
6.	Did you have any head injuries as a child?		Yes	No
	a) If yes, please explain:			
7.	Were you treated for emotional illness as a child?		Yes	No

HABITS:

8.	Do you drink alcohol?	Yes	No
	a) If yes, what kind and how much?		
	b) Does alcohol bring on or aggravate a headache?	Yes	No
9.	Do you smoke?	Yes	No
	a) If yes, how much? Pack and ½ a day		
	b) Does smoking or smoke-filled rooms cause or aggravate headaches?	Yes	No
10.	Do you drink caffeinated beverages?	Yes	No
	a) If yes, how much? very little		

MENSTRUAL HISTORY:

At what age did menses begin?______ Were they regular or irregular?______

How were they related to your headache?______

Are you or were you ever on Birth Control Pills?______ Did they affect your headache? ______

Have you had a hysterectomy, partial or total, and why?______

Are you in menopause, and if yes, how long?______

Are you on hormones, and if yes, which ones?______

HEADACHE ASSESSMENT FORM

HA PROFILE	INCAPACITATING #3	INTERFERING #2	IRRITATING #1
ONSET (Years ago and frequency)	1993 – 2 days after accident	N/A	N/A
CURRENT FREQUENCY	Every day	N/A	N/A
TIME OF ONSET	Awakens with	N/A	N/A
DURATION	20 – 30 minutes	N/A	N/A
CHARACTER	Throbbing	N/A	N/A
PRODROME OR AURA	N/A	N/A	N/A
ASSOCIATING FEATURES	Nausea; Vomiting; Sensitivity to Light? Noise? Odors? Do you get pale or flush? Do your eyes or nose run? Does your nose get stuffy? Does the white of your eyes get red? Does your eyelid droop? Do you pace, or go to bed?	Nausea; Vomiting; Sensitivity to Light? Noise? Odors? Do you get pale or flush? Do your eyes or nose run? Does your nose get stuffy? Does the white of your eyes get red? Does your eyelid droop? Do you pace, or go to bed?	Nausea; Vomiting; Sensitivity to Light? Noise? Odors? Do you get pale or flush? Do your eyes or nose run? Does your nose get stuffy? Does the white of your eyes get red? Does your eyelid droop? Do you pace, or go to bed?
PRECIPITATING OR AGGRAVATING FEATURES	Trying to concentrate	N/A	N/A

LOCATION: Mark the location for each tvne of headache with a different color pen.

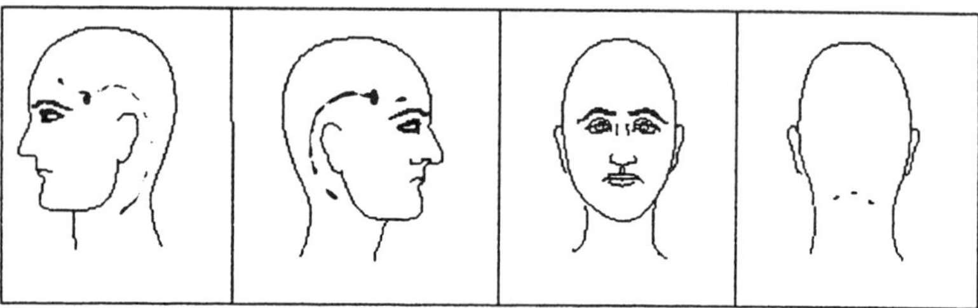

MEDICAL HISTORY:

Have you ever been or are you currently being treated for any of the following?

a) high blood pressure	Yes	No
b) stomach ulcers	Yes	No
c) asthma	Yes	No
d) allergies	Yes	No
e) pneumonia	Yes	No
f) kidney problems	Yes	No
g) low blood sugar	Yes	No
h) glaucoma	Yes	No
i) diabetes	Yes	No
j) heart problems	Yes	No

If you answered yes to any of the above, please describe:.

List all other medical problems you have had in the past. Include date diagnosed and treatment.
DO NOT LIST OPERATIONS

None.

SURGICAL HISTORY (List operations and dates performed)

1986 – Left kidney (infected). 1987 – Both forearms.

PSYCHIATRIC HISTORY (List visits with counselors, psychologists, etc., and type of treatment)

None.

ACCIDENTS IN ADULT LIFE (Briefly describe any accident that caused any blow to the head or that you feel is related to your headache)

1993 - Driving with seat belt. Brakes locked and I was rear-ended by another car. Thrown back over seat (seat had no neck support), and then thrown forward. Taken to emergency room, x-rayed, and released. Headaches began same day. No headaches before accident.

FAMILY HISTORY:

1.	Is your father living?	Yes	No
	Age 59		
	Cause of death		
	Was there a headache history?	Yes	No
2.	Is your mother living?	Yes	No
	Age 52		
	Cause of death		
	Was there a headache history?	Yes	No

3. Ages of brothers---Circle the ones with headache
 None
4. Ages of sisters---Circle the ones with headache
 34 37
5. List any other blood relatives with a history of severe headaches.
 None

MARITAL HISTORY:
List marriages:

1st marriage age 19 to 21	Did spouse have headaches?	Yes	No
2nd marriage age 24 to Present	Did spouse have headaches?	Yes	No
3rd marriage age _____ to _______	Did spouse have headaches?	Yes	No

Age of current spouse: 25

List ages and sex of all children:

Age 5 Sex M	Headaches?	Yes	No
Age 2 Sex M	Headaches?	Yes	No
Age ____ Sex _____	Headaches?	Yes	No
Age ____ Sex _____	Headaches?	Yes	No

STRESS FACTORS:

List any factors that may be affecting your headaches (money, loneliness, sexual problems, work, etc.)
 Fired from job because of accident. Money. Personal relations.

VEGETATIVE SIGNS:

1.	Do you have trouble falling asleep?	Yes	No
2.	Do you have trouble staying asleep?	Yes	No
3.	Has your appetite decreased?	Yes	No
4.	Have you gained or lost weight in the past year?	Yes	No
5.	Have you felt tearful or depressed lately?	Yes	No
6.	Have you had any thoughts of wanting to die?	Yes	No
7.	Have you been forgetful lately?	Yes	No
8.	Any other changes in your normal day-to-day living?		

Please list any medications you are allergic or sensitive to: None.

Please list any medications you are currently taking (including dosages and frequency per day):
 Hydrocodone 5 mg, 1 every 4 hours. Cyclobenzaprine (Flexeril), 1 three times a day.
 Ibuprofen.

PREVIOUS CARE:

1. List doctors who have treated you for headaches:____________________________________

____

____

____

2. List any tests you have had for your headache (e.g., EEG, CT scan, MRI, X-Ray, etc.):

X-rays.

____

____

____

____

3. List any other treatment you have had for your headache (e.g., biofeedback, acupuncture, chiropractic, or any other treatment you had):

____

____

____

MICHAEL
Category: Whiplash

This 27-year-old male came to Florida from New York looking for work, and while looking for employment he was involved in a significant auto accident in which he was driving without his seatbelt. He was stopped while waiting to make a left turn. He was rear-ended and shoved into oncoming traffic into another car. He said he was dazed, and was taken to the emergency room at a local hospital, x-rayed, and released, and stated his headaches began that day. He states that he had an occasional irritating (#1) headache before the accident.

The incapacitating (#3) headaches started 2 to 3 days after the accident, and he has been having these daily. The symptom is throbbing, and it starts in the posterior cervical region in the back of his neck and works its way forward to the frontal and periorbital, around the eyes and head. He states that when he has these headaches he sees "little bugs" and blurry vision. With this headache, he has nausea and vomiting, and must go to bed.

The interfering (#2) headaches, which are moderate to severe, started the day of the accident and he is having them daily, and eventually they will become incapacitating. They are constant and very similar to the incapacitating headaches.

Irritating (#1), or annoying, headaches: He has had these about once a month since his teens, but since he has the severe headaches, he doesn't have them anymore.

His past history was essentially normal, and medically there was nothing significant. There was no headache history in his family.

While seeing me, he saw a chiropractor and also a pain specialist for his back pain.

While examining this patient, he began to have a migraine attack, with his eyes becoming reddened and teary, and he began to have all the other features of a severe migraine. In order to make sure that there was no structural brain damage during the accident, an MRI was ordered.

Because the patient said he was dazed, it was difficult to ascertain whether he had hit his head, and this patient could be given a diagnosis of post traumatic incapacitating headaches, or both whiplash and incapacitating headaches. Also associated with that would be vascular headaches with aura (or migraine), and also daily muscle contraction headache component. The patient also had trigger points.

He had moved back to New York and I was unable to follow his course; but, based on his presentation, the prognosis is not good, and he probably will continue to have a chronic headache problem.

MEDICAL HEADACHE HISTORY

Name: Michael **Age:** 27 **Sex** M **Date:** 10/26/92

Date of Birth: 00/00/65 **Birthplace:** NY **Race:** C **Education:** Some college

Occupation: Unemployed **Accident:** 7/23/92

Armed Services & Type of Discharge: 1982-92 – U. S. Air Force

PAST HISTORY:

1.	Did you have a normal birth?	<u>Yes</u>	No
	a) forceps used?	Yes	<u>No</u>
	b) cesarean section?	Yes	<u>No</u>
2.	Did you have problems with bedwetting?	Yes	<u>No</u>
	a) If yes, age bedwetting stopped		______
3.	Were you car sick as a child (motion)?	Yes	<u>No</u>
	a) If yes, how severe? Slight	Moderate	Severe
4.	Did you have unexplained abdominal cramps as a child?	Yes	<u>No</u>
5.	Did you have any of the following illnesses in childhood?		
	a) meningitis	Yes	<u>No</u>
	b) encephalitis	Yes	<u>No</u>
	c) scarlet fever	Yes	<u>No</u>
	d) rheumatic fever	Yes	<u>No</u>
6.	Did you have any head injuries as a child?	Yes	<u>No</u>
	a) If yes, please explain: ______		
7.	Were you treated for emotional illness as a child?	Yes	<u>No</u>

HABITS:

8.	Do you drink alcohol?	<u>Yes</u>	No
	a) If yes, what kind and how much? 2 beers a week		
	b) Does alcohol bring on or aggravate a headache?	Yes	<u>No</u>
9.	Do you smoke?	Yes	<u>No</u>
	a) If yes, how much? ______		
	b) Does smoking or smoke-filled rooms cause or aggravate headaches?	Yes	<u>No</u>
10.	Do you drink caffeinated beverages?	<u>Yes</u>	No
	a) If yes, how much? Couple times a day		

MENSTRUAL HISTORY:

At what age did menses begin?______ Were they regular or irregular?______

How were they related to your headache?______

Are you or were you ever on Birth Control Pills?______ Did they affect your headache? ______

Have you had a hysterectomy, partial or total, and why?______

Are you in menopause, and if yes, how long?______

Are you on hormones, and if yes, which ones?______

HEADACHE ASSESSMENT FORM

HA PROFILE	INCAPACITATING #3	INTERFERING #2	IRRITATING #1
ONSET (Years ago and frequency)	2-3 days after accident, every night after accident	Day of accident Every day	Early teens, one a month
CURRENT FREQUENCY	Every day	Every day, increases to a #3 in evening	Not now
TIME OF ONSET	Later in the day	Awaken with	Anytime
DURATION	1 to 2 hours	Constant	1 hr. with OTC medication
CHARACTER	Throbbing	Throbbing	Dull ache
PRODROME OR AURA	Sees "little bugs" with #3 headache, blurred vision	Vision problem if turns head	N/A
ASSOCIATING FEATURES	Nausea; Vomiting; Sensitivity to Light? Noise? Odors? Do you get pale or flush? Do your eyes or nose run? Does your nose get stuffy? Does the white of your eyes get red? Does your eyelid droop? Do you pace, or go to bed?	Nausea; Vomiting; Sensitivity to Light? Noise? Odors? Do you get pale or flush? Do your eyes or nose run? Does your nose get stuffy? Does the white of your eyes get red? Does your eyelid droop? Do you pace, or go to bed?	Nausea; Vomiting; Sensitivity to Light? Noise? Odors? Do you get pale or flush? Do your eyes or nose run? Does your nose get stuffy? Does the white of your eyes get red? Does your eyelid droop? Do you pace, or go to bed?
PRECIPITATING OR AGGRAVATING FEATURES		N/A	N/A

LOCATION: Mark the location for each type of headache with a different color pen.

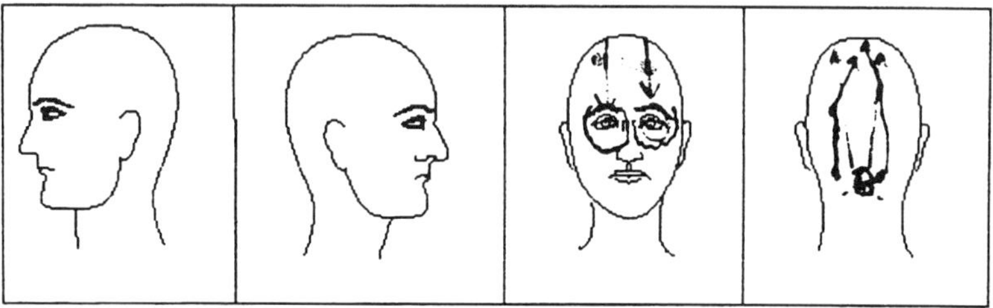

MEDICAL HISTORY:

Have you ever been or are you currently being treated for any of the following?

a) high blood pressure	Yes	No
b) stomach ulcers	Yes	No
c) asthma	Yes	No
d) allergies	Yes	No
e) pneumonia	Yes	No
f) kidney problems	Yes	No
g) low blood sugar	Yes	No
h) glaucoma	Yes	No
i) diabetes	Yes	No
j) heart problems	Yes	No

If you answered yes to any of the above, please describe: Gastritis last 10 years.

List all other medical problems you have had in the past. Include date diagnosed and treatment.
DO NOT LIST OPERATIONS

Stomach pain (gastritis) 1983 – 1991. Blood pressure increased since accident.

SURGICAL HISTORY (List operations and dates performed)

Cyst removed from back 1987.

PSYCHIATRIC HISTORY (List visits with counselors, psychologists, etc., and type of treatment)

ACCIDENTS IN ADULT LIFE (Briefly describe any accident that caused any blow to the head or that you feel is related to your headache)

Driving with seatbelt. Stopped to make a left turn, rear-ended and shoved into lane of oncoming traffic into another car. Dazed. Taken to ER, x-rayed, and released. Headaches began that day.

FAMILY HISTORY:

1. Is your father living? Yes No
   - Age________
   - Cause of death Heart, 55
   - Was there a headache history? Yes No
2. Is your mother living? Yes No
   - Age 49
   - Cause of death________
   - Was there a headache history? Yes No

3. Ages of brothers---Circle the ones with headache
   ___30___________________________
4. Ages of sisters---Circle the ones with headache
   ____
5. List any other blood relatives with a history of severe headaches.
   ___None_________________________

MARITAL HISTORY:
List marriages:

1st marriage age _22_ to _27_	Did spouse have headaches?	Yes	<u>No</u>
2nd marriage age ____ to ____	Did spouse have headaches?	Yes	No
3rd marriage age ____ to ____	Did spouse have headaches?	Yes	No

Age of current spouse:__________

List ages and sex of all children:

Age _5_ Sex _M_ Headaches?	Yes	<u>No</u>
Age ____ Sex ____ Headaches?	Yes	No
Age ____ Sex ____ Headaches?	Yes	No
Age ____ Sex ____ Headaches?	Yes	No

STRESS FACTORS:

List any factors that may be affecting your headaches (money, loneliness, sexual problems, work, etc.)
___Work problems___________________________
____

VEGETATIVE SIGNS:

1.	Do you have trouble falling asleep?	<u>Yes</u>	No
2.	Do you have trouble staying asleep?	Yes	<u>No</u>
3.	Has your appetite decreased?	<u>Yes</u>	No
4.	Have you gained or lost weight in the past year?	<u>Yes</u>	No
5.	Have you felt tearful or depressed lately?	Yes	<u>No</u>
6.	Have you had any thoughts of wanting to die?	Yes	<u>No</u>
7.	Have you been forgetful lately?	Yes	<u>No</u>
8.	Any other changes in your normal day-to-day living?__________		

Please list any medications you are allergic or sensitive to:___None.___________
____
____

Please list any medications you are currently taking (including dosages and frequency per day):
___Robaxin 750 mg. 2, twice a day. Lorcet, 1 three times a day. Relafen 1 three times a day.___
___Flexeril 1 three times a day.___
____

PREVIOUS CARE:

1. List doctors who have treated you for headaches: Dr. B, Dr. C.

2. List any tests you have had for your headache (e.g., EEG, CT scan, MRI, X-Ray, etc.):
X-rays. MRI.

3. List any other treatment you have had for your headache (e.g., biofeedback, acupuncture, chiropractic, or any other treatment you had):
Chiropractic (no help). Trigger point injections (no help).

PAULA
Category: Whiplash

On her headache intake form, this 26-year-old married, pregnant women reports that as the driver of her vehicle, she was waiting for a car in front of her to turn when she was struck from behind by a second vehicle traveling approximately 30 miles per hour. She was wearing seat restraints, with both hands on the wheel, looking straight ahead, and was unaware of the impending crash. The patient recalls her head snapping backward and forward, but does not remember striking any other part of the car interior. She did not lose consciousness and did not go to the hospital. She awoke the next day extremely sore, and was examined in a hospital where she was diagnosed as having severe muscle strain and was released. She was seeing a chiropractor for neck strain.

Interestingly enough, at the time of the accident she was 5 months pregnant, with no injury to the fetus; but, after she delivered the baby, she noticed that her headaches became more severe.

Incapacitating headaches: The patient stated that these started in her early twenties. They occurred only once in awhile, perhaps several times a year. Since the delivery of the baby, she had been having them for several weeks. They can last for 10 to 12 hours, and she has typical symptoms of a vascular or migraine-type headache, which is throbbing. It can start either on the right or the left and seems to begin in the posterior or back of her neck and work its way forward. Once it gets extremely severe, the entire head is involved and, again, she has symptoms of migraine with vomiting, nausea, light sensitivity, noise sensitivity, and her face becomes pale. She also has sensitivity to various odors that cause her headaches to get worse. Her eyes run or lacrimate. There is nasal stuffiness, her eyes become red, and she has to go to bed. Coughing and sneezing will make her headaches worse. These are all typical of the migraine sufferer.

Interfering headaches are moderate to severe. She says that these started in her teenage years, and she would have one perhaps every several weeks. However, since the birth of the baby, she has been having them daily. They are similar to the incapacitating headaches, except that she can perform certain duties even though the pain is severe. She does not complain of the irritating or annoying headaches.

Family history reveals that her mother suffered interfering headaches. This is a patient who again, like many other patients, has occasional migraine-type headaches, or migraine. As a result of the whiplash, the headaches increase in frequency. The patient who continues to have these chronic type problems might be classified in the category of cervicogenic headache, because there may have been an inflammation of the facet joint, as described in the chapter on cervicogenic headache, that will become a chronic situation.

MEDICAL HEADACHE HISTORY

Name: Paula **Age:** 26 **Sex** F **Date:** 10/15/92

Date of Birth: 00/00/66 **Birthplace:** MD **Race:** C **Education:** 2 yrs college

Occupation: Homemaker **Accident:** 4/12/91

Armed Services & Type of Discharge: N/A

PAST HISTORY:

1.	Did you have a normal birth?		Yes	No
	a) forceps used?		Yes	No
	b) cesarean section?		Yes	No
2.	Did you have problems with bedwetting?		Yes	No
	a) If yes, age bedwetting stopped		______	
3.	Were you car sick as a child (motion)?		Yes	No
	a) If yes, how severe?	Slight	Moderate	Severe
4.	Did you have unexplained abdominal cramps as a child?		Yes	No
5.	Did you have any of the following illnesses in childhood?			
	a) meningitis		Yes	No
	b) encephalitis		Yes	No
	c) scarlet fever		Yes	No
	d) rheumatic fever		Yes	No
6.	Did you have any head injuries as a child?		Yes	No
	a) If yes, please explain:			
7.	Were you treated for emotional illness as a child?		Yes	No

HABITS:

8.	Do you drink alcohol?	Yes	No
	a) If yes, what kind and how much?		
	b) Does alcohol bring on or aggravate a headache?	Yes	No
9.	Do you smoke?	Yes	No
	a) If yes, how much?		
	b) Does smoking or smoke-filled rooms cause or aggravate headaches?	Yes	No
10.	Do you drink caffeinated beverages?	Yes	No
	a) If yes, how much? 2 – 3 a day		

MENSTRUAL HISTORY:

At what age did menses begin? 14 Were they regular or irregular? WNL

How were they related to your headache? Increase headaches

Are you or were you ever on Birth Control Pills? Yes Did they affect your headache? No

Have you had a hysterectomy, partial or total, and why? No

Are you in menopause, and if yes, how long? No

Are you on hormones, and if yes, which ones? No

HEADACHE ASSESSMENT FORM

HA PROFILE	INCAPACITATING #3	INTERFERING #2	IRRITATING #1
ONSET (Years ago and frequency)	Early 20's, occasionally	As a child, occasionally	N/A
CURRENT FREQUENCY	1 – 2 a week	Every day since 10/91	N/A
TIME OF ONSET	Anytime	Awaken with	N/A
DURATION	10 – 12 hours	Constant	N/A
CHARACTER	Throbbing	Same, less intense	N/A
PRODROME OR AURA	N/A	N/A	N/A
ASSOCIATING FEATURES	Nausea: Vomiting: Sensitivity to Light? Noise? Odors? Do you get pale or flush? Do your eyes or nose run? Does your nose get stuffy? Does the white of your eyes get red? Does your eyelid droop? Do you pace, or go to bed?	Nausea: Vomiting: Sensitivity to Light? Noise? Odors? Do you get pale or flush? Do your eyes or nose run? Does your nose get stuffy? Does the white of your eyes get red? Does your eyelid droop? Do you pace, or go to bed?	Nausea: Vomiting: Sensitivity to Light? Noise? Odors? Do you get pale or flush? Do your eyes or nose run? Does your nose get stuffy? Does the white of your eyes get red? Does your eyelid droop? Do you pace, or go to bed?
PRECIPITATING OR AGGRAVATING FEATURES	Heat, coughing, sneezing	N/A	N/A

LOCATION: Mark the location for each type of headache with a different color pen.

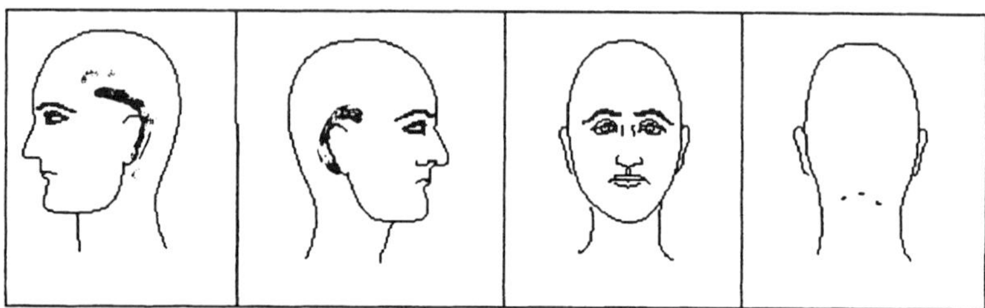

MEDICAL HISTORY:

Have you ever been or are you currently being treated for any of the following?

a) high blood pressure	Yes	No
b) stomach ulcers	Yes	No
c) asthma	Yes	No
d) allergies	Yes	No
e) pneumonia	Yes	No
f) kidney problems	Yes	No
g) low blood sugar	Yes	No
h) glaucoma	Yes	No
i) diabetes	Yes	No
j) heart problems	Yes	No

If you answered yes to any of the above, please describe: Asthma diagnosed as teenager. Allergies are environmental. Pneumonia as a child. Last kidney infection 1½ years ago.

List all other medical problems you have had in the past. Include date diagnosed and treatment. DO NOT LIST OPERATIONS

None

SURGICAL HISTORY (List operations and dates performed)

None.

PSYCHIATRIC HISTORY (List visits with counselors, psychologists, etc., and type of treatment)

None.

ACCIDENTS IN ADULT LIFE (Briefly describe any accident that caused any blow to the head or that you feel is related to your headache)

Car accident 4/91. Driving with seatbelt. Stopped in traffic and rear-ended by another car. Flexion-extension injury. No change in frequency of headaches until after birth of baby four months later.

FAMILY HISTORY:

1. Is your father living? Yes No
   - Age 62
   - Cause of death cancer
   - Was there a headache history? Yes No
2. Is your mother living? Yes No
   - Age 63
   - Cause of death
   - Was there a headache history? Yes No

3. Ages of brothers---Circle the ones with headache
   37 33
4. Ages of sisters---Circle the ones with headache
   242 41 35
5. List any other blood relatives with a history of severe headaches.
   None

MARITAL HISTORY:
List marriages:

1st marriage age 20 to Present	Did spouse have headaches?	Yes	No
2nd marriage age ______ to ______	Did spouse have headaches?	Yes	No
3rd marriage age ______ to ______	Did spouse have headaches?	Yes	No

Age of current spouse: 30

List ages and sex of all children:

Age 3	Sex F	Headaches? Yes	No
Age 1	Sex M	Headaches? Yes	No
Age _____	Sex ______	Headaches? Yes	No

STRESS FACTORS:

List any factors that may be affecting your headaches (money, loneliness, sexual problems, work, etc.)

____

____

VEGETATIVE SIGNS:

1.	Do you have trouble falling asleep?	Yes	No
2.	Do you have trouble staying asleep?	Yes	No
3.	Has your appetite decreased?	Yes	No
4.	Have you gained or lost weight in the past year?	Yes	No
5.	Have you felt tearful or depressed lately?	Yes	No
6.	Have you had any thoughts of wanting to die?	Yes	No
7.	Have you been forgetful lately?	Yes	No
8.	Any other changes in your normal day-to-day living?______		

Please list any medications you are allergic or sensitive to: NKA

____

Please list any medications you are currently taking (including dosages and frequency per day):
Naprosyn 375 mg twice a day; Amitriptyline 25 at bedtime.

____

PREVIOUS CARE:

1. List doctors who have treated you for headaches: Dr. S. , Dr. D., Dr. E.

2. List any tests you have had for your headache (e.g., EEG, CT scan, MRI, X-Ray, etc.):
CAT scan – several years ago.
MRI of brain – 3 months ago (normal).

3. List any other treatment you have had for your headache (e.g., biofeedback, acupuncture, chiropractic, or any other treatment you had):
Chiropractic (helps temporarily). Medication. TMJ splint (helps).

RICHARD
Category: Whiplash

This is a 28-year-old man who was in an accident almost a year before he saw me. He was driving, wearing a seatbelt, and was stopped due to a stalled vehicle and was rear-ended by another car. The patient felt that the other car was going about 45 mph. He did not hit his head, and this looked like a typical acceleration/deceleration or whiplash accident. He stated that prior to the accident he had an occasional mild headache.

Interfering headaches (moderate to severe): These headaches started the day of the accident. He states he currently gets these headaches daily and they are constant, throbbing, and pressure pain in the posterior occipital region on the right side, and radiate to the front of the head. He says that sometimes changing position might cause the headaches, but these headaches can start at any time and occasionally these headaches will become incapacitating for several minutes. This can happen multiple times during the day.

Although this patient's record is in the chapter on whiplash, this could also be placed in the chapter on cervicogenic headaches, because that is most likely the origin of the headache and why the headache has been persistent.

MEDICAL HEADACHE HISTORY

Name: Richard **Age:** 28 **Sex** M **Date:** 5/22/90

Date of Birth: 00/00/62 **Birthplace:** WV **Race:** W **Education:** High school

Occupation: Painter **Accident:** 6/89

Armed Services & Type of Discharge: N/A

PAST HISTORY:

1.	Did you have a normal birth?		Yes (underlined)	No
	a) forceps used?		Yes	No
	b) cesarean section?		Yes	No
2.	Did you have problems with bedwetting?		Yes	No (underlined)
	a) If yes, age bedwetting stopped		______	
3.	Were you car sick as a child (motion)?		Yes	No (underlined)
	a) If yes, how severe?	Slight	Moderate	Severe
4.	Did you have unexplained abdominal cramps as a child?		Yes	No (underlined)
5.	Did you have any of the following illnesses in childhood?			
	a) meningitis		Yes	No (underlined)
	b) encephalitis		Yes	No (underlined)
	c) scarlet fever		Yes	No (underlined)
	d) rheumatic fever		Yes	No (underlined)
6.	Did you have any head injuries as a child?		Yes	No (underlined)
	a) If yes, please explain:______			
7.	Were you treated for emotional illness as a child?		Yes	No (underlined)

HABITS:

8.	Do you drink alcohol?	Yes (underlined)	No
	a) If yes, what kind and how much? 3 – 4 beers a week or less		
	b) Does alcohol bring on or aggravate a headache?	Yes	No (underlined)
9.	Do you smoke?	Yes	No (underlined)
	a) If yes, how much?______		
	b) Does smoking or smoke-filled rooms cause or aggravate headaches?	Yes (underlined)	No
10.	Do you drink caffeinated beverages?	Yes (underlined)	No
	a) If yes, how much? Iced tea, 1 glass a day		

MENSTRUAL HISTORY:

At what age did menses begin?______ Were they regular or irregular?______
How were they related to your headache?______
Are you or were you ever on Birth Control Pills?______ Did they affect your headache? ______
Have you had a hysterectomy, partial or total, and why?______
Are you in menopause, and if yes, how long?______
Are you on hormones, and if yes, which ones?______

HEADACHE ASSESSMENT FORM

HA PROFILE	INCAPACITATING #3	INTERFERING #2	IRRITATING #1
ONSET (Years ago and frequency)		#2 "swells" to #3 occas. Lasts for seconds Day of accident Every day	N/A
CURRENT FREQUENCY		Every day	N/A
TIME OF ONSET		Constant	N/A
DURATION		Constant	N/A
CHARACTER		Throbbing, pressure	N/A
PRODROME OR AURA		N/A	N/A
ASSOCIATING FEATURES	Nausea; Vomiting; Sensitivity to Light? Noise? Odors? Do you get pale or flush? Do your eyes or nose run? Does your nose get stuffy? Does the white of your eyes get red? Does your eyelid droop? Do you pace, or go to bed?	Nausea; Vomiting; Sensitivity to Light? Noise? Odors? Do you get pale or flush? Do your eyes or nose run? Does your nose get stuffy? Does the white of your eyes get red? Does your eyelid droop? Do you pace, or go to bed?	Nausea; Vomiting; Sensitivity to Light? Noise? Odors? Do you get pale or flush? Do your eyes or nose run? Does your nose get stuffy? Does the white of your eyes get red? Does your eyelid droop? Do you pace, or go to bed?
PRECIPITATING OR AGGRAVATING FEATURES		Changing position Not taking medication	N/A

LOCATION: Mark the location for each type of headache with a different color pen.

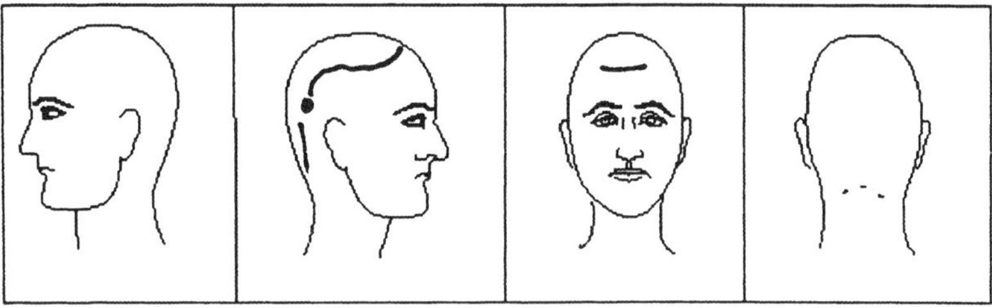

MEDICAL HISTORY:

Have you ever been or are you currently being treated for any of the following?

a) high blood pressure	Yes	No
b) stomach ulcers	Yes	No
c) asthma	Yes	No
d) allergies	Yes	No
e) pneumonia	Yes	No
f) kidney problems	Yes	No
g) low blood sugar	Yes	No
h) glaucoma	Yes	No
i) diabetes	Yes	No
j) heart problems	Yes	No

If you answered yes to any of the above, please describe: Ulcers diagnosed 2 years ago. No problem now.

List all other medical problems you have had in the past. Include date diagnosed and treatment.
DO NOT LIST OPERATIONS
Bad earaches as a child around 1972 to 1974.

SURGICAL HISTORY (List operations and dates performed)
Appendix removed at age 5.

PSYCHIATRIC HISTORY (List visits with counselors, psychologists, etc., and type of treatment)
None.

ACCIDENTS IN ADULT LIFE (Briefly describe any accident that caused any blow to the head or that you feel is related to your headache)
Rear end collision. Driving with seat belt. Stopped due to a stalled vehicle and was rear-ended. Flexion-tension injury. Taken to emergency room, x-rayed and released. Headaches began that day. Occasional headaches before the accident.

FAMILY HISTORY:

1. Is your father living? Yes No
   Age 54
   Cause of death ______
   Was there a headache history? Yes No
2. Is your mother living? Yes No
   Age 54
   Cause of death ______
   Was there a headache history? Yes No

3. Ages of brothers---Circle the ones with headache
   25
4. Ages of sisters---Circle the ones with headache
   21 26 29 31 33
5. List any other blood relatives with a history of severe headaches.
   Unknown

MARITAL HISTORY:

List marriages:

1st marriage age 22 to Present Did spouse have headaches? Yes <u>No</u>
2nd marriage age _____ to _______ Did spouse have headaches? Yes No
3rd marriage age _____ to _______ Did spouse have headaches? Yes No

Age of current spouse: 25

List ages and sex of all children:

Age 5 Sex M Headaches? Yes <u>No</u>
Age 10 mo Sex M Headaches? Yes ? <u>No</u>
Age _____ Sex _____ Headaches? Yes No
Age _____ Sex _____ Headaches? Yes No

STRESS FACTORS:

List any factors that may be affecting your headaches (money, loneliness, sexual problems, work, etc.)
Money, sexual problems.

VEGETATIVE SIGNS:

1. Do you have trouble falling asleep? <u>Yes</u> No
2. Do you have trouble staying asleep? Yes <u>No</u>
3. Has your appetite decreased? <u>Yes</u> No
4. Have you gained or lost weight in the past year? Yes <u>No</u>
5. Have you felt tearful or depressed lately? <u>Yes</u> No
6. Have you had any thoughts of wanting to die? Yes <u>No</u>
7. Have you been forgetful lately? <u>Yes</u> No
8. Any other changes in your normal day-to-day living?_______

Please list any medications you are allergic or sensitive to: None.

Please list any medications you are currently taking (including dosages and frequency per day):
Pamelor 25 mg. every night.

1. List doctors who have treated you for headaches: Dr. S., Dr. G.

2. List any tests you have had for your headache (e.g., EEG, CT scan, MRI, X-Ray, etc.):

X-rays.

CAT scan (without contrast) – 6 months ago (normal).

3. List any other treatment you have had for your headache (e.g., biofeedback, acupuncture, chiropractic, or any other treatment you had):

Physical therapy including massage, heat/cold packs and electrical stimulation (no help).

October 29, 1992

[Doctor's name and address omitted]

RE: BRIAN

Dear Dr. [...]:

Thank you for your referral of Brian [...].

This is a 21-year-old male, born in [...], now living in [...]. He has a high school education and works as a store manager for a convenience store.

The patient states on 00/00/92, he was in an automobile accident while driving with his seatbelt and stopped at a light and was rear-ended by another car. He was not unconscious. He evidently had a flexion extension injury, was taken to the emergency room, examined and released. His headaches began three months ago, almost four months after the accident. He states that he had an occasional irritating headache before the accident.

HEADACHE PROFILE

Incapacitating headaches: He has had two or three since the accident that last one to three days. At any time, it is a throbbing headache in the bilateral periorbital and frontal region. He has had two periods of weakness, blurred vision, amnesia for about fifteen minutes, and then the headaches began with associated features of nausea, photophobia, sonophobia, nasal stuffiness, and he needs to go to bed.

Interfering headaches (moderate to severe): He has been having them daily. He wakes up with them, and they increase during the day to constant pain. It is also somewhat throbbing and in the periorbital and frontal regions of his head. There is no aura, there is some photophobia, sonophobia, and he goes to bed if possible.

Irritating headaches (annoying): Started at age 15; they are rare. He gets one of these a month and he will abort them with over-the-counter medication. It is a slight pressure in the frontal part of his head. There are no associated features.

Past history: Birth was normal. There is no history of enuresis or unexplained abdominal cramps pre-puberty. There is no history of car sickness as a child. There is no history of meningitis. No history of encephalitis, scarlet fever, or rheumatic fever.

Habits: He does not drink; does not smoke.

Medical history: The patient has no history of high blood pressure, stomach ulcers, asthma, allergies, pneumonia, kidney problems, low blood sugar, glaucoma, diabetes, or heart problems.

Review of systems: Pulmonary negative, cardiovascular negative, gastrointestinal negative, urogenital negative.

Surgical history: The patient was operated on by Dr. [...], oral surgeon. He was operated on for what appears to be a temporomandibular joint problem; however, it was described by Dr. [...] as a bilateral sagittal ramus osteotomy rotation and set back and genioplasty augmentation. This was done on 00/00/91. The patient evidently had pain in opening his mouth prior to surgery, and since that time the problem has been corrected. The patient, other than the occasional irritating headache, did not complain of headaches and his surgery was not done for any headache problem.

Psychiatric history: Negative.

Family history: Father living, 44, no headache. Mother living, 41, no headache. There is a 15-year-old brother with no headaches.

Allergies to medication: NKA.

Current medications: Currently taking Hydrocodone 5 mg as needed. He had seen Dr. [...], who put him on Pamelor 10 mg three times a day and he was on that for three days. It did not help and he said it aggravated the back of his neck. He has also had Cafergot tablets, which he said helped at first. He says Midrin helps a little.

Previous work-up: He was seeing Dr. [...], chiropractor, and is having some chiropractic treatments and he sees him periodically now. There is some relief of the tension in his neck, but not of his headaches. He had an EEG, which was normal. He has had x-rays of the back of his neck and head. Dr. [...] read the x-rays of his neck and it revealed retrolisthesis of C3 on C4 and C4 on C5. AP view reveals pedicles intact, no fractures, dislocations, or gross osseous pathology noted. Extension view reveals increase of retrolisthesis of C3 on C4 and C4 on C5. Flexion view reveals majority of flexion occurring at C4–C5 and it read as cervical hyperextension flexion injury to the neck and headache syndrome. He also had lumbar x-rays which, according to Dr. [...], reveal a left antalgic listing and facet tropism to L5–S1, slight disc wedging on L3 on L4. Lateral view shows normal lumbar lordosis, slight decrease in disc height to L5-S1. No fractures, disc location, or gross osteopathology noted. AP thoracic view taken due to thoracolumbar pain and due to left antalgic listing of lumbar AP view. No further curvature noted in thoracics.

Physical examination: The patient is 6'4", 190 pounds, pulse 72, left BP 102/74, right BP 98/70. The face did not show any asymmetry. The temporomandibular joint area was grossly normal. The eyes appeared normal. Conjunctivae were clear and the pupils reacted equally to light and accommodation. Retinal fundus examination revealed no papilledema and no abnormalities with the arteries and veins. There were no bruits over the supraorbital region. The nose appeared normal. The auditory canals were clear and the tympanic membranes appeared intact. The mouth and throat appeared normal. Gums, tongue, buccal mucosa and teeth were grossly normal. The neck was supple and there were no masses felt in the thyroid gland. Carotid bruits could not be heard. Cervical nodes were not enlarged. The lungs were clear to auscultation and percussion. The heart had a regular sinus rhythm with no murmurs. The abdomen was soft and nontender. A rectal examination was not done.

Neurological examination: Cranial nerve II: Visual fields were grossly normal. III, IV and VI: No strabismus, nystagmus or ptosis. V: Normal sensation and corneal reflex. VII: Normal facial movements (wrinkle, frown, smile, and strength of eyelids). VIII: Normal Weber and Rinne. IX and X: Good gag reflex. XI: Normal sternocleidomastoid and trapezius. XII: Normal protrusion and strength of tongue. Cerebellar: Negative Rhomberg. Normal finger-to-nose, diadochokinesis, heel-shin, tandem, and heel and toes walking. Motor system: No atrophy, fasciculations, wasting, or tremors. Good muscle strength in arms, wrists, fingers and legs. Sensory system: Superficial tactile, pain, and vibrations (wrists, elbows, knees, and ankles) were normal. Normal motion and positions of fingers and toes. Normal 2-point discrimination. Reflexes: Normal 2+ reflexes of triceps, biceps, knee jerk, ankle jerk, etc. Normal pulses in dorsalis pedis, posterior tibial and popliteal.

DIAGNOSIS

1. Post traumatic (flexion/extension-whiplash) vascular headaches.
2. Rule out post traumatic (flexion/extension-whiplash) vascular headache with muscle contraction component.
3. Rule out post traumatic (flexion/extension-whiplash) intracranial structural lesion.

IMPRESSION

This is a pleasant 27-year-old male who had a flexion extension injury on 00/00/92. The patient did not start getting these headaches for some time after. The headaches that he has seem to mimic migraine-like headaches and he is having daily headaches that mimic vascular headaches with a muscle contraction component. However, he has discussed the fact that he has had with these headaches periods of weakness, blurred vision, amnesia for about 15 minutes before the headache began. I feel it is extremely important that we rule out any structural lesion as a result of this accident and MRI of his brain is ordered. Also I would like to see if there is any metabolic problem causing his headache and a blood profile will be drawn of a CBC, SMAC-20, ESR, TSH, B-12, folic acid, RPR.

I discussed with the patient that we would not start medication treatment with him until I have the results of all these tests, inasmuch as I am not sure why the headaches started almost four months after the accident. The patient will be seen as soon as the results of these tests are done and a more conclusive diagnosis will be made.

Thank you, once again, for your referral of this very nice patient. If you have any questions, please do not hesitate to call or write.

Sincerely,

BERNARD SWERDLOW, M.D.

These notes were dictated with the patient present.

MEDICAL HEADACHE HISTORY

Name: Brian **Age:** 21 **Sex** M **Date:** 10/29/92

Date of Birth: 00/00/71 **Birthplace:** KY **Race:** W **Education:** High School

Occupation: Store Manager **Accident:** 1992

Armed Services & Type of Discharge: N/A

PAST HISTORY:

1.	Did you have a normal birth?		Yes	No
	a) forceps used?		Yes	No
	b) cesarean section?		Yes	No
2.	Did you have problems with bedwetting?		Yes	No
	a) If yes, age bedwetting stopped			
3.	Were you car sick as a child (motion)?		Yes	No
	a) If yes, how severe?	Slight	Moderate	Severe
4.	Did you have unexplained abdominal cramps as a child?		Yes	No
5.	Did you have any of the following illnesses in childhood?			
	a) meningitis		Yes	No
	b) encephalitis		Yes	No
	c) scarlet fever		Yes	No
	d) rheumatic fever		Yes	No
6.	Did you have any head injuries as a child?		Yes	No
	a) If yes, please explain:			
7.	Were you treated for emotional illness as a child?		Yes	No

HABITS:

8.	Do you drink alcohol?	Yes	No
	a) If yes, what kind and how much?		
	b) Does alcohol bring on or aggravate a headache?	Yes	No
9.	Do you smoke?	Yes	No
	a) If yes, how much?		
	b) Does smoking or smoke-filled rooms cause or aggravate headaches?	Yes	No
10.	Do you drink caffeinated beverages?	Yes	No
	a) If yes, how much?		

MENSTRUAL HISTORY:

At what age did menses begin?______ Were they regular or irregular?______
How were they related to your headache?______
Are you or were you ever on Birth Control Pills?______ Did they affect your headache? ______
Have you had a hysterectomy, partial or total, and why?______
Are you in menopause, and if yes, how long?______
Are you on hormones, and if yes, which ones?______

HEADACHE ASSESSMENT FORM

HA PROFILE	INCAPACITATING #3	INTERFERING #2	IRRITATING #1
ONSET (Years ago and frequency)	2 – 3 since accident	1992, Every day	Age 15, rare
CURRENT FREQUENCY	Anytime	Every day	1 every other month
TIME OF ONSET	Starts anytime	Awakens with, increases during the day	Anytime
DURATION	1 to 3 days	Constant	1 hr. with OTC medication
CHARACTER	Throbbing	Same, less intense	Slight pressure
PRODROME OR AURA	2 periods of weakness, blurred vision, amnesia x 15 min. HA began	N/A	N/A
ASSOCIATING FEATURES	Nausea; Vomiting; Sensitivity to Light? Noise? Odors? Do you get pale or flush? Do your eyes or nose run? Does your nose get stuffy? Does the white of your eyes get red? Does your eyelid droop? Do you pace, or go to bed?	Nausea; Vomiting; Sensitivity to Light? Noise? Odors? Do you get pale or flush? Do your eyes or nose run? Does your nose get stuffy? Does the white of your eyes get red? Does your eyelid droop? Do you pace, or go to bed? If possible	Nausea; Vomiting; Sensitivity to Light? Noise? Odors? Do you get pale or flush? Do your eyes or nose run? Does your nose get stuffy? Does the white of your eyes get red? Does your eyelid droop? Do you pace, or go to bed?
PRECIPITATING OR AGGRAVATING FEATURES	N/A	N/A	N/A

LOCATION: Mark the location for each type of headache with a different color pen.

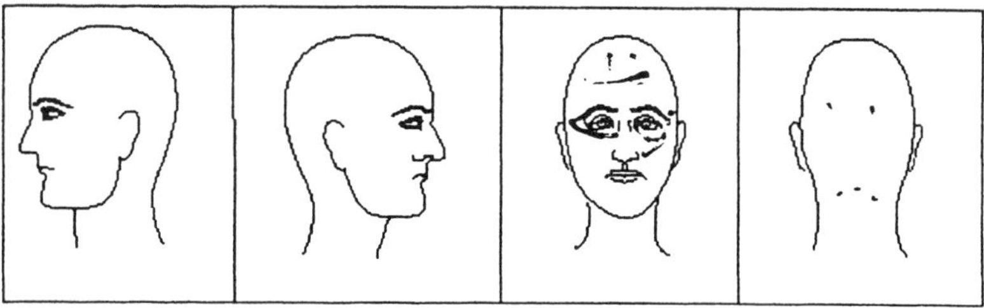

MEDICAL HISTORY:

Have you ever been or are you currently being treated for any of the following?

a) high blood pressure	Yes	No
b) stomach ulcers	Yes	No
c) asthma	Yes	No
d) allergies	Yes	No
e) pneumonia	Yes	No
f) kidney problems	Yes	No
g) low blood sugar	Yes	No
h) glaucoma	Yes	No
i) diabetes	Yes	No
j) heart problems	Yes	No

If you answered yes to any of the above, please describe:____________________

List all other medical problems you have had in the past. Include date diagnosed and treatment.
DO NOT LIST OPERATIONS

None.

SURGICAL HISTORY (List operations and dates performed)

Bilateral sagittal ramus osteotomy rotation and setback. Genioplasty augmentation.

PSYCHIATRIC HISTORY (List visits with counselors, psychologists, etc., and type of treatment)

None.

ACCIDENTS IN ADULT LIFE (Briefly describe any accident that caused any blow to the head or that you feel is related to your headache)

1992 - Driving with seat belt. Stopped at light and was rear-ended by another car. Not unconscious. Flexion-extension injury. Taken to emergency room, examined and released. Headaches began in July. Occasional #1 headache before accident.

FAMILY HISTORY:

1. Is your father living? Yes No
   - Age 44
   - Cause of death________________
   - Was there a headache history? Yes No
2. Is your mother living? Yes No
   - Age 41
   - Cause of death________________
   - Was there a headache history? Yes No

3. Ages of brothers---Circle the ones with headache
   15
4. Ages of sisters---Circle the ones with headache
   None
5. List any other blood relatives with a history of severe headaches.
   None

MARITAL HISTORY:
List marriages:

1st marriage age _____ to _______ Did spouse have headaches? Yes No
2nd marriage age _____ to _______ Did spouse have headaches? Yes No
3rd marriage age _____ to _______ Did spouse have headaches? Yes No
Age of current spouse: N/A

List ages and sex of all children:
Age _____ Sex ______ Headaches? Yes No
Age _____ Sex ______ Headaches? Yes No
Age _____ Sex ______ Headaches? Yes No
Age _____ Sex ______ Headaches? Yes No

STRESS FACTORS:

List any factors that may be affecting your headaches (money, loneliness, sexual problems, work, etc.)
____
____

VEGETATIVE SIGNS:

1. Do you have trouble falling asleep? Yes No
2. Do you have trouble staying asleep? Yes No
3. Has your appetite decreased? Yes No
4. Have you gained or lost weight in the past year? Yes No
5. Have you felt tearful or depressed lately? Yes No
6. Have you had any thoughts of wanting to die? Yes No
7. Have you been forgetful lately? Yes No
8. Any other changes in your normal day-to-day living?________________

Please list any medications you are allergic or sensitive to: None.
____
____

Please list any medications you are currently taking (including dosages and frequency per day):
Hydrocodone 5 mg, as needed.
____
____

PREVIOUS CARE:

1. List doctors who have treated you for headaches: Dr. R.

2. List any tests you have had for your headache (e.g., EEG, CT scan, MRI, X-Ray, etc.):

X-rays.

EEG.

3. List any other treatment you have had for your headache (e.g., biofeedback, acupuncture, chiropractic, or any other treatment you had):

Chiropractic.

July 19, 1993

[Doctor's name and address omitted)

RE: JENNIFER

Dear Dr. [...]:

Thank you for the referral of Ms. Jennifer [...].

This is a 17-year-old female born 00/00/75 in [...]. She has a high school education and was working at [...] until she had an accident on 00/00/93. Since that time, she has not been able to work because of her pain.

On 00/00/93, she was driving, wearing a seat belt. It was raining, and while slowing down for the car in front of her, she was rear-ended. This caused a chain reaction and her car was hit twice in the rear. She hit the car in front also. The patient had a flexion extension injury and was not unconscious. She went to the emergency room the next day, was x-rayed, treated, and released. The patient's headaches started the day of the accident, and she states that she did not have headaches prior to the accident.

HEADACHE PROFILE

Incapacitating headaches: These started the night of the accident, and she was getting them two days a week. The patient is currently getting them one day a week and they last for at least an hour. The character of the pain is throbbing and pressure, and the pain starts in the posterior occipital region and travels cephalad to the front of her head and also to the periorbital regions. There is no prodrome or aura. Associated features are nausea, photophobia, phonophobia, and she will go to bed. Any kind of exertion can make it worse.

Interfering headaches (moderate to severe): These started three months after the accident, and she would get these two to three days a week. The patient is currently getting these headaches daily. These attacks last thirty minutes to an hour, and they are somewhat less intense. The location of pain is the same as just described. There is no aura and associated features are sometimes photophobia, and she will go to bed if possible.

Irritating headaches (annoying): N/A.

Menstrual history: Began at age 14 and has always been irregular. The patient was on birth control pills at age 16 for one year, with no adverse effects.

Past history: The patient was most probably a normal delivery. There is no history of enuresis or unexplained abdominal cramps pre-puberty. There is no history of car sickness as a child. There is no history of meningitis, encephalitis, scarlet fever, or rheumatic fever. There were no head injuries as a child.

Habits: She does not drink and does not smoke.

Medical history: The patient was diagnosed as having asthma four years ago and is taking medications for that, and she has some environmental allergies. The rest of her medical history is essentially negative.

Review of systems: Cardiovascular negative, gastrointestinal negative, urogenital negative.

Surgical history: Negative.

Psychiatric history: Negative.

Family history: Her father is living, age 48, with no headache history. Her mother is living, age 49, with no headache history. There is a 20-year-old brother with no headache history. The patient is not married and does not have any children.

Current medications: The patient only takes medications for her asthma, Beconase, etc., and inhalers.

Doctors seen in the past for headaches: She sees a Dr. [...] for her asthma.

Treatments tried in the past: The patient is currently in physical therapy prescribed by you that seems to help her back, but does not help her headache.

Physical examination: Height 5'3", weight 108 pounds, pulse 78, left BP 122/80, right BP 122/82. The face did not show any asymmetry. The temporomandibular joint area was grossly normal. The eyes appeared normal. Conjunctivae were clear and the pupils reacted equally to light and accommodation. Retinal fundus examination revealed no papilledema and no abnormalities with the arteries and veins. There were no bruits over the supraorbital region. The nose appeared normal. The auditory canals were clear and the tympanic membranes appeared intact. The mouth and throat appeared normal. Gums, tongue, buccal mucosa and teeth were grossly normal. There were exquisitely tender myofascial trigger points in the upper left splenius capitis and longissimus capitis areas, and there were less painful trigger points in the right side in the same area. Carotid bruits could not be heard. Cervical nodes were not enlarged. The lungs were clear to auscultation and percussion. The heart had a regular sinus rhythm with no murmurs. The abdomen was soft and nontender.

Neurological examination: Cranial nerve II: Visual fields were grossly normal. III, IV and VI: No strabismus, nystagmus, or ptosis. V: Normal sensation and corneal reflex. VII: Normal facial movements (wrinkle, frown, smile, and strength of eyelids). VIII: Normal Weber and Rinne. IX and X: Good gag reflex. XI: Normal sternocleidomastoid and trapezius. XII: Normal protrusion and strength of tongue. Cerebellar: Negative Rhomberg. Normal finger-to-nose, diadochokinesis, heel-shin, tandem, and heel and toes walking. Motor system: No atrophy, fasciculations, wasting, or tremors. Good muscle strength in arms, wrists, fingers, and legs. Sensory system: Superficial tactile, pain, and vibrations (wrists, elbows, knees, and ankles) were normal. Normal motion and positions of fingers and toes. Normal 2-point discrimination. Reflexes: Normal 1+ reflexes of triceps, biceps, knee jerk, ankle jerk, etc. Normal pulses in dorsalis pedis, posterior tibial and popliteal.

DIAGNOSIS

1. Post traumatic (flexion/extension-whiplash) daily headache.
2. Post traumatic vascular headache.
3. Post traumatic muscle contraction headache with myofascial trigger points.
4. Rule out post whiplash-cervicogenic headache.

IMPRESSION

This pleasant 17-year-old woman comes in with daily headaches since she had an accident on 00/00/93. Her headaches have both components of being vascular with the throbbing and gastrointestinal and neurogenic features, and also muscle contraction with the myofascial trigger points.

I feel that the patient should be medicated to see if we can help reduce some of the headaches, and she will be placed on Cardizem 30 mg t.i.d., Parafon Forte t.i.d., and Midrin to help abort her headaches. The patient will also be set up to do a posterior cervical regional block of C1, 2 and 3 on the left side, which I think will be very beneficial in helping to reduce her pain and problems, and getting her back to functioning again. This will all be set up.

If the cervicogenic component is felt to be addressed, then consideration for a cervical facet block with fluoroscopic guidance would be considered.

Thank you once again for the referral of this very pleasant patient. If there are any questions, please do not hesitate to call or write, and further reports will be sent to you.

Sincerely,

BERNARD SWERDLOW, M.D.

These notes were dictated with the patient present.

MEDICAL HEADACHE HISTORY

Name: Jennifer **Age:** 17 **Sex** F **Date:** 7/19/93

Date of Birth: 00/00/75 **Birthplace:** FL **Race:** W **Education:** High school

Occupation: Not working at present **Accident:** 00/00/93

Armed Services & Type of Discharge: N/A

PAST HISTORY:

1.	Did you have a normal birth?		Yes	No
	a) forceps used?		Yes	No
	b) cesarean section?		Yes	No
2.	Did you have problems with bedwetting?		Yes	No
	a) If yes, age bedwetting stopped		______	
3.	Were you car sick as a child (motion)?		Yes	No
	a) If yes, how severe?	Slight	Moderate	Severe
4.	Did you have unexplained abdominal cramps as a child?		Yes	No
5.	Did you have any of the following illnesses in childhood?			
	a) meningitis		Yes	No
	b) encephalitis		Yes	No
	c) scarlet fever		Yes	No
	d) rheumatic fever		Yes	No
6.	Did you have any head injuries as a child?		Yes	No
	a) If yes, please explain: ______			
7.	Were you treated for emotional illness as a child?		Yes	No

HABITS:

8.	Do you drink alcohol?	Yes	No
	a) If yes, what kind and how much? ______		
	b) Does alcohol bring on or aggravate a headache?	Yes	No
9.	Do you smoke?	Yes	No
	a) If yes, how much? ______		
	b) Does smoking or smoke-filled rooms cause or aggravate headaches?	Yes	No
10.	Do you drink caffeinated beverages?	Yes	No
	a) If yes, how much? ______		

MENSTRUAL HISTORY:

At what age did menses begin? 14 Were they regular or irregular? Irregular
How were they related to your headache? N/A
Are you or were you ever on Birth Control Pills? Yes Did they affect your headache? No
Have you had a hysterectomy, partial or total, and why? No
Are you in menopause, and if yes, how long? No
Are you on hormones, and if yes, which ones? No

HEADACHE ASSESSMENT FORM

HA PROFILE	INCAPACITATING #3	INTERFERING #2	IRRITATING #1
ONSET (Years ago and frequency)	Night of the accident 2 days a week	3 months after accident 2 – 3 days a week	N/A
CURRENT FREQUENCY	1 a week	Every day 1 – 5 every day	N/A
TIME OF ONSET	Anytime	Anytime	N/A
DURATION	1 hour	30 min. – 1 hour	N/A
CHARACTER	Throbbing and pressure	Same, less intense	N/A
PRODROME OR AURA	N/A	N/A	N/A
ASSOCIATING FEATURES	Nausea; Vomiting; Sensitivity to Light? Noise? Odors? Do you get pale or flush? Do your eyes or nose run? Does your nose get stuffy? Does the white of your eyes get red? Does your eyelid droop? Do you pace, or go to bed?	Nausea; Vomiting; Sensitivity to Light? Noise? Odors? Do you get pale or flush? Do your eyes or nose run? Does your nose get stuffy? Does the white of your eyes get red? Does your eyelid droop? Do you pace, or go to bed?	Nausea; Vomiting; Sensitivity to Light? Noise? Odors? Do you get pale or flush? Do your eyes or nose run? Does your nose get stuffy? Does the white of your eyes get red? Does your eyelid droop? Do you pace, or go to bed?
PRECIPITATING OR AGGRAVATING FEATURES	Sneezing	N/A	N/A

LOCATION: Mark the location for each type of headache with a different color pen.

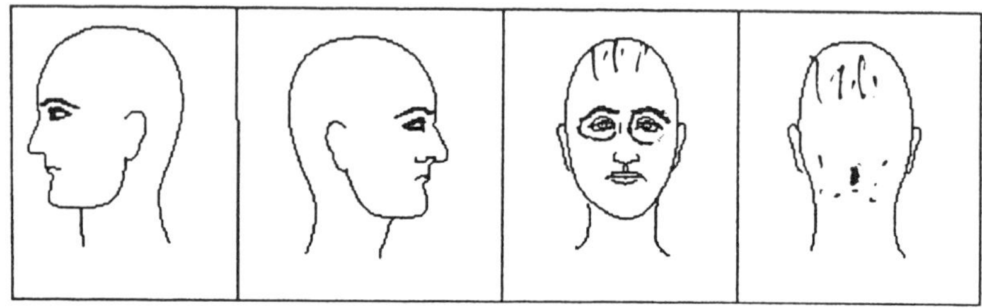

MEDICAL HISTORY:

Have you ever been or are you currently being treated for any of the following?

a) high blood pressure	Yes	No
b) stomach ulcers	Yes	No
c) asthma	Yes	No
d) allergies	Yes	No
e) pneumonia	Yes	No
f) kidney problems	Yes	No
g) low blood sugar	Yes	No
h) glaucoma	Yes	No
i) diabetes	Yes	No
j) heart problems	Yes	No

If you answered yes to any of the above, please describe: Asthma diagnosed 4 years ago. Taking medication. Environmental allergies.

List all other medical problems you have had in the past. Include date diagnosed and treatment.
DO NOT LIST OPERATIONS

Asthma.

SURGICAL HISTORY (List operations and dates performed)

None.

PSYCHIATRIC HISTORY (List visits with counselors, psychologists, etc., and type of treatment)

None.

ACCIDENTS IN ADULT LIFE (Briefly describe any accident that caused any blow to the head or that you feel is related to your headache)

Car accident 1993. Driving with seatbelt. Raining. While slowing down for car in front of me, I was rear-ended. This caused a chain reaction and my car was hit twice in rear. I hit car in front. Flexion extension injury. Went to emergency room the next day, x-rayed, treated, and released. Headaches started the day of the accident. No headaches before accident.

FAMILY HISTORY:

1. Is your father living? Yes No
   - Age 48
   - Cause of death __________
   - Was there a headache history? Yes No
2. Is your mother living? Yes No
   - Age 49
   - Cause of death __________
   - Was there a headache history? Yes No

3. Ages of brothers---Circle the ones with headache
   ____20____________________________________
4. Ages of sisters---Circle the ones with headache
   ____None__________________________________
5. List any other blood relatives with a history of severe headaches.
   ____None__________________________________

MARITAL HISTORY:
List marriages:

1st marriage age ______ to ______	Did spouse have headaches?	Yes	No
2nd marriage age ______ to ______	Did spouse have headaches?	Yes	No
3rd marriage age ______ to ______	Did spouse have headaches?	Yes	No

Age of current spouse:___________

List ages and sex of all children:

Age _____ Sex ______	Headaches?	Yes	No
Age _____ Sex ______	Headaches?	Yes	No
Age _____ Sex ______	Headaches?	Yes	No

STRESS FACTORS:

List any factors that may be affecting your headaches (money, loneliness, sexual problems, work, etc.)
____Tiredness, stress, when my back and neck hurts.______________________________
____

VEGETATIVE SIGNS:

1.	Do you have trouble falling asleep?	Yes	No (underlined)
2.	Do you have trouble staying asleep?	Yes (underlined)	No
3.	Has your appetite decreased?	Yes (underlined)	No
4.	Have you gained or lost weight in the past year?	Yes	No (underlined)
5.	Have you felt tearful or depressed lately?	Yes	No (underlined)
6.	Have you had any thoughts of wanting to die?	Yes	No (underlined)
7.	Have you been forgetful lately?	Yes	No (underlined)
8.	Any other changes in your normal day-to-day living?___________________		

Please list any medications you are allergic or sensitive to:___None_____________________
____

Please list any medications you are currently taking (including dosages and frequency per day):
____Beconase and inhaler for asthma.____
____

PREVIOUS CARE:

1. List doctors who have treated you for headaches: Dr. S.

2. List any tests you have had for your headache (e.g., EEG, CT scan, MRI, X-Ray, etc.):
None

3. List any other treatment you have had for your headache (e.g., biofeedback, acupuncture, chiropractic, or any other treatment you had):
Physical therapy.

October 6, 1993

[Doctor's name and address omitted]

RE: CHRISTINA

Dear Dr. [...]:

Thank you for the referral of Ms. Christina [...].

This is a 23-year-old female born 00/00/69 in Florida. She is a homemaker.

She was in an accident on 00/00/93, where she was driving, wearing her seat belt, and another car pulled out in front of her and hit her car in the passenger side. The patient was thrown sideways, did not hit her head. She saw a physician the next day. The patient states that she had rare annoying headaches prior to the accident. Her other type of headaches started immediately after the accident.

HEADACHE PROFILE

Incapacitating headaches: The patient had one attack in 00/93, while she was eight months pregnant. Since that attack, the patient has not had any further incapacitating headaches. At that time her headache lasted 12 hours. It was severe throbbing in the frontal and occipital portions of her head. There was no aura and there was some nausea, photophobia, phonophobia, pallor, and she went to bed. Movement made that headache worse.

Interfering headaches (moderate to severe): These headaches started the day of the accident on 00/00/93, and she has had them daily ever since. It is a constant headache, it is throbbing, and it is in the frontal and occipital regions and the cervical area. There is no aura. With these headaches, the patient has severe nausea, sometimes photophobia, phonophobia, sensitivity to odors, she passes out four to five times a week in any place, and she complains of dizziness. She will go to bed with these headaches. Any kind of quick movement or changing position can exacerbate these headaches.

Irritating headaches (annoying): These headaches started at age 17 and they were occasional. The patient has not had any of these headaches since 1991. The patient was able to abort these headaches with over-the-counter medication in one hour. It was a dull ache with no associated features.

Menstrual history: Began at age 12 and has been regular. The patient was on birth control pills from age 15 to age 16 with no adverse effects. She did not have a history of having headaches with her menstrual periods.

Past history: The patient was most probably a normal delivery. There is no history of enuresis or unexplained abdominal cramps pre-puberty. There is a history of some slight car sickness as a child. There is no history of meningitis, encephalitis, scarlet fever, or rheumatic fever. There were no head injuries as a child.

Habits: She does not drink and does not smoke.

Medical history: The patient had suffered with situational anxiety in 1987. She did discuss that she had some vascular headaches during her pregnancy one time and possibly at age 17, but she has had none of those headaches since 1991. The patient has some lower back pain from the accident. The rest of her medical history is essentially negative.

Review of systems: Pulmonary negative, cardiovascular negative, gastrointestinal negative, urogenital negative.

Surgical history: The patient had a D&C for a miscarriage in 1991.

Psychiatric history: Negative.

Family history: Her father is living, age 42, and has a history of severe headaches. Her mother is living, age 42, with no headache history. There is a 20-year-old brother with no headache history. The patient has been married from age 18 to present. There are two children, a 4-year-old boy with no headaches, and a 6-month-old girl.

Stress factors: The patient states that since the accident, she has been under stress because she cannot function as she did prior to the accident.

Allergies to medications: The patient stated that Inderal caused her "heart to stop." In 1988, the patient went to a walk-in clinic and was placed on Inderal. She hallucinated and she says that her heart stopped or she blacked out; she is not sure. Morphine causes nausea and vomiting.

Current medications: The patient is currently taking Roxicet as needed, which she says increases her headache, Tylenol #3 as needed, Flexeril as needed, and Tigan as needed. In previous years, she was on Doxepin. Since the accident, the patient has been on Flexeril, Percocet, Tylenol #3. She also had Midrin for the previous headache that she had and that helped.

Doctors seen in the past for headaches: She saw a Dr. [...] 5½ years ago and attended a clinic 4½ years ago. The patient also saw Dr. [...], orthopedic specialist, at the clinic and he ordered an MRI of her lower back. That was in 1993. She had an anxiety attack as a result of that test.

Tests done in the past: No other tests have been done.

Treatments tried in the past: The patient is currently having chiropractic treatment.

Physical examination: Height 5'4", weight 120 pounds, pulse 80, left BP 110/70, right BP 116/72. The face did not show any asymmetry. The temporomandibular joint area was grossly normal. The eyes appeared normal. Conjunctivae were clear and the pupils reacted equally to light and accommodation. Retinal fundus examination revealed no papilledema and no abnormalities with the arteries and veins. There were no bruits over the supraorbital region. The nose appeared normal. The auditory canals were clear and the tympanic membranes appeared intact. The mouth and throat appeared normal. Gums, tongue, buccal mucosa and teeth were grossly normal. There were multiple myofascial trigger points in the middle and upper trapezius region. Carotid bruits could not be heard. Cervical nodes were not enlarged. The lungs were clear to auscultation and percussion. The heart had a regular sinus rhythm with no murmurs. The abdomen was soft and nontender. A rectal or vaginal exam was not done.

Neurological examination: Cranial nerve II: Visual fields were grossly normal. III, IV, and VI: No strabismus, nystagmus, or ptosis. V: Normal sensation and corneal reflex. VII. Normal facial movements (wrinkle, frown, smile, and strength of eyelids). VIII: Normal Weber and Rinne. IX and X: Good gag reflex. XI: Normal sternocleidomastoid and trapezius. XII: Normal protrusion and strength of tongue. Cerebellar: Negative Rhomberg. Normal finger-to-nose, diadochokinesis, heel-shin, tandem, and heel and toes walking. Motor system: No atrophy, fasciculations, wasting, or tremors. Right hand appears to be weaker than the left. Good muscle strength in arms, wrists, fingers and legs. Sensory system: The patient states that her right hand and arm get numb with a heat sensation and then some paresthesia or tingling. Using a brush stroke, patient had more sensation in her left arm than her right arm, although there was some sensation in the right arm. Superficial tactile, pain, and vibrations (wrists, elbows, knees, and ankles) were normal. Normal motion and positions of fingers and toes. Normal 2-point discrimination. Reflexes: Normal 2+ reflexes of triceps, biceps, knee jerk, ankle jerk, etc. Normal pulses in dorsalis pedis, posterior tibial and popliteal.

DIAGNOSES

1. Post traumatic (flexion/extension-whiplash) daily vascular headache.
2. Post traumatic (flexion/extension-whiplash) daily muscle contraction headache with myofascial trigger points.
3. Post traumatic (flexion/extension-whiplash) exacerbation of pre-existing rare migraine.
4. Post traumatic (flexion/extension-whiplash) sensory changes in right arm.

IMPRESSION

This pleasant 23-year-old woman comes in who was in an accident on 00/00/93. There was evidently a flexion extension injury, and since that time she has been having daily vascular headaches and muscle contraction headaches that are anywhere from moderate to severe where she will have to lie down. There was a history of her having several migraine attacks previously, but they were very rare. According to the patient, she had one attack in 12/88 and that ran through the early part of 1991 and then stopped. Then, later on the patient was pregnant and miscarried and was upset about this and had stopped eating. She then had headaches for about two months and then they again went into remission in 1991. The patient has not had a headache since that time until 00/93, where she had one attack when she was pregnant with her current six-month-old child. After that attack in 1993, the patient did not have any headaches until 00/00/93, when she had this latest accident.

The patient presents with multiple problems, and I feel that further evaluation should be completed. As far as the fainting and dizziness is concerned, an EEG will be done and a headache profile of blood work will be done to rule out any metabolic reasons for these headaches. An MRI of the brain will be considered later on if we are not able to correct the situation. The patient will also have an MMPI and a stress test to evaluate any psychophysiologic distress problems. I also feel that we ought to do a somatic sensory examination of her right arm to see if there is any type of nerve involvement.

As far as treatment is concerned, I recommend biofeedback as a means of helping the patient reduce her stress problems and also her headaches. The patient will start on the following medications: Bellergal-S 1 b.i.d. q.12h., Amitriptyline 10 mg h.s., Midrin to help abort the moderate headaches, and Dihydroergotamine Nasal Spray for the severe headaches. The patient will maintain a headache log and will be seen in one month for re-evaluation. However, the patient will come in for trigger point injections and deep neuromuscular mobilization following the trigger point injections.

I explained to the patient that for the time being her chiropractic treatment should be limited to her low back, because the patient explains that after manipulations of her neck, she has severe headaches and some of her arm problems. This is not unusual for people with migraines who, upon using their necks in various motions, can create a vascular headache attack. Once, however, I think the myofascial trigger points are in a state of remission, she should continue with her chiropractic manipulations of her neck also.

Thank you very much for the referral of this pleasant patient. If there are any questions, please do not hesitate to call or write.

Sincerely,

BERNARD SWERDLOW, M.D.

MEDICAL HEADACHE HISTORY

Name: Christina **Age:** 23 **Sex** F **Date:** 10/6/93

Date of Birth: 00/00/69 **Birthplace:** FL **Race:** W **Education:** Some college

Occupation: Homemaker **Accident:** 00/00/93

Armed Services & Type of Discharge: N/A

PAST HISTORY:

1.	Did you have a normal birth?		<u>Yes</u>	No
	a) forceps used?		Yes	<u>No</u>
	b) cesarean section?		Yes	<u>No</u>
2.	Did you have problems with bedwetting?		Yes	<u>No</u>
	a) If yes, age bedwetting stopped		____	
3.	Were you car sick as a child (motion)?		<u>Yes</u>	No
	a) If yes, how severe?	<u>Slight</u>	Moderate	Severe
4.	Did you have unexplained abdominal cramps as a child?		Yes	<u>No</u>
5.	Did you have any of the following illnesses in childhood?			
	a) meningitis		Yes	<u>No</u>
	b) encephalitis		Yes	<u>No</u>
	c) scarlet fever		Yes	<u>No</u>
	d) rheumatic fever		Yes	<u>No</u>
6.	Did you have any head injuries as a child?		Yes	<u>No</u>
	a) If yes, please explain:			
7.	Were you treated for emotional illness as a child?		Yes	<u>No</u>

HABITS:

8.	Do you drink alcohol?	Yes	<u>No</u>
	a) If yes, what kind and how much?		
	b) Does alcohol bring on or aggravate a headache?	Yes	<u>No</u>
9.	Do you smoke?	Yes	<u>No</u>
	a) If yes, how much?		
	b) Does smoking or smoke-filled rooms cause or aggravate headaches?	Yes	No
10.	Do you drink caffeinated beverages?	<u>Yes</u>	No
	a) If yes, how much?		

MENSTRUAL HISTORY:

At what age did menses begin? 12 Were they regular or irregular? WNL
How were they related to your headache? N/A
Are you or were you ever on Birth Control Pills? Yes Did they affect your headache? No
Have you had a hysterectomy, partial or total, and why? No
Are you in menopause, and if yes, how long? No
Are you on hormones, and if yes, which ones? No

HEADACHE ASSESSMENT FORM

HA PROFILE	INCAPACITATING #3	INTERFERING #2	IRRITATING #1
ONSET (Years ago and frequency)	1993, one attack while 8 mos. pregnant	Day of accident	Age 17, occasionally
CURRENT FREQUENCY	Had only one	Every day	None since 1991
TIME OF ONSET	Awakened with	Anytime	Anytime
DURATION	12 hours	Constant	1 hour with OTC meds
CHARACTER	Severe throbbing	Throbbing	Dull ache
PRODROME OR AURA	N/A	N/A	N/A
ASSOCIATING FEATURES	Nausea; Vomiting; Sensitivity to Light? Noise? Odors? Do you get pale or flush? Do your eyes or nose run? Does your nose get stuffy? Does the white of your eyes get red? Does your eyelid droop? Do you pace, or go to bed?	Nausea; Vomiting; Sensitivity to Light? Noise? Odors? Do you get pale or flush? Do your eyes or nose run? Does your nose get stuffy? Does the white of your eyes get red? Does your eyelid droop? Do you pace, or go to bed?	Nausea; Vomiting; Sensitivity to Light? Noise? Odors? Do you get pale or flush? Do your eyes or nose run? Does your nose get stuffy? Does the white of your eyes get red? Does your eyelid droop? Do you pace, or go to bed?
PRECIPITATING OR AGGRAVATING FEATURES	Movement	Quick movement, changing position	N/A

LOCATION: Mark the location for each type of headache with a different color pen.

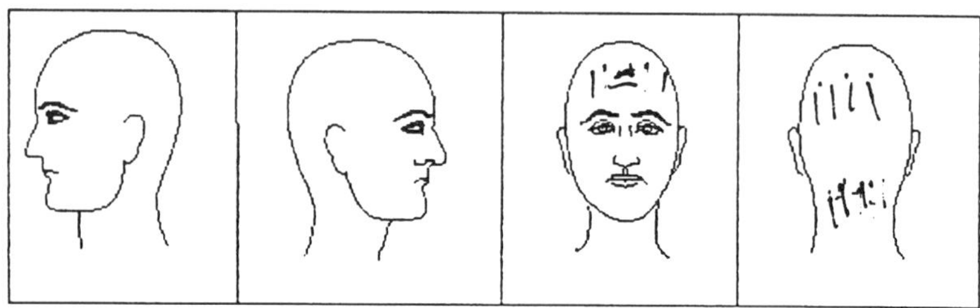

MEDICAL HISTORY:

Have you ever been or are you currently being treated for any of the following?

a) high blood pressure	Yes	No
b) stomach ulcers	Yes	No
c) asthma	Yes	No
d) allergies	Yes	No
e) pneumonia	Yes	No
f) kidney problems	Yes	No
g) low blood sugar	Yes	No
h) glaucoma	Yes	No
i) diabetes	Yes	No
j) heart problems	Yes	No

If you answered yes to any of the above, please describe:____________________

List all other medical problems you have had in the past. Include date diagnosed and treatment. DO NOT LIST OPERATIONS

Situational anxiety, 1987. Vascular headaches, 1987 and 1988. Lower back injury.

SURGICAL HISTORY (List operations and dates performed)

D&C after miscarriage, 1991.

PSYCHIATRIC HISTORY (List visits with counselors, psychologists, etc., and type of treatment)

None.

ACCIDENTS IN ADULT LIFE (Briefly describe any accident that caused any blow to the head or that you feel is related to your headache)

Car accident 1993. Driving with seatbelt. Another car pulled out in front of me and hit on passenger side. Thrown sideways. Did not hit head. Saw physician next day. Had rare headaches before accident. Headaches started immediately after accident.

FAMILY HISTORY:

1.	Is your father living?	Yes	No
	Age 42		
	Cause of death________________		
	Was there a headache history?	Yes	No
2.	Is your mother living?	Yes	No
	Age 42		
	Cause of death________________		
	Was there a headache history?	Yes	No

3. Ages of brothers---Circle the ones with headache
   20
4. Ages of sisters---Circle the ones with headache
   None
5. List any other blood relatives with a history of severe headaches.
   None

MARITAL HISTORY:
List marriages:

1st marriage age 18 to Now Did spouse have headaches?	Yes	No
2nd marriage age ______ to ______ Did spouse have headaches?	Yes	No
3rd marriage age ______ to ______ Did spouse have headaches?	Yes	No

Age of current spouse: 23

List ages and sex of all children:

Age 4 Sex M Headaches?	Yes	No
Age 6 mo. Sex F Headaches?	Yes	No
Age ______ Sex ______ Headaches?	Yes	No

STRESS FACTORS:

List any factors that may be affecting your headaches (money, loneliness, sexual problems, work, etc.)
Accident. Being unable to do everything I need to because of the pain in my body.

VEGETATIVE SIGNS:

1.	Do you have trouble falling asleep?	Yes	No
2.	Do you have trouble staying asleep?	Yes	No
3.	Has your appetite decreased?	Yes	No
4.	Have you gained or lost weight in the past year?	Yes	No
5.	Have you felt tearful or depressed lately?	Yes	No
6.	Have you had any thoughts of wanting to die?	Yes	No
7.	Have you been forgetful lately?	Yes	No
8.	Any other changes in your normal day-to-day living?______		

Please list any medications you are allergic or sensitive to: Inderal, Morphine

Please list any medications you are currently taking (including dosages and frequency per day):
Roxicet, as needed. Tylenol #3 as needed. Flexeril, as needed. Tigan, as needed.

PREVIOUS CARE:

1. List doctors who have treated you for headaches: Dr. X., Clinic

2. List any tests you have had for your headache (e.g., EEG, CT scan, MRI, X-Ray, etc.):
MRI, 1993.

3. List any other treatment you have had for your headache (e.g., biofeedback, acupuncture, chiropractic, or any other treatment you had):
None.

June 17, 1993

[Doctor's name and address omitted]

RE: JANE

Dear Dr. [...]:

Thank you for the referral of Ms. Jane [...].

This is a 48-year-old female born 00/00/45 in [...] and living in [...] for 25 years. She works at [...].

On 00/00/92, the patient was in a flexion extension accident. She was wearing her seat belt. The patient went to an orthopedic specialist the day after the accident. She had x-rays and was treated with medications. She had pain in her upper back, neck, head, etc. The patient stated that her head pain started immediately, but she considered a headache to be something that comes and goes. However, we were able to find that the headaches did start right after the accident. She had minor headaches prior to the accident.

HEADACHE PROFILE

Interfering headaches (moderate to severe): These started in 1992, and the pain is constant. The patient currently gets these headaches every seven to ten days since she has been placed on Inderal in March of this year. These headaches can last anywhere from three to four hours to three days. It is a sharp, stabbing pain in the occipital, parietal, and frontal part of her head and also the orbital region. Associated features are nausea, vomiting, photophobia, phonophobia, sensitivity to odors, and she goes to bed. She talks about visual disturbances, but they do not seem to be auras.

Irritating headaches (annoying): The patient has had these throughout her adult life. When she gets these on occasion, she will take aspirin and she can abort these headaches. These are generally in the frontal part of her head.

Menstrual history: Began at age 13 and has always been irregular with a heavy flow and cramps. The patient used to get headaches with her menstrual periods prior to her hysterectomy. In 1989, she had a complete hysterectomy for endometriosis and polycystic ovaries, etc. She is currently taking estrogen, but she is not sure of the dose.

Past history: The patient was most probably a forceps delivery. There is no history of enuresis or unexplained abdominal cramps pre-puberty. There is no history of car sickness as a child. There is no history of meningitis, encephalitis, or rheumatic fever. There were no head injuries as a child. The patient had scarlet fever as a child.

Habits: She drinks occasionally and will sometimes get a headache. She does not smoke.

Medical history: The patient has no history of high blood pressure, stomach ulcers, asthma, allergies, pneumonia, kidney problems, low blood sugar, glaucoma, diabetes, or heart problems.

Surgical history: The patient had an appendectomy in 1963, and an exploratory laparotomy at the same time. She had a tonsillectomy in 1948. She had a breast biopsy in 1964; cesarean section in 1977 and 1979, and a hysterectomy as described in 1989.

Psychiatric history: Negative.

Family history: Her father is living, age 77, with no headache history. Her mother is living, age 73, with no headache history. There are three brothers, ages 49, 43, and 40, and the youngest one may have some migraines. There is a 46-year-old sister with no headache history.

The patient has been married from age 21 to present. There are three children: two boys, ages 24 and 14, and a girl, age 16, all with no headache history.

Allergies to medications: She is allergic to Penicillin and Codeine.

Current medications: She is currently taking Inderal 20 mg at bedtime and 10 mg in the morning. She is taking Esgic plus and estrogen.

Doctors seen in the past for headaches: She has seen Dr. [...] a rehabilitation specialist, in March of this year.

Tests done in the past: She had an MRI in June or July of 1992. She states that there is something about three bulging discs. I do not have the report. She has also had some thermography.

Physical examination: Height 5’9”, weight 140 pounds, pulse 60, left BP 100/72, right BP 199/70. The face did not show any asymmetry. The temporomandibular joint area was grossly normal. The eyes appeared normal. Conjunctivae were clear and the pupils reacted equally to light and accommodation. Retinal fundus examination revealed no papilledema and no abnormalities with the arteries and veins. There were no bruits over the supraorbital region. The nose appeared normal. The auditory canals were clear and the tympanic membranes appeared intact. The mouth and throat appeared normal. Gums, tongue, buccal mucosa, and teeth were grossly normal. She has had four active trigger points in the posterior cervical region and there were no masses felt in the thyroid gland. Carotid bruits could not be heard. Cervical nodes were not enlarged. The lungs were clear to auscultation and percussion. The heart had a regular sinus rhythm with no murmurs. The abdomen was soft and nontender. A rectal or vaginal exam was not done.

Neurological examination: Cranial nerve II: Visual fields were grossly normal. III, IV and VI: No strabismus, nystagmus, or ptosis. V: Normal sensation and corneal reflex. VII: Normal facial movements (wrinkle, frown, smile, and strength of eyelids). VIII: Normal Weber and Rinne. IX and X: Good gag reflex. XI: Normal sternocleidomastoid and trapezius. XII: Normal protrusion and strength of tongue. Cerebellar: Negative Rhomberg. Normal finger-to-noise, diadochokinesis, heel-shin, tandem, and heel and toes walking. Motor system: No atrophy, fasciculations, wasting, or tremors. Good muscle strength in arms, wrists, fingers, and legs. Sensory system: Superficial tactile, pain, and vibrations (wrists, elbows, knees, and ankles) were normal. Normal motion and positions of fingers and toes. Normal 2-point discrimination. Reflexes: Normal 2+ reflexes of triceps, biceps, knee jerk, ankle jerk, etc. Normal pulses in dorsalis pedis, posterior tibial, and popliteal.

DIAGNOSES

1. Post traumatic (flexion extension-whiplash) headache.
2. Post traumatic vascular headache.
3. Rule out cervicogenic headache.

IMPRESSION

This pleasant 48-year-old woman comes in with severe headaches that started after an accident she had on 00/00/92, which has been described. The patient is currently taking Propranolol about 30 mg a day, which seems to help somewhat, but she still continues to have a headache plus some depression. She has significant pain, more in the left posterior cervical region than the right.

The patient will be put on Zoloft 50 mg q.a.m. and will be brought in for some trigger point injections and deep neuromuscular mobilization and kinetic activity to see if we can break that up. If that does not break up, then I recommend that she have a posterior cervical regional block of C1, 2, and 3, which we can do in this office quite easily.

If the cervicogenic component will be treated, then it will be done with cervical facet blocks using fluoroscopic guidance.

We will start the patient with this program and see how she is in the next few weeks.

Thank you once again for the referral of this very pleasant patient. If there are any questions, please do not hesitate to call or write.

Sincerely,

BERNARD SWERDLOW, M.D.

These notes were dictated with the patient present.

MEDICAL HEADACHE HISTORY

Name: Jane **Age:** 48 **Sex** F **Date:** 6/17/93

Date of Birth: 00/00/45 **Birthplace:** VT **Race:** C **Education:** 3 years college

Occupation: Lab Tech **Accident:** 00/00/92

Armed Services & Type of Discharge: N/A

PAST HISTORY:

1.	Did you have a normal birth?		Yes	No
	a) forceps used?		Yes	No
	b) cesarean section?		Yes	No
2.	Did you have problems with bedwetting?		Yes	No
	a) If yes, age bedwetting stopped			
3.	Were you car sick as a child (motion)?		Yes	No
	a) If yes, how severe?	Slight	Moderate	Severe
4.	Did you have unexplained abdominal cramps as a child?		Yes	No
5.	Did you have any of the following illnesses in childhood?			
	a) meningitis		Yes	No
	b) encephalitis		Yes	No
	c) scarlet fever		Yes	No
	d) rheumatic fever		Yes	No
6.	Did you have any head injuries as a child?		Yes	No
	a) If yes, please explain:			
7.	Were you treated for emotional illness as a child?		Yes	No

HABITS:

8.	Do you drink alcohol?	Yes	No
	a) If yes, what kind and how much? Occasional		
	b) Does alcohol bring on or aggravate a headache?	Yes	No
9.	Do you smoke?	Yes	No
	a) If yes, how much?		
	b) Does smoking or smoke-filled rooms cause or aggravate headaches?	Yes	No
10.	Do you drink caffeinated beverages?	Yes	No
	a) If yes, how much? 1 cup of coffee a day, or less		

MENSTRUAL HISTORY:

At what age did menses begin? 13 Were they regular or irregular? Heavy flow, cramps

How were they related to your headache? Yes, but not since hysterectomy

Are you or were you ever on Birth Control Pills? Yes Did they affect your headache? No

Have you had a hysterectomy, partial or total, and why? Yes, 1989, complete; endometriosis

Are you in menopause, and if yes, how long? -

Are you on hormones, and if yes, which ones? Estrogen

HEADACHE ASSESSMENT FORM

HA PROFILE	INCAPACITATING #3	INTERFERING #2	IRRITATING #1
ONSET (Years ago and frequency)	N/A	Since accident Constant	Throughout adult life
CURRENT FREQUENCY	N/A	1 every 7 to 10 days	Occasionally
TIME OF ONSET	N/A	When wake up in a.m.	Varied
DURATION	N/A	3 – 4 hours to 3 days	Went away with aspirin
CHARACTER	N/A	Sharp stabbing	Can't recall
PRODROME OR AURA	N/A	Have visual disturbances, but not sure if it precedes or accompanies HA pain	N/A
ASSOCIATING FEATURES	Nausea: Vomiting: Sensitivity to Light? Noise? Odors? Do you get pale or flush? Do your eyes or nose run? Does your nose get stuffy? Does the white of your eyes get red? Does your eyelid droop? Do you pace. or go to bed?	Nausea: Vomiting: Sensitivity to Light? Noise? Odors? Do you get pale or flush? Do your eyes or nose run? Does your nose get stuffy? Does the white of your eyes get red? Does your eyelid droop? Do you pace. or go to bed?	Nausea: Vomiting: Sensitivity to Light? Noise? Odors? Do you get pale or flush? Do your eyes or nose run? Does your nose get stuffy? Does the white of your eyes get red? Does your eyelid droop? Do you pace. or go to bed?
PRECIPITATING OR AGGRAVATING FEATURES	N/A	N/A	Menses

LOCATION: Mark the location for each type of headache with a different color pen.

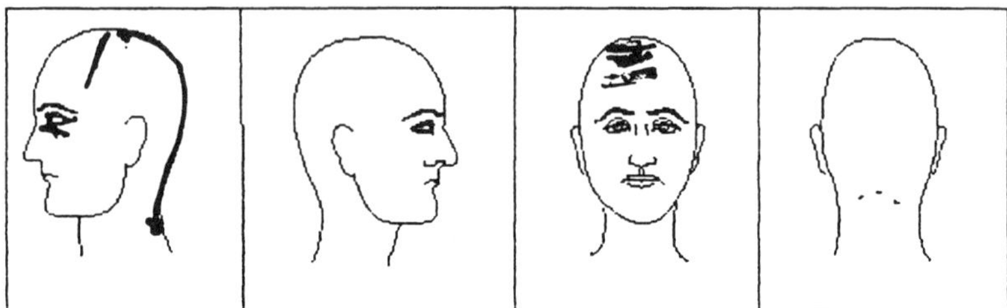

MEDICAL HISTORY:

Have you ever been or are you currently being treated for any of the following?

a) high blood pressure	Yes	No
b) stomach ulcers	Yes	No
c) asthma	Yes	No
d) allergies	Yes	No
e) pneumonia	Yes	No
f) kidney problems	Yes	No
g) low blood sugar	Yes	No
h) glaucoma	Yes	No
i) diabetes	Yes	No
j) heart problems	Yes	No

If you answered yes to any of the above, please describe:____________________

List all other medical problems you have had in the past. Include date diagnosed and treatment.
DO NOT LIST OPERATIONS

GYN – hormone replacement therapy.

SURGICAL HISTORY (List operations and dates performed)

Appendix and exploratory laparotomy, 1963. Tonsillectomy, 1948. Breast biopsy, 1964. Cesarean sections, 1977 and 1979. Hysterectomy (complete), 1989.

PSYCHIATRIC HISTORY (List visits with counselors, psychologists, etc., and type of treatment)

None.

ACCIDENTS IN ADULT LIFE (Briefly describe any accident that caused any blow to the head or that you feel is related to your headache)

Car accident 1992. Driving, wearing seatbelt. Sitting stopped in off ramp of freeway. Cars in front and back of me were also stopped. The driver behind me accelerated and hit the rear of my car, throwing me into the car in front of me. My head went back, and forward. Went to an orthopedic specialist the next day for x-rays, treatment, and medication. Had pain in upper back, neck, and head. Had constant pain in my head from the day of the accident.

FAMILY HISTORY:

1. Is your father living? Yes No
   Age 77
   Cause of death________________
   Was there a headache history? Yes No
2. Is your mother living? Yes No
   Age 73
   Cause of death________________
   Was there a headache history? Yes No

3. Ages of brothers---Circle the ones with headache
   49 43 (40)
4. Ages of sisters---Circle the ones with headache
   46
5. List any other blood relatives with a history of severe headaches.
   None

MARITAL HISTORY:
List marriages:

1st marriage age 21 to Now	Did spouse have headaches?	Yes	No
2nd marriage age ______ to ______	Did spouse have headaches?	Yes	No
3rd marriage age ______ to ______	Did spouse have headaches?	Yes	No

Age of current spouse: 46

List ages and sex of all children:

Age 24	Sex M	Headaches? Yes	No
Age 16	Sex F	Headaches? Yes	No
Age 14	Sex M	Headaches? Yes	No
Age ____	Sex ____	Headaches? Yes	No

STRESS FACTORS:

List any factors that may be affecting your headaches (money, loneliness, sexual problems, work, etc.)
Neck injury.

VEGETATIVE SIGNS:

1.	Do you have trouble falling asleep?	Yes	No
2.	Do you have trouble staying asleep?	Yes	No
3.	Has your appetite decreased?	Yes	No
4.	Have you gained or lost weight in the past year?	Yes	No
5.	Have you felt tearful or depressed lately?	Yes	No
6.	Have you had any thoughts of wanting to die?	Yes	No
7.	Have you been forgetful lately?	Yes	No
8.	Any other changes in your normal day-to-day living? ______		

Please list any medications you are allergic or sensitive to: Penicillin, Codeine

Please list any medications you are currently taking (including dosages and frequency per day):
Inderal, 20 mg q.h.s., 10 mg. q.a.m. Esgic Plus. Estrogen.

PREVIOUS CARE:

1. List doctors who have treated you for headaches: Dr. V.

2. List any tests you have had for your headache (e.g., EEG, CT scan, MRI, X-Ray, etc.):

MRI, 1992.

X-rays, 1993.

Thermography.

3. List any other treatment you have had for your headache (e.g., biofeedback, acupuncture, chiropractic, or any other treatment you had):

Chiropractic (currently in care).

January 25, 1995

[Doctor's name and address omitted]

RE: ELLA

Dear Dr. [...]:

Thank you for referring Ms. [...] for further headache evaluation and treatment. I had the pleasure of reviewing your records, and will encourage her to return to you for continued care after any treatment we might propose.

As you know, Ms. [...] is a 63-year-old female born 00/00/31 in [...]. She has completed a GED, has lived in [...] for one year, and is employed as a cashier for [...].

HEADACHE PROFILE

The patient was involved in a motor vehicle accident on 00/00/94, when she was driving an automobile, restrained with a seat belt. She stopped at a light and was rear-ended by another car. She did not suffer loss of consciousness; however, she was taken to an emergency room where she was x-rayed, treated, and released. The patient noted the immediate onset of headaches with only occasional headaches prior to this accident (1 to 2 per year).

Incapacitating headaches: None.

Interfering headaches (moderate to severe): The patient noted the onset of these headaches the day of the accident. They were daily at that time. She is now suffering four to five of these headaches per week. The onset of these headaches can be at any time of the day and the patient can awaken with these headaches. These headaches will last approximately one day in duration and are described as a vice-like pain in a band-like distribution around the head, and also in the periorbital areas of the eyes. There is no prodrome with these headaches. There are some nausea symptoms with no vomiting and some phonophobia. The patient will seek bed rest when possible. The patient notes that coughing will increase her symptoms.

Irritating headaches (annoying): The patient noted these headaches in 1948 and they occurred on a rare basis, 1 to 2 per year. She is not suffering any of these headaches at the current time. These headaches did occur at any time of the day and were relieved in one hour with over-the-counter medication. The pain was located in the nasal area and was described as a sinus-type pain.

Menstrual history: Began at age 13 and is reported as normal. No increase in symptoms with menstrual period. The patient had a partial hysterectomy in 1966 for fibroids. She currently has her ovaries. The patient is uncertain as to the time of menopause.

Past history: The patient was most probably a normal delivery. There is no history of enuresis or unexplained abdominal cramps pre-puberty. There is no history of car sickness as a child. There is no history of meningitis, encephalitis, scarlet fever, or rheumatic fever. There were no head injuries as a child.

Habits: The patient does not drink alcohol. She does smoke 1 to 1½ packs of cigarettes per day. The patient consumes 1 to 2 gallons of iced tea per day.

Medical history: The patient had toxemia after childbirth in 1954, easily resolved with medication. History of pneumonia, resolved. History of sinus infections, currently asymptomatic. The patient had a mild CVA in 1974 and was initially treated with anticoagulants. She is currently not treated. She suffered a fractured pelvis in 1994 after a fall.

Surgical history: Tonsillectomy and adenoidectomy in 1950; partial hysterectomy in 1966; left shoulder surgery, last operation in 1975; right inguinal hernia repair in 1992; foot surgery in 1990 and 1991; left arm surgery in 1993 and 1994 to repair fractured arm and shoulder.

Psychiatric history: The patient was hospitalized in 1976 for a nervous condition and treatment of alcohol consumption.

Family history: Her father is deceased at age 71, train accident. Her mother is deceased, no headache history. The patient has one brother and one sister, no headache history. The patient has a son with post traumatic headaches after injury. The patient is currently divorced and has 5 sons and 1 daughter; 3 of the children have a headache history.

Vegetative signs: The patient does not have trouble in falling or staying asleep. No depression, suicidal ideation, or memory difficulties.

Allergies to medications: Codeine — nausea and vomiting.

Current medications: The patient is currently taking ibuprofen p.r.n.

Doctors seen in the past for headaches: Previous treatment for headaches includes evaluation by Dr. [...], including EMG — negative. Also Dr. [...], who stated the patient had a "bulging" cervical disc.

Tests done in the past: The patient had a CT scan in 1994 which was negative, an MRI in 1994 which was negative, EEG in 1994 which was negative, and a brain scan, also negative.

Treatments tried in the past: The patient has had treatment by Dr. [...] with some improvement in symptoms.

Medications taken: Sinequan, which the patient states helped to a small degree; Cardizem, no help; Motrin, slight help; Valium and Flexeril, no improvement in symptoms; Midrin, some mild improvement. The patient has also been treated with multiple analgesics and anti-emetics. The patient did not have the Inderal prescription filled.

Physical examination: Height 5'6", weight 135 pounds, pulse 78, left BP 138/94, right BP 132/92. The face did not show any asymmetry. The temporomandibular joint area was grossly normal. The eyes appeared normal. Conjunctivae were clear and the pupils reacted equally to light and accommodation. Retinal fundus examination revealed no papilledema and no abnormalities with the arteries and veins. There were no bruits over the supraorbital region. The nose appeared normal. The auditory canals were clear and the tympanic membranes appeared intact. The mouth and throat appeared normal. Gums, tongue, buccal mucosa, and teeth were grossly normal. The neck was supple and there were no masses felt in the thyroid gland. Carotid bruits could not be heard. Cervical nodes were not enlarged. The lungs were clear to auscultation and percussion. The heart had a regular sinus rhythm with no murmurs. The abdomen was soft and nontender. A rectal or vaginal exam was not done.

Neurological examination: Cranial nerve II: Visual fields were grossly normal. III, IV and VI: No strabismus nystagmus, or ptosis. V: Normal sensation and corneal reflex. VII: Normal facial movements (wrinkle, frown, smile, and strength of eyelids). VIII: Normal Weber and Rinne. IX and X: Good gag reflex. XI: Normal sternocleidomastoid and trapezius. XII: Normal protrusion and strength of tongue. Cerebellar: Negative Rhomberg. Normal finger-to-nose, diadochokinesis, heel-shin, tandem and heel and toes walking. Motor system: No atrophy, fasciculations, wasting, or tremors. Good muscle strength in arms, wrists, fingers, and legs. Sensory system: Superficial tactile, pain, and vibrations (wrists, elbows, knees, and ankles) were normal. Normal motion and positions of fingers and toes. Normal 2-point discrimination. Reflexes: Normal 2+ reflexes of triceps, biceps, knee jerk, ankle jerk, etc. Normal pulses in dorsalis pedis, posterior tibial, and popliteal.

DIAGNOSIS

1. Post traumatic (flexion extension-whiplash) headache syndrome (chronic), with components of muscle contraction headache. International Headache Society diagnosis 5.2.
2. Extreme caffeine intake. The patient is advised to reduce this significantly, but slowly.
3. Tobacco use. The patient was counseled regarding discontinuing.

I would like to start her on:

1. Bellergal-S, 1 tablet q.h.s. with $^1/_2$ tablet at noon.
2. Zoloft 50 mg q.a.m. to increase the serotonin.
3. Continue Midrin. The patient will be instructed to take the Midrin with a Fioricet at the onset of headaches.
4. Cervical regional blocks. The patient states there is a trigger area in the left side that actually can reduce her symptoms, and I feel it would be beneficial to perform a cervical plexus regional block in this area to see if we can break her headache cycle. I would like to schedule her back for 2 to 3 blocks at her convenience and then evaluate the course of her care in 4 weeks.

Dr. [...], thank you for the opportunity to assist you in the care of your patient.

Sincerely,

[Doctor's name]

MEDICAL HEADACHE HISTORY

Name: Ella **Age:** 63 **Sex** F **Date:** 1/23/95

Date of Birth: 00/00/31 **Birthplace:** MO **Race:** C **Education:** G.E.D.

Occupation: Cashier **Accident:** 00/00/94

Armed Services & Type of Discharge: N/A

PAST HISTORY:

1.	Did you have a normal birth?		Yes	No
	a) forceps used?		Yes	No
	b) cesarean section?		Yes	No
2.	Did you have problems with bedwetting?		Yes	No
	a) If yes, age bedwetting stopped			
3.	Were you car sick as a child (motion)?		Yes	No
	a) If yes, how severe?	Slight	Moderate	Severe
4.	Did you have unexplained abdominal cramps as a child?		Yes	No
5.	Did you have any of the following illnesses in childhood?			
	a) meningitis		Yes	No
	b) encephalitis		Yes	No
	c) scarlet fever		Yes	No
	d) rheumatic fever		Yes	No
6.	Did you have any head injuries as a child?		Yes	No
	a) If yes, please explain:			
7.	Were you treated for emotional illness as a child?		Yes	No

HABITS:

8.	Do you drink alcohol?	Yes	No
	a) If yes, what kind and how much?		
	b) Does alcohol bring on or aggravate a headache?	Yes	No
9.	Do you smoke?	Yes	No
	a) If yes, how much? 1 to 1½ packs a day		
	b) Does smoking or smoke-filled rooms cause or aggravate headaches?	Yes	No
10.	Do you drink caffeinated beverages?	Yes	No
	a) If yes, how much? 1 to 2 gallons		

MENSTRUAL HISTORY:

At what age did menses begin? 13 Were they regular or irregular? WNL
How were they related to your headache? N/A
Are you or were you ever on Birth Control Pills? Yes Did they affect your headache? No
Have you had a hysterectomy, partial or total, and why? Partial 1966; Fibroids
Are you in menopause, and if yes, how long? No
Are you on hormones, and if yes, which ones? No

HEADACHE ASSESSMENT FORM

HA PROFILE	INCAPACITATING #3	INTERFERING #2	IRRITATING #1
ONSET (Years ago and frequency)	N/A	Day of accident Every day	1948, Rare
CURRENT FREQUENCY	N/A	4 – 5/week	None now
TIME OF ONSET	N/A	Anytime, can awaken with	Anytime
DURATION	N/A	1 day	1 hr. with OTC meds
CHARACTER	N/A	Vise-like	Ache
PRODROME OR AURA	N/A	N/A	N/A
ASSOCIATING FEATURES	Nausea: Vomiting: Sensitivity to Light? Noise? Odors? Do you get pale or flush? Do your eyes or nose run? Does your nose get stuffy? Does the white of your eyes get red? Does your eyelid droop? Do you pace, or go to bed?	Nausea: Vomiting: Sensitivity to Light? Noise? Odors? Do you get pale or flush? Do your eyes or nose run? Does your nose get stuffy? Does the white of your eyes get red? Does your eyelid droop? Do you pace, or go to bed?	Nausea: Vomiting: Sensitivity to Light? Noise? Odors? Do you get pale or flush? Do your eyes or nose run? Does your nose get stuffy? Does the white of your eyes get red? Does your eyelid droop? Do you pace, or go to bed?
PRECIPITATING OR AGGRAVATING FEATURES	N/A	Coughing	N/A

LOCATION: Mark the location for each type of headache with a different color pen.

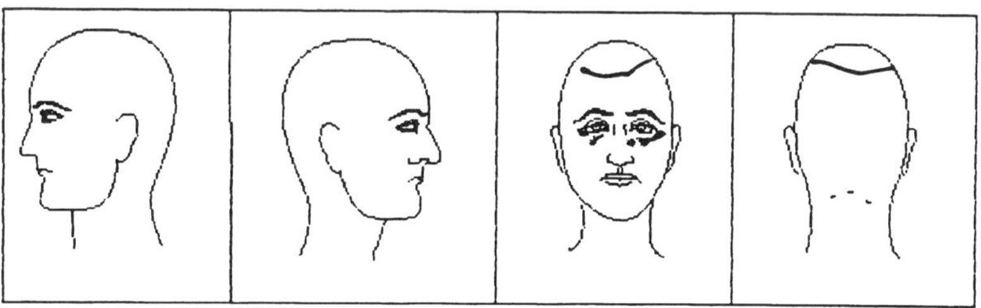

MEDICAL HISTORY:

Have you ever been or are you currently being treated for any of the following?

a) high blood pressure	Yes	<u>No</u>
b) stomach ulcers	Yes	<u>No</u>
c) asthma	Yes	<u>No</u>
d) allergies	Yes	<u>No</u>
e) pneumonia	<u>Yes</u>	No
f) kidney problems	Yes	<u>No</u>
g) low blood sugar	Yes	<u>No</u>
h) glaucoma	Yes	<u>No</u>
i) diabetes	Yes	<u>No</u>
j) heart problems	Yes	<u>No</u>

If you answered yes to any of the above, please describe: Pneumonia in 1970s.

List all other medical problems you have had in the past. Include date diagnosed and treatment.
DO NOT LIST OPERATIONS

Kidney poisoning after childbirth, 1954. Pneumonia, 1970s. Sinus. Broken bones. Stroke 1974. Fractured pelvis in fall, 1995.

SURGICAL HISTORY (List operations and dates performed)

Tonsils & Adenoids, 1950. Partial hysterectomy, 1966. Left shoulder, 1975. Right inguinal hernia, 1992. Left foot, 1990 and 1991. Left arm, 1993. Rod removal, fractured shoulder and arm, 1994.

PSYCHIATRIC HISTORY (List visits with counselors, psychologists, etc., and type of treatment)

X Hospital for nervous breakdown and alcohol abuse, 1976.

ACCIDENTS IN ADULT LIFE (Briefly describe any accident that caused any blow to the head or that you feel is related to your headache)

Car accident 1994. Driving with seatbelt. Stopped at light and rear-ended from behind. Not unconscious. Taken to emergency room, x-rayed, treated and released. Headaches began immediately. Occasional headaches before accident (approximately 1-2/year).

FAMILY HISTORY:

1.	Is your father living?	Yes	<u>No</u>
	Age ______		
	Cause of death Train accident, age 71		
	Was there a headache history?	Yes	<u>No</u>
2.	Is your mother living?	Yes	<u>No</u>
	Age 49		
	Cause of death 1990		
	Was there a headache history?	Yes	<u>No</u>

3. Ages of brothers---Circle the ones with headache
   52, deceased
4. Ages of sisters---Circle the ones with headache
   67
5. List any other blood relatives with a history of severe headaches.
   Son.

MARITAL HISTORY:

List marriages:

1st marriage age 17 to 41	Did spouse have headaches?	Yes	No
2nd marriage age ____ to ____	Did spouse have headaches?	Yes	No
3rd marriage age ____ to ____	Did spouse have headaches?	Yes	No

Age of current spouse: Don't have any, don't want any

List ages and sex of all children:

Age 43	Sex M	Headaches?	Yes	No
Age 40	Sex M	Headaches?	Yes	No
Age 39	Sex M	Headaches?	Yes	No
Age 37	Sex F	Headaches?	Yes	No
Age 35	Sex M	Headaches?	Yes	No
Age 34	Sex M	Headaches?	Yes	No
Age ____	Sex ____	Headaches?	Yes	No

STRESS FACTORS:

List any factors that may be affecting your headaches (money, loneliness, sexual problems, work, etc.)
None

VEGETATIVE SIGNS:

1.	Do you have trouble falling asleep?	Yes	No
2.	Do you have trouble staying asleep?	Yes	No
3.	Has your appetite decreased?	Yes	No
4.	Have you gained or lost weight in the past year?	Yes	No
5.	Have you felt tearful or depressed lately?	Yes	No
6.	Have you had any thoughts of wanting to die?	Yes	No
7.	Have you been forgetful lately?	Yes	No
8.	Any other changes in your normal day-to-day living? ____		

Please list any medications you are allergic or sensitive to: Codeine

Please list any medications you are currently taking (including dosages and frequency per day):
Ibuprofen as needed

PREVIOUS CARE:

1. List doctors who have treated you for headaches: Dr. J., Dr. C.

2. List any tests you have had for your headache (e.g., EEG, CT scan, MRI, X-Ray, etc.):

CAT scan, 1994 (negative)

MRI, 1994 (negative)

EEG, 1994 (negative).

Brain scan, (negative).

3. List any other treatment you have had for your headache (e.g., biofeedback, acupuncture, chiropractic, or any other treatment you had):

Chiropractic.

May 11, 1994

[Doctor's name and address omitted]

RE: JOHN

Dear Dr. [...]:

Thank you very much for the referral of Mr. John [...] for headache and chronic pain management.

The patient is a 64-year-old male born 00/00/29 in [...]. He has lived in [...] for the last 22 years and is currently retired after a career with the federal government.

The patient was involved in a motor vehicle accident 00/00/93. At that time, the patient was the driver of a motor vehicle, wearing his seat belt, and was stopped at a red light. There was a two-car collision behind his automobile, and the second automobile ran into the back of his car. The patient did not suffer loss of consciousness or strike his head. The patient had no headache history prior to this event and noted that his headaches developed a few days after this motor vehicle accident.

HEADACHE PROFILE

Incapacitating headaches: None.

Interfering headaches (moderate to severe): These headaches developed, as noted above, two to three days after the motor vehicle accident and have been daily since the injury. These headaches will occur generally at 3:00 a.m. and 3:00 p.m. and are noted to be constant unless medication is taken. The patient describes his pain as a constant dull aching pain in the bilateral frontal, occipital and cervical area of the head. There is no prodrome with these headaches, nor any associated gastrointestinal or sensory changes with these headaches. The patient will sit quietly during a headache.

Irritating headaches (annoying): The patient noted the onset of these headaches as a young adult and they were rare at that time. These headaches resolved spontaneously as he aged, and the patient has not suffered from these headaches for 20 to 30 years.

The patient has been extensively evaluated for this problem by Dr. [...] at the clinic, reports of which have been forwarded to this office to facilitate the patient's medical care here. The patient has been treated with nonsteroidal anti-inflammatory medications, physical therapy, and oral analgesics under limited prescription.

X-ray evaluation showed "AP, lateral and odontoid views of the cervical spine today indicate a certain amount of degenerative disease in the cervical area particularly at C5/6, C6/7 levels. Alignment satisfactory. No evidence of bony injury." MRI performed 00/00/94 shows "multi-level spondylitic changes including osteophytes indenting dural sac."

Due to persistence of symptoms despite these measures, the patient is referred for further pain management treatment.

Past history: The patient was most probably a normal delivery. There is no history of enuresis or unexplained abdominal cramps pre-puberty. There is no history of car sickness as a child. There is no history of meningitis, encephalitis, scarlet fever, or rheumatic fever. There were no head injuries as a child.

Habits: The patient does not consume alcohol and does not smoke. The patient consumes two cups of coffee per day.

Medical history: Hypertension diagnosed 24 years ago, not currently treated. Environmental allergies.

Surgical history: None.

Psychiatric history: None.

Head injuries in adult life: As noted above.

Family history: His father is deceased, at age 60, of myocardial infarction, with no headache history. His moving is living, age 89. The patient has one brother and four sisters with no headache history. The patient is currently married and has one son and one daughter, with no headache history.

Stress factors: None listed.

Vegetative signs: The patient denies any difficulty in falling asleep; however, he does note trouble in staying asleep.

Allergies to medications: The patient is allergic to Penicillin.

Current medications: The patient is currently taking Tylenol-PM one every day, and Darvocet 1 to 2 per day on a p.r.n. basis.

Physical examination: Height 5'10", weight 180 pounds, pulse 68, respirations 16, left BP 146/82, right BP 136/88. The face did not show any asymmetry. The temporomandibular joint area was grossly normal. The eyes appeared normal. Conjunctivae were clear and the pupils reacted equally to light and accommodation. Retinal fundus examination revealed no papilledema and no abnormalities with the arteries and veins. There were no bruits over the supraorbital region. The nose appeared normal. The auditory canals were clear and the tympanic membranes appeared intact. The mouth and throat appeared normal. Gums, tongue, buccal mucosa, and teeth were grossly normal. The neck was supple and there were no masses felt in the thyroid gland. Carotid bruits could not be heard. Cervical nodes were not enlarged. The lungs were clear to auscultation and percussion. The heart had a regular sinus rhythm with no murmurs. The abdomen was soft and nontender. A rectal exam was not done.

Neurological examination: Cranial nerve II: Visual fields were grossly normal. III, IV and VI: No strabismus, nystagmus, or ptosis. V: Normal sensation and corneal reflex. VII: Normal facial movements (wrinkle, frown, smile, and strength of eyelids). VIII: Normal Weber and Rinne. IX and X: Good gag reflex. XI: Normal sternocleidomastoid and trapezius. XII: Normal protrusion and strength of tongue. Cerebellar: Negative Rhomberg. Normal finger-to-nose, diadochokinesis, heel-shin, tandem and heel and toes walking. Motor system: No atrophy, fasciculations, wasting, or tremors. Good muscle strength in arms, wrists, fingers, and legs. Sensory system: Superficial tactile, pain, and vibrations (wrists, elbows, knees, and ankles) were normal. Normal motion and positions of fingers and toes. Normal 2-point discrimination. Reflexes: Normal 2+ reflexes of triceps, biceps, knee jerk, ankle jerk, etc. Normal pulses in dorsalis pedis, posterior tibial, and popliteal.

DIAGNOSES

1. Post traumatic (flexion extension-whiplash) headache.
2. Cervicogenic headache secondary to motor vehicle accident.

While the patient does have degenerative disk disease that predated the accident, nonetheless he was completely asymptomatic prior to this and his symptoms developed immediately after his injury. This temporal course is certainly consistent with post traumatic headache syndrome. I feel that his headaches are also exacerbated by his cervical pain, and this has certainly been increased also by the injury.

I would suggest for this patient:

1. Very low dose of Amitriptyline 10 mg q.h.s. to regulate his sleep pattern.
2. Bellergal 1 tablet p.o. q.h.s. and $^1/_2$ tablet at noon in an effort to abort his 3:00 a.m. and 3:00 p.m. headaches.
3. Trial of cervical epidural steroids for relief of his cervicogenic pain.

Hopefully the combination of both the medical and block therapy will assist the patient in returning to his previous symptom-free state.

4. If necessary, cervical facet blocks using fluoroscopic guidance would be considered.
5. We will also obtain a baseline headache profile to rule out any metabolic causes of his headaches and to establish a baseline.

Dr. [...], I greatly appreciate your confidence and the kind referral of this most pleasant patient. I will keep you informed as to his progress, and if there are any questions, or anything further I can do, please contact me.

Sincerely,

[Doctor's name omitted]

These notes were dictated with the patient present.

MEDICAL HEADACHE HISTORY

Name: John **Age:** 64 **Sex** M **Date:** 5/11/94

Date of Birth: 00/00/29 **Birthplace:** DC **Race:** W **Education:** ______

Occupation: Retired **Accident:** 00/00/93

Armed Services & Type of Discharge: 1946-49 – Navy

PAST HISTORY:

1.	Did you have a normal birth?		Yes (underlined)	No
	a) forceps used?		Yes	No
	b) cesarean section?		Yes	No
2.	Did you have problems with bedwetting?		Yes	No (underlined)
	a) If yes, age bedwetting stopped		______	
3.	Were you car sick as a child (motion)?		Yes	No (underlined)
	a) If yes, how severe?	Slight	Moderate	Severe
4.	Did you have unexplained abdominal cramps as a child?		Yes	No (underlined)
5.	Did you have any of the following illnesses in childhood?			
	a) meningitis		Yes	No (underlined)
	b) encephalitis		Yes	No (underlined)
	c) scarlet fever		Yes	No (underlined)
	d) rheumatic fever		Yes	No (underlined)
6.	Did you have any head injuries as a child?		Yes	No (underlined)
	a) If yes, please explain: ______			
7.	Were you treated for emotional illness as a child?		Yes	No (underlined)

HABITS:

8.	Do you drink alcohol?	Yes	No (underlined)
	a) If yes, what kind and how much? ______		
	b) Does alcohol bring on or aggravate a headache?	Yes	No
9.	Do you smoke?	Yes	No (underlined)
	a) If yes, how much? ______		
	b) Does smoking or smoke-filled rooms cause or aggravate headaches?	Yes	No
10.	Do you drink caffeinated beverages?	Yes (underlined)	No
	a) If yes, how much? 2 cups of coffee per day		

MENSTRUAL HISTORY:

At what age did menses begin? ______ Were they regular or irregular? ______
How were they related to your headache? ______
Are you or were you ever on Birth Control Pills? ______ Did they affect your headache? ______
Have you had a hysterectomy, partial or total, and why? ______
Are you in menopause, and if yes, how long? ______
Are you on hormones, and if yes, which ones? ______

HEADACHE ASSESSMENT FORM

HA PROFILE	INCAPACITATING #3	INTERFERING #2	IRRITATING #1
ONSET (Years ago and frequency)	N/A	Few days after accident Every day	Young adult, Rare
CURRENT FREQUENCY	N/A	Every day	None now
TIME OF ONSET	N/A	Awakens with, 3:00 a.m.	Anytime
DURATION	N/A	Constant without meds	1 hr. with OTC medication
CHARACTER	N/A	Constant dull ache	?
PRODROME OR AURA	N/A	N/A	N/A
ASSOCIATING FEATURES	Nausea: Vomiting: Sensitivity to Light? Noise? Odors? Do you get pale or flush? Do your eyes or nose run? Does your nose get stuffy? Does the white of your eyes get red? Does your eyelid droop? Do you pace, or go to bed?	Nausea: Vomiting: Sensitivity to Light? Noise? Odors? Do you get pale or flush? Do your eyes or nose run? Does your nose get stuffy? Does the white of your eyes get red? Does your eyelid droop? Do you pace, or go to bed? Sit quietly	Nausea: Vomiting: Sensitivity to Light? Noise? Odors? Do you get pale or flush? Do your eyes or nose run? Does your nose get stuffy? Does the white of your eyes get red? Does your eyelid droop? Do you pace, or go to bed?
PRECIPITATING OR AGGRAVATING FEATURES	N/A	N/A	N/A

LOCATION: Mark the location for each type of headache with a different color pen.

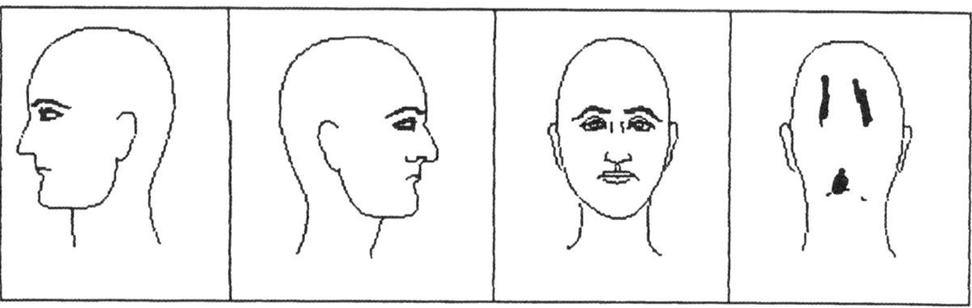

MEDICAL HISTORY:

Have you ever been or are you currently being treated for any of the following?

a) high blood pressure	<u>Yes</u>	No
b) stomach ulcers	Yes	<u>No</u>
c) asthma	Yes	<u>No</u>
d) allergies	<u>Yes</u>	No
e) pneumonia	Yes	<u>No</u>
f) kidney problems	Yes	<u>No</u>
g) low blood sugar	Yes	<u>No</u>
h) glaucoma	Yes	<u>No</u>
i) diabetes	Yes	<u>No</u>
j) heart problems	Yes	<u>No</u>

If you answered yes to any of the above, please describe: High BP diagnosed 24 years ago, no meds. Environmental Allergies.

List all other medical problems you have had in the past. Include date diagnosed and treatment.
DO NOT LIST OPERATIONS

SURGICAL HISTORY (List operations and dates performed)
None.

PSYCHIATRIC HISTORY (List visits with counselors, psychologists, etc. and type of treatment)
None.

ACCIDENTS IN ADULT LIFE (Briefly describe any accident that caused any blow to the head or that you feel is related to your headache)
Auto accident 00/00/93. Driving with seatbelt. Stopped at a light and rear-ended by another car. Not unconscious. Sought medical treatment the next day with back pain. No back pain before the accident. Headaches began a few days later. Rare #1 headaches before accident.

FAMILY HISTORY:

1. Is your father living? Yes <u>No</u>
   Age________
   Cause of death MI, age 60
   Was there a headache history? Yes <u>No</u>
2. Is your mother living? <u>Yes</u> No
   Age 89
   Cause of death________
   Was there a headache history? Yes <u>No</u>

3. Ages of brothers---Circle the ones with headache
   58
4. Ages of sisters---Circle the ones with headache
   50, 66, 68, 70
5. List any other blood relatives with a history of severe headaches.
   None

MARITAL HISTORY:
List marriages:

1st marriage age 25 to 65	Did spouse have headaches?	Yes	No
2nd marriage age ____ to ____	Did spouse have headaches?	Yes	No
3rd marriage age ____ to ____	Did spouse have headaches?	Yes	No

Age of current spouse:__________

List ages and sex of all children:

Age 32 Sex M	Headaches?	Yes	No
Age 30 Sex F	Headaches?	Yes	No
Age ____ Sex ____	Headaches?	Yes	No
Age ____ Sex ____	Headaches?	Yes	No

STRESS FACTORS:

List any factors that may be affecting your headaches (money, loneliness, sexual problems, work, etc.)

VEGETATIVE SIGNS:

1.	Do you have trouble falling asleep?	Yes	No
2.	Do you have trouble staying asleep?	Yes	No
3.	Has your appetite decreased?	Yes	No
4.	Have you gained or lost weight in the past year?	Yes	No
5.	Have you felt tearful or depressed lately?	Yes	No
6.	Have you had any thoughts of wanting to die?	Yes	No
7.	Have you been forgetful lately?	Yes	No
8.	Any other changes in your normal day-to-day living?__________		

Please list any medications you are allergic or sensitive to: Penicillin – rash.

Please list any medications you are currently taking (including dosages and frequency per day):
Tylenol-PM – 1 per day. Darvocet, 1 – 2 per day as needed.

PREVIOUS CARE:

1, List doctors who have treated you for headaches: Dr. N.

2. List any tests you have had for your headache (e.g., EEG, CT scan, MRI, X-Ray, etc.):

X-rays. MRI.

3. List any other treatment you have had for your headache (e.g., biofeedback, acupuncture, chiropractic, or any other treatment you had):

Physical Therapy.

Chapter 15

Biomechanics of Whiplash (Cervical Acceleration/Deceleration Syndrome)

A constant argument that intrigues all of those involved in observing a patient who continues to suffer from a whiplash accident is, why so much pain from a low speed accident with relatively little damage to the automobile? Foreman and Croft in their excellent book *Whiplash Injuries — The Cervical Acceleration/Deceleration Syndrome*,[1] spend a great deal of effort reviewing the literature and the development of information from Savery's work in the 1950s to the present. They take great pains to include all the arguments concerning the pros and cons of the research done. For those readers who are interested in the ramifications of this complex issue, I would suggest reading their book.

On the question of continued pain following a low-speed accident, it was hypothesized that the occupants of these vehicles may be subjected to acceleration forces greater than the forces imparted to the vehicle that was struck. Both human volunteers and anthropometric dummies were used. These subjects were seated in nonmoving, standard-sized vehicles with no brakes applied, while a similar sized vehicle at low speed struck the car with the humans or the dummies. Using electronic and mechanical accelerometers and high-speed motion pictures, data were collected of the rear end collisions. What was discovered was that at 8 mph in a rear impact collision the head and neck were exposed to acceleration forces up to $2^1/_2$ times that of the vehicle itself, and at higher-speed collisions this acceleration force may increase 4 to 10 times higher. This then begins to explain why injuries of this magnitude occur in low-speed accidents. This may also explain why the driver in the striking car does not suffer an injury of the same intensity.

Of course, since the 1950s there have been many changes in the weight and the construction of automobiles, plus the addition of seat belts, shoulder harnesses and head rests, which require additional research. It is interesting to note that a great deal of effort to save the life of the occupant of the car using seat belts, shoulder harnesses and head restraints has not really been successful in preventing whiplash or cervical acceleration/deceleration (CAD) injuries.

The reasons for this observed by researchers are the following:

The struck vehicle and the occupant behave differently.

1. The vehicle accelerates and the occupant is forced into the seat in 0 to 100 milliseconds. After 100 milliseconds the shoulder, caught up in the vehicle's acceleration, also accelerates.

2. At this point the head is not accelerating and instead of moving forward is moving rearward and is moving into extension and not flexion. This results in shear stress and axial stretch in the cervical spine. If there is a head rest, the extension of the head will continue until it hits the head rest. If there is no head rest, then the head could extend until there is no more limit to the muscles and ligaments.

Foreman and Croft discuss the sequence of events in time and in phases.

Initial phase (0–100 milliseconds). The vehicle moved forward beneath the test subject, compressing the seat cushion. This caused an initial forward and vertical motion of the hips and low back. Simultaneously the upper part of the seat back began to flex rearward under the load of the torso, which remained nearly stationary at this stage (Figure 15.1A).

Principal forward acceleration (100–200 milliseconds). During the first 100 milliseconds the seat back reaches the maximal rearward movement of 10 degrees. The subject moves upward and forward. The neck is compressed. The cervical spine is straightened and moves upward and rearward. The head in a chin-up position begins to rotate rearward. By 160 milliseconds the vertical motion of the torso begins to pull the neck forward as the head continues into extension. During this phase there are significant shearing forces. Ramping may start at this phase (vertical rotation) (Figure 15.1B).

Head overspeed/torso recovery (200–300 milliseconds). At 200 milliseconds maximal vertical motion has taken place. At 250 milliseconds the head starts its forward motion. The seat back returns to its original position while the trunk descends back down the seat back (Figure 15.1C).

Head deceleration/torso rest (300–400 milliseconds). At 300 milliseconds the descent of the trunk is now complete and the torso is moving at the same velocity as the vehicle. At 400 milliseconds there is active deceleration of the neck (Figure 15.1D).

Restitution phase (400–600 milliseconds). All parts of the body are moving at the vehicle velocity, and impact-related motions are essentially complete at 400 milliseconds.

Foreman and Croft[1] synthesize a great deal of the existing research and describe the sequence of events in a cervical CAD or whiplash accident in four separate phases.

Phase I: They describe this as a nonelastic or plastic collision in that the vehicle in front attains the common velocity after being struck by the vehicle from behind. Therefore, the greater the impact speed, the greater the deformation of the vehicles, and therefore the more plastic the collision. First the torso is forced backward into the seat back. There is an abrupt upward movement of the torso while the head and neck remain fixed and there is a straightening of the cervical, thoracic and possibly the lumbar spines. Because of this, the cervical spine becomes compressed and at the end of this phase the head and neck begin to extend. This also may be a time when there are ruptures of the discs (Figure 15.2A).

Phase II: It is during this phase that the temporomandibular joint can be injured. TMJ injury and dysfunction are discussed in Chapter 18. The seat back will now return to its previous position and at this point the torso begins its forward movement and acceleration. The head is still moving in the opposite direction (extension), and the vehicle is at its peak acceleration. This all adds to the shear strain of the lower cervical spine. There is some slack in the lap belt and shoulder restraint system because the torso rises and moves rearward in the seat. This will cause the foot to be drawn away from the brake pedal which may cause the vehicle to accelerate. By the end of this phase both the torso and vehicle will be at their peak acceleration, while the head is just beginning its acceleration phase (Figure 15.2B).

Phase III: During this phase the head and the torso are at peak acceleration, while the vehicle's acceleration is decreasing. If there is any slack left in the restraint system, then this will permit some more forward movement of the torso, pelvis, and head, increasing the potential for injury. Foreman and Croft feel that at this phase there will be reapplied pressure to the brake (if it was lost during Phase II) and therefore increase the deceleration process, causing greater flexion rotation forces in the neck and cervical spine (Figure 15.2C).

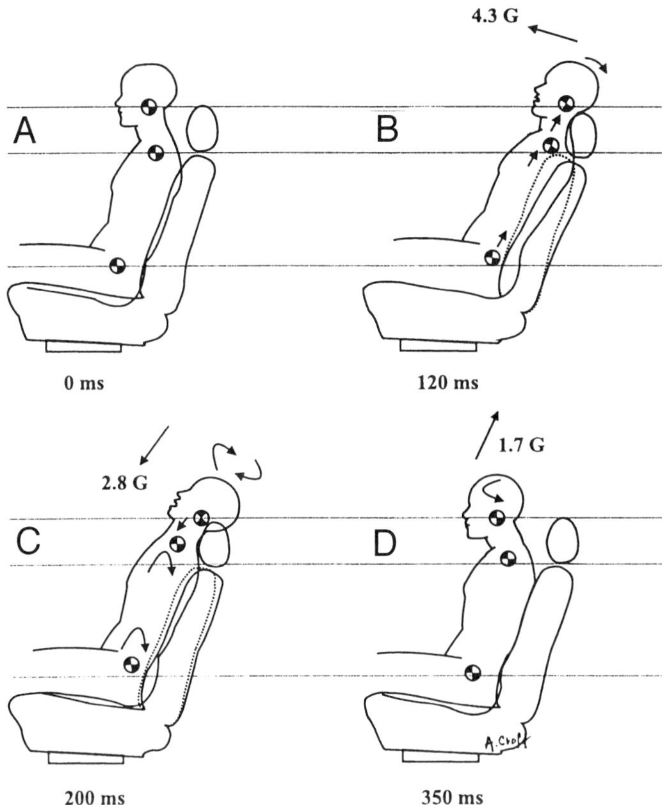

Figure 15.1 The sequence of events in a rear-end collision. (From Foreman, S.M., Croft, A.C., *Whiplash Injuries of Cervical Acceleration/Deceleration Syndrome,* 2nd ed., Williams & Wilkins, Baltimore, 1995. With permission.)

Phase IV: The vehicle is no longer accelerating, while the head and neck are at full deceleration. The torso may be abruptly restrained from the shoulder harness, but the head continues to decelerate unrestrained in a forward arc and this acute and violent bending may be responsible for much of the ligament and muscular soft tissue injury (Figure 15.2D).

It is beyond the scope of this book to describe the mathematical forces that are calculated in determining the biomechanics of cervical injury. Again, I refer the reader, if interested, to read Foreman and Croft[1] and the other literature.

Forces generated in the head and neck are usually expressed in G force. One G is equivalent to the acceleration resulting from the earth's gravity, 9.81 m/sec^2 (32.2 feet/sec^2). The forces that develop in the head are 2 to $2^1/_2$ times that of the struck vehicle and these forces increase as the collision speed increases over 10 mph. Linear velocity described after rear-end impact is usually expressed in feet per second or as meters per second. Angular velocity is also expressed in radians per second, which is measured as a unit of plane angular measurement that is equal to the angle at the center of a circle subtended by an arc equal in length to the radius, which is then measured to determine the velocity to determine damage. What is really important to understand is that as a result of impact there is severe movement that causes hyperflexion, hyperextension, compression on the vertebrae, shearing forces and rotational acceleration that damage the various types of tissue (muscle, nervous, connective and bone). The interesting aspect is that all this happens within 300 milliseconds. The other interesting aspect is that the vast majority of these people recover fully in a matter of weeks to months.

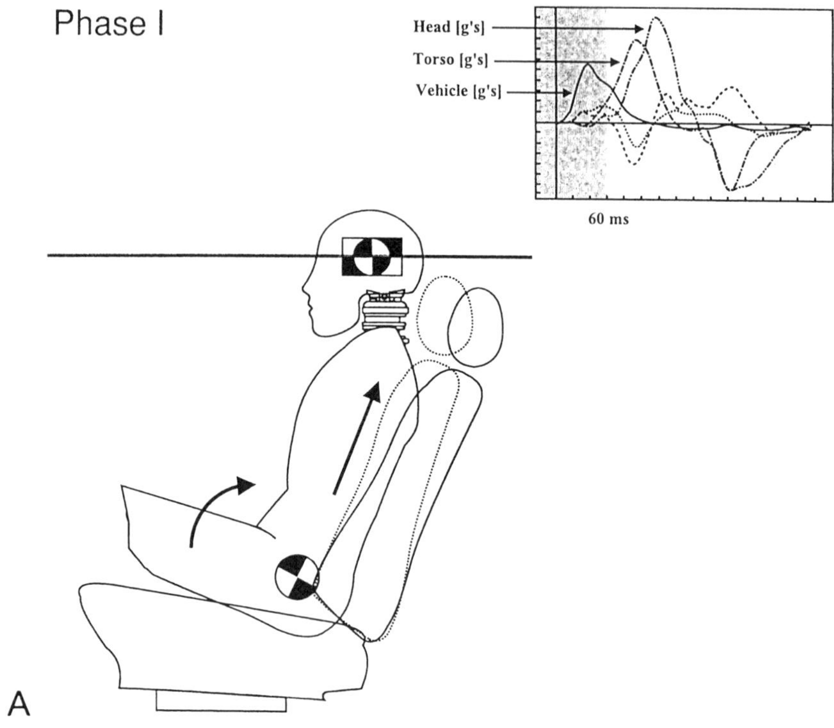

Figure 15.2 Four phases in which injuries can occur. (From Foreman, S.M., Croft, A.C., *Whiplash Injuries of Cervical Acceleration/Deceleration Syndrome,* 2nd ed., Williams & Wilkins, Baltimore, 1995. With permission.)

As mentioned in Chapter 13, it is not always necessary to have head contact to have a post concussion syndrome. Many experiments have been done with rhesus monkeys and skulls with gel that simulated brain tissue and were exposed to accidents. Some monkeys had electroencephalograms (EEG) after whiplash trauma and evidence of concussion was found although the animals did not lose consciousness. Other experiments were done on these animals that would simulate side impact (coronal) and rear end impact (saggital). The side impact accident seemed to cause the more severe of the brain injuries. The animal studies showed that there was more brain injury (DAI, diffuse axonal injury) from side injuries than rear end injuries. Other work has demonstrated that DAI is not necessarily only the result of shearing forces, but may also be secondary to a reactive degeneration caused by the accident.

Chapter 19 discusses the injury to the cervical region from whiplash. The most severe injuries to the cervical spine are C4 to C5 in hyperextension and C5 to C6 in hyperflexion.

As a result of a great deal of research, various alterations in the design of automobiles have been made in order to reduce the number of injuries. Head restraints became mandatory equipment in 1969 in the United States. It appears that the intregal restraints at the right height has been shown to reduce rear-end collisions by 24.5%.

A problem called ramping, which is vertical displacement during the acceleration phase in a whiplash accident, may occur because of a combination of rear impact and typical slight inclination of the seat back. When a car is struck from the rear, it tends to lift up in front, thus lowering itself at the center of gravity. To control ramping, alterations in the automobile have been made by changing the seat back angle, correcting occupant position, correcting impact severity, correcting seat back/occupant friction, correcting vertical motion of the vehicle at impact, and adding seat belts to hold the pelvis down to prevent ramping (Figure 15.3).

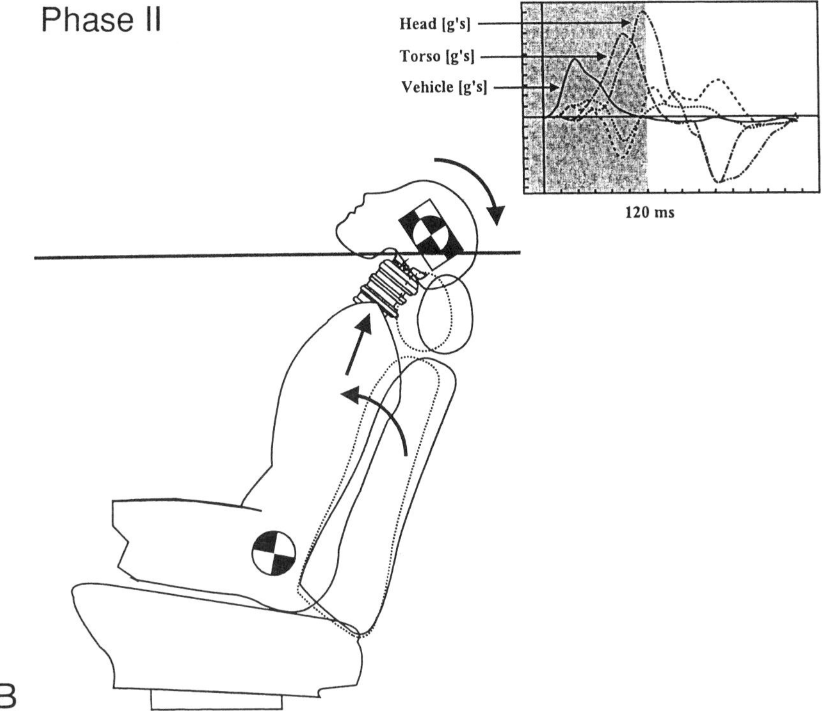

Figure 15.2 (continued)

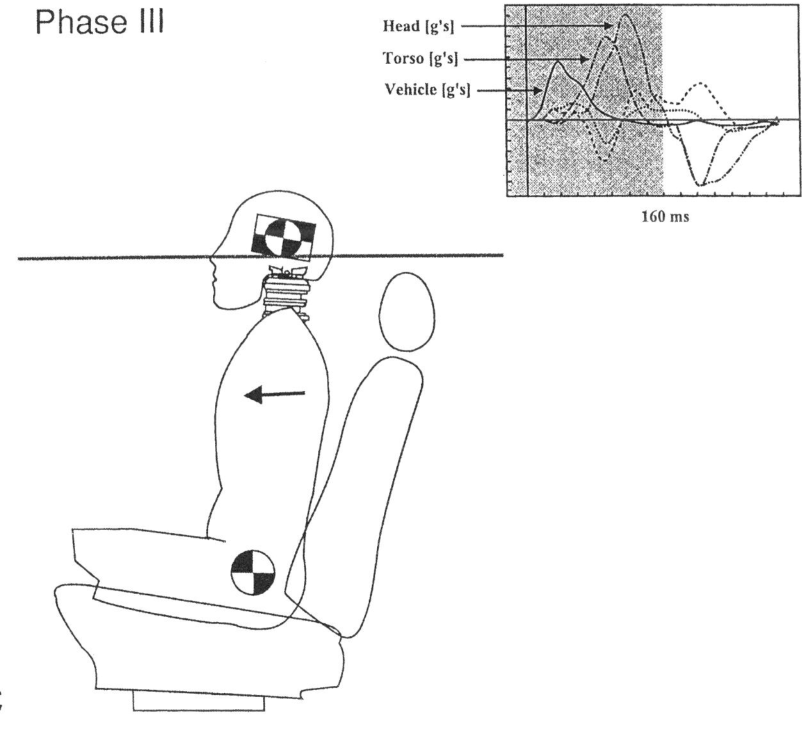

Figure 15.2 (continued)

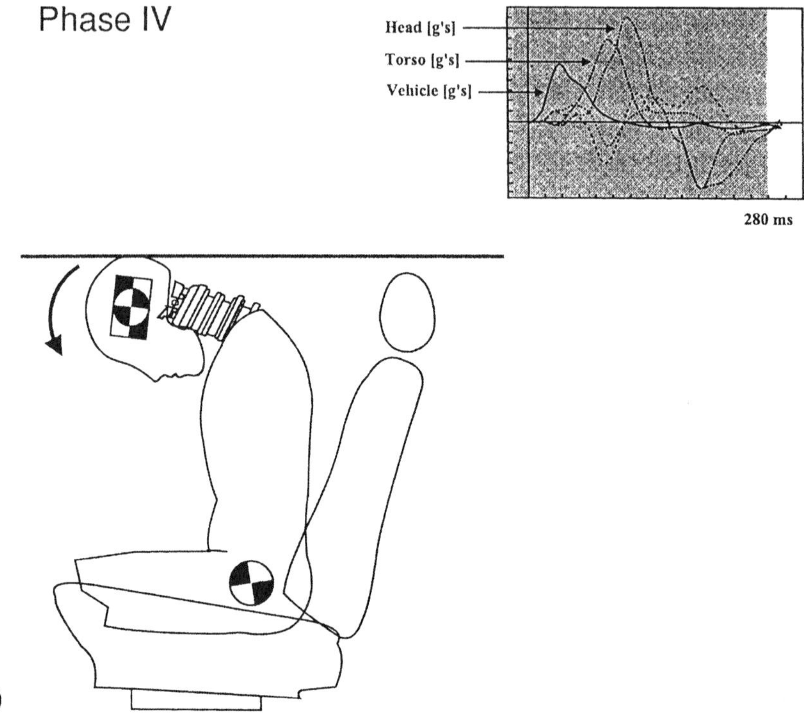

Figure 15.2 (continued)

Seat belts and shoulder harnesses have had significant impact on reducing automobile accident deaths and severe injury. Ironically, these same safety mechanisms sometimes create an increased cervical injury.

A harness that has some slack may potentiate the forward motion of the torso and cause injury to the cervical, thoracic, and lumbar spines (Figure 15.4).

Head injury has caused more deaths in the past 12 years than all the deaths from all the wars this country has been in. Automobile accidents are the leading cause of death for Americans younger than 35, and the major cause of paraplegia and quadriplegia. Headache is the leading cause of lost work days and it has been estimated that proper protection to avoid these injuries would save more than $25 billion each year. Input and pressure from safety engineers, the medical profession, the legal profession, the insurance companies, and the general public will help the auto manufacturers create a vehicle that will minimize the amount of damage inflicted on drivers and passengers in a collision.

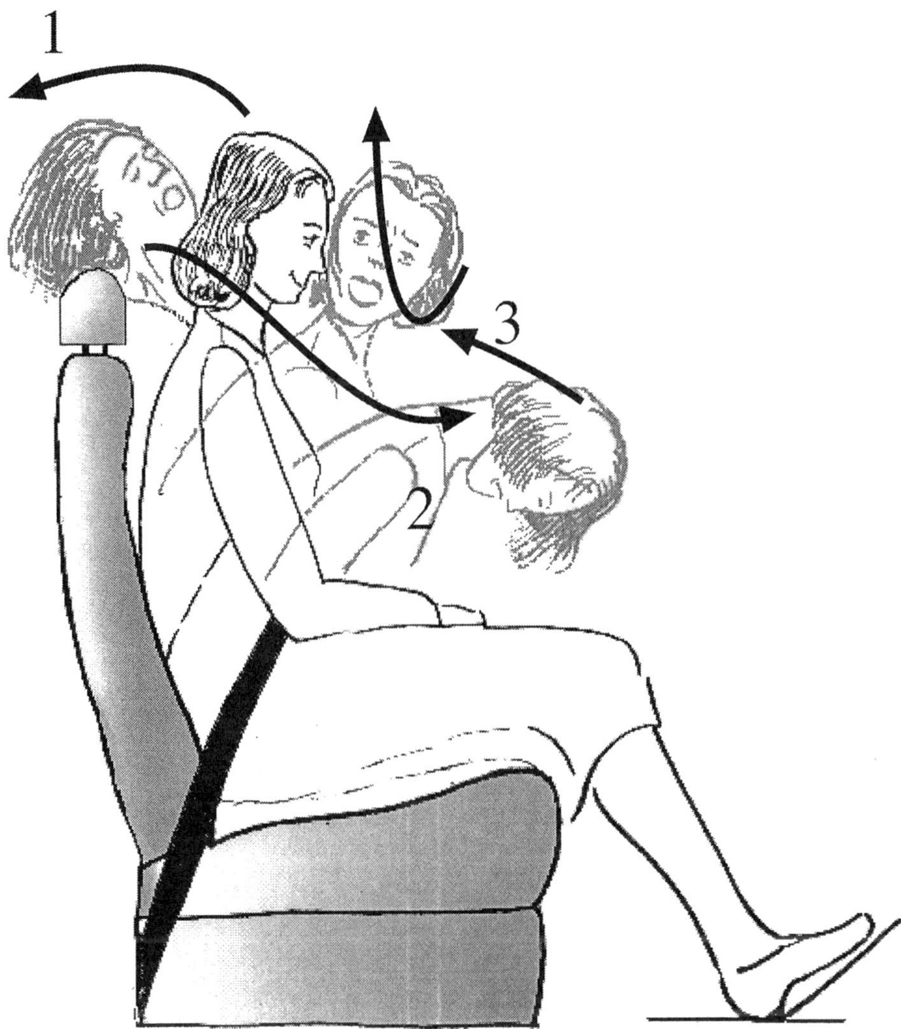

Figure 15.3 During the flexion-extension phase, there is also a vertical displacement called "ramping." This is caused by altering the center of gravity when the car is struck from the rear. Often during this ramping phase, the head will hit the roof of the internal car without the patient's even being aware of striking the head against this surface.

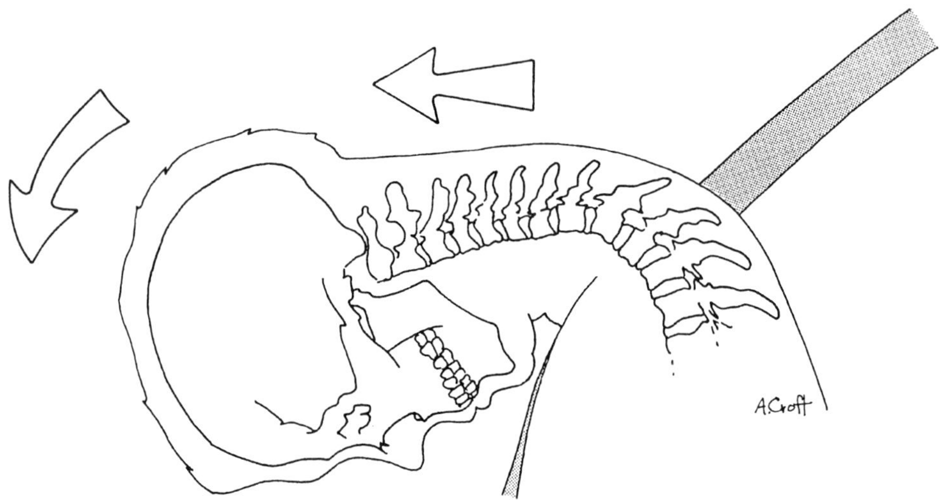

Figure 15.4 Shoulder harnesses restrain the decelerating trunk of the occupant while the head's inertia carries it forward unrestrained. This may be a reason that neck injuries could be accentuated as a result of these restraining systems. (From Foreman, S.M., Croft, A.C., *Whiplash Injuries of Cervical Acceleration/Deceleration Syndrome,* 2nd ed., Williams & Wilkins, Baltimore, 1995. With permission.)

REFERENCES

1. Foreman, S.M., Croft, A.C., *Whiplash Injuries — The Cervical Acceleration/Deceleration Syndrome,* Williams & Wilkins, Baltimore, 1995.

Chapter 16

Anatomy of the Neck and Head

The anatomical structures involved in whiplash are many and can be rather complex. An attempt will be made to discuss the major anatomical areas that are affected in a whiplash injury without the intricate detail that may overwhelm the reader.

Although there are hundreds of different anatomical structures in the head and neck, they all fall into four major categories of tissue types: (1) muscle tissue, (2) nervous tissue, (3) epithelium, and (4) connective tissue.[1]

1. *Muscle tissue:* These are connected cells that have the ability to contract. The three forms are: (a) skeletal muscles, which are striated or striped cells; (b) smooth muscle, or non-striped; and (c) cardiac muscle, which is striped but acts differently than skeletal muscle. Skeletal muscles are under voluntary control and we are familiar with these muscles because we consciously make these muscles work for us. Smooth muscles are always working for us without our knowledge and control organs such as our digestive tract and the dilatation or constriction of our blood vessels, etc. Cardiac muscle, although striped, is not under our voluntary control.
2. *Nervous tissue:* Is a collection of cells that eventually become neurons. Neurons form pathways that send electrical messages that conduct either sensory or motor signals. There are some tissues called glial cells, that support the neurons.
3. *Epithelium:* Is a class of tissue that lines cavities, covers surfaces, or forms glands. These cells can function in absorption or secretion of different materials. They vary in shape and may be simple or stratified. They may line the intestines or respiratory systems, or they may form tubules in organs like the kidney. When they are stratified they cover the oral mucosa and form the skin.
4. *Connective tissue:* Is a very diverse class of tissue and because of the different shapes and chemicals that compose it, the structures it forms can be very strong. These are the cells that form connective tissue, adipose (fat), bone, cartilage, and blood.

Injury to the head and neck not only causes headache, but may also have an effect on the other systems in the body. Therefore, it is important to understand some of the functions of these systems and what organs are associated with them.

The outline shown in Table 16.1, though not complete, will help you to understand the relationship of the systems, their organs, and their function.

When medical reports are sent to the insurance carriers and lawyers, there are medical terms that are clearly understood by clinicians that are difficult to change and still have the exact same meaning. Table 16.2 shows some common terms and their definitions that will help to make medical reports easier to understand.

Table 16.1

System		Organs/Tissues	Major Functions
Cardiovascular		Heart, arteries, arterioles, veins, venules, capillaries, blood	The arterial system distributes nutrients, the venous system collects waste, and both help in temperature regulation
Digestive		Mouth, esophagus, stomach, small and large intestine, liver, gall bladder, pancreas, and salivary glands	Starts digestion and breaks down food for nutrient absorption and elimination of wastes
Endocrine		Ductless glands that secrete hormones — pituitary, thyroid, parathyroid, pancreas, adrenals, ovaries or testes	Secretes hormones into the bloodstream
Integumentary		Skin (epidermis and dermis), hair, lashes and nails, sweat, oil, wax glands	Protects body, maintains temperature, and helps in excretion of wastes
Lymphatic		Spleen, thymus, tonsils, lymph nodes, lymph vessels, lymphocytes	Produces white blood cells for defense against disease and returns plasma and proteins to the blood
Muscular	1.	Skeletal muscles and their tendons anchor them to bones	By contraction they cause and restrict movement of most of the skeleton and help to generate heat
	2.	Smooth Muscle is found in the walls of the many organs	Gastrointestinal, respiratory, and many glands
	3.	Cardiac muscle is found only in the heart	Pumps blood through the heart and vascular system
Nervous		Brain, spinal cord, nerves, ganglia, and the organs of the special senses	Controls body by conduction of impulses, which includes both the motor and sensory systems
Reproductive		Female: ovaries, uterus, vagina, mammaries Testes, prostate, scrotum, penis	Reproduction and sexual relations
Respiratory		Nose, mouth, pharynx, larynx, trachea, bronchi and lungs	Absorbs O_2, eliminates CO_2 and regulates acid/base of body; voice control
Skeletal		There are 206 bones and corresponding ligaments, plus joints and cartilage	They act as support, protection, provide movement, and store minerals, plus help manufacture blood products
Urinary		Kidneys, ureters, bladder and urethra	Adjusts chemical content and volume of blood, excretes waste and water; regulates acid/base of body

Table 16.2

	Anatomical Names		Positional Landmarks
1.	Calvaria — skull cap	1.	Superior — closer to the top of the head
2.	Cephalic — head	2.	Inferior — closer to the bottom of the feet
3.	Cervical — neck	3.	Medial — closer to the body midline
4.	Glossal — tongue	4.	Lateral — further away from the midline
5.	Orbital — eye	5.	Anterior — closer to the front, ventral
6.	Oral — mouth	6.	Posterior — closer to the back, dorsal
7.	Nasal — nose	7.	Internal — on the inside, deep
8.	Pharynx — back of throat	8.	External — on the outside, superficial
9.	Larynx — voice box	9.	Proximal — closer to the trunk
10.	Auditory — ear	10.	Distal — further from the trunk

Adapted from Porta, D.J., in *Head and Neck Injury,* Levine, R.S., Ed., Society of Automotive Engineers, 1994.

Anatomical, surgical, pathological and radiological (CT, MRI) descriptions of the body are related to *sections* in various planes, called coronal (frontal), horizontal (cross-sectional) and sagittal.

1. Frontal or coronal sections are seen when a person faces you. The body is sliced into front and back portions (Figures 16.1 and 16.2).
2. Horizontal (cross-sectional) sections view the body that is cut into superior (to top of head) and inferior portions (Figure 16.3).
3. Sagittal images appear passing from the front to back while looking at a person from his/her side (Figure 16.4 and 16.5).

Other terms that describe motion during an accident are the following: (1) flexion (when the head and/or neck rocks forward, moving the chin closer to the chest); (2) extension (the opposite of flexion, when the head moves toward the back); (3) rotation (when the head moves about a vertical axis); and (4) lateral bending (this brings the ear closer to the shoulder) (Figure 16.6).

Because the jaw is a joint and has movement and is the only movable bone in the skull, the various movements are described as the following: depression (when the jaw is dropped or lowered); elevation with the opposite movements; protracted (slides forward); and retracted (when it is withdrawn).

When reviewing medical reports there are terms that describe injuries to the various systems. Many of the more common terms will be addressed. Injuries to the skin are described in the following terms:

1. Lacerations (cuts)
2. Abrasions (scrapes)
3. Contusions (bruises)
4. Burns
   a. First degree (like sunburn, damages the epidermis)
   b. Second degree (blistering of epidermis and dermis)
   c. Third degree (damage to epidermis, dermis, subcutaneous layer and sometimes chars the organs below. More than 30% of the body can be life threatening. Head and neck in adult is 8 to 10% of the surface of the body and 20% in the infant.)

Injuries to bones, cartilage, and ligaments are described in the following terms:

Bones: Fracture (break or crack). This can be (a) incomplete (cracked, but unbroken); or (b) complete (broken into separate pieces) and either displaced (not in original position) or nondisplaced (still in original position).
Displaced (dislocated)

Cartilage: Fracture (break or crack; similar to bone).
Displaced.

Ligaments: Overstretched or sprained (not strained, which occurs in muscles or tendons).

Injuries to the brain have the following terms:

Contusion (bruised) may be caused by fracture of the skull or the brain striking the skull (i.e., acceleration/deceleration, shearing or rotational forces).

Laceration (cuts) may be caused as above.

Diffuse axonal injury (DAI) is a lesion (disrupted tissue) of numerous neurons caused by acceleration/deceleration.

Concussion is a brief loss of consciousness (see Chapter 13)

Coma is seen in a person rendered unconscious who cannot be aroused.

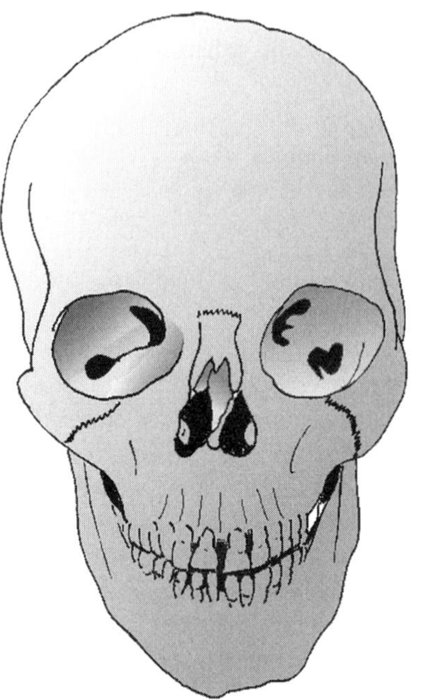

Figure 16.1 The frontal part of the skull.

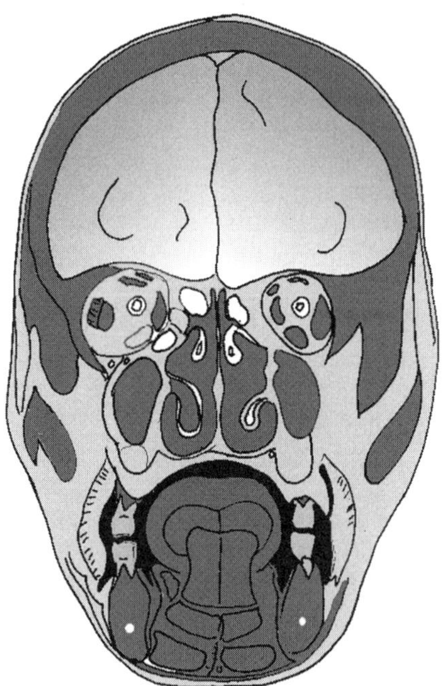

Figure 16.2 A coronal section is a cut through the head showing the interior from a frontal view, but inside the skull.

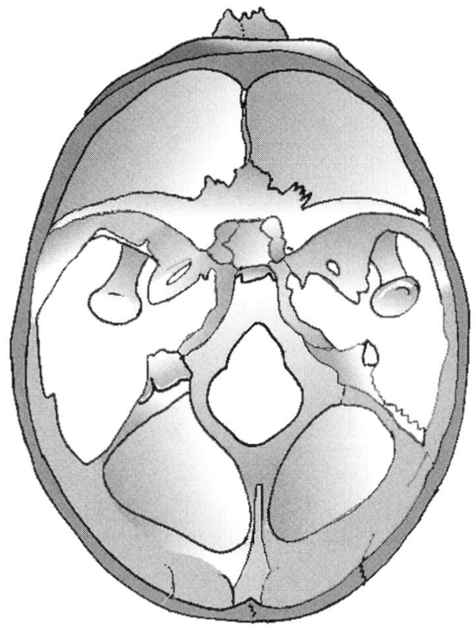

Figure 16.3 A horizontal view showing the interior of either the inferior or the superior portions.

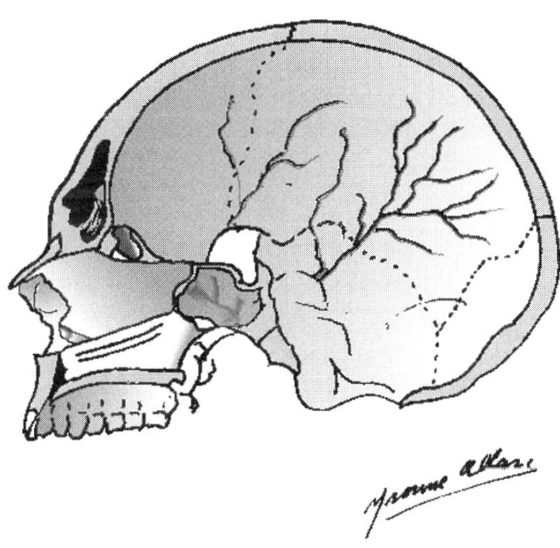

Figure 16.4 A sagittal image of the skull.

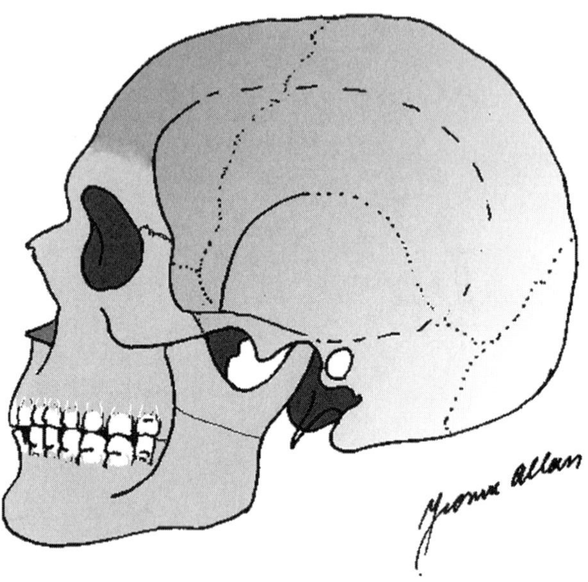

Figure 16.5 A side view of the skull.

Infarct is a focal area of nervous tissue that may be injured and die as a result of ischemia (loss of blood supply).

Transient ischemic attacks (TIA) are temporary losses of blood supply, causing brief lost brain function.

Cerebrovascular accident (CVA) or stroke is caused by sudden ischemia (loss of blood supply), causing permanent neurologic damage.

Cerebrovascular hemorrhage is caused by bleeding.

Embolism is a blockage of a vessel by a clot, fat, air, etc.

Aneurysm is a thinning of the wall of a blood vessel that results in a bulging portion of that vessel. Untreated, the aneurysm may rupture and bleed massively.

Hematoma is a collection of blood from a broken blood vessel. These hematomas can invade or create a space between the layers of the meninges (coverings of the brain); epidural, subdural, or subarachnoid.

Contusion, laceration, and DAI may also occur in the spinal cord.

BONES OF THE HEAD AND NECK

Before birth all the bones in the head develop as pairs. After birth some of these paired bones become fused (frontal, occipital, and mandibular bones) and the joints (synostosis) between the two parts form a suture line which can be very difficult to find and are often considered unpaired.

There are 29 bones of the head and they are divided into 8 cranial bones, 6 auditory bones, 14 facial bones, and 1 hyoid bone, grouped as shown in Table 16.3.

Cranial bones (8 bones): They cover the superior of the brain (cranial vault) and the underside of the brain (cranial base or basilar). In the basilar portion, there are foramina (holes) that transmit nerves and blood vessels. The bones include the frontal bone, two parietal bones, two temporal bones, one occipital bone, one ethmoid bone and one sphenoid bone.

Auditory ossicles (6 bones): These bones, in three pairs, are housed in the temporal bones and vibrate when sound waves strike the eardrum. They are called the incus, stapes, and the malleus bones.

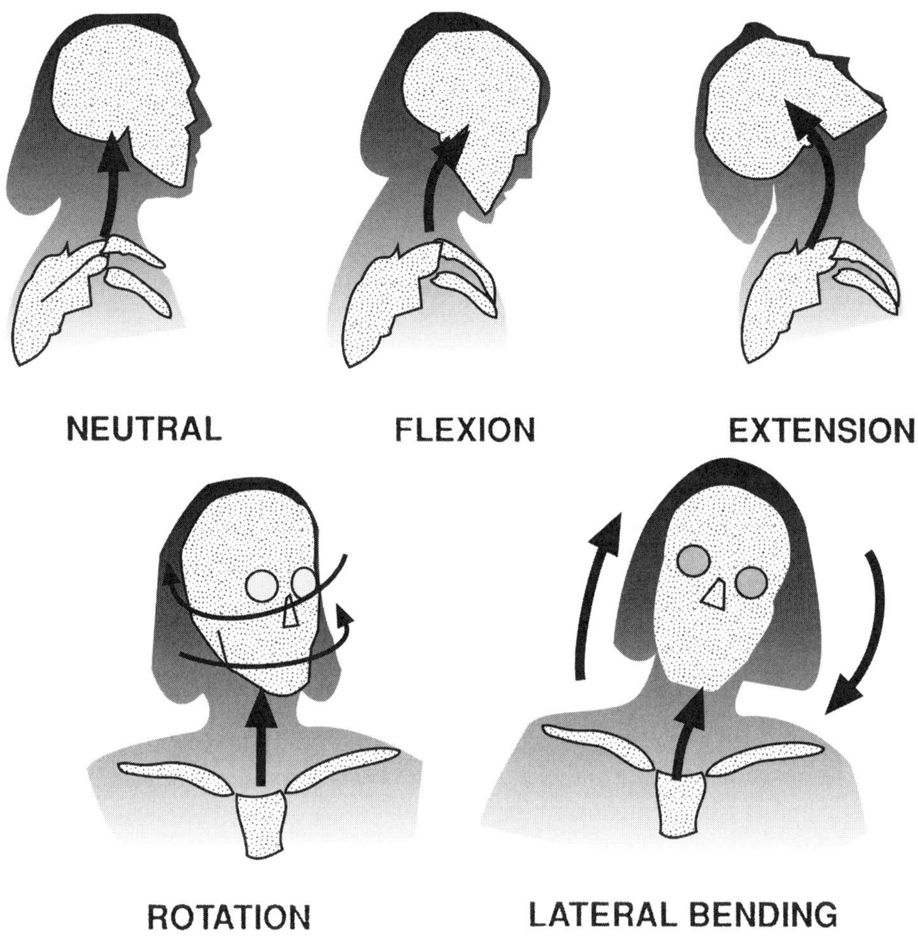

Figure 16.6 Anatomical descriptions of head motion.

Table 16.3 The Bones of the Head

Cranial vault	Frontal, temporalis, parietal and occipital bones
Cranial base (basilar)	Frontal, ethmoid, temporalis, sphenoid, and occipital bones
Auditory region	Temporal with auditory ossicles (incus, stapes, and malleus)
Orbital cavity	Frontal, zygomatic, maxilla, lacrimal, ethmoid, sphenoid and palatine bones
Nasal cavity	Nasals, maxillae, ethmoid, inferior nasal conchae, sphenoid and palatines
Nasal septum	Ethmoid, vomer, maxillae, and palatine bones
Oral cavity	Maxillae, palatines, sphenoid, and mandible
Paranasal sinuses	Found inside the frontal, ethmoid, sphenoid, and maxillary bones

From Travell, J.G., Simons, D.G., *Myofascial Pain and Dysfunction: The Trigger Point Manual,* Williams & Wilkins, Baltimore, 1983. With permission.

Facial bones (14 bones): Six pairs of facial bones are nasal bones (bridge only, the rest are cartilage), lacrimal bones, zygomatic bones (cheek bones), maxillary bones, inferior nasal conchae, and the palatine bones. The two unpaired facial bones are the vomer and the mandible. Several of the bones around the nasal cavity contain large air pockets and are lined with mucous membranes. These pockets open into the nasal cavity and are called the paranasal sinuses. They seem to decrease the weight of the skull and affect the resonant characteristics of vocalization. The mandible is the

1- Ethmoid
2- Frontal
3- Inferior Nasal Concha
4- Lacrimal
5- Mandible
6- Nasal
7- Parietal
8- Sphenoid
9- Temporal
10- Vomer
11- Maxilla
12- Zygomatic

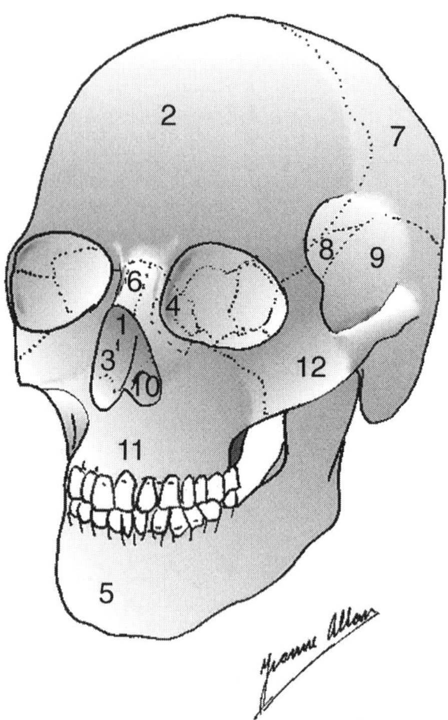

Figure 16.7 Anterior view of skull bones. (Adapted from Travell, J.G., Simons, D.G., *Myofascial Pain and Dysfunction: The Trigger Point Manual*, Williams & Wilkins, Baltimore, 1983.)

only voluntary movable bone of the skull. The joint that allows this movement is called the temporomandibular joint (TMJ). Proper alignment of the teeth in the mandible and maxilla is termed occlusion. Misalignment is called malocclusion (Figure 16.7).

Hyoid bone (1 bone): This bone does not articulate directly with the other skull bones, but is connected by long ligaments to the styloid process of the temporal bone. Muscles attached to it are associated with the tongue and neck.

The bones of the neck consist of seven cervical vertebrae and are often referred to from superior to inferior, as C1 to C7. The anterior portion of the vertebra is called the body or centrum. A ring of bone encloses the spinal cord and that opening is called the vertebral foramen. The posterior portion of this foramen is called the neural or vertebral arch. These arches have pedicles that lead to laminae. The vertebra articulates with the vertebrae above and below it on flat surfaces called facets which create a joint, called the facet joint or apophysial or zygapophyseal joints. Tranverse processes are lateral protrusions that spring from the arch and a spinous process is directed posteriorly. The transverse process of the cervical vertebrae have additional openings that protect the vertebral arteries that supply the brain.

C1, or the first cervical vertebra, is called the *atlas*. The entire head rests on the atlas. This vertebrae is a simple ring of bone almost lacking a body. C2 is called the *axis* and its body is fused to the atlas. The body of C2 extends up into the ring of C1 and is called the odontoid process, and has facets both on the anterior and posterior sides. This body is similar to an axle in a wheel and when we rotate our heads, the head and atlas pivot around the body of the axis.

The vertebral column is flexible and has normal curves that support and balance our weight. In the upper cervical region the curvature is convex (looking from the anterior) to center our head over our body. Important in whiplash injuries is to understand the role of the ligaments (supporting bone to bone) that may be injured and cause pain. There are numerous ligaments interconnecting portions of the vertebral arches of neighboring vertebrae whose names are beyond the scope of

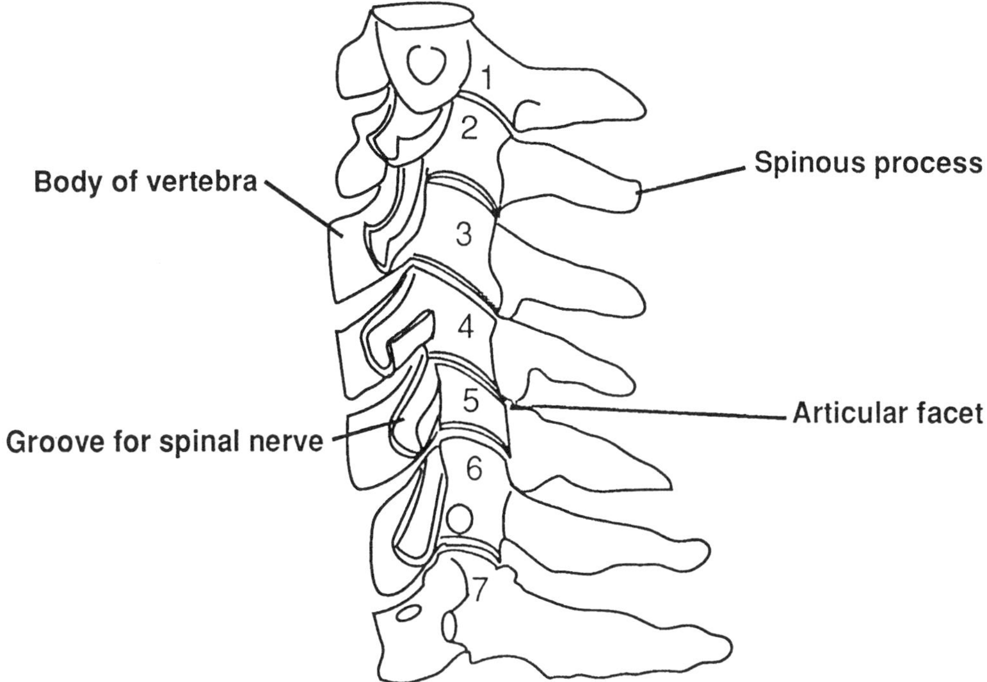

Figure 16.8 The 2nd to 7th cervical vertebrae.

this book, but are often referred to as interspinous ligaments, interlaminary ligaments, supraspinous ligaments, etc. There are longitudinal ligaments that span the anterior and posterior portions of the vertebral bodies. These longitudinal ligaments are the anterior longitudinal ligament, the posterior longitudinal ligament, the tectorial membrane, anterior and posterior atlanto-occipital ligament, atlanto-epistrophic ligament and the ligamentum nuchae (Figure 16.8).

JOINTS OF THE NECK AND HEAD

There is more evidence that ongoing neck and head pain may be related to the joints in the neck and mandible in the face. A joint or articulation is a union of two or more bones. Rarely do bones touch each other, and the joints are usually separated and classified as fibrous, cartilaginous and synovial.

Fibrous joints have tough fibrous connective tissue between the bones, making the joint virtually immovable (synarthroses). Before birth the fetus has very wide and dense connective tissue causing soft spots (fontanels) between several of the cranial bones. Usually within two years the soft spots are replaced by bone and suture lines remain. Gomphoses are peg-and-socket style joints between the teeth and the jaw. The connective tissue holds the teeth firmly in their sockets (alveoli).

Cartilaginous joints are somewhat movable (amphiarthroses) due to a disc of fibrocartilage between the bones. The bodies of the cervical vertebrae are connected to one another via fibrocartilage pads called intervertebral discs. These discs have some motion and act like a shock absorber. The center of the disc is called the nucleus palposus and contains glycosaminoglycans or GAGs that bind water. When injured or compressed, there is release of water and the disc stiffens.

Other areas of the head and neck that are made up of cartilage but are not joints are the epiglottis, most of the external ear, and the auditory or eustachian tube, which are made up of elastic cartilage.

Hyaline cartilage makes up the majority of the nose and also the tips of the facets of the vertebrae, parts of the TMJ, most of the larynx, the tracheal rings, and the thyroid cartilage (Adam's apple).

Synovial joints are extremely important and have been implicated in cervicogenic headache. These joints are fluid-filled cavities between the bones that allow them to move freely. In the jaw the synovial fluid joint allows the temporomandibular joint (TMJ) to move so we may chew and talk. In the neck, there are synovial joints between the articular facets of one cervical vertebra with another.

These joints, together with the cartilaginous intervertebral disc joint between the bodies of the vertebrae, provide a considerable range of motion for the spine.

MUSCLES OF THE HEAD AND NECK

There are huge numbers of muscles related to the head and neck. They serve many functions: facial expression, mastication, posture, position of the head, position of the eye, position of the glossal (swallowing), position of the pharynx, position of the palate, and position of the larynx. This section discusses the various muscles of the head and neck that are often mentioned as a cause of headache as a result of a whiplash accident. The cause of headache may be due to spasm of the muscle or trigger points that have referred pain to the head.

Travell and Simons,[2] in their landmark volume on trigger points have developed a muscle pain guide and mention specific areas that hurt from trigger points (Figure 16.9). The pain guide breaks the areas into the following groups:

1. Vertex pain
2. Back of head pain
3. Temporal headache
4. Frontal headache
5. Ear and temporomandibular joint pain
6. Eye and eyebrow pain
7. Cheek and jaw pain
8. Toothache
9. Back of neck pain
10. Throat and front of neck pain

The muscles that refer pain to these areas are listed in Table 16.4. The letter (s) refers to muscles that are spillover pattern to the region.

A discussion of all the attachments and the neural innervations of these muscles is beyond the scope of this book and I advise the reader to refer to Travell and Simon's book *Myofascial Pain and Dysfunction. The Trigger Point Manual*[2] for an excellent explanation of this information. A brief description of these muscles is provided below. Trigger points are discussed in more detail in Chapter 17.

Sternocleidomastoid muscle: This muscle has two divisions, the sternal and the clavicular. The sternal division attaches from the manubrium sterni to the mastoid process and the nuchal line of the occipital bone. The clavicular section attaches from the anterior surface of the clavicle to the same structures as the sternal section. The action of one muscle alone rotates the face to the opposite side and lifts it toward the ceiling, and the action of the muscles working together flex the head and act as auxiliary muscles of inspiration (Figure 16.10).

Masseter muscle: This muscle attaches above to the zygomatic arch and maxilla and below to the outer surface of the mandible. Its innervation comes from the mandibular division of the trigeminal nerve (C-V). The actions are to elevate the mandible and to retrude (to force inward or backward) it (Figure 16.11).

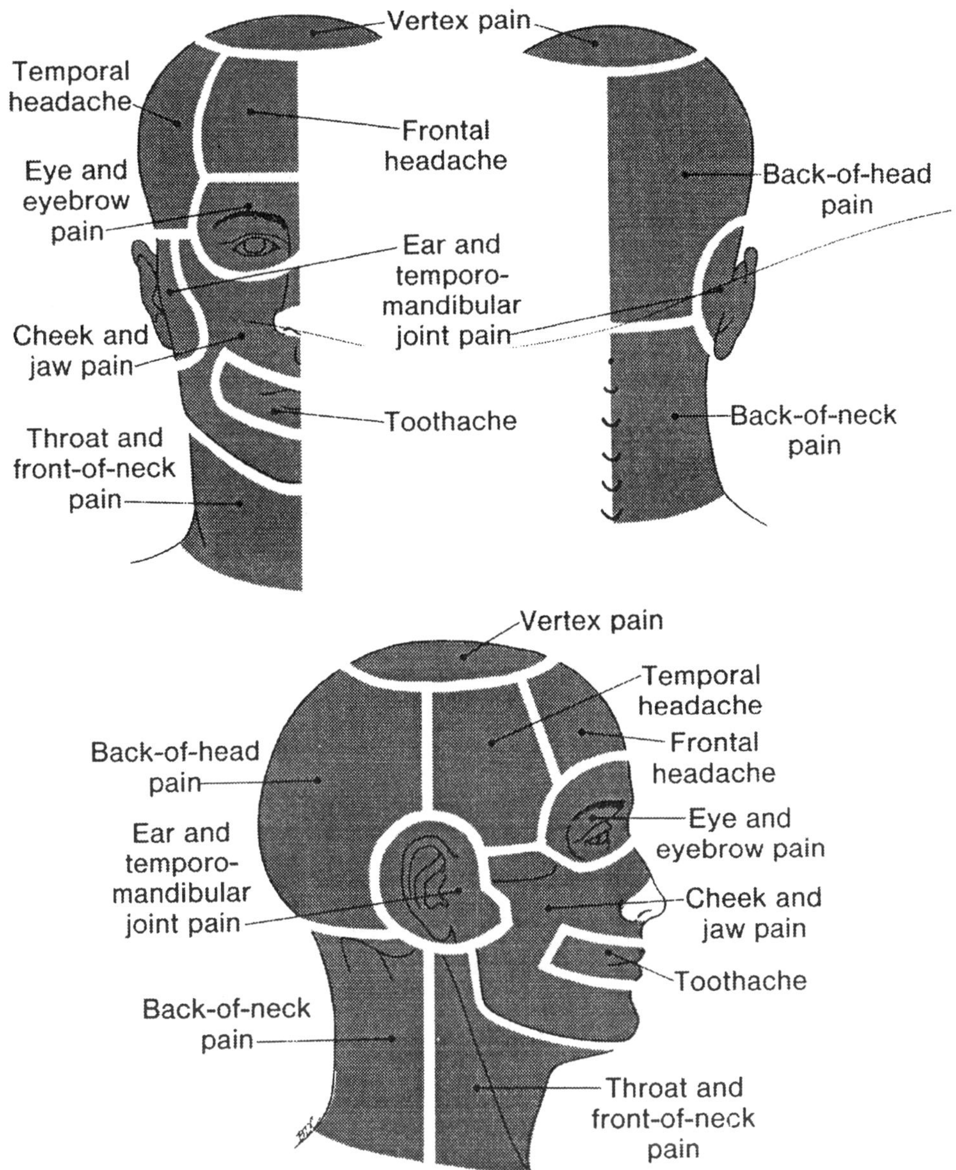

Figure 16.9 Pain guide to the head and neck region. (From Travell, J.G., Simons, D.G., *Myofascial Pain and Dysfunction: The Trigger Point Manual*, Williams & Wilkins, Baltimore, 1983. With permission.)

Temporalis muscle: This muscle attaches above to the temporal bone and below to the coronoid process of the mandible. The innervation comes from the mandibular division of the trigeminal nerve (C-V). The action of the muscle is to close the jaw and retrude the mandible (Figure 16.12).

Medial (internal) pterygoid muscle: This muscle attaches from the angle of the mandible and to the lateral pterygoid plate and forms a sling with the masseter muscle. The innervation comes from the mandibular division of the trigeminal nerve (C-V). The action is to elevate the mandible and to laterally deviate it (Figure 16.13).

Lateral (external) pterygoid muscle: There are two divisions of this muscle. The superior division attaches to the sphenoid bone and to the articular disc and capsule of the TMJ. The inferior division attaches to the lateral pterygoid plate and to the neck of the mandible. This muscle is

Table 16.4 Muscles that Refer Pain in the Head and Neck

1. Vertex pain
    - Sternocleidomastoid (sternal portion)
        - (s) Splenius capitis

2. Back of head pain
    - Trapezius
    - Sternocleidomastoid (sternal portion)
    - Sternocleidomastoid (clavicular portion)
        - (s) Semispinalis capitis
        - (s) Semispinalis cervicus
        - (s) Splenius cervicis
        - (s) Suboccipital group
        - (s) Occipitalis
        - (s) Digastric
        - (s) Temporalis

3. Temporal headache
    - Trapezius
    - Sternocleidomastoid (sternal portion)
    - Temporalis
        - (s) Splenius cervicis
        - (s) Suboccipital group
    - Semispinalis capitis

4. Frontal headache
    - Sternocleidomastoid (clavicular portion)
    - Sternocleidomastoid (sternal portion)
        - (s) Semispinalis capitis
    - Frontalis
    - Zygomaticus major

5. Ear and temporomandibular joint pain
    - Lateral pterygoid
    - Masseter (deep portion)
    - Sternocleidomastoid (clavicular portion)
    - Medial pterygoid

6. Eye and eyebrow pain
    - Sternocleidomastoid (sternal portion)
    - Temporalis
    - Spenius cervicis
    - Masseter (superficial portion)
        - (s) Suboccipital group
    - Occiptalis
    - Orbicularis oculi
        - (s) Trapezius

7. Cheek and jaw pain
    - Sternocleidomastoid (sternal portion)
    - Masseter (superficial portion)
    - Lateral pterygoid
    - Trapezius
        - (s) Masseter
        - (s) Digastric
        - (s) Medial pterygoid
    - Platysma
    - Orbicularis oculi
    - Zygomaticus major

Table 16.4 Muscles that Refer Pain in the Head and Neck (continued)

8.	Toothache
	Temporalis
	Masseter (superficial)
	Digastric (anterior portion)
9.	Back of neck pain
	Trapezius (various portions)
	Multifidi
	(s) Levator scapulae
	(s) Spenius cervicis
	(s) Infraspinatus
10.	Throat and front of neck pain
	Sternocleidomastoid (sternal portion)
	Digastric
	(s) Medial pterygoid

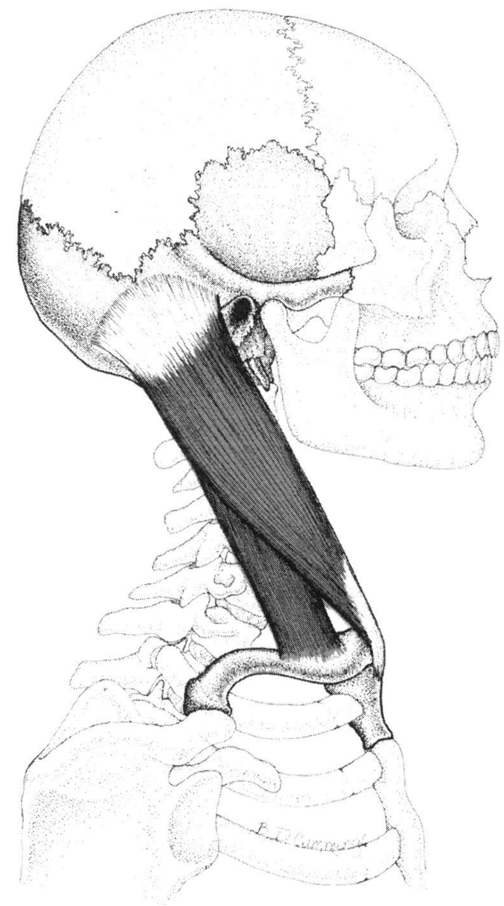

Figure 16.10 Attachments of the sternocleidomastoid muscle. (From Travell, J.G., Simons, D.G., *Myofascial Pain and Dysfunction: The Trigger Point Manual*, Williams & Wilkins, Baltimore, 1983. With permission.)

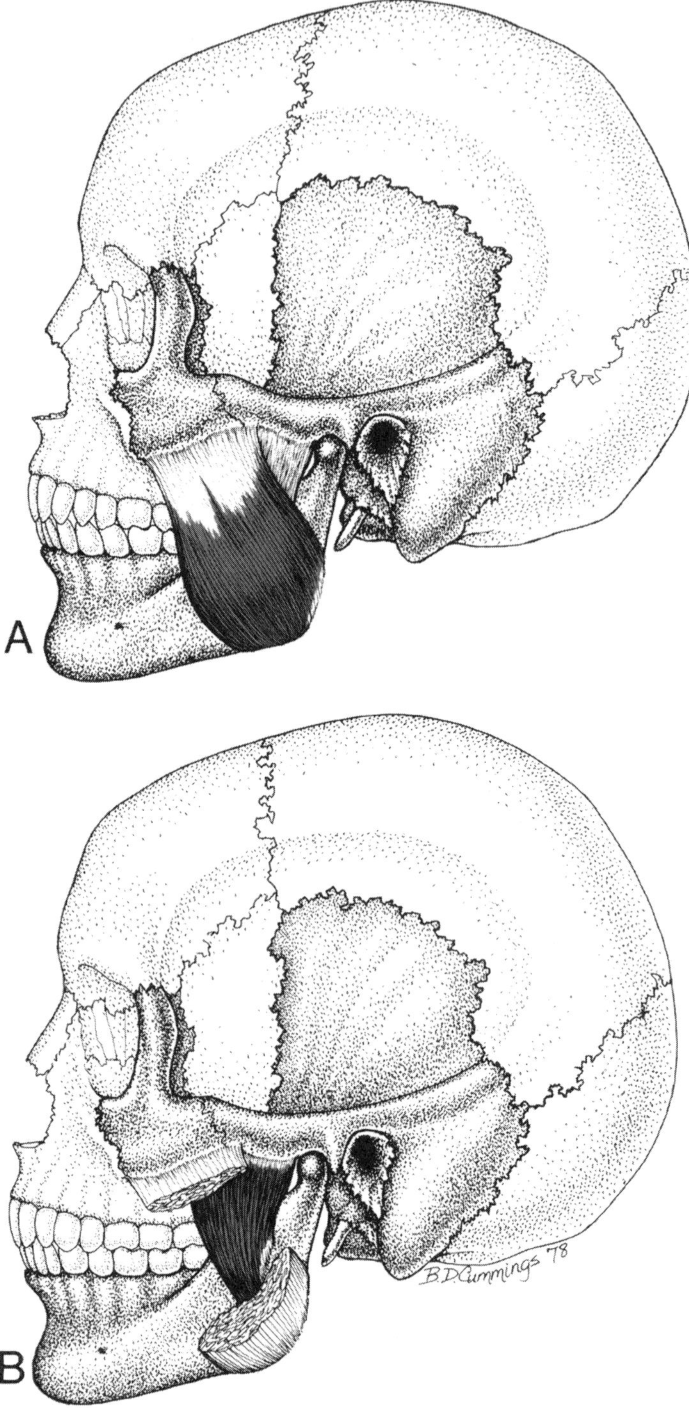

Figure 16.11 Attachments of the masseter muscle. (A) Superficial layer, (B) deep layer, with superficial layer removed. (From Travell, J.G., Simons, D.G., *Myofascial Pain and Dysfunction: The Trigger Point Manual*, Williams & Wilkins, Baltimore, 1983. With permission.)

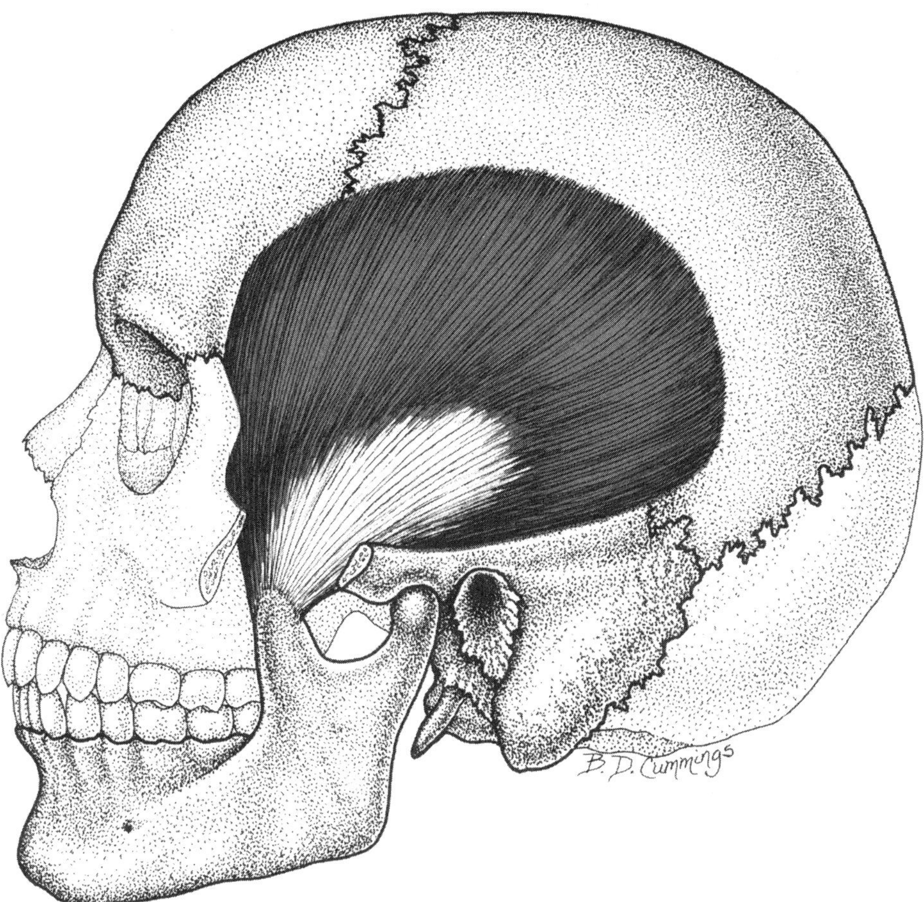

Figure 16.12 Attachments of the temporalis muscle to the coronoid process of the mandible and, above, to the temporal bone. (From Travell, J.G., Simons, D.G., *Myofascial Pain and Dysfunction: The Trigger Point Manual*, Williams & Wilkins, Baltimore, 1983. With permission.)

primarily supplied by the mandibular division of the trigeminal nerve (C-V). The action of this muscle is to act on the disc and assist in mandibular elevation, and the inferior division protrudes and depresses the mandible (Figure 16.14).

Digastric muscle: This muscle has two bellies, the anterior, which attaches the symphysis of the mandible to the hyoid bone, and the posterior belly, from the hyoid bone to the mastoid notch. The innervation to the anterior belly comes from offshoots of the mandibular division of the trigeminal nerve (C-V) and the posterior belly from a branch of the facial nerve (C-VII). The action of both bellies assists in the depression and retrusion of the mandible (Figure 16.15).

Facial muscles (orbicularis oculi, zygomaticus major, and platysma): These muscles are involved in facial expression. These muscles are rarely attached to bone and are mostly attached to fascia (fibrous membrane coverings, supporting and separating muscles). These muscles are supplied by the facial nerve (C-VII). The action of the orbicularis oculi is to close the eye. The zygomaticus major draws the corners of the mouth upward and backward. The platysma tenses the skin of the anterior neck and pulls the corner of the mouth downward (Figure 16.16).

Occipitofrontalis: These muscles are not attached to bone and are innervated by the facial nerve (C-VII). Their action is to wrinkle the forehead (Figure 16.17).

The muscles in the back of the neck lie in five layers of increasing depth: (1) the trapezius, (2) the splenius capitis and cervicis, (3) the semispinalis capitis, semispinalis cervicis, and the

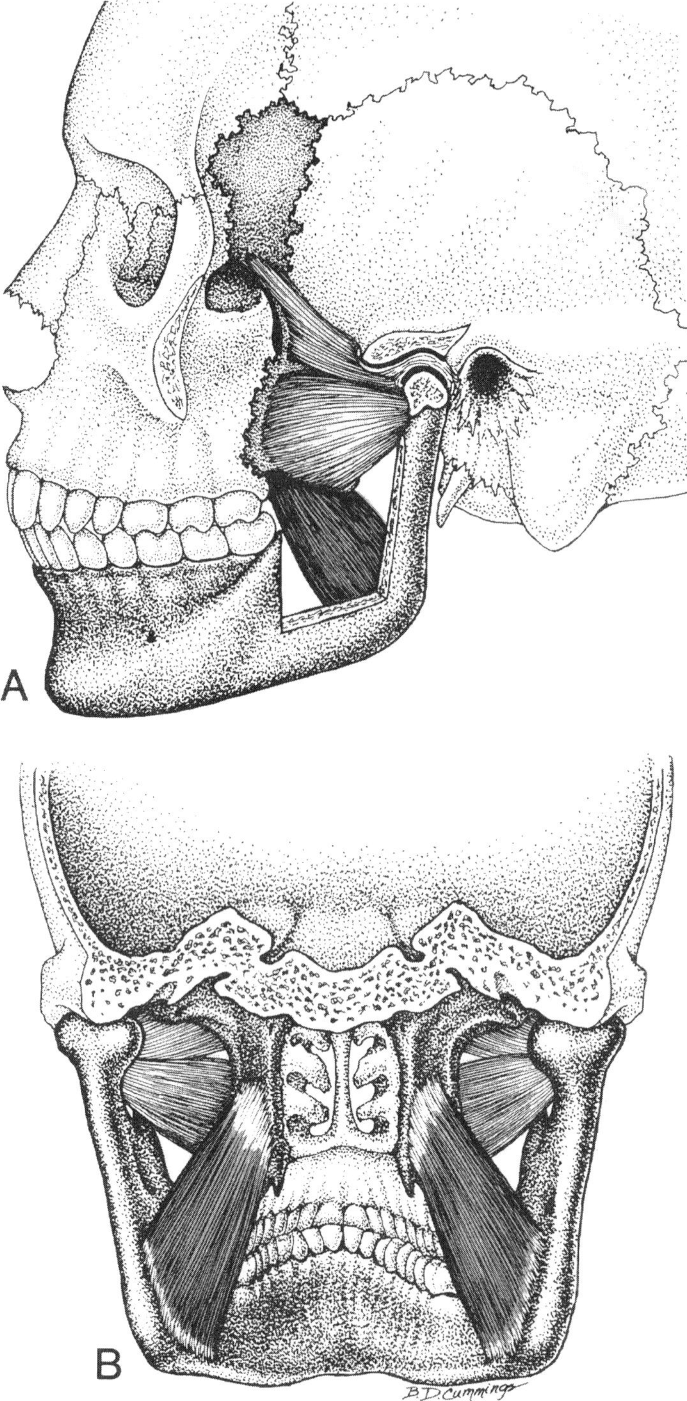

Figure 16.13 Attachments of the medial pterygoid muscle. (A) See text for attachments. (B) Coronal section of the skull, just behind the temporomandibular joint looking forward inside the mouth. Attachments are, above, to the lateral pterygoid plate of the sphenoid bone and, below, to the medial surface of the mandible. (From Travell, J.G., Simons, D.G., *Myofascial Pain and Dysfunction: The Trigger Point Manual*, Williams & Wilkins, Baltimore, 1983. With permission.)

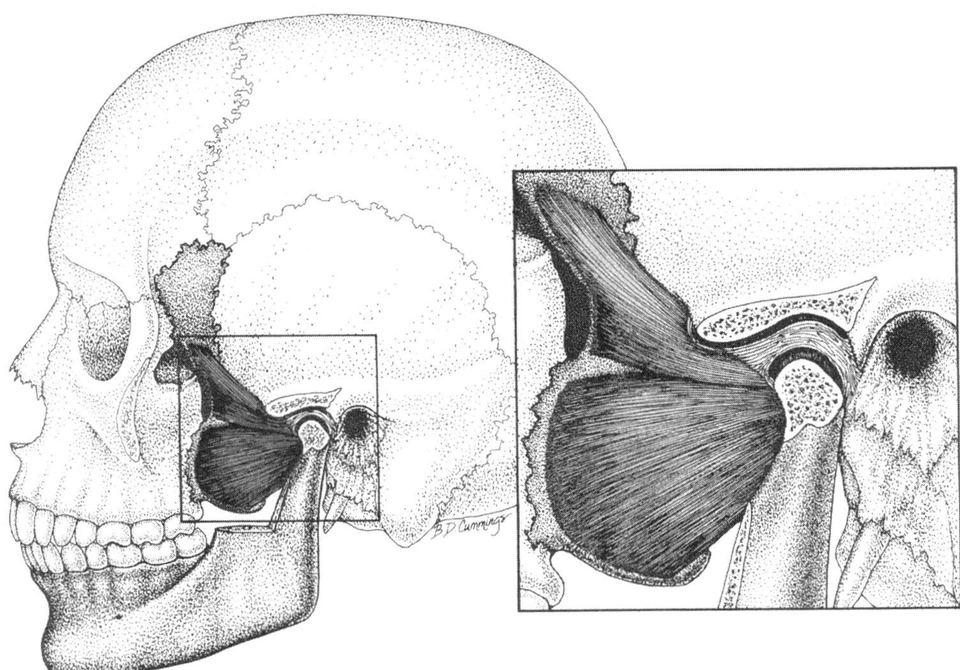

Figure 16.14 Attachments of the lateral or external pterygoid muscle. (From Travell, J.G., Simons, D.G., *Myofascial Pain and Dysfunction: The Trigger Point Manual*, Williams & Wilkins, Baltimore, 1983. With permission.)

longissimus capitis, (4) the multifidi, rotatores, and small suboccipital muscles that connect the occiput with the first two cervical vertebrae, and (5) the recti capitis posterior major and minor, and the obliquus capitis inferior and superior.

Trapezius muscle: This muscle has three divisions, upper, middle, and lower fibers. They are diamond-shaped and attach from the occiput to T12 and laterally to the front of the clavicle and the back of the spine of the scapula. The spinal accessory or cranial nerve XI supplies the motor fibers and the 2nd to 4th cervical nerves supply the sensory fibers. The action of the upper trapezius elevates the shoulders and rotates the glenoid fossa so that the socket of the shoulder joint faces upward. The lower trapezius assists in this rotation, and the middle trapezius adducts (retracts) the scapula (Figure 16.18).

Splenius capitis and splenius cervicis muscles: These attachments are from the spinous processes of the lower cervical and upper thoracic vertebrae and to the transverse processes of the upper cervical vertebrae and to the mastoid process of the skull. The innervation of these muscles is from the lateral branches of the dorsal primary division of spinal nerves C2 to C4. Some may come from C1, C5, and rarely C6. The actions of these muscles are to extend the head and neck and to rotate them, turning the face toward the same side (Figure 16.19).

Posterior cervical muscles (semispinalis capitis, semispinalis cervicis, and multifidi and rotatores): The semispinalis capitis and semispinalis cervicis muscles attach from below to the transverse processes of thoracic vertebrae (T1 to T6) and from the cervical vertebrae (C3 to C6) and above to the nuchal lines of the occiput and to the spinous processes of C2 to C5. The cervical multifidi attach above to the spinous processes of vertebrae C2 to C5 and below to the articular processes of C4 to C7. The rotatores have similar attachments but are shorter and connect adjacent or alternate vertebrae. These muscles lie beneath the multifidi and have the same functions. The innervation is from the posterior primary divisions of the first four or five cervical nerves. The

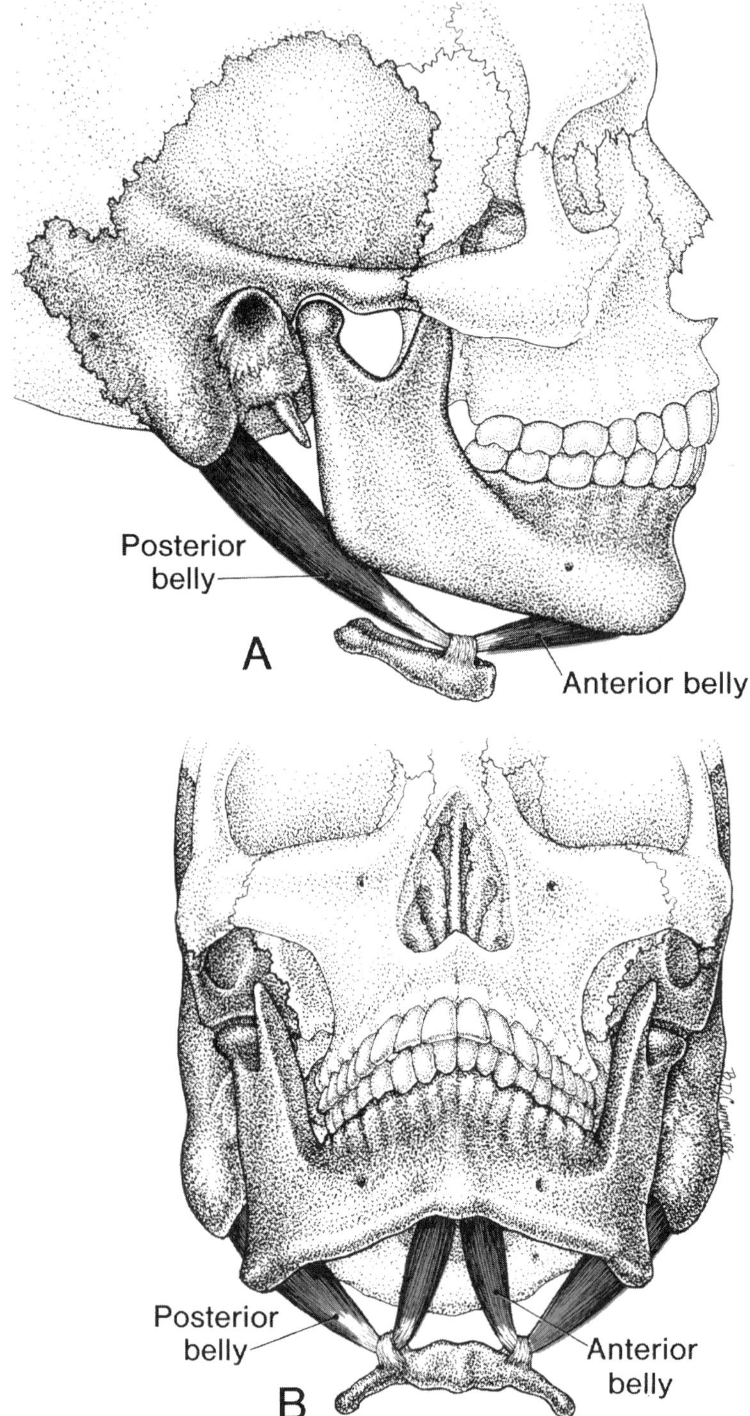

Figure 16.15 Attachments of the digastric muscle. The posterior belly attaches to the mastoid notch above, and below to the tendon of the hyoid bone. The anterior belly attaches above to the mandible, and below to the common tendon of the hyoid bone. (From Travell, J.G., Simons, D.G., *Myofascial Pain and Dysfunction: The Trigger Point Manual*, Williams & Wilkins, Baltimore, 1983. With permission.)

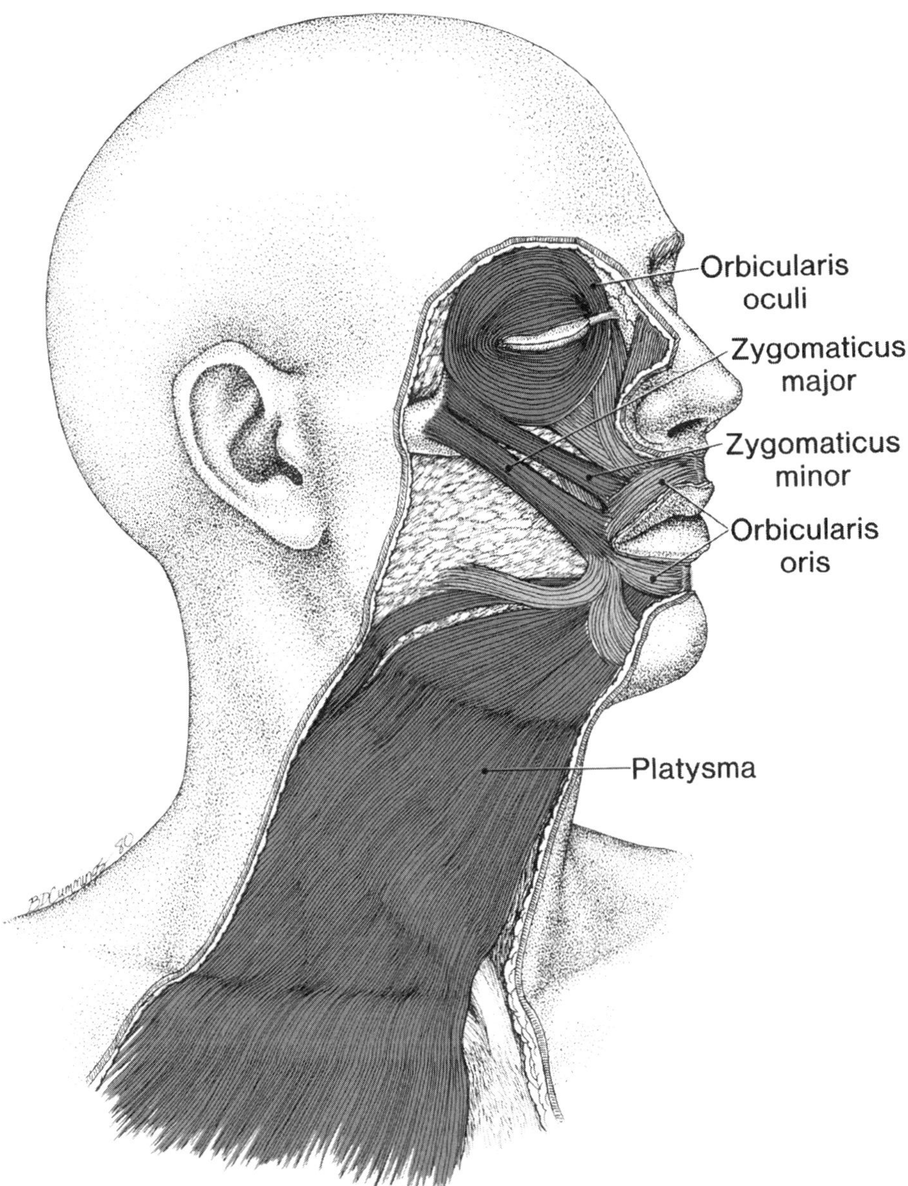

Figure 16.16 Attachments of selected facial muscles and face-related cutaneous muscles. The muscles are the orbicularis oculi, the zogomaticus major, the zygomaticus minor, orbicularis oris, and the platysma. See text for attachments and function. (From Travell, J.G., Simons, D.G., *Myofascial Pain and Dysfunction: The Trigger Point Manual*, Williams & Wilkins, Baltimore, 1983. With permission.)

actions of the posterior cervical muscles are primarily extension and rotation of the head and neck (Figure 16.20).

Suboccipital muscles (recti capitis posterior major and minor and obliquus capitis superior and inferior): These muscles attach from the tubercle on the posterior arch of the atlas and the first two cervical vertebrae with the occipital bone. The innervation of these muscles is supplied by branches of the dorsal primary division of the suboccipital nerve (C1). The actions of these muscles are to extend, rotate and tilt the head to the same side (Figure 16.21).

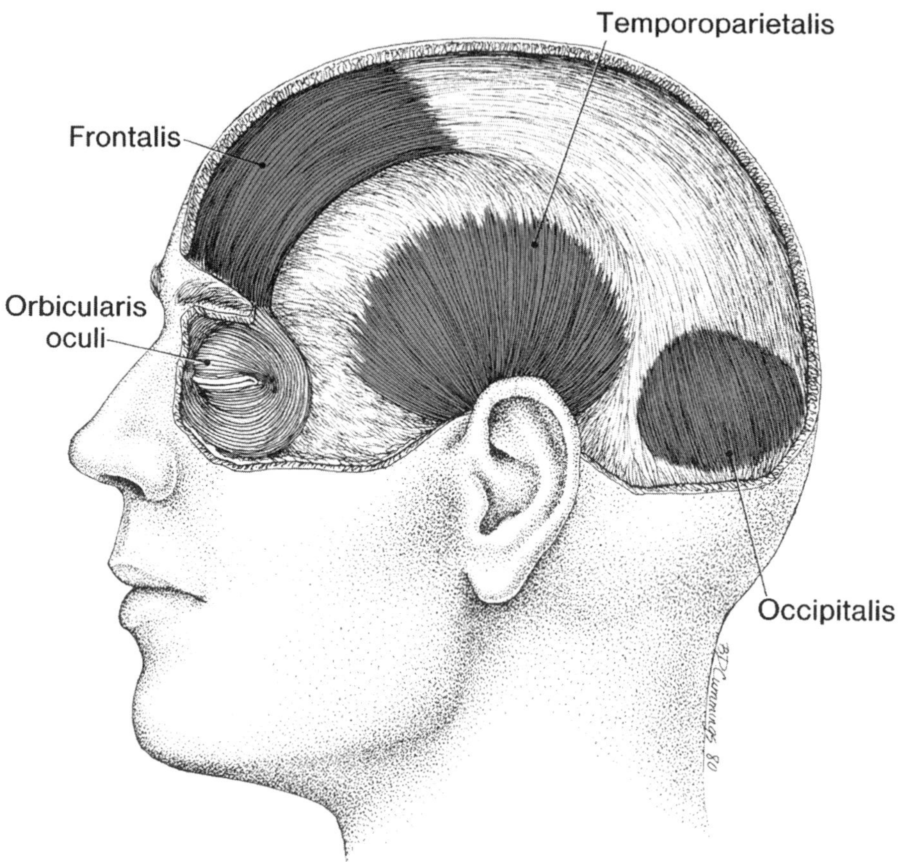

Figure 16.17 Orbicularis oculi and fontalis. These muscles are not attached to bone, but instead to tendons. The occipitalis anchors to the bone along the superior nuchal line of the occipital bone. See text for their actions. (From Travell, J.G., Simons, D.G., *Myofascial Pain and Dysfunction: The Trigger Point Manual*, Williams & Wilkins, Baltimore, 1983. With permission.)

THE NERVOUS SYSTEM OF THE HEAD AND NECK

It is the nervous system that controls all systems of our body. The system is divided into a central nervous system (CNS) and a peripheral nervous system (PNS). CNS includes the brain, brainstem, cerebellum, and spinal cord, while the PNS includes all the other nerves that emanate from the CNS. These nerves are made up of chains of neurons that are called pathways. There are motor and sensory pathways. Motor pathways almost always originate in the brain and descend to the muscles and glands. The sensory pathways originate from the skin or other organs and ascend to the brain.

The Central Nervous System

The largest portion of the CNS is the *cerebrum*, which is supported by the brainstem leading to the spinal cord. Off the back or posterior part is the cerebellum. The entire brain weighs about 3 to 4 pounds, or about 2% of the body weight. The cerebrum is a highly convoluted mass of nervous tissue and has ridges (gyri) and grooves (sulci) and are consistent from one person to the next. The cerebrum is incompletely divided into hemispheres by longitudinal fissure in the

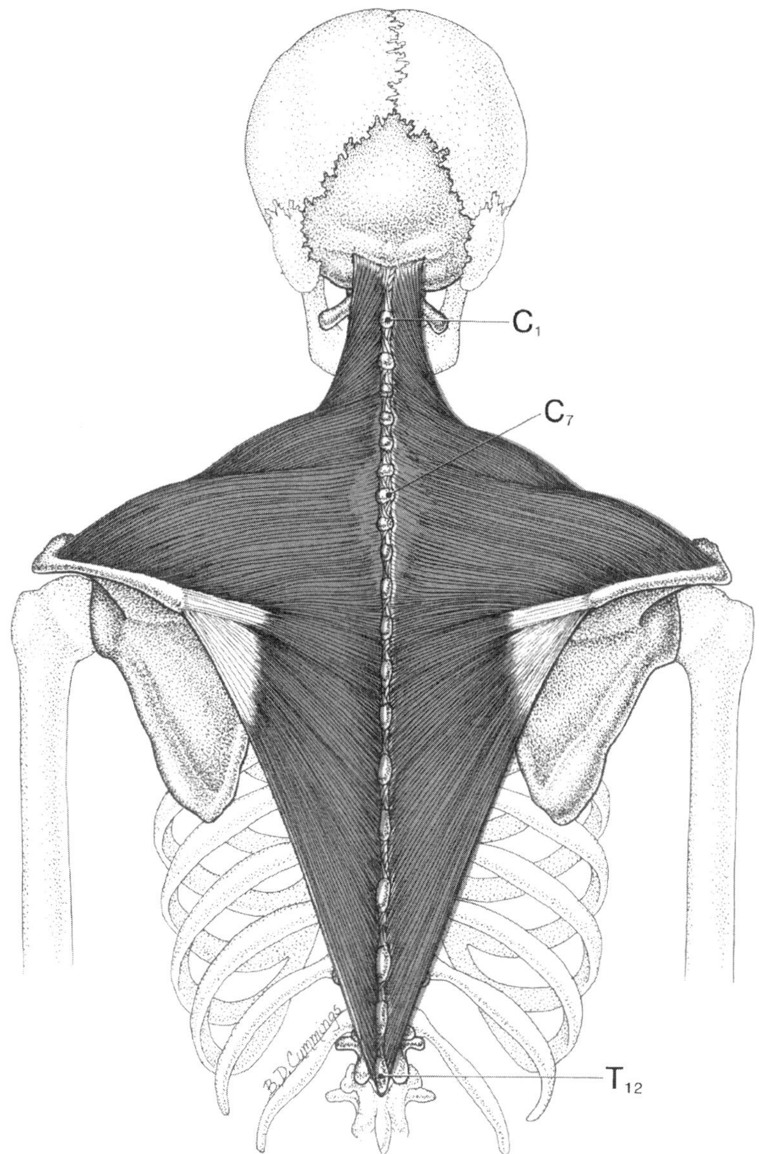

Figure 16.18 Attachments of the trapezius muscles. See text for attachments and function. (From Travell, J.G., Simons, D.G., *Myofascial Pain and Dysfunction: The Trigger Point Manual*, Williams & Wilkins, Baltimore, 1983. With permission.)

midsagittal plane. The hemispheres are further divided into lobes that are named after the portion of the bone under which they lie, thus the names frontal, temporal, parietal, and occipital lobes. The general functions of the lobes are the following: frontal — motor control and personality traits; parietal — the ultimate destination for most sensory pathways; temporal — process auditory stimuli and play a role in memory; and the occipital — visual senses. Intellect and language, etc. result from the interaction of different parts of the brain. Areas that control smell or olfaction and emotions are deeper in the brain and have other names, such as the olfactory lobe, the limbic lobe, etc.

The motor and sensory pathways cross at some point and therefore the left side of the brain will send and receive signals from the right side of the body. This is the same for the right side of the brain. When dissecting the brain, one sees white matter and gray matter. The white appearance

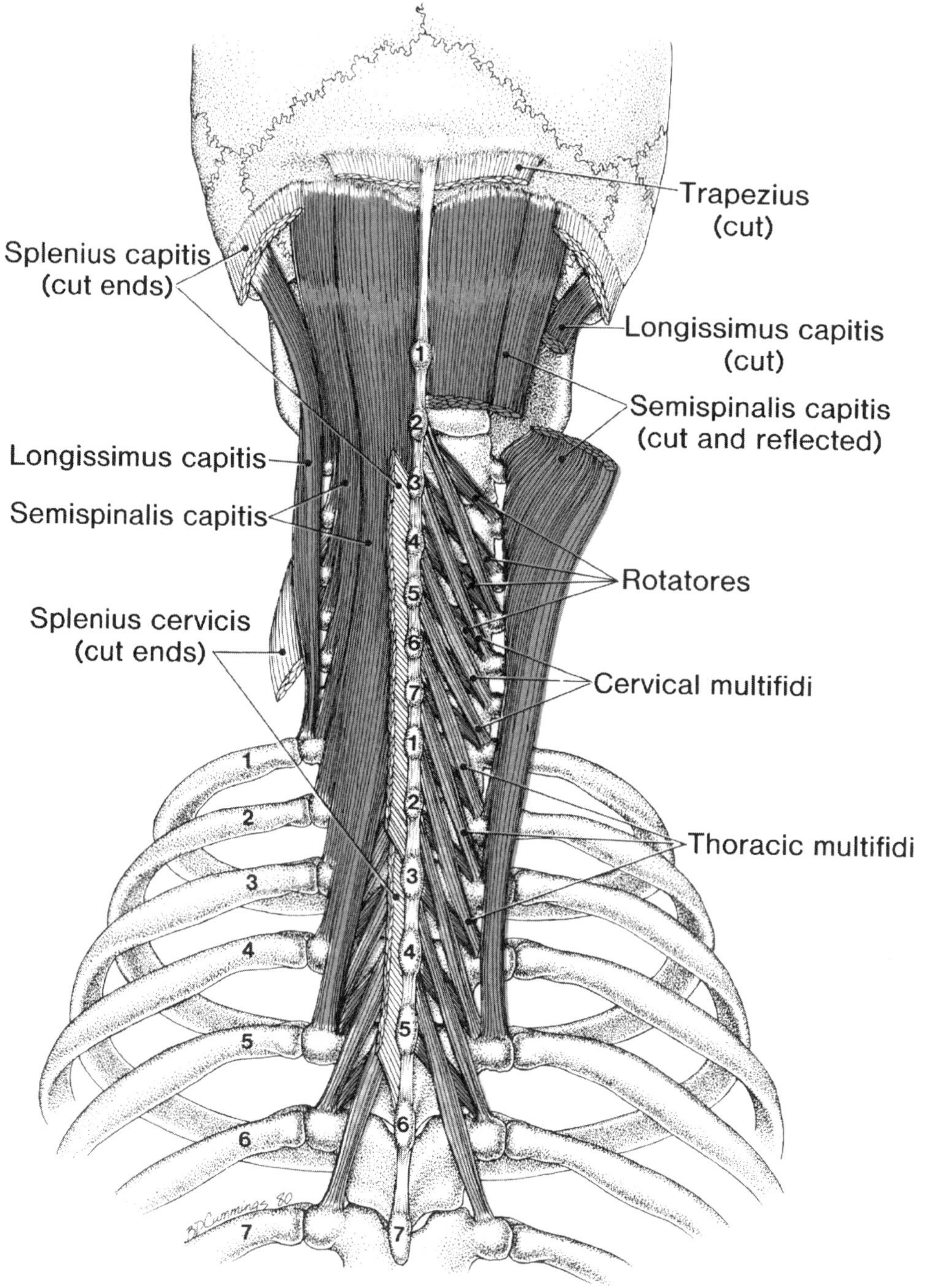

Figure 16.19 Longissimus capitis, splenius capitis, semispinalis capitis, splenius cervicis, semispinalis cervicis, cervical multifidi, thoracic multifidi, rotatores, and trapezius muscles. See text for the innervations and actions of these muscles. (From Travell, J.G., Simons, D.G., *Myofascial Pain and Dysfunction: The Trigger Point Manual*, Williams & Wilkins, Baltimore, 1983. With permission.)

is due to the nerves, which are covered with an insulating material called myelin. The gray matter is a collection of cell bodies that lack the myelin. The coupling of one neuron to the next usually occurs in the gray matter.

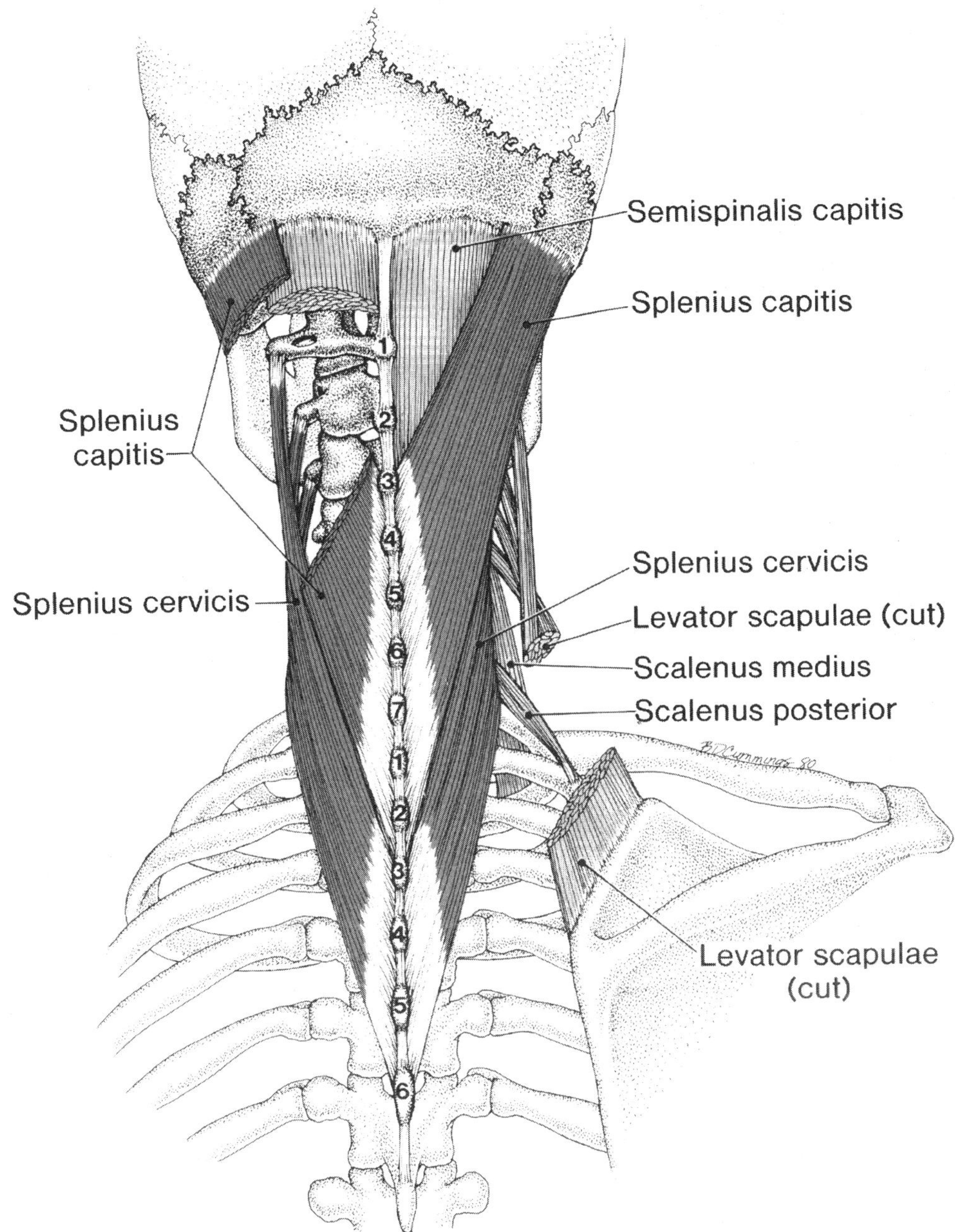

Figure 16.20 Splenius capitis, semispinalis capitis, splenius cervicis, levator scapulae, scalenus medius, and scalenus posterior muscles. See text for attachments and innervations of these muscles. (From Travell, J.G., Simons, D.G., *Myofascial Pain and Dysfunction: The Trigger Point Manual*, Williams & Wilkins, Baltimore, 1983. With permission.)

The *brainstem* rests between the cerebrum and the spinal cord. All messages using the neuron pathways into or out of the brain will pass through the brainstem. Almost all of the motor and sensory pathways cross sides in the lower brainstem, including fine touch, vibration signals and proprioception (awareness of posture, movement, equilibrium, and the relation of the body to position, weight, etc.). The brainstem is the center of vital reflexes that deal with heart rate, respirations, blood pressure, consciousness, and basically the life support system. The brainstem

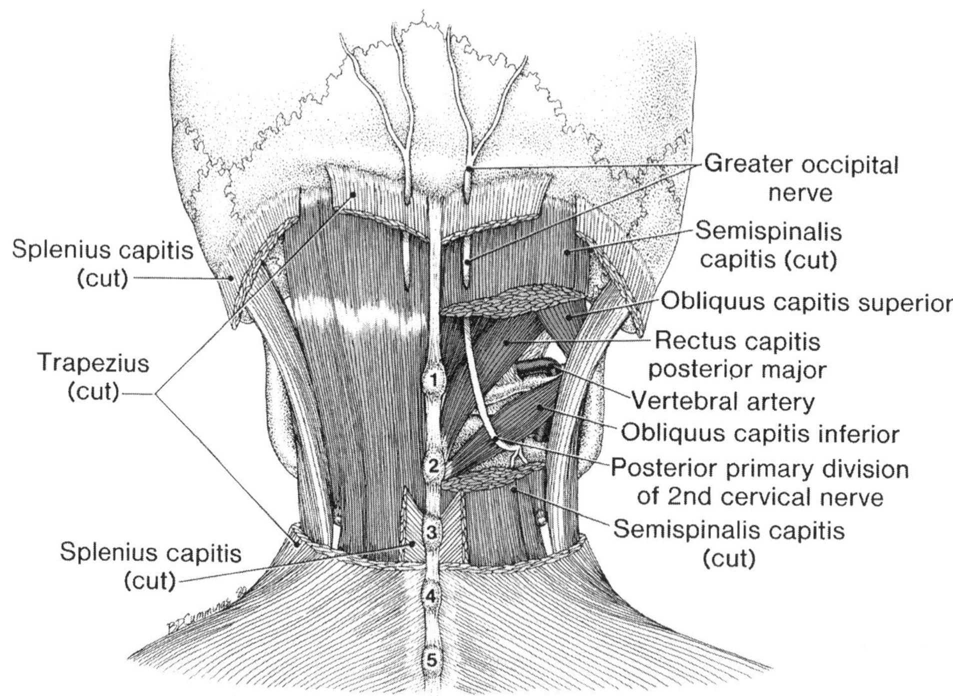

Figure 16.21 Suboccipital muscles. Obliquus capitis inferior and superior, rectus capitis posterior major and minor. See text for attachments and innervations of these muscles. (From Travell, J.G., Simons, D.G., *Myofascial Pain and Dysfunction: The Trigger Point Manual*, Williams & Wilkins, Baltimore, 1983. With permission.)

also contains the nuclei of most of the cranial nerves, except C1 and C2 (see Table 16.5) and then becomes the spinal cord after passing out of the cranium (Figure 16.22).

During a head trauma there may be injury to the bones that have a foramen that the cranial nerves pass through, or injury to the nerve or nerves themselves. Table 16.5 gives a simple explanation of the functions of the cranial nerves. Figure 16.23 shows the origin and termination of cranial nerves I through XII. The complex anatomy of these nerves is not discussed.

The cerebellum is mounted on the posterior aspect of the brainstem and is situated just inferior to the occipital lobe of the cerebrum. The cerebellum modulates motor signals to many muscle groups, which allows for smooth, coordinated muscle performance.

The spinal cord continues from the brainstem and passes down the vertebral canal. The spinal cord has a gray area shaped like an H and is a mass of neuron cell bodies. Surrounding this area of gray matter are organized tracts of white matter sending axons up (sensory) and down (motor). Sensory pathways dealing with pain, temperature, pressure, and crude touch generally cross sides near the level at which they enter the cord and then ascend in the white matter to reach the appropriate site in the cerebral hemisphere. The white matter containing the motor pathways has already crossed in the brainstem.

The CNS has various protective sources, such as the cranium or bony structures, and various coverings and cerebral spinal fluid. The meninges are three layers of connective tissue surrounding the brain and spinal cord. There is also the cerebrospinal fluid (CSF) that helps to protect the brain.

The outer layer is tough and splits into two sheets and is termed *dura mater.* The outer or osteal layer is bound to the bone with a separate fibrous layer underneath that forms cavities at certain points called venous sinuses. These venous sinuses are the major veins of the cranium and are full of blood. These sinuses will eventually drain into the internal jugular vein and drain to the heart and the lungs.

Table 16.5 The Functions of the Cranial Nerves

Nerve Name	Bone[a]	Sensory Functions[b]	Motor Functions
C-I Olfactory	Ethmoid	Olfaction	None known
C-II Optic	Sphenoid	Vision	None known
C-III Oculomotor	Sphenoid	Proprioception	Some movements of the eye and lid; constricts pupil, accommodates lens
C-IV Trochlear	Sphenoid	Proprioception	Moves eye down and out
C-V Trigeminal	Sphenoid	Proprioception	
V-1 Ophthalmic	V-1	GS forehead[c]	V-1 none known
V-2 Maxillary	V-2	GS cheek and upper jaw[c]	V-2 none known
V-3 Mandibular	V-3	GS lower jaw and neck[c]	V-3 Mastication
C-VI Abducens	Sphenoid	Proprioception	Move eye laterally
C-VII Facial	Temporal	Proprioception, taste from anterior 2/3 of tongue	None known
C-VIII Vestibulocochlear	Temporal	Equilibrium (balance) Hearing	None known
C-IX Glossopharyngeal	Occipital	Proprioception, taste from posterior 1/3 of tongue and much of pharynx	Secretion from parotid gland, some pharyngeal motion
C-X Vagus	Occipital	GS from many organs[c] Proprioception	Speech, swallowing, contraction of gut Decreases heart rate
C-XI Accessory	Occipital	Proprioception	Assists in swallowing, turns and flexes head
C-XII Hypoglossal	Occipital	Proprioception	Tongue movement

[a] Passes through the foramen in this bone to exit the cranium.
[b] Proprioception is the sensory signals sent to the CNS informing it of the position of a muscle.
[c] GS, general sensations such as touch, temperature, and pain.

From Porta, D.J., in *Head and Neck Injury*, Levine, R.S., Ed., Society of Automotive Engineers, 1994. With permission.

The next layer is called the *arachnoid mater* and has spidery projections to the third meningeal covering. Within this layer is the subarachnoid space where CSF circulates, and most of the blood vessels travel. The CSF has some nutrient value, but its primary function is to protect and support the brain. The CSF forms a cushion between the brain and the bones of the skull so that the brain actually floats. The CSF is manufactured within the brain.

Within the brain are four ventricles and inside these ventricles are small structures, called *choroid plexuses*, that produce the cerebrospinal fluid. The CSF circulates through the ventricles, then around the brain and spinal cord within the subarachnoid space. There is some arachnoid mater that protrudes into the venous sinuses that was made from dura mater. These bits of arachnoid mater are called arachnoid granulations and their function is to remove or absorb CSF and filter it into venous blood. The fact that the CSF is produced in the brain and absorbed outside the brain creates a circulation and a pressure.

The third meningeal layer, the *pia mater*, adheres to the brain and spinal cord and permits blood vessels to pass through it to service the brain (Figures 16.24 and 16.25).

The Peripheral Nervous System

This system is comprised of the cranial nerves and the spinal nerves. The cranial nerves have already been discussed. The spinal nerves emerge from the spinal cord. These nerves are formed from the dorsal (back) and from the ventral (frontal) nerve roots on both sides of the cord within the vertebral canal. The nerves exit through the intervertebral foramina between the pedicles of the vertebrae to all the parts of the body. Out of 31 pairs of nerves, 8 are cervical and 7 of these nerves travel above the pedicles of the vertebrae. Their names are the same as that of the vertebrae, i.e., C2 arises above C2 vertebrae. However, C8 exits between C7 and T1 (thoracic) vertebrae.

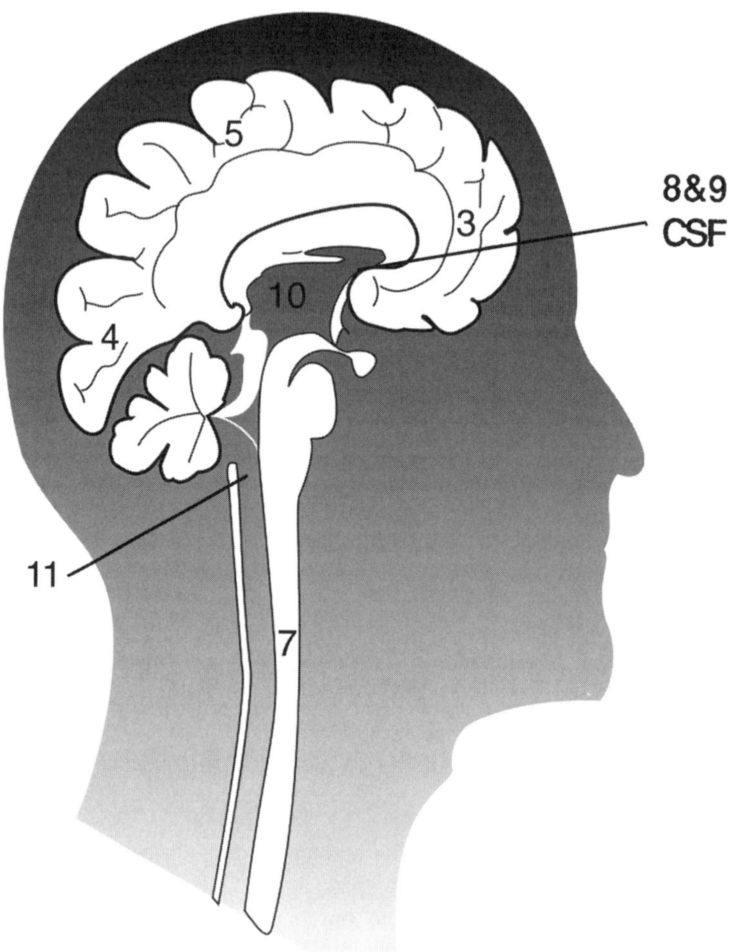

Figure 16.22 Midsagittal view of central nervous system. **1**, brainstem; **2**, cerebellum; **3**, frontal lobe of cerebrum; **4**, occipital lobe; **5**, parietal lobe; **6**, pituitary gland; **7**, spinal cord; **8**, **9**, lateral ventricles; **10**, 3rd ventricle; **11**, 4th ventricle.

These nerves carry proprioceptive sensations (positional, etc.) and motor and sensory sensations. Sensory signals are sent into the CNS from the periphery, while motor signals are sent from the CNS to the rest of the body through this peripheral system.

The actions of these nerves are quite complex; simply stated, they act in the following way. Sensory fibers of the cervical nerves are involved with touch, pain, pressure, and temperature sensations from the skin. Dermatomes are areas of distribution to different cervical nerves. Roughly, the following nerves supply these areas: C8, C7, and C6 supply the different parts of the hand; C6 also supplies the lateral forearm; C5 the shoulder; C4 the superior thorax and inferior neck; C3 the rest of the neck; C2 the chin and the scalp above and behind the ear; and C1 is disputed.

Sensations are special or general. Special senses are vision, hearing, taste, smell and balance. General senses are touch, pressure, pain, and temperature. General senses are divided into visceral vs. somatic. Visceral general sensations are felt from organs within the body, e.g. blood pressure, body temperature, and pain from organs. Somatic general senses are those received from the body wall or limbs and provide information about the outside of the body.

Proprioception is the general sensation that allows one to be aware of the position of different parts of the body. As an example, one would know where to locate parts of the body without looking

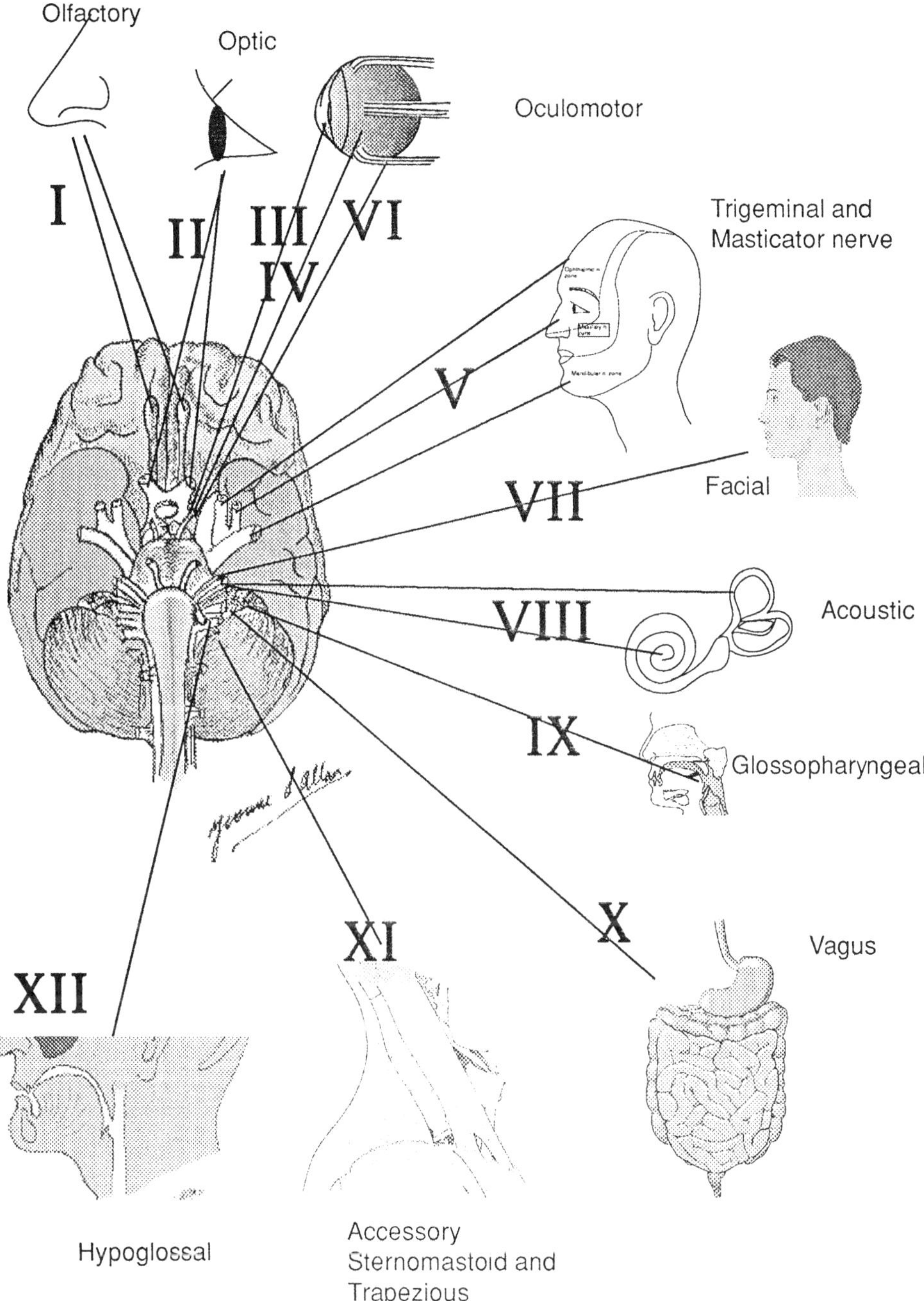

Figure 16.23 Cranial nerves. This demonstrates the origin and termination of cranial nerves I through XII.

at them, or to walk and not touch items on the floor without having to measure them as one walks, etc. These nerves and the brain can calculate these exact positions without conscious thinking.

Motor pathways supply muscle groups, as follows: C1 to C5 supply the deep neck muscles. C1 to C3 supply most of the muscles associated with the thyroid cartilage and hyoid bone. C3 to C5 supplies the diaphragm after forming the phrenic nerve. C5 to T1 supply the muscles of the shoulder, arm, and hand after forming the brachial plexus.

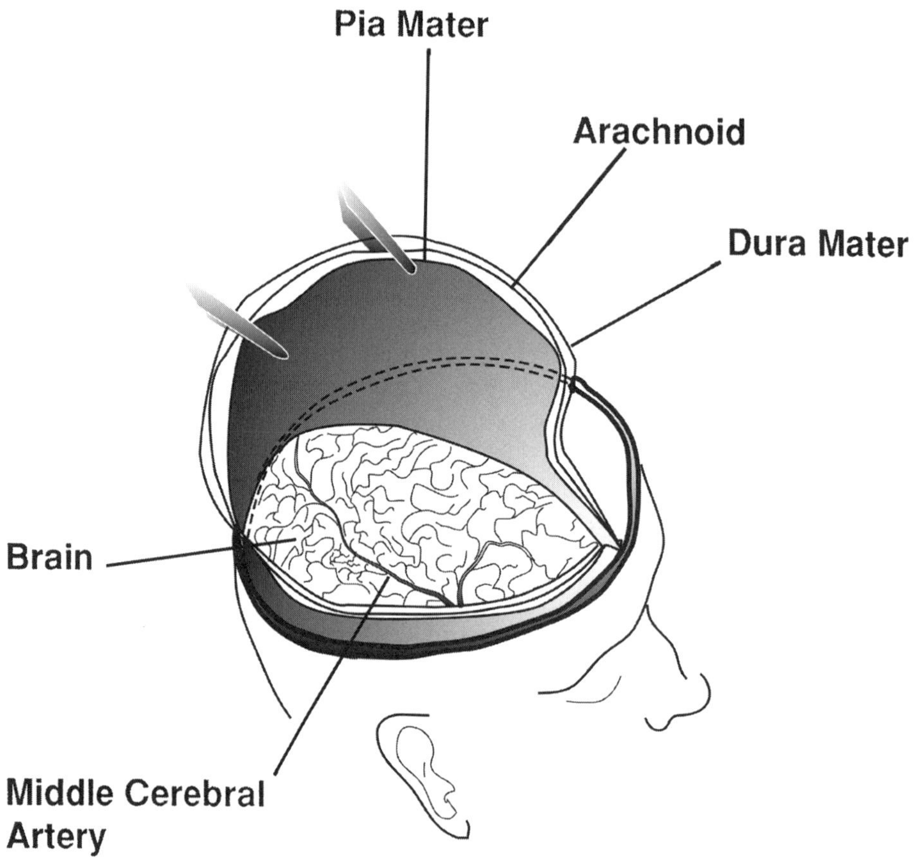

Figure 16.24 The layer covering the brain, called the *pia mater*, and above that the *arachnoid membrane*. Above that is the *dura mater*. Other than some parts of the dura mater, the layers are not pain sensitive; however, some of the large blood vessels traversing through these membranes can cause pain. The dura mater is a dense, fibrous structure with an inner and an outer layer. These layers are generally fused, except where they separate to provide space for the venous sinuses. The outer layer attaches to the inner surface of the cranial bones and sends vascular and fibrous extensions into the bone. The inner layer encloses some of the venous sinuses and forms partitions within the brain. The pia mater is a thin connective tissue membrane close to the brain and it carries blood vessels supplying the nervous tissues. It extends into the sulci and fissures throughout the brain. The arachnoid is a delicate nonvascular membrane between the dura and pia maters. It is separated from the overlying dura by a subdural space, and from the underlying pia mater by the subarachnoid space, which contains cerebrospinal fluid.

Motor control gives off signals that are divided into voluntary and involuntary control. Voluntary or somatic signals travel from the CNS to muscles.

Involuntary signals go to organs that must work all the time, such as cardiac muscles, smooth muscles (e.g., intestines), and glands. This system is controlled by the autonomic nervous system which is divided into the sympathetic and parasympathetic systems.

The sympathetic system originates from the spinal cord, from the first thoracic to the second lumbar levels (T1 to L2) or the thoracolumbar area. The sympathetic autonomic motor signals travel to smooth muscles and glands all over the body and also to the heart. These signals travel in spinal nerves along with the voluntary motor and general sensory signals. Because these nerves must reach all the smooth muscles and glands over the whole body, there are way-stations that are called sympathetic chain ganglia and they are placed on either side of the vertebral column from the base of the skull to the pelvis. From these ganglia the nerves then travel to their destinations.

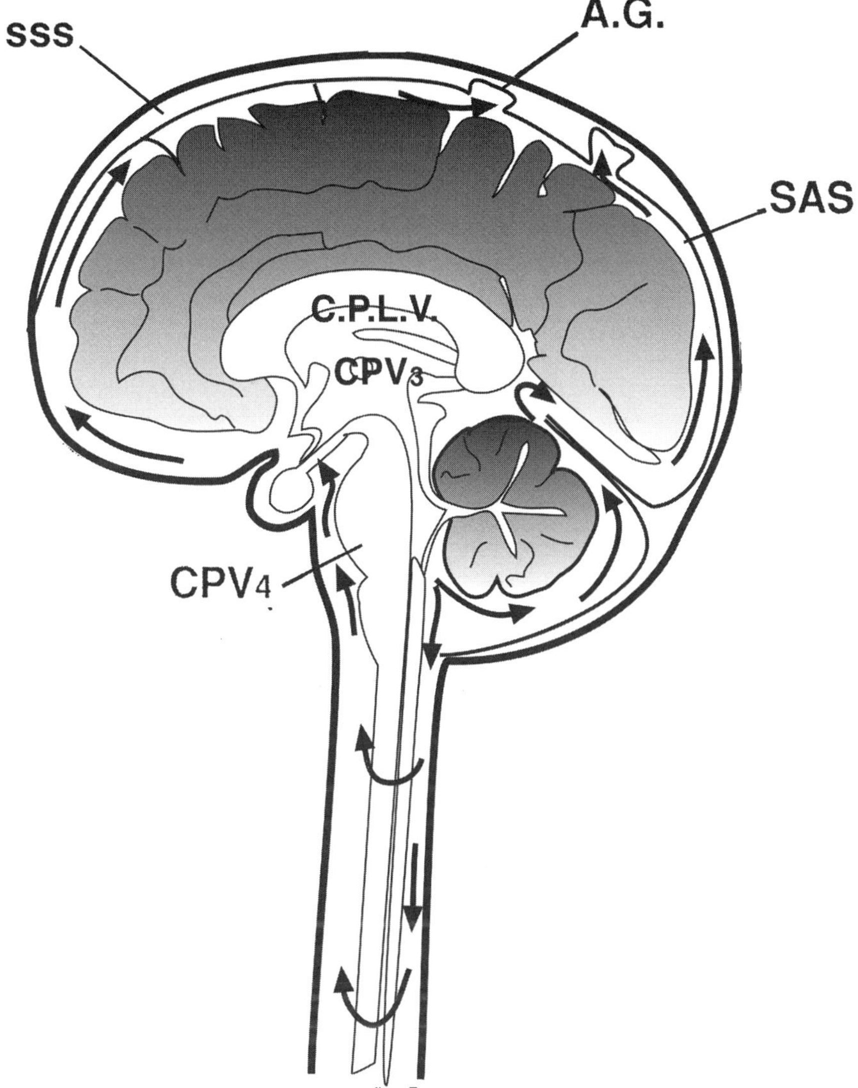

Figure 16.25 Cerebrospinal fluid circulation. The cerebrospinal fluid is produced by the choroid plexus in the ventricles of the brain and may also be produced in the central canal of the spinal cord. The arrows indicate the flow of the cerebrospinal fluid in the brain and spinal cord. The cerebrospinal fluid is processed in the arachnoidal villae and then emptied into the superior sagittal sinus and some of the smaller sinuses. CSF is a clear liquid that protects the cavities in the brain and spinal cord. Samples of the fluid may be obtained by a lumbar puncture and used to diagnose certain diseases. C.P.L.V., choroid plexus lateral ventricle; CPV_3, choroid plexus 3rd ventricle; CPV_4, choroid plexus space; sss, superior sagittal sinus.

The sympathetic system is always preparing us for stressful situations — "fight or flight." This system increases our heart rate, respirations, sweat glands, increases blood flow to the muscles and decreases the rate of our digestive system and its blood supply.

The parasympathetic autonomic nervous system originates from the craniosacral areas with certain cranial nerves and between the second and fourth sacral spinal levels. The parasympathetic system maintains the body equilibrium by acting opposite to the sympathetic system.

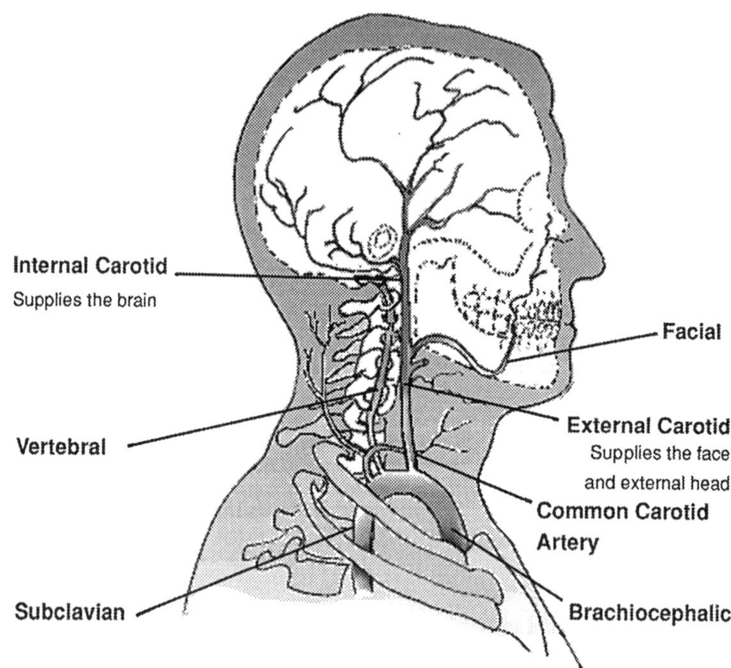

Figure 16.26 The arteries of the head.

THE BLOOD SUPPLY OF THE HEAD AND NECK

The three major types of blood vessels are arteries, veins, and capillaries. Arteries carry blood enriched with oxygen and nutrients from the heart to the rest of the body. Veins bring blood that needs oxygen and contains waste products back to the heart and lungs. Capillaries are one-celled tubes that bridge the arteries and the veins where the exchange of oxygen and nutrients takes place. For the most part, veins parallel arteries.

The blood to the neck and head originates from the paired common carotid and the subclavian arteries. These supply all the structures previously discussed. The subclavian arteries supply the thyrocervical and costocervical trunks and the vertebral artery. The vertebral arteries enter the skull through the foramen magnum to supply the brain.

The heart gives off the aorta, and on the left side the aorta gives off the left common carotid, while on the right side the aorta gives off the innominate artery, which then gives off the right common carotid artery. The common arteries on each side give off the external and internal carotids at the level of the thyroid cartilage. The internal carotids are the major blood supply to the brain. The external carotids supply the face and much of the neck and give off these major branches: superior thyroid, lingual (tongue), facial, maxillary and the superior temporal. The meninges are supplied by the middle meningeal artery, a branch of the maxillary artery.

The brain receives its blood supply from the internal carotids and the vertebrals. Branches of the internal carotids and vertebrals supply the entire superior portion of the central nervous system. On the base of the brain these two arteries join and form a loop that is called the circle of Willis. From the circle of Willis comes the anterior, middle, and posterior cerebral arteries that supply the cerebrum. The vertebral artery gives off the cerebellar, spinal, and brainstem arteries (Figure 16.26).

The veins of the brain drain into the venous sinuses (discussed before) within the folds of the dura matter. The sinuses drain through the jugular foramen and into the jugular vein. The meninges also have their veins drain into the venous sinuses. Most of the veins of the brain drain into the jugular vein to form the brachiocephalic. The right and left brachiocephalic veins combine to form the superior vena cava, which then empties into the right atrium of the heart to be oxygenated and start the cycle all over again.

Although this has been a very basic description of the anatomy of the head and neck, many of these terms will appear in medical reports and hopefully it will help the reader to understand some of the anatomical terms frequently used. This chapter may also add information that can clarify some of the other chapters on injuries of these areas.

REFERENCES

1. Porta, D.J., Introduction to head and neck anatomy, in *Head and Neck Injury,* Levine, R.S., Ed., Society of Automotive Engineers, 1994.
2. Travell, J.G., Simons, D.G., *Myofascial Pain and Dysfunction: The Trigger Point Manual*, Williams & Wilkins, Baltimore, 1983.

Chapter 17

Injuries to the Muscles, Tendons, and Ligaments of the Head and Neck

Barnsley, Lord, and Bogduk[1] state, "There are grounds, therefore, to believe that what may have been misrepresented as cervical trigger points after whiplash actually represent painful, tender zygapophyseal joints.

"Whatever might be written or believed about myofascial pain in general, there is no explicit, reliable data on its occurrence after whiplash, yet there is data that casts doubt on the reliability of diagnosis of trigger points in general, and of trigger points in the neck in particular."

I had the pleasure of attending a seminar that Nikolai Bogduk gave on cervicogenic headache and am convinced that Dr. Bogduk is a scientific purist and is correct in the above statements. However, few doctors are trained to do zygapophyseal blocks and at the present time there is no long-term treatment of this problem. Therefore, the clinician has a responsibility to diagnose and to treat a suffering patient with the tools that he or she has in his or her armamentarium.

As described in Chapter 15, whiplash occurs when the individual's torso is accelerated while the unrestrained head and neck are thrust backward and rotate into extension. When the rate of stretch of these muscles is rapid and they are overstretched and the muscle fibers do not have sufficient time to relax, they may rupture. If, at the same time, the victim's vehicle strikes an object such as another car in front and there is rapid deceleration, there may also be damage during the flexion phase. Researchers have produced grossly visible tears and ruptures in muscles in primates subjected to these forces[2] (Figure 17.1). These tears have been given grades as to their severity. Muscle tears have been described as strains and these strains will generally heal in a few weeks. The question is whether this condition will develop into another condition called myofascial pain disorder (MPD) and whether muscle or myofascial trigger points develop.

Dr. Janet Travell was one of the leading investigators in the diagnoses and treatment of myofascial trigger points, and had the honor of treating President John Kennedy, who suffered back problems as a result of his heroic actions on PT 109 during World War II. For decades she labored to document the scientific work she has done on myofascial pain and dysfunction, and with the collaboration of Dr. David Simons, published the landmark work, *Myofascial Pain and Dysfunction: The Trigger Point Manual.*[3]

Unfortunately, even today with the term "trigger points" constantly being used, my experience has been that few doctors know how to examine them and even fewer know how to treat them. For some reason unknown to me, doctors do not seem to have an interest in muscle and almost deny muscle involvement as the cause of pain. Other than pain pills or anti-inflammatory drugs, they

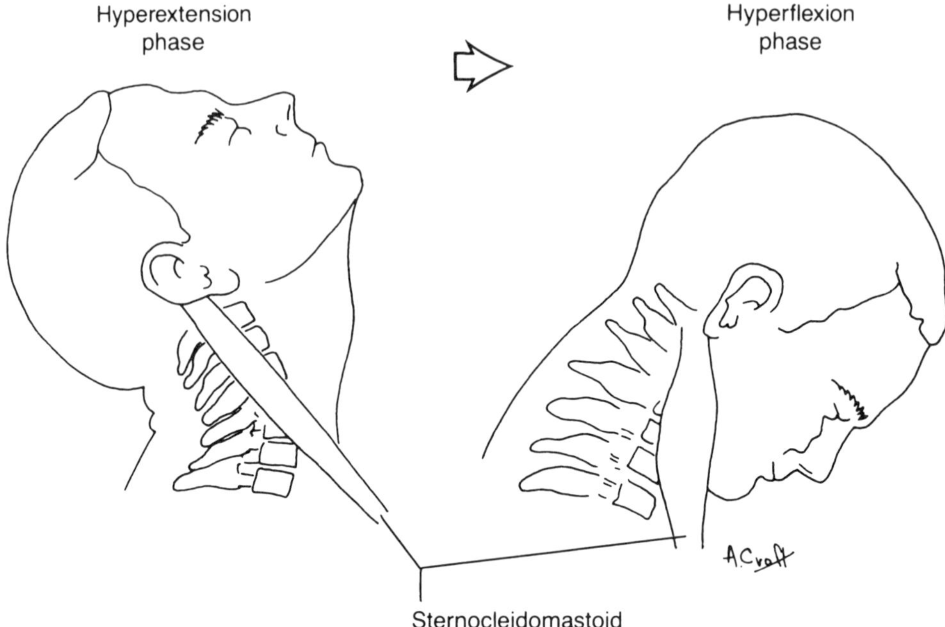

Figure 17.1 The hyperflexion phase of injury that, after the preceding hyperextension phase, subjects the muscles to injury. This muscle is the sternocleidomastoid muscle as a demonstration, but all the muscles of the neck that are involved with flexion-extension are subject to the same problem. (From Foreman, S.M., Croft, A.C., *Whiplash Injuries: The Cervical Acceleration/Deceleration Syndrome*, Williams & Wilkins, Baltimore, 1995. With permission.)

seem to stop short of any other treatment. Yet after injury, simple treatments can offer pain relief. After whiplash injury with acute pain from overstretching of the muscles, looking for and treating these trigger points could reduce pain enormously. Once pain becomes chronic, then one should consider the possibility of other causes for the pain problem.

Travell and Simons[3] define a myofascial trigger point as a "hyperirritable locus within a taut band of skeletal muscle and/or its associated fascia. The spot is painful on compression and can evoke characteristic *referred* pain and autonomic phenomena." Myofascial trigger points, TPs, are classified as active or latent. An active TP causes the patient to have pain and referred pain to another area, while a latent TP does not cause pain but may cause restriction of movement of the muscle.

Active TPs have referred target areas, depending on the specific muscle that contains the TP. The referred pain can range from dull to incapacitating. The pain does not follow a familiar neurological pattern. Trigger points are activated by overload and direct trauma. They can also be activated by arthritic joints and other triggering mechanisms. The intensity of the TP may vary at different times and a latent TP can be activated. A TP can also guard a muscle from being overactivated. Often with adequate rest an active TP can become a latent TP.

The active TP is often found by a sudden onset during an acute overload, characteristic patterns of pain, weakness and restriction in the stretch range in the affected muscle, a taut or palpable band in the affected muscle, exquisite pain in the band of taut muscle, a local twitch response to needling, and a jump sign when palpating the trigger point.

In Chapter 16 on the anatomy of the head and neck, a list of muscles was given that may cause pain in the neck, face, and head. Only the muscles that refer pain to the head that would be considered headache will be discussed here. The actions of the muscles were discussed in Chapter 16.

In each of the drawings (Figures 17.2 to 17.9), the Xs identify the trigger points and areas of referred pain. The method of treating trigger points is discussed in Chapter 25.

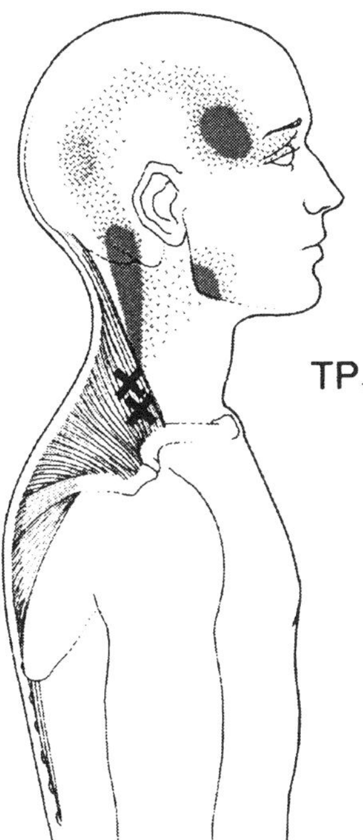

Figure 17.2 The trapezius muscle: active trigger points in the upper trapezius muscle where the Xs are located, and the area of referred pain when palpation of these trigger points is done. This pain can travel from the posterior aspect of the neck all the way to the frontal part of the head. (From Travell, J.G., Simons, D.G., *Myofascial Pain and Dysfunction: The Trigger Point Manual*, Williams & Wilkins, Baltimore, 1983. With permission.)

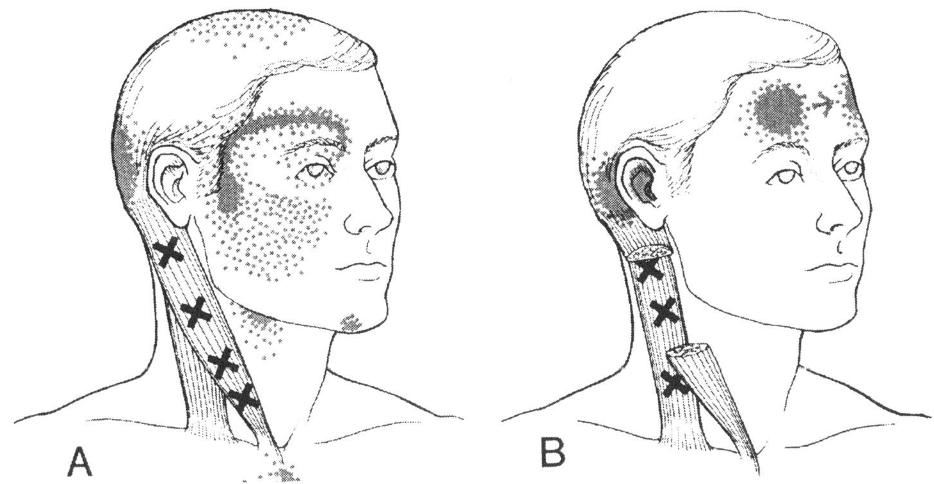

Figure 17.3 The sternocleidomastoid muscle: the sternocleidomastoid muscle has few muscle structures. The active trigger points are marked by Xs. In the right sternocleidomastoid muscle (A) is the external division and (B) is the clavicular (deep) division. The stippled and dark areas demonstrate where there will be referred pain with palpation of these muscles. (From Travell, J.G., Simons, D.G., *Myofascial Pain and Dysfunction: The Trigger Point Manual*, Williams & Wilkins, Baltimore, 1983. With permission.)

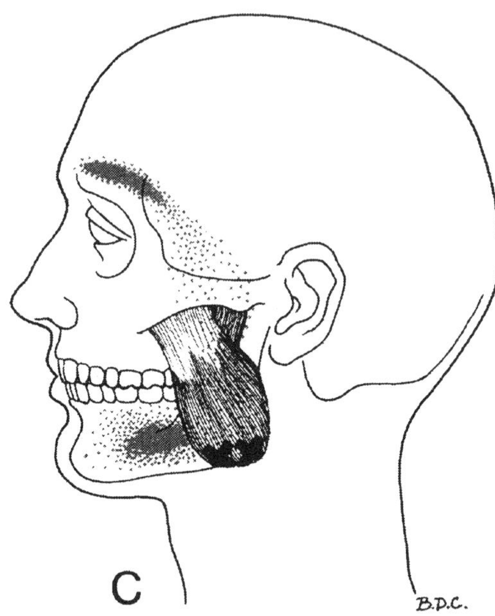

Figure 17.4 The masseter muscle: the Xs, which are the active trigger points of the masseter muscle, demonstrate with the stippled areas and the deeper dark areas, where the referred pain would be. (From Travell, J.G., Simons, D.G., *Myofascial Pain and Dysfunction: The Trigger Point Manual*, Williams & Wilkins, Baltimore, 1983. With permission.)

Ligaments are bands of fibers that connect bones or cartilage, serving to support and strengthen joints. Tears in ligaments have been reported in animal experiments and in cadaver experiments and also have been found at operations and at postmortem examinations.

Ligament injuries are not diagnosable clinically but have been found with MRI (magnetic resonance imaging) when the injury is severe. Because ligaments are highly elastic, their damage with tears would reflect severe trauma involving destruction of the cervical vertebrae resulting most often in death of the occupant.

The anterior longitudinal ligament merges with the anterior annulus of the intervertebral disc indicating that an injury to this structure may come as a result of a disc injury (Figure 17.10). Whiplash injury in experimental injury to animals, has produced damage to the posterior longitudinal ligament and the ligamentum flavum, but has not been reported with imaging studies or at surgery in humans after a whiplash injury.

Unless there is obvious physical destruction of the ligament, which would be treated with surgery, all other therapy would be based on the assumption that there is damage to the ligament. Although treatments called sclerotherapy, prolotherapy, proliferative and reconstructive (all the same) therapy are used to help the growth of new tissue of the ligaments, I have not seen these to be helpful in post whiplash headache. Perhaps this may be explained by the fact that these injuries are not the direct cause of the headache. There may be some patients who respond positively to these treatments, but I have not seen any literature that statistically supports this therapy for whiplash headaches. Although I have seen that small doses of cortisone have helped for short periods of time (hours to weeks), I am not sure that it is not the cortisone that is reducing the inflammation around the nerves (C1, 2, 3 and part of C4) that is in fact helping and this treatment has nothing to do with the ligaments.

For further reading on these anatomical structures, see the bibliography at the end of this book.

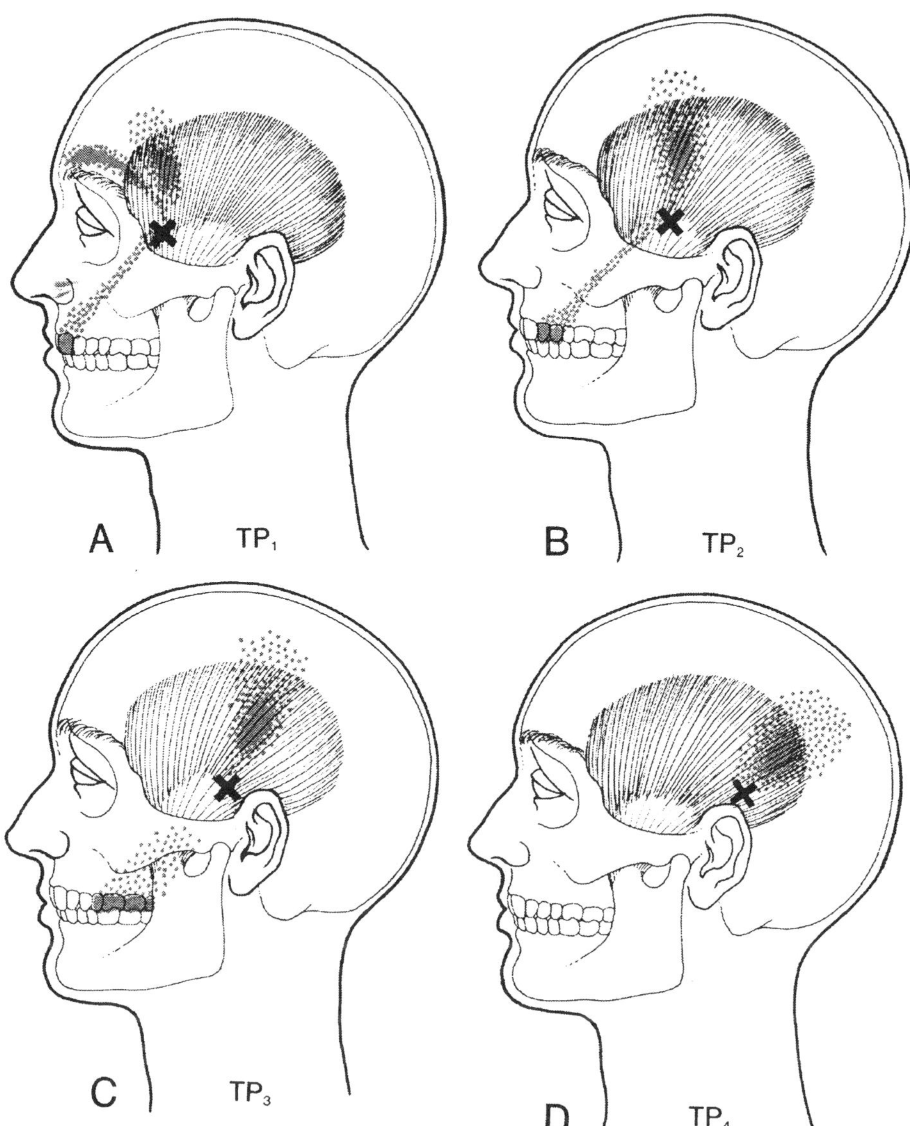

Figure 17.5 The temporalis muscle: the X demonstrates the active trigger point with referred pain to the stippled areas. (From Travell, J.G., Simons, D.G., *Myofascial Pain and Dysfunction: The Trigger Point Manual*, Williams & Wilkins, Baltimore, 1983. With permission.)

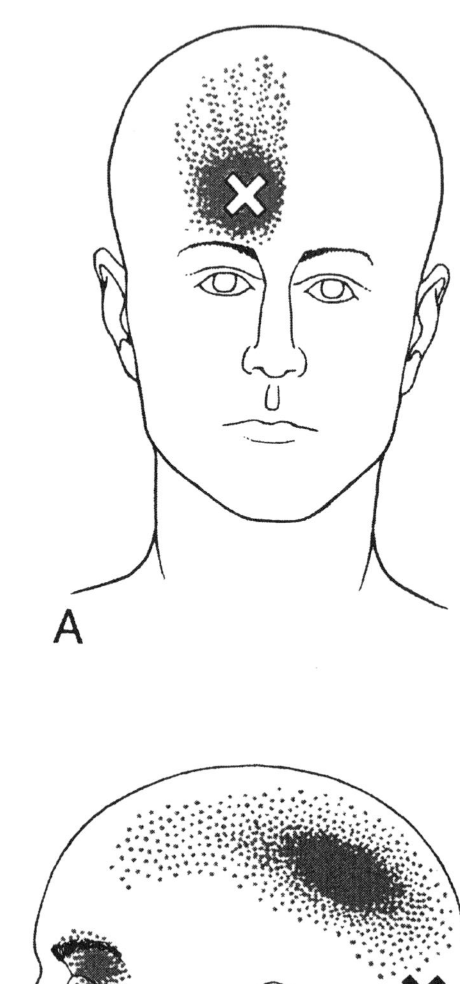

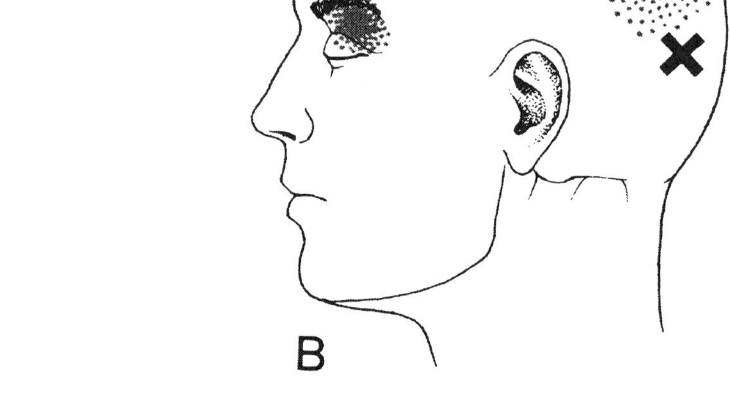

Figure 17.6 The occipitofrontalis muscle: the Xs demonstrates the active trigger point. The stippled and deeper and darker areas show where the referred pain is. (From Travell, J.G., Simons, D.G., *Myofascial Pain and Dysfunction: The Trigger Point Manual*, Williams & Wilkins, Baltimore, 1983. With permission.)

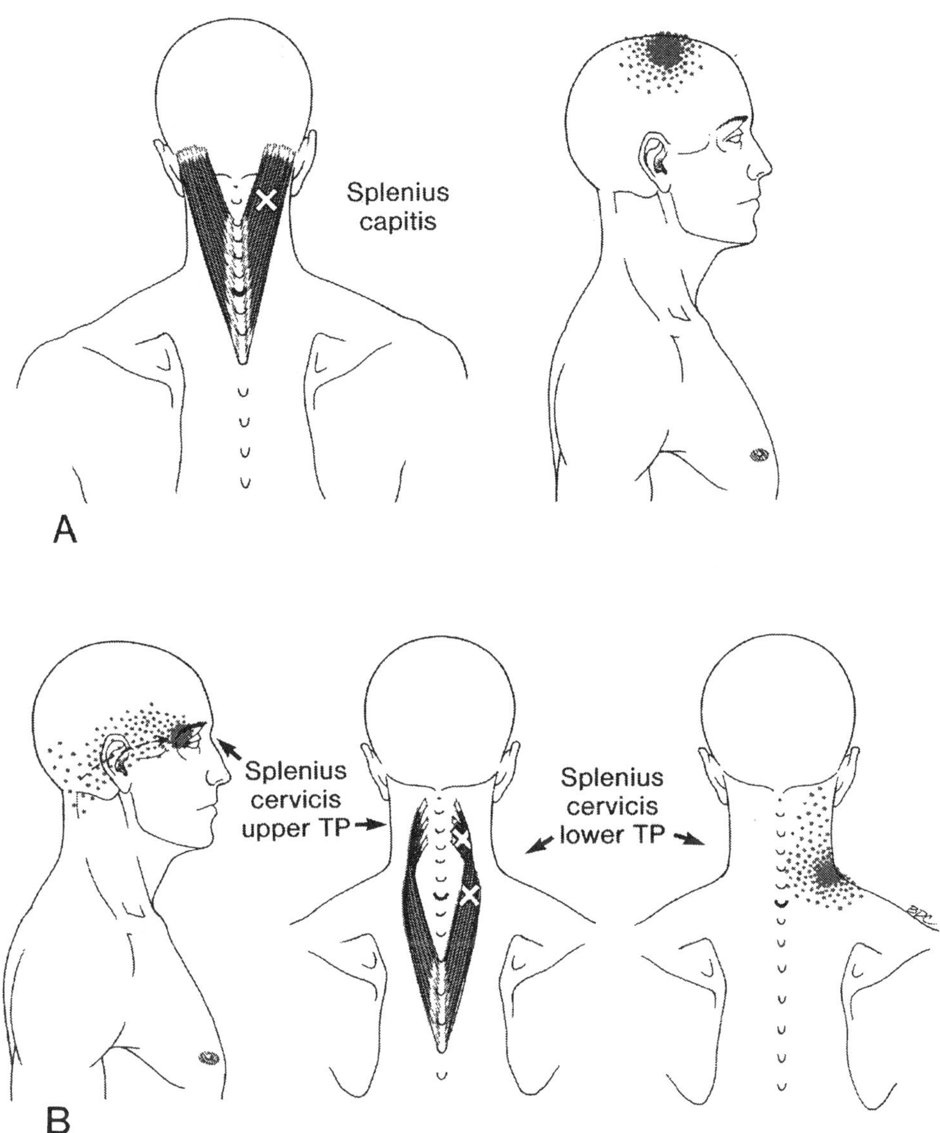

Figure 17.7 The splenius capitis and splenius cervicis muscle: these show the active trigger points which are rather common in these muscles after whiplash injury. They show where the referred pain would be, going all the way from the occipital portion to the top of the head to the frontal part of the head. (From Travell, J.G., Simons, D.G., *Myofascial Pain and Dysfunction: The Trigger Point Manual*, Williams & Wilkins, Baltimore, 1983. With permission.)

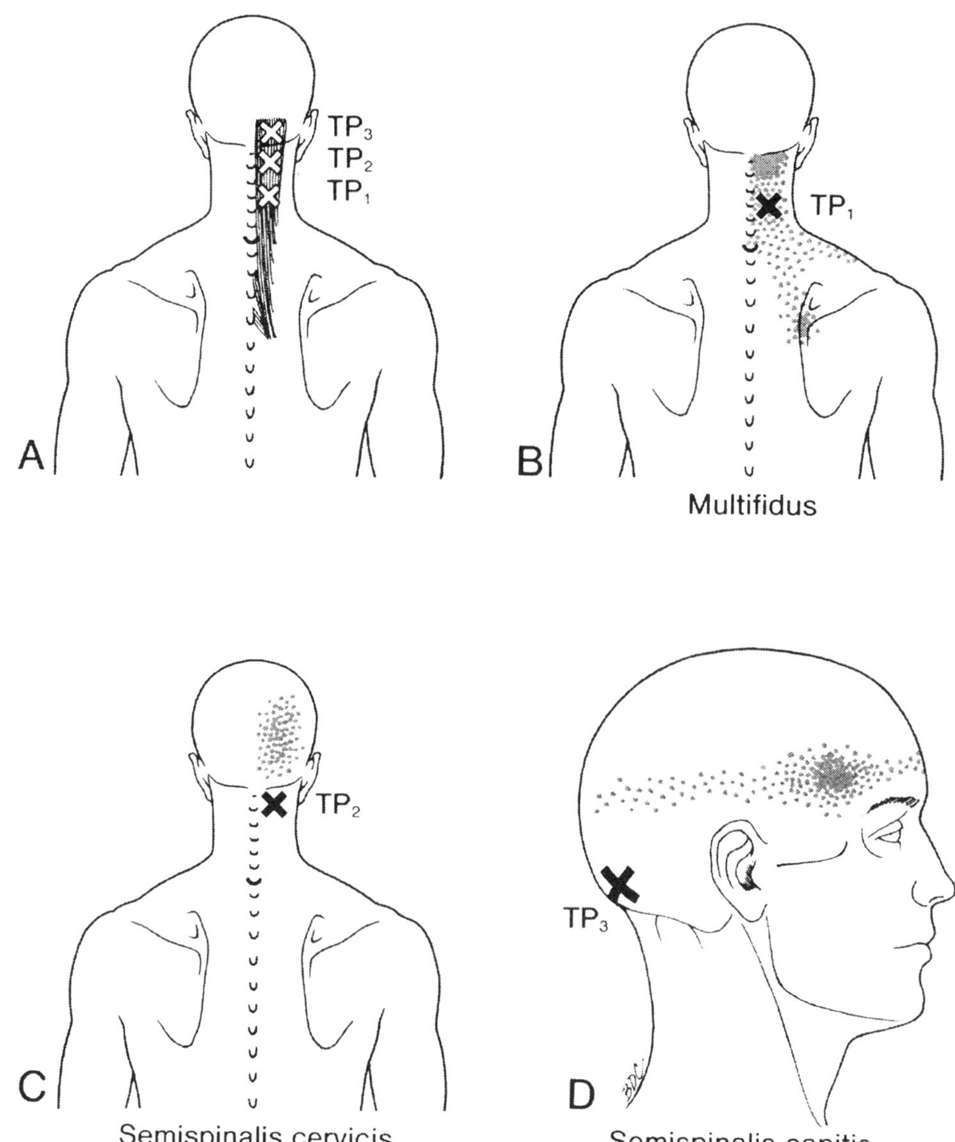

Figure 17.8 The posterior cervical muscles: these illustrations show that in the very deep muscles, trigger points also can refer pain to the occipital portion of the head and the temporal frontal portion of the head. (From Travell, J.G., Simons, D.G., *Myofascial Pain and Dysfunction: The Trigger Point Manual*, Williams & Wilkins, Baltimore, 1983. With permission.)

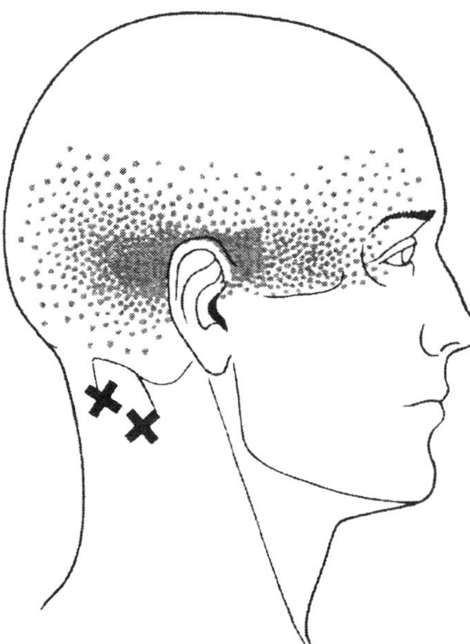

Figure 17.9 The suboccipital muscles: this illustration demonstrates the active trigger points, (Xs), and the darker and stippled areas demonstrate where the pain would be. (From Travell, J.G., Simons, D.G., *Myofascial Pain and Dysfunction: The Trigger Point Manual*, Williams & Wilkins, Baltimore, 1983. With permission.)

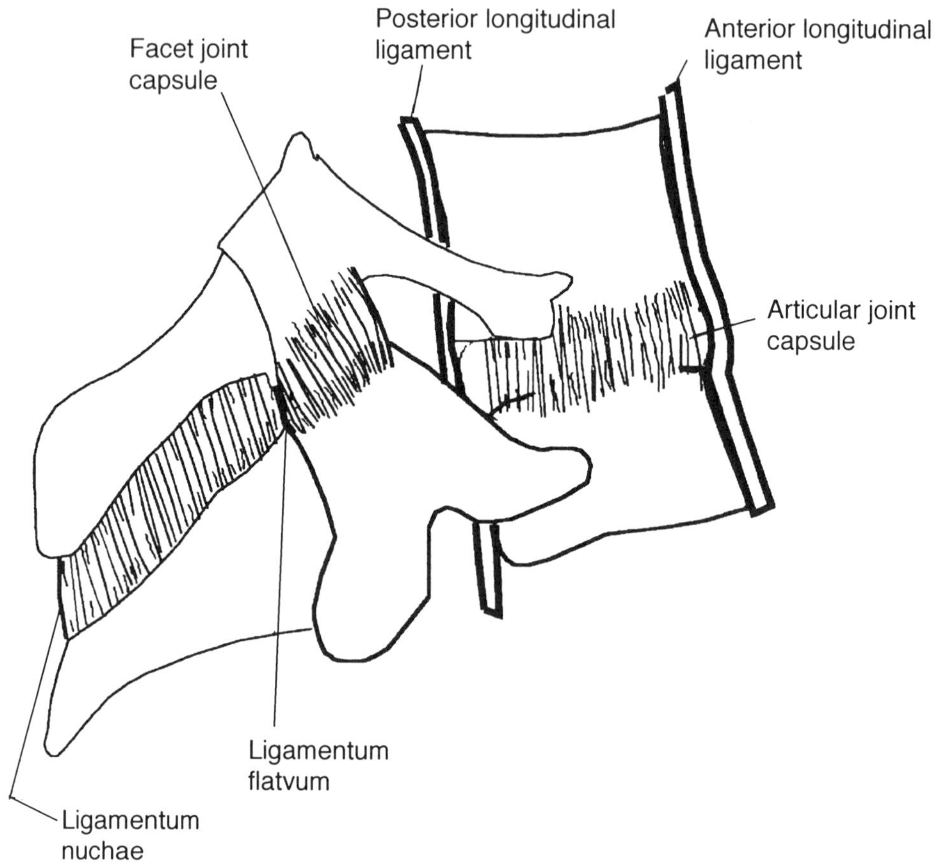

Figure 17.10 The anatomical relationship of the ligaments surrounding the cervical vertebrae. (From Foreman, S.M., Croft, A.C., *Whiplash Injuries: The Cervical Acceleration/Deceleration Syndrome*, Williams & Wilkins, Baltimore, 1983. With permission.)

REFERENCES

1. Barnsley, L., Lord, S., Bogduk, N., Clinical review: whiplash injury, *Pain*, 58, 283–307, 1994.
2. Foreman, S.M., Croft, A.C., *Whiplash Injuries: The Cervical Acceleration/Deceleration Syndrome*, Williams & Wilkins, Baltimore, 1995.
3. Travell, J.G., Simons, D.G., *Myofascial Pain and Dysfunction: The Trigger Point Manual*, Williams & Wilkins, Baltimore, 1983.

Chapter 18

Injury to the Temporomandibular Joint

Thomas P. Hand, D.S.S., F.A.C.D., F.I.C.D.

Crash dummies used in tests don't chew, yawn, grind their teeth, or whistle. They can't do this because crash dummies don't have jaws. They have wrists, knees, necks, but no temporomandibular joints. The extensive research into flexion-extension injuries has focused little on injuries to the temporomandibular joint (TMJ) and its associated structures and the impact on the musculature and the vascular aspects of the retrodiscal tissue of the TMJ. The complex interaction of the muscles of mastication and the muscles of the cervical pain in many cases can prolong the symptoms and pain secondary to acceleration-deceleration injuries (Figure 18.1).

The interaction of the muscles of mastication and the cervical spine is unique in the musculoskeletal system. The influence combination of the fixation forces of the muscles of the cervical spine applied to the primary movement of the mandible is seldom appreciated. These two systems, the cervical spine, the muscles of the jaw, and the TMJs should be looked upon as a single entity.

The TMJ is a complex joint. It not only rotates, as other joints in the body, but also translates as the mouth opens (Figure 18.2). This translation consists of the head of the condyle or the articulating portion of the mandible sliding across the skull. This is necessary so the mouth can open without impinging on the subject's airway.

This complex action is dictated primarily by a muscle directly in front of the TMJ, the external pterygoid muscle. It moves both the articulating head of the mandible (condyle) and a cartilaginous disc that separates the upper and lower chambers of the TMJ.

In accidents that suddenly and violently hyperextend the head, the infrahyoid muscles (Figure 18.3) can maintain the mandible in a fixed position. This causes excessive translation of the condyle forward (Figure 18.4), which can impact the external pterygoid muscle (Figure 18.5) at its insertion and tear or dislodge the ligaments of the temporomandibular joints (Figure 18.6). It can cause a hemarthrosis (joint dysfunction) and hemorrhage (bleeding in the joint) from the retrodiscal tissue, a highly vascular and innervated (supplied by nerves) tissue behind the condyle. This tissue actually is a shunt that allows the filling of the space behind the condyle when the jaw opens.

The lack of investigation into this problem has generated a great deal of controversy in the dental literature. Various studies have been done that attempt to either prove or disprove these contentions. This makes it difficult for the clinician, or an attorney in litigation, to establish if, indeed, there is a direct relationship between acceleration-deceleration trauma and injury to the temporomandibular joint.

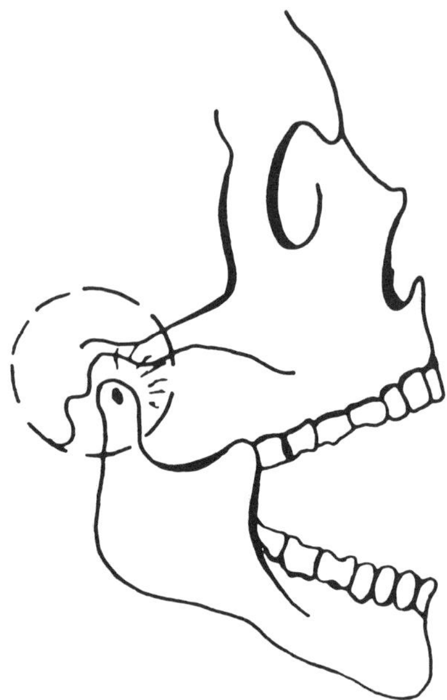

Figure 18.1 The temporomandibular joint.

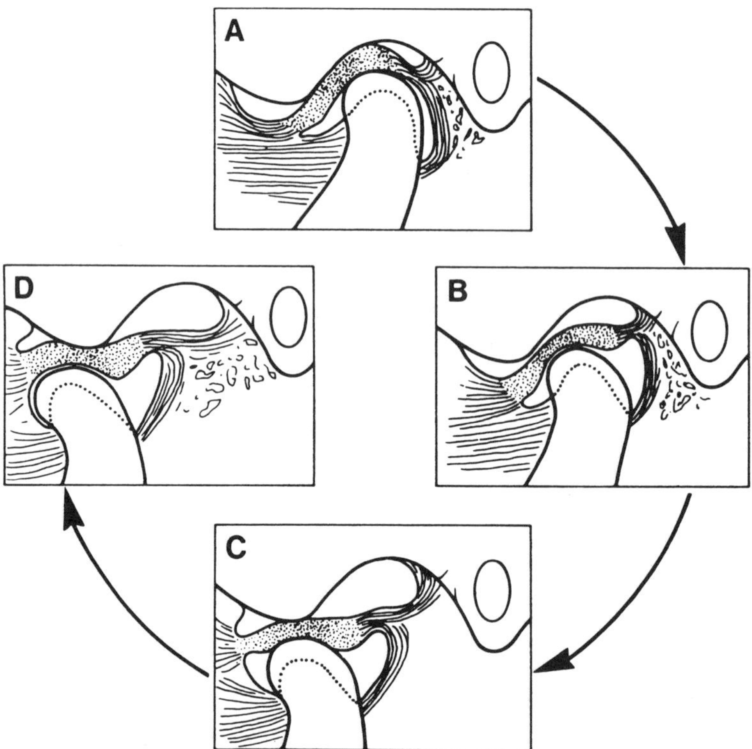

Figure 18.2 Normal temporomandibular joint function during opening movement. The disc is the stippled structure between the condyle below and the temporal bone above. (A) The mandible in the closed position. (B) to (D) Progressive changes in opening. The disc slides forward with the condyle as it translates to and sometimes over the articular eminence. (From Travell, J.G., Simons, D.G., *Myofascial Pain and Dysfunction: The Trigger Point Manual*, Williams & Wilkins, Baltimore, 1983, p. 175. With permission.)

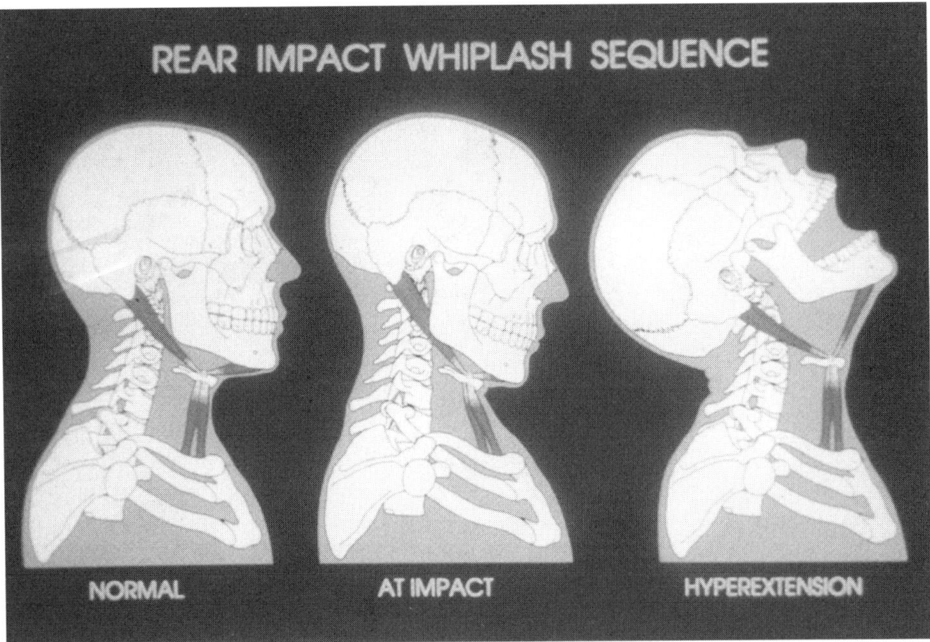

Figure 18.3 Rear impact whiplash sequence.

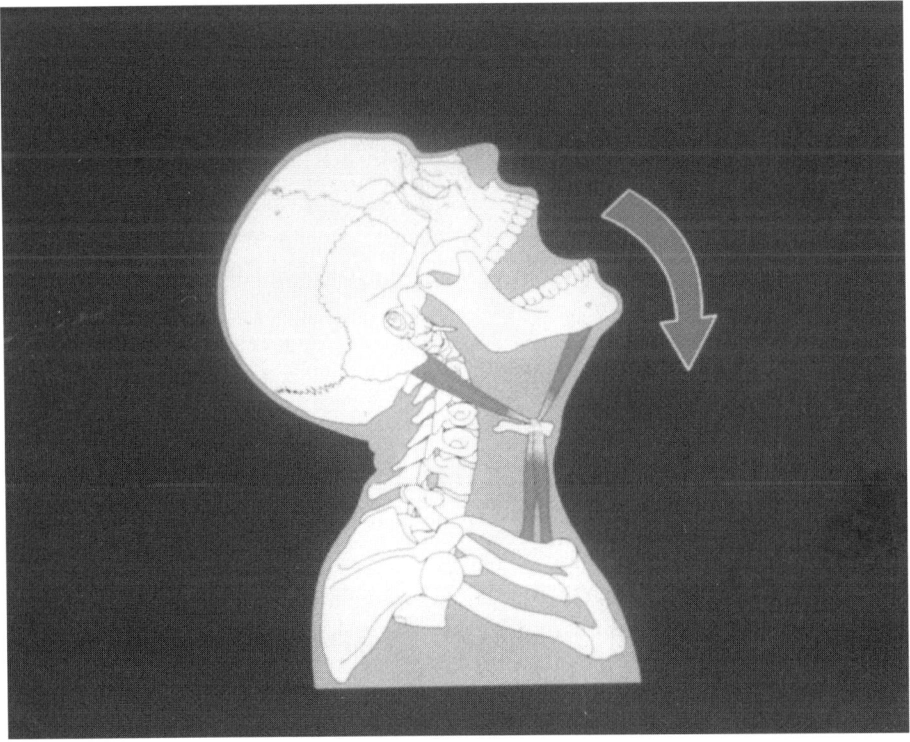

Figure 18.4 Disc causes excessive translation of the condyle forward.

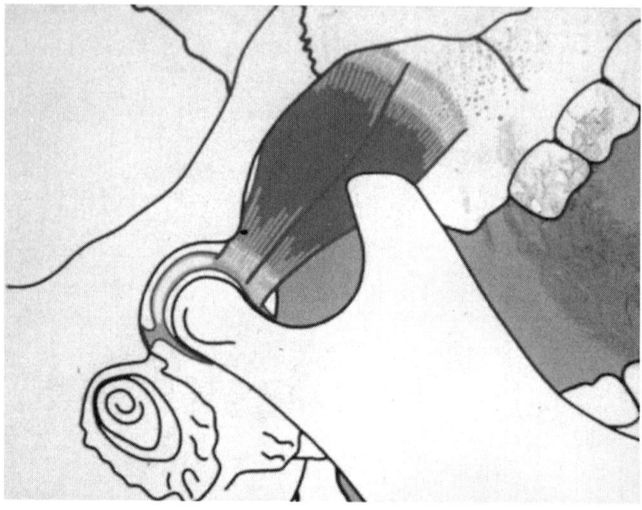

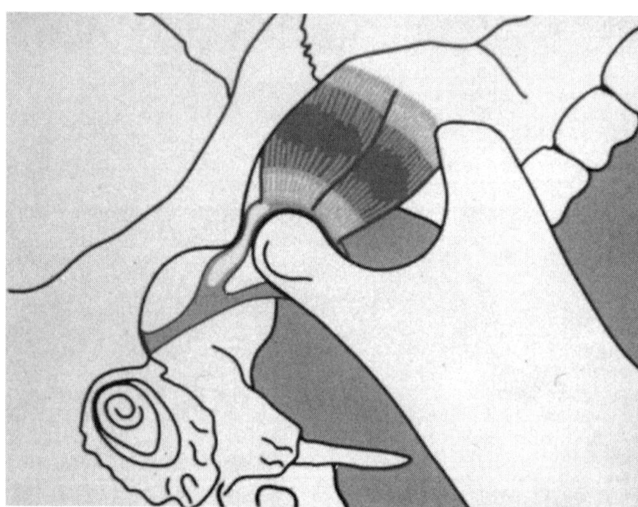

Figure 18.5 The external pterygoid can be impacted at its insertion. (A) Normal condyle position. (B) Hyperextension of the condylar head impacting the external pterygoid muscle. This can tear or dislodge ligaments of the temporomandibular joint and can cause a hemarthrosis and hemorrhage in the joint space.

Although the actual biomechanics are still in question, I feel common sense would tell us that the violent forces received from acceleration-deceleration accidents could, indeed, injure soft tissue and the ligaments of these structures.

In a rear-impact collision that produces acceleration of 12 Gs, the resulting horizontal acceleration of the head is greater than 50 Gs for a period of 40 milliseconds. In a 20 G acceleration, the maximal potential load on the cervical spine may exceed 700 foot-pounds, which is in excess of the average potential breaking load of cervical vertebrae which is 244 foot-pounds, and in cervical intervertebral discs, 194 foot-pounds. The tissues of the head and neck are, indeed, subjected to significant trauma.

The occupants in most car seats are offered little protection to lateral acceleration forces and the initial response to impact is lateral flexion toward the striking vehicle with compression of spinal structures on the concave and stretching of the myofascial structures in the neck on the

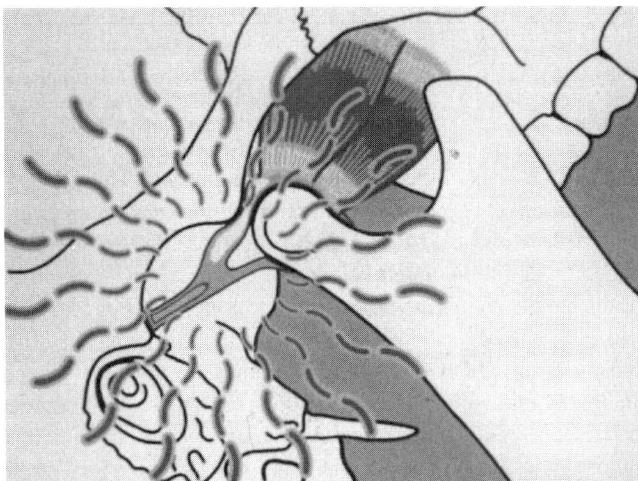

Figure 18.6 When the head is carried in a normal position, the muscles of the cervical spine are at rest. In a head forward position, the excessive forward weight of the skull generates stress on the intrinsic muscles of the cervical spine and indirectly causes stress to the muscles of mastication.

convex side. It is unlikely that these same shearing, torquing forces would not generate a shearing force to the freely movable mandible. The interplay of these forces can be severe.

In my clinical experience, we have found that even low-grade impact accidents can generate accident-related headaches and facial pain that are amenable to treatment of the associated masticatory structures and temporomandibular joint.

Studies have shown there is a high incidence of infusions seen in MRIs of the temporomandibular joints taken after flexion-extension injuries. These infusions demonstrate increased vascularity and hemorrhage in the joint itself secondary to trauma. The inflammation and swelling of the TMJ (hemarthrosis) can lead to associated muscle dysfunction and adhesions with the joint, resulting in a limitation of jaw movement.

The onset of pain can be delayed or become apparent in other regions after several weeks. In musculoskeletal pain, the patient will protect the region where the pain arises either by muscle guarding or restriction of motion. When a muscle becomes painful, other muscles tend to assume an attitude in space that relieves the tension on the involved painful muscle and restricts its functional movement. Thus, muscle splinting, much as a leg would be splinted to reduce movement, accompanies many painful conditions involving the cervical and masticatory muscles. Sustained splinting can develop into muscle spasm and protracted long-term muscle spasm can produce contractile or degenerative changes in muscle. Understanding this explains why facial pain can occur some time after the initiating event and lead to a permanent alteration in function.

This sustained muscle splinting can be enhanced by injury to the cervical tissue or by overloading the masticatory system with dental interferences that alters the normal course of mandibular function. Excessive tooth grinding (bruxism) can apply overloads to muscles. This is habitual in nature and is generally present prior to the accident. However, this can maintain and sustain the myofascial pain (muscle tension pain) that is symptomatic of long-term headaches and facial pain associated with these traumatic incidents.

Over the course of 30 years, I have been treating temporomandibular joint dysfunction problems. TMJ, as it is commonly termed, is a collective term for many separate problems. These range from arthritides of the joint to dislocations of the disc in the joint itself, or more commonly, the dysfunction of the muscles of mastication and the associated muscles of the cervical spine. Ninety percent (90%) of temporomandibular joint complaints are muscle related. This is a complex subject, and the clinician should provide a specific diagnosis, not utilize an umbrella term as nonspecific as "TMJ."

If patients do not respond appropriately to the usual conservative treatment for cervical injuries and the patient continues to complain of persistent headache and facial pain, a dental consultation should be considered.

The treating dentist should examine the patient thoroughly. The exam should include the evaluation of mandibular range of motion. If there is any limitation of opening or limitation in the side-to-side movement of the mandible, this should be assessed. Lateral range of motion both with the teeth apart and together should be noted. When the teeth are together and the subject is unable to slide the jaw from side to side, that is an indication of muscle guarding and/or muscle dysfunction. Wear facets present on the subject's dentition are an indication of a bruxism habit that may be present and may sustain the muscular component of pain.

The temporomandibular joint should be auscultated utilizing a stethoscope to see if there are any crepitotic sounds in the joint itself or if there are signs of popping and clicking on mandibular opening and lateral movement. It must be kept in mind that a third of the population has clicking and popping temporomandibular joints, and these sounds in the temporomandibular joint in and of themselves are not an indication for treatment. Crepitation or a coarse gravelly sound on opening and closing of the temporomandibular joints is indicative of a deterioration of the articular surfaces of the joint itself.

The muscles of mastication and the neck should be palpated. This is done by using moderate finger pressure on the masseters, the temporalis, the sternomastoids, the trapezius, and medial pterygoids and the insertion of the temporalis intraorally. Also, the external pterygoid muscle can be palpated behind the hamular notch or the posterior of the upper jaw. This muscle cannot be palpated directly; however, it can be indirectly palpated by exerting pressure in that area. In a patient who is suffering from chronic or acute muscle spasm, the palpation of these muscles elicits a painful response. This should be graded in its severity.

We have used for many years a stretch and spray technique in which we utilize Fluori-Methane spray applied across the stretched muscles of mastication. Fluori-Methane spray applied in this way will interrupt a spinal reflex arch between the muscle spindle and the spinal cord, which maintains chronic muscle spasm. Often the patient will experience immediate although temporary relief from their complaint of pain. When this happens, it is a firm indication that the patient has primary myofascial pain and no injury to the internal structures of the temporomandibular joint itself. The question then is to determine whether the muscles of mastication or the muscles of the cervical spine primarily generate the myofascial pain.

An aid toward a differential diagnosis is the fabrication of a centric relation splint. This is an appliance fitted to either the upper or lower teeth, which allows the mandible to move freely from side to side and forward; and when the teeth are clenched together, it allows the jaw to move to centric relation. This is an anatomic position of the TMJ in which the condyles are seated firmly in the uppermost and most medial portion of the glenoid fossae. If this position can be attained without pain, that is an indication that the joint is patent. With such an appliance, the patient can continue to clench their teeth (bruxism) without insult to the already traumatized musculature. If the appliance is made carefully and precisely, parafunctional movements (movements out of the normal range of function) of the mandible will be less stressful. Without opposing interferences, the muscles cannot generate enough force to maintain the continued aggravation that these habits generate.

As the muscles of mastication become more relaxed, the condyle tends to settle in a more normal anatomic position requiring alteration of the appliance surface. This therapy should be continued over a period of six to eight weeks and if there is no significant remission in the patient's complaint of pain, then other avenues should be considered.

Injury to the temporomandibular joint, with the exception of an acute dislocation, is not considered a time-sensitive procedure.

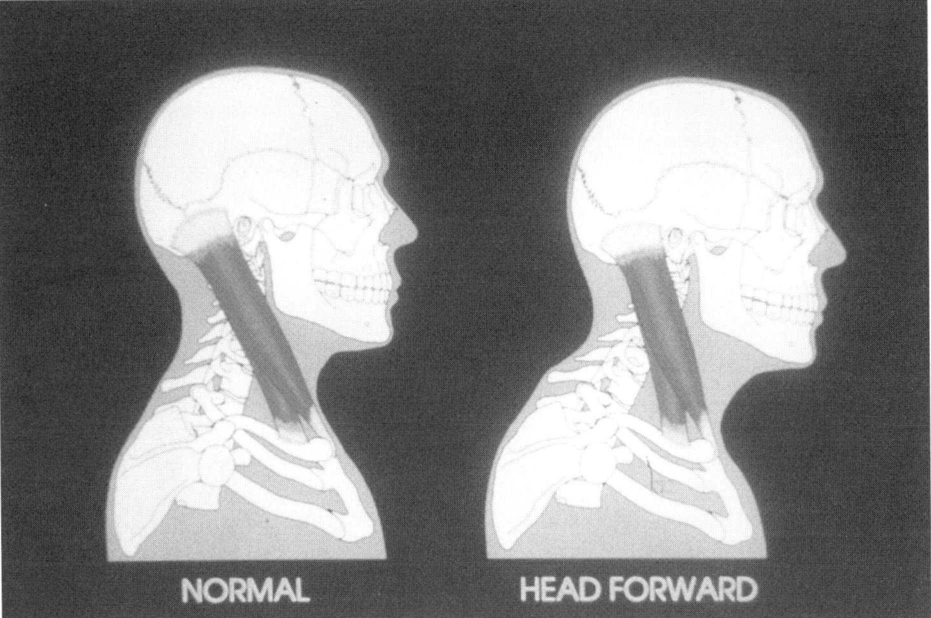

Figure 18.7 The head in an altered position can create abnormal muscle stress.

If a patient has a primary arthrosis of the joint or inflammation and tenderness in the joint itself, it is best to treat this conservatively. Anti-inflammatory medications and muscle relaxants (to reduce muscle tension) such as tricyclic antidepressants or diazepam (Valium) are effective muscle relaxants.

Immediate conservative physical therapy should be instituted consisting of heat, electrical stimulation, evaluation of cervical range of motion, massage and iontophoresis to the temporomandibular joints. If attempts to eliminate the patient's complaint of pain with conservative dental measures are not productive, then a cervical evaluation should be considered if myofascial pain is still suspected.

Many patients present with a head forward position in which the head is carried well forward and constantly stresses the supporting muscles and structure of the cervical spine. The human head (Figure 18.7) weighs approximately as much as a bowling ball and, if carried in an altered position over time, can create abnormal muscle stress. Ergonomic habits such as continued computer use, cradling a telephone on the shoulder, or sustained, stressful work positions can contribute to abnormal muscle loading.

These factors can maintain and sustain the complaint of pain initiated by the cervical acceleration-deceleration injury.

If the utilization of conservative physical therapy, ice, heat, massage, range of motion, manipulation, and ultrasound, is not productive and the patient has passed the acute phase of injury, we have had success utilizing specific strengthening of the cervical spine. We find in our studies that if the intrinsic muscles of the cervical spine are strengthened, it can decrease the complaint of pain. Specific muscle strengthening is preferred, as normal weight training programs challenge the functional muscles of the cervical spine but do not challenge the compromised intrinsic muscles of the cervical spine.

The relationship of the muscles to mastication and the TMJ to its importance in cervical acceleration-deceleration injuries often goes unrecognized.

Studies have shown that the use of a cervical collar can actually add to TMJ stress and cause further injury to the temporomandibular system. If the cervical collar is indicated, a soft collar should be used and this only for a short time.

The primary goal of treatment is gentle mobilization as soon as possible.

Anti-inflammatory medication and the use of muscle relaxants and tricyclic antidepressants are indicated in the early course of treatment.

Although there is some disagreement as to the extent of injury to the temporomandibular joint and the muscles of mastication in cervical acceleration-deceleration injuries, in my experience clinically, I have no question the temporomandibular structure is involved. Often the simple use of a bite splint can eliminate the patient's ongoing complaint of pain.

CASE 1

Cindy, a 21-year-old women who was involved in a rear-end collision, would generally become worse with stress, and at times the pain could be incapacitating. She had complaints of persistent headaches and pain for six months after the traumatic incident. She was seen by several practitioners and was unable to obtain relief through conventional physical therapy and medication. When seen in this office, the muscles of mastication were extremely tender to palpation. A centric relation appliance was fabricated and inserted for Cindy. She returned in 48 hours for an adjustment and stated she was pain free. This is not always the case, but demonstrates how the interruption of cyclic muscle spasm can markedly eliminate pain.

More often treatment rendered is a slower process associated with physical therapy and medication. However, appliance therapy should be markedly effective in six to eight weeks or the patient reevaluated.

CASE 2

Paula received a blow on the back of the neck and was essentially incapacitated. She was a prominent figure and was seen in many centers throughout the country. When seen in this office, she had an undiagnosed temporomandibular joint problem which had been present over a period of years post trauma.

Utilizing a centric relation appliance, trigger point injections, and appropriate medication in a period of 48 hours she was able to function in an acceptable manner. After the stabilization of her immediate symptoms, her occlusion was then altered to a more stable relationship, and following specific strengthening of the cervical musculature, she obtained almost complete relief of this problem, which had previously interrupted her career. When seen several years later, she said, "No one ever looked at my jaw or teeth."

After splint therapy is accomplished, finalization should be considered often through the use of occlusal equilibration of the patient's dentition. This is a procedure where the chewing surfaces of the teeth are reshaped so they hit together evenly and destructive interferences are removed in functional movements. This also has become a controversial issue in dentistry. However, it is my firm opinion that proper occlusal stabilization is a significant adjunct to long-term resolution of occluso-muscle pain. This is a technique that requires considerable skill and judgment by the practitioner. The patient should be referred to someone who has an adequate knowledge of this treatment modality.

Since temporomandibular joint surgery is indicated in only 3% to 5% of the patients involved, the practice of primary referral to an oral surgeon should be questioned. Also, few patients need direct orthodontic interception, as in most cases a functional occlusion can be attained even though there may be some existing occlusal disharmonies. A functional occlusion can usually be generated with relatively simple procedures.

If the patient has lost many teeth or has had such drifting and position change of their teeth that a functional occlusion cannot be obtained by equilibration procedures, then restorative dental procedures should be considered. When this is done, these restorative dental procedures should be considered a direct result of the traumatic incident the patient was involved in.

Over the years I have seen many patients complaining of pain secondary to whiplash-type injuries. Often concurrent treatment of the muscles of mastication and the cervical spine can lead to a quicker, more effective, and less costly resolution of these problems.

CASE 3

Category: Preexisting facial pain symptoms exacerbated by cervical and temporomandibular joint trauma.

Annette is a 52-year-old women who had ongoing facial pain complaints who was involved in a motor vehicle accident in which she was hit from the side. She suffered trauma from the steering wheel to her chest, a broken anterior tooth, and complained of exacerbated headaches and pain.

When seen, she was restricted to a soft diet, had constant pain, which increased with both stress and mastication, had been diagnosed with fibromyalgia, and had a long course of medical care for chronic pain complaints. Her complaint of pain exacerbated after the accident and became incapacitating.

Examination: She had a normal opening of the mandible. There were no sounds in either temporomandibular joint, and she had full range of mandibular motion to the right and left. There were excessive wear facets present on the anterior teeth, and the muscles of mastication were exquisitely tender to palpation. Both temporomandibular joints could be loaded in centric relation without the complaint of pain. Doppler auscultation elicited some mild retrodiscal hyperemia in the left temporomandibular joint. Vapocoolant spray applied to the muscles of mastication markedly reduced her complaint of pain from the stated 8 at the time to 2. She presented with a great deal of restorative dentistry. She complained that she felt her bite was off and had a positive occlusal sense.

Utilization of a centric relation appliance decreased her complaint of pain from 8 to 2. The altered occlusal sense in the closed vertical dimension maintained and sustained the soft tissue trauma. After splint therapy, rehabilitation of her dentition to optimize her occlusion is indicated. However, she will still have some resultant cervical pain and specific rehabilitation of the intrinsic muscles of the cervical spine would be indicated in this case.

Prognosis: The prognosis is guarded. The patient has preexisting complaint of fibromyalgia and chronic pain. However, restorative dental procedures markedly reduced her complaint of pain.

CASE 4

Juanita is a 42-year-old women who presented with persistent pain in the left preauricular and zygomatic area. She complained of retro-orbital pain and headaches that were in the area of the left occiput and down the neck. She was involved in a motor vehicle accident in which she was hit from the left side by an unseen vehicle and had immediate facial pain and complaint of persistent headaches after the incident.

Examination: She presented with a restricted opening of the mandible; however, with moderate pressure, it could be opened to a normal opening, and that was associated with a complaint of pain. Doppler auscultation elicited marked retrodiscal hyperemia in the right temporomandibular joint. Conservative appliance therapy was not productive in this case and an auricular temporal block (a diagnostic block that deadens the nerve that supplies the temporomandibular joint) markedly eliminated her complaint of pain. She was referred to a maxillofacial surgeon for consideration of temporomandibular joint surgery. This was performed and the patient had complete relief of her pain. However, she was involved in a second accident and after conservative appliance therapy she did not improve. Again an auricular temporal block was utilized and she was referred for temporomandibular joint surgery. This reduced her complaint of pain, but did not eliminate it. Unfortunately, she was involved in a third accident and at this time is considering additional temporomandibular joint surgery.

Prognosis: The prognosis in this case is guarded. Additional surgery in the temporomandibular joint is not predictable and is utilized only in cases of interfering or incapacitating complaints of pain. This is an example of primary trauma to the temporomandibular joint and demonstrates the difficulty in treating a patient with a prior condition generated by trauma after the second traumatic event.

CASE 5

Linda is a 48-year-old woman who was involved in a motor vehicle accident in which she was hit from the rear. She was rendered unconscious. When she recovered, she advised her jaws were locked shut. She complained of immediate headache, neck pain, and associated pain in the thoracic and lumbar areas. She suffered three dislocated vertebral discs in this accident. She was given a cervical collar for two or three weeks, was treated with physical therapy and was seen by many practitioners. She had long-term facial pain over a period of several years and was limited to a soft and liquid diet. She had headaches daily. On a lineal digital scale of 1 to 10, it could vary from 6 to 8 or 9. It generally occurred in the occipital area, radiating to the vertex of the skull in the temporal area and became global when they were severe. She advised she had pain in the right and left preauricular areas and more severe on the left side than the right.

Utilization of a centric relation splint markedly eliminated her complaint of pain. She presented with a worn dentition, an unsatisfactory partial denture prosthesis in which the anterior guidance or the length of the anterior teeth was compromised.

After appliance therapy, Linda's dentition was restored utilizing a more stable prosthesis (fixed bridgework) and the incisal guidance was altered to eliminate any occlusal interference. This markedly reduced her complaint of pain approximately 60%. She is now able to eat a regular diet. Her headaches have diminished, and although she still has complaint of occasional headaches, she is markedly improved.

This is a case of acute trauma to the soft tissues that is maintained and sustained by occlusal disharmony. This points out the need for restoration of a preexisting occluso-muscle problem that is exacerbated by trauma and can be significantly reduced by occlusal rehabilitation.

In extensive treatment for temporomandibular joint disorders, including splint therapy, surgical intervention, orthodontics and restorative procedures, there is a significant input of cervical musculature into the same complaints of pain as temporomandibular joint disorders.

It also strongly suggests that the evaluation of cervical disorder should be considered prior to invasive treatment modalities utilizing temporomandibular joint disorders and concurrent use of specific muscle strengthening of the cervical spine coupled with traditional treatment of temporomandibular joint disorders is an effective treatment modality.

CASE 6

Category: Post traumatic temporomandibular joint dysfunction.

John is a 37-year-old nurse who was injured in restraining a psychiatric patient. While restraining the patient, he was hit in the side of the neck. He stated he had immediate pain in the neck and this worsened over four to six months. He was seen by his physician and referred to a neurologist for ongoing complaint of facial pain.

He was referred for a dental examination, and at that time we noted a normal opening of the mandible and no sounds in the temporomandibular joints. However, he was unable to make functional movements of the mandible to the right or left but had full range of mandibular motion with the teeth apart. There were marked wear facets on the right cuspid teeth. Both temporomandibular joints could be loaded in centric relation without the complaint of pain. The patient presented with a severe head forward posture.

Doppler auscultation exhibited retrodiscal hyperemia on the contralateral side.

Vapocoolant spray applied to the muscles of mastication completely eliminated his complaint of pain.

A centric relation appliance was fabricated and inserted, and the patient returned one week later, stating that he had had complete remission of his complaint of pain. Occlusal equilibration was performed to eliminate any parafunctional occlusal disharmonies, and the patient was advised to continue using a centric relation splint nocturnally.

This is an example of a soft tissue injury that is sustained and maintained by parafunctional habits and bruxism, and the myofascial pain patterns that he displays can generate facial pain symptoms although the temporomandibular joints are patent.

CASE 7

Cathy, a 37-year-old office worker, was involved in a motor vehicle accident in which she was hit from behind and her auto then hit a restraining rail. She complained of immediate neck pain, arm and shoulder pain. The complaint of pain became more severe after several weeks. She experienced pain bilaterally and along the border of the mandible and through the neck. She had a popping sound in the temporomandibular joints, which became worse when associated with pain and had difficulty with mandibular opening. Her pain level on a digital level of 1 to 10 was a 5 to 6. The pain was constant, and she experienced pain, tingling and numbness in the left extremity.

She presented with a reciprocal click in both temporomandibular joints. These sounds were on very late opening and very late closing. The opening sounds were sharp and the closing sounds dull. She had a limited range of lateral mandibular motion, and the muscles of mastication were exquisitely sensitive to palpation. Both temporomandibular joints could be loaded in centric relation.

Her facial pain became apparent after several weeks. Vapocoolant spray applied to the muscles of mastication demonstrated no remarkable change.

A centric relation appliance was fabricated, inserted, and the patient had a remission of her complaint of pain of 50%. She returned after wearing the appliance for occlusal equilibration and after this was performed, she still complained of lessened but significant facial pain.

The patient was then referred for a specific exercise protocol to strengthen the intrinsic muscles of the cervical spine. This again lessened her complaint of pain, although she still had a residual complaint of pain.

The popping and clicking of the temporomandibular joints was not significant, as the sound was late in the opening movement. The temporomandibular joints could be loaded and were patent. However, the patient generated muscle dysfunction associated with cervical myospasm, and the secondary onset of masticatory pain is most likely due to altered cervical function and its influence on its shared muscles, the muscles of mastication.

Elimination of occluso-muscle pain was significant but not complete. Exercise/strengthening therapy also decreased her complaint of pain. This patient presents with a chronic cervical myospasm that indirectly generates myofascial pain patterns and masticatory muscle dysfunction. Her problem did not respond totally to therapy.

CASE 8

Wendy is an 18-year-old student who was involved in a motor vehicle accident. The vehicle she was in impacted the vehicle in front of her. She did not wear a seat belt. She received a contusion of the head, and one month after the accident she experienced clicking and popping in the temporomandibular joints, and concurrent neck pain. There was no complaint of clicking or popping prior to this accident. She complained of pain in the right temporomandibular joint and had interfering headaches in the frontal area and along the sides of the neck.

The temporomandibular joints could be loaded in centric relation. Vapocoolant spray applied to the muscles of mastication eliminated her complaint of pain and the accompanying click in the temporomandibular joints on mandibular opening.

A centric relation appliance was fabricated and inserted, and the patient received immediate relief in 24 hours. This elimination of pain continued as long as the appliance was worn. When removed after several hours, her complaint of pain would return.

This was an example of a soft tissue injury secondary to trauma that could be eliminated with occlusal therapy. The patient received immediate relief utilizing appliance therapy, and this was maintained by occlusal equilibration and nocturnal appliance wear. In this case a lateral pole dislocation of the disc of the temporomandibular joint was reduced by eliminating muscle dysfunction.

REFERENCES

1. Travell, J.G., Simons, D.J., *Myofascial Pain and Dysfunction: The Trigger Point Manual*, Williams & Wilkins, Baltimore, 1983.
2. Teasell, R.W., Shapiro, A.P., Eds., *State of the Art Reviews: Spine, Cervical Flexion-Extension-Whiplash Injuries*, Hanley & Belfus, Philadelphia, 1993.
3. Foreman, S.M., Croft, A.C. *Whiplash Injuries, The Cervical Acceleration-Deceleration Syndrome,* 2nd ed., Williams & Wilkins, Baltimore, 1995.
4. Dawson, P.E., *Evaluation, Diagnosis, and Treatment of Occlusal Problems*, Peter E. Dawson, DDS, C. V. Mosby, St. Louis: 1989.
5. Okeson, J.P., *Management of Temporomandibular Disorders and Occlusion*, C. V. Mosby, St. Louis: 1989.
6. Porterfield, J.A., DeRosa, C., *Mechanical Neck Pain*, W. B. Saunders, Philadelphia, 1995.
7. McNeill, C. *Temporomandibular Disorders*, Quintessence, 1993.
8. Shore, N.A., *Occlusal Equilibration and Temporomandibular Joint Dysfunction*, Lippincott, Philadelphia, 1959.
9. Mahan, P.E., Alling, C.C., Lea & Febiger, Philadelphia, 1991.
10. Bell, W., *Clinical Management of Temporomandibular Disorders*, Yearbook Medical Publishers, Chicago, 1983.
11. Irby, W.B., *Current Advances in Oral Surgery*, C. V. Mosby, St. Louis, 1980.
12. Bell, W.E., *Orofacial Pains, Differential Diagnosis*, Yearbook Medical Publishers, Chicago, 1979.
13. Rocabado, M., *Musculoskeletal Approach to Maxillofacial Pain*, J. Lippincott, Philadelphia, 1991.
14. Tenaca, T.T., Ed., *Head, Neck and TMJ Pain Management Seminar*, University of California-San Diego, 1992.
15. Hand, T.P., *Exercise Rehabilitation of the Spine*, University of Florida, 1997.

Chapter 19

A Newer Concept — The Cervicogenic Headache

Although the history of headache dates back thousands of years, the relationship of headache and the neck is a relatively newer concept. It has only been in the last 20 to 25 years that significant research has been published to make a connection between problems of the neck and the cause of chronic headache. The anatomical and neurophysiological research that has been done has now given us a logical and scientific explanation of how the two problems of head and neck are related.

Patients who complain of headache will often identify the neck as an area that is also part of the pain picture. They may identify that the pain starts in the neck and travels up and to the front of the head and face, or that the pain starts in the front of the head and travels down to the back of the neck. They may say that the pain in the neck is bilateral, that is, on both sides of the neck, or that the pain in the neck is one-sided and that the continued pain in the head and face is also one-sided. Those patients who have suffered head trauma, or whiplash (cervical acceleration/deceleration) injuries and continue to complain of chronic pain may now have a physical explanation of this condition. However, this problem does not have to be associated with injury to the neck.

Although the International Headache Society (IHS) has not yet given cervicogenic headache an official classification, the enormous input from well-respected medical centers around the world appears to be making ground in changing that classification. Hopefully, the IHS will accept this term.

Sjaastad, Fredriksen, and Pfaffenrath[1] have proposed the following criteria for cervicogenic headache.

Major symptoms and signs

1. Unilaterality of the head pain, without sideshift. (The pain is on one side of the head and the pain does not shift to the other side. Only during severe episodes, the pain may be felt vaguely across the midline, but it is always worse on the usual side.)
2. Symptoms and signs of neck involvement:
   (a) Provocation of attacks:
      A. Pain, seemingly of a similar nature, triggered by neck movement and/or sustained awkward head positioning.
      B. Pain similar in distribution and character to the spontaneously occurring pain elicited by external pressure over the ipsilateral (same side) upper, posterior neck region or occipital region. (The areas from which attacks may be precipitated can be rather clearly defined, i.e., along the major occipital nerve and immediately behind the mastoid process.)
   (b) Ipsilateral neck, shoulder, and arm pain of a rather vague, non-radicular nature.
   (c) Reduced range of motion in the cervical spine.

Pain characteristics

3. Nonclustering pain episodes. (Unlike cluster headache, these pains do not come at different times of the year for a certain period of time.)
4. Pain episodes of varying duration (they can last from a few hours to a few days to a few weeks; these pains are usually longer than the episode of common migraine), or fluctuating continuous pain (that is, the intensity of the pain varies, not the duration).
5. Moderate, non-excruciating pain, usually of a non-throbbing nature.
6. Pain starting in the neck, eventually spreading to oculo (eye)-frontal-temporal areas, where the maximum pain is often located. (It has been suggested that the pain below the eye may result from neck involvement from the cervical roots lower than the C2 root.)

Other important criteria

7. Anesthetic blockades of the major occipital nerve and/or of the C2 root on the symptomatic side abolish the pain transiently. (This is not considered a mandatory component of the routine diagnostic workup.)
8. There is a preponderance among females of almost 4:1.
9. Head and/or neck trauma (whiplash) by history.

Nonobligatory symptoms and signs. Various attack-related phenomena:

10. Autonomic symptoms and signs:
    (a) Nausea
    (b) Vomiting
    (c) Ipsilateral edema (same-side swelling)
    (d) Flushing (mostly around the eyes)
11. Dizziness
12. Phono and photophobia
13. Blurred vision in the eye on the same side of the pain
14. Difficulties on swallowing

Sjaastad et al. feel that points (1) and (2) are obligatory for the diagnosis. In point (2) either (A) or (B) is obligatory. The other points are strong supportive evidence for the diagnosis.

Within the neck there are many anatomical structures that may be responsible for causing pain, both in the neck and the head.

These cervical structures are bones, muscles, ligaments, nerves, and arteries.

1. The bones of the vertebral column include the following structures:
   a. Joints, that are called facets, apophyseal, and zygapophyseal
   b. Intervertebral discs
   c. Spinous ligaments
   d. Periosteum (specialized connective tissue covering the bones of the body with bone forming potential)
2. There are numerous cervical muscles and their tendons that may be responsible for this pain.
3. The cervical nerves and their tributaries and the roots of these nerves and their relationship to the trigeminal system that send messages to the front of the head.
4. Irritation of the vertebral arteries may also be responsible for this pain.

Enormous work has been done to study the relationship of the joints of the vertebrae and how this may explain the continued pain following head and neck injuries. A great deal of this work was done by a group of doctors in Australia (Bogduk and coworkers[2]), and a list of their articles I have reviewed is at the end of this chapter (Figure 19.1).

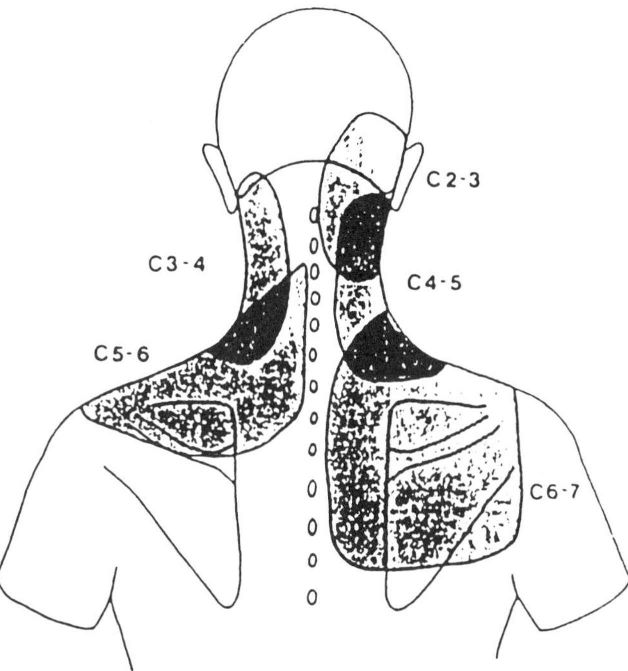

Figure 19.1 A composite map of zygapophyseal joint patterns showing the characteristic distribution of pain from the zygapophyseal joints at segments C2–3 to C6–7. (From Dwyer, A. et al., *Spine*, 15, 453–457, 1990. With permission.)

In their studies they have concluded that cervical **zygapophyseal joint** pain was the most common source of chronic pain after whiplash. It is beyond the scope of this book to demonstrate the intricate neurophysiological and neuroanatomical details of their work. Those who wish to learn more may benefit from reviewing the references listed.

They conclude that whiplash injury has done a great deal to polarize views in the medical community. One side argues that chronic pain after whiplash injuries is maintained by psychological factors either for financial gain or because there were preexisting psychological factors. The other side argues that the continued pain can be explained by organic lesions.

After some of the earlier papers suggested that these patients were primarily malingerers, newer studies that had much better scientific designs and data have revealed that there is little evidence to support such a proposition. Another study by Radonov et al.[3] refutes the hypothesis that chronic symptoms after whiplash arise from preexisting psychological problems.

Bogduk et al.[2] continue to say that data supporting an organic basis for chronic pain is compelling and this information has been derived from many different sources, including experimental studies on animals and cadavers, plus descriptive studies on postmortem and clinical findings. They go on to say that these different approaches have been consistent in their findings, revealing that a number of these pathologic lesions are capable of producing chronic pain after a cervical acceleration/deceleration (whiplash) injury to the neck. These lesions include injuries to the discs, ligaments, and the zygapophyseal joints (Figure 19.2).

Both clinical and experimental studies of whiplash patients have revealed tears of the joint capsules, hemarthrosis (bleeding into a joint or its synovial cavity), and fractures of the joint cartilage or bone beneath the cartilage. The problem is that it is extremely difficult to detect these injuries in the living specimen (*in vivo*). Conventional x-ray and clinical examination do not permit identification of injury to the zygapophyseal joint. This is why the pain from this area has not been known. The studies conducted by Bogduk et al. were to develop an anesthetic block of the joint

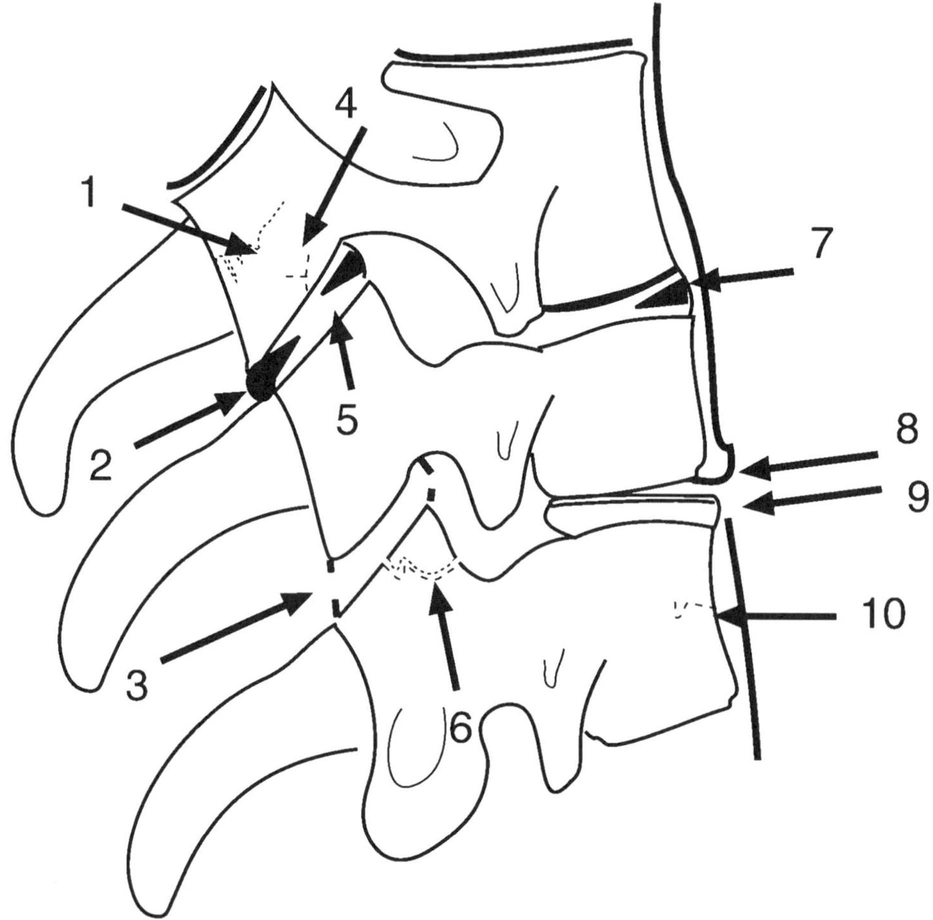

Figure 19.2 A sketch of the more common lesions affecting the cervical spine following whiplash: (**1**) articular pillar fracture; (**2**) hemarthrosis of the zygapophysial joint; (**3**) rupture or tear of the zygapophyseal joint capsule; (**4**) fracture of the subchondral plate; (**5**) contusion of the intra-articular meniscus of the zygapophysial joint; (**6**) fracture involving the articular surface; (**7**) tear of the annulus fibrosus of the intervertebral disc; (**8**) tear of the anterior longitudinal ligament; (**9**) endplate avulsion/fracture; (**10**) vertebral body fracture. (Adapted from Barnsley, L. et al., *Pain*, 58, 283–307, 1994.)

or the nerves that supply this joint that relieves the pain, and therefore infers that this target joint is the source of the pain. In a 1995 publication, a study was done using 38 patients from a 50 patient selection injecting a long- and short-acting anesthetic and seeing whether the patient could differentiate the effect of the two different anesthetics. The results were extremely interesting in that they showed a positive response to these blocks in eliminating the pain for the time the anesthetics would work.

They were positive over 50% of the time. Now that there is an identification of the problem, attempts are being made to treat of this condition. What has to be understood is that a negative response in a minority of these tests only excludes one possible diagnosis, that is zygapophyseal joint pain, and does not rule out genuine pain from other sources.

Injury to the **intervertebral disc** has also been shown to be a source of continued pain after cervical acceleration/deceleration (whiplash) accidents. Tears or avulsions of the disc from its end plate or tears of the annulus fibrosus (a ring between) of the disc and separation of the disc from the vertebrae or fracture of of the vertebral end plate may be responsible for the continued pain. These injuries have been found at postmortem examinations, at surgery, reproduced experimentally and some of them found with x-ray and MRI. Some of these postmortem examinations have been done after the victim survived the initial injury before dying. There have been careful studies on cadavers who were then exposed to whiplash injuries and producing anterior disc lesions, especially after hyperextension. The patients who survived and had ongoing symptoms after ten years all developed degenerative changes in the area of injury. A study comparing degenerative changes between whiplash persons and controlled groups showed a significant prevalence in the whiplash victims.

Injury to the **ligaments** is another source of pain. Injuries to the anterior longitudinal ligament have also been reported in animal experiments, surgical procedures on humans, postmortem examinations and in cadaver experiments. Although special MRI imaging has confirmed some of these tears, physical examination does not lend itself to making that diagnosis. Because anatomically the anterior longitudinal ligament merges with the anterior annulus of the intervertebral disc, injuries to the ligament may also be associated with disc injuries (see Figure 17.10). Injuries to the posterior longitudinal ligament have been reported in animal experiments, postmortem examination, and cadaver experiments, but are never seen at operations. The probable explanation is that in order to damage this ligament, which is very flexible, the injury has to be so severe that survival is highly unlikely.

The **atlanto-axial joints** in severe injury can be fractured and the ligaments attached to them can be torn, which can create ongoing pain. Some of these damages can be found on x-ray, and in some cases of specialized CT scanning, disruption of the alar ligaments may be detected. Again, these injuries have been detected as above in postmortem and experimental design (Figure 19.3).

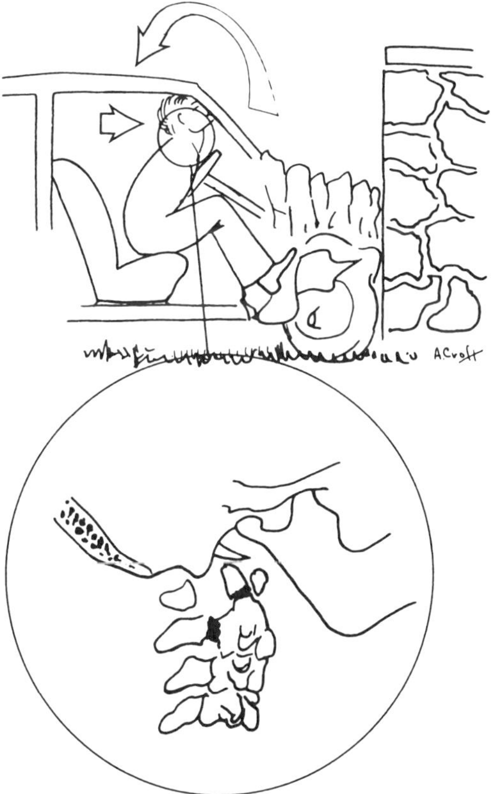

Figure 19.3 This illustrates that with severe flexion-extension a fracture of the atlanto-axial joint can be produced. See text. (From Foreman, S.M., Croft, A.C., *Whiplash Injuries: The Cervical Acceleration/Deceleration Syndrome,* 2nd ed., Williams & Wilkins, Baltimore, 1995.)

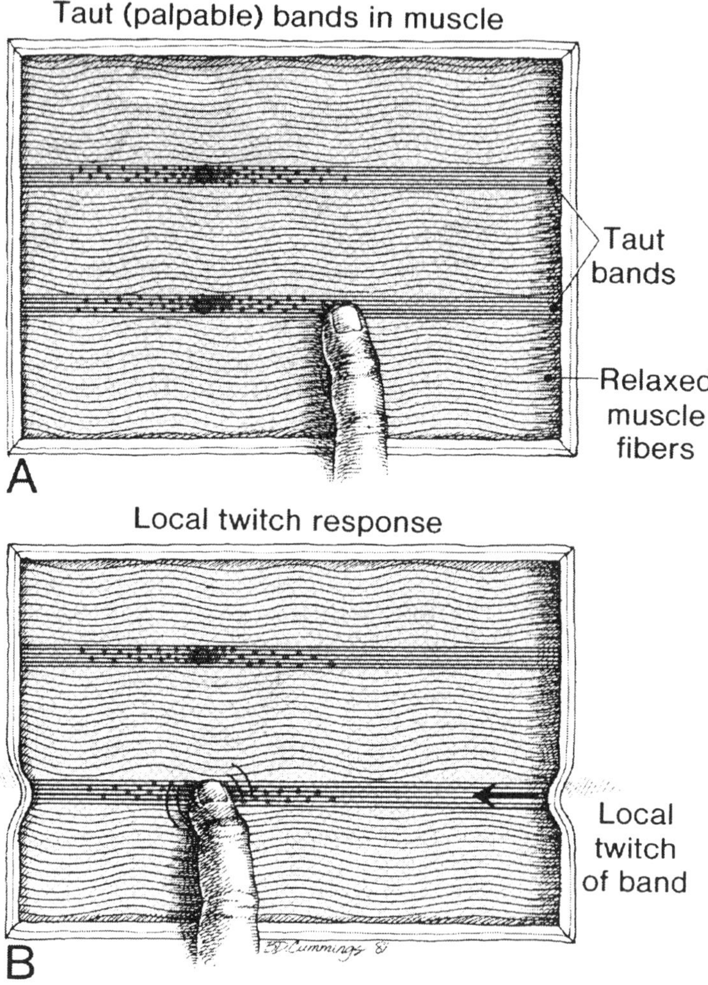

Figure 19.4 This illustration demonstrates the taut bands in the muscle that are caused by trigger points. When one palpates the actual trigger point, there can be referred pain to another area and automatically the patient will jump, even if they don't want to. This is an easy and accessible diagnostic criteria for trigger points. (From Travell, J.G., Simons, D.G., *Myofascial Pain and Dysfunction: The Trigger Point Manual*, Williams & Wilkins, Baltimore, 1983. With permission.)

After a whiplash (cervical acceleration/deceleration) accident there may also be damage to the **cervical vertebrae**. If there is an overt fracture of the vertebrae below C2, then conventional x-ray or CT scan may be used to recognize this problem. However, fractures of the pedicles, and laminae, or the transverse process, and compression fractures of the vertebral bodies are difficult to visualize, and only specialized views will reveal these fractures. Again, these fractures have been demonstrated in experimental studies on animals and cadavers, as well as in postmortem examinations.

Muscle tears may also lead to pain and these also have been seen in animal experiments and postmortem examinations on humans. Clinical examination and ultrasound have revealed muscle tears and hemorrhage. Most muscle tears will eventually heal, leaving scar tissue with little or no pain. Muscle tears do not seem to be the cause of continued chronic pain and headache.

Trigger points and myofascial pain were discussed in Chapter 17. Although statistical research has not produced the kind of data necessary in proving medical theory, the clinician will often find trigger points after whiplash injury. Treating these trigger points will often give some to total relieve for a period of time. Travell and Simons[4] have been very explicit in defining trigger points. Unfortunately, many physicians have misinterpreted the specific criteria and this diagnosis has been used in instances where true active trigger points were not found. If in fact a patient has an active trigger point, then with palpation a headache can be produced.

The headache may vary from a tension-type headache to a migraine-like headache. The major criterion of an active trigger point is that it refers pain to another area, that is from somewhere in the neck to somewhere in the head. On palpation there should be a palpable taut band and a "jump sign." Finding these signs does not exclude the presence of other conditions previously discussed (Figure 19.4).

Unfortunately, the term "trigger points" have been misused in the area of both medical treatments and in the legal arena. There were many clinicians who claimed that trigger points could be identified using thermography. Swerdlow and Dieter[5] could not correlate in their research the relationship between trigger points and "hot spots."

Properly diagnosed, myofascial trigger points that are active may be responsible for producing headaches, and if properly treated may give relief for some period of time to this condition of chronic headache.

Treatments for this disorder are discussed in Chapter 25.

Although it has been over a hundred years since the relationship between the neck and the head was made, the actual attempt to define the relationship between the neural structures from the cervical region to the head and face is relatively new. The anatomic and functional overlap between the trigeminal nucleus caudalis and the cervical sensory area has been experimentally defined. The significance is that impulses giving rise to sensations of pain (nociceptive) from the upper two or three cervical roots could potentially activate the trigeminal nociceptive system, producing pain in the trigeminal distribution of the face and head. Pain can also be expressed to the back of the head in the occipital and suboccipital areas. This pain can also be directed from the C1, C2, and C3 to the skin and muscles of the suboccipital and occipital regions via the greater and lesser occipital nerves.

Even though it is sometimes impossible to visualize these physical problems using radiographic techniques, there is certainly enough evidence to support physical reasons for ongoing chronic pain following whiplash accidents.

REFERENCES

1. Sjaastad, O., Fredriksen, T.A., Pfaffenrath, V., Cervicogenic headache: diagnostic criteria, *Headache*, 30, 725–726, 1990.
2. Barnsley, L., Lord, S., Bogduk, N., Clinical review: whiplash injury, *Pain*, 58, 283–307, 1994.
3. Radonov, P.R., Stefano, G., Schnidrig, A., Ballinari, P., Role of psychological stress in recovery from common whiplash, *Lancet*, 338, 712–715, 1991.
4. Travell, J.G., Simons, D.G., Myofascial pain and dysfunction: the trigger point manual, Williams & Wilkins, Baltimore, 1983.
5. Swerdlow, B., Dieter, J.N. An evaluation of medical thermography for the documentation of myofascial trigger points, *Pain*, 48(2), 205–213, 1992.

ARTICLES REVIEWED

Aprill, C., Bogduk, N., The prevalence of cevical zygapophyseal joint pain: a first approximation, *Spine*, 17(7), 1992.

Aprill, C., Dwyer, A., Bogduk, N., Cervical zygapophyseal joint pain patterns. II. A clinical evaluation, *Spine*, 15(6), 1990.

Barnsley, L., Bogduk, N., Medial branch blocks are specific for the diagnosis of cervical zygapophyseal joint pain, *Reg Anesthesia*, 18(6), 1993.

Barnsley, L., Lord, S., Bogduk, N., Clinical review: whiplash injury, *Pain*, 58, 283–307.

Barnsley, L., Lord, S., Bogduk, N., Comparative local anesthetic blocks in the diagnosis of cervical zygapophysial joint pain, *Pain*, 55, 99–106, 1993.

Barnsley, L., Lord, S., Wallis, B., Bogduk, N., False-positive rates of cervical zygapophysial joint blocks, *Clinical Journal of Pain*, 9, 124–130, 1993.

Barnsley, L., Lord, S.M., Wallis, B.J., Bogduk, N., Lack of effect of intraarticular corticosteroids for chronic pain in the cervical zygapophyseal joints, *New England Journal of Medicine*, 330(15), 1994.

Barnsley, L., Lord, S.M., Wallis, B.J., Bogduk, N., The prevalence of chronic cervical zygapophysial joint pain after whiplash, *Spine*, 20(1), 20–26, 1995.

Bogduk, N., Aprill, C., On the nature of neck pain, discography and cervical zygapophysial joint blocks, *Pain*, 54, 213–217, 1993.

Bogduk, N., Corrigan, B., et al., Cervical headache, *Medical Journal of Australia*, 143(5), 1985.

Bogduk, N., Lambert, G.A., Duckworth, J.W., The anatomy and physiology of the vertebral nerve in elation to cervical migraine, *Cephalalgia*, 1981.

Bogduk, N., Marsland, A., On the concept of third occipital headache, *Journal of Neurology Neurosurgery and Psychiatry*, 49, 775–780, 1986.

Bogduk, N., Marsland, A., The cervical zygopophysial joints as a source of neck pain, *Spine*, 13(6), 1988.

Bogduk, N., Windsor, M., Inglis, A., The innervation of the cervical interbertebral disks, *Spine*, 13(1), 1988.

Bogduk, N., Headaches and the cervical spine. An editorial, *Cephalalgia Editorial*, 4, 7, 1984.

Bogduk, N., Neck pain: an update, *Australian Family Physician*, 17(2), 1988.

Bogduk, N., The argument for discography, *Neurosurgery Quarterly*, 6(2), 1996.

Bogduk, N., The clinical anatomy of the cervical dorsal rami, *Spine*, 7(4), 1982.

Dwyer, A., Aprill, C., Bogduk, N., Cervical zygapophyseal joint pain patterns. I. A study in normal volunteers, *Spine*, 15(6), 1990.

Lord, S.M., Barnsley, et al., Percutaneous radio-frequency neurotomy for chronic cervical zygapophyseal-joint pain, *New England Journal of Medicine*, 335(23), 1996.

Lord, S.M., Barnsley, L., Wallis, B.J., Bogduk, N., Percutaneous radiofrequency neurotomy in the treatment of cervical zygapophysial joint pain: a caution, *Neurosurgery*, 36(4), 1995.

Lord, S.M., Barnsley, L., Wallis, B.J., Bogduk, N., Third occipital nerve headache: a prevalence study, *Journal of Neurology, Neurosurgery, and Psychiatry*, 57, 1187–1190, 1994.

CASE HISTORIES*

* On the headache assessment forms that accompany these case histories, incapacitating headaches are indicated with solid black lines, interfering headaches with dotted lines, and irritating headaches with gray shading.

MEDICAL HEADACHE HISTORY

Name: Sue **Age:** 40 **Sex** F **Date:** 12/21/93

Date of Birth: 0/00/53 **Birthplace:** WV **Race:** C **Education:** High School

Occupation: Hair Stylist **Accident:** 1993

Armed Services & Type of Discharge: N/A

PAST HISTORY:

1.	Did you have a normal birth?		Yes (underlined)	No
	a) forceps used?		Yes	No (underlined)
	b) cesarean section?		Yes	No (underlined)
2.	Did you have problems with bedwetting?		Yes	No (underlined)
	a) If yes, age bedwetting stopped		______	
3.	Were you car sick as a child (motion)?		Yes	No (underlined)
	a) If yes, how severe?	Slight	Moderate	Severe
4.	Did you have unexplained abdominal cramps as a child?		Yes	No (underlined)
5.	Did you have any of the following illnesses in childhood?			
	a) meningitis		Yes	No (underlined)
	b) encephalitis		Yes	No (underlined)
	c) scarlet fever		Yes	No (underlined)
	d) rheumatic fever		Yes	No (underlined)
6.	Did you have any head injuries as a child?		Yes	No (underlined)
	a) If yes, please explain: ______			
7.	Were you treated for emotional illness as a child?		Yes	No (underlined)

HABITS:

8.	Do you drink alcohol?	Yes (underlined)	No
	a) If yes, what kind and how much? Moderately		
	b) Does alcohol bring on or aggravate a headache?	Yes	No (underlined)
9.	Do you smoke?	Yes (underlined)	No
	a) If yes, how much? About 7 to 11 a day		
	b) Does smoking or smoke-filled rooms cause or aggravate headaches?	Yes	No (underlined)
10.	Do you drink caffeinated beverages?	Yes (underlined)	No
	a) If yes, how much? 2 to 3 cups of coffee a day		

MENSTRUAL HISTORY:

At what age did menses begin? 11 Were they regular or irregular? WNL
How were they related to your headache? Not related
Are you or were you ever on Birth Control Pills? No Did they affect your headache? N/A
Have you had a hysterectomy, partial or total, and why? Yes, 1988, Total; Fibroids, endometriosis
Are you in menopause, and if yes, how long? No
Are you on hormones, and if yes, which ones? No

HEADACHE ASSESSMENT FORM

HA PROFILE	INCAPACITATING #3	INTERFERING #2	IRRITATING #1
ONSET (Years ago and frequency)	Age 23, occasionally None for last 5 years	Day of accident Every day	N/A
CURRENT FREQUENCY	2 to 3/week since accident	Every day	N/A
TIME OF ONSET	Anytime, can awaken with	Awakens with; better in a.m.; increases during day	N/A
DURATION	1 to 2 days	Constant	N/A
CHARACTER	Severe pressure	Throbbing	N/A
PRODROME OR AURA	N/A	N/A	N/A
ASSOCIATING FEATURES	Nausea; Vomiting; Sensitivity to Light? Noise? Odors? Do you get pale or flush? Do your eyes or nose run? Does your nose get stuffy? Do the whites of your eyes get red? Does your eyelid droop? Do you pace, or go to bed?	Nausea; Vomiting; Sensitivity to Light? Noise? Odors? Do you get pale or flush? Do your eyes or nose run? Does your nose get stuffy? Do the whites of your eyes get red? Does your eyelid droop? Do you pace, or go to bed?	Nausea; Vomiting; Sensitivity to Light? Noise? Odors? Do you get pale or flush? Do your eyes or nose run? Does your nose get stuffy? Do the whites of your eyes get red? Does your eyelid droop? Do you pace, or go to bed?
PRECIPITATING OR AGGRAVATING FEATURES	Any movement	Exertion	N/A

LOCATION: Mark the location for each type of headache with a different color pen.

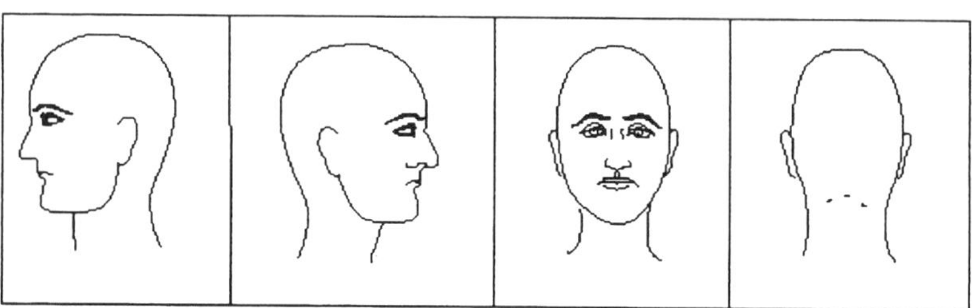

MEDICAL HISTORY:

Have you ever been or are you currently being treated for any of the following?

a) high blood pressure	Yes	No
b) stomach ulcers	Yes	No
c) asthma	Yes	No
d) allergies	Yes	No
e) pneumonia	Yes	No
f) kidney problems	Yes	No
g) low blood sugar	Yes	No
h) glaucoma	Yes	No
i) diabetes	Yes	No
j) heart problems	Yes	No

If you answered yes to any of the above, please describe: Ulcers diagnosed 1 year ago, on Zantac. Kidney infections.

List all other medical problems you have had in the past. Include date diagnosed and treatment. DO NOT LIST OPERATIONS

Migraines 1980. Gallbladder 1975. Endometriosis, fibroid tumors. Car accident 1993.

SURGICAL HISTORY (List operations and dates performed)

Gallbladder, 1984. Hysterectomy and appendectomy, 1988.

PSYCHIATRIC HISTORY (List visits with counselors, psychologists, etc., and type of treatment)

None.

ACCIDENTS IN ADULT LIFE (Briefly describe any accident that caused any blow to the head or that you feel is related to your headache)

Car accident, 1993. Passenger, wearing lap seatbelt. Another car pulled out in front of us and we hit it. Hit head on windshield. Not unconscious. Taken to ER, x-rayed and released. Headaches began that day. Had occasional migraine before accident, although no headaches for 5 years prior to accident.

FAMILY HISTORY:

1.	Is your father living?	Yes	No
	Age 67		
	Cause of death		
	Was there a headache history?	Yes	No
2.	Is your mother living?	Yes	No
	Age 60		
	Cause of death		
	Was there a headache history?	Yes	No

3. Ages of brothers---Circle the ones with headache
   43 (41)

4. Ages of sisters---Circle the ones with headache
 39 (33)
5. List any other blood relatives with a history of severe headaches.
 Paternal cousin.

MARITAL HISTORY:
List marriages:

1st marriage age 17 to 22	Did spouse have headaches?	Yes	No
2nd marriage age 27 to 32	Did spouse have headaches?	Yes	No
3rd marriage age ___ to ___	Did spouse have headaches?	Yes	No

Age of current spouse: N/A

List ages and sex of all children:

Age 22 Sex F Headaches?	Yes	No
Age 20 Sex F Headaches?	Yes	No
Age 13 Sex M Headaches?	Yes	No
Age ___ Sex ___ Headaches?	Yes	No

STRESS FACTORS:

List any factors that may be affecting your headaches (money, loneliness, sexual problems, work, etc.)
 None except for accident.

VEGETATIVE SIGNS:

1.	Do you have trouble falling asleep?	Yes	No
2.	Do you have trouble staying asleep?	Yes	No
3.	Has your appetite decreased?	Yes	No
4.	Have you gained or lost weight in the past year?	Yes	No
5.	Have you felt tearful or depressed lately?	Yes	No
6.	Have you had any thoughts of wanting to die?	Yes	No
7.	Have you been forgetful lately?	Yes	No
8.	Any other changes in your normal day-to-day living?		

Please list any medications you are allergic or sensitive to: Morphine, Codeine

Please list any medications you are currently taking (including dosages and frequency per day):
 Bellergal-S, 3 times a day. Flexeril.

PREVIOUS CARE:

1. List doctors who have treated you for headaches: Dr. V.

2. List any tests you have had for your headache (e.g., EEG, CT scan, MRI, X-Ray, etc.):
CAT scan 1980.

3. List any other treatment you have had for your headache (e.g., biofeedback, acupuncture, chiropractic, or any other treatment you had):
Occipital nerve block.

The following is an actual medical report that will help you identify how the physician makes his diagnosis.

December 21, 1993

Dr. V.
N. Orange Avenue
Orlando, FL 32804

RE: SUE

Dear Dr. V.:

Thank you for the referral of Ms. Sue for headache evaluation.

The patient is a 40-year-old female born 00/00/53 in West Virginia. She has lived in Florida for the last years and has attained a high school education. She is employed as a hair stylist and is currently working part-time.

HEADACHE PROFILE

The patient states that she did have occasional migraine-like headaches starting at age 23; however, she was completely headache-free for the last five years until she was involved in a motor vehicle accident on 00/00/93. At that time, the patient was a passenger in an automobile, wearing a lap belt. Another car pulled out in front of her automobile, and they hit. The patient states that she hit her head on the windshield, denies loss of consciousness. She was evaluated in the emergency room, including x-rays, and was released. The patient notes that headache symptoms began the day of the accident. After the motor vehicle accident, the patient also noted complaints of neck pain, right knee pain, left ankle pain, and shoulder pain. X-rays of these areas were noted and no acute process was shown.

Incapacitating Headaches: The patient notes the onset of these headaches at age 23 and they were occasional in nature, with no headaches over the last five years. She currently has these headaches two to three times per week since the above-noted motor vehicle accident. These headaches can occur at any time of the day, and the patient can awaken with them. These headaches will last for 24 to 48 hours and are described as a severe pressure sensation in the right occipital cervical area, radiating to the right eye. There is no prodrome. These headaches are associated with nausea, vomiting, photophobia, phonophobia, sensitivity to odors and pallor. The patient will seek bed rest if possible and notes that any movement will increase symptoms.

Interfering Headaches (moderate to severe): The patient notes the onset of these headaches on the day of the accident and they have continued on a daily basis since then. The patient awakens with these headaches, and they resolve to some degree and then get worse as the day progresses. These headaches are essentially constant and the pain is described as a throbbing pain in the occipital cervical region, radiating to the frontal region of the head. There is no prodrome or nausea, vomiting or photophobia. The patient does not have phonophobia and will seek bed rest if possible. These headaches are exacerbated by exertion.

Irritating Headaches (annoying): None.

Menstrual History: Began at age 11 and is reported to be normal with no relationship to headaches. The patient had a total hysterectomy in 1988 for endometriosis, including oophorectomy.

PAST HISTORY: The patient was most probably a normal delivery. There is no history of enuresis or unexplained abdominal cramps pre-puberty. There is no history of car sickness as a child. There is no history of meningitis, encephalitis, scarlet fever, or rheumatic fever. The patient did sustain head injuries in two motor vehicle accidents as a child, without any sequelae.

Habits: The patient has a moderate consumption of alcohol which does not increase headache symptoms. The patient smokes approximately half a pack of cigarettes per day without any increase in headache symptoms. She drinks two to three cups of caffeinated beverages per day.

Medical History: Peptic ulcer disease diagnosed one year ago and currently treated with Zantac. History of recurrent renal infection. Complaints of orthopedic concerns in the lower extremities as a result of a motor vehicle accident.

The patient has no history of high blood pressure, stomach ulcers, asthma, allergies, pneumonia, kidney problems, low blood sugar, glaucoma, diabetes, or heart problems.

REVIEW OF SYSTEMS: Pulmonary negative, cardiovascular negative, gastrointestinal negative, urogenital negative.

Surgical History: The patient had a cholecystectomy in 1984, a hysterectomy in 1988, and an appendectomy.

Psychiatric History: None.

Head Injuries in Adult Life: See headache profile above.

Family History: Her father is living, age 67, with multiple myeloma, no headache history. Her mother is living, age 60, with a history of incapacitating headaches. The patient has two brothers and two sisters; one brother and one sister have headache histories. There is a fraternal cousin with a headache history. The patient is currently divorced with three children, two daughters and one son without a headache history.

Stress Factors: The patient denies stress factors, except for association with motor vehicle accident.

Vegetative Signs: The patient does not complain of trouble falling and staying asleep and does complain of depression, but denies suicidal or homicidal ideation. No decrease in memory.

Allergies to Medications: The patient is allergic to Morphine and Codeine.

Current Medications: The patient is currently taking Bellergal-S t.i.d. and Flexeril. The patient notes that these medications initially were effective, but are not currently effective.

Doctors Seen in the Past for Headaches: The patient has been evaluated for headache symptoms by Dr. V.

Tests Done in the Past: The patient was evaluated in 1980 for her migraine history with a CT scan as reported to be normal.

Treatments Tried in the Past: The patient underwent an occipital nerve block which provided excellent symptom relief for two to three hours.

Physical Examination: Height 5'4", weight 185 pounds, pulse approximately 60 and regularly irregular, left BP 132/100, right BP 130/100. The face did not show any asymmetry. The temporomandibular joint area was grossly normal. The eyes appeared normal. Conjunctivae were clear and the pupils reacted equally to light and accommodation. Retinal fundus examination revealed no papilledema and no abnormalities with the arteries and veins. There were no bruits over the supraorbital region. The nose appeared normal. The auditory canals were clear and the tympanic membranes appeared intact. The mouth and throat appeared normal. Gums, tongue, buccal mucosa and teeth were grossly normal. Neck: There was exquisite tenderness over the occipital nerve region, especially the right greater than the left. Carotid bruits could not be heard. Cervical nodes were not enlarged. The lungs were clear to auscultation and percussion. The heart had a regular sinus rhythm with no murmurs. The abdomen was soft and nontender. A rectal or vaginal exam was not done.

Neurological Examination: Cranial nerve II: Visual fields were grossly normal. III, IV and VI: No strabismus, nystagmus, or ptosis. V: Normal sensation and corneal reflex. VII: Normal facial movements (wrinkle, frown, smile, and strength of eyelids). VIII: Normal Weber and Rinne. IX and X: Good gag reflex. XI: Normal sternocleidomastoid and trapezius. XII: Normal protrusion and strength of tongue. Cerebellar: Negative Rhomberg. Normal finger-to-noise, diadochokinesis, heel-shin, tandem, and heel and toes walking. Motor System: No atrophy, fasciculations, wasting, or tremors. Good muscle strength in arms, wrists, fingers, and legs. Sensory System: Superficial tactile, pain, and vibrations (wrists, elbows, knees, and ankles) were normal. Normal motion and positions of fingers and toes. Normal 2-point discrimination. Reflexes: Normal 2+ reflexes of triceps, biceps, knee jerk, ankle jerk, etc. Normal pulses in dorsalis pedis, posterior tibial and popliteal.

DIAGNOSES:
1. Post traumatic vascular headache.
2. Post traumatic cervicogenic headache.

The headaches by history are temporally related to a motor vehicle accident where there was evidence of flexion extension injury to the patient based on a history of hitting her head on the windshield. The pain distribution from the occipital cervical region radiating to the temple would be in the region of the C2 nerve root, which is commonly effected with these types of injuries. This would account for the cervicogenic symptoms. The patient also has post traumatic symptoms with her incapacitating headaches. The association with G.I. symptoms of nausea and vomiting, also photophobia, phonophobia, and sensitivity to odors is consistent with the vascular type headache. Also, the duration of 24 to 48 hours and increase in symptoms with movement are also suggestive.

I would suggest:

1. Laboratory work via headache profile to rule out any metabolic causes for this problem.

2. MRI of the brain to rule out any structural lesions.

3. Electrocardiogram with irregular heart beat noted on physical exam before beginning any medications that are cardioactive.

Since the patient has had this essentially constant headache for three months, the headache cycle will have to be broken before any type of oral medication will be of value. This can be done as an in-patient in the hospital with continuous DHE-45 infusion, or it can be done in an ambulatory setting with a percutaneously inserted central catheter and continuous ambulatory infusion device with, of course, close monitoring by our office. When some measure of control is obtained, then oral medications would be instituted and hopefully prove effective.

The cervicogenic component will also need to be addressed and consideration for cervical facet blocks with fluoroscopic guidance would be a most reasonable option. Unless the cervicogenic component is addressed, the patient will remain symptomatic. When neck symptoms are resolving, then deep neuromuscular mobilization and trigger point injections, if necessary, could be added.

Thank you again for the kind referral of this patient. As we are authorized only for an evaluation today, we would be happy to proceed with treatment pending insurance clearance. If there are any questions or anything further I can do, please contact me.

Sincerely,

R. , M.D.

/rao

GWEN
Category: Cervicogenic headaches

This is a 32-year-old woman who was in an accident approximately 10 months before she was seen in my office. She was stopped at a red light and was rear-ended by another car. She sustained a flexion-extension injury. She went to the emergency room the next day, where she was x-rayed and released. The headaches began the day of the accident. The patient reports there were no headaches prior to the accident.

Incapacitating headaches: These started the day of the accident and the patient had them daily for two months. She is no longer having these headaches. They came on at anytime, lasting three to four hours with pain medication. The character of the pain was "grabbing," which was located in the posterocervical region. Associated features were nausea, photophobia, sonophobia, and the patient went to bed. There was no aura with this headache.

Interfering headaches (moderate to severe): These started two months after the accident, after the incapacitating headaches stopped. Currently the patient experiences these two to three times a week, coming on at any time. The character of the pain is constant, also "grabbing" and similar to the incapacitating headaches.

Irritating headaches (annoying): These started two months after the accident. The patient has them daily. They are constant, with a dull ache in the occipital region.

Although this patient's record could be placed in the chapter on whiplash headaches, I put this in the chapter on cervicogenic headaches because I think the origin of her headache is in the cervicogenic region.

Her diagnoses would be

1. Flexion-extension post acceleration/deceleration vascular headaches.
2. Post acceleration/deceleration muscle tension headaches.
3. Cervicogenic headaches.
4. Myofascial trigger points.

MEDICAL HEADACHE HISTORY

Name: Gwen **Age:** 32 **Sex** F **Date:** 5/7/90

Date of Birth: 0/00/57 **Birthplace:** TX **Race:** W **Education:** High school

Occupation: Inventory Clerk **Accident:** 1989

Armed Services & Type of Discharge: N/A

PAST HISTORY:

1.	Did you have a normal birth?		<u>Yes</u>	No
	a) forceps used?		Yes	<u>No</u>
	b) cesarean section?		Yes	<u>No</u>
2.	Did you have problems with bedwetting?		Yes	<u>No</u>
	a) If yes, age bedwetting stopped		______	
3.	Were you car sick as a child (motion)?		Yes	<u>No</u>
	a) If yes, how severe?	Slight	Moderate	Severe
4.	Did you have unexplained abdominal cramps as a child?		Yes	<u>No</u>
5.	Did you have any of the following illnesses in childhood?			
	a) meningitis		Yes	<u>No</u>
	b) encephalitis		Yes	<u>No</u>
	c) scarlet fever		Yes	<u>No</u>
	d) rheumatic fever		Yes	<u>No</u>
6.	Did you have any head injuries as a child?		Yes	<u>No</u>
	a) If yes, please explain: ______			
7.	Were you treated for emotional illness as a child?		Yes	<u>No</u>

HABITS:

8.	Do you drink alcohol?	<u>Yes</u>	No
	a) If yes, what kind and how much? Maybe 2 a month		
	b) Does alcohol bring on or aggravate a headache?	Yes	<u>No</u>
9.	Do you smoke?	<u>Yes</u>	No
	a) If yes, how much? 1 pack a day		
	b) Does smoking or smoke-filled rooms cause or aggravate headaches?	Yes	<u>No</u>
10.	Do you drink caffeinated beverages?	<u>Yes</u>	No
	a) If yes, how much? 3 or 4 cups of coffee a day		

MENSTRUAL HISTORY:

At what age did menses begin? 12 Were they regular or irregular? WNL
How were they related to your headache? N/A
Are you or were you ever on Birth Control Pills? Yes Did they affect your headache? No
Have you had a hysterectomy, partial or total, and why? No
Are you in menopause, and if yes, how long? No
Are you on hormones, and if yes, which ones? No

HEADACHE ASSESSMENT FORM

HA PROFILE	INCAPACITATING #3	INTERFERING #2	IRRITATING #1
ONSET (Years ago and frequency)	Day of accident Every day for 2 months	2 months after accident 2 – 3 a week	2 months after accident Every day
CURRENT FREQUENCY	0	2 – 3 a week	Every day
TIME OF ONSET	Anytime	Anytime	Constant
DURATION	3 – 4 hours with pain medication	All day	Constant
CHARACTER	Grabbing	Constant "grabbing"	Dull ache
PRODROME OR AURA	N/A	N/A	N/A
ASSOCIATING FEATURES	Nausea; Vomiting; Sensitivity to Light? Noise? Odors? Do you get pale or flush? Do your eyes or nose run? Does your nose get stuffy? Do the whites of your eyes get red? Does your eyelid droop? Do you pace, or go to bed?	Nausea; Vomiting; Sensitivity to Light? Noise? Odors? Do you get pale or flush? Do your eyes or nose run? Does your nose get stuffy? Do the whites of your eyes get red? Does your eyelid droop? Do you pace, or go to bed?	Nausea; Vomiting; Sensitivity to Light? Noise? Odors? Do you get pale or flush? Do your eyes or nose run? Does your nose get stuffy? Do the whites of your eyes get red? Does your eyelid droop? Do you pace, or go to bed?
PRECIPITATING OR AGGRAVATING FEATURES	Movement	Movement	N/A

LOCATION: Mark the location for each type of headache with a different color pen.

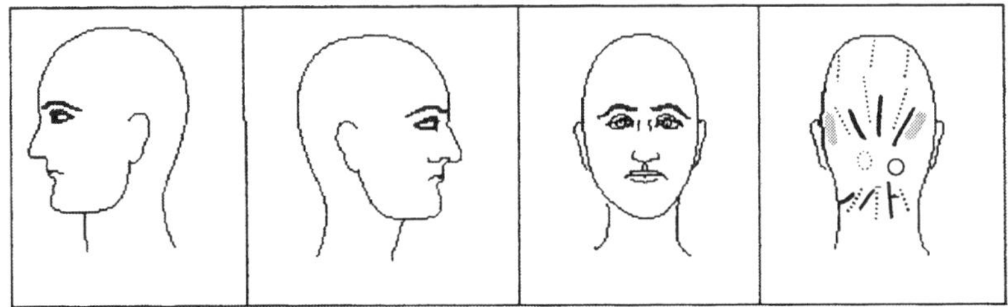

MEDICAL HISTORY:

Have you ever been or are you currently being treated for any of the following?

a) high blood pressure	Yes	No
b) stomach ulcers	Yes	No
c) asthma	Yes	No
d) allergies	Yes	No
e) pneumonia	Yes	No
f) kidney problems	Yes	No
g) low blood sugar	Yes	No
h) glaucoma	Yes	No
i) diabetes	Yes	No
j) heart problems	Yes	No

If you answered yes to any of the above, please describe:____________________

List all other medical problems you have had in the past. Include date diagnosed and treatment.
DO NOT LIST OPERATIONS

Hepatitis 1982.

SURGICAL HISTORY (List operations and dates performed)

None.

PSYCHIATRIC HISTORY (List visits with counselors, psychologists, etc., and type of treatment)

None.

ACCIDENTS IN ADULT LIFE (Briefly describe any accident that caused any blow to the head or that you feel is related to your headache)

Car accident August, 1989. Driving with seat belt. Stopped at red light, rear-ended by another car. Flexion-extension injury. Went to ER next day, x-rayed and released. Headaches began day of accident. No headaches prior to accident.

FAMILY HISTORY:

1. Is your father living? Yes No
   - Age 61
   - Cause of death________________
   - Was there a headache history? Yes No
2. Is your mother living? Yes No
   - Age________
   - Cause of death 63, heart attack
   - Was there a headache history? Yes No

3. Ages of brothers---Circle the ones with headache
 34 36
4. Ages of sisters---Circle the ones with headache
 None
5. List any other blood relatives with a history of severe headaches.
 None

MARITAL HISTORY:

List marriages:

1st marriage age 20 to 21 Did spouse have headaches?	Yes	No
2nd marriage age 26 to Present Did spouse have headaches?	Yes	No
3rd marriage age ____ to ____ Did spouse have headaches?	Yes	No

Age of current spouse: 33

List ages and sex of all children:

Age 6 Sex M Headaches?	Yes	No
Age ____ Sex ____ Headaches?	Yes	No
Age ____ Sex ____ Headaches?	Yes	No

STRESS FACTORS:

List any factors that may be affecting your headaches (money, loneliness, sexual problems, work, etc.)

VEGETATIVE SIGNS:

1.	Do you have trouble falling asleep?	Yes	No
2.	Do you have trouble staying asleep?	Yes	No
3.	Has your appetite decreased?	Yes	No
4.	Have you gained or lost weight in the past year?	Yes	No
5.	Have you felt tearful or depressed lately?	Yes	No
6.	Have you had any thoughts of wanting to die?	Yes	No
7.	Have you been forgetful lately?	Yes	No
8.	Any other changes in your normal day-to-day living?		

Please list any medications you are allergic or sensitive to: None

Please list any medications you are currently taking (including dosages and frequency per day):

Clinoril – 200 mg 2 to 4 a day.

PREVIOUS CARE:

1. List doctors who have treated you for headaches: Dr. R., Dr. S.

2. List any tests you have had for your headache (e.g., EEG, CT scan, MRI, X-Ray, etc.):
None.

3. List any other treatment you have had for your headache (e.g., biofeedback, acupuncture, chiropractic, or any other treatment you had):
Chiropractic.

CHRISTEN
Category: Cervicogenic headaches

This interesting case most likely is the result of a cervicogenic headache. This is a 16-year-old boy whose headaches started 8 months ago after a wrestling match while he was on the wrestling team at school.

Incapacitating headaches: He has had four of these attacks since then. They can last one to three days. It is a throbbing and pressure headache. The pain is in the bilateral orbital regions, the frontal, occipital, and also in the cervical region. He complains of numbness on the top of his head. Sometimes with the headache he will have blurred vision and some nausea. Associated features with the headache are nausea, photophobia, sonophobia, sensitivity to odors, nasal stuffiness, and he will have to go to bed.

Interfering headaches (moderate to severe): These also started after the wrestling match, and he was getting them 3 times a week. Currently he is getting them once a week. They can last 45 minutes to 90 minutes and there is also throbbing and pressure and the location is the same as above.

Irritating headaches (annoying): These started at age 10. They were occasional. Since his wrestling accident, he is getting them 3 or 4 times a week, coming on at any time. He generally can abort them with over-the-counter medications, but there are no associated features.

His diagnoses then would be a cervicogenic headache (1) associated with migraine, and (2) associated with muscle tension headache; (3) preexisting irritating headaches on occasion.

MEDICAL HEADACHE HISTORY

Name: Christen **Age:** 16 **Sex** M **Date:** 9/9/91

Date of Birth: 00/00/75 **Birthplace:** NY **Race:** C **Education:** High School

Occupation: Student **Accident:** N/A

Armed Services & Type of Discharge: N/A

PAST HISTORY:

1.	Did you have a normal birth?		Yes	No
	a) forceps used?		Yes	No
	b) cesarean section?		Yes	No
2.	Did you have problems with bedwetting?		Yes	No
	a) If yes, age bedwetting stopped			
3.	Were you car sick as a child (motion)?		Yes	No
	a) If yes, how severe?	Slight	Moderate	Severe
4.	Did you have unexplained abdominal cramps as a child?		Yes	No
5.	Did you have any of the following illnesses in childhood?			
	a) meningitis		Yes	No
	b) encephalitis		Yes	No
	c) scarlet fever		Yes	No
	d) rheumatic fever		Yes	No
6.	Did you have any head injuries as a child?		Yes	No
	a) If yes, please explain: Head injury age 12			
7.	Were you treated for emotional illness as a child?		Yes	No

HABITS:

8.	Do you drink alcohol?	Yes	No
	a) If yes, what kind and how much?		
	b) Does alcohol bring on or aggravate a headache?	Yes	No
9.	Do you smoke?	Yes	No
	a) If yes, how much?		
	b) Does smoking or smoke-filled rooms cause or aggravate headaches?	Yes	No
10.	Do you drink caffeinated beverages?	Yes	No
	a) If yes, how much? Once a month		

MENSTRUAL HISTORY:

At what age did menses begin?_______ Were they regular or irregular?____________________
How were they related to your headache?____________________
Are you or were you ever on Birth Control Pills?______ Did they affect your headache? _______
Have you had a hysterectomy, partial or total, and why?____________________
Are you in menopause, and if yes, how long?____________________
Are you on hormones, and if yes, which ones?____________________

HEADACHE ASSESSMENT FORM

HA PROFILE	INCAPACITATING #3	INTERFERING #2	IRRITATING #1
ONSET (Years ago and frequency)	8 months ago Has had only 4	8 months ago 3 a week	Age 10, occasionally
CURRENT FREQUENCY	Only had 4	1 a week	3 to 4 a week
TIME OF ONSET	Anytime	Anytime	Anytime
DURATION	1 to 3 days	45 to 90 minutes	1 hour with OTC medication
CHARACTER	Throbbing and pressure	Same, less intense	Slight throb
PRODROME OR AURA	Blurred vision and nausea Headache 5 to 10 minutes later	N/A	N/A
ASSOCIATING FEATURES	Nausea: Vomiting; Sensitivity to Light? Noise? Odors? Do you get pale or flush? Do your eyes or nose run? Does your nose get stuffy? Does the white of your eyes get red? Does your eyelid droop? Do you pace, or go to bed?	Nausea: Vomiting: Sensitivity to Light? Noise? Odors? Do you get pale or flush? Do your eyes or nose run? Does your nose get stuffy? Does the white of your eyes get red? Does your eyelid droop? Do you pace, or go to bed?	Nausea: Vomiting: Sensitivity to Light? Noise? Odors? Do you get pale or flush? Do your eyes or nose run? Does your nose get stuffy? Does the white of your eyes get red? Does your eyelid droop? Do you pace, or go to bed?
PRECIPITATING OR AGGRAVATING FEATURES	Any movement	Sneezing Head movement	N/A

LOCATION: Mark the location for each type of headache with a different color pen.

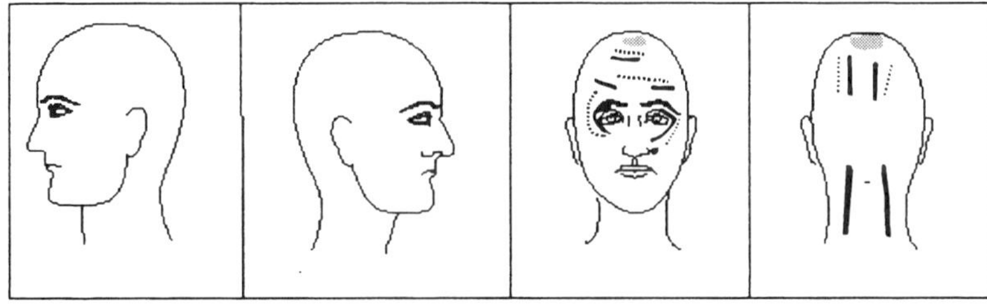

MEDICAL HISTORY:

Have you ever been or are you currently being treated for any of the following?

a) high blood pressure	Yes	No
b) stomach ulcers	Yes	No
c) asthma	Yes	No
d) allergies	Yes	No
e) pneumonia	Yes	No
f) kidney problems	Yes	No
g) low blood sugar	Yes	No
h) glaucoma	Yes	No
i) diabetes	Yes	No
j) heart problems	Yes	No

If you answered yes to any of the above, please describe: Asthma diagnosed as an infant. No attacks in 6 years.

List all other medical problems you have had in the past. Include date diagnosed and treatment. DO NOT LIST OPERATIONS

Neck injury during wrestling, age 12. Going to chiropractic.

SURGICAL HISTORY (List operations and dates performed)

None.

PSYCHIATRIC HISTORY (List visits with counselors, psychologists, etc., and type of treatment)

None

ACCIDENTS IN ADULT LIFE (Briefly describe any accident that caused any blow to the head or that you feel is related to your headache)

Neck injury during wrestling, age 12. Headaches increased 2 to 3 weeks later.

FAMILY HISTORY:

1. Is your father living? Yes No
   - Age 36
   - Cause of death ______
   - Was there a headache history? Yes No
2. Is your mother living? Yes No
   - Age 40
   - Cause of death ______
   - Was there a headache history? Yes No

3. Ages of brothers---Circle the ones with headache
____
4. Ages of sisters---Circle the ones with headache
24
5. List any other blood relatives with a history of severe headaches.
Paternal aunt.

MARITAL HISTORY:
List marriages:

1st marriage age _____ to _______ Did spouse have headaches?	Yes	No
2nd marriage age _____ to _______ Did spouse have headaches?	Yes	No
3rd marriage age _____ to _______ Did spouse have headaches?	Yes	No

Age of current spouse:____________

List ages and sex of all children:

Age _____ Sex ______ Headaches?	Yes	No
Age _____ Sex ______ Headaches?	Yes	No
Age _____ Sex ______ Headaches?	Yes	No
Age _____ Sex ______ Headaches?	Yes	No

STRESS FACTORS:

List any factors that may be affecting your headaches (money, loneliness, sexual problems, work, etc.)
Money, Car, Work, Family.
____

VEGETATIVE SIGNS:

1.	Do you have trouble falling asleep?	Yes	No (underlined)
2.	Do you have trouble staying asleep?	Yes (underlined)	No
3.	Has your appetite decreased?	Yes	No (underlined)
4.	Have you gained or lost weight in the past year?	Yes	No (underlined)
5.	Have you felt tearful or depressed lately?	Yes	No (underlined)
6.	Have you had any thoughts of wanting to die?	Yes	No (underlined)
7.	Have you been forgetful lately?	Yes	No (underlined)
8.	Any other changes in your normal day-to-day living?____________		

Please list any medications you are allergic or sensitive to: No known allergies
____
____

Please list any medications you are currently taking (including dosages and frequency per day):
None.
____

PREVIOUS CARE:

1. List doctors who have treated you for headaches: Dr. D., Dr. M., Dr. D.

2. List any tests you have had for your headache (e.g., EEG, CT scan, MRI, X-Ray, etc.):

CAT scan – 1991 (normal).

X-rays (neck).

3. List any other treatment you have had for your headache (e.g., biofeedback, acupuncture, chiropractic, or any other treatment you had):

Chiropractic (helped a little).

Acupuncture.

The following is an example of an actual medical report demonstrating the diagnoses.

October 4, 1994

[Doctor's name and address omitted]

RE: DON

Dear Dr. [...]:

Thank you for the referral of Mr. Don [...].

This is a 46-year-old male born 00/00/46 in [...], and living in [...] since [...]. He works at [...].

On 00/00/92, the patient was at work and 20 sheets of pegboard fell from a truck. The patient tried to catch the pegboard and felt a sharp pain in his right shoulder. He saw a doctor the next day, and he had injured that shoulder. There was a previous injury on the same shoulder eight months earlier. The patient had surgery on that shoulder in 00/92 and states that his headaches began after the second surgery and the intensity has been increasing.

HEADACHE PROFILE

Incapacitating headaches: The patient had these headaches rarely in his teens. Prior to the accident on 00/00/92, the patient would have these headaches once or twice a year, maximum. After the accident on 00/00/92, the patient began to notice that the frequency of his headaches was increasing. After his surgery in 00/92, the headaches continued to increase in frequency, and since two months ago, the patient has been getting these headaches daily. The patient describes this pain as stabbing and pressure type, which starts in the upper cervical region and works itself cephalad through the occipital and frontal region of his head. There is no aura. There is sometimes some nausea, photophobia, pallor, and he will go to bed. Whenever the patient uses his right shoulder, it seems to increase his headaches.

Interfering headaches (moderate to severe): These headaches started in his teens and they were occasional. The patient does not get these headaches now.

Irritating headaches (annoying): These headaches started in his teens, and he get them once a week. The patient can abort these headaches with over-the-counter medication. It is a dull ache in the frontal part of his head.

Past history: The patient was most probably a normal delivery. There is no history of enuresis or unexplained abdominal cramps pre-puberty. There is no history of car sickness as a child. There is no history of meningitis, encephalitis, scarlet fever, or rheumatic fever. There were no head injuries as a child.

Habits: He does not drink and does no smoke.

Medical history: The patient's medical history has been essentially negative.

Review of systems: Pulmonary negative, cardiovascular negative, gastrointestinal negative, urogenital negative.

Surgical history: The patient had some nasal surgery in 1965, and he had a back operation in 1968 which was a herniated disk in his lower back. The patient had two shoulder operations, one in 1992 and one in 1993. Both of these surgeries were for the 00/00/92 accident.

Psychiatric history: Negative

Family history: His father is living, age 73, and has a history of severe headaches. His mother is living, age 74, with no headache history. There is a 49-year-old brother and a 42-year-old sister with no headache history. The patient has been married from age 22 to present. There are three children, two boys, ages 24 and 20 with no headaches, and an 18-year-old daughter who has headaches.

The patient is currently working, but every time he has to use his right arm and shoulder, he gets more pain.

Allergies to medications: The patient stated that Penicillin causes a rash. He cannot take typhoid medication. Codeine causes convulsions. The patient is also allergic to Demerol.

Current medications: The patient is currently taking ibuprofen 800 mg 2 to 3 times a day and daily for the last 3 weeks, Butalbital 1 or 2 twice daily, and Nortriptyline 25 mg 4 to 5 times a day. The patient has been on Pamelor, Anaprox, Motrin, etc.

Doctors seen in the past for headaches: The patient saw a Dr. [...], neurologist.

Tests done in the past: The patient had an MRI of the brain in 1993 and that was negative.

Physical examination: Height 6'2", weight 204 pounds, pulse 90, left BP 160/88. We could not do the right BP because of moving the patient's shoulder. The face did not show any asymmetry. The temporomandibular joint area was grossly normal. The eyes appeared normal. Conjunctivae were clear and the pupils reacted equally to light and accommodation. Retinal fundus examination revealed no papilledema and no abnormalities with the arteries and veins. There were no bruits over the supraorbital region. The nose appeared normal. The auditory canals were clear and the tympanic membranes appeared intact. The mouth and throat appeared normal. Gums, tongue, buccal mucosa and teeth were grossly normal. There was some stiffness and spasm of the upper right trapezius muscle. Carotid bruits could not be heard. Cervical nodes were not enlarged. The lungs were clear to auscultation and percussion. The heart had a regular sinus rhythm with no murmurs. The abdomen was soft and nontender. A rectal exam was not done.

Neurological examination: Cranial nerve II: Visual fields were grossly normal. III, IV and VI: No strabismus, nystagmus, or ptosis. V: Normal sensation and corneal reflex. VII: Normal facial movements (wrinkle, frown, smile, and strength of eyelids.) VIII: Normal Weber and Rinne. IX and X: Good gag reflex. XI: Normal sternocleidomastoid and trapezius. XII: Normal protrusion and strength of tongue. Cerebellar: Negative Rhomberg. Normal finger-to-nose, diabochokinesis, heel-shin, tandem, and heel and toes walking. Motor system: No atrophy, fasciculations, wasting, or tremors. Good muscle strength in arms, wrists, fingers, and legs. Sensory system: Superficial tactile, pain and vibrations (wrists, elbows, knees, and ankles) were normal. Normal motion and positions of fingers and toes. Normal 2-point discrimination. Reflexes: Normal 1+ reflexes of triceps, biceps, knee jerk, ankle jerk, etc. Normal pulses in dorsalis pedis, posterior tibial and popliteal.

DIAGNOSES

1. Post traumatic daily vascular headache.
2. Rule out post traumatic cervicogenic headache.
3. Preexisting rare vascular and irritating headaches.

IMPRESSION

This pleasant 46-year-old gentleman comes in who had rare headaches prior to an accident he suffered on 00/0092. There was another accident which was previously described. Since that accident on

00/00/92, his headaches have been increasing, and since his surgery on 00/93, his headaches have become very frequent. There is some gastrointestinal and neurogenic features to his headache, and there is a history of headache with the patient's father, which were probably migraine.

I suggest that the patient be placed on Propranolol 20 mg t.i.d., Parafon Forte t.i.d., and Midrin plus Darvocet N-100 to help his severe pain, and a posterior cervical regional block of C1, 2, and 3 on the right side should be done. This will be arranged. If this works well then we will consider having a block done on C5/6 also, which might prevent some of these muscle spasms he is having. The patient will be given a headache log and will be seen in one month, but prior to that we will do the posterior cervical regional block of C1, 2, and 3.

The treatment of the cervicogenic component will be addressed and consideration for cervical facet blocks with fluoroscopic guidance would be a mot reasonable option. If this is a cervicogenic headache and is not treated, then the patient will most likely remain symptomatic. This facet treatment would be considered after he has the regional blocks, which have been recommended. Also, neuromuscular mobilization (muscle massaging) and trigger point injections will be considered as part of is treatment if necessary.

I have also discontinued the Nortriptyline, the Butalbital and the Ibuprofen 800.

Thank you for referring this patient. If there are any questions, please do not hesitate to call or write.

Sincerely,

BERNARD SWERDLOW, M.D.

These notes were dictated with the patient present.

MEDICAL HEADACHE HISTORY

Name: Don **Age:** 46 **Sex** M **Date:** 10/4/93

Date of Birth: 00/00/46 **Birthplace:** IL **Race:** W **Education:** 2 years college

Occupation: Auto Parts **Accident:** 00/00/92

Armed Services & Type of Discharge: N/A

PAST HISTORY:

1.	Did you have a normal birth?		Yes	No
	a) forceps used?		Yes	No
	b) cesarean section?		Yes	No
2.	Did you have problems with bedwetting?		Yes	No
	a) If yes, age bedwetting stopped		______	
3.	Were you car sick as a child (motion)?		Yes	No
	a) If yes, how severe?	Slight	Moderate	Severe
4.	Did you have unexplained abdominal cramps as a child?		Yes	No
5.	Did you have any of the following illnesses in childhood?			
	a) meningitis		Yes	No
	b) encephalitis		Yes	No
	c) scarlet fever		Yes	No
	d) rheumatic fever		Yes	No
6.	Did you have any head injuries as a child?		Yes	No
	a) If yes, please explain:______			
7.	Were you treated for emotional illness as a child?		Yes	No

HABITS:

8.	Do you drink alcohol?		Yes	No
	a) If yes, what kind and how much?______			
	b) Does alcohol bring on or aggravate a headache?		Yes	No
9.	Do you smoke?		Yes	No
	a) If yes, how much?______			
	b) Does smoking or smoke-filled rooms cause or aggravate headaches?		Yes	No
10.	Do you drink caffeinated beverages?		Yes	No
	a) If yes, how much?______			

MENSTRUAL HISTORY:

At what age did menses begin?_______ Were they regular or irregular?______
How were they related to your headache?______
Are you or were you ever on Birth Control Pills?______ Did they affect your headache? _______
Have you had a hysterectomy, partial or total, and why?______
Are you in menopause, and if yes, how long?______
Are you on hormones, and if yes, which ones?______

HEADACHE ASSESSMENT FORM

HA PROFILE	INCAPACITATING #3	INTERFERING #2	IRRITATING #1
ONSET (Years ago and frequency)	In teens, rare	In teens, occasionally	In teens
CURRENT FREQUENCY	1 to 2/week every 2 mos. Before this 1/month	None now	1/week
TIME OF ONSET	Anytime	N/A	Anytime
DURATION	3 to 4 hours	N/A	1 hour with OTC meds
CHARACTER	Stabbing-pressure	N/A	Dull ache
PRODROME OR AURA	N/A	N/A	N/A
ASSOCIATING FEATURES	Nausea; Vomiting; Sensitivity to Light? Noise? Odors? Do you get pale or flush? Do your eyes or nose run? Does your nose get stuffy? Does the white of your eyes get red? Does your eyelid droop? Do you pace, or go to bed?	Nausea; Vomiting; Sensitivity to Light? Noise? Odors? Do you get pale or flush? Do your eyes or nose run? Does your nose get stuffy? Does the white of your eyes get red? Does your eyelid droop? Do you pace, or go to bed?	Nausea; Vomiting; Sensitivity to Light? Noise? Odors? Do you get pale or flush? Do your eyes or nose run? Does your nose get stuffy? Does the white of your eyes get red? Does your eyelid droop? Do you pace, or go to bed?
PRECIPITATING OR AGGRAVATING FEATURES	Using right shoulder	N/A	N/A

LOCATION: Mark the location for each type of headache with a different color pen.

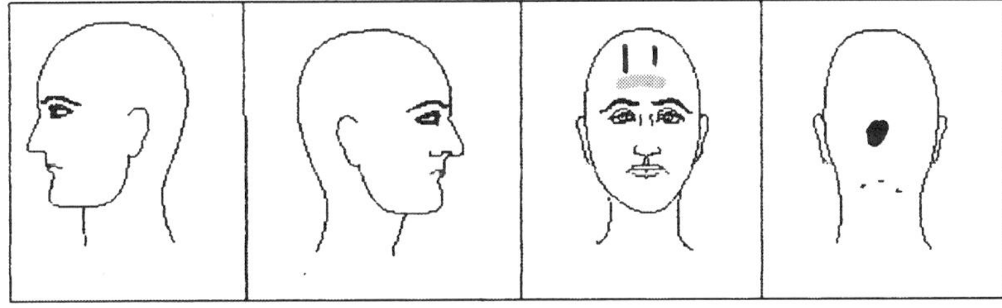

MEDICAL HISTORY:

Have you ever been or are you currently being treated for any of the following?

a) high blood pressure	Yes	No
b) stomach ulcers	Yes	No
c) asthma	Yes	No
d) allergies	Yes	No
e) pneumonia	Yes	No
f) kidney problems	Yes	No
g) low blood sugar	Yes	No
h) glaucoma	Yes	No
i) diabetes	Yes	No
j) heart problems	Yes	No

If you answered yes to any of the above, please describe:________________________

List all other medical problems you have had in the past. Include date diagnosed and treatment.
DO NOT LIST OPERATIONS

None other than surgeries listed.

SURGICAL HISTORY (List operations and dates performed)

Nose surgery, 1965. Back surgery, 1968. Shoulder surgery, 1992 and 1993.

PSYCHIATRIC HISTORY (List visits with counselors, psychologists, etc., and type of treatment)

None.

ACCIDENTS IN ADULT LIFE (Briefly describe any accident that caused any blow to the head or that you feel is related to your headache)

1992 – At work, 20 sheets pegboard dropped from a truck and I caught them. Felt sharp in right shoulder. Saw doctor next day. Had injured same shoulder 8 months earlier. Had surgery in 1993. Headaches began after this, then increased in intensity after second surgery.

FAMILY HISTORY:

1. Is your father living? Yes No
   - Age 73
   - Cause of death____________________
   - Was there a headache history? Yes No
2. Is your mother living? Yes No
   - Age 74
   - Cause of death____________________
   - Was there a headache history? Yes No

3. Ages of brothers---Circle the ones with headache
   49
4. Ages of sisters---Circle the ones with headache
   42
5. List any other blood relatives with a history of severe headaches.
   None

MARITAL HISTORY:
List marriages:

1st marriage age 22 to Present	Did spouse have headaches?	Yes	<u>No</u>
2nd marriage age ____ to ____	Did spouse have headaches?	Yes	No
3rd marriage age ____ to ____	Did spouse have headaches?	Yes	No

Age of current spouse: 43

List ages and sex of all children:

Age 24	Sex M	Headaches?	Yes	<u>No</u>
Age 20	Sex M	Headaches?	Yes	<u>No</u>
Age 18	Sex F	Headaches?	<u>Yes</u>	No
Age ____	Sex ____	Headaches?	Yes	No

STRESS FACTORS:

List any factors that may be affecting your headaches (money, loneliness, sexual problems, work, etc.)
Work. Using right shoulder causes pain, which eventually causes my headaches.

VEGETATIVE SIGNS:

1.	Do you have trouble falling asleep?	Yes	<u>No</u>
2.	Do you have trouble staying asleep?	Yes	<u>No</u>
3.	Has your appetite decreased?	Yes	<u>No</u>
4.	Have you gained or lost weight in the past year?	Yes	<u>No</u>
5.	Have you felt tearful or depressed lately?	<u>Yes</u>	No
6.	Have you had any thoughts of wanting to die?	<u>Yes</u>	No
7.	Have you been forgetful lately?	Yes	<u>No</u>
8.	Any other changes in your normal day-to-day living? ____		

Please list any medications you are allergic or sensitive to: Penicillin, Typhoid vaccine, Codeine, Tetanus vaccine, Demerol.

Please list any medications you are currently taking (including dosages and frequency per day):
Ibuprofen, 800 mg 2 to 3 times a day; Butalbital 1 or 2 twice daily; Nortriptyline 25 mg 4 to 5 times a day.

PREVIOUS CARE:

1, List doctors who have treated you for headaches: Dr. C.

2, List any tests you have had for your headache (e.g., EEG, CT scan, MRI, X-Ray, etc.):
MRI, 1993. Negative.

3, List any other treatment you have had for your headache (e.g., biofeedback, acupuncture, chiropractic, or any other treatment you had):
None.

December 17, 1993

[Doctor's name and address omitted]

RE: Katherine

Dear Dr. [...]:

Thank you for the referral of Ms. Katherine [...] for chronic headache evaluation.

The patient is a 35-year-old female born [...] in [...]. She has attained a high school education and has lived in Florida for the last [...] years. The patient is currently unemployed.

The patient was involved in a motor vehicle accident on 00/00/93. She was driving at approximately 35 to 40 mph when a car pulled in front of her. She was wearing only a lap restraint and struck the windshield, sustaining a hematoma of the forearm. There was no loss of consciousness. The patient did hit her head on the windshield and sustained a skin abrasion and small laceration over the left forehead. The patient noted at the scene of the accident changes in hearing, vision, and a headache at the scene. She was later evaluated at [...] Hospital with x-rays of the cervical spine and a CT scan of the brain showing no acute process. She was treated with Lortab and Robaxin in the emergency room. The patient noted mild "stress" headaches prior to this motor vehicle accident; however, these current headaches are stated to be entirely of a different nature than those previous mild "stress" headaches. The patient also complains of left arm pain and neck pain with also recurrence of chronic low back pain.

The patient has been treated with occipital nerve blocks and also medical management with Bellergal, Naprosyn, Pamelor, and Robaxin, all without any significant improvement.

HEADACHE PROFILE

Incapacitating headaches: The patient initially suffered a #2 or interfering headache at the scene of the accident and within one week after the motor vehicle accident she developed #3 or incapacitating headaches. She suffered six in the first week and is currently suffering one to four of these headaches per week. The patient wakes up with the headache and the headache will last anywhere from one to six days continuously. The patient can obtain transient, i.e. two hours, relief with Bellergal and Robaxin; however, the symptoms will return after that. The pain is characterized by a throbbing pressure sensation mostly in the right cervical and temporal region of the head. The patient will also get an intermittent sharp shooting or lancing pain. There is no prodrome associated with these headaches. The patient does note nausea, vomiting, photophobia, phonophobia and lacrimation with these headaches. She will seek bed rest when possible and there are no specific aggravating factors.

Interfering headaches (moderate to severe): The patient notes the onset of these headaches immediately after the motor vehicle accident and they are currently appearing approximately every other day. The patient will awaken with these headaches and can get transient relief with Bellergal and Robaxin; however, they will return in two hours or so. She characterizes this pain as a pressure sensation in the supraorbital areas bilaterally. There is no prodrome associated with these headaches. The patient does note photophobia and lacrimation with these headaches and will seek bed rest.

Irritating headaches (annoying): None.

Menstrual history: Relationship to menstruation — none. Began at age 11 and is reported to be normal except for severe dysmenorrhea in the first two days. No hysterectomy or oral contraceptive use at this time.

Past history: The patient was most probably a normal delivery. There is a history of some enuresis as a child. There is no history of unexplained abdominal cramps pre-puberty. There is no history of car sickness as a child. There is no history of meningitis, encephalitis, scarlet fever, or rheumatic fever. There were no head injuries as a child.

Habits: The patient will consume one to two drinks one to two times per week. Alcohol does not increase headache symptoms. The patient does smoke one to two packs of cigarettes a day without increase in headache symptoms. She drinks approximately two caffeinated beverages per day.

Medical history:

1. History of bronchitis and reactive airway disease and four episodes of pneumonia.
2. History of endometriosis since age 25.

The patient has no history of high blood pressure, stomach ulcers, asthma, allergies, kidney problems, low blood sugar, glaucoma, diabetes, or heart problems.

Review of systems: Pulmonary negative, cardiovascular negative, gastrointestinal negative, urogenital negative.

Surgical history:

1. Tonsillectomy in 1964.
2. Appendectomy in 1966.
3. Bilateral mastectomy in 1984 for multiple fibroid cysts.
4. Arthroscopy of the right knee in 1990 and also two additional arthroscopies in 1991.

Psychiatric history: The patient saw [...] for depression counseling. This was five years ago and related to a loss of business. No psychiatric problem since that time.

Head injuries in adult life:

1. Motor vehicle accident 00/00/93 as described above.
2. Previous accident in approximately 1985 with no headache or other trauma after that.
3. Slipped, injuring knee with no headache or head injuries. This was in 1990.

Family history: Her father is living, age 60, with no headache history. Her mother is living, age 59, with no headache history. The patient has two brothers and one sister without headache history. The patient is currently divorced with no children.

Stress factors: The patient denies any stress factors to her life at current.

Vegetative signs: The patient currently complains of trouble both falling and staying asleep. She complains of mild situational depression due to her current pain state and complications of life with recent motor vehicle accident. She denies homicidal or suicidal ideations.

Allergies to medications: Codeine — welts and itching. Sumycin antibiotic and also urticarial edema.

Current medications: The patient is currently taking Robaxin p.r.n., Bellergal p.r.n., Zantac q.d., Naprosyn b.i.d., and Pamelor 10 mg q.h.s.

Doctors seen in the past for headaches: The patient has been treated by Dr. [...] with occipital nerve blocks, which provided relief for a few days.

Tests done in the past: Evaluation by Dr. [...] included CT scan as noted above.

Physical examination: Height 5'2", weight 189 pounds, pulse 80, respirations 16, left BP 108/88, right BP 114/92. The face did not show any asymmetry. The temporomandibular joint area was grossly normal. The eyes appeared normal. Conjunctivae were clear and the pupils reacted equally to light and accommodation. Retinal fundus examination revealed no papilledema and no abnormalities with the arteries and veins. There were no bruits over the supraorbital region. The nose appeared normal. The auditory canals were clear and the tympanic membranes appeared intact. The mouth and throat appeared normal. Gums, tongue, buccal mucosa, and teeth were grossly normal. Neck: There were multiple trigger points in the splenius capitis muscle group and at the occipital cervical junction. Negative axial loading test. Carotid bruits could not be heard. Cervical nodes were not enlarged. Lungs: There are mild diffuse scattered wheezes. The heart had a regular sinus rhythm with no murmurs. The abdomen was soft and nontender. A rectal or vaginal exam was not done.

Neurological examination: Cranial nerve II: Visual fields were grossly normal. III, IV and VI: No strabismus, nystagmus, or ptosis. V: Normal sensation and corneal reflex. VII: Normal facial movements (wrinkle, frown, smile, and strength of eyelids). VIII: Normal Weber and Rinne. IX and X: Good gag reflex. XI: Normal sternocleidomastoid and trapezius. XII: Normal protrusion and strength of tongue. Cerebellar: Negative Rhomberg. Normal finger-to-nose, diadochokinesis, heel-shin, tandem, and heel and toes walking. Motor system: No atrophy, fasciculations, wasting, or tremors. Good muscle strength in arms, wrists, fingers, and legs. Sensory system: Superficial tactile, pain, and vibrations (wrists, elbows, knees, and ankles) were normal. Normal motion and positions of fingers and toes. Normal 2-point discrimination. Reflexes: Normal 2+ reflexes of triceps, biceps, knee jerk, ankle jerk, etc. Normal pulses in dorsalis pedis, posterior tibial and popliteal.

DIAGNOSES

1. Post traumatic vascular headache.
2. Post traumatic migraine headache.
3. Post traumatic cervicogenic headache.

The patient has clear components of vascular-migraine headache with a throbbing pain primarily unilateral, that is associated with nausea, vomiting, and photophobia. This new type of headache developed temporally after her motor vehicle accident.

Recommendations

1. Headache profile — fasting. Rule out any metabolic causes for her problem
2. Continuous DHE-45 infusion to abort the patient's headache cycle. Once this is accomplished, then oral medications would then hopefully be of value. With the patient's history of reactive airway disease, increasing Inderal to very high doses would certainly not be prudent. Oral medications that would be effective are not found to be effective unless the headache cycle is broken with medication and, in this case, with the patient's vascular component of throbbing headache pain, DHE would be an excellent choice.
3. We will start Inderal at a very low dose. The patient was advised to immediately discontinue if any signs of wheezing occur.
4. Midrin and Ergopak as abortive measures.
5. Certainly continue the Pamelor.
6. Once a course of intravenous DHE is started, then deep neuromuscular mobilization and trigger point injections to address the cervicogenic component of the patient's pain would be of value.
7. The cervicogenic component will also need to be addressed and consideration for cervical facet blocks with fluoroscopic guidance would be a most reasonable option.

We will also offer the patient parenteral DHE and Reglan, judge response, and further use this to evaluate her suitability for a continuous DHE infusion.

Coordination through her insurance carrier will be made by this office.

Dr. [...], thank you again for allowing us to see this most pleasant patient.

Sincerely,

[Doctor's name omitted]

MEDICAL HEADACHE HISTORY

Name: Katherine **Age:** 35 **Sex** F **Date:** 12/17/93

Date of Birth: 0/00/58 **Birthplace:** AL **Race:** W **Education:** High School

Occupation: Unemployed **Accident:** 1993

Armed Services & Type of Discharge: N/A

PAST HISTORY:

1.	Did you have a normal birth?		Yes	No
	a) forceps used?		Yes	No
	b) cesarean section?		Yes	No
2.	Did you have problems with bedwetting?		Yes	No
	a) If yes, age bedwetting stopped			
3.	Were you car sick as a child (motion)?		Yes	No
	a) If yes, how severe?	Slight	Moderate	Severe
4.	Did you have unexplained abdominal cramps as a child?		Yes	No
5.	Did you have any of the following illnesses in childhood?			
	a) meningitis		Yes	No
	b) encephalitis		Yes	No
	c) scarlet fever		Yes	No
	d) rheumatic fever		Yes	No
6.	Did you have any head injuries as a child?		Yes	No
	a) If yes, please explain:			
7.	Were you treated for emotional illness as a child?		Yes	No

HABITS:

8.	Do you drink alcohol?	Yes	No
	a) If yes, what kind and how much? 1 to 2 drinks 1 to 2 times a week		
	b) Does alcohol bring on or aggravate a headache?	Yes	No
9.	Do you smoke?	Yes	No
	a) If yes, how much? 1 to 2 packs a day		
	b) Does smoking or smoke-filled rooms cause or aggravate headaches?	Yes	No
10.	Do you drink caffeinated beverages?	Yes	No
	a) If yes, how much? 1 to 2 cups per day		

MENSTRUAL HISTORY:

At what age did menses begin? 11 Were they regular or irregular? Severe dysmenorrhea
How were they related to your headache? Not related
Are you or were you ever on Birth Control Pills? No Did they affect your headache? No
Have you had a hysterectomy, partial or total, and why? No
Are you in menopause, and if yes, how long? No
Are you on hormones, and if yes, which ones? No

HEADACHE ASSESSMENT FORM

HA PROFILE	INCAPACITATING #3	INTERFERING #2	IRRITATING #1
ONSET (Years ago and frequency)	Within a week after accident; 6 in first month	At scene; constant	N/A
CURRENT FREQUENCY	1 to 4/week	Every other day	N/A
TIME OF ONSET	Wakes with	Same as #3	N/A
DURATION	Meds will relieve for 1-2 hours; 1 day to 1 week	Same as #3	N/A
CHARACTER	Throbbing, pressure	Pressure	N/A
PRODROME OR AURA	N/A	N/A	N/A
ASSOCIATING FEATURES	Nausea; Vomiting; Sensitivity to Light? Noise? Odors? Do you get pale or flush? Do your eyes or nose run? Does your nose get stuffy? Do the whites of your eyes get red? Does your eyelid droop? Do you pace, or go to bed?	Nausea; Vomiting; Sensitivity to Light? Noise? Odors? Do you get pale or flush? Do your eyes or nose run? Does your nose get stuffy? Do the whites of your eyes get red? Does your eyelid droop? Do you pace, or go to bed?	Nausea; Vomiting; Sensitivity to Light? Noise? Odors? Do you get pale or flush? Do your eyes or nose run? Does your nose get stuffy? Do the whites of your eyes get red? Does your eyelid droop? Do you pace, or go to bed?
PRECIPITATING OR AGGRAVATING FEATURES	N/A	Flash from polaroid pictures increases headache	N/A

LOCATION: Mark the location for each type of headache with a different color pen.

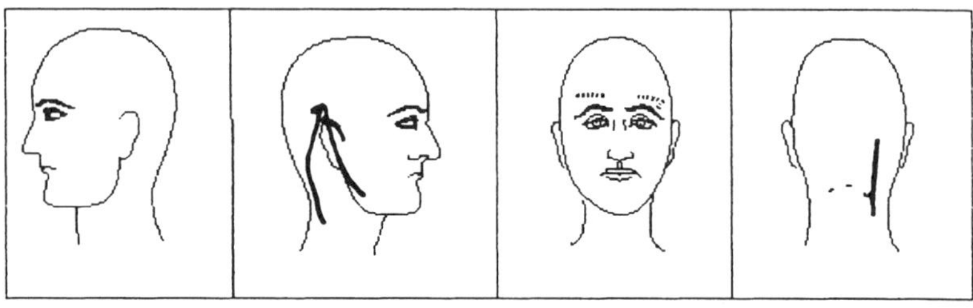

MEDICAL HISTORY:

Have you ever been or are you currently being treated for any of the following?

a) high blood pressure	Yes	<u>No</u>
b) stomach ulcers	Yes	<u>No</u>
c) asthma	<u>Yes</u>	No
d) allergies	Yes	<u>No</u>
e) pneumonia	<u>Yes</u>	No
f) kidney problems	Yes	<u>No</u>
g) low blood sugar	Yes	<u>No</u>
h) glaucoma	Yes	<u>No</u>
i) diabetes	Yes	<u>No</u>
j) heart problems	Yes	<u>No</u>

If you answered yes to any of the above, please describe: Chronic bronchial asthma. Pneumonia 4 times, most recently age 19.

List all other medical problems you have had in the past. Include date diagnosed and treatment. DO NOT LIST OPERATIONS

Lateral release of patella. Lower left back pain. Pain in left forearm and wrist. Pain in neck and shoulders. Endometriosis since age 25.

SURGICAL HISTORY (List operations and dates performed)

Tonsillectomy, 1964. Appendectomy, 1966. Mastectomy, 1984. Arthroscopy right knee, 1990, 1991.

PSYCHIATRIC HISTORY (List visits with counselors, psychologists, etc., and type of treatment)

Counseling for depression, about 5 years ago.

ACCIDENTS IN ADULT LIFE (Briefly describe any accident that caused any blow to the head or that you feel is related to your headache)

Car accident, 1993. Driving, wearing lap seatbelt. Car pulled in front of me and hit. Hit head on windshield. One previous accident in 1985. Fell asleep at wheel, was driving wearing seatbelt. Hit lip on steering wheel. Slipped in grease in 1990 and fell and injured knee.

FAMILY HISTORY:

1.	Is your father living?	<u>Yes</u>	No
	Age 60		
	Cause of death ______		
	Was there a headache history?	<u>Yes</u>	No
2.	Is your mother living?	<u>Yes</u>	<u>No</u>
	Age 59		
	Cause of death ______		
	Was there a headache history?	Yes	<u>No</u>

3. Ages of brothers---Circle the ones with headache
   37 31
4. Ages of sisters---Circle the ones with headache
   30
5. List any other blood relatives with a history of severe headaches.
   None

MARITAL HISTORY:
List marriages:

1st marriage age 19 to 21	Did spouse have headaches?	Yes	No
2nd marriage age _____ to ______	Did spouse have headaches?	Yes	No
3rd marriage age ______to _______	Did spouse have headaches?	Yes	No

Age of current spouse: N/A

List ages and sex of all children:

Age ______	Sex ______ Headaches?	Yes	No
Age ______	Sex ______ Headaches?	Yes	No
Age ______	Sex ______ Headaches?	Yes	No

STRESS FACTORS:

List any factors that may be affecting your headaches (money, loneliness, sexual problems, work, etc.)
N/A.

VEGETATIVE SIGNS:

1.	Do you have trouble falling asleep?	Yes (underlined)	No
2.	Do you have trouble staying asleep?	Yes (underlined)	No
3.	Has your appetite decreased?	Yes	No (underlined)
4.	Have you gained or lost weight in the past year?	Yes (underlined)	No
5.	Have you felt tearful or depressed lately?	Yes	No (underlined)
6.	Have you had any thoughts of wanting to die?	Yes	No (underlined)
7.	Have you been forgetful lately?	Yes	No (underlined)
8.	Any other changes in your normal day-to-day living?________________		

Please list any medications you are allergic or sensitive to: Sumycin, Codeine

Please list any medications you are currently taking (including dosages and frequency per day):
Robaxin, as needed. Bellegal, as needed. Zantac, 1/day. Naprosyn, 1/twice a day. Pamelor, 1 at bedtime.

PREVIOUS CARE:

1. List doctors who have treated you for headaches: Dr. V.

2. List any tests you have had for your headache (e.g., EEG, CT scan, MRI, X-Ray, etc.):
CAT scan 1993.

3. List any other treatment you have had for your headache (e.g., biofeedback, acupuncture, chiropractic, or any other treatment you had):
Shots – 3 injections at base of skull. Not helpful for more than a few days.

September 14, 1994

[Doctor's name and address omitted]

RE: SANDY

Dear Dr. [...]:

Thank you for the kind referral of Ms. Sandy [...] for headache evaluation and treatment.

The patient is a 58-year-old female born 00/00/35 in [...]. She has lived in Florida for the last [...] years and is currently employed in the insurance industry.

The patient's headache history dates back to 00/00/94 when she was a passenger in a car that was rear-ended by a truck, and her car was pushed into the car in front of her. The patient felt a flexion/extension movement of her neck. She was immediately taken to the emergency room at [...] Hospital and evaluated and released with instructions to wear a rib belt for torn cartilage and a cervical collar. X-rays were also performed at that time which were negative for cervical fracture.

HEADACHE PROFILE

Incapacitating headaches: None

Interfering headaches (moderate to severe): The patient stated that she noted these headaches approximately one month after the motor vehicle accident; however, the pain of her rib injuries was predominant, probably by patient history covering up the pain sensation of her headaches. These headaches have been on an every-other-day basis, will occur at any time of the day, including the patient will possibly wake up with these headaches. These headaches last 24 to 48 hours and the pain is described as a piercing pain sensation in the cervical and occipital region of the head bilaterally. There is no prodrome with these headaches. However, they are associated with some flushing, phonophobia, lacrimation, and the patient will seek bed rest when possible. There are no gastrointestinal symptoms with these headaches and the patient denies any precipitating or aggravating factors.

Irritating headaches (annoying): The patient has suffered from these headaches since the time she was a young adult, with approximately one headache per month at that time. She is currently noting one irritating headache every two weeks, described as a dull aching pain in the same location as her #2 or interfering headaches. There is no prodrome with these headaches, and they are associated only with sweating in the face There are no precipitating or aggravating factors noted with these headaches. These headaches can be relieved by Extra Strength Tylenol and muscle relaxants.

Menstrual history: Began at age 11 and is reported to be normal. There is no relationship of menstruation to headache symptoms. The patient did have a total hysterectomy in 1971 and has been on Premarin hormone replacement since 1993.

Past history: The patient was most probably a normal delivery. There is no history of enuresis or unexplained abdominal cramps pre-puberty. There is no history of car sickness as a child. There is no history of meningitis, encephalitis, scarlet fever, or rheumatic fever. There were no head injuries as a child.

Habits: The patient does not consume alcohol and does not smoke. She does, however, consume 2 to 3 caffeinated beverages per day.

Medical history:
1. History of duodenal ulcers 10 years ago, currently asymptomatic.
2. Compression fracture of T9 in 1991 when she was pushing a car and felt a pain sensation and was treated conservatively with back brace and bed rest.

Surgical history:
1. Uterine suspension in 1962.
2. Appendectomy in 1968.
3. Cholecystectomy in 1990.

Psychiatric history: None

Head injuries in adult life: See history of headache profile.

Family history: Her father is deceased of cerebral aneurysm in 1943, no headache history. Her mother is deceased, age 78 of congestive heart failure, no headache history. The patient has two brothers and two sisters, none with headache history. The patient is currently married and has two daughters. No headache history in the family.

Stress factors: The patient denies any stress factors exacerbating her headaches.

Vegetative signs: No sleep disturbance, depression, or memory difficulties.

Allergies to medications: Codeine causes urticaria.

Current medications: The patient is currently taking Soma t.i.d., p.r.n., Premarin as prescribed. The patient also takes ibuprofen for headaches on occasion.

Doctors seen in the past for headaches: The patient has been evaluated fully by Dr. [...], including cervical x-rays, which are negative.

Physical examination: Height 5'5", weight 140 pounds, pulse 76, respirations 18, left BP 110/72, right BP 130/72. The face did not show any asymmetry. Temporomandibular joint area was grossly normal. The eyes appeared normal. Conjunctivae were clear and the pupils reacted equally to light and accommodation. Retinal fundus examination revealed no papiledema and no abnormalities with the arteries and veins. There were no bruits over the supraorbital region. The nose appeared normal. The auditory canals were clear and the tympanic membranes appeared intact. The mouth and throat appeared normal. Gums, tongue, buccal mucosa, and teeth were grossly normal. Neck: The patient had exquisite trigger points at the occipital cervical junction bilaterally consistent with out cervical plexus regional blocks. Carotid bruits could not be heard. Cervical modes were not enlarged. The lungs were clear to auscultation and percussion. The heart had a regular sinus rhythm with no murmurs. The abdomen was soft and nontender. A rectal or vaginal exam was not done.

Neurological examination: Cranial nerve II: Visual fields were grossly normal. III, IV and VI: No strabismus, nystagmus, or ptosis. V: Normal sensation and corneal reflex. VII: Normal facial movements (wrinkle, frown, smile, and strength of eyelids). VIII: Normal Weber and Rinne. IX and X: Good gag reflex. XI: Normal sternocleidomastoid and trapezius. XII: Normal protrusion and strength of tongue. Cerebellar: Negative Rhomberg. Normal finger-to-nose, diadochokinesis, heel-shin, tandem, and heel and toes walking. Motor system: No atrophy, fasciculations, wasting, or tremors. Good muscle strength in arms, wrists, fingers, and legs. Sensory system: Superficial tactile, pain, and vibrations (wrists, elbows, knees, and ankles) were normal. Normal motion and positions of fingers and toes. Normal 2-point discrimination. Reflexes: Normal 2+ reflexes of triceps, biceps, knee jerk, ankle jerk, etc. Normal pulses in dorsalis pedis, posterior tibial and popliteal.

DIAGNOSES

1. Post traumatic cervicogenic headache secondary to motor vehicle accident with flexion/extension injury.
2. Cervical sprain/strain syndrome.

RECOMMENDED TESTS

1. Headache profile to rule out any metabolic cause of patient's symptoms or any metabolic cause that could be exacerbating the patient's symptoms.
2. CT scan of the brain with and without contrast to rule out any structural lesion in this patient who has now had 6 months of every-other-day headaches.

INITIAL THERAPY

1. Amitriptyline 10 mg q.h.s. for its effect on chronic pain and the serotonin system.
2. Continue the Soma as prescribed by Dr. [...].
3. As abortive measures for headache, Midrin and Fioricet.
4. For the patient's morning headaches, we will start Bellergal-S one tablet q.h.s. and one-half tablet every noon.
5. The patient will also be scheduled for bilateral cervical plexus regional blocks with exquisite pain in this area, hoping to break the pain cycle.
6. Consideration will be given to cervical facet blocks with fluoroscopic guidance.
7. Physical therapy and trigger point injections if needed to enhance the effectiveness of the cervical regional blocks.
8. The patient will be given a headache log and a headache diet to observe.

Thank you for the referral of this pleasant patient. If there are any questions, please do not hesitate to call or write.

Sincerely,

BERNARD SWERDLOW, M.D.

These notes were dictated with the patient present.

MEDICAL HEADACHE HISTORY

Name: Sandy **Age:** 58 **Sex** F **Date:** 9/14/94

Date of Birth: 0/00/35 **Birthplace:** FL **Race:** W **Education:** High School

Occupation: Insurance **Accident:** 1994

Armed Services & Type of Discharge: N/A

PAST HISTORY:

1.	Did you have a normal birth?		**Yes**	No
	a) forceps used?		Yes	**No**
	b) cesarean section?		Yes	**No**
2.	Did you have problems with bedwetting?		Yes	**No**
	a) If yes, age bedwetting stopped			
3.	Were you car sick as a child (motion)?		Yes	**No**
	a) If yes, how severe?	Slight	Moderate	Severe
4.	Did you have unexplained abdominal cramps as a child?		Yes	**No**
5.	Did you have any of the following illnesses in childhood?			
	a) meningitis		Yes	**No**
	b) encephalitis		Yes	**No**
	c) scarlet fever		Yes	**No**
	d) rheumatic fever		**Yes**	No
6.	Did you have any head injuries as a child?		Yes	**No**
	a) If yes, please explain:			
7.	Were you treated for emotional illness as a child?		Yes	**No**

HABITS:

8.	Do you drink alcohol?	Yes	**No**
	a) If yes, what kind and how much?		
	b) Does alcohol bring on or aggravate a headache?	Yes	**No**
9.	Do you smoke?	Yes	**No**
	a) If yes, how much?		
	b) Does smoking or smoke-filled rooms cause or aggravate headaches?	Yes	**No**
10.	Do you drink caffeinated beverages?	**Yes**	No
	a) If yes, how much? 2 –3 cups coffee per day		

MENSTRUAL HISTORY:

At what age did menses begin? 11 Were they regular or irregular? WNL

How were they related to your headache? Not related

Are you or were you ever on Birth Control Pills? Yes Did they affect your headache? No

Have you had a hysterectomy, partial or total, and why? 1971, Total

Are you in menopause, and if yes, how long? No

Are you on hormones, and if yes, which ones? Premarin

HEADACHE ASSESSMENT FORM

HA PROFILE	INCAPACITATING #3	INTERFERING #2	IRRITATING #1
ONSET (Years ago and frequency)	N/A	Approx. 6 mos. ago Every other day	Young adult, approx. 1/month
CURRENT FREQUENCY	N/A	Every other day	2/week
TIME OF ONSET	N/A	Varies, May wake up with	Varies
DURATION	N/A	24 to 48 hours	Approx. 1 hour
CHARACTER	N/A	Excruciating piercing pain	Dull ache
PRODROME OR AURA	N/A	N/A	N/A
ASSOCIATING FEATURES	Nausea; Vomiting; Sensitivity to Light? Noise? Odors? Do you get pale or flush? Do your eyes or nose run? Does your nose get stuffy? Do the whites of your eyes get red? Does your eyelid droop? Do you pace, or go to bed?	Nausea; Vomiting; Sensitivity to Light? Noise? Odors? Do you get pale or flush? Do your eyes or nose run? Does your nose get stuffy? Do the whites of your eyes get red? Does your eyelid droop? Do you pace, or go to bed?	Nausea; Vomiting; Sensitivity to Light? Noise? Odors? Do you get pale or flush? Do your eyes or nose run? Does your nose get stuffy? Do the whites of your eyes get red? Does your eyelid droop? Do you pace, or go to bed? Sweat
PRECIPITATING OR AGGRAVATING FEATURES	N/A	N/A	N/A

LOCATION: Mark the location for each type of headache with a different color pen.

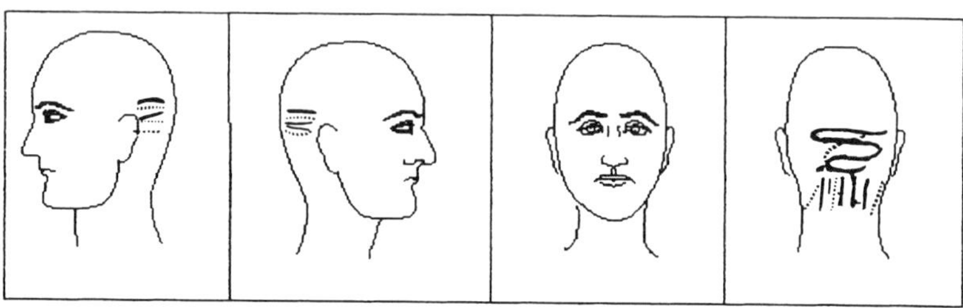

MEDICAL HISTORY:

Have you ever been or are you currently being treated for any of the following?

a) high blood pressure	Yes	No (underlined)
b) stomach ulcers	Yes (underlined)	No
c) asthma	Yes	No (underlined)
d) allergies	Yes	No (underlined)
e) pneumonia	Yes	No (underlined)
f) kidney problems	Yes	No (underlined)
g) low blood sugar	Yes	No (underlined)
h) glaucoma	Yes	No (underlined)
i) diabetes	Yes	No (underlined)
j) heart problems	Yes	No (underlined)

If you answered yes to any of the above, please describe: Ulcer 10 yrs. ago, presently not active.

List all other medical problems you have had in the past. Include date diagnosed and treatment.
DO NOT LIST OPERATIONS

Compression fracture T-9, 1991. Pushed stalled car off the road and felt strain in back. Off work for 4 months, in back brace and on bed rest.

SURGICAL HISTORY (List operations and dates performed)

Total hysterectomy, 1971. Gall bladder, 1970. Appendectomy, 1968. Uterine suspension, 1962.

PSYCHIATRIC HISTORY (List visits with counselors, psychologists, etc., and type of treatment)

None.

ACCIDENTS IN ADULT LIFE (Briefly describe any accident that caused any blow to the head or that you feel is related to your headache)

Car accident, 1994. Driving with seat belt. Stopped at a light, rear-ended by Wells Fargo truck and hit the cars in front of me. Felt a whiplash injury occur. Taken to emergency room, released and instructed to wear rib belt and C-collar.

FAMILY HISTORY:

1. Is your father living? Yes No (underlined)
   - Age________
   - Cause of death Brain aneurysm, age 43
   - Was there a headache history? Yes No (underlined)
2. Is your mother living? Yes No (underlined)
   - Age________
   - Cause of death Congestive heart failure, age 78
   - Was there a headache history? Yes No (underlined)

3. Ages of brothers---Circle the ones with headache
   65 51
4. Ages of sisters---Circle the ones with headache
   60 51
5. List any other blood relatives with a history of severe headaches.
   None

MARITAL HISTORY:
List marriages:

1st marriage age 25 to 45	Did spouse have headaches?	Yes	No
2nd marriage age 47 to Present	Did spouse have headaches?	Yes	No
3rd marriage age ______ to ______	Did spouse have headaches?	Yes	No

Age of current spouse: 58

List ages and sex of all children:

Age 30 Sex F	Headaches?	Yes	No
Age 26 Sex F	Headaches?	Yes	No
Age ______ Sex ______	Headaches?	Yes	No

STRESS FACTORS:

List any factors that may be affecting your headaches (money, loneliness, sexual problems, work, etc.)
N/A.

VEGETATIVE SIGNS:

1.	Do you have trouble falling asleep?	Yes	No
2.	Do you have trouble staying asleep?	Yes	No
3.	Has your appetite decreased?	Yes	No
4.	Have you gained or lost weight in the past year?	Yes	No
5.	Have you felt tearful or depressed lately?	Yes	No
6.	Have you had any thoughts of wanting to die?	Yes	No
7.	Have you been forgetful lately?	Yes	No
8.	Any other changes in your normal day-to-day living?		

Please list any medications you are allergic or sensitive to: Codeine

Please list any medications you are currently taking (including dosages and frequency per day):
Soma, 3 times a day as needed. Premarin, every day for 5 days, off 2, on 5.

PREVIOUS CARE:

1. List doctors who have treated you for headaches: Dr. R.

2. List any tests you have had for your headache (e.g., EEG, CT scan, MRI, X-Ray, etc.):
X-rays,

3. List any other treatment you have had for your headache (e.g., biofeedback, acupuncture, chiropractic, or any other treatment you had):
None.

The following is an example of an actual medical report demonstrating the diagnoses.

January 14, 1994

[Doctor's name and address omitted]

RE: MELISSA

Dear Dr. [...]:

Thank you for the referral of Ms. Melissa [...]

This is a 22-year-old female born in [...], and living in [...] for years. She is currently seeking employment. The patient states that she was in a significant accident on 00/00/93.

She was driving with a shoulder seat belt only, was stopped in a line of cars, and was rear-ended, causing her to hit the car in front of her. She does not remember hitting her head, but her glasses were twisted on her face. There was a flexion/extension injury and she sought medical treatment about $1^1/_2$ weeks later. Her headaches began the day after the accident. The patient states that she had no headaches prior to the accident.

HEADACHE PROFILE

Incapacitating headaches: The patient has had two of these headaches since the accident. These headaches come on any time and last a full day. It is severe pressure and the location of pain is the posterior cervical region, the occipital portion of her head, and also travels cerphalad to the parietal regions. There is some nausea and photophobia associated with the headache, and she has to go to bed. Quick movements make this headache worse.

Interfering headaches (moderate to severe): These headaches started the day after the accident, and she now gets these three times a week. This headache starts with shoulder pain; it is constant, she can awaken with it, and it will last all day. It is a sharp piercing pain and throbbing in the head and severe tightness in the same locations just described plus the periorbital regions. She has photophobia and will go to bed if possible.

Irritating headaches (annoying): N/A.

Menstrual history: Began at age 13 and her menstrual periods have been irregular. The patient was on birth control pills from age 19 to age 22. She stopped the birth control pills seven months ago, the month after the accident, and she did not have her period again until December. This is often seen after head injuries post trauma.

Past history: The patient was most probably a normal delivery. There is no history of enuresis or unexplained abdominal cramps pre-puberty. There is no history of car sickness as a child. There is no history of meningitis, encephalitis, scarlet fever, or rheumatic fever. There were no head injuries as a child.

Habits: She does not drink and does not smoke.

Medical history: The patient's medical history is essentially negative.

Review of systems: Pulmonary negative, cardiovascular negative, gastrointestinal negative, urogenital negative.

Surgical history: Negative

Psychiatric history: Negative

Head injuries in adult life: See above for details.

Family history: Her father is living, age 46, with no headache history. Her mother is living, age 60, with no headache history. There is a 31-year-old half-brother and a 33-year-old half-sister, with no headache history, and 24-year-old brother, with no headache history. The patient is not married and does have any children.

Allergies to medications: NKA.

Tests done in the past: The patient had some x-rays of her neck in [a doctor's] office.

Treatments tried in the past: The patient had some acupuncture which seemed to help temporarily; she had some physical therapy which made her feel worse; and she had some muscular therapy on Nautilus.

Physical examination: Height 5'2", weight 106 pounds, pulse 80, left BP 102/60, right BP 94/60. The face did not show any asymmetry. Temporomandibular joint area was grossly normal. The eyes appeared normal. Conjunctivae were clear and the pupils reacted equally to light and accommodation. Retinal fundus examination revealed no papiledema and no abnormalities with the arteries and veins. There were no bruits over the supraorbital region. The nose appeared normal. The auditory canals were clear and the tympanic membranes appeared intact. The mouth and throat appeared normal. Gums, tongue, buccal mucosa, and teeth were grossly normal. Neck: The patient had exquisite trigger points at the occipital cervical junction bilaterally consistent with out cervical plexus regional blocks. Carotid bruits could not be heard. Cervical modes were not enlarged. The lungs were clear to auscultation and percussion. The heart had a regular sinus rhythm with no murmurs. The abdomen was soft and nontender. A rectal or vaginal exam was not done.

Neurological examination: Cranial nerve II: Visual fields were grossly normal. III, IV and VI: No strabismus, nystagmus, or ptosis. V: Normal sensation and corneal reflex. VII: Normal facial movements (wrinkle, frown, smile, and strength of eyelids). VIII: Normal Weber and Rinne. IX and X: Good gag reflex. XI: Normal sternocleidomastoid and trapezius. XII: Normal protrusion and strength of tongue. Cerebellar: Negative Rhomberg. Normal finger-to-nose, diadochokinesis, heel-shin, tandem, and heel and toes walking. Motor system: No atrophy, fasciculations, wasting, or tremors. Good muscle strength in arms, wrists, fingers, and legs. Sensory system: Superficial tactile, pain, and vibrations (wrists, elbows, knees, and ankles) were normal. Normal motion and positions of fingers and toes. Normal 2-point discrimination. Reflexes: Normal 2+ reflexes of triceps, biceps, knee jerk, ankle jerk, etc. Normal pulses in dorsalis pedis, posterior tibial and popliteal.

DIAGNOSES

1. Post traumatic headache.
2. Rule out post traumatic vascular headache.
3. Post traumatic muscle contraction headache with occipital neuralgia.
4. Rule out cervicogenic headache.

IMPRESSION

This pleasant 22-year-old woman comes in who was headache-free until an accident she suffered on 00/00/93. It appears that the patient has some occipital neuralgia and this causes the headaches both in back of her head and in front of her head. There may be a mild vascular component. I think the patient should have a regional bock of C1, 2 and 3, and mild neuromuscular mobilization to help reduce the muscle spasm. The patient did not do well with deep neuromuscular mobilization and I would try to avoid that.

She will be given some Midrin and Lorcet as a means of aborting her headache, but I will hold back on putting her on daily preventative medication at this time, because I think this might be improved just with mechanical intervention.

The cervicogenic component will also need to be addressed and consideration for cervical blocks with fluoroscopic guidance would be of consideration in her treatment. If this is a cervicogenic headache, then the patient will remain symptomatic unless treated properly.

Again, thank you for the referral of this pleasant patient. If there are any questions, please do not hesitate to call or write.

Sincerely,

BERNARD SWERDLOW, M.D.

These notes were dictated with the patient present.

MEDICAL HEADACHE HISTORY

Name: Melissa **Age:** 22 **Sex** F **Date:** 1/14/94

Date of Birth: 0/00/71 **Birthplace:** OH **Race:** W **Education:** 1 year college

Occupation: Seeking employment **Accident:** 1993

Armed Services & Type of Discharge: N/A

PAST HISTORY:

1.	Did you have a normal birth?		Yes	No
	a) forceps used?		Yes	No
	b) cesarean section?		Yes	No
2.	Did you have problems with bedwetting?		Yes	No
	a) If yes, age bedwetting stopped		______	
3.	Were you car sick as a child (motion)?		Yes	No
	a) If yes, how severe?	Slight	Moderate	Severe
4.	Did you have unexplained abdominal cramps as a child?		Yes	No
5.	Did you have any of the following illnesses in childhood?			
	a) meningitis		Yes	No
	b) encephalitis		Yes	No
	c) scarlet fever		Yes	No
	d) rheumatic fever		Yes	No
6.	Did you have any head injuries as a child?		Yes	No
	a) If yes, please explain:			
7.	Were you treated for emotional illness as a child?		Yes	No

HABITS:

8.	Do you drink alcohol?	Yes	No
	a) If yes, what kind and how much?		
	b) Does alcohol bring on or aggravate a headache?	Yes	No
9.	Do you smoke?	Yes	No
	a) If yes, how much?		
	b) Does smoking or smoke-filled rooms cause or aggravate headaches?	Yes	No
10.	Do you drink caffeinated beverages?	Yes	No
	a) If yes, how much? 4 times a week		

MENSTRUAL HISTORY:

At what age did menses begin? 13 Were they regular or irregular? Irregular

How were they related to your headache? N/A

Are you or were you ever on Birth Control Pills? Yes Did they affect your headache? No

Have you had a hysterectomy, partial or total, and why? No

Are you in menopause, and if yes, how long? No

Are you on hormones, and if yes, which ones? No

HEADACHE ASSESSMENT FORM

HA PROFILE	INCAPACITATING #3	INTERFERING #2	IRRITATING #1
ONSET (Years ago and frequency)	Have had 2 since accident	Day after accident	N/A
CURRENT FREQUENCY	N/A	3 a week	N/A
TIME OF ONSET	Anytime	Can awaken with	N/A
DURATION	1 day	All day	N/A
CHARACTER	Severe pressure	Sharp piercing pain and throbbing in head	N/A
PRODROME OR AURA	N/A	N/A	N/A
ASSOCIATING FEATURES	<u>Nausea</u>; Vomiting; <u>Sensitivity to Light</u>? Noise? Odors? Do you get pale or flush? Do your eyes or nose run? Does your nose get stuffy? Do the whites of your eyes get red? Does your eyelid droop? Do you pace, or <u>go to bed</u>?	Nausea; Vomiting; <u>Sensitivity to Light</u>? Noise? Odors? Do you get pale or flush? Do your eyes or nose run? Does your nose get stuffy? Do the whites of your eyes get red? Does your eyelid droop? Do you pace, or <u>go to bed</u>?	Nausea; Vomiting; Sensitivity to Light? Noise? Odors? Do you get pale or flush? Do your eyes or nose run? Does your nose get stuffy? Do the whites of your eyes get red? Does your eyelid droop? Do you pace, or go to bed?
PRECIPITATING OR AGGRAVATING FEATURES	Quick movement	N/A	N/A

LOCATION: Mark the location for each type of headache with a different color pen.

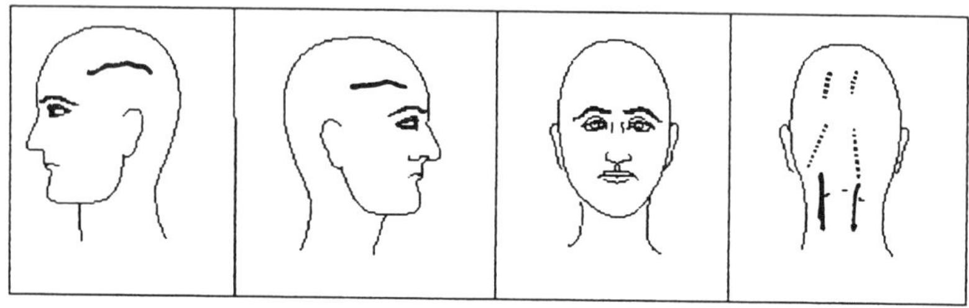

MEDICAL HISTORY:

Have you ever been or are you currently being treated for any of the following?

a) high blood pressure	Yes	No
b) stomach ulcers	Yes	No
c) asthma	Yes	No
d) allergies	Yes	No
e) pneumonia	Yes	No
f) kidney problems	Yes	No
g) low blood sugar	Yes	No
h) glaucoma	Yes	No
i) diabetes	Yes	No
j) heart problems	Yes	No

If you answered yes to any of the above, please describe:____________________

List all other medical problems you have had in the past. Include date diagnosed and treatment.
DO NOT LIST OPERATIONS

None.

SURGICAL HISTORY (List operations and dates performed)

None.

PSYCHIATRIC HISTORY (List visits with counselors, psychologists, etc., and type of treatment)

None.

ACCIDENTS IN ADULT LIFE (Briefly describe any accident that caused any blow to the head or that you feel is related to your headache)

Car accident, 1993. Driving with shoulder seat belt. Stopped in a line of cars and rear-ended, causing my car to hit car in front of me. Don't remember hitting head, but glasses were twisted on my face. Flexion extension injury. Sought medical treatment 1 ½ weeks later. Headaches began day after accident. No headaches before accident.

FAMILY HISTORY:

1.	Is your father living?	Yes	No
	Age 46		
	Cause of death__________		
	Was there a headache history?	Yes	No
2.	Is your mother living?	Yes	No
	Age 60		
	Cause of death__________		
	Was there a headache history?	Yes	No

3. Ages of brothers---Circle the ones with headache
   31 24
4. Ages of sisters---Circle the ones with headache
   33
5. List any other blood relatives with a history of severe headaches.
   None.

MARITAL HISTORY:

List marriages:

1st marriage age _____ to ______ Did spouse have headaches?	Yes	No
2nd marriage age _____ to ______ Did spouse have headaches?	Yes	No
3rd marriage age _____ to ______ Did spouse have headaches?	Yes	No

Age of current spouse: N/A

List ages and sex of all children:

Age _____ Sex _____ Headaches?	Yes	No
Age _____ Sex _____ Headaches?	Yes	No
Age _____ Sex _____ Headaches?	Yes	No

STRESS FACTORS:

List any factors that may be affecting your headaches (money, loneliness, sexual problems, work, etc.)
None.

VEGETATIVE SIGNS:

1.	Do you have trouble falling asleep?	Yes	<u>No</u>
2.	Do you have trouble staying asleep?	<u>Yes</u>	No
3.	Has your appetite decreased?	<u>Yes</u>	No
4.	Have you gained or lost weight in the past year?	Yes	<u>No</u>
5.	Have you felt tearful or depressed lately?	Yes	<u>No</u>
6.	Have you had any thoughts of wanting to die?	Yes	<u>No</u>
7.	Have you been forgetful lately?	Yes	<u>No</u>
8.	Any other changes in your normal day-to-day living? ______		

Please list any medications you are allergic or sensitive to: NKA

Please list any medications you are currently taking (including dosages and frequency per day):
None.

PREVIOUS CARE:

1. List doctors who have treated you for headaches: Dr. D.; Physical Therapy.

2. List any tests you have had for your headache (e.g., EEG, CT scan, MRI, X-Ray, etc.):
X-Rays.

3. List any other treatment you have had for your headache (e.g., biofeedback, acupuncture, chiropractic, or any other treatment you had):
Acupuncture, physical therapy, muscular therapy, Nautilus.

November 4, 1993

[Doctor's name and address omitted]

RE: SHEILA

Dear Dr. [...]:

Thank you for the referral of Ms. Sheila [...].

This is a 42-year-old female born 00/00/59 in [...]. She works for [...] County as a [...].

The patient states that on 00/00/93, she was driving, wearing a seatbelt, was stopped at a red light and was rear-ended by another car. She had a flexion-extension injury. She saw the family physician the next day, and her headaches began that night. The patient stated that she had an occasional irritating or annoying headache prior to the accident.

HEADACHE PROFILE

Incapacitating headaches: The headaches started the week of the accident, and she had one every 7 to 10 days. The patient still gets one of these headaches every 7 to 10 days, and it lasts 2 to 3 hours. It is a throbbing headache and it starts in the posterior cervical region and works its way cephalad up the occipital, around the frontal and periorbital regions. It is a throbbing headache. There is no aura. Associated features are nausea, photophobia, phonophobia, sensitivity to odors, pallor, nasal stuffiness, and she will go to bed. Exertion and movement make these headaches worse.

Interfering headaches (moderate to severe): These headaches started the day of the accident. The patient currently gets these headaches four to five times a week and they last all day. It is a throbbing headache, again in the same location as previously described. There is no aura. There is some nausea, photophobia, and the patient has difficulty working with this headache.

Irritating headaches (annoying): These headaches started in her twenties and they were occasional. The patient does not have these headaches now since the accident, because of the severity of the other headaches. These headaches used to last an hour and the patient was able to abort then with over-the-counter medication. It was a dull ache in the frontal part of her head.

Menstrual history: Began at age 12 and has always been irregular. The patient was on birth control pills from age 19 to present on an "on and off' basis and with no adverse effects.

Past history: The patient was most probably a normal delivery. There is no history of enuresis or unexplained abdominal cramps pre-puberty. There is no history of car sickness as a child. There is no history of meningitis, encephalitis, scarlet fever, or rheumatic fever. There were no head injuries as a child.

Habits: The patient rarely drinks and does not get a headache with it. She does not smoke, but smoke-filled rooms now will aggravate her headache.

Medical history: The patient's medical history is essentially negative.

Review of systems: Pulmonary negative, cardiovascular negative, gastrointestinal negative, urogenital negative.

Surgical history: The patient had operations in 1985 and 1986 for a rectal vaginal fissure which was repaired. She had a tubal ligation in 1986.

Psychiatric history: Negative

Head injuries in adult life: See above for details.

Family history: Her father is living, age 73, with a history of headaches. Her mother is living, age 73, with no headache history. There is a 54-year-old brother and a 37-year-old sister, both with no headache history. The patient was married four times, and is currently married. There are three children, all boys, ages 24, 18 and 8, all with no headache history.

Allergies to medications: NKA.

Current medications: The patient currently takes Motrin, Skelaxin, and Tagament. She was on Prozac for four days and it made her feel "weird."

Tests done in the past: In 1993, the patient had an MRI of her neck which was negative and a bone scan which was negative.

Treatments tried in the past: The patient has had physical therapy with minimum success.

Physical examination: Height 5'6", weight 145 pounds, pulse 84, left BP 104/68, right BP 108/72. The face did not show any asymmetry. Temporomandibular joint area was grossly normal. The eyes appeared normal. Conjunctivae were clear and the pupils reacted equally to light and accommodation. Retinal fundus examination revealed no papiledema and no abnormalities with the arteries and veins. There were no bruits over the supraorbital region. The nose appeared normal. The auditory canals were clear and the tympanic membranes appeared intact. The mouth and throat appeared normal. Gums, tongue, buccal mucosa, and teeth were grossly normal. Neck: The patient had exquisite trigger points at the occipital cervical junction bilaterally consistent with out cervical plexus regional blocks. Carotid bruits could not be heard. Cervical modes were not enlarged. The lungs were clear to auscultation and percussion. The heart had a regular sinus rhythm with no murmurs. The abdomen was soft and nontender. A rectal or vaginal exam was not done.

Neurological examination: Cranial nerve II: Visual fields were grossly normal. III, IV and VI: No strabismus, nystagmus, or ptosis. V: Normal sensation and corneal reflex. VII: Normal facial movements (wrinkle, frown, smile, and strength of eyelids). VIII: Normal Weber and Rinne. IX and X: Good gag reflex. XI: Normal sternocleidomastoid and trapezius. XII: Normal protrusion and strength of tongue. Cerebellar: Negative Rhomberg. Normal finger-to-nose, diadochokinesis, heel-shin, tandem, and heel and toes walking. Motor system: No atrophy, fasciculations, wasting, or tremors. Good muscle strength in arms, wrists, fingers, and legs. Sensory system: Superficial tactile, pain, and vibrations (wrists, elbows, knees, and ankles) were normal. Normal motion and positions of fingers and toes. Normal 2-point discrimination. Reflexes: Normal 2+ reflexes of triceps, biceps, knee jerk, ankle jerk, etc. Normal pulses in dorsalis pedis, posterior tibial and popliteal.

DIAGNOSES

1. Post traumatic cervicogenic headaches.
2. Post traumatic migraine-like headaches.
3. Post traumatic muscle contraction with myofascial trigger points.
4. Rule out metabolic cause of headache.
5. Preexisting (now nonexisting) rare muscle tension headache.

IMPRESSION

This pleasant 42-year-old woman comes in who had relatively minor headaches on rare occasions prior to an accident she suffered on 99/00/93. As a result of a flexion-extension injury that was significant, she now has ongoing chromic headaches. The headaches seem to originate from the cervical region and she appears to have a post traumatic cervicogenic vascular and muscle contraction-like headache.

The patient has a migraine-like headache because she has the throbbing qualities plus the gastrointestinal and neurogenic features of a migraine. For this, the patient will be placed on Propranolol 20 mg t.i.d., and to prevent her early morning headaches. She will be placed on Bellergal-S.h.s. To abort her headaches as a first line of defense, she will have Midrin, and as a second line of defense she will have Ergopak with 25 mg of Promethazine suppositories. For the cervicogenic headache, she will get regional blocks of C1, 2 and 3, which should help to reduce the inflammatory response, and for her trigger points, she will have trigger point injections with deep neuromuscular mobilization at the same movement to break up the spasms. if this approach is not successful, then the cervicogenic component will be addressed by giving cervical facet blocks with fluoroscopic guidance.

The patient will maintain a headache log and will be seen for a regular visit in about a month for reevaluation. However, the other treatments will continue as soon as possible.

Thank you very much for the referral of this pleasant patient. If there are any questions, please do not hesitate to call or write.

Sincerely,

BERNARD SWERDLOW, M.D.

These notes were dictated with the patient present.

MEDICAL HEADACHE HISTORY

Name: Sheila **Age:** 42 **Sex** F **Date:** 11/4/93

Date of Birth: 0/00/50 **Birthplace:** FL **Race:** W **Education:** High School

Occupation: Food Service **Accident:** 1992

Armed Services & Type of Discharge: N/A

PAST HISTORY:

1.	Did you have a normal birth?		Yes (underlined)	No
	a) forceps used?		Yes	No
	b) cesarean section?		Yes	No
2.	Did you have problems with bedwetting?		Yes	No (underlined)
	a) If yes, age bedwetting stopped		________	
3.	Were you car sick as a child (motion)?		Yes	No (underlined)
	a) If yes, how severe?	Slight	Moderate	Severe
4.	Did you have unexplained abdominal cramps as a child?		Yes	No (underlined)
5.	Did you have any of the following illnesses in childhood?			
	a) meningitis		Yes	No (underlined)
	b) encephalitis		Yes	No (underlined)
	c) scarlet fever		Yes	No (underlined)
	d) rheumatic fever		Yes	No (underlined)
6.	Did you have any head injuries as a child?		Yes	No (underlined)
	a) If yes, please explain: ________			
7.	Were you treated for emotional illness as a child?		Yes	No (underlined)

HABITS:

8.	Do you drink alcohol?	Yes (underlined)	No
	a) If yes, what kind and how much? Sometimes, very little		
	b) Does alcohol bring on or aggravate a headache?	Yes	No (underlined)
9.	Do you smoke?	Yes	No (underlined)
	a) If yes, how much? ________		
	b) Does smoking or smoke-filled rooms cause or aggravate headaches?	Yes (underlined)	No
10.	Do you drink caffeinated beverages?	Yes (underlined)	No
	a) If yes, how much? ________		

MENSTRUAL HISTORY:

At what age did menses begin? 12 Were they regular or irregular? WNL

How were they related to your headache? N/A

Are you or were you ever on Birth Control Pills? Yes Did they affect your headache? No

Have you had a hysterectomy, partial or total, and why? No

Are you in menopause, and if yes, how long? No

Are you on hormones, and if yes, which ones? No

HEADACHE ASSESSMENT FORM

HA PROFILE	INCAPACITATING #3	INTERFERING #2	IRRITATING #1
ONSET (Years ago and frequency)	Week of the accident 1 every 7 to 10 days	Day of accident 2 to 3 a week	In 20's, occasionally
CURRENT FREQUENCY	1 every 7 to 10 days	4 to 5 a week	None now
TIME OF ONSET	Later in the day	Can awaken with	Anytime
DURATION	2 to 3 hours	All day	1 hr. with OTC meds
CHARACTER	Throbbing	Throbbing	Dull ache
PRODROME OR AURA	N/A	N/A	N/A
ASSOCIATING FEATURES	Nausea; Vomiting; Sensitivity to Light? Noise? Odors? Do you get pale or flush? Do your eyes or nose run? Does your nose get stuffy? Do the whites of your eyes get red? Does your eyelid droop? Do you pace, or go to bed?	Nausea; Vomiting; Sensitivity to Light? Noise? Odors? Do you get pale or flush? Do your eyes or nose run? Does your nose get stuffy? Do the whites of your eyes get red? Does your eyelid droop? Do you pace, or go to bed?	Nausea; Vomiting; Sensitivity to Light? Noise? Odors? Do you get pale or flush? Do your eyes or nose run? Does your nose get stuffy? Do the whites of your eyes get red? Does your eyelid droop? Do you pace, or go to bed?
PRECIPITATING OR AGGRAVATING FEATURES	Movement	Lying down	N/A

LOCATION: Mark the location for each type of headache with a different color pen.

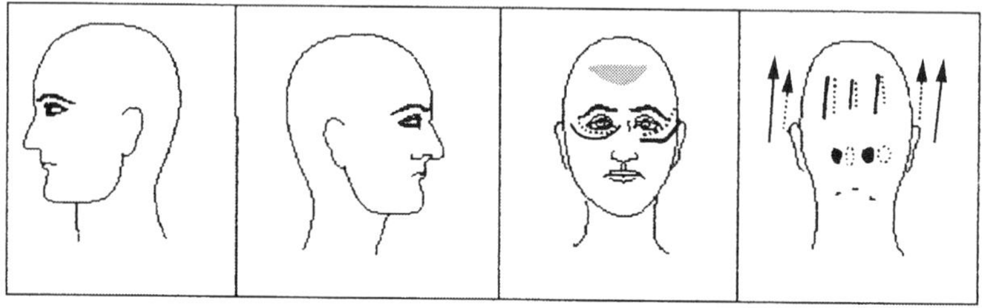

MEDICAL HISTORY:

Have you ever been or are you currently being treated for any of the following?

a) high blood pressure	Yes	No
b) stomach ulcers	Yes	No
c) asthma	Yes	No
d) allergies	Yes	No
e) pneumonia	Yes	No
f) kidney problems	Yes	No
g) low blood sugar	Yes	No
h) glaucoma	Yes	No
i) diabetes	Yes	No
j) heart problems	Yes	No

If you answered yes to any of the above, please describe:____________________

List all other medical problems you have had in the past. Include date diagnosed and treatment.
DO NOT LIST OPERATIONS

Colds, female problems.

SURGICAL HISTORY (List operations and dates performed)

Rectovaginal fistula repairs, 1985 and 1986. Tubal, 1986.

PSYCHIATRIC HISTORY (List visits with counselors, psychologists, etc., and type of treatment)

None.

ACCIDENTS IN ADULT LIFE (Briefly describe any accident that caused any blow to the head or that you feel is related to your headache)

Car accident, 1992. Driving with seat belt. Stopped at red light and rear-ended by another car. Flexion extension injury. Saw family physician next day. Headaches began that night. Had occasional #1 headaches before accident.

FAMILY HISTORY:

1.	Is your father living?	Yes	No
	Age 73		
	Cause of death__________		
	Was there a headache history?	Yes	No
2.	Is your mother living?	Yes	No
	Age 73		
	Cause of death__________		
	Was there a headache history?	Yes	No

3. Ages of brothers---Circle the ones with headache
 54
4. Ages of sisters---Circle the ones with headache
 37
5. List any other blood relatives with a history of severe headaches.
 ?

MARITAL HISTORY:
List marriages:

1st marriage age _____ to ______	Did spouse have headaches?	Yes	No
2nd marriage age _____ to ______	Did spouse have headaches?	Yes	No
3rd marriage age _____ to ______	Did spouse have headaches?	Yes	No
4th marriage age _____ to ______	Did spouse have headaches?	Yes	No

Age of current spouse: 31

List ages and sex of all children:

Age 24 Sex M	Headaches?	Yes	No
Age 18 Sex M	Headaches?	Yes	No
Age 8 Sex M	Headaches?	Yes	No
Age _____ Sex _____	Headaches?	Yes	No

STRESS FACTORS:

List any factors that may be affecting your headaches (money, loneliness, sexual problems, work, etc.)
None.

VEGETATIVE SIGNS:

1.	Do you have trouble falling asleep?	Yes	No
2.	Do you have trouble staying asleep?	Yes	No
3.	Has your appetite decreased?	Yes	No
4.	Have you gained or lost weight in the past year?	Yes	No
5.	Have you felt tearful or depressed lately?	Yes	No
6.	Have you had any thoughts of wanting to die?	Yes	No
7.	Have you been forgetful lately?	Yes	No
8.	Any other changes in your normal day-to-day living?		

Please list any medications you are allergic or sensitive to: NKA

Please list any medications you are currently taking (including dosages and frequency per day):
Motrin, Skelaxin, Tagamet.

PREVIOUS CARE:

1. List doctors who have treated you for headaches: Dr. T. , Dr. M.

2. List any tests you have had for your headache (e.g., EEG, CT scan, MRI, X-Ray, etc.):
MRI 1993, negative. Bone scan, 1993, negative.

3. List any other treatment you have had for your headache (e.g., biofeedback, acupuncture, chiropractic, or any other treatment you had):
Physical therapy. TENS unit.

[Doctor's name and address omitted]

RE: BARBARA

Dear Dr. [...]:

Thank you for your referral of Barbara [...]. This is a 44-year-old female born 00/00/48 in [...], living in Florida [...] years. She works at [...].

On 00/00/92 the patient was in an accident in which she was driving with a seat belt. She was starting to move through an intersection when she was rear-ended by another car. She had a flexion-extension injury. She saw a physician four days after the accident. Her headaches began two days after the accident. The patient states that she was not a headache sufferer before the accident.

HEADACHE PROFILE

Interfering headaches (moderate to severe): These started two days after the accident. She has been having them daily and finds that these headaches will come about if there is any motion of her body, such as dancing, or anywhere where there seems to be movement of the cervical vertebra. They seem to stop an hour after she stops this motion. She discusses the pain as being a constant sharp pain in the occipital portions of her head and the frontal portions of her head. She says that if she drives for awhile she will become nauseous and that at times she will have blurred vision with the headache. She will go to bed if she can.

Menstrual history: Began at age 11 and is within normal limits. She was on birth control pills at age 30-31. In 1987 she had a total hysterectomy because of precancerous cells.

Past history: The patient was most probably a normal delivery. She had rheumatic fever as a child and this has resolved with no after-effects. There is no history of enuresis or unexplained abdominal cramps pre-puberty. There is no history of car sickness as a child. There is no history of meningitis, encephalitis, scarlet fever. There were no head injuries as a child.

Habits: She has a drink of alcohol a week and this does not affect her headache. She does not smoke.

Medical history: The patient has no history of high blood pressure, stomach ulcers, asthma, allergies, pneumonia, kidney problems, low blood sugar, glaucoma, diabetes, or heart problems.

Review of systems: Pulmonary, negative. Cardiovascular, negative. Gastrointestinal, negative. Urogenital, negative.

Surgical history: Total hysterectomy in 1987 for precancerous cells plus an appendectomy.

Psychiatric history: Patient was treated for depression in 1988 and this is in remission.

Family history: Father living, age 70 without headache history. Mother living, age 65 without headache history. There is a 35-year-old brother and 46-year-old sister with no headaches.

Marital history: Patient is married and there are four children, three girls, ages 29, 25 and 12, the oldest one has some headaches, and a 27-year-old son without headaches.

Allergies to medications: NKA.

Medications: She currently takes aspirin and Tylenol as needed.

Previous work-up: The patient has had x-rays of her neck and she had an MRI of the brain 00/00/92, which is read as normal. She also had dermatomal somatosensory evoked potentials of the upper extremities which were also read as normal.

Physical exam: Height 5'5", weight 195 pounds, pulse is 62, left BP is 132/80, right BP 128/82. The face did not show any asymmetry. The temporomandibular joint area was grossly normal. The eyes appeared normal. Conjunctivae were clear and the pupils reacted equally to light and accommodation. Retinal fundus examination revealed no papilledema and no abnormalities with the arteries and veins. There were no bruits over the supraorbital region. The nose appeared normal. The auditory canals were clear and the tympanic membranes appeared intact. The mouth and throat appeared normal. Gums, tongue, buccal mucosa, and teeth were grossly normal. The neck has 3 to 5 myofascial trigger points in the right upper trapezius and right splenius capitis muscles. There were no masses felt in the thyroid gland. Carotid bruits could not be heard. Cervical nodes were not enlarged. The lungs were clear to auscultation and percussion. The heart had a regular sinus rhythm with no murmurs. The abdomen was soft and nontender. A rectal or vaginal examination was not done.

Neurological examination: Cranial nerve II: Visual fields were grossly normal. III, IV and VI: No strabismus, nystagmus, or ptosis. V: Normal sensation and corneal reflex. VII: Normal facial movements (wrinkle, frown, smile, and strength of eyelids). VIII: Normal Weber and Rinne. IX and X: Good gag reflex. XI: Normal sternocleidomastoid and trapezius. XII: Normal protrusion and strength of tongue. Cerebellar: Negative Rhomberg. Normal finger-to-nose, diadochokinesis, heel-shin, tandem, and heel and toes walking. Motor system: No atrophy, fasciculations, wasting, or tremors. Good muscle strength in arms, wrists, fingers, and legs. Sensory system: Superficial tactile, pain, and vibrations (wrists, elbows, knees, and ankles) were normal. Normal motion and positions of fingers and toes. Normal 2-point discrimination. Reflexes: Normal 2+ reflexes of triceps, biceps, knee jerk, ankle jerk, etc. Normal pulses in dorsalis pedis, posterior tibial and popliteal.

DIAGNOSES

1. Post traumatic cervicogenic headache.
2. Rule out vascular headache with muscular contraction component and myofascial trigger points.

IMPRESSION/RECOMMENDATIONS

This pleasant 44-year-old woman comes in who has suffered an accident on 00/00/92 and suffers moderate to severe headaches whenever motion is involved. The patient has some obvious objective trigger points that have to be injected and use of deep neuromuscular kinetic activity to break the spasm. Hopefully, this would be the only treatment the patient needs at this moment. However, consideration for cervical facet blocks with fluoroscopic guidance would be considered if the diagnosis of cervicogenic headache is the major cause of her problems. Hopefully, she would need very few treatments to resolve this problem. Arrangements will be made for treating the patient.

Thank you once again for this referral of this pleasant woman. If there are any questions, please do not hesitate to call or write.

Sincerely,

BERNARD SWERDLOW, M.D.

These notes were dictated with the patient present.

MEDICAL HEADACHE HISTORY

Name: Barbara **Age:** 44 **Sex** F **Date:** 11/5/92

Date of Birth: 0/00/48 **Birthplace:** MS **Race:** W **Education:** GED

Occupation: Graphic Arts **Accident:** 1992

Armed Services & Type of Discharge: N/A

PAST HISTORY:

1.	Did you have a normal birth?		**Yes**	No
	a) forceps used?		Yes	No
	b) cesarean section?		Yes	No
2.	Did you have problems with bedwetting?		Yes	**No**
	a) If yes, age bedwetting stopped			
3.	Were you car sick as a child (motion)?		Yes	**No**
	a) If yes, how severe?	Slight	Moderate	Severe
4.	Did you have unexplained abdominal cramps as a child?		Yes	**No**
5.	Did you have any of the following illnesses in childhood?			
	a) meningitis		Yes	**No**
	b) encephalitis		Yes	**No**
	c) scarlet fever		Yes	**No**
	d) rheumatic fever		**Yes**	No
6.	Did you have any head injuries as a child?		Yes	**No**
	a) If yes, please explain:			
7.	Were you treated for emotional illness as a child?		Yes	**No**

HABITS:

8.	Do you drink alcohol?	**Yes**	No
	a) If yes, what kind and how much? Glass of wine a week		
	b) Does alcohol bring on or aggravate a headache?	Yes	**No**
9.	Do you smoke?	Yes	**No**
	a) If yes, how much?		
	b) Does smoking or smoke-filled rooms cause or aggravate headaches?	Yes	**No**
10.	Do you drink caffeinated beverages?	**Yes**	No
	a) If yes, how much? 2 glasses per day		

MENSTRUAL HISTORY:

At what age did menses begin? 11 Were they regular or irregular? WNL

How were they related to your headache? N/A

Are you or were you ever on Birth Control Pills? Yes Did they affect your headache? No

Have you had a hysterectomy, partial or total, and why? 1987, Total, precancerous

Are you in menopause, and if yes, how long? No

Are you on hormones, and if yes, which ones? No

HEADACHE ASSESSMENT FORM

HA PROFILE	INCAPACITATING #3	INTERFERING #2	IRRITATING #1
ONSET (Years ago and frequency)	N/A	2 days after accident Every day	N/A
CURRENT FREQUENCY	N/A	Every day, only with motion	N/A
TIME OF ONSET	N/A	Anytime driving or riding	N/A
DURATION	N/A	1 hour after stopping car	N/A
CHARACTER	N/A	Constant sharp pain	N/A
PRODROME OR AURA	N/A	Blurred vision with headache	N/A
ASSOCIATING FEATURES	Nausea: Vomiting: Sensitivity to Light? Noise? Odors? Do you get pale or flush? Do your eyes or nose run? Does your nose get stuffy? Do the whites of your eyes get red? Does your eyelid droop? Do you pace, or go to bed?	Nausea: Vomiting; Sensitivity to Light? Noise? Odors? Do you get pale or flush? Do your eyes or nose run? Does your nose get stuffy? Do the whites of your eyes get red? Does your eyelid droop? Do you pace, or go to bed?	Nausea; Vomiting; Sensitivity to Light? Noise? Odors? Do you get pale or flush? Do your eyes or nose run? Does your nose get stuffy? Do the whites of your eyes get red? Does your eyelid droop? Do you pace, or go to bed?
PRECIPITATING OR AGGRAVATING FEATURES	N/A	N/A	N/A

LOCATION: Mark the location for each type of headache with a different color pen.

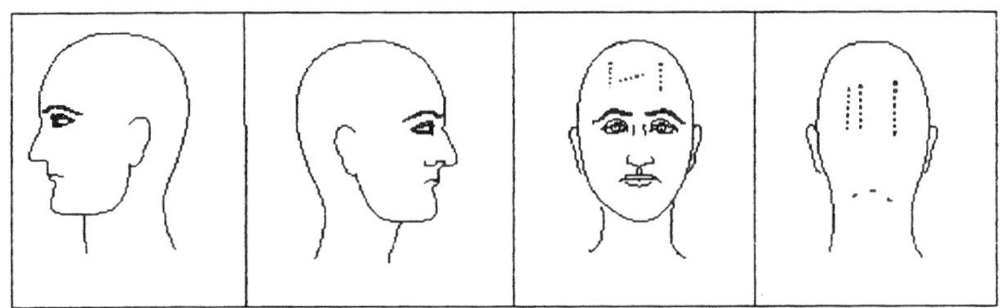

MEDICAL HISTORY:

Have you ever been or are you currently being treated for any of the following?

a) high blood pressure	Yes	No
b) stomach ulcers	Yes	No
c) asthma	Yes	No
d) allergies	Yes	No
e) pneumonia	Yes	No
f) kidney problems	Yes	No
g) low blood sugar	Yes	No
h) glaucoma	Yes	No
i) diabetes	Yes	No
j) heart problems	Yes	No

If you answered yes to any of the above, please describe:____________________

List all other medical problems you have had in the past. Include date diagnosed and treatment.
DO NOT LIST OPERATIONS

SURGICAL HISTORY (List operations and dates performed)

Total hysterectomy and appendectomy, 1978.

PSYCHIATRIC HISTORY (List visits with counselors, psychologists, etc., and type of treatment)

1988 – depression.

ACCIDENTS IN ADULT LIFE (Briefly describe any accident that caused any blow to the head or that you feel is related to your headache)

Car accident, 1992. Driving with seat belt. Starting to move through intersection. Rear-ended by another car. Flexion extension injury. Saw doctor 4 days later. Headaches began 2 days later. No headaches before accident.

FAMILY HISTORY:

1. Is your father living? Yes No
   - Age 70
   - Cause of death____________________
   - Was there a headache history? Yes No
2. Is your mother living? Yes No
   - Age 65
   - Cause of death____________________
   - Was there a headache history? Yes No

3. Ages of brothers---Circle the ones with headache
   (35)
4. Ages of sisters---Circle the ones with headache
   (46)
5. List any other blood relatives with a history of severe headaches.
   Daughter

MARITAL HISTORY:

List marriages:

1st marriage age 13 to 39	Did spouse have headaches?	Yes	No
2nd marriage age ____ to ____	Did spouse have headaches?	Yes	No
3rd marriage age ____ to ____	Did spouse have headaches?	Yes	No

Age of current spouse: N/A

List ages and sex of all children:

Age 29	Sex F	Headaches?	Yes	No
Age 27	Sex M	Headaches?	Yes	No
Age 25	Sex F	Headaches?	Yes	No
Age 12	Sex F	Headaches?	Yes	No
Age ____	Sex ____	Headaches?	Yes	No

STRESS FACTORS:

List any factors that may be affecting your headaches (money, loneliness, sexual problems, work, etc.)
Sometimes stress at work.

VEGETATIVE SIGNS:

1.	Do you have trouble falling asleep?	Yes	No
2.	Do you have trouble staying asleep?	Yes	No
3.	Has your appetite decreased?	Yes	No
4.	Have you gained or lost weight in the past year?	Yes	No
5.	Have you felt tearful or depressed lately?	Yes	No
6.	Have you had any thoughts of wanting to die?	Yes	No
7.	Have you been forgetful lately?	Yes	No
8.	Any other changes in your normal day-to-day living? ____		

Please list any medications you are allergic or sensitive to: None

Please list any medications you are currently taking (including dosages and frequency per day):
Aspirin, Tylenol, as needed.

PREVIOUS CARE:

1. List doctors who have treated you for headaches: Dr. R.

2. List any tests you have had for your headache (e.g., EEG, CT scan, MRI, X-Ray, etc.):
X-rays, MRI.

3. List any other treatment you have had for your headache (e.g., biofeedback, acupuncture, chiropractic, or any other treatment you had):

August 16, 1993

[Doctor's name and address omitted]

RE: ELIZABETH

Dear Dr. [...]:

Thank you for your referral of Ms. Elizabeth [...].

This is a 43-year-old woman born 00/00/49 in [...], and living in [...] for [...] years. She was in an accident on 00/00/93, in which she was a passenger, wearing a seat belt. She was stopped and rear-ended in a seven-car pile up. The patient had a flexion-extension injury, and she sought medical treatment two days later. She states that her headaches began immediately after the accident. The patient states that she just had some minor headaches before the accident.

HEADACHE PROFILE

Incapacitating headaches: These started one day after the accident, and the patient had these headaches every day for three months. She is currently getting these headaches several times a week, and they last a full day. It is a throbbing and pressure-type headache. The pain is in the periorbital regions, the front of her head, and the posterior cervical region. The pain seems to start in the posterior cervical region and works cephalad around to her eyes. There is no aura, but it is extremely severe pain, and there is nausea, photophobia, phonophobia, sensitivity to odors, lacrimation, and she must go to bed. Any kind of head movement with this headache will make it worse.

Interfering headaches (moderate to severe): These started the day of the accident, and the patient has had these headaches every day since the accident. She can awaken with them, and they last all day, sometimes waxing and waning, but mostly it is all day. It is also throbbing with severe pressure, and the pain is in the same location as just described. There is no prodrome or aura, and there is also nausea, photophobia, phonophobia, lacrimation, and she will go to bed, if possible.

Irritating headaches (annoying): These started in her twenties, and they were occasional. The patient has not had any of these headaches since the accident, because they are all interfering and incapacitating headaches. She was able to abort these headaches prior to the accident with over-the-counter medication. It was a dull ache in the frontal part of her head.

Menstrual history: Began at age 14 and was within normal limits. The patient never got headaches during her menstrual periods. She was on birth control pills at age 20 for six months with no adverse effects. In 1978, the patient had a partial hysterectomy for cysts in her uterus and still has her ovaries.

Past history: The patient was most probably a cesarean section delivery. There is no history of enuresis or unexplained abdominal cramps pre-puberty. There is no history of car sickness as a child. There is no history of meningitis, encephalitis, scarlet fever or rheumatic fever. There were no head injuries as a child.

Habits: She does not drink, and she smokes one pack of cigarettes in two days.

Medical history: The patient has been treated for high blood pressure since 1990 and is on Tenormin 50 mg a day for her blood pressure. She also has been diagnosed as having mitral valve prolapse, she has an enlarged heart, and she has angina occasionally. The patient had a back injury in 1988, which was a work-related injury. Other than that, the patient's medical history is essentially negative.

Review of systems: Pulmonary, negative, gastrointestinal, negative, urogenital, negative.

Surgical history: The patient had a T&A at age 14, and a bunionectomy in 1991, both left and right. She had a fibrous dysplasia, left check, in 1989, and a partial hysterectomy in 1978 as discussed before.

Psychiatric history: Negative.

Family history: Her father is living, age 70 with no headache history. Her mother living, age 72 with no headache history. There is a brother, age 46, and four sisters ages 50, 49, 48, and 44, all with no headache history. The patient was married from age 41 to present. There are five children, three boys ages 25, 23, and 21, and two girls ages 24 and 22 all with no headache history.

Current medications: The patient is currently taking Carisoprodol 350 mg one tablet 3 times a day, Hydrocodone 5 mg one tablet 3 times a day, which she has been taking daily for two to three weeks, and Tenormin 50 mg for her blood pressure. The patient has previously taken Corgard for her heart problem. She has been a bunch of non-steroidal anti-inflammatories, Naprosyn, Orudis, Voltaren, Feldene, Motrin, and Indocin (for the back problem).

Doctors seen in the past for headaches: I received a note form [...], her orthopedic doctor, who diagnosed her as having occipital headaches with visual blurring. The patient also saw an ophthalmologist and her work-up was negative.

Tests done in the past: The patient had a cervical MRI which showed an abnormal cervical bending as in ligament tear at one level.

Treatments tried in the past: The patient had biofeedback for her back problem, which helps her to relax.

Physical examination: Height 5'5$^1/_2$", weight 145 pounds, pulse 72, left BP 130/84, right BP 130/86. The face did not show any asymmetry. The temporomandibular joint area was grossly normal. The eyes appeared normal. Conjunctivae were clear and the pupils reacted equally to light and accommodation. Retinal fundus examination revealed no papilledema and no abnormalities with the arteries and veins. There were no bruits over the supraorbital region. The nose appeared normal. The auditory canals were clear and the tympanic membranes appeared intact. The mouth and throat appeared normal. Gums, tongue, buccal mucosa, and teeth were grossly normal. The neck was supple and there were no masses felt in the thyroid gland. Carotid bruits could not be heard. Cervical nodes were not enlarged. The lungs were clear to auscultation and percussion. The heart had a regular sinus rhythm with no murmurs. The abdomen was soft and nontender. A rectal or vaginal exam was not done.

Neurological examination: Cranial nerve II: Visual fields were grossly normal. III, IV and VI: No strabismus, nystagmus, or ptosis. V: Normal sensation and corneal reflex. VII: Normal facial movements (wrinkle, frown, smile, and strength of eyelids). VIII: Normal Weber and Rinne. IX and X: Good gag reflex. XI: Normal sternocleidomastoid and trapezius. XII: Normal protrusion and strength of tongue. Cerebellar: Negative Rhomberg. Normal finger-to-nose, diadochokinesis, heel-shin, tandem, and heel and toes walking. Motor system: No atrophy, fasciculations, wasting, or tremors. Good muscle strength in arms, wrists, fingers, and legs. Sensory system: Superficial tactile, pain, and vibrations (wrists, elbows, knees, and ankles) were normal. Normal motion and positions of fingers and toes. Normal 2-point discrimination. Reflexes: Normal 1+ to 2+ reflexes of triceps, biceps, knee jerk, ankle jerk, etc. Normal pulses in dorsalis pedis, posterior tibial and popliteal.

DIAGNOSES

1. Post traumatic migraine-like headache.
2. Post traumatic cervicogenic headache.
3. Preexisting annoying muscle tension headache.

IMPRESSION

This pleasant 43-year-old woman had a significant accident on 00/00/93, as previously described. Since that time, she has been having moderate to incapacitating headaches almost a daily basis. The pain seems to start in the posterior cervical region and runs cephalad to the frontal and periorbital regions.

I suggested to the patient that she have a posterior cervical regional block of C1, 2, and 3, and also ambulatory infusion of Dihydroergotamine via a PICC line.

Because of her previous history of having mitral valve prolapse, I called her doctor, Dr. [...], who is a cardiologist, but he was out and I spoke to her nurse. I told the nurse that I wanted to start this therapy of a medication that is a venoconstrictor, not a vasoconstrictor, and I want clearance from Dr. [...] to go ahead with this treatment. However, we will start her off with a posterior cervical regional block of C1, 2, and 3, as soon as possible.

The cervicogenic component will also need to be addressed and consideration for cervical facet blocks with fluoroscopic guidance would be a reasonable option. If in fact this is a cervicogenic headache problem, then unless it is addressed, the patient will remain symptomatic.

After we are to break the cycle of everyday headaches, the patient will then be placed on the appropriate medication to prevent them from coming back.

Thank you once again for referring this pleasant patient. If there are any questions, please do not hesitate to call or write.

Sincerely,

BERNARD SWERDLOW, M.D.

MEDICAL HEADACHE HISTORY

Name: Elizabeth **Age:** 43 **Sex** F **Date:** 8/16/93

Date of Birth: 0/00/49 **Birthplace:** SC **Race:** B **Education:** 1 yr. college

Occupation: Unemployed **Accident:** 1993

Armed Services & Type of Discharge: N/A

PAST HISTORY:

1.	Did you have a normal birth?		Yes	No
	a) forceps used?		Yes	No
	b) cesarean section?		<u>Yes</u>	No
2.	Did you have problems with bedwetting?		Yes	<u>No</u>
	a) If yes, age bedwetting stopped		______	
3.	Were you car sick as a child (motion)?		Yes	<u>No</u>
	a) If yes, how severe?	Slight	Moderate	Severe
4.	Did you have unexplained abdominal cramps as a child?		Yes	<u>No</u>
5.	Did you have any of the following illnesses in childhood?			
	a) meningitis		Yes	<u>No</u>
	b) encephalitis		Yes	<u>No</u>
	c) scarlet fever		Yes	<u>No</u>
	d) rheumatic fever		Yes	<u>No</u>
6.	Did you have any head injuries as a child?		Yes	<u>No</u>
	a) If yes, please explain: ______			
7.	Were you treated for emotional illness as a child?		Yes	<u>No</u>

HABITS:

8.	Do you drink alcohol?	Yes	<u>No</u>
	a) If yes, what kind and how much? ______		
	b) Does alcohol bring on or aggravate a headache?	Yes	No
9.	Do you smoke?	<u>Yes</u>	No
	a) If yes, how much? 1 pack every 2 days		
	b) Does smoking or smoke-filled rooms cause or aggravate headaches?	Yes	<u>No</u>
10.	Do you drink caffeinated beverages?	<u>Yes</u>	No
	a) If yes, how much? ______		

MENSTRUAL HISTORY:

At what age did menses begin? 14 Were they regular or irregular? WNL
How were they related to your headache? N/A
Are you or were you ever on Birth Control Pills? Yes Did they affect your headache? No
Have you had a hysterectomy, partial or total, and why? Partial, 1978. Cysts
Are you in menopause, and if yes, how long? No
Are you on hormones, and if yes, which ones? No

HEADACHE ASSESSMENT FORM

HA PROFILE	INCAPACITATING #3	INTERFERING #2	IRRITATING #1
ONSET (Years ago and frequency)	1 day after accident Every day for 3 months	Day of accident, every day since 3 mo. after accident	Since 20s, occasionally
CURRENT FREQUENCY	1 – 2/week	Every day	None since accident
TIME OF ONSET	Anytime	Anytime, can awaken with	Anytime
DURATION	2 hrs to 12 hrs	All day, off and on	1 hr. with OTC meds
CHARACTER	Throbbing and severe pressure	Same, less intense	Dull ache
PRODROME OR AURA	N/A	N/A	N/A
ASSOCIATING FEATURES	Nausea; Vomiting; Sensitivity to Light? Noise? Odors? Do you get pale or flush? Do your eyes or nose run? Does your nose get stuffy? Do the whites of your eyes get red? Does your eyelid droop? Do you pace, or go to bed?	Nausea; Vomiting; Sensitivity to Light? Noise? Odors? Do you get pale or flush? Do your eyes or nose run? Does your nose get stuffy? Do the whites of your eyes get red? Does your eyelid droop? Do you pace, or go to bed?	Nausea; Vomiting; Sensitivity to Light? Noise? Odors? Do you get pale or flush? Do your eyes or nose run? Does your nose get stuffy? Do the whites of your eyes get red? Does your eyelid droop? Do you pace, or go to bed?
PRECIPITATING OR AGGRAVATING FEATURES	Head movement	N/A	N/A

LOCATION: Mark the location for each type of headache with a different color pen.

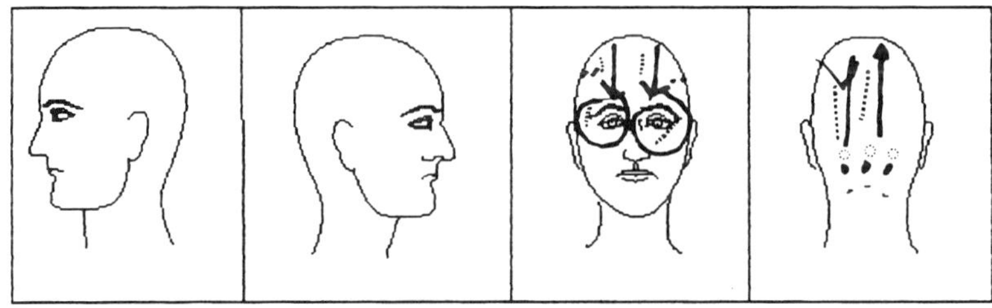

MEDICAL HISTORY:

Have you ever been or are you currently being treated for any of the following?

a) high blood pressure	Yes (underlined)	No (underlined)
b) stomach ulcers	Yes	No
c) asthma	Yes	No (underlined)
d) allergies	Yes	No (underlined)
e) pneumonia	Yes	No (underlined)
f) kidney problems	Yes	No (underlined)
g) low blood sugar	Yes	No (underlined)
h) glaucoma	Yes	No (underlined)
i) diabetes	Yes	No (underlined)
j) heart problems	Yes (underlined)	No

If you answered yes to any of the above, please describe: High blood pressure diagnosed 1990, take medication. Angina occasionally, MVP, enlarged heart, 1986.

List all other medical problems you have had in the past. Include date diagnosed and treatment. DO NOT LIST OPERATIONS

Back injury, 1988. MVP.

SURGICAL HISTORY (List operations and dates performed)

None.

PSYCHIATRIC HISTORY (List visits with counselors, psychologists, etc., and type of treatment)

Tonsillectomy & adenoidectomy, age 14. 1991, bunionectomy. Fibrous dysplasia left cheeck, 1989. Partial hysterectomy, 1978.

ACCIDENTS IN ADULT LIFE (Briefly describe any accident that caused any blow to the head or that you feel is related to your headache)

Car accident, 1993. Passenger with seat belt. Stopped and rear-ended in a 7-car pileup. Flexion extension injury. Sought medical treatment 2 days later. Headaches began immediately after accident. Had occasional #1 headache after accident.

FAMILY HISTORY:

1. Is your father living? Yes (underlined) No
   - Age 70
   - Cause of death ____
   - Was there a headache history? Yes No (underlined)
2. Is your mother living? Yes (underlined) No
   - Age 72
   - Cause of death ____
   - Was there a headache history? Yes No (underlined)

3. Ages of brothers---Circle the ones with headache
   46
4. Ages of sisters---Circle the ones with headache
   50 49 48 44
5. List any other blood relatives with a history of severe headaches.
   None

MARITAL HISTORY:
List marriages:

		Did spouse have headaches?		
1st marriage age 41	to Present	Did spouse have headaches?	Yes	No
2nd marriage age ____	to ____	Did spouse have headaches?	Yes	No
3rd marriage age ____	to ____	Did spouse have headaches?	Yes	No

Age of current spouse: 50

List ages and sex of all children:

Age	Sex	Headaches?		
25	M	Headaches?	Yes	No
24	F	Headaches?	Yes	No
23	M	Headaches?	Yes	No
22	F	Headaches?	Yes	No
21	M	Headaches?	Yes	No
____	____	Headaches?	Yes	No

STRESS FACTORS:

List any factors that may be affecting your headaches (money, loneliness, sexual problems, work, etc.)
Physical conditions limited.

VEGETATIVE SIGNS:

1.	Do you have trouble falling asleep?	Yes	No
2.	Do you have trouble staying asleep?	Yes	No
3.	Has your appetite decreased?	Yes	No
4.	Have you gained or lost weight in the past year?	Yes	No
5.	Have you felt tearful or depressed lately?	Yes	No
6.	Have you had any thoughts of wanting to die?	Yes	No
7.	Have you been forgetful lately?	Yes	No
8.	Any other changes in your normal day-to-day living? ____		

Please list any medications you are allergic or sensitive to: Codeine.

Please list any medications you are currently taking (including dosages and frequency per day):
Carisoprodol, 350 mg t.i.d., Hydrocodone, 5 mg t.i.d., Tenormin 50 mg q.d.

PREVIOUS CARE:

1. List doctors who have treated you for headaches: Dr.B.

2. List any tests you have had for your headache (e.g., EEG, CT scan, MRI, X-Ray, etc.):
MRI (normal).

3. List any other treatment you have had for your headache (e.g., biofeedback, acupuncture, chiropractic, or any other treatment you had):
Biofeedback.

January 11, 1993

[...] Insurance Company

[Address omitted]

ATTN: Adjuster, Ms. [...]

RE: Robert

Dear Ms. [...]:

Thank you for your referral of Robert [...], who is being seen for evaluation only.

This is a 46-year-old male born on 00/00/47 in [...]. He has been living in [...] for [...] years. He is an ex-marine, who served from 1965 to 1976 with an honorable discharge. He currently works as a general manager for [...]. The patient states that he had a significant accident on 00/00/85 in which he lifted a 55-gallon drum that fell over and pulled muscles in his neck. He states that the drum fell and that as he tried to push it up, he got a severe headache and passed out. He was taken to a chiropractor. He stated that he had occasional annoying headaches prior to the accident.

HEADACHE PROFILE

Incapacitating headaches: These started the day of the accident. He had them 2 or 3 times per week for a period of time and currently gets these attacks 2 to 4 times per month. They can last from 3 hours to half a day. It is a sharp, steady pain in the posterior cervical, occipital, temporal and lateral orbital regions. There is no aura. He has associated features of nausea, photophobia, pallor, and he has to go to bed. Coughing or movement of his neck will aggravate the situation.

Interfering headaches (moderate to severe): These started weeks after the accident. He gets 4 to 5 attacks a week and they also can last 3 hours to half a day. The pain is similar to the incapacitating headache and the location is also the same. Associated features are also nausea, photophobia, pallor, and he will go to bed.

Irritating headaches (annoying): These started in his 20s, but he does not have these headaches now. He was able to abort these headaches in the past, prior to the accident, with over-the-counter medications. It was a dull ache in the frontal part of his head.

Past history: The patient was most probably a normal delivery. There is no history of enuresis or unexplained abdominal cramps pre-puberty. There is no history of car sickness as a child. There is no history of meningitis, encephalitis, scarlet fever or rheumatic fever. There were no head injuries as a child.

Habits: He does not drink or smoke.

Medical history: He was diagnosed as having hypertension 15 years ago and is currently taking medications, described later. He was also diagnosed as having gastric ulcers 20 years ago. This has resolved. He had pneumonia at age 2. He had some renal calculi in 1990 and 1991 that was treated with Lythotrip.

Review of systems: Pulmonary, negative. Cardiovascular, negative. Gastrointestinal, negative.

Surgical history: He had an appendectomy in 1960. He had some knee surgery in 1989. T&A at age 2.

Psychiatric history: Negative.

Family history: His father is deceased, age 44, of a coronary with no headache history. His mother is living at age 67 without headaches.

Marital history: The patient has been married from age 21 to present. His wife is 43. There are three children, two boys, 22 and 20, and a girl 17, with no headaches.

Allergies to medications: The patient cannot take Nubain which causes nausea and vomiting. Dimethylamine, Dioxy, dimethyltetracycline, tetracycline, Vibramycin, Vectrin, and mynacine cause shortness of breath.

Medications: He is currently taking Minoxidil 10 mg per day for his blood pressure, Furosemide 80 mg twice a day, Topraxl 100 mg per day, K-Dur 20 mg per day, and allopurinol 300 mg per day. He also takes 3 to 4 Butalbital pain pills per day. He also takes Nizoral one per day for fungi. He has been given Percocet for his headaches. He has taken Inderal in the past which he believes helped his headache. When the Inderal stopped working, he was placed on another type of beta-blocker but he does not know the name. He has been on Flexeril and Parafon Forte.

Previous work-up: He has seen [four doctors named]. He has had CT scans in 1991, without contrast, which were normal. An MRI of his head in January 1993 was normal. He saw a chiropractor who used weights or traction for his neck, and physical therapy, with which he did not have much success.

Physical exam: Height 5'11$^1/_2$", weight 210 pounds, pulse 80, left arm BP 168/104, right arm BP 162/106. The face did not show any asymmetry. The temporomandibular joint area was grossly normal. The eyes appeared normal. Conjunctivae were clear and the pupils reacted equally to light and accommodation. Retinal fundus examination revealed no papilledema and no abnormalities with the arteries and veins. There were no bruits over the supraorbital region. The nose appeared normal. The auditory canals were clear and the tympanic membranes appeared intact. The mouth and throat appeared normal. Gums, tongue, buccal mucosa, and teeth were grossly normal. In the neck there were multiple myofascial trigger points in the right upper trapezius and splenius capitis regions. There were no masses felt in the thyroid gland. Carotid bruits could not be heard. Cervical nodes were not enlarged. The lungs were clear to auscultation and percussion. The heart had a regular sinus rhythm with no murmurs. The abdomen was soft and nontender. A rectal examination was not done.

Neurological examination: Cranial nerve II: Visual fields were grossly normal. III, IV and VI: No strabismus, nystagmus, or ptosis. V: Normal sensation and corneal reflex. VII: Normal facial movements (wrinkle, frown, smile, and strength of eyelids). VIII: Normal Weber and Rinne. IX and X: Good gag reflex. XI: Normal sternocleidomastoid and trapezius. XII: Normal protrusion and strength of tongue. Cerebellar: Negative Rhomberg. Normal finger-to-nose, diadochokinesis, heel-shin, tandem, and heel and toes walking. Motor system: No atrophy, fasciculations, wasting, or tremors. Good muscle strength in arms, wrists, fingers, and legs. Sensory system: Superficial tactile, pain, and vibrations (wrists, elbows, knees, and ankles) were normal. Normal motion and positions of fingers and toes. Normal 2-point discrimination. Reflexes: Normal 1+ reflexes of triceps, biceps, knee jerk, ankle jerk, etc. Normal pulses in dorsalis pedis, posterior tibial and popliteal.

DIAGNOSES

1. Post traumatic headache.
2. Rule out post traumatic vascular headache.
3. Post traumatic cervicogenic headache with myofascial trigger points.

IMPRESSION/RECOMMENDATION

This pleasant 46-year-old gentleman comes in with moderate to incapacitating headaches that started after an accident (described above) on 00/00/85. The patient appears to have had a cervicogenic strain and since that time has been having these headaches. The headaches appear to have a vascular component in that there is some nausea, photophobia and pallor with the headaches. The patient has been treated with a beta-blocker and has had some improvement some time in the past, according to his history. In examining the patient, there were obvious trigger points with the patient having a "jump sign" that precipitated pain in his head.

I recommend that the patient be placed on calcium channel blockers as a means of controlling the vascular component of his headache and that he have myofascial trigger points with deep neuromuscular mobilization and kinetic activity in order to break these spasms.

The cervicogenic component will also need to be addressed and consideration for cervical facet blocks with fluoroscopic guidance would be a reasonable option. If this is a cervicogenic headache, then unless this component is addressed properly, the patient will remain symptomatic.

Thank you for permitting me to see this patient. If there are any questions, please do not hesitate to call or write.

Sincerely,

BERNARD SWERDLOW, M.D.

MEDICAL HEADACHE HISTORY

Name: Robert **Age:** 46 **Sex** M **Date:** 1/11/93

Date of Birth: 00/00/47 **Birthplace:** PA **Race:** W **Education:** High school

Occupation: General Manager **Accident:** 00/00/85

Armed Services & Type of Discharge: Marines, 1965-1976.

PAST HISTORY:

1.	Did you have a normal birth?		Yes	No
	a) forceps used?		Yes	No
	b) cesarean section?		Yes	No
2.	Did you have problems with bedwetting?		Yes	No
	a) If yes, age bedwetting stopped		________	
3.	Were you car sick as a child (motion)?		Yes	No
	a) If yes, how severe?	Slight	Moderate	Severe
4.	Did you have unexplained abdominal cramps as a child?		Yes	No
5.	Did you have any of the following illnesses in childhood?			
	a) meningitis		Yes	No
	b) encephalitis		Yes	No
	c) scarlet fever		Yes	No
	d) rheumatic fever		Yes	No
6.	Did you have any head injuries as a child?		Yes	No
	a) If yes, please explain:________			
7.	Were you treated for emotional illness as a child?		Yes	No

HABITS:

8.	Do you drink alcohol?	Yes	No
	a) If yes, what kind and how much?________		
	b) Does alcohol bring on or aggravate a headache?	Yes	No
9.	Do you smoke?	Yes	No
	a) If yes, how much?________		
	b) Does smoking or smoke-filled rooms cause or aggravate headaches?	Yes	No
10.	Do you drink caffeinated beverages?	Yes	No
	a) If yes, how much? Pepsi or coke, 1 or 2/day		

MENSTRUAL HISTORY:

At what age did menses begin?______ Were they regular or irregular?________
How were they related to your headache?________
Are you or were you ever on Birth Control Pills?______ Did they affect your headache? ______
Have you had a hysterectomy, partial or total, and why?________
Are you in menopause, and if yes, how long?________
Are you on hormones, and if yes, which ones?________

HEADACHE ASSESSMENT FORM

HA PROFILE	INCAPACITATING #3	INTERFERING #2	IRRITATING #1
ONSET (Years ago and frequency)	Day of accident 2 to 3/week	Several weeks after accident	In 20s, occasionally
CURRENT FREQUENCY	1 every 2 to 4 months	4 to 5/week	None now
TIME OF ONSET	Anytime	Anytime	Anytime
DURATION	1 to 3 hours	1 to 3 hours	1 hour with OTC meds
CHARACTER	Same as #2, more intense	Sharp, steady pain like "eating ice ream too fast"	Dull ache
PRODROME OR AURA	N/A	N/A	N/A
ASSOCIATING FEATURES	Nausea: Vomiting: Sensitivity to Light? Noise? Odors? Do you get pale or flush? Do your eyes or nose run? Does your nose get stuffy? Does the white of your eyes get red? Does your eyelid droop? Do you pace, or go to bed?	Nausea: Vomiting: Sensitivity to Light? Noise? Odors? Do you get pale or flush? Do your eyes or nose run? Does your nose get stuffy? Does the white of your eyes get red? Does your eyelid droop? Do you pace, or go to bed?	Nausea; Vomiting; Sensitivity to Light? Noise? Odors? Do you get pale or flush? Do your eyes or nose run? Does your nose get stuffy? Does the white of your eyes get red? Does your eyelid droop? Do you pace, or go to bed?
PRECIPITATING OR AGGRAVATING FEATURES	Coughing	Coughing	N/A

LOCATION: Mark the location for each type of headache with a different color pen.

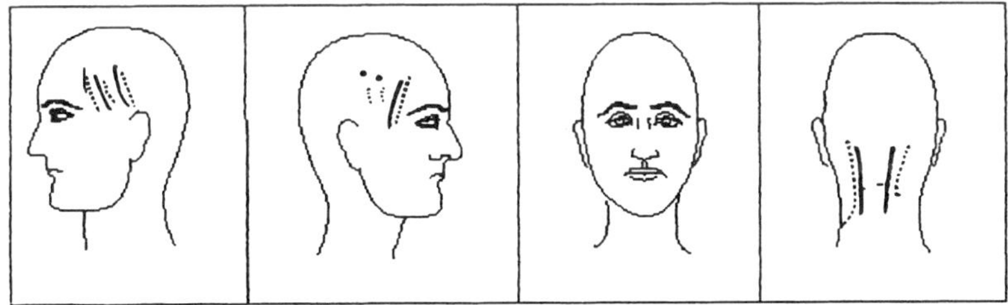

MEDICAL HISTORY:

Have you ever been or are you currently being treated for any of the following?

a) high blood pressure	Yes	No
b) stomach ulcers	Yes	No
c) asthma	Yes	No
d) allergies	Yes	No
e) pneumonia	Yes	No
f) kidney problems	Yes	No
g) low blood sugar	Yes	No
h) glaucoma	Yes	No
i) diabetes	Yes	No
j) heart problems	Yes	No

If you answered yes to any of the above, please describe: High blood pressure diagnosed 15 yrs. ago, take medication. Ulcers diagnosed 20 yrs. ago, resolved. Pneumonia, age 2. Kidney stones 2 yrs. ago, lithotripsy.

List all other medical problems you have had in the past. Include date diagnosed and treatment.
DO NOT LIST OPERATIONS

See above.

SURGICAL HISTORY (List operations and dates performed)

Appendix and bowel scraping in 1960. Knee surgery in 1989. Tonsillectomy, age 2.

PSYCHIATRIC HISTORY (List visits with counselors, psychologists, etc., and type of treatment)

None.

ACCIDENTS IN ADULT LIFE (Briefly describe any accident that caused any blow to the head or that you feel is related to your headache)

1985 – Lifted 55 gallon drum that fell over and it pulled muscles in neck. After that, severe headaches and passing out. Headaches began that evening. Saw chiropractor. Had occasional #1 headache before accident.

FAMILY HISTORY:

1. Is your father living? Yes No
   Age_________
   Cause of death 44, coronary heart attack
   Was there a headache history? Yes No
2. Is your mother living? Yes No
   Age 67
   Cause of death_________
   Was there a headache history? Yes No

3. Ages of brothers---Circle the ones with headache
   None
4. Ages of sisters---Circle the ones with headache
   None
5. List any other blood relatives with a history of severe headaches.
   None

MARITAL HISTORY:
List marriages:

1st marriage age 21 to Present Did spouse have headaches?	Yes	No
2nd marriage age _____ to _______ Did spouse have headaches?	Yes	No
3rd marriage age _____ to _______ Did spouse have headaches?	Yes	No

Age of current spouse: 43

List ages and sex of all children:

Age 22 Sex M Headaches?	Yes	No
Age 20 Sex M Headaches?	Yes	No
Age 17 Sex F Headaches?	Yes	No
Age _____ Sex ______ Headaches?	Yes	No

STRESS FACTORS:

List any factors that may be affecting your headaches (money, loneliness, sexual problems, work, etc.)
Some stress in managerial problems.

VEGETATIVE SIGNS:

1.	Do you have trouble falling asleep?	Yes	No
2.	Do you have trouble staying asleep?	Yes	No
3.	Has your appetite decreased?	Yes	No
4.	Have you gained or lost weight in the past year?	Yes	No
5.	Have you felt tearful or depressed lately?	Yes	No
6.	Have you had any thoughts of wanting to die?	Yes	No
7.	Have you been forgetful lately?	Yes	No
8.	Any other changes in your normal day-to-day living?________		

Please list any medications you are allergic or sensitive to: Nubain, Dimethylamine, Dioxy, Dimethyltetracycline, Hydrochloride, Tetracycline, Vibramycin, Vectrin, and mynacine.

Please list any medications you are currently taking (including dosages and frequency per day):
Minoxidil, 10 mg q.d., Furosemide, 80 mg b.i.d., Topraxl, 100 mg q.d., K-Dur, 20 mg q.d., Allopurinol, 300 mg q.d., Butalbital, q.6-8h., Nizoral q.d. for fungus, Percocet, p.r.n., Fiorinal 4-5/wk.

PREVIOUS CARE:

1, List doctors who have treated you for headaches: Dr. P, Dr. L, Dr. H, Dr. O.

2, List any tests you have had for your headache (e.g., EEG, CT scan, MRI, X-Ray, etc.):
CT scan – normal (1991), X-rays, MRI of head normal (1993).

3, List any other treatment you have had for your headache (e.g., biofeedback, acupuncture, chiropractic, or any other treatment you had):
Chiropractic. Physical therapy.

July 6, 1994

[Doctor's name and address omitted]

RE: VICKIE

Dear Dr. [...]:

Thank you for the referral of Ms. Vickie [...] for headache evaluation and treatment.

The patient is a 29-year-old female born 00/00/64 in [...]. She has completed a high school education and is currently employed as a secretary.

HEADACHE PROFILE

The patient was involved in a motor vehicle accident on 00/00/93 when she was driving an automobile and restrained with a seat belt. She was stopped at a red light and was rear-ended by another car. The patient suffered a flexion/extension injury of the neck. She did not suffer loss of consciousness nor direct head trauma. The next day the patient noticed cervical pain and headache and was seen at your office. She does note that immediately after the accident she had cervical and headache symptoms. Prior to the motor vehicle accident, she had only rate #3 or incapacitating headaches that are consistent with migraine-type headaches.

Incapacitating headaches: The patient developed these headaches as a child and they were noted to be rare in frequency, approximately one to two times per year. Frequency has persisted, i.e., one to two headaches per year. The patient can awaken with these headaches and they will last anywhere from 42 to 72 hours. The pain is characterized as a severe pressure with throbbing sensations localized in the left periorbital and temporal region. There is no prodrome with these headaches. They are, however, associated with nausea, vomiting, photophobia, phonophobia, sensitivity to odors, pallor, and the patient will seek bed rest if possible. The patient notes that movement or exertion will increase her headache symptoms.

Interfering headaches (moderate to severe): These headaches were noted the day of the accident and the patient has suffered from these headaches daily since. The patient will awaken with these headaches and they are constant in duration. The patient describes the pain as a constant dull ache located in the right occipital cervical junction and bilateral occipital region of the head. There is no prodrome with these headaches and they are associated with nausea, some photophobia and some phonophobia. The patient will seek bed rest if possible and notes that exertion will increase symptoms.

Irritating headaches (annoying): The patient noted these headaches began when she was in her teens and they have essentially resolved as she has grown older. These headaches occurred at any time of the day and they were easily relieved with over-the-counter medication.

Menstrual history: Began at age 13 and is reported to be normal except for heavy flow. The patient does not note any increase in headache symptoms with her menstrual cycle.

Past history: The patient was most probably a normal delivery. There is no history of enuresis or unexplained abdominal cramps pre-puberty. There is no history of car sickness as a child. There is no history of meningitis, encephalitis, scarlet fever or rheumatic fever. There were no head injuries as a child.

Habits: The patient does not drink alcohol and she does not smoke, but she does note that secondary smoke will increase her headache symptoms. The patient consumes 2 caffeinated beverages per day.

Medical history: The patient has no history of high blood pressure, stomach ulcers, asthma, allergies, pneumonia, kidney problems, low blood sugar, glaucoma, diabetes, or heart problems.

Review of systems: Pulmonary negative, cardiovascular negative, gastrointestinal negative, urogenital negative.

Surgical history: Cesarean sections in 1981 and 1982.

Psychiatric history: Monthly visit with psychologist and treatment with Prozac for depression.

Family history: Her father is living, age 62, with no headache history. Her mother is living, age 56, with a history of #3 or incapacitating headaches. The patient has 2 brothers and 3 sisters, one of whom is deceased from a massive heart attack, and this sister did have a severe headache history. The patient is currently married and has one son and daughter. Her 12-year-old son does have a headache history.

Stress factors: The patient notes work as a stress factor that increases her symptoms.

Vegetative signs: The patient notes no sleep disturbance, but does note depression without suicidal ideation.

Allergies to medications: NKA.

Current medications: The patient is currently taking Prozac 20 mg q.d.

Doctors seem in the past for headaches: Previous care for headaches includes Dr. [...] and chiropractic medicine, which is of help, but unfortunately the symptoms return. Neuromuscular massage also helps, but unfortunately the symptoms return.

Physical examination: Height 5'4", weight 115 pounds, pulse 72, respirations 18, left BP 110/64, right BP 118/70. The face did not show any asymmetry. The temporomandibular joint area was grossly normal. The eyes appeared normal. Conjunctivae were clear and the pupils reacted equally to light and accommodation. Retinal fundus examination revealed no papilledema and no abnormalities with the arteries and veins. There were no bruits over the supraorbital region. The nose appeared normal. The auditory canals were clear and the tympanic membranes appeared intact. The mouth and throat appeared normal. Gums, tongue, buccal mucosa, and teeth were grossly normal. Neck: The patient has exquisite tenderness on palpation of the right occipital cervical junction with radiation down the splenius capitis muscle group and forward into the frontal region of the head. Carotid bruits could not be heard. Cervical nodes were not enlarged. The lungs were clear to auscultation and percussion. The heart had a regular sinus rhythm with no murmurs. The abdomen was soft and nontender. A rectal or vaginal exam was not done.

Neurological examination: Cranial nerve II: Visual fields were grossly normal. III, IV and VI: No strabismus, nystagmus, or ptosis. V: Normal sensation and corneal reflex. VII: Normal facial movements (wrinkle, frown, smile, and strength of eyelids). VIII: Normal Weber and Rinne. IX and X: Good gag reflex. XI: Normal sternocleidomastoid and trapezius. XII: Normal protrusion and strength of tongue. Cerebellar: Negative Rhomberg. Normal finger-to-nose, diadochokinesis, heel-shin, tandem, and heel and toes walking. Motor system: No atrophy, fasciculations, wasting, or tremors. Good muscle strength in arms, wrists, fingers, and legs. Sensory system: Superficial tactile, pain, and vibrations (wrists, elbows, knees, and ankles) were normal. Normal motion and positions of fingers and toes. Normal 2-point discrimination. Reflexes: Normal 2+ reflexes of triceps, biceps, knee jerk, ankle jerk, etc. Normal pulses in dorsalis pedis, posterior tibial and popliteal.

DIAGNOSES

1. Post traumatic headache syndrome by history. The patient headaches that originate in the cervical region and then move forward into the midline in the forehead area. These headaches are constant and described as a dull ache. These are clearly different from her preexisting migraine headaches.
2. Cervicogenic headaches secondary to cervical sprain and strain.
3. History of migraine headaches, 1 to 2 per year. The patient does not give classic history of migraine headache with throbbing periorbital pain associated with gastrointestinal and sensory changes and exacerbated by movement or straining. These headaches are clearly different from her post traumatic accident headaches.

I would recommend:

1. CT scan of the brain to rule out any structural lesions since the patient has been symptomatic for essentially a year with a constant, unremitting headache.
2. Headache profile to rule out any metabolic causes of the patient's symptoms.

THERAPY

1. I would begin with Bellergal-S q.h.s. to attempt to prevent the headaches that the patient awakens with.
2. Increase Prozac to 40 mg b.i.d. at 8:00 a.m. and noon to increase serotonin and hopefully reduce symptoms via the serotonergic mechanism.
3. Series of 3 cervical plexus regional blocks in an attempt to break the pain cycle and also to facilitate the treatment of Dr. [...], which I have recommended to her to continue.
4. Consideration for cervical facet blocks with fluoroscopic guidance will be considered.

The patient will be seen on a weekly basis for blocks and formally evaluated in 4 weeks in the context of an office visit where further medical management and evaluation will occur.

Dr. [...], thank you again for the kind referral of this most pleasant patient. If there are any questions or anything further I can add, please contact me. I will keep you updated regarding the patient's progress.

Sincerely,

[Doctor's name omitted]

MEDICAL HEADACHE HISTORY

Name: Vickie **Age:** 29 **Sex** F **Date:** 7/6/94

Date of Birth: 0/00/64 **Birthplace:** FL **Race:** W **Education:** High school

Occupation: Secretary **Accident:** 1993

Armed Services & Type of Discharge: N/A

PAST HISTORY:

1.	Did you have a normal birth?		Yes (underlined)	No
	a) forceps used?		Yes	No (underlined)
	b) cesarean section?		Yes	No (underlined)
2.	Did you have problems with bedwetting?		Yes	No (underlined)
	a) If yes, age bedwetting stopped		______	
3.	Were you car sick as a child (motion)?		Yes	No (underlined)
	a) If yes, how severe?	Slight	Moderate	Severe
4.	Did you have unexplained abdominal cramps as a child?		Yes	No (underlined)
5.	Did you have any of the following illnesses in childhood?			
	a) meningitis		Yes	No (underlined)
	b) encephalitis		Yes	No (underlined)
	c) scarlet fever		Yes	No (underlined)
	d) rheumatic fever		Yes	No (underlined)
6.	Did you have any head injuries as a child?		Yes	No (underlined)
	a) If yes, please explain:______			
7.	Were you treated for emotional illness as a child?		Yes	No (underlined)

HABITS:

8.	Do you drink alcohol?	Yes	No (underlined)
	a) If yes, what kind and how much?______		
	b) Does alcohol bring on or aggravate a headache?	Yes	No
9.	Do you smoke?	Yes	No (underlined)
	a) If yes, how much?______		
	b) Does smoking or smoke-filled rooms cause or aggravate headaches?	Yes (underlined)	No
10.	Do you drink caffeinated beverages?	Yes (underlined)	No
	a) If yes, how much? 2 a day		

MENSTRUAL HISTORY:

At what age did menses begin? 13 Were they regular or irregular? WNL, heavy flow

How were they related to your headache? N/A

Are you or were you ever on Birth Control Pills? No Did they affect your headache? N/A

Have you had a hysterectomy, partial or total, and why? No

Are you in menopause, and if yes, how long? No

Are you on hormones, and if yes, which ones? No

HEADACHE ASSESSMENT FORM

HA PROFILE	INCAPACITATING #3	INTERFERING #2	IRRITATING #1
ONSET (Years ago and frequency)	As a child, rare 1 to 2/year	Day of accident	In teens, resolved
CURRENT FREQUENCY	1 to 2/year	Every day	N/A
TIME OF ONSET	Can awaken with	Can awaken with	N/A
DURATION	42 to 72 hours	Constant	N/A
CHARACTER	Severe pressure with throbbing sensations	Constant dull ache	N/A
PRODROME OR AURA	N/A	N/A	N/A
ASSOCIATING FEATURES	Nausea; Vomiting; Sensitivity to Light? Noise? Odors? Do you get pale or flush? Do your eyes or nose run? Does your nose get stuffy? Do the whites of your eyes get red? Does your eyelid droop? Do you pace, or go to bed?	Nausea; Vomiting; Sensitivity to Light? Noise? Odors? Do you get pale or flush? Do your eyes or nose run? Does your nose get stuffy? Do the whites of your eyes get red? Does your eyelid droop? Do you pace, or go to bed?	Nausea; Vomiting; Sensitivity to Light? Noise? Odors? Do you get pale or flush? Do your eyes or nose run? Does your nose get stuffy? Do the whites of your eyes get red? Does your eyelid droop? Do you pace, or go to bed?
PRECIPITATING OR AGGRAVATING FEATURES	Movement Exertion	Exertion	N/A

LOCATION: Mark the location for each type of headache with a different color pen.

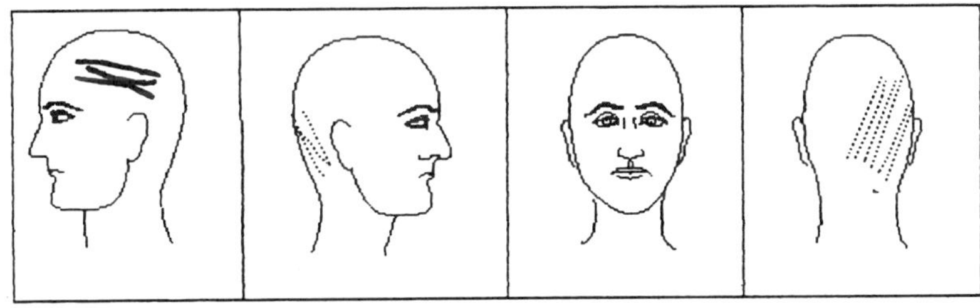

MEDICAL HISTORY:

Have you ever been or are you currently being treated for any of the following?

a) high blood pressure	Yes	No
b) stomach ulcers	Yes	No
c) asthma	Yes	No
d) allergies	Yes	No
e) pneumonia	Yes	No
f) kidney problems	Yes	No
g) low blood sugar	Yes	No
h) glaucoma	Yes	No
i) diabetes	Yes	No
j) heart problems	Yes	No

If you answered yes to any of the above, please describe:____________________

List all other medical problems you have had in the past. Include date diagnosed and treatment.
DO NOT LIST OPERATIONS

None.

SURGICAL HISTORY (List operations and dates performed)

Cesarean sections, 1981 and 1982..

PSYCHIATRIC HISTORY (List visits with counselors, psychologists, etc., and type of treatment)

See Dr. X., monthly for depression. Prozac.

ACCIDENTS IN ADULT LIFE (Briefly describe any accident that caused any blow to the head or that you feel is related to your headache)

Car accident 1993. Driving with seat belt. Stopped at red light, rear-ended by another car.
Flexion-extension injury of neck. No loss of conscious. Went to doctor's office the next day.
Headaches began immediate after accident. Prior to accident had rare #3 headaches.

FAMILY HISTORY:

1. Is your father living? Yes No
   Age 62
   Cause of death____________________
   Was there a headache history? Yes No
2. Is your mother living? Yes No
   Age 56
   Cause of death____________________
   Was there a headache history? Yes No

3. Ages of brothers---Circle the ones with headache
   38 36
4. Ages of sisters---Circle the ones with headache
   39 32 (31) – deceased.
5. List any other blood relatives with a history of severe headaches.
   None

MARITAL HISTORY:

List marriages:

1st marriage age 16 to Present	Did spouse have headaches?	Yes	No
2nd marriage age ___ to ___	Did spouse have headaches?	Yes	No
3rd marriage age ___ to ___	Did spouse have headaches?	Yes	No

Age of current spouse: 32

List ages and sex of all children:

Age 13	Sex F	Headaches?	Yes	No
Age 12	Sex M	Headaches?	Yes	No
Age ___	Sex ___	Headaches?	Yes	No

STRESS FACTORS:

List any factors that may be affecting your headaches (money, loneliness, sexual problems, work, etc.)
Work.

VEGETATIVE SIGNS:

1.	Do you have trouble falling asleep?	Yes	No
2.	Do you have trouble staying asleep?	Yes	No
3.	Has your appetite decreased?	Yes	No
4.	Have you gained or lost weight in the past year?	Yes	No
5.	Have you felt tearful or depressed lately?	Yes	No
6.	Have you had any thoughts of wanting to die?	Yes	No
7.	Have you been forgetful lately?	Yes	No
8.	Any other changes in your normal day-to-day living?		

Please list any medications you are allergic or sensitive to: NKA.

Please list any medications you are currently taking (including dosages and frequency per day):
Prozac, 20 mg q.d.

PREVIOUS CARE:

1. List doctors who have treated you for headaches: Dr. W.

2. List any tests you have had for your headache (e.g., EEG, CT scan, MRI, X-Ray, etc.):
None.

3. List any other treatment you have had for your headache (e.g., biofeedback, acupuncture, chiropractic, or any other treatment you had):
Chiropractic, helps. Neuromuscular massage, helps.

October 3, 1993

[Doctor's name and address omitted]

RE: DIANE

Dear Dr. [...]:

Thank you for the referral of Ms. Diane [...].

This is a 27-year-old woman born 00/00/66 in [...] and living in [...]. She has a BA in [...]. She is a secretary.

She was in an accident on 00/00/92 in which she was driving, with her seat belt. She was going through an intersection when another car ran a stoplight and hit her car and spun it around. She had a flexion-extension injury and was not unconscious. She saw physicians two days later and states her headaches have increased dramatically since the accident.

HEADACHE PROFILE

Incapacitating headaches: This started at age 18 but she only had two in the past 9 years and the ones she had prior to the accident were years before that. Since the accident, she said she is having them two to three times a month. They can last two to three days. It is severe pressure and throbbing 95% on the left side in the periorbital, frontal, occipital, and cervical area. She states that the pain starts in the posterior cervical region and works its way up cephalad. There is no aura. Associated features are some nausea, photophobia, phonophobia, sensitivity to odors, pallor, and movement will make it worse.

Interfering headaches (moderate to severe): This also started at age 18 and they were occasional. Prior to the accident, she might have been getting one every two months. Currently she is getting two to three a week, again coming on at any time, and can last from hours to three days. It is also pressure and throbbing and the location of pain is the same as just described. There is some photophobia, phonophobia, and she will go to bed, if possible.

Irritating headaches (annoying): N/A.

Menstrual history: Began at age 13 andhas been within normal limits. She has not noticed any headaches during this time.

Past history: The patient was most probably a normal delivery. There is no history of enuresis or unexplained abdominal cramps pre-puberty. There is no history of car sickness as a child. There is no history of meningitis, encephalitis, scarlet fever or rheumatic fever. There were no head injuries as a child.

Habits: She says that since the accident she occasionally will drink some wine and will get a headache. She does not smoke.

Medical history: She was diagnosed as having gastric ulcers a year ago and is taking medication on an as-needed basis. She takes Pepcid. She was also diagnosed as having a seizure disorder in 1986. Her first seizure was at age 19, and the last one was four years ago and was diagnosed as petit mal. She currently takes Dilantin 200 mg h.s. and she is being followed by Dr. [...]. This diagnosis was made up at [...] Hospital while she was a college student. The rest of her medical history is essentially negative.

Review of systems: Pulmonary negative, cardiovascular negative, gastrointestinal negative, urogenital negative.

Surgical history: Negative.

Psychiatric history: Negative.

Family history: Her father is living, age 53, with no headaches. Her mother is living, age 52, with no headaches. There are two brothers, ages 35 and 24, with no headaches, and three sisters, ages 40, 39, and 56. The middle one has severe headaches.

Patient is not married and his no children.

Allergies to medications: Ibuprofen causes itchiness and rash.

Current medications: Currently she is taking Esgic when the migraines ocur. She has taken Ergostat in the past, which did not help. She has been on multiple analgesic medications.

Doctors seem in the past for headaches: Her current doctor is Dr. [...].

Tests done in the past: Because of the seizure disorder in 1986, she had a CT scan, MRI, spinal tap, and EEG, and all were normal.

Physical examination: Height 5'7", weight 124 pounds, pulse 74, left BP 118/78, right BP 110/72. The face did not show any asymmetry. The temporomandibular joint area was grossly normal. The eyes appeared normal. Conjunctivae were clear and the pupils reacted equally to light and accommodation. Retinal fundus examination revealed no papilledema and no abnormalities with the arteries and veins. There were no bruits over the supraorbital region. The nose appeared normal. The auditory canals were clear and the tympanic membranes appeared intact. The mouth and throat appeared normal. Gums, tongue, buccal mucosa, and teeth were grossly normal. There were active myofascial trigger points, more on the left than the right, in the middle and upper trapezius region. Carotid bruits could not be heard. Cervical nodes were not enlarged. The lungs were clear to auscultation and percussion. The heart had a regular sinus rhythm with no murmurs. The abdomen was soft and nontender. A rectal or vaginal exam was not done.

Neurological examination: Cranial nerve II: Visual fields were grossly normal. III, IV and VI: No strabismus, nystagmus, or ptosis. V: Normal sensation and corneal reflex. VII: Normal facial movements (wrinkle, frown, smile, and strength of eyelids). VIII: Normal Weber and Rinne. IX and X: Good gag reflex. XI: Normal sternocleidomastoid and trapezius. XII: Normal protrusion and strength of tongue. Cerebellar: Negative Rhomberg. Normal finger-to-nose, diadochokinesis, heel-shin, tandem, and heel and toes walking. Motor system: No atrophy, fasciculations, wasting, or tremors. Good muscle strength in arms, wrists, fingers, and legs. Sensory system: Superficial tactile, pain, and vibrations (wrists, elbows, knees, and ankles) were normal. Normal motion and positions of fingers and toes. Normal 2-point discrimination. Reflexes: Normal 2+ reflexes of triceps, biceps, knee jerk, ankle jerk, etc. Normal pulses in dorsalis pedis, posterior tibial and popliteal.

DIAGNOSES

1. Post traumatic exacerbation of preexisting rare headache.
2. Post traumatic cervicogenic migraine without aura.
3. Post traumatic muscle contraction headache with active myofascial trigger points.
4. Preexisting rare (two attacks in nine years) migraine.
5. Preexisting rare (one attack every two months) vascular headache.
6. Petit mal.

IMPRESSION

This pleasant 27-year-old woman was in a significant accident on 00/00/92. She suffered a flexion-extension injury, was described in the first paragraph. The patient had rare migraine attacks prior to the accident, two in nine years, and some vascular headaches, one every two months. Currently her headaches are almost daily, ranging from moderate to severe to incapacitating. On examination, she had multiple myofascial trigger points that I am going to recommend injections for, plus deep neuromuscular mobilization and kinetic activity. I also suggest that we do a regional block of C1, 2, and 3 on the left side for the cervicogenic migraine that she is having.

The cervicogenic component will also need to be addressed and consideration for cervical facet blocks with fluoroscopic guidance would be a most reasonable option. If this is a headache syndrome secondary to a cervicogenic origin, then unless this component is addressed, the patient may remain symptomatic.

As far as medications are concerned, as preventative medication, she will be placed on Propranolol 20 mg t.i.d. and Amitriptyline 10 mg h.s. To abort her headaches, she will receive Ergopak suppositories with 25 mg of Promethazine. She will be given a log and also a diet, and hopefully we will be able to get her started as soon as possible. With this approach, I would hope that we would break the cycle and give her a significant amount of relief

Again, thank you again for the referral of this very pleasant patient. If there are any questions, please do not hesitate to call or write.

Sincerely,

BERNARD SWERDLOW, M.D.

MEDICAL HEADACHE HISTORY

Name: Diane **Age:** 27 **Sex** F **Date:** 10/8/93

Date of Birth: 0/00/66 **Birthplace:** MA **Race:** B **Education:** BA

Occupation: Secretary **Accident:** 1992

Armed Services & Type of Discharge: N/A

PAST HISTORY:

1.	Did you have a normal birth?		Yes	No
	a) forceps used?		Yes	No
	b) cesarean section?		Yes	No
2.	Did you have problems with bedwetting?		Yes	No
	a) If yes, age bedwetting stopped			
3.	Were you car sick as a child (motion)?		Yes	No
	a) If yes, how severe?	Slight	Moderate	Severe
4.	Did you have unexplained abdominal cramps as a child?		Yes	No
5.	Did you have any of the following illnesses in childhood?			
	a) meningitis		Yes	No
	b) encephalitis		Yes	No
	c) scarlet fever		Yes	No
	d) rheumatic fever		Yes	No
6.	Did you have any head injuries as a child?		Yes	No
	a) If yes, please explain:			
7.	Were you treated for emotional illness as a child?		Yes	No

HABITS:

8.	Do you drink alcohol?	Yes	No
	a) If yes, what kind and how much? Little, special occasions		
	b) Does alcohol bring on or aggravate a headache?	Yes	No
9.	Do you smoke?	Yes	No
	a) If yes, how much?		
	b) Does smoking or smoke-filled rooms cause or aggravate headaches?	Yes	No
10.	Do you drink caffeinated beverages?	Yes	No
	a) If yes, how much? 2 or 3 cokes a week		

MENSTRUAL HISTORY:

At what age did menses begin? 13 Were they regular or irregular? WNL

How were they related to your headache? Increased headaches

Are you or were you ever on Birth Control Pills? No Did they affect your headache? No

Have you had a hysterectomy, partial or total, and why? No

Are you in menopause, and if yes, how long? No

Arc you on hormones, and if yes, which ones? No

HEADACHE ASSESSMENT FORM

HA PROFILE	INCAPACITATING #3	INTERFERING #2	IRRITATING #1
ONSET (Years ago and frequency)	Age 18, only had 2 until accident	Age 18, occasional until accident, 1 every 2 months	N/A
CURRENT FREQUENCY	2 – 3/month	2 – 3/week	N/A
TIME OF ONSET	Anytime	Anytime, can awaken with	N/A
DURATION	2 – 3 days	3 days, hours with meds	N/A
CHARACTER	Severe pressure and throbbing	Same, less intense	N/A
PRODROME OR AURA	N/A	N/A	N/A
ASSOCIATING FEATURES	Nausea; Vomiting; Sensitivity to Light? Noise? Odors? Do you get pale or flush? Do your eyes or nose run? Does your nose get stuffy? Do the whites of your eyes get red? Does your eyelid droop? Do you pace, or go to bed?	Nausea; Vomiting; Sensitivity to Light? Noise? Odors? Do you get pale or flush? Do your eyes or nose run? Does your nose get stuffy? Do the whites of your eyes get red? Does your eyelid droop? Do you pace, or go to bed?	Nausea; Vomiting; Sensitivity to Light? Noise? Odors? Do you get pale or flush? Do your eyes or nose run? Does your nose get stuffy? Do the whites of your eyes get red? Does your eyelid droop? Do you pace, or go to bed?
PRECIPITATING OR AGGRAVATING FEATURES	Movement	N/A	N/A

LOCATION: Mark the location for each type of headache with a different color pen.

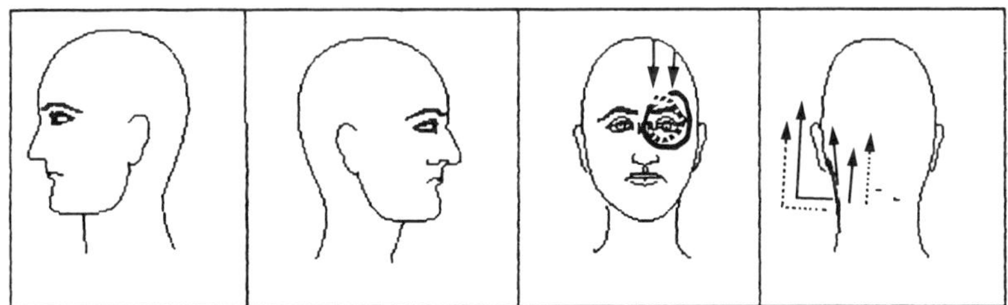

MEDICAL HISTORY:

Have you ever been or are you currently being treated for any of the following?

a) high blood pressure	Yes	No
b) stomach ulcers	Yes	No
c) asthma	Yes	No
d) allergies	Yes	No
e) pneumonia	Yes	No
f) kidney problems	Yes	No
g) low blood sugar	Yes	No
h) glaucoma	Yes	No
i) diabetes	Yes	No
j) heart problems	Yes	No

If you answered yes to any of the above, please describe: Ulcers diagnosed 1 yr. ago, take meds as needed.

List all other medical problems you have had in the past. Include date diagnosed and treatment.
DO NOT LIST OPERATIONS

Seizure disorder, 1986. Take dilantin 200 mg h.s.

SURGICAL HISTORY (List operations and dates performed)

None.

PSYCHIATRIC HISTORY (List visits with counselors, psychologists, etc., and type of treatment)

None.

ACCIDENTS IN ADULT LIFE (Briefly describe any accident that caused any blow to the head or that you feel is related to your headache)

Car accident, 1992. Driving with seat belt. Going through an intersection. Another car ran a stoplight and hit my car and spun me around. Had flexion extension injury. Not unconscious. Saw doctor 2 days later. Headaches dramatically increased since accident.

FAMILY HISTORY:

1. Is your father living? Yes No
   - Age 53
   - Cause of death ____
   - Was there a headache history? Yes No
2. Is your mother living? Yes No
   - Age 52
   - Cause of death ____
   - Was there a headache history? Yes No

3. Ages of brothers---Circle the ones with headache
   24 35
4. Ages of sisters---Circle the ones with headache
   36 (39) 40
5. List any other blood relatives with a history of severe headaches.
   None

MARITAL HISTORY:

List marriages:

1st marriage age _____ to _______	Did spouse have headaches?	Yes	No
2nd marriage age _____ to _______	Did spouse have headaches?	Yes	No
3rd marriage age ______to _______	Did spouse have headaches?	Yes	No

Age of current spouse: N/A

List ages and sex of all children:

Age ______ Sex _____	Headaches?	Yes	No
Age ______ Sex _____	Headaches?	Yes	No
Age ______ Sex _____	Headaches?	Yes	No

STRESS FACTORS:

List any factors that may be affecting your headaches (money, loneliness, sexual problems, work, etc.)
Work, leaving for school.

VEGETATIVE SIGNS:

1.	Do you have trouble falling asleep?	Yes	No
2.	Do you have trouble staying asleep?	Yes	No
3.	Has your appetite decreased?	Yes	No
4.	Have you gained or lost weight in the past year?	Yes	No
5.	Have you felt tearful or depressed lately?	Yes	No
6.	Have you had any thoughts of wanting to die?	Yes	No
7.	Have you been forgetful lately?	Yes	No
8.	Any other changes in your normal day-to-day living?_______		

Please list any medications you are allergic or sensitive to: Ibuprofen

Please list any medications you are currently taking (including dosages and frequency per day):
Dilantin, 200 mg at bedtime. Esgic, when migraines occur.

PREVIOUS CARE:

1. List doctors who have treated you for headaches: Dr. M.

2. List any tests you have had for your headache (e.g., EEG, CT scan, MRI, X-Ray, etc.):
CT scan, 1986 (normal). MRI, 1986 (normal). EEG, 1986 (normal). Spinal tap, 1986 (normal).

3. List any other treatment you have had for your headache (e.g., biofeedback, acupuncture, chiropractic, or any other treatment you had):
None.

March 15, 1994

[Doctor's name and address omitted]

RE: JEFF

Dear Dr. [...]:

Thank you for the referral of Mr. Jeff [...]. This letter is being sent to you at his request.

The patient is a 21-year-old male born 00/00/72 in [...]. He has completed one year of college and is currently a student.

The patient was involved in a motor vehicle accident 00/00/93 when, while driving and wearing his seat belt, he crossed an intersection and another car ran a red light and hit his car broadside on the driver's side. The patient did not suffer loss of consciousness, but did hit the left side of his head on the window. He was taken to the emergency room where he was evaluated and released. The patient noted the onset of incapacitating and interfering headaches the day of the accident. His headache history prior to this motor vehicle accident is a rare irritating headache.

HEADACHE PROFILE

Incapacitating headaches: As noted above, these headaches began on the day of the accident and occur approximately once per month. The onset of these headaches is late in the day; they last three to four hours; and the pain is described as a throbbing pain localized in the periorbital, occipital, and cervical areas. There is no prodrome with these headaches. There is some phonophobia and sensitivity to odors noted. The patient will seek bed rest if possible.

Interfering headaches (moderate to severe): These headaches occurred two to three weeks after the accident as described above and the patient notes these headaches one to two times per week. These headaches will occur later in the day, last two to three hours, and the pain has the same character and location as the incapacitating headaches. There is no prodrome and these headaches are associated with some phonophobia and odor sensitivity. The patient will seek bed rest if possible. There are no precipitating or aggravating features noted with the incapacitating or interfering headaches.

Irritating headaches (annoying): The patient noted the onset of these headaches when he was in his teens and they were rare at that time. He is currently suffering from these headaches one to two times per week, and they will occur anytime of the day, will last one hour, and are aborted with over-the-counter medications. The pain is described as a dull aching pain in the temporal regions bilaterally. There are no prodrome, associated features or aggravating factors.

Past history: The patient was most probably a normal delivery. There is no history of enuresis or unexplained abdominal cramps pre-puberty. There is a history of slight car sickness as a child. There is no history of meningitis, encephalitis, scarlet fever or rheumatic fever. There were no head injuries as a child.

Habits: The patient does not consume alcohol and does not smoke. He does consume one caffeinated beverage per day.

Medical history: The patient has no history of high blood pressure, stomach ulcers, asthma, allergies, pneumonia, kidney problems, low blood sugar, glaucoma, diabetes, or heart problems.

Review of systems: Pulmonary negative, cardiovascular negative, gastrointestinal negative, urogenital negative.

Surgical history: Negative

Psychiatric history: Negative.

Head injuries in adult life: As described above.

Family history: His father is living, age 50, with no headache history. His mother is living, age 40, with a history of occasional interfering headaches. The patient has one brother and two sisters with no headache history. The patient is not married and has one son, age 5, with no headache history.

Stress factors: The patient denies any stress factors.

Vegetative signs: No sleep disturbance, depression to suicidal ideation.

Allergies to medications: NKA.

Current medications: None

Doctors seen in the past: The patient had, by history, both cervical and thoracic spine x-rays in the emergency room and also by Dr. [...]. The patient has been followed by Dr. [...] and reports improvement in symptoms in his back. However, his headache symptoms persist.

Treatments tried in the past: Medications previously taken include Flexeril.

Physical examination: Height 5'11", weight 150 pounds, pulse 74, respirations 16, left BP 92/62, right BP 92/64. The face did not show any asymmetry. The temporomandibular joint area was grossly normal. The eyes appeared normal. Conjunctivae were clear and the pupils reacted equally to light and accommodation. Retinal fundus examination revealed no papilledema and no abnormalities with the arteries and veins. There were no bruits over the supraorbital region. The nose appeared normal. The auditory canals were clear and the tympanic membranes appeared intact. The mouth and throat appeared normal. Gums, tongue, buccal mucosa, and teeth were grossly normal. There was some tenderness on palpation at both the left and right occipital cervical junction. Carotid bruits could not be heard. Cervical nodes were not enlarged. The lungs were clear to auscultation and percussion. The heart had a regular sinus rhythm with no murmurs. The abdomen was soft and nontender. A rectal examination was not done.

Neurological examination: Cranial nerve II: Visual fields were grossly normal. III, IV and VI: No strabismus, nystagmus, or ptosis. V: Normal sensation and corneal reflex. VII: Normal facial movements (wrinkle, frown, smile, and strength of eyelids). VIII: Normal Weber and Rinne. IX and X: Good gag reflex. XI: Normal sternocleidomastoid and trapezius. XII: Normal protrusion and strength of tongue. Cerebellar: Negative Rhomberg. Normal finger-to-nose, diadochokinesis, heel-shin, tandem, and heel and toes walking. Motor system: No atrophy, fasciculations, wasting, or tremors. Good muscle strength in arms, wrists, fingers, and legs. Sensory system: Superficial tactile, pain, and vibrations (wrists, elbows, knees, and ankles) were normal. Normal motion and positions of fingers and toes. Normal 2-point discrimination. Reflexes: Normal 2+ reflexes of triceps, biceps, knee jerk, ankle jerk, etc. Normal pulses in dorsalis pedis, posterior tibial and popliteal.

DIAGNOSES

1. Post traumatic vascular headache, migraine-like. Rule out structural root lesion. Rule out metabolic etiology.
2. Post traumatic cervicogenic headache.

RECOMMENDED TESTS

1. MRI to rule out any structural lesion in this patient with prolonged headache symptoms.
2. Metabolic profile to rule out any metabolic etiologies for patient's symptoms.

Suggested therapy would include:

1. Cervical regional block to address the area of patient's pain in the cervical region, hoping to break the headache cycle for the cervicogenic headache.
2. Prophylactic medication, since the patient is having approximately 8 to 10 interfering to incapacitating headaches per month. I would initially start out with a tricyclic antidepressant, nonsteroidal anti-inflammatory medication, and beta-blocker.
3. Abortive medication for the vascular component to consist of Midrin and an Ergotamine preparation.
4. The cervicogenic component will also need to be addressed and consideration for cervical facet blocks with fluoroscopic guidance would be a reasonable option.

I also discussed with the patient his continuing with you for treatment of his cervical complaints. Hopefully this, in combination with our treatment, will give additional benefit.

Thank you for the referral of this pleasant patient. If I can be of further assistance in this case, please contact me.

Sincerely,

[Doctor's name omitted]

MEDICAL HEADACHE HISTORY

Name: Jeff **Age:** 21 **Sex** M **Date:** 3/15/94

Date of Birth: 00/00/72 **Birthplace:** FL **Race:** W **Education:** 1 yr. College

Occupation: Student **Accident:** 00/00/93

Armed Services & Type of Discharge: N/A

PAST HISTORY:

1.	Did you have a normal birth?		Yes	No
	a) forceps used?		Yes	No
	b) cesarean section?		Yes	No
2.	Did you have problems with bedwetting?		Yes	No
	a) If yes, age bedwetting stopped			
3.	Were you car sick as a child (motion)?		Yes	No
	a) If yes, how severe?	Slight	Moderate	Severe
4.	Did you have unexplained abdominal cramps as a child?		Yes	No
5.	Did you have any of the following illnesses in childhood?			
	a) meningitis		Yes	No
	b) encephalitis		Yes	No
	c) scarlet fever		Yes	No
	d) rheumatic fever		Yes	No
6.	Did you have any head injuries as a child?		Yes	No
	a) If yes, please explain:			
7.	Were you treated for emotional illness as a child?		Yes	No

HABITS:

8.	Do you drink alcohol?	Yes	No
	a) If yes, what kind and how much?		
	b) Does alcohol bring on or aggravate a headache?	Yes	No
9.	Do you smoke?	Yes	No
	a) If yes, how much?		
	b) Does smoking or smoke-filled rooms cause or aggravate headaches?	Yes	No
10.	Do you drink caffeinated beverages?	Yes	No
	a) If yes, how much? Once a day		

MENSTRUAL HISTORY:

At what age did menses begin?_______ Were they regular or irregular?_______
How were they related to your headache?_______
Are you or were you ever on Birth Control Pills?_______ Did they affect your headache? _______
Have you had a hysterectomy, partial or total, and why?_______
Are you in menopause, and if yes, how long?_______
Are you on hormones, and if yes, which ones?_______

HEADACHE ASSESSMENT FORM

HA PROFILE	INCAPACITATING #3	INTERFERING #2	IRRITATING #1
ONSET (Years ago and frequency)	Day of accident	2 to 3 weeks after accident	In teens, rare
CURRENT FREQUENCY	1/month	1 to 2/week	1 to 2/week
TIME OF ONSET	Later in the day	Later in day	Anytime
DURATION	3 to 4 hours	2 to 3 hours	1 hour with OTC meds
CHARACTER	Throbbing	Same, less intense	Dull ache
PRODROME OR AURA	N/A	N/A	N/A
ASSOCIATING FEATURES	Nausea; Vomiting; Sensitivity to Light? Noise? Odors? Do you get pale or flush? Do your eyes or nose run? Does your nose get stuffy? Does the white of your eyes get red? Does your eyelid droop? Do you pace, or go to bed?	Nausea; Vomiting; Sensitivity to Light? Noise? Odors? Do you get pale or flush? Do your eyes or nose run? Does your nose get stuffy? Does the white of your eyes get red? Does your eyelid droop? Do you pace, or go to bed?	Nausea; Vomiting; Sensitivity to Light? Noise? Odors? Do you get pale or flush? Do your eyes or nose run? Does your nose get stuffy? Does the white of your eyes get red? Does your eyelid droop? Do you pace, or go to bed?
PRECIPITATING OR AGGRAVATING FEATURES	N/A	N/A	N/A

LOCATION: Mark the location for each type of headache with a different color pen.

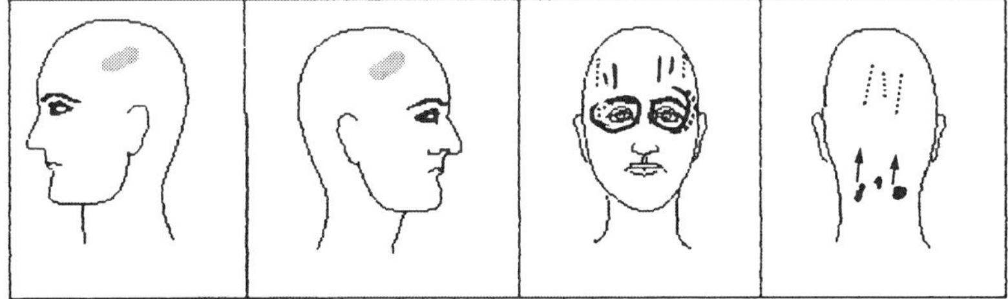

MEDICAL HISTORY:

Have you ever been or are you currently being treated for any of the following?

a) high blood pressure	Yes	No
b) stomach ulcers	Yes	No
c) asthma	Yes	No
d) allergies	Yes	No
e) pneumonia	Yes	No
f) kidney problems	Yes	No
g) low blood sugar	Yes	No
h) glaucoma	Yes	No
i) diabetes	Yes	No
j) heart problems	Yes	No

If you answered yes to any of the above, please describe:____________________

List all other medical problems you have had in the past. Include date diagnosed and treatment.
DO NOT LIST OPERATIONS

None.

SURGICAL HISTORY (List operations and dates performed)

None.

PSYCHIATRIC HISTORY (List visits with counselors, psychologists, etc., and type of treatment)

None.

ACCIDENTS IN ADULT LIFE (Briefly describe any accident that caused any blow to the head or that you feel is related to your headache)

1993 – Driving with seat belt. Crossing intersection. Another car ran a light and hit me in driver's side. Not unconscious. Taken to ER, treated and released. Headaches began that day. (Hit left side of head on window.) Had rare #1 headache before accident.

FAMILY HISTORY:

1.	Is your father living?	Yes	No
	Age 50		
	Cause of death__________		
	Was there a headache history?	Yes	No
2.	Is your mother living?	Yes	No
	Age 50		
	Cause of death__________		
	Was there a headache history?	Yes	No

3. Ages of brothers---Circle the ones with headache
   ___31___________________________________
4. Ages of sisters---Circle the ones with headache
   ___14 30________________________________
5. List any other blood relatives with a history of severe headaches.
   ___None_________________________________

MARITAL HISTORY:
List marriages:

1st marriage age _____ to _______	Did spouse have headaches?	Yes	No
2nd marriage age _____ to _______	Did spouse have headaches?	Yes	No
3rd marriage age _____ to _______	Did spouse have headaches?	Yes	No

Age of current spouse:____________

List ages and sex of all children:

Age __5__ Sex __M__	Headaches?	Yes	No
Age _____ Sex ______	Headaches?	Yes	No
Age_____ Sex ______	Headaches?	Yes	No
Age _____ Sex ______	Headaches?	Yes	No

STRESS FACTORS:

List any factors that may be affecting your headaches (money, loneliness, sexual problems, work, etc.)
___None.____
____

VEGETATIVE SIGNS:

1.	Do you have trouble falling asleep?	Yes	No
2.	Do you have trouble staying asleep?	Yes	No
3.	Has your appetite decreased?	Yes	No
4.	Have you gained or lost weight in the past year?	Yes	No
5.	Have you felt tearful or depressed lately?	Yes	No
6.	Have you had any thoughts of wanting to die?	Yes	No
7.	Have you been forgetful lately?	Yes	No
8.	Any other changes in your normal day-to-day living?____________________		

Please list any medications you are allergic or sensitive to:___NKA.___________________
____
____

Please list any medications you are currently taking (including dosages and frequency per day):
___None.____
____

PREVIOUS CARE:

1, List doctors who have treated you for headaches:________________________

2, List any tests you have had for your headache (e.g., EEG, CT scan, MRI, X-Ray, etc.):

X-rays.

3, List any other treatment you have had for your headache (e.g., biofeedback, acupuncture, chiropractic, or any other treatment you had):

Chiropractic (helped back, not headaches).

BERNARD
Category: Cervicogenic headache

After reviewing this chart, I feel that this patient probably would have been diagnosed as a post traumatic cervicogenic headache. At the time that he was seen, that diagnosis was not yet a working diagnosis.

This 28-year-old male, fully employed, had an accident approximately a year before he saw me. He was running across a parking lot and tripped on a handicapped ramp which was not marked, and he states that when he hit the ramp he "flew about 12 or 15 feet and landed with outstretched hands." He stated he did not hit his head and he said his headaches began immediately.

He did have a fractured skull when he was age 12 and had headaches for a short period of time, but he said they resolved. At the time that he saw me, he was in litigation with the owner of the parking lot.

Incapacitating headaches: These started after this accident and he had them four to five times a week. The headaches started the day immediately following the accident, and they seem to get worse as they day progresses. Sometimes it becomes so severe that he must be taken from work to go home. He says that he cannot function when he gets these terrible headaches and the character of the pain is severe pressure. They start in the posterocervical region, or the back of the neck, where he states that it radiates around to where his eye sockets are. Associated features are typical of vascular or migraine-like headaches, which are nausea, vomiting, photophobia, and then he must go to bed.

At the time that I saw him, I recorded that I felt there may have been a tearing of some ligaments or structures in the cervical region. This is also a situation in which a previous accident where there were headaches that went into remission may have been exacerbated or this is a new condition. However, seeing him one year later, the condition being the same, the region of the area that the pains start in would make one think that this resulted eventually in a cervicogenic headache in which there is both inflammation and perhaps an arthritic condition in the cervical region as suggested in this chapter. Although this was not an automobile accident, I would assume that the type of injury he had would be similar to a flexion-extension injury.

MEDICAL HEADACHE HISTORY

Name: Bernard **Age:** 28 **Sex.** M **Date:** 5/24/90

Date of Birth: 00/00/61 **Birthplace:** FL **Race:** W **Education:** High School

Occupation: Management **Accident:** 6/2/89

Armed Services & Type of Discharge: N/A

PAST HISTORY:

1.	Did you have a normal birth?		Yes	No
	a) forceps used?		Yes	No
	b) cesarean section?		Yes	No
2.	Did you have problems with bedwetting?		Yes	No
	a) If yes, age bedwetting stopped		______	
3.	Were you car sick as a child (motion)?		Yes	No
	a) If yes, how severe?	Slight	Moderate	Severe
4.	Did you have unexplained abdominal cramps as a child?		Yes	No
5.	Did you have any of the following illnesses in childhood?			
	a) meningitis		Yes	No
	b) encephalitis		Yes	No
	c) scarlet fever		Yes	No
	d) rheumatic fever		Yes	No
6.	Did you have any head injuries as a child?		Yes	No
	a) If yes, please explain: Head injury age 12			
7.	Were you treated for emotional illness as a child?		Yes	No

HABITS:

8.	Do you drink alcohol?	Yes	No
	a) If yes, what kind and how much? Maybe 1 drink a month		
	b) Does alcohol bring on or aggravate a headache?	Yes	No
9.	Do you smoke?	Yes	No
	a) If yes, how much?______		
	b) Does smoking or smoke-filled rooms cause or aggravate headaches?	Yes	No
10.	Do you drink caffeinated beverages?	Yes	No
	a) If yes, how much? 1 to 2 12 oz. drinks a day		

MENSTRUAL HISTORY:

At what age did menses begin?_______ Were they regular or irregular?__________

How were they related to your headache?__________

Are you or were you ever on Birth Control Pills?______ Did they affect your headache? _______

Have you had a hysterectomy, partial or total, and why?__________

Are you in menopause, and if yes, how long?__________

Are you on hormones, and if yes, which ones?__________

HEADACHE ASSESSMENT FORM

HA PROFILE	INCAPACITATING #3	INTERFERING #2	IRRITATING #1
ONSET (Years ago and frequency)	1 every 2 weeks	N/A	Headaches begin as #1 and progress to #3
CURRENT FREQUENCY	4 to 5 a week	N/A	N/A
TIME OF ONSET	Later in the day, can awaken with	N/A	N/A
DURATION	Hours	N/A	N/A
CHARACTER	Severe pressure	N/A	N/A
PRODROME OR AURA	N/A	N/A	N/A
ASSOCIATING FEATURES	Nausea; Vomiting; Sensitivity to Light? Noise? Odors? Do you get pale or flush? Do your eyes or nose run? Does your nose get stuffy? Does the white of your eyes get red? Does your eyelid droop? Do you pace, or go to bed? Diarrhea	Nausea; Vomiting; Sensitivity to Light? Noise? Odors? Do you get pale or flush? Do your eyes or nose run? Does your nose get stuffy? Does the white of your eyes get red? Does your eyelid droop? Do you pace, or go to bed?	Nausea; Vomiting; Sensitivity to Light? Noise? Odors? Do you get pale or flush? Do your eyes or nose run? Does your nose get stuffy? Does the white of your eyes get red? Does your eyelid droop? Do you pace, or go to bed?
PRECIPITATING OR AGGRAVATING FEATURES	N/A	N/A	N/A

LOCATION: Mark the location for each type of headache with a different color pen.

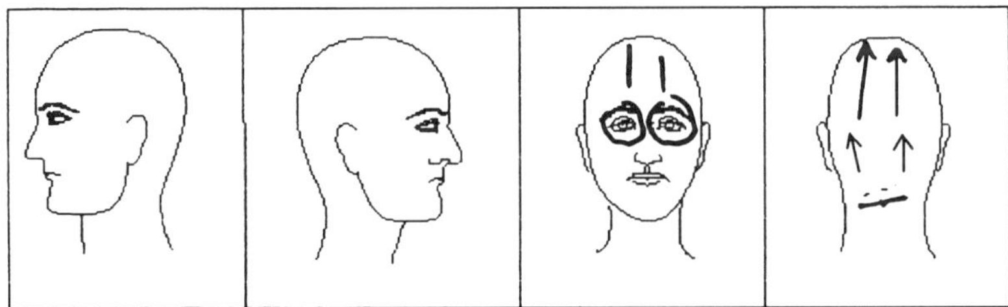

MEDICAL HISTORY:

Have you ever been or are you currently being treated for any of the following?

a) high blood pressure	Yes	**No**
b) stomach ulcers	Yes	**No**
c) asthma	Yes	**No**
d) allergies	Yes	**No**
e) pneumonia	**Yes**	No
f) kidney problems	**Yes**	No
g) low blood sugar	Yes	**No**
h) glaucoma	Yes	**No**
i) diabetes	Yes	**No**
j) heart problems	Yes	**No**

If you answered yes to any of the above, please describe: Pneumonia at age 4. Kidney stones for four years. Passed 13 stones. None for 2 years.

List all other medical problems you have had in the past. Include date diagnosed and treatment. DO NOT LIST OPERATIONS

Fractured skull age 12, playing baseball. Fractured left ankle. Fractured ribs in high school. Both feet crushed in accidents. Fractured nose twice.

SURGICAL HISTORY (List operations and dates performed)

Appendectomy, 1984.

Urinary tract, 1987.

PSYCHIATRIC HISTORY (List visits with counselors, psychologists, etc., and type of treatment)

None

ACCIDENTS IN ADULT LIFE (Briefly describe any accident that caused any blow to the head or that you feel is related to your headache)

1989 – Was running across a parking lot and tripped on a handicap ramp and "flew about 12-15. Feet." Landed on outstretched hands. Did not hit head. Headaches began immediately. Had headaches after fractured skull at age 12, but they resolved.

FAMILY HISTORY:

1.	Is your father living?	**Yes**	No
	Age 65		
	Cause of death________		
	Was there a headache history?	Yes	**No**
2.	Is your mother living?	**Yes**	No
	Age 57		
	Cause of death________		
	Was there a headache history?	Yes	**No**

3. Ages of brothers---Circle the ones with headache
   36 27 23
4. Ages of sisters---Circle the ones with headache
   (38) 35
5. List any other blood relatives with a history of severe headaches.
   None

MARITAL HISTORY:
List marriages:

1st marriage age 20 to 23	Did spouse have headaches?	Yes	No
2nd marriage age _____ to _______	Did spouse have headaches?	Yes	No
3rd marriage age _____ to _______	Did spouse have headaches?	Yes	No

Age of current spouse:____________

List ages and sex of all children:

Age _____ Sex ______	Headaches?	Yes	No
Age _____ Sex ______	Headaches?	Yes	No
Age _____ Sex ______	Headaches?	Yes	No
Age _____ Sex ______	Headaches?	Yes	No

STRESS FACTORS:

List any factors that may be affecting your headaches (money, loneliness, sexual problems, work, etc.)
None.

VEGETATIVE SIGNS:

1.	Do you have trouble falling asleep?	Yes	No
2.	Do you have trouble staying asleep?	Yes	No
3.	Has your appetite decreased?	Yes	No
4.	Have you gained or lost weight in the past year?	Yes	No
5.	Have you felt tearful or depressed lately?	Yes	No
6.	Have you had any thoughts of wanting to die?	Yes	No
7.	Have you been forgetful lately?	Yes	No
8.	Any other changes in your normal day-to-day living?__________		

Please list any medications you are allergic or sensitive to: None

Please list any medications you are currently taking (including dosages and frequency per day):
Aspirin and muscle relaxers.

PREVIOUS CARE:

1. List doctors who have treated you for headaches: Dr. C.

2. List any tests you have had for your headache (e.g., EEG, CT scan, MRI, X-Ray, etc.):
None.

3. List any other treatment you have had for your headache (e.g., biofeedback, acupuncture, chiropractic, or any other treatment you had):
Chiropractic (helps temporarily).

Chapter 20

Introduction to Neuropsychology

John N.I. Dieter

AN OVERVIEW OF NEUROPSYCHOLOGY

Neuropsychology is a specialization of clinical psychology that studies the relationship between the brain and behavior. These brain-behavior relationships are usually examined through standardized psychological tests (e.g., those that measure intelligence, motor functions, reasoning, etc.). The discipline incorporates elements of neuroscience, neurological medicine, psychological assessment, and clinical intervention.[1]

When considering the history of modern neuropsychology, the work of nineteenth century scientists such as Paul Broca, Pierre Flourens, John Hughlings-Jackson, and Carl Wernicke was seminal.[2] Through ablation studies with animals, human autopsy, or the examination of persons who had sustained serious brain injury, these investigators determined that damage to specific brain regions resulted in the loss of specific behavioral functions. Broca localized the expressive language center within the left frontal-temporal region and Wernicke found the receptive language center in the left posterior temporal lobe (see below). Such findings were further substantiated with the acceptance of the *neuron hypothesis*, which proposed that the nervous system is composed of autonomous cells that interact, but are separated by, a small space called the *synapse*.[3] In addition, Hughlings-Jackson argued that the nervous system was arranged as a functional hierarchy whereby lower anatomical regions were more simple, and higher brain regions more complex.

Between 1920 and 1950, Karl Lashley introduced such important concepts as *mass action* and *equipotentiality*.[3] Mass action is the idea that the entire *neocortex* (i.e., the youngest, in terms of evolution, and most complex part of the brain) participates in every behavior. This concept is important to the study of head injury because it maintains that the overall complexity and quality of behavior is the function of the total amount of healthy brain tissue. The notion of equipotentiality proposes that the brain is flexible and that regions can adopt new functions. This idea is also relevant to head injury and probably underlies the restoration of behaviors following brain trauma.

The 1940s and 1950s saw the application of psychometric research to the study of brain-behavior relationships. Hebb administered the first IQ tests to brain-damaged people and Ward Halstead published a monograph based on observations of several hundred cases of persons with frontal lobe damage.[2,4] Later, Halstead and his student, Ralph Reitan, developed and modified the first *neuropsychological test battery*: a group of psychological tests used to document the effects of different cortical *lesions* (i.e., pathology arising from either damage or disease) on specific behaviors.[4]

During the 1960s, the pioneer Russian neuropsychologist Aleksandr Luria believed the two goals of neuropsychology were: (1) to develop means for the early diagnosis and location of brain lesions; and (2) to enhance our understanding of which brain areas are responsible for complex psychological functions.[5] While these goals are still pertinent today, the last decade has seen a shift in focus from attempts to localize specific brain lesions, to a more comprehensive approach that assesses brain-behavior relationships within a much broader context.[4] This approach arose from research findings that showed that damage to one brain region can have ramifications for psychological functioning across a number of domains, and that complex psychological behavior arises from the integration of numerous interdependent structures throughout the brain. Furthermore, the effects of brain damage are more often evaluated within the structure of a biopsychosocial model that considers the whole person, including his or her developmental history, premorbid functioning, and past and current social environment.

Other recent trends in neuropsychology include the debate over relying upon comprehensive test batteries vs. more individualized approaches towards assessment; the application of neuropsychological research results and clinical findings to the cognitive rehabilitation and retraining of brain-damaged persons; and the establishment of special training programs, licensing, and boarding demands for those practicing neuropsychology.[4] Neuropsychologists are also playing an important role in the legal arena and are frequently called upon to testify in court cases. It is likely that the discipline of clinical neuropsychology will continue to be one of the most dynamic and growing fields in mental health care.

FUNCTIONAL NEUROANATOMY

Previous chapters provide a more thorough introduction to the neuroanatomy of whiplash and chronic headache. This section is directed toward the functional anatomy of the central nervous system that is most relevant to topics of neuropsychology and head injury.

The Central Nervous System and Neurons

The *central nervous system* (CNS) is composed of the brain and spinal cord. The human CNS represents the highest form of biological evolution on earth. The CNS allows us to gather information about the world and respond to it in a flexible way, which is most important to both adaptation and survival.

The brain and spinal cord are composed of billions of unique nerve cells called *neurons*. Neurons differ from all other cells in the body because of their ability to communicate with each other through electrochemical signals. Figure 20.1 presents a "typical" neuron.

The main divisions of the neuron consist of the *cell body* and its extensions.[3] The cell body or *soma* contains the nucleus and produces the energy required for the transmission of electrochemical information. From the soma arise appendages that are involved with the reception and transmission of information. *Dendrites* specialize in receiving neural information from *neurotransmitters*, chemical messages released by neurons. The *axon* is a long fiber that extends from the soma and conducts the electrical impulses that promote the release of neurotransmitters into the synapse (i.e., the small space that separates the axon of one neuron and the dendrites of another).

Neural Transmission

The process of neural transmission is one of the most wondrous events in nature. From a neighboring nerve cell, a chemical message is sent across the synapse and received by the dendrites of a neuron. The quality of this neurotransmitter is of either an *excitatory* or *inhibitory* nature. The combination of excitatory (i.e., promoting the electrical discharge of the neuron) and inhibitory (i.e., blocking the electrical discharge of the neuron) messages from other neurons determine

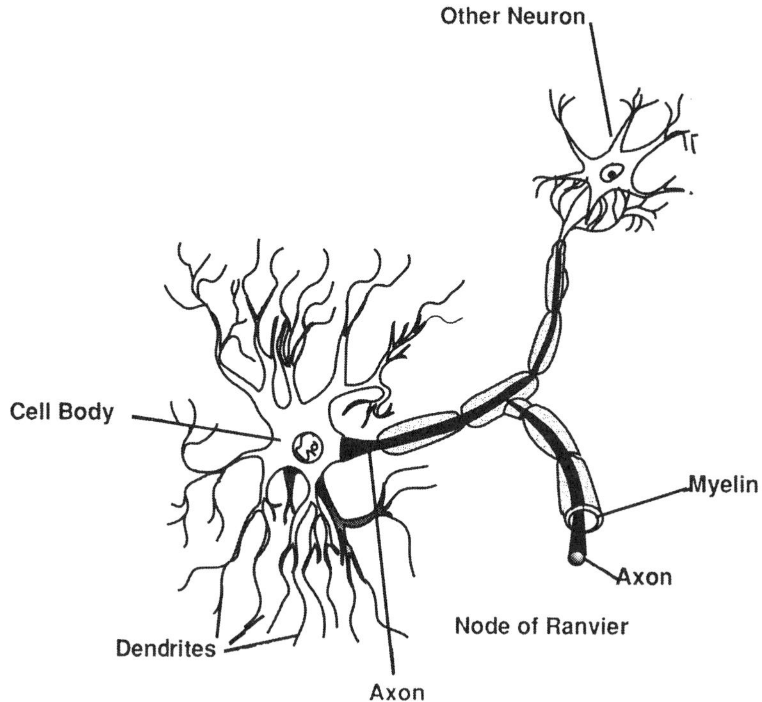

Figure 20.1 A "typical" neuron of the brain.

whether *saltatory conduction* will occur. Saltatory conduction results when the proportion of excitatory messages outnumber the proportion of inhibitory messages. The process begins when the chemical environment of the axon changes so that the arrangement of sodium and potassium ions is such that an electrical charge is produced (much as occurs in an automobile battery), a threshold is crossed, and the axon *fires*. The firing of a neuron involves the generation of an electric spark that "jumps" along the outside surface of the axon. Electrical transmission down the axon is accelerated by the presence of *myelin*, a fatty sheath or covering that, ironically, does not conduct the electric spark. Along the axon there are gaps in the myelin that are called *nodes of Ranvier*. Electrical transmission is accelerated because the spark does not travel down the entire length of the axon: instead, it skips from node of Ranvier to node of Ranvier. At the end of the axon are *telodendria* or *axonal endings*. These multibranching fibers form the synapse with the dendrites, cell bodies, and, on occasion, the axon of other neurons.[3] It is from the axonal endings that neurotransmitters are released into the synapse, interact with the next neighboring neuron(s), and continue the process of neurotransmission.

Neurotransmitters have received considerable attention because of the role that they play in consciousness, and particularly, mental illness. For instance, depression has been linked to *serotonin*, and drugs like Prozac (i.e., fluoxetine hydrochloride[6]) increase the effect of this neurotransmitter upon neurons by prolonging its stay in the synapse. Dopamine, a neurotransmitter that affects muscle control, is produced in an area of the brain called the *substantia nigra*. An excess of dopamine has been implicated in Tourette's syndrome and schizophrenia. Parkinson's disease is believed to arise from a dysfunction of the substantia nigra that leads to a decrease in the production of dopamine. Drugs such as L-dopa increase the presence of dopamine in the CNS and reduce Parkinsonian symptoms. There are at least eight known and suspected neurotransmitters.[3] The study of these chemicals, and their impact upon behavior, continues to be a central focus of neuroscience research.

Neuron Death and Brain Damage

All cells in the body eventually die from age, injury, or disease. Usually, when a cell dies, it is replaced through the cell division (i.e., mitosis) of the remaining cells. This does not occur in the central nervous system. Dead neurons are not replaced.[3] This has powerful implications for CNS injury. The reason a person who suffers a serious spinal cord injury experiences permanent paralysis is because those neurons that were damaged never recover and are never replaced. In the brain, normal neuronal death is compensated for in two ways: first, we are all born with an excess of neurons which provide us with "a backup army of neural forces than can be pressed into service at any time";[3] second, because of the phenomenon of equipotentiality (see above), neighboring neurons can adopt the function of the lost neurons. It is only when insult upon the brain is great enough, or function cannot be mimicked by other neural regions, that behavioral deficits arise.

Brain Structures and Their Functions

The brain sits within the skull with the spinal cord attached to its posterior underside. When contemplating the brain, it is important to view it as a three-dimensional structure. One must consider *anterior* (towards the front), *posterior* (towards the back), *lateral* (away from the middle), *medial* (towards the middle), *dorsal/superior* (towards the top), and *inferior/ventral* (underside) aspects.

For conceptual purposes, the brain is often subdivided into the forebrain, midbrain, and hindbrain.[3] Figure 20.2 presents these three subdivisions.

The Hindbrain

The hindbrain is within the inferior posterior region, is connected directly to the spinal cord, and divided into the *medulla* and *pons*.[3] These two structures, along with the midbrain (see below),

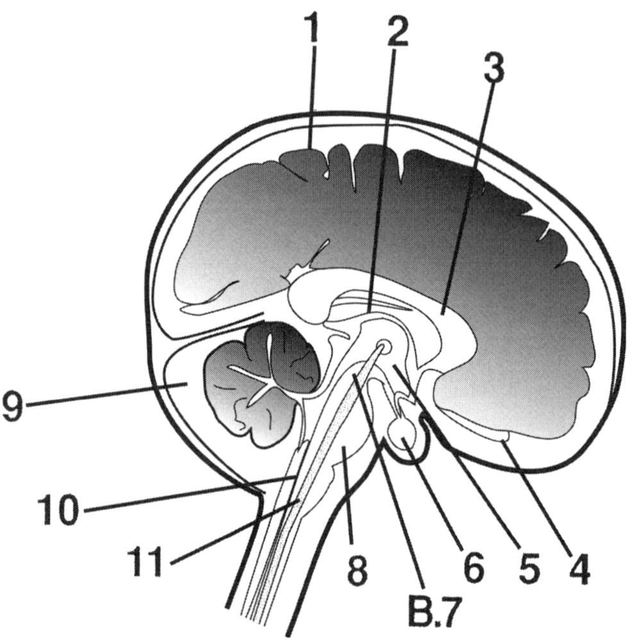

Figure 20.2 The forebrain comprises (**1**) cerebral hemisphere; (**2**) thalamus; (**3**) corpus callosum; (**4**) olfactory bulbs; (**5**) hypothalamus; and (**6**) pituitary gland. The midbrain (**B.7**) contains the superior and inferior colliculus, the substantia negra, and the red nucleus. The hindbrain structures are (**8**) pons; (**9**) cerebellum; (**10**) medulla; and (**11**) reticular formation.

collectively form the *brainstem*.[7] The medulla controls autonomic physiological functions, such as heart rate and respiration. Damage to the medulla can result in immediate death. The pons is composed of numerous sensory and motor pathways that channel incoming information to the brain and behavioral commands from the brain to the rest of the body. From the pons extend two important structures, the *cerebellum*, which maintains body balance and muscle coordination, and the *reticular activating system* (RAS). The RAS projects sensory pathways through the upper parts of the brain and has two main purposes: the first is to screen out non-important sensory information in an effort to avoid sensory overload; the second is to alert the higher brain centers of incoming information.[3] Other related hindbrain structures include the *raphe nuclei*, which are important to the control of pain suppression, sleep, and emotion, and the locus ceruleus, which also plays a role in controlling sleep and emotion.

The Midbrain

Also involved in the transmission of information to higher brain centers, the midbrain contains a number of important structures, including the *superior colliculus*, *inferior colliculus*, substantia nigra, and *red nucleus*. The superior colliculus is associated with the control of eye movement, the inferior colliculus with the startle reaction to sound, and the red nucleus with motor control.[3] As discussed above, the substantia nigra, or "black body," is involved in both the production of the neurotransmitter dopamine and the control of muscular activity.

The Forebrain

The forebrain is divided into the *cerebral hemispheres* and includes such important neural structures as the *hypothalamus*, *basal ganglia*, *thalamus*, *limbic system*, and *cortex*.[3] It is from the forebrain that complex human experiences such as emotion and thought arise.

The hypothalamus is of great importance in maintaining the body's homeostatic balance and serving as a link between the nervous and endocrine (i.e., hormonal) systems. Hypothalamic functions include control of heart rate, blood pressure, and hunger, as well as the movements and glandular secretions of the stomach and intestines; regulation of arousal, body temperature, and weight, as well as water and electrolyte balance, and production of neurosecretory substances that stimulate the pituitary gland to release hormones.[7]

Between the hypothalamus and cortex lie a number of brain regions important to motor movement.[3] The basal ganglia, consisting of the *putamen*, *globus pallidus*, and *caudate nucleus*, coordinates muscle movement through the transmission of information received from the cortex and directing it to the spinal cord. The basal ganglia have been implicated in the motor symptoms observed in persons with schizophrenia, as well as Parkinson's disease.

Superior to the hypothalamus is the thalamus. This collection of neurons serves as a "sensory way station" by transmitting sensory information from the *peripheral nervous system* (i.e., those portions of the nervous system outside the brain and spinal cord, e.g., the nerves of the arms and legs) to the cortex. The *lateral geniculate* transmits visual information to the vision centers of the cortex. The *medial geniculate* relays auditory information to the hearing centers of the cortex. The *ventrobasal complex* sends information about touch, pressure, temperature, and pain to the feeling centers of the cortex.

The limbic system forms a crude border around the brainstem and consists of portions of the *frontal cortex*, *temporal cortex*, thalamus, hypothalamus, *fornix*, *amygdala*, *hippocampus*, and *mammillary bodies*.[3] Collectively, this group of structures contribute to the control of aggression, fear, pleasure, and pain. Additionally, the limbic system has been implicated in memory processing (particularly the hippocampus and mammillary bodies).

Much could be said about the role of the limbic system in the regulation of emotion and motivation, and this brain region is currently a significant focus of neuroscience research. The limbic system is sometimes referred to as the *reptilian brain* because it first evolved in lower species such as amphibians and reptiles.[2] Many consider the limbic system to be the seat of our more "primitive emotions." Psychoanalytically oriented thinkers interested in functional neuroanatomy have suggested that the limbic system is the residence of the psychic structure, the *id* (i.e., the mental representations of instinctual drives such as sex and aggression, as well as some of the contents of the unconscious), first proposed by Sigmund Freud.

The Cerebral Hemispheres

Essentially identical right and left halves of the forebrain, each cerebral hemisphere is divided into four functional lobes, the *frontal*, *temporal*, *parietal*, and *occipital* (see below).[3] The hemispheres of the brain are connected by a large bundle of nerve fibers called the *corpus collosum*. These fibers are a communication pathway that permits the flow of information from one hemisphere to the other. In rare cases, persons with extreme forms of epilepsy have their corpus collosum surgically severed in order to stop the march of a seizure from one side of the brain to the other.

The cortex is the layer of gray matter on the surface of the cerebral hemispheres that has a convoluted appearance marked by ridges and valleys. A ridge is referred to as a *gyrus*, and the grove between one gyrus and another is called a *sulcus* or *fissure*. The convolutions of the cerebral cortex provide for a much greater cellular density than if the surface was smooth. Essentially, regions of neurons are compressed together so as to occupy a relatively small space, and it is this bunching that gives rise to the sulci and gyri.

Cerebral Functional Asymmetry

Much has been said about the differences between the functional qualities of the right and left hemispheres. Since the last decade, people often refer to themselves as being "right-brained" or "left-brained". "Left-brain people" are considered more logical, conservative, and goal-oriented, while "right-brain people" are described as being more spontaneous, emotional, and artistic. Neuroscience research has consistently found that the two cerebral hemispheres process different types of information and do possess unique qualities unto themselves. However, it is very important to remember that the complex brain physiology that underlies human experience relies upon the joint operation of both cerebral hemispheres, as well as the mid- and hindbrain, the spinal cord, and peripheral nervous system.

In most persons, the left cerebral hemisphere is associated with language and verbal abilities such as speech, reading, writing, and arithmetic. Left hemisphere functioning also appears to be more conscious, rational, and oriented to concepts such as the past, present, and future. Contrarily, the right hemisphere more commonly processes nonverbal or *visual-spatial* (i.e., the relationship of objects in space) information. Furthermore, current research has shown that the right hemisphere has a stronger connection to the limbic system, and therefore, plays a greater role in emotional experience. While left hemisphere thought is more reality-based and logical, right hemisphere thinking appears more unconscious and dream-like, relying heavily upon the use of fantasy. Psychoanalytically oriented thinkers have recently proposed that the right hemisphere specializes in *primary process thinking* (a more primitive type of thinking that seeks immediate gratification and relies upon the use of wishes[8]) and the left hemisphere, in *secondary process thinking* (a more mature form of thinking oriented towards the outside world and directed towards achieving goals[8]). Furthermore, these researchers suggest that many of the conflicts that we experience in our mental lives reflect the differing demands and modes of operations of the two cerebral hemispheres.

The relationship between cerebral hemisphere and function is further complicated by the phenomenon of *contralateral representation*: each hemisphere of the brain controls the side of the body that is opposite to it. For instance, the right hand is under the influence of the left hemisphere, and the left hand is directed by the right hemisphere. Furthermore, in many cases, an injury to a particular brain region will lead to a sensory or motor deficit in that part of the body that is opposite to the side of the lesion. While a number of scientists have hypothesized why the relationship between the brain and body is crossed, the phenomenon of contralateral representation remains a mystery.

The Lobes of the Brain

While consciousness arises from the symphonic operation of the entire brain, neuroscience research has found that the four lobes of the two cerebral hemispheres are fairly specialized in function. Figure 20.3 presents the lobes of the brain as viewed from the lateral aspect. Our examination of the four cortical lobes will proceed from the posterior to the anterior regions.

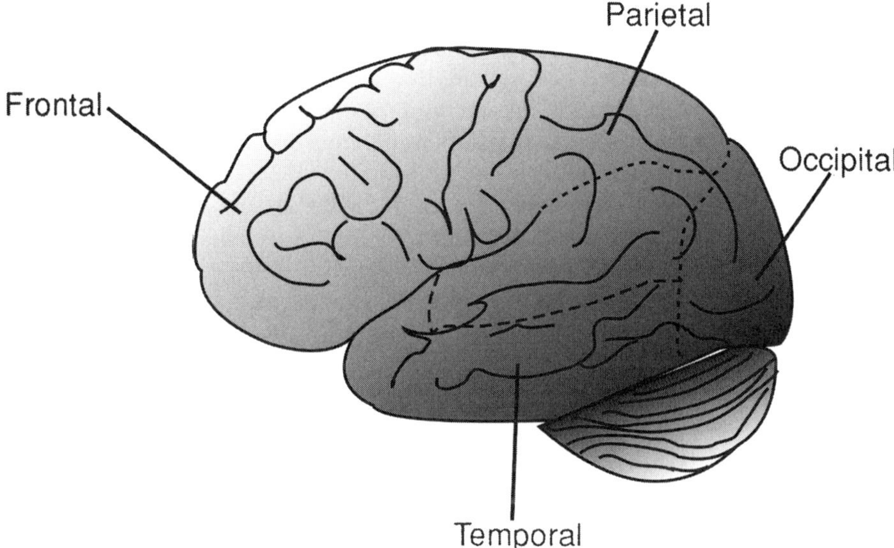

Figure 20.3 Lateral view of the brain.

Occipital Lobe

Located at the posterior end of the cerebral hemispheres, the occipital lobe is predominately responsible for our sense of sight. Every visual experience arises from the functioning of the 100 million neurons that compose the occipital cortex.[10] Sensory experience received by the eyes reaches the right and left occipital lobes via the thalamus.[9] In general, visual information received by the left eye is sent to the right hemisphere, and information received by the right eye is sent to the left hemisphere. The exception is the outer part of the visual field (i.e., nearer the temples) which does not cross.[3]

Visual information sent to either hemisphere is first processed by the *striate* (so named because of its striped appearance) or *primary visual cortex*. Neurons in the primary visual cortex specialize in the detection of the basic features of visual stimuli, such as brightness, darkness, and the perception of edges.[10] The perceptual complexity of a visual image increases as visual stimuli are processed by the anterior regions of the occipital lobe.

Occipital Lobe Damage

Damage to the striate cortex leads to a loss of vision that is proportional to the amount of injured tissue. Injury to more anterior regions of the occipital lobe results in more subtle visual impairment. As will be discussed in greater detail in the next chapter, the types of visual problems that follow mild head injury often involve subtle perceptual disturbances. Such impairment does not readily indicate what area of the occipital lobe is affected: mild deficits could arise from the posterior or anterior visual cortex, as well as the neural connections which link the occipital lobe to other brain regions.

Parietal Lobe

Lying between the occipital lobe and the *central sulcus* (the large groove separating the frontal lobe from the rest of the brain[3]), the parietal lobe specializes in the processing of *somatosensory* (i.e., body sense) information. Such information arises from touch receptors, muscle-stretch receptors, and joint receptors.[9] It is through the functioning of the parietal lobe that we are able to identify objects merely by touch, coordinate information received from different sensory channels, and navigate our way through the world. Somatosensory information from the right side of the body is processed by the left hemisphere, and somatosensory information from the left side of the body is processed by the right hemisphere.

The cortex immediately behind the central sulcus is known as the *postcentral gyrus* or *primary somatosensory area*. This brain region includes four bands of cells that receive tactile information from various body parts. Two cell bands specialize in mostly light-touch information, one in deep pressure information, and the last, a combination of the two.[9] Interestingly, the amount of primary somatosensory cortex (or as it is often called the *sensory strip*) devoted to a particular body region is not equally distributed across the body. For instance, in humans, a larger section of the postcentral gyrus is dedicated to processing sensory stimuli gathered by the hands since it is through the hands, that we obtain our most relevant tactile information.

Research has shown that the function of the parietal lobe is not limited to the processing of incoming body sensations arising from touch, or the position of a limb in space. Beyond the postcentral gyrus, the posterior regions of the parietal cortex specialize in integrating sensory input from the somatic, visual, and auditory brain regions. One type of complex information processing mediated by the anterior parietal cortex is *cross-modal matching*. This is our ability to gather information from one sensory modality (e.g., touch), and then transfer that information to another sensory system (e.g., sight). For instance, through cross-modal matching we are able to hold an object in our hands and then later identify it solely by sight.[2] Reading is another complex behavior mediated by the cross-modal matching abilities of the left posterior parietal lobe. Neuroscientists such as Norm Geshwind and Aleksandr Luria have proposed that language arises from the integration of auditory, visual, and somatic information mediated by the *angular gyrus* and *supramarginal gyri*, left hemisphere parietal structures that border on the temporal and occipital lobes.[2]

The processing of visual-spatial information (i.e., the visual perception of an object in space, or in relation to other objects) is another important integrating function of the parietal lobe. Specific right hemisphere parietal cells are probably responsible for our ability to acknowledge an object as being the same, regardless from which angle we view it.[9] This function should not be underestimated, for it plays an important role in our capacity to draw and read maps, as well as describe how to get somewhere.

Parietal Lobe Damage

Damage to the postcentral gyrus seldom results in a complete lose of the sensations coming from touch, muscle, or joint receptors. Instead, the most common complaint is in the interpretation of somatosensory information and using it to control movement behavior.

Because the functioning of the parietal lobe is central to the integration of information coming from visual, auditory and somatosensory channels, parietal lobe damage can lead to very significant neuropsychological impairment. Common difficulties include deficits in the ability to identify objects by touch or sight; clumsiness or inability to carry out actions on the side of the body opposite to the region of damage (i.e., *apraxia*); *contralateral neglect* (i.e., the person fails to acknowledge an area of the body or object [e.g., the person fails to read the right side of the page, or shave the right side of his face] on the side opposite to the brain damage); language problems (e.g., *alexia, aphasia*); difficulty with arithmetic; short-term memory problems; and deficits in visual-spatial abilities such as drawing and assembling objects from their component parts (i.e., *constructional abilities*).[2,9] The parietal lobe deficits indicative of minor head injury are discussed in the next chapter.

Temporal Lobe

Positioned laterally and near the temples in each cerebral hemisphere, the temporal lobe is responsible for processing information arising in the ears and the vestibular organs (i.e., those dealing with balance, equilibrium, and the sensation of movement in space).[9] As with the eyes, information received by the right ear is processed by the left temporal lobe, and information received by the left ear is processed by the right temporal lobe.

As with the other lobes, the temporal cortex has secondary functions beyond the primary role it plays in hearing and equilibrium. These include contributing to the perception of complex visual patterns (e.g., the recognition of faces [a right temporal lobe function]), the understanding of language (a left temporal lobe function), and the experience of emotion and motivation. The temporal lobe is also involved in the long-term memory of sensory information.[2] The hippocampus (see above), a deep temporal lobe structure, appears to effect the storage and retrieval of sensory information.

The temporal lobe is part of the limbic system (see above) and is involved in assigning affective qualities to stimuli in order to infuse them with motivational significance. Essentially, the temporal lobe labels an experience as having a positive, negative, or neutral consequence. This is particularly relevant to learning because if experience lacked an emotional valence, all stimuli would be treated equally and would be responded to indifferently.[2]

Temporal Lobe Damage

Persons with temporal lobe injury or disease may experience a wide range of symptoms, some which can have devastating consequences. The principal temporal lobe deficits include trouble with both auditory sensation and perception; language disturbances; problems with selectively attending to auditory and visual stimuli; impaired memory; changes in sexual behavior, emotional experience, and personality.[2]

Temporal lobe damage rarely leads to complete hearing loss. Instead, the capacity to recognize different forms of auditory stimuli occurs. Such deficits include *amusia* (i.e., problems with the perception of music, e.g., tone deafness, disorders of rhythm, measure, or tempo) and *agnosia for sounds* (i.e., an inability to identify the meaning of nonverbal sounds).[2] Both of these disorders are most often associated with damage to the right temporal lobe.

Lesions of the temporal lobes beyond those areas that specialize in audition produce deficits that affect complex cognitive functions and personality. Left temporal injuries have been associated with an inability to recognize spoken words despite being able to hear pure tones (i.e., *word deafness*). Left temporal lobe lesions have also been found to produce disturbances in memory, which include difficulty in recalling verbal material regardless of whether it was presented aurally or visually.

Right temporal lobe damage has been associated with a severe condition called *temporal lobe personality*. This *neuropsychological syndrome* (i.e., a collection of neuropsychological symptoms related to one another by anatomical, physiological, or behavioral qualities) is marked by child-like speech, perseveration over personal problems, paranoia, preoccupation with religion, and aggressive outbursts.[2] While few patients demonstrate this syndrome, a more common and less severe condition is *temporal lobe epilepsy*. This disorder manifests in personality characteristics such as an emphasis on the trivial and a significant decrease in sexual interest.

Frontal Lobe

Extending from the central sulcus to the anterior limit of the brain, the frontal lobe specializes in motor behavior and consciousness. While the rest of the brain focuses upon the sensation and perception of incoming stimuli from the outside world, it is the frontal lobe that mobilizes us towards action and allows us to respond to the demands of life. Much of who we are, with respect to personality and sense of self, arises from the complexities of the left and right frontal lobes. Furthermore, damage to no other cerebral structure produces such a wide range of neuropsychological symptoms.[2]

As with the other lobes of the brain, the frontal cortex is not anatomically homogeneous. The posterior region terminating at the central sulcus is labeled the *precentral gyrus* and is the motor counterpart to the postcentral gyrus, or sensory strip (see above). The precentral gyrus is the brain's primary motor cortex and it specializes in the control of the body's movements. The left precentral gyrus predominately controls the right side of the body, and the right precentral gyrus is primarily responsible for the left side of the body. Specific areas of the *motor strip* are devoted to the movement of each body part. As with the sensory strip, the amount of precentral gyrus dedicated to a body region is proportional to the complexity of the behavior that it controls. For example, the area of the primary motor cortex responsible for controlling the complexities of speech (e.g., movements of the mouth, tongue, and jaw) is comparable to the amount of the motor strip devoted to the entire torso and legs.

Human experience is most closely linked to the anterior regions of the frontal lobes referred to as the *prefrontal cortex*. This large portion of the frontal lobe is the only cortical area that receives information from all other sensory modalities, including smell.[9] It is within the prefrontal cortex, particularly those most anterior regions labeled the *preorbital cortex* (located essentially above the orbit of both eyes) where information from all brain areas is synthesized to create consciousness.

Frontal Lobe Damage

The most common disorders of movement that result from injury to the frontal lobe include *apraxia* and *hemiplegia*.[2] Apraxia is the inability to carry out purposeful movements that were known in the past.[11] This condition usually arises from damage to more anterior frontal lobe regions.[2] Hemiplegia, which most often follows a lesion to the primary motor cortex, is complete or partial paralysis to one side of the body contralateral to the side of the brain injury.[2] While hemiplegia is a severe form of paralysis, the loss of movement in any part of the body may follow an injury to the precentral gyrus. However, unlike the permanent paralysis that usually follows spinal cord damage, loss of movement after injury to the primary motor cortex is often temporary because of equipotentiality (see above).

Lesions to the more anterior areas of the frontal lobe are associated with impairment of a wide variety of complex behaviors. Some of the most common symptoms of persons with frontal lobe damage are the inability to inhibit behavior, problems with attention, and tendencies towards behavioral inflexibility and perseveration.[2] Persons with these symptoms are often labeled as suffering from *frontal lobe syndrome.* This disorder can be quite severe and can lead to very disturbed psychological functioning. Frontal lobe syndrome patients may appear psychotic in that their thinking can appear bizarre and obsessional. They may repeat certain words, phrases, or motor behaviors over and over again. Persons with frontal lobe damage may have trouble inhibiting themselves and often demonstrate socially inappropriate behavior. Contrarily, frontal lobe patients may exhibit flat affect, a limited range of emotions, a lack of spontaneous behavior, and very concrete thinking. Unfortunately, persons with frontal lobe syndrome usually experience permanent neuropsychological impairment.

Other deficits common to prefrontal lobe damage include problems with memory and spatial orientation. Frontal lobe lesions do not usually interfere with the long-term storage of material; rather, impairment is most often to *memory for recency.*[2] Patients with frontal lesions commonly have difficulty remembering the order of events, with the right frontal lobe being more important for nonverbal or pictorial recency, and the left frontal lobe for the order of events coded verbally. The type of spatial difficulty associated with frontal lobe damage is for the accurate assessment of one's body orientation in space. Contrary to the rule that the right hemisphere dominates spatial ability, problems with personal orientation appear to arise from damage to the left frontal lobe.

NEUROPSYCHOLOGICAL EVALUATION

The neuropsychological evaluation consists of a comprehensive assessment of the patient's current level of cognitive, emotional, and psychosocial functioning. These evaluations are conducted in private practice, out-patient clinic, or hospital settings with a wide variety of patients. Patients referred for "neuropsych testing" include those who are experiencing cognitive-emotional symptoms as a result of motor vehicle accidents (MVA), cerebral vascular accidents (i.e., stroke [CVA]), head injuries, various diseases (e.g., AIDS), and old age. The primary goals of neuropsych testing are the documentation of brain dysfunction and recommendations for appropriate treatment. Such information is most often presented to the referring clinician through a detailed written report (see below).

Training and Practice in Neuropsychology

The practice of neuropsychology is demanding and requires the full attention of the clinician. More and more, neuropsychological evaluations are being conducted by clinical psychologists whose scholastic and clinical training has predominately revolved around the study of brain-behavior relationships and comprehensive psychometric assessment. Persons interested in neuropsychology usually seek a Ph.D. clinical psychology program that offers a specialized track in the discipline. Such programs often have close relationships with medical schools. During graduate school, future neuropsychologists take additional courses in neuroanatomy and neurophysiology outside the psychology department. Their clinical practicum is directed more towards neuropsychological assessment and less towards traditional psychotherapy. Following graduate school, clinical Ph.D. candidates are required by the American Psychological Association (APA) to complete a one-year internship program of in-depth clinical training. Those interested in neuropsychology seek internships that focus on the evaluation and treatment of persons with neuropsychological disorders. In order to be considered a neuropsychologist, internship must be followed by a one- or two-year period of formal postdoctoral training in neuropsychology. Some neuropsychologists then seek boarding through the American Board of Profession Psychology (ABPP).

Conducting a neuropsychological evaluation is both time-demanding and labor-intensive. Most assessments take between 4 and 8 hours. If the patient is especially impaired, an evaluation is completed over a number of days. The examination also requires very specialized testing material and equipment that is expensive to purchase. Such factors demand that clinicians devote the majority of their professional energies to neuropsychology. It is very difficult to be a good "part-time" neuropsychologist without either the general clinical practice or neuropsychological element of the practice suffering.[11]

The Neuropsychological Evaluation

Neuropsychological tests are structured tasks that require the patient to make a particular response depending on the domain of functioning being assessed. Performance on a specific test usually yields a numerical score. This score may reflect any one of a variety of test variables, including the number of correct responses, mistakes, or time to complete the task. Individual test scores are usually compared against *standardized norms*. These norms reflect typical or expected performance on a particular task and are gathered through the standardized administration of the test to both clinical and nonclinical populations. Standardized scores are often broken down by age, gender, and clinical condition.

Regardless of whether the neuropsychologist administers the same test battery to each patient, or selects tests specific to the referral question, each evaluation addresses functioning across a number of cognitive and emotional domains. These commonly include general intellectual functioning, academic achievement, memory and attentional abilities, language, motor skills, executive functioning, as well as personality and emotional functioning. As with every clinical evaluation, assessment begins with a thorough history of the patient's account of his or her problems. Each aspect of the neuropsychological evaluation is addressed below, and the most common tests applied to the measurement of the various functional domains are reviewed.

History Taking

Upon their arrival, most patients are asked to complete a structured "fill-in-the-blank" questionnaire that inquires about personal history, past and present medical history, developmental history, educational and occupational history, family and social history, as well as possible neuropsychological symptoms related to the presenting condition. For many patients, relevant medical records are forwarded to the neuropsychologist for review.

Upon completion of initial paperwork, the neuropsychologist meets with the patient for an extended interview. The gathering of a competent history is a skill that requires, in addition to a broad knowledge of neuropsychology, neurology, psychology, and general medicine, an awareness of the subtleties that occur during the clinical interview process. Patients are often tense and nervous about their conditions and the job of the clinician is to establish a rapport that is conducive to the acquisition of vital diagnostic information. Because the presentation style, and level of impairment, differs across patients, the neuropsychologist must possess a flexible interview approach. Therefore, history taking does not follow a fixed format; rather, the choice of questions and their presentation order are guided by the patient's account of his or her problems.[12]

The clinical interview is not limited to gathering historical information relevant to the patient's presenting problems. Through behavioral observation, very important data are obtained about the patient's general appearance (e.g., amount of eye contact, modulation of verbal and emotional expression, hygiene, and style of dress), motor activity (e.g., motor abnormalities, hyperkinesis, psychomotor retardation), mood, level of cooperation, and behavioral abnormalities of language, prosody, or memory.[12]

General Intellectual Functioning

Intelligence is a complex phenomenon thought to arise from both verbal and nonverbal abilities. Intellectual functioning is often defined as a person's general aptitude for performing cognitive tasks.[13] *Cognition* refers to mental processes by which knowledge is acquired.[6] Gardner maintains there are multiple intelligences including linguistic, musical, logical-mathematic, spatial, bodily-kinesthetic, and personal.[14] While this intriguing notion would account for achievement in such diverse fields as football, playing the piano, writing books, building skyscrapers, and understanding psychology, it has not been widely accepted.

Another interesting way that cognitive abilities have been described is through the concepts of *crystallized* and *fluid* intelligence. Fluid intelligence is seen as the person's ability to acquire and manipulate new knowledge; in other words, an aptitude for learning. Crystallized intelligence reflects the person's storehouse of knowledge from which they can draw for adaptation. The depth of a person's crystallized intelligence depends on his or her fluid abilities. Head injury has a different impact upon these two cognitive structures: crystallized knowledge such as vocabulary is more commonly spared, while fluid intelligence, such as the ability to solve logic puzzles that demand learning new concepts, or involves actively manipulating facts, is more frequently affected by brain injury.

General intelligence or "*g*" is defined through the *intelligence quotient*, or *IQ*, which indicates how an individual scored relative to other persons of comparable age.[14] On most scales the exact average IQ is 100. IQ is measured through standardized test batteries that are frequently composed of subtests which address specific verbal and nonverbal/spatial abilities. Verbal abilities are usually viewed as reflecting left hemisphere functioning, and spatial abilities are thought to reflect right hemisphere functioning.

IQ Tests

While many IQ tests exist, those developed by David Wechsler have been the most frequently used measures of intelligence. Wechsler's tests were adapted from the Stanford-Binet Intellectual Scale, as well as the Army Alpha and Beta Tests developed to evaluate recently inducted soldiers earlier this century. Most neuropsychological test batteries incorporate one of Wechsler's three scales: the Wechsler Adult Intelligence Scale – Revised (WAIS-R [for ages 16 to 74]), the Wechsler Intelligence Scale for Children – III (WISC-III [for ages 6 to 16]), and the Wechsler Preschool and Primary Scale of Intelligence – Revised (WPPSI-R [for ages 3 to 7]).[12] At the time of this writing, a new edition of the WAIS is being prepared.

Because most minor head injuries that lead to neuropsychological sequelae occur in adults, our focus will be upon the WAIS-R. Besides Full-Scale IQ, Wechsler divides intelligence into Verbal and Performance IQ scores. Verbal IQ is derived from scores on six subtests that include Information (i.e., knowledge of facts about general topics such as history, science, and literature), Digit Span (i.e., a measure of attention examined through the recall of aurally presented strings of numbers, both forwards and backwards), Vocabulary (i.e., knowledge of word definitions), Arithmetic (i.e., tasks that range from counting blocks to solving aurally presented word problems), Comprehension (i.e., knowledge of societal rules and norms, and practical reasoning), and Similarities (i.e., abstract verbal ability measured through knowledge of how paired-associates are alike). While not inclusive, a number of the Verbal Subtests are directed more towards crystallized intelligence (e.g., Information, Vocabulary, Comprehension). Performance IQ, or nonverbal intelligence, is measured through five subtests: Picture Completion (i.e., attention to visual detail measured through the identification of the missing part of pictures), Picture Arrangement (i.e., social/visual abstract ability measured through the proper placement of sequences of pictures that tell stories), Block Design (i.e., visual-spatial constructional abilities measured through the arrangement of red- and white-sided blocks into patterns), Object Assembly (i.e., visual-spatial constructional abilities measured through the placement of puzzle pieces that form meaningful objects), and Digit Symbol (i.e., grapho-motor skill measured through the timed transferring of number cues into geometric symbols). Most of the Performance IQ Subtests reflect fluid intelligence.

The Wechsler intelligence tests divide IQ into seven categories that reflect a spectrum spanning from mental impairment to intellectual superiority. Each category is defined by a range of IQ scores:

Very Superior	130 and above
Superior	120–129
High Average	110–119
Average	90–109
Low Average	80–89
Borderline	70–79
Intellectually Deficient	69 and below

IQ Test Performance and Brain Injury

The arrangement of Verbal and Performance Subscale scores provides important diagnostic information to the neuropsychologist. In general, Performance IQ is more commonly affected by head injury. Because the Vocabulary Subtest is an excellent measure of crystallized ability, performance on this scale is a good indicator of a person's premorbid intelligence. A significant discrepancy between Verbal and Performance IQ often reflects left vs. right hemisphere pathology. Deficits of attention are evident through poor scores on a number of subtests, including Digit Span and Arithmetic. Problems with attention are often related to frontal lobe damage. Visual-spatial problems, suggestive of right parietal lobe involvement, become obvious through low scores on the Block Design and Object Assembly subtests. Abstract thinking, another frontal lobe function, is measured through the Similarities (left hemisphere) and Picture Arrangement (right hemisphere) subtests. The next chapter describes specific research findings of the effect of minor head injury on general intellectual functioning.

Academic Achievement

Aptitude refers to a person's inherent intellectual abilities. Achievement is a person's storehouse of knowledge and skills obtained through education. These concepts are somewhat analogous to the computer terms "hardware (hard drive)" and "software (programs)". The computer's hardware is the wiring and circuitry that allows it to process and store information. Much like a person's intellect, the capabilities of this hardware ultimately determine the complexity and quality of information the computer can process and store. Software are the various skills or "applications" that are "copied" (a computer analogue to learning) onto the hard drive, thus giving the computer the abilities to carry out specific tasks, just as education permits a person to reach his or her intellectual potential.

As with IQ testing, there are a number of popular assessment batteries that evaluate a person's academic achievement. What is common to most batteries is that their scoring systems are arranged so as to provide meaningful information about a person's level of achievement in relation to their intellectual aptitude, as measured with an IQ test. This is accomplished through the use of a *standard score* that reflects the conversion of the *raw score* (i.e., the number of correct answers for a subtest) to the scale adopted for IQ values (see above): Once again, a standard score of 100 is considered the exact average. The use of standard scores provides valuable information to the neuropsychologist. Of itself, a person's standard score on a particular subtest (e.g., arithmetic), reveals his or her level of knowledge and ability for that area of academic achievement. When compared to IQ, the standard score indicates whether the person's level of achievement within an academic area is commensurate with his or her intellectual aptitude.

Recently, much has been said about *learning deficits* or *disabilities*. These conditions reflect deficient academic achievement in one or more areas that is not related to mental retardation, emotional problems, poor education, or sensory or motor problems.[15] Unfortunately, the diagnosis of a learning disability is often made arbitrarily, without proper neuropsychological evaluation, and has become somewhat of a "catch-all" label when a child or adult is having scholastic difficulties. Fortunately, most states now require a formal evaluation prior to the provision of social or academic services. Such evaluations usually include IQ and academic assessment, along with tests that evaluate complaints related to the specific problem, as well as the possible contribution of emotional factors. Two important criteria that often must be fulfilled prior to the assignment of a formal learning disability are: (1) the person must have an average IQ or higher (i.e., generally, a score of 90 or above); (2) there must be at least a 15-point discrepancy (i.e., a full standard deviation) between the achievement standard score and the person's Full-Scale IQ score. For example, if a person has been having difficulty with mathematics and his or her IQ is 105, a formal diagnosis of a learning disorder is dependent upon an arithmetic standard score of 90 or below.

Achievement tests also provide *grade scores* which indicate at what grade level a person's current abilities are for a certain academic area. These scores are very useful for determining the impact of head injury on academic performance. For instance, if a person with head trauma following an MVA had a premorbid IQ of 115, and graduated from college with an above average GPA (i.e., grade point average), we would expect his or her grade scores to be at least 13 (i.e., one year or more past high school). Scores lower than these, along with other supportive test findings, would suggest that the head injury impacted the person's level of academic achievement.

Achievement Tests

Of the various achievement tests, three in particular are used widely: the Woodcock-Johnson Psychoeducational Battery – Revised (WJ-R), the Peabody Individual Achievement Test – Revised (PIAT-R), and the Wide Range Achievement Test – Revision 3 (WRAT 3).[12] Growing in popularity is the Wechsler Individual Achievement Test (WIAT) whose advantage is that the design of the subscales and test scores more closely correspond to the parameters of the WISC-III and WAIS-R, the most widely used IQ tests (see above).

The PIAT-R is a popular screening test of achievement for children from kindergarten to the 12th grade and measures ability in the areas of mathematics, reading recognition, reading comprehension, spelling, and general information.[12] The WRAT 3 is another popular academic screen that provides standard and grade scores in the general areas of reading, spelling, and arithmetic. The WRAT 3 is commonly administered when academic achievement is not a major focus of assessment, or time restraints prohibit a more thorough evaluation. The Woodcock-Johnson may be the most widely used comprehensive inventory of academic achievement. The test battery measures achievement in the areas of reading, mathematics, written language, and general knowledge of science, social studies, and humanities.[12] The WJ-R is applicable to both handicapped and nonhandicapped persons from the ages of 2 to 90 years.

While academic achievement is clearly influenced by brain trauma, psychoeducational batteries are not as sensitive for documenting the range of deficits, or location of brain injury, as are other neuropsychological tests. The most apparent reason for this is that the skills measured by most achievement tests load more heavily onto functions that are principally language-based and predominately mediated by the left hemisphere.

Memory and Attention

Attention and memory are very complex constructs. *Attention* is the cognitive mechanism that selects some relevant material from the environment for further processing and excludes the rest.[16] Attention is commonly viewed as a frontal lobe function. As indicated above, frontal lobe damage can lead to a condition whereby a person has problems focusing his or her attention; contrarily, the person may perseverate upon a stimulus beyond its relevance to a current situation.

Within the context of *information processing theory* (i.e., the notion that information flows through a multistage memory system), memory is generally thought to be composed of three distinct constructs: *sensory memory*, *short-term memory*, and *long-term memory*.[16] Sensory memory is our retention of environmental sights and sounds as mere sense impressions. Sensory memory allows us to survey the environment for important stimuli that might be selected for further attention and memory processing. Sensory memory is very brief, lasting only about one second. The two forms of sensory memory are called *echoic* and *iconic*. Echoic memory is for auditory impressions and iconic memory is for visual impressions.

The fraction of incoming information that we attend to via sensory memory enters short-term memory.[16] Short-term memory holds information for about fifteen to thirty seconds. This holding of information is referred to as *coding*. The persistence of stimuli in short-term memory arises from *acoustic* (sound or language-based) and *semantic* (meaning or category-based) coding. Short-term memory is limited by the amount of information it can process before it fades away. Consistently, research has found that the *memory span* is limited to seven items (e.g., seven letters, numbers, or words), plus or minus two (i.e., 5 or 9).

Long-term memory involves the more permanent storage of information through the process of *encoding*. Encoding transforms information into a form that can be handled and stored by the long-term memory system.[16] *Rehearsal* and *retrieval* are the two processes that permit us to store and access long-term information. *Maintenance rehearsal* is when we repeat an item over and over, as when we look up a phone number and rehearse it prior to dialing. *Elaborative rehearsal* is when we relate an item to be remembered to other times or items with which it can be associated.[16] For instance, we might remember a phone number by associating the arrangement of numbers to some other meaningful numerical sequence (e.g., a birthday, birth year, or historical event). Research has shown that the more elaborate the approach for memorizing material, the more likely it will be encoded into the long-term memory system.[16]

Retrieval is the process of calling information up from long-term memory. It is believed that during retrieval, the process of encoding is reversed and information reenters short-term memory.[16] Some have argued that all encoded long-term memory is retained and potentially *available* for information processing. Why memory is not readily retrievable is a problem of *accessibility*, for instance, the *tip-of-the-tongue phenomenon* whereby we are unable to recall a normally remembered fact.[16]

With respect to neuroanatomy, memory does not appear to be stored in one area of the brain, but is distributed throughout the entire cortex. Presumably, those forms of memory that are related to a specific function are stored in those brain regions dedicated to it. For instance, verbal memory is distributed throughout the left hemisphere, and nonverbal memory throughout the right. Therefore, damage to one brain region may hinder one form of memory, while leaving other types of memory intact.

Tests of Attention and Memory

As is discussed in the next chapter, memory disturbance is a very common complaint following minor head injury. Problems include trouble attending to stimuli, as well as deficits in retaining and retrieving information. Evaluation of memory functioning should assess immediate or short-term retention, the rate and pattern of acquiring new information, the efficiency with which recently learned information and long-standing memory are retrieved, and the impact of interfering stimuli, across both the verbal and nonverbal domains.[12]

When assessing memory, most neuropsychologists use an assortment of tests. Tests of verbal attention and memory often rely upon lists of numbers or words, as well as groups of sentences and paragraphs. During these tests, patients are presented the verbal stimuli in either spoken or written forms and asked to attend to and memorize them. These tests frequently include measures of immediate and long-term recall and recognition, and increased sensitivity to *proactive* (i.e., earlier learning that interferes with the later recall of newly learned material[16]) and *retroactive interference* (i.e., interference arising from learning that occurs between the acquisition and recall of previously learned material[16]).[12] Common tests of verbal attention and memory include the Digit Span Subtest from the WAIS-R, the Rey Auditory Verbal Learning Test, the Nonsense Syllable Learning Test, the California Verbal Learning Test, and the Sentence Repetition Test.[11,12]

Evaluation of visual-spatial attention and memory is usually accomplished through the brief presentation of visual designs followed by recognition (e.g., choosing the design out of a set of stimuli) or recall (i.e., reproducing the design, usually through drawing) at varying lengths of delay (e.g., immediate, 5 minutes, 10 minutes, 30 minutes).[12] Popular tests of visual-spatial attention and memory include the Benton Visual Retention Test – Revised, the Tactile Performance Test, the Rey Visual Learning Test, and the Rey-Osterrieth Complex Figure Test.[11,12]

Specific Tests of Attention and Memory

There are myriad tests of attention and memory. This section will provide more detailed presentation of a number of the most popular tests used for both clinical assessment and research.

Wechsler Memory Scale – Revised (WMS-R): The WMS-R is the most widely used battery of memory tests.[12] The battery is intended for persons ranging in age from 16 to 74 years and provides good normative data based upon a large representative sample of persons from the U.S. population. The Wechsler Memory Scale yields a number of Memory Indexes including those that represent global memory functioning, attention and concentration, verbal and nonverbal memory, as well as an index of delayed recall. As with the other Wechsler batteries (e.g., the WAIS-R and WIAT), a score of 100 represents the exact average.

The WMS-R consists of thirteen subtests.[12] Information and Orientation inquires about topics such as the patient's name, birthday, and who are current political officials (e.g., "Who is President of the United States?"). Other questions ask about the day, date, time, and patient's location. The first WMS-R subtest gathers information common to a *Mental Status Examination* (MSE).[11] A MSE is usually part of a psychiatric evaluation and obtains diagnostic material about the patient's presenting symptoms, appearance, language functions, thought processes, emotional functioning, insight, and judgment. The Information and Orientation subtest is used for screening the patient's general ability for completing the remainder of the battery. The subtest does not yield a scale score and is not included in the calculation of the Memory Indexes.

Mental Control is the second subtest of the Wechsler Memory Scale. The patient is asked to count backwards, recite the alphabet, and count a sequence of numbers by fours. This subtest measures automatic responding and the ability to engage in a sequence of mental operations.[12]

Figural Memory is the third WMS-R subtest. This is a measure of visual memory recognition whereby the patient is asked to briefly examine abstract figures and then identify them from a group of other abstract stimuli.[12]

The fourth subtest, Logical Memory I, measures the immediate recall of two aurally presented stories. Patients are assigned a score based on the number of key verbal details they are able to recall from both tales.[11]

Memory for material related by association is measured with the next two subtests.[12] On Visual Paired Associates I, the patient is presented six abstract drawings paired with six colors. Test trials consist of identifying the correct color associated with each figure. During Verbal Paired Associates I, the patient is read a group of eight word pairs up to six times; on test trials only the first word is presented and the patient must provide the second word.

Immediate recall of visual stimuli is assessed with the Visual Reproduction I subtest.[12] Patients are briefly presented geometric designs and then asked to draw them.

A measure of verbal memory span is obtained through a Digit Span subtest similar to that found on the WAIS-R.[12] Visual memory span is assessed by having the patient tap patterned sequences upon colored squares. Across trials, the length of the sequences increase. As with Digit span, separate trials measure forwards and backwards recall.

Approximately 30 minutes after the presentation of the Logical Memory I subtest, during which time a number of other subtests have been administered, the patient is given the Logical Memory II, Visual Paired Associates II, Verbal Paired Associates II, and Visual Reproduction II subtests. The presentation of these subtests is identical to the first trial except no learning trials occur. The patient is just asked to remember, as best they can, and either recognize or reproduce the various visual and verbal stimuli.

The WMS-R is an excellent global assessment of verbal and nonverbal memory functioning. While most neuropsychologists agree that the WMS-R is a very valuable instrument, it should not be the sole measure of memory obtained during a comprehensive evaluation. Some researchers argue that the verbal and nonverbal memory indexes are not sensitive enough to infer that poor performance on a scale is related to dysfunction within the corresponding hemisphere (e.g., poor verbal memory performance arising from left hemisphere dysfunction).[12] Additionally, WMS-R index scores are commonly skewed in relationship to IQ scores obtained on the Wechsler intelligence batteries. It has been this author's clinical experience that in person's with average or above-average IQs, WMS-R index scores are often much higher than anticipated.

Paced Auditory Serial Addition Test (PASAT): The PASAT is a serial-addition task that assesses sustained attention.[12] This measure of concentration and information processing has received considerable application within both clinical and research environments. The task itself can be quite challenging to many patients: a prerecorded tape presents a series of 61 numbers from 1 to 9, and the patient is asked to add pairs of numbers so that each number is added to the one immediately proceeding it (e.g., 2 and 7 are added equaling 9; if the next number is 4, this is added to 7 giving 11).[12] The numbers can be presented across four trials. The presentation rate of the numbers increases across trials and ranges from 2.4 seconds to 1.2 seconds.

The PASAT has been shown to be a very sensitive test of information processing difficulties in persons with mild brain trauma such as mild concussion. Research has demonstrated that the PASAT is a better measure of post traumatic memory problems than post traumatic amnesia (see the next chapter), and test performance can indicate a person's readiness to return to work.[12]

Concentration Endurance Test (d2 Test): Like the PASAT, the d2 Test is also a measure of sustained attention. While the PASAT is presented aurally, the d2 Test involves visual scanning. The d2 is a *cancellation test* whereby the patient is asked to scan 14 lines of letters and circle the letter "d" whenever two slashes (i.e., ") appear above it.[12] The patient is allowed 20 seconds per line. The task is made more difficult through the omission of slashes, the use of only one slash, and the placement of slashes below the "d's". Additionally, slashes are also placed above and below many of the letter "p's" that appear in the 14 lines.

The d2 is only one of many cancellation tests. Another that is commonly administered by neuropsychologists is the Finding A's test. Along with testing sustained attention, cancellation tasks measure visual scanning, response speed, ability to shift responses, and unilateral spatial neglect.[12]

Benton Visual Retention Test – Revised (BVRT-R): The revised BVRT tests visual perception and memory, and visuoconstructive abilities through drawing.[12] While the "Benton" has a number of administration formats, all rely upon presenting the patient a geometric figure for 5 or 10 seconds and asking him or her to reproduce it by drawing or distinguish it from other figures. The patient is asked to respond either immediately or following a 15-second delay.

The Benton is a widely used and valuable instrument. It is sensitive for detecting brain damage usually within the right posterior hemisphere. Test performance may also aid the neuropsychologist in discriminating between perceptual, motor, and memory problems. The BVRT is useful for detecting persons who are attempting to exaggerate their symptoms. Research has shown that persons attempting to feign symptoms produce more distortions, fewer perseverations, and fewer errors than brain-damaged patients.[12]

California Verbal Learning Test (CVLT): The CVLT is a popular test of verbal memory and learning, including the patient's ability for categorical thinking, the effects of proactive and retroactive interference, as well as the effect of time on retention of verbal material.[17] Across five trials, the patient is read a list of words said to represent a shopping list ("Monday list") that includes items of clothing, fruit, and spices. After each trial, the patient is asked to recall as many words as they can. Following the five trials, the patient is introduced to another shopping list ("Tuesday list") which they attempt to memorize. Free recall and cued recall trials of the Monday list then measure the effects of a short-delay and interfering stimuli on verbal memory. During the cued trials, the patient is asked to recall the words by category (i.e., fruits, clothes, spices). Following a 20-minute delay, during which time *nonverbal* tests are given, the patient is once again asked to recall the Monday list. This trial assesses longer-term integration of verbal stimuli into memory.

The CVLT provides a number of valuable memory scores that assess recall, recognition, perseveration, and semantic memory. Because the test is well-normed on both clinical and research populations it is included in most neuropsychological batteries.

Rey-Osterrieth Complex Figure Test: The Complex Figure (CF) is perhaps the most widely used measure of visual construction (i.e., drawing) ability and memory, and is an essential component of almost every neuropsychological evaluation. The test consists of presenting the patient with a card on which is printed an abstract design consisting of a large central rectangle and an arrangement of details including squares, triangles, lines, crosses, and a circle that forms a unified figure (the CF is intentionally not reproduced here in an effort to maintain the instrument's integrity). The patient is then asked to copy the figure as best he or she can using an arrangement of colored pencils. The presentation of the pencils in an ordered sequence (e.g., red followed by green, blue, and orange) allows the neuropsychologist to document the strategy with which the patient reproduced the figure. The approach towards drawing the figure reveals important information about the patient's nonverbal cognitive processes including planning, organizational and problem-solving skills.[12] Without warning, the patient is then asked to reproduce the CF to the best of his or her ability (immediate recall). The Immediate Recall trial is usually followed by a Delay Recall trial that ranges in time span from 3 to 45 minutes. Most examiners rely upon a 30-minute delay during which tests of *verbal* ability are administered. The amount of time taken by the patient to reproduce the CF is usually timed during the Copy, Immediate Recall, and Delayed-Recall trials.

A number of scoring systems have been developed to evaluate CF performance. They are based upon the correctness of the details and their placement.[12] The figure is broken down into component parts and a numerical score is assigned to the quality with which the patient produced each segment.

Interpretation of a patient's drawings is based upon both the global CF scores for copying and recall, as well as qualitative aspects of performance.[12] As indicated above, the patient's approach taken towards reproducing the figure reveals important information on his or her nonverbal cognitive abilities. Research on normal individuals has shown that the strategy taking towards copying the CF evolves during childhood. Young children usually take a *piecemeal approach* whereby elements of the CF are drawn in a haphazard manner. By age 13 the normal strategy becomes more configurational: the child begins with the large central rectangle and the details are added on in relation to it.[12] During recall trials, it is rare for a child to use the piecemeal approach after age 9.[12] The use of the piecemeal approach by an adult is suggestive of a deficit in visual-spatial planning, organization, and execution. It is not uncommon that a person's approach towards reproducing the CF switches from configurational to piecemeal as a result of a significant head injury, cerebral vascular accident, or dementia. This is an example of an important neuropsychological phenomena: compromising neurological conditions arising from trauma or disease often lead to a state of neuropsychological regression where a person exhibits behavior common to a younger developmental period. For instance, seriously head injured persons sometimes show certain muscular reflexes normally seen in very young infants that then disappear during the first year of life.

The Rey-Osterrieth Complex Figure is an excellent instrument for detecting problems of visual-spatial constructional ability and memory. In many cases, poor performance does reflect a right hemisphere deficit. Research has shown that persons with right-frontal lobe lesions are more likely to show planning problems when attempting the task, whereas right parietal-occipital lesions contribute to difficulties with the spatial organization of the figure.[12] Of interest is that the piecemeal approach is shown by persons with both left and right hemisphere brain damage. However, right hemisphere lesions are associated with less accurate and more highly distorted reproductions. Furthermore, persons with right hemisphere damage perform more poorly on recall trials.

Rey Auditory-Verbal Learning Test (RAVLT): The RAVLT is a measure of verbal learning and memory.[12] The format of the RAVLT is quite similar to that of the CVLT (see above). The patient is asked to remember and recall a word list administered aurally across five trials. A different list is then presented for the purpose of interference, followed by another attempt by the patient to recall the first list. Following a 20-minute delay, the patient is again asked to recall the first list. This is followed by a recognition trial where the patient is presented a printed list of the words and asked to circle those from the first list.

The RAVLT is a brief, easily administered test, that measures immediate memory span, learning, susceptibility to interference, and recognition memory.[12] The instrument is sensitive to left-hemisphere problems in a variety of patient groups and has been shown to differentiate memory disorders.

Tactile Performance Test (TPT): This interesting neuropsychological test assesses a variety of functions, including recognition of forms through touch, memory for shapes, and spatial location, as well as psychomotor problem solving.[12] The TPT is an excellent measure of cross-modal matching (see above). Patients are required to gather information through the sense of touch and then use it to operate upon a visual-spatial domain, all without the aid of vision. The TPT consists of a Form Board upon which geometric-shaped blocks fit into same-shaped spaces, much in the manner with which puzzle pieces fit in a background board. For persons aged 15 years and older, the Form Board has 10 blocks; for children under age 15, the Form Board has 6 blocks. During each of the three test trials, the patient is blind-folded and attempts to place each block into its corresponding space. For the first trial, patients are allowed to use only their preferred hand; the second trial is for the nonpreferred hand; during the final trial, the patient is permitted to use both hands. After the last trial, and the blindfold is removed, patients are asked to draw the face of the Form Board as best as they can with respect to both the shape and placement of the blocks. The TPT yields a variety of scores: (1) total time on each placement trial, (2) the total number of correctly drawn shapes, and (3) the number of correctly drawn block locations.[12]

Language

Normal language depends on a complex interaction between systems of symbolic association, motor skills, learned syntactic patterns, sensory integration, and verbal memory.[2] In most persons, the complexities of language arise predominately from the functioning of two areas in the left hemisphere. *Broca's area* is a left frontal lobe region believed to be involved in language production (i.e., the ability to talk).[2] *Wernicke's area*, a region in the left posterior portion of the superior temporal lobe, is thought to underlie the comprehension of language and the person's ability to arrange sounds into coherent speech.[2]

There are many language disorders. In general, they can be arranged under two broad categories: *disorders of comprehension* and *disorders of production*.[2] Disorders of comprehension entail difficulties with understanding language in either the spoken or written form. Disorders of production include problems with articulation, writing, verbal fluency, grammar and syntax.

Aphasia is another term commonly used to denote different classes of language deficit.[2] In *Broca's* or *motor aphasia* the patient has trouble speaking, although he or she continues to understand speech. *Wernicke's aphasia* consists of an inability to comprehend words or arrange sounds into coherent speech. *Conduction aphasia* is an unusual disorder where the patient can engage in all aspects of speech except he or she cannot repeat words. With *isolation syndrome* the patient retains all language abilities, but is either unable to produce spontaneous speech, or he or she can repeat words but is unable to comprehend them. *Anomic aphasia* entails difficulty finding the names of objects. Patients with this disorder commonly compensate by describing the function of the object whose name they cannot recall. *Paraphasias* are mistakes in speech such as the production of unintended syllables, words, or phrases.

Testing Language Abilities

Neuropsychological testing assesses language function across both the comprehension and production domains. During a neuropsychological evaluation, patients are asked to speak, read, and write. Assessment occurs through both formal and informal approaches. Many measures of language function exist. While an exhaustive list is not included, several of the most commonly used tests are described below.

Aphasia Screening Test (AST): The AST is perhaps the most widely used test for assessing aphasia.[11] The test asks the patient to engage in a variety of tasks, including drawing simple shapes, naming shapes and objects, spelling words, repeating words, writing a simple sentence, and solving math problems. Several versions of the test exist. They differ in the number of items that they contain, ranging from only 4 to 51.[11] The emphasis of the test is upon determining the presence and, to a lesser extent, the nature of communication problems.[11] Test findings are predominately handled in a descriptive fashion, although some examiners use a six-point rating scale to indicate the severity of the aphasic disorder.

While the AST is good at determining the presence of language problems, it is limited by its qualitative approach and lack of strong normative data. Persons with left hemisphere disorders are expected to have difficulty completing verbally based tasks while persons with right hemisphere lesions should have trouble performing the drawing tasks.[11]

Boston Naming Test (BNT): This test assesses the patient's ability to name pictured objects, a task that entails transforming nonverbal information into a verbal response. One at a time, the patient is presented 60 cards, each of which contains a drawing. The name for each item becomes more difficult as the set progresses (e.g., an early card shows a "tree," while a later card presents an "abacus"[12]). The patient is instructed to spontaneously respond to each card. If the patient fails to respond to the card after 20 seconds, one or two cues are given. A *semantic cue* provides a hint about the function of the target object.[12] For instance, if the target object was a "piece of cake," a semantic cue might be "something you eat." The examiner gives a *phonemic cue* by speaking the initial phoneme of the object's name. A variety of scores are generated, including: (1) the number of spontaneous correct answers, (2) the number of cues provided, (3) the number of correct responses following cues, (4) the number of phonemic cues given, and (5) the number of correct and incorrect responses following phonemic cues.[12] Along with typical normative data, the BNT manual includes mean performance scores for persons diagnosed with aphasias of differing severity, as determined by the Boston Diagnostic Aphasia Examination.[12]

Because of the high frequency of naming problems in aphasia, most assessments of language function will include a naming test.[12] The Peabody Picture Vocabulary Test – Revised (PPVT-R) is another popular test similar in design to the BNT. The crucial difference between the two tests is that the revised PPVT reverses the information processing pathway assessed by the BNT. Rather than speaking the name of the object shown on the stimulus card, the patient must pick out the picture of the object whose name is spoken by the examiner. The different approaches taken by these two instruments warrant the inclusion of both tests in a neuropsychological evaluation, particularly if anomic aphasia or isolation syndrome is suspected (see above).

Controlled Oral Word Association (Word Fluency/FAS Test): The Word Fluency test measures the patient's spontaneous production of words that begin either with a certain letter or are from a specific class (e.g., foods) within a limited amount of time (i.e., 1 minute).[12] The assessment is commonly called the FAS Test because these three letters have been the most commonly used. During administration, the patient is merely asked to provide as many words as they can beginning with the target letter. It is requested that they give no proper names (e.g., "Fred") or repeat a word with a different ending (e.g., "sing" and "singing"). The patient's score reflects the number of correct words for the three letters (or categories).

In many cases, persons with right hemisphere damage do not have impaired FAS Test performance. However, a number of studies suggest that word fluency is affected by lesions in either hemisphere, especially if damage is to the left or right frontal cortex.[12] When assessing word fluency, it is important to consider that psychological symptoms such as anxiety and depression can significantly hinder performance.

Sentence Repetition Test: This measure assesses the patient's ability to immediately repeat a list of sentences that increase in length.[12] The patient is administered either Forms A or B, each set consisting of 22 sentences. Some examiners use a tape recorded administration. The test is discontinued if the patient makes five consecutive mistakes. One point is given for each correctly repeated sentence.

The Sentence Repetition Test has been well studied in brain damaged persons and good normative data are available. Poorest performance has been associated with left hemisphere lesions in persons who have experienced either a CVA or closed head injury. The test is most sensitive for detecting isolation syndrome.

Motor Functioning

As is evident from the above descriptions, many neuropsychological tests include a motor component (e.g., TPT, Complex Figure, WAIS Block Design, etc.). Specific motor tests are useful for making inferences about the functional integrity of the two hemispheres of the brain, as well as those areas of the frontal lobes dedicated to movement. This is most often accomplished by comparing the performance of one hand to the other. When administering and interpreting motor tests it is always crucial to account for the inherent differences between a person's *dominant* (usually the hand with which they write), and *nondominant hand.* Three of the more widely used motor tests are presented below.

Finger Tapping Test (FTT): The FTT measures the motor speed of the index finger of both hands through the use of an apparatus that looks like a Morse code key pad. A counter registers each time the patient strikes the key. With the patient's palm down, fingers extended, and index finger on the key pad, he or she is asked to strike the pad as quickly as possible for 10 seconds. Three to five 10-second trials are administered for each hand. The score for each hand represents the average number of taps across the trials.

When examining FTT findings, two strategies are used. The number of taps provided by each of the patient's hands is compared against age-, sex-, and education-based norms. Then the performances of the two hands are directly examined to determine if one hand consistently demonstrated a fewer number of taps. This comparison takes into account that, on average, people will perform about 10 percent better with their preferred hand.[12]

Poor FTT performance in one hand is expected to reflect a lesion in the contralateral cerebral hemisphere; however, FTT findings should be interpreted with caution. It is not uncommon for a person to exhibit a performance with their nonpreferred hand that is equal or superior to that of their preferred hand.[12] Therefore, any diagnosis of a motor deficit must depend on consistent findings across several motor tasks.

Hand Dynamometer (Grip Strength): The dynamometer is an instrument that measures the voluntary strength and intensity of movement of both hands. With arm held at side, the patient is instructed to squeeze the stirrup-shaped dynamometer as hard as he or she can, taking as much time as needed.[12] Alternating between hands, two or three test trials are administered.

The approach to evaluating and interpreting grip strength is the same as with the Finger Tapping Test. Again, large discrepancies between hands are not uncommon. It has been suggested that grip strength performance can more accurately identify the lateralization of a brain lesion (i.e., being in either the right or left hemisphere) than either the FTT or Tactile Performance Test.

Grooved Pegboard: The Grooved Pegboard measures finger and hand dexterity.[17] The test involves the patient placing metal pegs into a grid of holes as quickly and accurately as he or she can. Rather than being cylindrical, each peg contains a ridge along one side so that the shape of both ends is irregular. The task is made more difficult because the orientation of the each peg hole, with respect to the location of the groove, changes across the grid. Most administrations of the test include separate trials for the preferred hand, nonpreferred hand, and both hands. Each trial is timed and mistakes, such as dropping pegs, are recorded. Length of time to complete each trial is compared to sex- and age-based norms. Similar interpretive strategies used for other motor tasks apply to the Grooved Pegboard.

Executive Functioning

Executive functions are those most often associated with the anterior frontal lobes and include abstract reasoning, conceptual thought, planning, and the ability to regulate a level and focus of attention that is appropriate for the task at hand. The management of attention is not limited to just focusing on a particular stimulus. The efficient processing of information depends on the ability to alter attention and plan of action as the stimulus environment changes.

Many persons with brain injury have difficulty changing their *cognitive set*. The notion of cognitive set includes the strategy a person assumes for solving a particular problem. For instance the approach a person takes for driving to the store remains unaltered if there is little traffic, and no road construction. However, if traffic is congested, there is road construction, or an accident occurs, the driver must quickly alter cognitive set and mentally reroute his or her course in order to reach his or her destination. An unexpected event, such as this one, can be quite difficult for someone with a frontal lobe injury. As detailed above, frontal lobe conditions are often marked by the inability to inhibit behavior, problems with attention and abstract thought, and tendencies towards behavioral inflexibility and perseveration. Tests of executive function evaluate how well patients can maintain and change their cognitive set, often as they attempt to solve abstract problems that tax conceptual thinking.

Trail Making Test (Trails A & B): The Trail Making Test has been widely used as a measure of attention, mental flexibility, and visual-conceptual/visuomotor tracking.[11] The task itself is much like the "connect-the-dots" games of children. In Trails A, the patient is asked to draw lines connecting consecutively numbered circles printed on a worksheet (i.e., 1 to 2, 2 to 3, etc.). Trails B is more challenging and demands that the patient change cognitive set: the task consists of alternating responding between connecting numbers and letters. The patient begins with "1" and draws a line to the letter "A"; this is followed by drawing a line from "A" to the number "2", then to the letter "B", and so on. The patient continues to alternate letters and numbers until he or she reaches the end of the list. Each trial is timed and mistakes are pointed out to the patient and corrected if they occur. Performance on both Trails A and B is compared against norms based on age for time to completion.

The Trail Making Test is very sensitive to brain damage, particularly if the time to complete Trails B is longer than expected in relation to the time it took the patient to complete Trails A. While the simplicity of the test implies that it would be easy to fake impairment by just lengthening the time to complete Trails A and B, research has shown this not to be the case.[12] When normal persons were asked to behave as if they were brain damaged, they greatly underestimated the amount of time needed by real patients to complete the test, especially Trails B.

Category Test: This test of abstract reasoning and concept formation can be quite difficult for many persons.[12] The goal of the test is to find the underlying principle across a set of visual stimuli.

For instance, number of objects, finding a missing part of a sequence, or understanding the position of an object in relation to the entire set of stimuli. One at a time, the patient views each stimulus composing the set. No clues are given as to what the underlying principle is for each of the seven stimuli categories. Instead, patients use feedback they receive from the examiner about whether each of their responses is correct.[12] Thus, through trial and error, the patient attempts to learn the principle that unifies the set of stimuli.

Three sets of the Category Test exist. The adult version, for ages 15 years, 8 months and up, consists of 208 items. The intermediate version, consisting of 168 items, is for ages 9 years to 15 years, 8 months. The child version, for ages 8 and up, contains 80 items across 5 stimulus categories. Scoring for each version entails summing the total number of errors.

The Category Test is very sensitive to neurological damage, particularly when it includes brain centers involved in abstract thought. While originally developed to exclusively measure frontal lobe functioning, research has determined that the Category Test is not sensitive to determining the specific location or laterality of brain damage.[12]

Wisconsin Card Sorting Test (WCST): Conceptually similar to the Category Test, the WCST has received considerable attention from researchers, and is widely used by clinicians. The purpose of the test is to evaluate the patient's ability to form abstract concepts, as well as shift and maintain cognitive set.[12] Unlike the Category Test, the Wisconsin Card Sort is sensitive to frontal lobe lesions.

The test materials consist of four stimulus cards, each showing a different arrangement of colored geometric shapes (e.g., four blue circles, two green stars), and two packs of 64 response cards. Each response card contains a design similar to those on the stimulus cards, but varies in color, geometric form, and number. The patient is simply told to match each of the response cards to one of the four stimulus cards arranged in a line in front of him or her. The examiner then informs the patient if each response is correct or incorrect. Without any foreknowledge, the patient's task is to comprehend whether the color, shape, or number of geometric items on each card determines where the card is placed. For example, if the current category is "color", and the response card contains two *blue* triangles, the correct reply is to place the response card on the stimulus card containing four *blue* circles. The WCST is made more difficult because the response categories change six times throughout the test (e.g., from color to number of items, from number of items to specific shape, etc.). A change in category follows 10 consecutive correct responses.

The WCST can be quite frustrating. Patients usually have little difficulty obtaining the first and second categories. As the test progresses, it is common for brain-injured persons to "loose set". This entails either a return to the previous category, or a haphazard search for cues to the category, even though the patient may have just made a series of correct responses.

The WCST scoring system is fairly complicated and yields a number of measures including "categories achieved", "perseverative responses", "perseverative errors", and "nonperseverative errors".[12] Categories achieved indicate how many of the six stimulus categories (i.e., those based on color, form, number, etc.) the patient successfully completed. The two perseverative scores document the patient's inability to change cognitive set in response to the changing categories. The measures of perseveration are very useful for predicting the presence or absence of brain damage and the presence of frontal lobe involvement.

While the Category Test and WCST are not identical, both measure the patient's ability to deduce a classification principle by means of "response-contingent feedback", use it when it is relevant, and abandon the principle when it becomes obsolete.[12] If problems with abstract thought are suspected, both tests should be part of the neuropsychological evaluation. The Category Test is particularly suited for measuring perceptual abstraction abilities. The WCST is a better measure of perseveration, a symptom common to frontal lobe syndrome. If both tests are given, the WCST should precede the Category Test in order to reduce order effects.[12]

Personality and Emotional Functioning

Personality refers to those persistent traits, patterns of behavior, and ways of thinking that distinguish one person from another. There is little doubt that genetic, congenital, developmental, and experiential factors all contribute to the formation and maintenance of one's personality. While there is considerable debate over how much a personality changes over time, it is clear that neuropsychological conditions can have a serious impact on personality functioning and emotional state. As will be discussed in the next chapter, minor head injury and chronic pain can lead to persistent psychological symptoms such as depression and anxiety. These symptoms themselves can exacerbate an ongoing cognitive disorder, which in turn, can further promote the patient's emotional distress. On a deeper level, any serious illness or medical condition reduces one's psychological defenses so that long-standing psychological concerns and conflicts often become more apparent. Therefore, an assessment of the patient's current psychological and emotional functioning is a very important part of the neuropsychological evaluation. Having some understanding of the patient's premorbid personality speaks to how he or she might cope with the current situation, as well as providing some hypotheses on how the patient will deal with symptoms that may persist for some time. Furthermore, knowledge of the patient's psychology aids in the formation of treatment approaches that can result in less resistance, and best target the patient's particular concerns and life problems.

Personality and Psychological Testing

There are many tests of psychological functioning. The tests usually involve one of three approaches that include asking the patient to complete a "paper and pencil" questionnaire, examine ambiguous visual stimuli, or draw. Psychological tests are often classified as being either *objective* or *projective*.

Objective tests, usually in the form of questionnaires, are directed as measuring specific symptoms, traits, or personality constructs. The approach taken towards interpreting these tests is quantitative and empirical. Specific numerical scores are derived and often a patient's responses are compared to norms based on demographic variables. Examples of objective psychological tests include the Minnesota Multiphasic Personality Inventory II (see below), the Symptom Checklist 90 – Revised, and the California Personality Inventory.

Projective tests ask the patient to respond to ambiguous stimuli with little or no guidance from the examiner. The principles behind projective testing arose from classical psychoanalytic theory and the belief that the human mind is composed of both conscious and unconscious psychological processes. One psychoanalytic concept particularly pertinent to projective tests is that unconscious wishes and personality aspects of the person are not expressed directly, but manifest through various forms of symbolic communication such as dreams, slips of the tongue, and *defense mechanisms*. One of these defense mechanisms is *projection*, which is the idea that a person will transfer or "project" unconscious wishes or conflicts onto others when they become unacceptable. It is believed that when one undergoes projective testing, the ambiguity of the stimuli lowers or "tricks" the person's psychological defenses so that he or she projects his or her unconscious personality structure and psychological conflicts and issues onto the projective stimuli.

There are a number of popular projective tests, including the Rorschach Ink Blot Test, Thematic Apperception Test (TAT), Bender Gestalt, and House-Tree-Person Drawing Test (H-T-P). With the exception of the Rorschach, the scoring systems of most projective tests are qualitative and rely upon the symbolic interpretation of elements of the patient's visual perceptions, verbal responses, or drawings. For instance, if a patient's drawing of a person depicts the figure as having very short arms, it is frequently interpreted that the patient feels powerless or inadequate about his or her attempts to control some aspect of the environment. While academic researchers frequently criticize projective tests as being "unscientific," the wide use of these instruments by practicing clinicians will undoubtedly continue. As with all psychological testing, no global assessment of functioning, or assignment of diagnoses, should be made from the results of a single test. Projective tests do add valuable information to the clinical picture and frequently reveal important psychological issues that are not easily accessed through more objective measures or structured approaches.

While there are many tests of personality and emotional functioning, most neuropsychological reports include one, if not all, of the following, the MMPI-II, the Rorschach Ink Blot Test, and the TAT. Each is described in turn.

Minnesota Multiphasic Personality Inventory II: Now in its second edition, the MMPI measures personality across 10 dimensions through the use of over 500 "true/false" questions. The test has been the most widely administered personality instrument for over forty years. It is simple to give, quick to score (especially with the aid of computer scoring programs), and fairly easy to interpret. Administration entails no more than asking the patient to complete each item at his or her own pace. In general, patients with little neuropsychological impairment finish the test in about 1 hour.

The different MMPI items contribute to three Validity and ten Clinical Scales. Each scale reflects a t score that equates the values across the 13 standard scales. In general, a scale is considered to be "clinically elevated" if the t value is 65 or higher. The higher the Clinical Scale score, the greater the psychological distress along that particular personality dimension.

L, F, and K are the three MMPI Validity Scales.[19] The L Scale is a measure of the patient's attempt to present him or herself in a good light through the denial of personal and social transgressions that most people make (e.g., "I never lie."). A high score on the F Scale is associated with an invalid profile; often because the patient failed to understand the instructions, or made little attempt to answer the questions in a realistic fashion. A high F score can also indicate significant psychological distress and the possibility of "psychiatric decompensation". The K Scale reflects the level of the patient's guardedness or defensiveness during test-taking. The relationship of the F Scale score to the K Scale score (F minus K) is another measure of the patient's attempt to present him or herself in a good or bad light. Positive scores are associated with "faking bad" and negative scores with "faking good".

The following are the ten Clinical Scales of the MMPI-II.[12,19] Each is accompanied by a brief description of personality aspects that the scale measures.

1. Hypochondriasis (Hs): Reflects abnormal concern over bodily health.
2. Depression (D): Physical, social, and psychological symptoms associated with depression.
3. Hysteria (Hy): Reflects level of psychological sophistication and the patient's propensity to use more primitive psychological defenses (e.g., repression, denial, conversion reaction).
4. Psychopathic Deviate (Pd): Characteristics associated with disregard for social conventions.
5. Masculinity-Femininity (Mf): Measures traits traditionally associated with men and women. Higher scores indicate that the person expresses interests more common to the opposite sex.
6. Paranoia (Pa): Symptoms of persecution and suspiciousness.
7. Psychasthenia (Pt): Symptoms of anxiety, self-concern, self-doubt, and obsessive-compulsive style.
8. Schizophrenia (Sz): Symptoms of thought disorder, including social alienation, bizarre thoughts and feelings, delusions, and somatic complaints.
9. Hypomania (Ma): Symptoms of excessive psychological or physical energy.
10. Social Introversion (Si): Symptoms of social inhibition.

While not widely used, there are other MMPI scales besides the three Validity and ten Clinical Scales. These supplementary scales measure a wide variety of symptoms and personality characteristics, including hostility, ego strength, and additional measures of depression.

One concern with MMPI-II data obtained from neurological or pain patients is that scores on Scales 1, 3, and 8 are often inflated due to the patients' accurate report of their real somatic symptoms. The next chapter will provide in-depth discussion of the use of the MMPI with head injured and post concussive headache patients.

Rorschach Ink Blot Test: This famous projective instrument has been used widely by clinicians for over 60 years. The test consists of 10 stimulus cards, on each of which appears a symmetrical ink blot of either black, black and red, or several colors.[12] Administration consists of a "free association" and "inquiry" phase. During Free Association, the patient is presented each card, one at a time, and is asked "What might this be?". The patient then relays what the ink blot looks like to him or her. Patients are allowed up to five responses per card. During the inquiry, the examiner reviews the patient's responses in an effort to determine what elements of the blot contributed to the patient's perceptions. In general, it takes about 30 minutes to one hour to administer the Rorschach.

Rorschach scoring systems can be quite complex and time consuming. Most systems derive interpretations of the patient's personality based on what area(s) and qualities of the blot (e.g., form, color, shading) are used to construct the perceptions. The contents of the patient's perceptions (e.g., humans, animals, sex, etc.) also contribute to interpretation. Of the various scoring systems, the one developed by Exner and colleagues (i.e., the Comprehensive System) is the most widely accepted.[12] This system, based on actuarial data obtained from the Rorschachs of clinical and nonclinical populations, is highly quantified and yields numerous scores. The Exner system requires considerable training and experience to master. Scoring and interpretation has been made somewhat easier through the recent introduction of a computerized scoring program.

Many clinicians choose to forsake the quantified Ink Blot scoring systems in favor of a more qualitative interpretation based on observations of the patient's cognitive processes, perceptual themes, emotional reactions to the stimuli, and tendencies towards perseveration. With regard to neuropsychological conditions, the Rorschach is a secondary measure of patients' perceptual abilities, processing of ambiguous stimuli, and reaction time.[12] Although many academically oriented psychologists continue to question the validity of the Rorschach, it retains its status as the premiere projective test.

Thematic Apperception Test (TAT): Second in popularity only to the Rorschach, the TAT is a projective test that measures thought content, emotions, and conflicts through stories that the patient provides in response to pictures.[12] Patients are usually presented with 10 of the 31 stimulus cards. Some cards are specified for men, some for women, and some for both genders. Often the choice of cards depends on the psychological issues the clinician wishes to examine. The pictures primarily depict individuals or couples engaged in some ambiguous activity; therefore, the patient's interpretations of events are thought to reflect personality characteristics and psychological issues.

Patient instructions are limited to the request that they create a story depicting what is occurring in the picture, that they include how the main character is feeling, as well as the events which lead up to the scene, and what the consequences of the events will be. Administration can usually be accomplished within 30 to 40 minutes.

While efforts have been taken to structure and quantify TAT interpretation, most clinicians rely upon a qualitative approach based on the symbolic meaning of the patient's narratives. The presence of conflicts, depiction of major characters, emotional tone, and defense mechanisms, are usually the focus of interpretation. Furthermore, each TAT card is believed to "pull" for certain psychological material (e.g., achievement drives, family relations, gender identity, heterosexual relations, etc.).

Many psychological evaluations will include both the TAT and Rorschach. The Rorschach provides valuable information about a person's perceptual and thinking processes, and the TAT reveals how the patient deals with other people and what social and interpersonal issues are most relevant. As is the case with the Rorschach, the TAT is a secondary neuropsychological measure. It does provide information about patients' ability to organize a story sequentially, their tendency towards concrete vs. abstract thinking, ability to integrate the entire visual stimulus, and word fluency.[12]

Recent years have seen the development of new apperception tests for a variety of populations. At present, these include children (CAT), adolescents (AAT), and senior citizens (SAT). Like the Rorschach, it is probable that the TAT will continue to receive wide clinical application, despite criticism from academics.

Psychiatric Diagnoses

When a neuropsychological evaluation is conducted, a patient is assigned a number of diagnoses based upon the diagnostic criteria established by the American Psychiatric Association in the *Diagnostic and Statistical Manual of Mental Disorders, fourth edition* (DSM-IV).[18] The DSM uses a multiaxial approach for assigning diagnoses across five spheres of functioning.

Axis I diagnoses are clinical disorders or other conditions that are the current major focus of clinical attention. These conditions are the primary psychological complaints of the patient and usually manifest as acute and specific symptoms. Axis I diagnoses entail many of the conditions that we think of as mental illness, including major depression, bipolar disorder (i.e., manic-depression), and schizophrenia. However, many Axis I diagnoses are less severe and reflect emotional and behavioral symptoms in reaction to life stressors. Such reactions often fall under the diagnosis of an adjustment disorder. Axis I diagnoses cover the full life-span and range from disorders first seen in infancy and childhood (e.g., autistic disorder) to those experienced by the elderly (dementia of the Alzheimer's type).

Axis II diagnoses are assigned when the person is found to have a *personality disorder.* Personality disorders are problems of functioning that stem from the person's global character structure. Axis II disorders are serious, long-standing, and usually have their origins in the person's early development. Personality-disordered persons often have a great deal of trouble getting along with others and frequently exhibit a low level of adjustment. The presence of a personality disorder complicates the treatment of Axis I diagnoses and can have a very significant impact on neuropsychological conditions. Common Axis II diagnoses include paranoid personality disorder, antisocial personality disorder, narcissistic personality disorder, and borderline personality disorder.

Axis III diagnoses are general medical conditions that coincide with the psychiatric disorders. Axis III diagnoses may impact, or be influenced by, the psychiatric conditions, revealing the complicated interplay between mind and body.

Axis IV documents the patient's psychosocial and environment problems that may exacerbate psychiatric conditions. Axis IV diagnoses include housing, educational, and financial troubles.

The patient's *Global Assessment of Functioning* (GAF) is documented on *Axis V.* The GAF Scale places the person's psychological, social, and occupational functioning on a hypothetical continuum of mental health. The scale ranges from 0 to 100. Lower values reflect more improvised functioning and a greater degree of mental illness. Scores below 71 reflect some mild psychiatric symptoms. A GAF of 51 to 60 indicates moderate symptoms. Scores below 50 suggest serious psychiatric symptoms.

DSM-IV Axis I and II diagnoses are assigned if the patient demonstrates a number of core psychological symptoms or criteria for a particular condition. The range of criteria reflects the clinical views and research findings of experts on a particular disorder. Most Axis I and II criteria demand that the patient exhibit between two and five of the core symptoms or behavioral characteristics prior to receiving a formal diagnosis.

DSM-IV and Head Injury

Although the diagnosis of post concussive syndrome has existed for many years, it remains very controversial. At present, it does not even appear in DSM-IV as an Axis I disorder. Instead, it is relegated to the appendix as a diagnosis that remains under review for possible future inclusion.[20] This presents the neuropsychologist with somewhat of a quandary when assigning diagnoses to patients exhibiting cognitive and emotional symptoms suspected to have arisen following head trauma. Commonly, cognitive deficits receive diagnoses such as delirium, dementia, and amnestic and other cognitive disorders. Common diagnoses include dementia due to head trauma and cognitive disorder not otherwise specified. In addition, these patients then receive an Axis III diagnosis of Head Trauma. This limitation also frequently demands another Axis I diagnosis to account for the psychological symptoms that commonly accompany post concussive syndrome (e.g., depression and anxiety [see the next chapter]). Hopefully, these problems will be reconciled in the next edition of the DSM by including post concussive syndrome as a formal Axis I diagnosis.

The Neuropsychological Report

Upon completion of testing, scoring, clinical interviews, review of charts, and consultations, the neuropsychologist composes an evaluation report. The presentation of the report is often quite extensive, and generally provides test findings and interpretation within each of the major functional domains described above.

The following is a mock report that reflects a consolidation of several cases seen by the author. All personal and organizational names have been changed in order to protect confidentiality.

CONFIDENTIAL NEUROPSYCHOLOGICAL EVALUATION

PATIENT'S NAME: Raymond Clifton
DATE OF BIRTH: 6/19/54
AGE: 44-2
ETHNICITY: European American
SEX: Male
DATE OF EVALUATION: 1/23/98
REFERRED BY: James McLean, MD
Rhonda Clarkston,
American Insurance Incorporated

TESTS & PROCEDURES ADMINISTERED:

Review of Available Records
Clinical Interview and Behavioral Observations
California Verbal Learning Test (CVLT)
Controlled Oral Word Association Test
Finger Tapping
Go-No Go and Contrasting Motor Paradigms
Grooved Pegboard
Hand Grip Strength (Hand Dynamometer)
Mental Status Exam
Minnesota Multiphasic Personality Inventory - 2 (MMPI-2)
Rey Memorization Task
Rey-Osterrieth Complex Figure Test
Rorschach Ink Blot Test
Sentence Repetition Test
Speech Sounds Perception Test
Tactile Performance Test (TPT)
Thematic Apperception Test (TAT)
Trail Making Tests A & B (Trails A & B)
Visual Naming Test

Wechsler Adult Intelligence Scale - Revised (WAIS-R)
Wechsler Memory Scale (WMS) Logical Memory I & II, Visual Reproduction I & II
Wisconsin Card Sorting Test (WCST)

REASON FOR REFERRAL:

Mr. Raymond Clifton was referred to assess his neuropsychological functioning in relationship to an automobile accident that occurred October 18, 1993. The evaluation was directed towards determining Mr. Clifton's level of impairment and whether he has reached maximum medical improvement from a psychiatric or psychological standpoint.

RELEVANT HISTORY:

According to Mr. Clifton's report and that of past medical records, he was injured 10/18/93 when his automobile was rear-ended at an intersection and projected into another vehicle. Contrary to medical reports, Mr. Clifton stated that he lost consciousness at the point of impact and has little memory for the accident. Medical records indicated that he sustained three fractured ribs and a flexion/extension injury to the neck. A CT scan of the head was normal. The patient spent one day in Harris Memorial Hospital. Upon his return home, Mr. Clifton indicated that he experienced persistent feelings of derealization, body pain, difficulty walking and balance problems. He also reported significant psychological distress including feelings of anxiety and bouts of crying.

Since the accident, Mr. Clifton has been treated by a number of physicians, has received several medical and psychological evaluations, and has been under the care of a clinical psychologist. In March 1994, Dr. Jamison, an orthopedic surgeon, failed to indicate that Mr. Clifton suffered from any significant neurological or psychological impairment. Dr. Jamison assigned Mr. Clifton a four percent impairment rating. In September 1994, Mr. Clifton was referred by his family physician, Dr. Stevens, to Dr. Richards, a neurologist. Dr. Richards diagnosed Mr. Clifton with a post concussion syndrome. An MRI in October 1994 was negative. Complaining of blurred vision, derealization, and some dizziness, Mr. Clifton was referred by Dr. Richards to Dr. Giovanni for a psychological evaluation. Dr. Giovanni reported that Mr. Clifton was experiencing a general memory disturbance, problems with math skills, some psychomotor retardation, and reduction in mental processing speed. Since February 1995, Mr. Clifton has received individual psychotherapy from Dr. Pensky, a clinical psychologist. Focus of treatment has been upon the reduction of Mr. Clifton's reported symptoms of depression and anxiety. Medical evaluations in 1996 and 1997 have raised some questions over how impaired Mr. Clifton was. Both Drs. Packard and Sherrington maintained that Mr. Clifton was not permanently disabled and was not experiencing significant psychological distress related to the accident.

At present, Mr. Clifton reported that he continues to experience constant feelings of derealization that he describes as a "mild intoxication." He further reported that he often finds himself staring and feeling "spaced out." He also acknowledged continued depression and that he commonly feels "blue." He indicated that his symptoms of depression exacerbate if he does not take nortriptyline (Pamelor). Mr. Clifton stated that he often awakens during the night and has some trouble returning to sleep. He indicated that his eating is good. He denied any suicidal or homicidal ideation. He reported to smoke one-half pack of cigarettes a day.

Mr. Clifton reported that he still has problems with concentration and has trouble remembering things. As present, his work as a delivery person entails driving a specific route and making frequent stops. Mr. Clifton stated that he has trouble learning a new route and can become confused while driving and looses his sense of time. He also reported that he has trouble finding the right words when talking and cannot think as quickly as he once did.

Mr. Clifton currently acknowledged daily headaches that he described as moderate to severe. He reported that the pain is bilateral, both dull and throbbing, and commonly includes tightness in the neck and scalp. He indicated that when his headaches are severe, they are accompanied by nausea and photophobia. He denied that his headaches are preceded by a prodromal phase. Mr.

Clifton stated that he had few headaches prior to his accident. He did report a positive family history of migraine.

With respect to Mr. Clifton's life history, he is currently separated from his wife. He reported that this separation is related to the effect of the auto accident on his behavior and his relationship with his wife. Mr. Clifton is a father to three children. All of the children currently live with their mother.

Mr. Clifton has a college degree in management. For 16 years he worked as an area manager of a furniture company. He stated that he left this position because of memory problems related to his auto accident. As indicated, Mr. Clifton is currently employed as a delivery person for the Richmond Corporation. He has been at this position for 11 months. Mr. Clifton denied any significant medical history outside of his head injury.

Mr. Clifton reported that he currently maintains his household responsibilities and is able to care for himself and manage his own finances. He stated that his social activities involve church, visiting friends, and shopping.

BEHAVIORAL OBSERVATIONS & MENTAL STATUS EXAM:

Mr. Clifton drove himself to the evaluation. He was dressed appropriately and demonstrated good grooming. His gait was normal and he appeared free of any gross motoric abnormalities. He did seem to have some difficulty when asked to carry out motor sequences with his hands. While Mr. Clifton did not make excessive mistakes, he was slow and often needed to self-correct his initial efforts to present the appropriate response. Mr. Clifton's speech was fluid, he did not appear to have any difficulty finding words, nor did he exhibit any other symptoms suggestive of an expression disorder.

Mr. Clifton was well oriented to person, place, and time. He failed to show signs suggestive of a thought disorder. He denied any hallucinations and did not appear to maintain any delusions. His insight into his medical condition was good and his judgment with respect to social and personal issues was considered fair to good.

Mr. Clifton's predominate mood was somewhat anxious. He exhibited a full and appropriate range of affect. He denied any current significant psychological distress and expressed no suicidal or homicidal ideation.

Mr. Clifton was highly cooperative and friendly throughout the examination. He appeared to exhibit consistent and good effort across the tests. He had no difficulty understanding instructions. He worked carefully and was not impulsive. Mr. Clifton was not judged to be malingering. The results of this evaluation are considered to be a valid estimate of Mr. Clifton's current neuropsychological functioning.

TEST RESULTS

Intellectual: On the WAIS-R, Mr. Clifton obtained a Full Scale IQ of 117, which is in the High Average range of intellectual functioning. His Verbal IQ was 123 and his Performance IQ was 106. His scale scores were as follows:

Subtest					
Verbal	**Score**	**Percentile**	**Performance**	**Score**	**Percentile**
Information	16	98	Picture Completion	11	63
Similarities	16	98	Digit Symbol	8	25
Arithmetic	11	63	Picture Arrangement	11	63
Vocabulary	14	90	Block Design	6	9
Comprehension	14	90	Object Assembly	8	25

Mr. Clifton's performance was quite similar to that reported by Dr. Giovanni in 1994. That his scores were better either suggests some improvement in his condition or greater ease with the testing situation. The current findings also indicate that Mr. Clifton's intellectual functioning is not deteriorating.

Mr. Clifton does retain the significant difference between his verbal and nonverbal aptitude that was observed in 1994. While this difference in aptitude might be clinically relevant, it is important to consider that Mr. Clifton's nonverbal abilities are at the high end of the average range of functioning. Additionally, it is difficult to say whether this split is a consequence of his head injury, or reflects an endemic difference between his verbal and nonverbal abilities. In support of Mr. Clifton's complaints about concentration, his arithmetic skills and ability to recall a span of numbers are not commensurate with his other verbal abilities. In further agreement with Dr. Giovanni's findings, Mr. Clifton had difficulty in constructing a whole from its constitute parts (scale score = 8), as well as problems with visual-motor integration (scale score = 6), and visual-spatial reasoning. Thus, his difficulties learning and remembering new routes in his present employment is consistent with current intellectual test results.

Memory: In general, Mr. Clifton's verbal memory is within the average to above average range of function. On both the CVLT and Logical Memory I WMS subtest, his ability to learn and immediately recall verbal material was within the average to high average range (CVLT 1st trial correct = 6 [M = 6.8, SD = 1.3], 5th trial correct = 12 [M = 12.1, SD = 1.7]; Logical Memory I = 66th percentile). His tendency to perseverate, while greater than average, was within normal limits (CVLT Total Preservations = 8 [M = 4.2, SD = 5.5]). Completing information did not significantly interfere with his recall (CVLT Total Intrusions = 2 [M = 2.4, SD = 2.5]). Mr. Clifton's ability to recall a list of words following both a short and long time delay was normal for his age (CVLT Short Delay Free Recall = 8 [M = 10.2, SD = 2.5]; CVLT Long Delay Free Recall = 10 [M = 11.4, SD = 2.9]). His delayed recall was substantially better when involving information structured as a story (WMS Logical Memory II = 78th percentile).

Mr. Clifton failed to exhibit any significant deficit in nonverbal/spatial memory. Both his immediate and delayed recall of the Rey-Osterrieth Complex Figure earned a scale score of 9 (M = 10, SD = 3). While he did retain much of the gestalt of the figure, he was prone to forgetting and confabulating internal details. Mr. Clifton's WMS Visual Reproduction I and II performance was within the superior range of functioning (98th percentile).

Language: As indicated by Mr. Clifton's WAIS-R performance, he has a superior vocabulary (scale score = 14) and excellent abstract verbal reasoning abilities (scale score = 16). He exhibited no problems in repeating complex verbal material (Sentence Repetition Test) or naming visual stimuli (Visual Naming Test). Contrary to Mr. Clifton's complaint of word finding problems, his verbal fluency performance was slightly above that expected for his age. He did exhibit some moderate impairment in his ability to understand nonsense words presented via audiotape (Speech-Sounds Perception Test = 11 errors [Moderate Range = 8 – 14]). In general, Mr. Clifton appears to have no significant language deficits.

Executive Functioning and Motor Skills: Mr. Clifton exhibited excellent performance on the WCST. He demonstrated fewer errors (Z = –0.70), fewer perseverative responses (Z = –0.91) and errors (Z = –0.77), and a greater number of completed categories (n = 6, Z = 0.36) than would be expected for his age. He never failed to maintain set. While his WCST findings indicate that Mr. Clifton's higher abstract functioning is intact and that his thinking is flexible, he did have some difficulty with both Trails A and B, and the Go-No Go Paradigm. His time to complete Trails A was over one standard deviation above what would be expected for his age (A = 53" [M = 36.73", SD = 13.68"). His Trails B performance was marked by mistakes and a very delayed time to completion (B = 2'12" [M = 76.97", SD = 30.52"]). Although Mr. Clifton did not exhibit a large number of mistakes on the Go-No Go Paradigm (total errors = 5), his performance was slow and peppered by numerous self-corrections. These findings suggest some inflexibility in Mr. Clifton's executive functioning when it involves more complex visual-spatial and motor behaviors. This apparent problem supports Mr. Clifton's complaint that he has difficulty in learning new driving routes in his job as a delivery person and that he becomes easily confused. Further difficulty in spatial-motor ability was evident in Mr. Clifton's TPT performance. His time to complete the task was long regardless if he used his right (8'19"), left (5'33"), or both hands (3'17"). Mr. Clifton exhibited some right-sided neglect of the stimuli board and was somewhat disorganized in his strategy and clumsy in his approach. His ability to draw the stimuli board following his blindfolded efforts was also poor.

Mr. Clifton is right hand dominant. Bilateral scores on Finger Tapping were as expected for his age, as was his hand grip strength. Mr. Clifton demonstrated a deficit in speeded motor accuracy. His Grooved Pegboard performance was considerably below that expected for his age (R = 95" [M = 69.5, SD = 11], L = 90" [M = 74.2", SD = 12.6"]) and he made several mistakes and occasionally dropped pegs. This finding further supports some problem in executing more complex motor patterns.

Personality: While Mr. Clifton's responses to the MMPI-2 appear to accurately reflect his current psychological state, he appears prone towards defensiveness. At present, Mr. Clifton exhibits some preoccupation with somatic concerns and a tendency to manifest psychological distress as physical symptoms. However, the labels of histrionic or hypochondriacal should be avoided in that some of the patient's responses probably reflect an accurate presentation of the cognitive and somatic complaints inherent to his condition. MMPI findings fail to indicate major depression, but do suggest that Mr. Clifton is exhibiting a low energy level and psychomotor retardation. TAT and Rorschach findings suggest that Mr. Clifton is probably somewhat psychologically naive, inhibits aggressive feelings, and may avoid some social situations. He may have some lowered self esteem.

SUMMARY AND RECOMMENDATIONS:

Results of this evaluation indicate that Mr. Clifton has many strengths that enhance his current level of neuropsychological functioning. He has an above average intelligence and superior verbal aptitude. This is commensurate with his educational history. He has good verbal and nonverbal memory abilities, and in general, fluid executive functioning and excellent abstract reasoning.

There is considerable support that Mr. Clifton has a deficit of motor functioning that entails not only psychomotor retardation, but problems in executing and inhibiting complex motor behaviors. He also appears to have some visual-spatial-motor difficulties that may contribute to his current complaints. These motor problems appear to underlie the significant difference between his verbal and nonverbal IQ scores.

While his motor deficits are consistent with nondominant hemisphere involvement, it is difficult to determine the etiology of his current symptoms. It is possible that his difficulties are a result of his motor vehicle accident. Deficits related to closed head injury often impact nonverbal, visual-spatial, and motor functions while leaving well-rehearsed and integrated verbal abilities relatively intact. Regardless of etiology, Mr. Clifton does currently exhibit some neuropsychological deficits that could significantly interfere with his ability to carry out his job as a delivery person. Considering Mr. Clifton's excellent verbal and abstract abilities, employment that is suited to these strengths would probably be more appropriate. One aspect of further psychological intervention should be directed at exploring the possibility of Mr. Clifton returning to a managerial position. Such intervention may entail disputing his fears that he is unable to efficiently carry out intellectually demanding tasks within the verbal/abstract domain. He may need to develop compensatory strategies that will allay his anxieties and assist him when he is experiencing difficulties. These might include notions such as needing extra time to complete tasks and avoiding environments that include a potentially overwhelming degree of sensory stimulation. He will also need guidance and support throughout the process if he chooses to seek other employment.

In consideration that Mr. Clifton has reported his cognitive symptoms for some time, and that the findings of this assessment generally agree with those of his previous psychological evaluation, it is suspected that he will continue to experience his visual-spatial and motor difficulties. Furthermore, these deficits might not lead themselves well to cognitive rehabilitation.

While Mr. Clifton no longer appears clinically depressed, he does demonstrate some tendency towards over-concern for his physical condition. Preoccupation with health is commonly seen in persons who have experienced a significant head trauma. His tendency to manifest psychological distress as physical symptoms reflects some degree of psychological unsophistication that might best be addressed in individual psychotherapy. Because of the length of time since the accident, and the impact that it has had on his life, it is difficult to tease out what current psychological concerns are directly related to his injury. What may have initially arisen from issues related to the accident are probably now maintained through less direct psychosocial contingencies. Once again, these factors are probably best addressed through continued psychotherapy. The issue of Mr. Clifton's marriage is also important and the possibility of reconciliation should be explored. Such exploration may include the initiation of couples psychotherapy.

On a case as this, concern for malingering is quite high, especially given Mr. Clifton's level of education. However, as noted previously, he does not appear to be particularly sophisticated psychologically. Further, his pattern of test performance is very consistent with his presenting problem. It is highly unlikely that Mr. Clifton could fake such a consistent neuropsychological profile. Noteworthy also is what appears to be a significant disparity and probable decline in nonverbal visual-spatial reasoning and complex psychomotor skills. As indicated above, it is not expected that these deficits will resolve with time.

In general, Mr. Clifton is a fairly high functioning individual. Although he has some difficulties, there appears no reason why he should not be employed, even if it entails a change in duties and possible retraining.

DIAGNOSTIC IMPRESSION:

The results of this evaluation suggest the following DSM-IV diagnoses:

Axis I: (294.9)	Cognitive Disorder Not Otherwise Specified
(309.28)	Adjustment Disorder With Mixed Anxiety and Depressed Mood, Chronic
Axis II: (V71.09)	No Diagnosis
Axis III:	History of Head Trauma
Axis IV:	Marital separation and employment stress
Axis V:	GAF = 60 (current)

Thank you for referring Mr. Clifton to our office. If we may be of further assistance, please contact our office at [telephone number].

____________________________ ____________________________

Licensed Clinical Psychologist
State License # [...]

Psychometrician

FORENSIC ISSUES AND MALINGERING

The number of neuropsychologists involved in forensic work has increased dramatically. A recent national survey of almost 500 practitioners found that over 50% have testified in court at least once, and nearly 20% had testified more than 10 times.[21] The rise of neuropsychology's role in the legal arena is partially explained by the increased activity of the legal profession in personal injury litigation, especially in those cases involving mild to moderate head injury.[21]

A number of essential questions are addressed in most forensic neuropsychological assessments. These include:

1. In what areas of function is the patient demonstrating deficits?
2. Is the patient able to work?
3. Are there neuropsychological or psychiatric disabilities?
4. Is the patient able to live independently and attend to duties of daily life?
5. Is there a need for supervision and, if so, in what areas?
6. Has the patient's intellectual functioning returned to premorbid levels?[20]

Answering these questions within the adversarial environment of the courtroom can prove quite challenging to the neuropsychologist. As an expert witness, the clinician must be well prepared; it is common that many attorneys are well read in the area of neuropsychology, and are adept at raising potential shortcomings in both the specific evaluation, as well as more global concerns inherent to the discipline of neuropsychological assessment. Therefore, the neuropsychologist must be able to demonstrate the validity of his or her clinical opinions. These opinions must be based on objective scientific evidence and cannot be influenced by the practitioner's loyalty to the retained attorney or plaintiff.[21] Common challenges to the expert witness include questions regarding reliability, validity, and normative data of the test employed; the level of the clinician's experience; and issues of the relationship between test findings and the patient's actual level of functioning.[21]

The Issue of Malingering

One of the most common questions an expert witness receives is whether the patient is malingering. The issue of malingering is complex and fueled by the emotionally charged opinions held by both legal and health care professionals.

A popular definition of malingering entails "pretending to be ill or injured in order to avoid duty or work."[22] Like all diagnostic statements, the label of malingering serves both clinical and social functions. Clinically, a diagnosis suggests a particular approach to treatment. Socially, a diagnosis defines the role the patient plays and evokes the granting or withholding of certain privileges.[22] Need-be-said, the diagnosis of malingering carries little benefit to the patient and usually leads to negative consequences.

The label malingering is conceptualized somewhat differently by legal, medical, and psychiatric professionals.[22] The question from the legal community revolves around whether the person is entitled to some form of compensation. Therefore, the legal system's sole interest is whether the person is self-consciously undertaking efforts to mislead financial, medical, or legal representatives for personal gain. Physicians often make the diagnosis of malingering when there are inconclusive physical findings and no obvious psychiatric diagnosis. The medical definition of malingering is not clear cut and the symptoms that the patient is suspected of feigning can result from several sources, including (1) pure invention; (2) continuing to complain of previously real symptoms; (3) exaggerating real symptoms; and (4) attributing real symptoms to another cause.[22] Some argue that mental health professionals seldom give a formal diagnosis of malingering, partly due to the absence of confirmatory tests, and the potential for assigning another diagnosis.[22] In the DSM-IV, malingering appears in a minor section titled Additional Conditions That May Be a Focus of Clinical Attention.[18] Assignment of the diagnosis is based upon objective evidence that the patient is intentionally inventing or exaggerating physical or emotional symptoms for the purpose of achieving external incentives. The diagnosis should be strongly suspected if the patient is involved in litigation, there is a marked discrepancy between the patient's complaints and objective test findings, the patient is uncooperative or noncompliant with assessment or treatment demands, or there is an Axis II diagnosis of Antisocial Personality Disorder.

The Neuropsychological Detection of Malingering

Erickson argues that the goal of mental health practitioners is to deliver services and avoid the diagnostic label of malingering, especially for those patients they cannot help.[22] While this recommendation is warranted in the clinical and treatment milieu, the forensic neuropsychologist is in the unavoidable predicament of having to make a judgment about whether a particular patient is faking or exaggerating his or her cognitive and psychological symptoms.

The prevailing consensus has been that it is very difficult to detect malingering, and that the diagnosis rests upon "chancy and undeveloped technology."[22] Clinical interview alone has been found to be untrustworthy.[21] In recent years, researchers have begun to tackle the problem of detecting malingering by neuropsychological patients. The focus of this research has been upon isolating the response styles and test performance patterns of persons actively malingering, as well as developing specific neuropsychological tests that aid in detecting malingering behavior.

Response Styles

Using the Halstead-Reitan Neuropsychological Test Battery, Goebel studied 141 persons who were instructed to fake brain injury and compared their performance to 52 patients with actual brain damage, as well as 61 normal participants not attempting deception.[23] Those persons trying to deceive used a variety of strategies; the most common included giving the wrong answer when they knew the correct response, slowing down performance or looking dull or confused, and showing motor incoordination or clumsiness. In reviewing the literature, Hall and Pritchard provide the following generic summary of the strategies persons use to feign believable deficits on neuropsychological evaluations:[24] (1) present realistic symptoms using common sense or popular notions of what brain-damaged persons act like; (2) distribute errors across the evaluation rather than missing only more difficult test items; (3) protest that the tasks are too difficult and/or feign confusion and frustration; (4) attempt to perform at a level below actual aptitude (e.g., slowing motor speed).

Detection Strategies

With the above findings in mind, the neuropsychological examiner must remain vigilant. Fortunately, lay persons' perceptions of the behavior of brain-damaged patients are often naive and exaggerated. Most neuropsychological tests are constructed so that simple items precede difficult ones; therefore, mistakes equally distributed throughout a test are highly suspect.

The neuropsychologist must be well trained in the presentation of neurological and psychological disorders. With such knowledge, it becomes more easy to determine whether there is a "lack of neurological fit" between the patient's presenting symptoms, test performance, and established behavioral patterns associated with specific neuropsychological syndromes.[24]

Examining the patient's test performance within and across tests is also a useful detection strategy.[24] An effective neuropsychological test battery includes several measures of the same neurobehavioral function, for example verbal memory. If the findings across two or more tests (e.g., the CVLT and the RAVLT [see above]) are grossly different, the patient's performance should be suspected. Likewise, it becomes suspicious if the patient fails to demonstrate improved performance across a test that has a number of learning trials (e.g., the CVLT). Retesting patients at another time is also a good detection strategy. Most malingering patients have difficulty incorporating the expected increase in performance that would accompany retesting. Those that do show a practice effect, often exhibit one greater than would be expected if their first performance reflected their true abilities.

Tests Useful for Detecting Malingering

Researchers have taken efforts to either create specific tests to detect malingering, or have sought out response patterns within established instruments that indicate faking. While the psychometric detection of malingering is in its early stage, this area of research continues to receive focused attention.

The MMPI has long been regarded as a measure for detecting malingering. The F minus K Index (see above), the Gough Dissimulation Scale, and the Obvious and Subtle subscales should be examined for clinical elevations in all patients suspected of symptom exaggeration.[21] High F Scale scores and elevations on six or more Clinical Scales are also associated with malingering.[24]

Hall and Pritchard list the following tests as useful for differentiating malingerers from persons with actual brain damage: Speech-Sounds Perception Test, Finger Tapping (see above), Finger Anosia, Sensory Suppressions, Grip Strength (see above), and WAIS Digit Span (see above).[24] Malingering persons have been shown to demonstrate a poorer performance on these measures in comparison to scores expected from brain damaged persons.

In recent years, specific tests have been developed to actively detect malingering, including the Symptom Validity Test, the Digit Recognition Test, and Rey's 15-Item Visual Memory Test. The format of these instruments is similar to other tests encountered during the neuropsychological examination. The tests are constructed with the appearance of being difficult; they are, however, fairly easy. Patients whose performance is below cut-off scores should be suspected of symptom exaggeration. A more detailed presentation of the relationship of minor head injury and tests of malingering appears in the next chapter.

REFERENCES

1. Walsh, K., *Neuropsychology: A Clinical Approach,* 3rd ed., Churchill Livingstone, New York, 1994.
2. Kolb, B., Whishaw, I.Q., *Fundamentals of Human Neuropsychology,* W.H. Freeman, San Francisco, 1980.
3. Schneider, A.M., Tarshis, B., *An Introduction to Physiological Psychology,* 3rd ed., Random House, New York, 1986.
4. Hartlage, L.C., Neuropsychology: definition and history, in, Hartlage, L.C., Asken, M.J., and Hornsby, J.L., Eds., *Essentials of Neuropsychological Assessment,* Springer, New York, 1987.
5. Luria, A.R., *Higher Cortical Functions in Man,* Basic Books, New York, 1980.
6. Thomas, C.L., Ed., *Taber's Cyclopedic Medical Dictionary,* 17th ed., F.A. Davis, Philadelphia, 1989.
7. Hole, J.W., *Human Anatomy and Physiology,* 2nd ed., Wm. C. Brown Company Publishers, Dubuque, IA, 1981.
8. Moore, B.E., Fine, B.D., Eds., *Psychoanalytic Terms and Concepts,* Yale University Press, New Haven, 1990.
9. Kalat, J.W., *Biological Psychology,* 3rd ed., Wadsworth, Belmont, CA, 1988.
10. Coren, S., Porac, C., Ward, L.M., *Sensation and Perception,* 2nd ed., Academic Press, Orlando, 1984.
11. Berg, R., Franzen, M., Wedding, D., *Screening for Brain Impairment: A Manual for Mental Health Practice,* Springer, New York, 1987.
12. Spreen, O., Strauss, E., *A Compendium of Neuropsychological Tests Administration, Norms, and Commentary,* Oxford University Press, New York, 1991.
13. Bourne, L.E., Ekstrand, B.R., Psychology Its Principles and Meanings, 4th ed., Holt, Rinehart, and Winston, New York, 1982.
14. Brody, N., *Intelligence,* 2nd ed., Academic Press, San Diego, 1992.
15. Frazen, M., Berg, R., *Screening Children for Brain Impairment,* Springer, New York, 1989.
16. Kimble, G.A., Garmezy, N., Zigler, E., *Principles of Psychology,* 6th ed., John Wiley & Sons, New York, 1984.
17. Freides, D., *Emory Neuropsychology Laboratory Manual of Tests,* Emory University, Atlanta, 1994.

18. *Diagnostic and Statistical Manual of Mental Disorders*, 4th ed., American Psychiatric Association, Washington D.C., 1994.
19. Kaplan, H.I., Freedman, A.M., Sadock, B.J., *Comprehensive Textbook of Psychiatry*, Vol. 3, Williams & Wilkins, Baltimore, 1980.
20. Lees-Haley, P.R., Dunn, J.T., Forensic issues in the neuropsychological assessment of patients with postconcussive syndrome, in, *Head Injury and Postconcussive Syndrome*, Rizzo, M., Tranel, D., Eds., Churchill Livingstone, New York, 1996, 469–497.
21. Guilmette, T.J., Giuliano, A.J., Taking the stand: Issues and strategies in forensic neuropsychology, *Clinical Neuropsychologist*, 5, 197–219, 1991.
22. Pankratz, L., Erickson, R.C., Two views of malingering, *Clinical Neuropsychologist*, 4, 379–389, 1990.
23. Goebel, R., Detection of faking on the Halstead-Retain Neuropsychological Test Battery, *Journal of Clinical Psychology,* 39, 731–742, 1989.
24. Hall, H.V., Pritchard, D.A., *Detecting Malingering and Deception Forensic Distortion Analysis (FDA),* St. Lucie Press, Delray Beach, FL, 1996.

CASE HISTORIES*

JOANNA
Category: Psychological conditions

This patient's history is put into the chapter on psychological conditions of the whiplash patient not because these headaches are psychological in nature, but because of what happens to the person's personality as a result of her injury. She is 30 years old and was working in [...] a year before I saw her.

She states that she was working on a ship and fell 15 feet and hit several objects and landed half on her back in an awkward position. She felt she hit her head "on something." She was not unconscious. She was taken to the emergency room at the local hospital, x-rayed and released, and she says that her headaches began immediately. She states there were no headaches prior to the accident.

Incapacitating headaches: These started the day of the accident. She was getting them daily, and when I saw her she was getting them about 4 times a week. The pain would last 2 to 4 hours. Again, she would have the typical symptoms of a vascular headache, in that the throbbing starts in the back or posterocervical and occipital regions of the back of the head, and also in the temporal regions on the side of the head. She gets nauseous, light sensitivity, noise sensitivity, sensitivity to odors, must go to bed, and any kind of excessive movement will make it worse.

Interfering headaches (moderate to severe): These started after the accident and she has been having them daily since. It is constant, waxes and wanes, and is similar to the incapacitating headaches, but less intense. The location is the same.

Irritating headaches: She does not complain of this type of headache.

She came from a large family with no headaches, except one older sister who she said had severe headaches. It is rather important to always find out if there is a history of headaches in the family to see whether there is any kind of possible genetic relationship between the patient's family and her headaches.

She had an extensive workup, and there was no evidence of any brain damage or abnormalities. When I examined the patient, she had many myofacial and muscle trigger points that would make her headache worse. A psychological test was done, the MMPI (Minnesota Multiphase Personality Inventory), and this suggested significant psychophysiologic distress patterns. These patterns are often seen with patients attempting to cope with their pain.

This patient would be classified as having a post traumatic intractable, daily headache, and also post traumatic migraine-like headache. Muscle contraction would be used in relationship to her trigger points. (See Chapter 17 concerning trigger points.)

* On the headache assessment forms that accompany these case histories, incapacitating headaches are indicated with solid black lines, interfering headaches with dotted lines, and irritating headaches with gray shading.

MEDICAL HEADACHE HISTORY

Name: JoAnna **Age:** 30 **Sex** F **Date:** 7/10/90

Date of Birth: 00/00/59 **Birthplace:** NY **Race:** B **Education:** 2 yrs college

Occupation: Unemployed **Accident:** 1989

Armed Services & Type of Discharge: N/A

PAST HISTORY:

1.	Did you have a normal birth?		Yes (underlined)	No
	a) forceps used?		Yes	No (underlined)
	b) cesarean section?		Yes	No (underlined)
2.	Did you have problems with bedwetting?		Yes	No (underlined)
	a) If yes, age bedwetting stopped		______	
3.	Were you car sick as a child (motion)?		Yes	No (underlined)
	a) If yes, how severe?	Slight	Moderate	Severe
4.	Did you have unexplained abdominal cramps as a child?		Yes	No (underlined)
5.	Did you have any of the following illnesses in childhood?			
	a) meningitis		Yes	No (underlined)
	b) encephalitis		Yes	No (underlined)
	c) scarlet fever		Yes	No (underlined)
	d) rheumatic fever		Yes	No (underlined)
6.	Did you have any head injuries as a child?		Yes	No (underlined)
	a) If yes, please explain: ______			
7.	Were you treated for emotional illness as a child?		Yes	No (underlined)

HABITS:

8.	Do you drink alcohol?	Yes (underlined)	No
	a) If yes, what kind and how much? 1 to 2 beers a week, glass of wine a month		
	b) Does alcohol bring on or aggravate a headache?	Yes (underlined)	No
9.	Do you smoke?	Yes	No (underlined)
	a) If yes, how much? ______		
	b) Does smoking or smoke-filled rooms cause or aggravate headaches?	Yes (underlined)	No
10.	Do you drink caffeinated beverages?	Yes (underlined)	No
	a) If yes, how much? Pepsi or iced tea daily		

MENSTRUAL HISTORY:

At what age did menses begin? 12 Were they regular or irregular? WNL

How were they related to your headache? N/A

Are you or were you ever on Birth Control Pills? Yes Did they affect your headache? N/A

Have you had a hysterectomy, partial or total, and why? No

Are you in menopause, and if yes, how long? No

Are you on hormones, and if yes, which ones? No

HEADACHE ASSESSMENT FORM

HA PROFILE	INCAPACITATING #3	INTERFERING #2	IRRITATING #1
ONSET (Years ago and frequency)	Day of accident Every day	After accident Every day	N/A
CURRENT FREQUENCY	4 a week	Every day	N/A
TIME OF ONSET	Anytime	Anytime	N/A
DURATION	2 to 4 hours	Constant, can wax and wane	N/A
CHARACTER	Throbbing	Same, less intense	N/A
PRODROME OR AURA	N/A	N/A	N/A
ASSOCIATING FEATURES	Nausea; Vomiting; Sensitivity to Light? Noise? Odors? Do you get pale or flush? Do your eyes or nose run? Does your nose get stuffy? Does the white of your eyes get red? Does your eyelid droop? Do you pace, or go to bed?	Nausea; Vomiting; Sensitivity to Light? Noise? Odors? Do you get pale or flush? Do your eyes or nose run? Does your nose get stuffy? Does the white of your eyes get red? Does your eyelid droop? Do you pace, or go to bed?	Nausea; Vomiting; Sensitivity to Light? Noise? Odors? Do you get pale or flush? Do your eyes or nose run? Does your nose get stuffy? Does the white of your eyes get red? Does your eyelid droop? Do you pace, or go to bed?
PRECIPITATING OR AGGRAVATING FEATURES	Coughing Movement	Exertion	N/A

LOCATION: Mark the location for each type of headache with a different color pen.

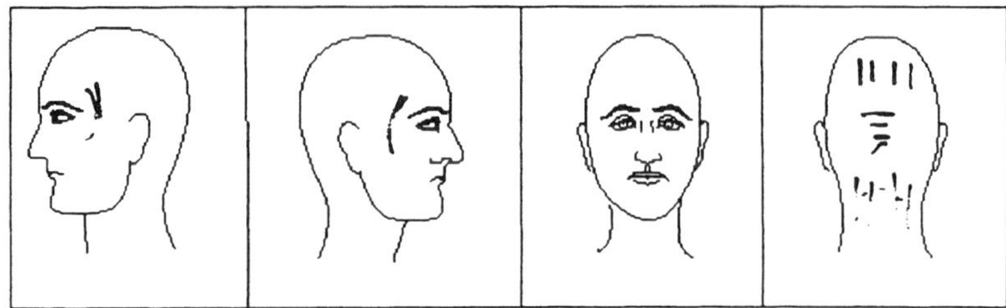

MEDICAL HISTORY:

Have you ever been or are you currently being treated for any of the following?

a) high blood pressure	Yes	No
b) stomach ulcers	Yes	No
c) asthma	Yes	No
d) allergies	Yes	No
e) pneumonia	Yes	No
f) kidney problems	Yes	No
g) low blood sugar	Yes	No
h) glaucoma	Yes	No
i) diabetes	Yes	No
j) heart problems	Yes	No

If you answered yes to any of the above, please describe:________________

List all other medical problems you have had in the past. Include date diagnosed and treatment.
DO NOT LIST OPERATIONS

Carpal tunnel syndrome in right hand. Herniated disk in lower back. Bulging disk in neck.

SURGICAL HISTORY (List operations and dates performed)

Cesarean section 1984.

PSYCHIATRIC HISTORY (List visits with counselors, psychologists, etc., and type of treatment)

ACCIDENTS IN ADULT LIFE (Briefly describe any accident that caused any blow to the head or that you feel is related to your headache)

Installing insulation on a ship in 1989. Fell 15 feet, and hit several objects on the way down. Landed half on rear and half on back. Hit head on something. Not unconscious. Taken to emergency room, x-rayed and released. Headaches began immediately. No headaches before accident.

FAMILY HISTORY:

1. Is your father living? — Yes / No
   - Age________
   - Cause of death TB, age 37
   - Was there a headache history? — Yes / No
2. Is your mother living? — Yes / No
   - Age 50
   - Cause of death________
   - Was there a headache history? — Yes / No

3. Ages of brothers---Circle the ones with headache
   31 32
4. Ages of sisters---Circle the ones with headache
   (29) 27 19
5. List any other blood relatives with a history of severe headaches.
   None

MARITAL HISTORY:
List marriages:

1st marriage age 23 to Present Did spouse have headaches?	Yes	<u>No</u>
2nd marriage age ____ to ______ Did spouse have headaches?	Yes	No
3rd marriage age ____ to ______ Did spouse have headaches?	Yes	No

Age of current spouse:__________

List ages and sex of all children:

Age 6 Sex F Headaches?	Yes	<u>No</u>
Age 4 Sex F Headaches?	Yes	<u>No</u>
Age 1 Sex F Headaches?	Yes	<u>No</u>
Age ____ Sex _____ Headaches?	Yes	No

STRESS FACTORS:

List any factors that may be affecting your headaches (money, loneliness, sexual problems, work, etc.)

____

____

VEGETATIVE SIGNS:

1.	Do you have trouble falling asleep?	<u>Yes</u>	No
2.	Do you have trouble staying asleep?	<u>Yes</u>	No
3.	Has your appetite decreased?	<u>Yes</u>	No
4.	Have you gained or lost weight in the past year?	<u>Yes</u>	No
5.	Have you felt tearful or depressed lately?	Yes	<u>No</u>
6.	Have you had any thoughts of wanting to die?	Yes	<u>No</u>
7.	Have you been forgetful lately?	Yes	<u>No</u>
8.	Any other changes in your normal day-to-day living?__________		

Please list any medications you are allergic or sensitive to: None known.

____

____

Please list any medications you are currently taking (including dosages and frequency per day):
None.

____

PREVIOUS CARE:

1. List doctors who have treated you for headaches: None.

2. List any tests you have had for your headache (e.g., EEG, CT scan, MRI, X-Ray, etc.):

X-rays at time of fall.

MRI of brain and back. Bulging disk cervical lumbar area.

EMG – abnormal on right side.

3. List any other treatment you have had for your headache (e.g., biofeedback, acupuncture, chiropractic, or any other treatment you had):

None.

JAMES
Category: Psychological conditions

This is a most interesting case in which a 31-year-old man was seen a year and a half after his significant accident.

According to the patient and his mother, who was with him, he was cutting off a beam on a double-wide trailer and as he was crawling out from under the trailer, the beam fell, pinning his head. The patient states the beam hit him on the left side of the head and face. He was rendered unconscious. He was taken to the hospital. He was hospitalized, then transferred to the [...] hospital for neurological surgery.

As a result of his surgery (which was to clip the left internal carotid artery to the ophthalmic artery as it exited the cavernous sinus) and because of his behavior, he was sent for psychological testing. This could not be done because he would have a headache or walk out of the testing area, or was unresponsive, and he continued to demand medication. The notes from the psychologist indicate that the patient's concentration skills seem diminished, and he has severe trouble with focusing his attention as well. His headache history states the following:

Incapacitating headaches: The patient states that since the accident, he has been experiencing daily incapacitating headaches. He wakes up with them, and the duration is constant. The character of the pain is severe pressure which is located in the right temporal region radiating down the parietal and cervical regions. There is no aura and associated features are sometimes nausea, vomiting, photophobia, sonophobia, and the patient has to go to bed or remain in a sitting position.

Interfering headaches (moderate to severe): The patient states that this headache is exactly the same as the incapacitating headache, with less intensity because he takes a pain pill, sometimes as much as 6 to 8 daily.

The working diagnoses is post traumatic migraine-like headaches. The patient has had extensive and excellent workup. The surgeon recorded that the patient "is dull, somewhat apathetic, and has slow thought processes, concentration, attention, with decreased memory and mentation. He had poor recall. He has poor calculations and abstractions." There was also some right-sided hemiparesis of a spastic variety with hyperflexion. He also noted that there were neurological problems in which the patient could not fulfill certain neurological testings, such as hopping in one place, etc.

Another neurologist stated that the patient became angry at the neurologist because the neurologist was trying to get him back to work. It was noted that he had limited brain skills and had a rigid way of thinking.

Another physician noted the patient watched a lot of television, and the mother stated he was tired all the time. The patient would go fishing and become exhausted. Several months prior to that, he went out to mow the lawn and passed out. According to the mother, he was never like this prior to the accident. The mother also stated he has little outside interests, and he is taking anywhere from 8 to 10 pain pills a day.

Another doctor noticed the patient tends to draw conclusions or he becomes angry at what is being said and what the possibilities are. He draws conclusions on what he thinks, and tends to misinterpret this and then becomes angry. The doctor suggested this is probably a personality problem, in which the patient cannot adapt to his disability. He states, "He concentrates on what he cannot do and does not tune into what he can do."

I was able to have the patient leave the room and sit outside while I spoke to his mother, who gave me a history of the patient prior to his accident and neurosurgery. She stated that prior to the accident he was an extremely capable individual. She said that out of all her sons, who are all in the mobile home transporting business, this patient was the best. He was able to give orders to 30-odd people involved in their business and had no difficulty with executive decisions. He was planning to marry and was living with a woman. Evidently, according to the mother, they had a very good relationship and there were no problems in his social or personal areas. Since the accident, she states he has lost all interest in socializing, and has withdrawn from this woman. She states that at times before the accident he would become somewhat frustrated and angry, but would quickly recover and then he would be able to deal with and resolve all issues, whereas now, he seems to overreact, is much more irritable, depressed, and tends not to function anywhere near the capacity he had prior to the accident.

My report back to the physician who sent the patient to me was that I did not feel that his behavior was because of a personality or psychodynamic conflicts as a result of his pain, but rather his inability to use his forebrain because of injury to it. This has been called in the past "frontal lobe syndrome" in which certain nerve tracts are damaged that go from the thalamus of the brain to the frontal part of the brain, and the interpretation of the frontal part of the brain cannot be completed. All the behavior described is often seen with this frontal lobe syndrome. The other interesting thing about the patient was that he lacked affect, which means that he did not seem to display the proper emotion with the content of the conversation, which is also seen in frontal lobe syndrome. There appears to be an apathy and lack of interest in his appearance and the whole response is generally a depressed response.

Also in frontal lobe syndrome, the motor activities diminish and personal habits are decreased and perseverations (repetition of behavior) noted.

Also in frontal lobe syndrome, the cognitive function becomes impaired, often affecting abstract thinking and memory. Eventually even the orientation to time and place are disturbed. What is important to note is that psychological phenomena are a significant change from the patient's previous status. Sometimes the change can be just an exaggeration of the former personality; but, in the case of this patient, according to the mother, this is a total change in the patient's personality.

The unfortunate part of this situation is that the prognosis is extremely poor, and probably this damage will not be able to be corrected.

MEDICAL HEADACHE HISTORY

Name: James **Age:** 31 **Sex** M **Date:** 10/18/89

Date of Birth: 00/00/58 **Birthplace:** KY **Race:** W **Education:** 10th Grade

Occupation: Unemployed **Accident:** 3/88

Armed Services & Type of Discharge: N/A

PAST HISTORY:

1.	Did you have a normal birth?		Yes (underlined)	No
	a) forceps used?		Yes	No
	b) cesarean section?		Yes	No
2.	Did you have problems with bedwetting?		Yes	No (underlined)
	a) If yes, age bedwetting stopped		______	
3.	Were you car sick as a child (motion)?		Yes	No (underlined)
	a) If yes, how severe?	Slight	Moderate	Severe
4.	Did you have unexplained abdominal cramps as a child?		Yes	No (underlined)
5.	Did you have any of the following illnesses in childhood?			
	a) meningitis		Yes	No (underlined)
	b) encephalitis		Yes	No (underlined)
	c) scarlet fever		Yes	No (underlined)
	d) rheumatic fever		Yes	No (underlined)
6.	Did you have any head injuries as a child?		Yes	No (underlined)
	a) If yes, please explain: ______			
7.	Were you treated for emotional illness as a child?		Yes	No (underlined)

HABITS:

8.	Do you drink alcohol?	Yes (underlined)	No
	a) If yes, what kind and how much? ______		
	b) Does alcohol bring on or aggravate a headache?	Yes	No (underlined)
9.	Do you smoke?	Yes (underlined)	No
	a) If yes, how much? 1 pack		
	b) Does smoking or smoke-filled rooms cause or aggravate headaches?	Yes	No (underlined)
10.	Do you drink caffeinated beverages?	Yes	No (underlined)
	a) If yes, how much? ______		

MENSTRUAL HISTORY:

At what age did menses begin? ______ Were they regular or irregular? ______
How were they related to your headache? ______
Are you or were you ever on Birth Control Pills? ______ Did they affect your headache? ______
Have you had a hysterectomy, partial or total, and why? ______
Are you in menopause, and if yes, how long? ______
Are you on hormones, and if yes, which ones? ______

HEADACHE ASSESSMENT FORM

HA PROFILE	INCAPACITATING #3	INTERFERING #2	IRRITATING #1
ONSET (Years ago and frequency)	Since accident	Keep headaches at a #2 level with Fiorinal daily	N/A
CURRENT FREQUENCY	Every day		N/A
TIME OF ONSET	Wakes up with		N/A
DURATION	Constant		N/A
CHARACTER	Severe pressure		N/A
PRODROME OR AURA	N/A		N/A
ASSOCIATING FEATURES	Nausea; Vomiting; Sensitivity to Light? Noise? Odors? Do you get pale or flush? Do your eyes or nose run? Does your nose get stuffy? Does the white of your eyes get red? Does your eyelid droop? Do you pace, or go to bed?	Nausea; Vomiting; Sensitivity to Light? Noise? Odors? Do you get pale or flush? Do your eyes or nose run? Does your nose get stuffy? Does the white of your eyes get red? Does your eyelid droop? Do you pace, or go to bed?	Nausea; Vomiting; Sensitivity to Light? Noise? Odors? Do you get pale or flush? Do your eyes or nose run? Does your nose get stuffy? Does the white of your eyes get red? Does your eyelid droop? Do you pace, or go to bed?
PRECIPITATING OR AGGRAVATING FEATURES	Sneezing Sun		N/A

LOCATION: Mark the location for each type of headache with a different color pen.

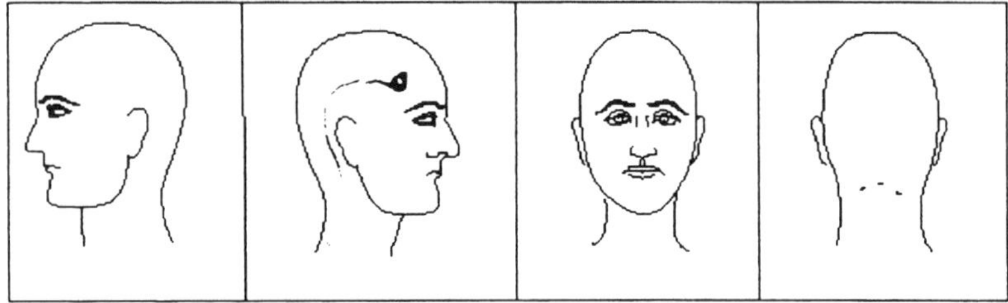

MEDICAL HISTORY:

Have you ever been or are you currently being treated for any of the following?

a) high blood pressure	Yes	No
b) stomach ulcers	Yes	No
c) asthma	Yes	No
d) allergies	Yes	No
e) pneumonia	Yes	No
f) kidney problems	Yes	No
g) low blood sugar	Yes	No
h) glaucoma	Yes	No
i) diabetes	Yes	No
j) heart problems	Yes	No

If you answered yes to any of the above, please describe:.____________________

List all other medical problems you have had in the past. Include date diagnosed and treatment.
DO NOT LIST OPERATIONS

Diminished hearing in both ears, sense of taste. CVA 4 days after the accident.

SURGICAL HISTORY (List operations and dates performed)

None.

PSYCHIATRIC HISTORY (List visits with counselors, psychologists, etc., and type of treatment)

None.

ACCIDENTS IN ADULT LIFE (Briefly describe any accident that caused any blow to the head or that you feel is related to your headache)

3/88 – Cutting off beam on double-wide trailer. Crawling out from under trailer and beam dropped, pinning head. Beam hit left side of head and face. Unconscious. Taken to hospital, then transferred to Shands Hospital for neurological surgery. Have "shunt" in right side of head.

FAMILY HISTORY:

1. Is your father living? Yes No
   Age 58
   Cause of death____________________
   Was there a headache history? Yes No

2. Is your mother living? Yes No
   Age__56_____
   Cause of death________________________________
   Was there a headache history? Yes No
3. Ages of brothers---Circle the ones with headache
   __35__34______________________________________
4. Ages of sisters---Circle the ones with headache
   __36__33__29__27__26__________________________
5. List any other blood relatives with a history of severe headaches.
   ___None______________________________________

MARITAL HISTORY:
List marriages:

1st marriage age __23__ to __26___ Did spouse have headaches? Yes No
2nd marriage age _____ to ______ Did spouse have headaches? Yes No
3rd marriage age _____ to ______ Did spouse have headaches? Yes No
Age of current spouse:__________

List ages and sex of all children:
Age __7__ Sex __F__ Headaches? Yes No
Age _____ Sex _____ Headaches? Yes No
Age_____ Sex _____ Headaches? Yes No

STRESS FACTORS:

List any factors that may be affecting your headaches (money, loneliness, sexual problems, work, etc.)
___Sexual problems, loneliness.____

VEGETATIVE SIGNS:

1. Do you have trouble falling asleep? Yes No
2. Do you have trouble staying asleep? Yes No
3. Has your appetite decreased? Yes No
4. Have you gained or lost weight in the past year? Yes No
5. Have you felt tearful or depressed lately? Yes No
6. Have you had any thoughts of wanting to die? Yes No
7. Have you been forgetful lately? Yes No
8. Any other changes in your normal day-to-day living?______________________

Please list any medications you are allergic or sensitive to:__Penicillin (rash).______________

Please list any medications you are currently taking (including dosages and frequency per day):
___Dilantin, 100 mg. - 3 times a day. Buspar, 10 mg. – 3 times a day. Fioricet, 5 – every day.______

PREVIOUS CARE:

1. List doctors who have treated you for headaches:

2. List any tests you have had for your headache (e.g., EEG, CT scan, MRI, X-Ray, etc.):
CAT scan,
EEG.
X-rays.

3. List any other treatment you have had for your headache (e.g., biofeedback, acupuncture, chiropractic, or any other treatment you had):
Chiropractic (no help).

Chapter 21

Neuropsychology of Minor Head Injury

John N.I. Dieter, Ph.D.

THE POST CONCUSSION AND WHIPLASH SYNDROMES

Introduction

The neuropsychology of minor head injury and whiplash is a complex field of study. This chapter addresses topics related to the description of the *post concussion* and *whiplash syndromes*, particularly their constellation and course of symptoms, as viewed from a neuropsychological perspective. Research findings are integrated in an effort to demonstrate that minor head injury and whiplash can have a profound effect on the global functioning of the individual. Evidence will be offered that the post concussion syndrome is frequently associated with significant neuropsychological impairment suggestive of underlying brain pathology. The interaction between cognitive impairment, chronic pain, and emotional distress will be discussed. The important issue of malingering in post concussion and whiplash patients will be addressed, including a review of neuropsychological tests commonly used to assess persons feigning neurocognitive symptoms. Finally, topics related to the psychological treatment of head injured persons will be reviewed.

Comprehending the impact that injuries to the head and neck have upon intellectual and emotional functioning requires an understanding of brain anatomy, consideration of the biopsychosocial dynamics of the patient, as well as an appreciation of the complexities of neuropsychological evaluation. As these issues are addressed below, reference to the previous chapter will prove helpful, particularly when neuroanatomy and neuropsychological test findings are discussed.

Minor Head Injury, Whiplash, and Symptoms of the Post Traumatic Syndrome

It has been estimated that between 750,000 and 3 million head traumas occur each year. Although mild head trauma frequently does not lead to hospitalization, 60,000 persons per year experience some degree of disability.[1] Of those head trauma patients seen in hospital emergency rooms, approximately 75% to 90% have minor head injury.[2] From their 1986 study of over 1000 minor head injury patients, Alves and colleagues found approximately 66% were men.[2] Over 80% of the patients were white and their average age was about 29 years. Forty-seven percent of these patients were injured in motor vehicle accidents, 20% were injured from falls, 10% from violent attack, and the remainder from idiosyncratic events.[2]

Minor head injury (MHI) can be defined as being marked by: (1) a transient loss of consciousness or other neurologic function (e.g., memory, language, or vision), (2) an initial *Glasgow Coma*

Scale score between 13 and 15, and (3) negative neurologic and neurodiagnostic findings at admission.[2,6] These criteria are fairly well accepted by both clinicians and researchers.

The Glasgow Coma Scale is a convenient and objective measure for rating the level of a person's consciousness.[3] The scale evaluates three areas of function in response to a verbal command or applied pain (e.g., administering a knuckle to a person's sternum): eye opening, motor responding, and verbal responding. Each area of function is scored and summed. Summed scores can range from 3 to 15. Patients who achieve a score of 7 and below are considered to be comatose. The Glasgow Coma Scale scores of persons with minor head injury reflect little disturbance in consciousness. Common symptoms include some disorientation and perhaps minor verbal mistakes.

Despite subtle neuropsychological symptoms, minor head injured persons usually perform within normal limits on preliminary neurologic and mental status examinations (see the previous chapter). Furthermore, they rarely demonstrate obvious anatomical damage when imagery studies (e.g., MRI, CT scan, x-ray) are conducted.

Many people who suffer minor head injury do not experience an actual loss of consciousness; if they do it is of short duration. Commonly, MHI patients are merely stunned and the alteration in consciousness is limited to a period of disorientation. Regardless of whether the injured person loses consciousness, minor head injury is often accompanied by a period of post traumatic amnesia (PTA) or disorientation. The duration of PTA is a very useful indicator of the severity of a patient's head injury, as well as a good predictor of when he or she might return to work.[3] Post traumatic amnesia can include both *antrograde* and *retrograde* components. Antrograde amnesia leads to memory problems related to events following the trauma. Retrograde amnesia is a memory deficit for events that occurred pre-trauma.[1] The total duration of post traumatic amnesia is measured from the time of the injury until the person is capable of continuous awareness and memory.[3] Often a person's retrograde amnesia "shrinks" so that he or she begins to progressively remember events leading up to the trauma. Persons considered to have a minor head injury experience post traumatic amnesia of less than one hour.[3]

Whiplash is a traumatic injury resulting from cervical sprain or strain due to hyperflexion/hyperextension. Unlike MHI, it does not involve a traumatic loss or alteration of consciousness.[4] Despite unique differences in the biomechanics of minor head injury and whiplash, both types of trauma result in a constellation of symptoms that is quite similar. Therefore, both conditions will be subsumed under the general rubric of the *post traumatic syndrome*.

Many researchers maintain that the post traumatic syndrome arises from both organic and psychosocial factors, and that symptoms are unrelated to the severity of the trauma or length of post traumatic amnesia.[1] The post concussive and whiplash syndromes consist of a set of somatic, psychophysiological, and psychosocial complaints that include: (1) headaches, (2) dizziness, (3) memory and concentration problems, (4) weakness and fatigue, (5) nausea, (6) numbness, (7) diplopia (i.e., double vision), (8) tinnitus (i.e., ringing in the ears), (9) hearing problems, (10) anxiety, depression, irritability, and (11) personality changes.[2]

While the neurological symptoms of minor head injury and whiplash are often emphasized initially, ensuing psychological symptoms and cognitive problems may determine the severity and duration of impairment. Neuropsychological symptoms can range from mild disturbances in perception, information processing, and general reasoning to very significant emotional or intellectual dysfunction. Such symptoms add to the patients' psychological distress as they perceive that their post trauma functioning is below premorbid levels. Common personality changes that accompany even mild head trauma include emotional lability, decreased impulse control, apathy, and indifference. Personality change often accompanies intellectual impairment. As will be discussed below, premorbid personality, preexisting psychopathology, and life stressors can influence the severity of the psychological and physical symptoms, and the overall level of disability, associated with post traumatic syndrome.

Debate over the veracity of post traumatic symptoms has persisted since the late 18th century.[2] Currently, there is no single explanation of the etiology of the post concussion or whiplash syndromes. Many suggest that the evidence of anatomical damage is insufficient to account for the severity of symptoms; furthermore, the onset and duration of symptoms can vary greatly across persons. Some authors argue that there is less than adequate evidence that the symptom spectrum associated with minor head injury and whiplash is consistent enough to qualify as a distinct syndrome.[2] As discussed in the previous chapter, the *Diagnostic and Statistical Manual of Mental Disorders*, 4th edition, of the American Psychiatric Association does not recognize post concussive or whiplash syndrome as a formal Axis I diagnosis. The view of the authors of this text is that there is overwhelming evidence that minor head injury and whiplash are associated with a distinct diagnostic syndrome that is far-reaching in its impact upon the individual and his or her social and personal environment.

THE COURSE AND DURATION OF POST CONCUSSION AND WHIPLASH SYMPTOMS

The natural course of post traumatic symptoms has not been studied extensively; nor have the roles of organic, psychological, or motivational factors been clearly delineated. As indicated, there is considerable variability to how long after the injury post concussion or whiplash symptoms arise. That symptoms begin at different times is probably further support for an etiological model that reflects the confluence of neurological, psychological, and social factors.[2] For instance, irritability, a common symptom, often occurs some time after the trauma and is probably a reaction to the social and emotional consequences of the ensuing neuropsychological deficits and chronic pain. Organic factors such as the person's age and general health, and psychosocial factors such as family and work stress, clearly interact to exacerbate and prolong post traumatic symptoms.

In general, the majority of post traumatic symptoms occur within three months of the accident. Early onset symptoms are often less recalcitrant; late onset symptoms are often associated with substantial social morbidity and sometimes malingering.[2] Symptoms that persist for two or three months are likely to continue for some time.[4] Post traumatic symptoms that persist past six months are sometimes labeled "late whiplash syndrome."

In general, many minor head injury and whiplash patients report only one or two somatic or psychophysiologic symptoms. Alves and colleagues arbitrarily decided that patients were at risk for post traumatic syndrome if at any time they exhibited two or more symptoms.[2] Using this criterion, as many as 50% of minor head injury patients may be at risk for post traumatic syndrome.

The Occurrence and Persistence of Post Traumatic Symptoms

The impact of minor head injury and whiplash on a person's life can be ubiquitous. Findings across the limited number of studies that examined the course of post traumatic symptoms indicate that they begin soon after the trauma and very often persist for years. This section will integrate these research findings in an effort to document the course of the syndrome. Table 21.1 provides a list of the most commonly reported symptoms and their frequency of occurrence across the first year post trauma.

The First Week

From their large-scale longitudinal study of minor head injury patients, Alves et al.[3] found that at discharge, the distribution of post traumatic symptoms was as follows: headaches (45.8%), dizziness (14.2%), memory problems (13.0%), weakness (10.4%), nausea (7.9%), numbness (5.8%), double vision (4.7%), tinnitus (2.2%), and hearing problems (2%). Approximately 75% of patients reported one or no symptoms at discharge. Less than 10% of patients reported three or more symptoms when leaving the hospital.

The above findings suggest that the prognosis for most post traumatic patients is very good, as indicated by the fairly few persons who report symptoms when they are discharged from the hospital. Unfortunately, this is not the case: a remarkable phenomenon common to the post traumatic syndrome is that the occurrence of symptoms often increases during the first three months following the trauma, and most dramatically during the first week. In a recent study, Ettlin et al.[7] examined 21 consecutive whiplash patients. The patients had a mean age of about 29 years; none of their injuries reflected direct head trauma, and none of the patients had a previous history of cervical injury. The investigators found that with the exception of nausea and irritability, every post traumatic symptom increased during the first three days following the trauma (see Table 21.1).[7] The most striking increases were in areas of neuropsychological and emotional functioning. During the first post traumatic week, nearly 50% of patients reported impaired memory, and over 60% of patients indicated difficulty concentrating. Whereas none of the patients reported anxiety immediately following their injuries, nearly 50% of the individuals became anxious during the first week post trauma. Symptoms of depression increased from approximately 14% to over 40%.

The results of the Ettlin et al. study begin to shed light on how biopsychosocial factors contribute to the occurrence of post traumatic symptoms. The delayed onset of neuropsychological and emotional symptoms may result from subtle neuroanatomical and neurochemical changes whose impact on functioning is not experienced until several days after the accident. Furthermore, as patients attempt to return to the normal routines of life, activity probably exacerbates physical symptoms. Additionally, a return to work promotes awareness of new problems with attention, concentration, and information processing. The natural psychological reaction to such events includes depression, in response to concerns over how current functioning compares to premorbid levels, and anxiety, in relation to fears that neuropsychological and somatic symptoms might persist into the future.

Six Weeks to Three Months

Table 21.1 presents an overview of the post traumatic symptoms reported by minor head injury and whiplash patients at six weeks and three months. Collective findings indicate that during this period post traumatic symptoms often continue to increase in frequency and intensity.

Table 21.1 Range of Somatic, Neuropsychological, and Emotional Symptoms Experienced by Whiplash Patients During the First Year

Symptom	Immediate	3 Days Post Injury	At 6 weeks	At 3 months	At 1 year
Somatic					
Headache	58.33%	85.71%	78.33%	57.89%	41.18%
Neck pain	76.19%	95.24%	N/A	63.16%	35.29%
Arm pain	42.86%	71.43%	N/A	31.58%	9.52%
Vertigo	38.10%	76.19%	N/A	42.11%	23.53%
Nausea	47.62%	14.29%	N/A	21.05%	0%
Visual symptoms	14.29%	42.86%	16.67%	36.84%	0%
Sleep disturbance	14.29%	85.71%	70.00%	52.63%	5.88%
Neuropsychological					
Impaired concentration	23.81%	61.90%	N/A	52.63%	29.41%
Impaired memory	4.76%	47.62%	N/A	47.37%	23.53%
Emotional					
Depression	14.29%	42.86%	N/A	42.11%	11.76%
Anxiety	0%	47.62%	N/A	36.84%	5.88%
Irritability	95.24%	61.90%	N/A	57.89%	17.65%

Data from References 2 and 7.

With the exception of headache (decreasing to 41.1%), Alves et al.[2] found that the frequency of each post traumatic symptom was greater at the three-month check-up. For those persons who returned to work, many become unemployed during this period. At three months, almost 34% of patients examined by the Ettlin et al. study had not returned to work.[7] Only 5 of the original 21 patients (23.81%) reported a complete recovery at three months post trauma.

Patients who exhibited the most substantial disability were most often married persons of middle age, individuals with semiskilled occupations, and lower socioeconomic status (SES), as well as those with prior psychiatric history.[1] Again this reflects the confluence of psychosomatic and environmental variables.

The impact of head and neck injury is usually greater in persons over 40 years of age. With respect to neuropsychological symptoms, this represents the increased vulnerability of the central nervous system that accompanies aging. As a person grows older, the brain loses *plasticity*, or the ability to adapt through equipotentiality (see the previous chapter) to injury or disease.

Married persons frequently have additional life stress as a result of both preexisting problems, as well as how the patient's post traumatic symptoms affect family relationships. Persons of lower SES often have jobs that require physical exertion and include closer scrutiny from bosses. Neurocognitive deficits and emotional reactions are often intensified by preexisting psychological problems and underlying personality structure. In addition, for those persons involved in litigation, the stress associated with an uncertain outcome may exacerbate post traumatic symptoms.[1]

At One Year

In most cases, the trend of symptom increase common to the first three months post trauma reverses during the remainder of the first year (see Table 21.1).[2,7,8] However, almost one half of patients continue to report somatic, neuropsychological, and emotional complaints.

At 12 months, somewhere between 30% and 40% of patients still experience head and neck pain. While decreasing, somatic symptoms such as dizziness (13%), vertigo (23.53%), and tinnitus (10.3%) are still fairly common.

At the end of the first year, neuropsychological and emotional symptoms remain persistent. Patients continue to complain of problems with concentration (29.41%) and memory (23.53%). While anxiety decreases substantially, symptoms of depression and irritability are reported by nearly 20% of post trauma patients.

Alves and colleagues found that the average number of post trauma symptoms across the first year rarely exceeded two. There was a positive relationship between the number of symptoms reported at discharge and those reported at 6 and 12 months.[2]

Beyond the First Year

Ettlin and colleagues conducted detailed follow-up examinations of patients two years post trauma.[7] In general, findings revealed that the course of post traumatic symptoms changed little after the first year. While 10 of 17 patients (58.82%) did indicate complete recovery, almost 30% of the sample still reported problems with concentration and subjective memory problems. Over 40% continued to have chronic or intermittent headaches at the two-year mark. Six patients (35.29%) continued to have neck pain, four (23.53%) vertigo, and two (11.76%) depression.

With respect to employment, over 75% of patients had returned to work full-time by the second year. Of the five patients who were not working full-time, four suffered from persistent cognitive dysfunction, and one from head and neck pain. Repeated neuropsychological testing of these patients showed no significant improvement after the first year.

Klonoff and associates evaluated the quality of life in patients two to four years after closed head injury.[9] Information was gathered through patient self-reports and supplemental information obtained from relatives and significant others. "Quality of life" was defined across four areas:

"emotional functioning", "social role functioning", including employment, home management, and social and family relationships; "daily living activities" (i.e., self-care skills and mobility); and the "ability to engage in enjoyable hobbies and other recreational pastimes".

Seventy-eight persons were assessed. While many of these patients had more serious closed head injuries, 60% had a Glasgow Coma Scale Rating between 11 and 14. Therefore, a fair amount of this subsample would probably meet the accepted criteria for minor head injury (see above). Over 60% (61.5%) of patients reported limb weakness, reduced strength and power, pain, and stiffness. The other most frequent somatic symptoms included sensory loss (37.5%), headache (22.9%), fatigue (14.6%), dizziness (12.5%), motor slowing and incoordination (12.5%), and alcohol intolerance (10.4%).

Almost 60% of patients (57.7%) indicated neuropsychological and emotional symptoms, including memory problems (60%), irritability (53.3%), trouble with concentration (24.4%), other cognitive problems (17.8%), and depression (15.6%). Patients demonstrated the greatest impairment on psychosocial subscales that measured social interaction, alertness, emotional behavior, and difficulties engaging in recreational activities and pastimes. Findings obtained from relatives and significant others indicated that they perceived closed head injury patients as being significantly more belligerent, motorically slowed, socially withdrawn, negative, suspicious, confused, more talkative, and socially obstreperous, than age-matched non-trauma persons.

Summary and Conclusions

Findings across a number of studies strongly indicate that post concussion and whiplash injuries are associated with a persistent symptom pattern. The most common complaints are headache and neck pain, problems with concentration and memory, and symptoms of depression and anxiety. Most patients report less than three post concussive symptoms at any one time. Regardless, as many as 50% of patients may be at risk for post traumatic syndrome. The course of the syndrome reflects a confluence of biological, psychological, and social factors. Patients who exhibit the most substantial disability are often married persons of middle age, individuals with semiskilled occupations, and lower socioeconomic status (SES), as well as those with prior psychiatric history.

While many patients experience few symptoms immediately following the trauma, somatic, cognitive, and emotional complaints increase during the first week. Furthermore, symptoms often exacerbate, to their height, over the next three months. Less than one quarter of patients with post traumatic symptoms report full recovery at three months. Over the remainder of the first post traumatic year, symptoms begin to decrease and commonly reach a plateau that then persists. At the one-year mark, most persons have returned to full employment, but almost one half of patients continue to wrestle with their somatic and psychological problems. About one quarter have memory and concentration problems. Between 35% and 40% report continued head and neck pain, and over 10% indicate that they are depressed.

Consistent findings suggest that the amount of recovery experienced by the patient at one year may be the maximum level he or she can expect for the next several years. Research has shown that the occurrence of symptoms changes little when patients are assessed at or beyond the second year, post trauma. Limited research findings demonstrate that post traumatic symptoms persist up to four years, clearly indicating a long-term disruption of the patient's life.

POSSIBLE NEUROLOGICAL MECHANISMS UNDERLYING POST TRAUMATIC SYMPTOMS

Evidence for Anatomical Damage

As indicated above, some critics argue that the failure by the majority of post traumatic patients to exhibit objective signs of brain or spinal cord damage is support against the existence of the syndrome. Although this is often the case, it has been demonstrated that post traumatic patients show evidence of functional nervous system abnormalities. Ettlin et al. examined whiplash patients during the acute injury period.[7] At insult, 21 consecutive patients had a full neurological examination, as well as cervical x-rays, an electroencephalograph (EEG), brainstem auditory evoked potentials (BEAP), and an MRI. While the BEAPs, x-rays, and MRIs of this sample were grossly normal, neurological examinations conducted within 14 days of the accident revealed that all the patients reported tenderness over the cervical region and reduced range of cervical spine motion. Sensory loss was also common and generally included more than one dematomal segment of the upper extremities. More impressive data came from EEG examinations that were performed within 7 to 8 days after the accident. EEGs reflect the electrical activity of the brain, that is, the firing of neurons within different brain areas (see the previous chapter). Eight of 18 patients examined (44.44%) had normal EEGs (i.e., the type of electrical activity that is expected for that region of the brain examined). Eight patients (44.44%) showed unilateral focally slow brain wave patterns in either the occipital, temporal-occipital, or parietal-occipital regions (see the previous chapter). One patient had mild diffuse slowing and another paroxysmal (i.e., seizure-like) bifrontal theta waves.

Most scientists who study post concussion and whiplash patients believe that the traumas these persons experience do result in actual brain damage. That it is not clearly evident on measures of gross anatomy, such as MRI and CT scan, is because the injuries often occur at the microscopic neuronal level.

Brain damage suspected to arise from MHI and whiplash probably results from the acceleration/deceleration forces that frequently accompany head and neck injuries, particularly those that occur from motor vehicle accidents. The brain is especially sensitive to the effects of inertia because it is not firmly attached to the skull and floats in cerebrospinal fluid. When an automobile strikes, or is struck by another object, the person's head is often projected forward and then back (or vice versa). Once moving, the brain has a tendency to continue its forward course, often until it makes contact with the inner wall of the skull. It can then "bounce" back and strike the opposite wall of the skull. Such motion can result in several forms of brain damage. When the brain directly hits the anterior, lateral, or posterior walls of the skull, this can lead to a *focal brain lesion* (i.e., a specific area of brain damage). As the brain is propelled forward and back, or side to side, it can also scrape along the bony ridges within the skull, causing more diffuse damage. Finally, the force with which the brain is propelled within the skull can lead to microscopic "tears" in brain tissue whereby neurons, particularly their axons, are injured. Most MHI and whiplash neuropsychological and emotional symptoms probably arise from this widespread *shearing* and stretching of neuron fibers which is greatest in the frontal and temporal lobes of the brain.

While autopsy studies of patients with mild head injury patients are rare, some findings indicate that damage to white matter axonal tracts underlie the long-term neuropsychological symptoms. Rimel and colleagues reported that diffuse microscopic neuronal loss has been observed during postmortem examination of persons in whom the only head injury was concussion and where there was no clinical evidence of brain damage.[6]

Levin and Grossman[10] have proposed a number of other mechanisms that may be responsible for behavioral changes associated with head injury. These include altered neurotransmitter metabolism, neuroendocrine disturbance related to involvement of the pituitary gland, reduced cerebral blood flow, and disruption of the reticular activating system that is associated with the regulation of arousal (see the previous chapter).

Cognitive Problems

Deficits of information processing that follow MHI or whiplash can arise from focal brain damage or shearing effects to a variety of hindbrain, midbrain, and forebrain structures. The type of cognitive problems experienced by the patient is usually related to the specific region of the brain that is damaged. For example, right-sided cortical lesions leading to problems of visual-spatial processing and left-sided lesions resulting in verbal processing deficits (see the previous chapter).

Parker[11] emphasizes that effects upon the amygdala (see the previous chapter) are especially important since this brain structure contributes to heightened arousal, which enhances sensory information processing. Furthermore, the amygdala is involved in linking sensory information with emotional reactions, especially the associations between stimuli and rewards, as well as in controlling autonomic changes associated with affect. These functions of the amygdala are essential to the learning process and understanding the consequences of our actions.

Lesions to the dorsolateral prefrontal cortex (see the previous chapter) probably affect information processing functions such as planning, anticipation, and judgment.[11] Damage to the orbitofrontal cortex, with its many connections to the limbic system, may underlie the impulsiveness, disinhibition, and misunderstanding of other's behavior commonly seen in head injured persons.[11]

Crossen and Wiens argue that acceleration/deceleration injuries result in a *divided attention deficit* whereby the damaged brain experiences a reduction in information processing capacity, either in terms of speed of processing, or the amount of information that can be handled simultaneously.[13] They suggest possible pathophysiological mechanisms of this condition include diffuse white matter lesions, brainstem dysfunction, or a disruption in the frontal-limbic reticular activating system (see the previous chapter).

Head and neck trauma may also contribute to cognitive problems through persistent alterations in a patient's state of consciousness including symptoms of *derealization* and *depersonalization*.[11] Derealization is a psychiatric symptom whereby the patient perceives the outside world as not quite real, or dream-like. Depersonalization involves the patient perceiving an alteration in self, for instance, that a part of his or her body is foreign, or has changed shape or size.[12] Feelings of derealization or depersonalization probably reflect a complex deficit in the integration of perceptual, visceral, affective, and cognitive information, and may be related to the hyperarousal that often follows trauma.[11] Disturbance of vestibular function (see the previous chapter) can also contribute to feelings of unreality. With such conditions, reality testing (i.e., the ability to differentiate reality from fantasy) is spared.

Memory

Memory disturbance is the most commonly reported neuropsychological symptom of the post traumatic syndrome. Different types of injuries may result in different forms of memory deficit since it is believed that memory functions are not unitary, and are dispersed throughout the brain.[6] Head injury patients appear to have particular difficulty in the active use of semantic organizational strategies. This function involves assigning information to different categories based upon some meaningful component.

The temporal poles and components of the limbic system, including connections with the orbitalfrontal surface of the frontal cortex, are especially sensitive to minor head injury.[6] This is due to the diffuse damage that occurs to these regions as inertial forces propel the underside of the brain across the bony surface of the skull's interior cavity (see above). MHI damage to these regions may be comparable to that experienced from severe head trauma. Auerbach (1986) has described two frontolimbic symptoms that are particularly vulnerable to MHI.[6] The basolateral limbic system includes the orbitofrontal cortex, insular temporal and anterotemporal cortex, along with their functional interconnections with the dorsomedial nucleus of the thalamus and the amygdala (see the previous chapter). The medial limbic system includes the dorsolateral prefrontal cortex, in connection with the Papez circuit, including the hippocampus, hypothalamus, anterior nuclei of the thalamus, and the cingulate gyrus.[6]

Emotional and Personality Changes

Depression is very common in mild, moderate, and severe head trauma. Frontal and temporal lobe damage has been implicated most frequently in post traumatic depression.[1] Rotational shear forces and minor impact particularly affect personality by influencing the functioning of the temporal lobes, the amygdala, and the tip of the frontal lobes, especially the parasagittal areas. It has been argued that frontal lesions are associated with depression due to damage to the norepinephrine projections from the locus ceruleus (see the previous chapter). Furthermore, cognitive deficits may compound or mask depressive symptoms.

Frontal lobe lesions often manifest as an inability to inhibit behavior.[1] Temporal lobe lesions can manifest as the *Kluver-Bucy syndrome* which includes passivity, hyperorality, hypersexuality, visual agnosia, and memory impairment. Both frontal and temporal lobe lesions can result in reduced control of aggressive impulses.[1] Stress and alcohol can further foster irritability. Violence behavior may be common in persons with preexisting antisocial personality characteristics.

Summary

Many investigators believe that MHI and whiplash lead to brain injury, despite few signs of gross anatomical damage on imaging tests such as MRI, CT scan, and x-ray. Such brain damage is most often linked to the acceleration/deceleration forces that accompany accidents such as automobile collisions. While specific focal brain lesions occur, researchers argue that the emotional and neuropsychological symptoms of post traumatic syndromes more often result from shear force effects. At impact, inertia propels the brain within the skull, leading to small microscopic "tears" in neuro-tissue whereby nerve cells, and particularly their axons, are injured. While shear forces can cause injury throughout the brain, the frontal and temporal lobes, and underlying midbrain structures, appear most vulnerable. Because these brain regions account for higher cortical functions and emotion, persons with minor head injury and whiplash frequently experience problems with information processing, memory, and depression that are the hallmark neuropsychological symptoms of the post traumatic syndrome.

NEUROPSYCHOLOGICAL FINDINGS SUPPORTIVE OF UNDERLYING BRAIN PATHOLOGY

Introduction

This section examines some of the literature strongly suggesting that persons with post traumatic syndrome demonstrate neuropsychological impairment indicative of either structural or functional brain pathology. Findings are examined across functional domains (e.g., intelligence, attention, and memory) and results from neuropsychological research are reviewed. Again, familiarity with the previous chapter will be helpful when specific neuropsychological tests are discussed.

Findings Obtained from Test Batteries

A *neuropsychological test battery* is a group of psychometric instruments that measures a variety of behaviors across several functional domains. Some batteries consist of an invariant group of tests, other batteries are arranged in response to specific diagnostic questions.

One of the first indications that MHI patients may have documentable neuropsychological deficits was presented by Barth and colleagues in 1983.[15] Seventy patients (mean age = 25.3 years; 39 men; mean education = 11.5 years; mean IQ = 100.4), who predominately experienced MVAs, were assessed at three months with the Halstead-Reitan Neuropsychological Test Battery.

The Halstead-Reitan consists of a number of measures that include the Trail Making Test (Trails A & B), Category Test, Tactile Performance Test (TPT), Finger Tapping, Hand Grip Strength, Seashore Rhythm Test, Speech-sounds Perception Test and several others, as well as the Wechsler Adult Intelligence Scale (WAIS), and Minnesota Multiphasic Personality Inventory (MMPI) (see the previous chapter for descriptions of tests).[3] When completed, the test scores yield the *Halstead-Reitan Impairment Index* that reflects the person's total level of neuropsychological dysfunction. Degree of impairment is proportionally related to the value of the index, which ranges from 0 to 1.0.

Barth et al.[15] found that 22 of the 70 participants (31.43%) exhibited a Halstead Impairment Index rating greater than 0.7 (i.e., moderate to severe); 22 patients (31.43%) demonstrated indexes between 0.3 and 0.6 (i.e., mild), and 26 persons (37.14%) exhibited impairment ratings below 0.3 (i.e., minimal). The median rating for the entire sample was 0.4 or greater. In addition, there was a moderate correlation between persons' impairment rating and trouble returning to work three months post trauma ($r = 0.41$, $p < .001$). Of importance is that a patient's previous work history did not influence injury-related job problems.

With respect to emotional functioning, 32% of the sample had at least one elevated MMPI scale. Scale 2 elevations (i.e., depression) were significantly correlated with a patient's Halstead Impairment Rating ($r = 0.22$, $p < .01$). While this relationship is fairly small, it does document the negative impact that neuropsychological impairment has upon a person's emotional adjustment.

The mean performance by this group of MHI patients met or exceeded the criteria for clinical significance on the following test measures: time to complete the TPT, difficulty with TPT location, Trails B, and Finger Tapping with both dominant and nondominant hands. These findings suggest that MHI patients have particular problems with spatial reasoning, cross-modal matching, motor speed, and changing cognitive set (see the previous chapter).

Other interesting and important findings indicated that older and less educated persons experienced the greatest cognitive impairment. Surprisingly, length of post traumatic amnesia and duration of unconsciousness did not affect the degree of a person's cognitive impairment.

A similar study was conducted by Leininger et al. in 1990.[16] An important difference is that these investigators examined MHI patients and compared findings against a control group of noninjured persons. A specific goal was to determine whether loss of consciousness influenced the severity of a person's neuropsychological deficits.

Thirty-one of the 53 patients (58.49%) experienced a brief loss of consciousness (defined as a concussion). Twenty-two patients (41.51%) experienced dazing, disorientation, or confusion after the trauma. There were also 23 control volunteers comparable to the MHI patients on demographic variables. Participants were administered the following tests: (1) Category Test (reasoning ability), (2) Trail Making Test Part B (mental flexibility, attention, visual search, and motor function), (3) Auditory Verbal Learning Test (language learning and memory), (4) Complex Figure Test: Copy Trial and Memory Trials (visuospatial constructional ability and visual memory), (5) Controlled Oral Word Association (FAS Test [language fluency and accessibility]), (6) Paced Auditory Serial Addition Task- Revised (PASAT-R [information processing speed and attention]). Minor head injury patients scored significantly poorer ($p < .05$) than control participants on 4 of the 6 neuropsychological tests including the Category Test (MHI M = 49.5, control M = 25.3), PASAT-R (MHI M

= 78.9, control M = 86.1), Auditory Verbal Learning Test (MHI M = 54.4, control M = 57.7), and the copy (MHI M = 32.3, control M = 34.4) and the memory (MHI M = 18.2, control M = 22.1) trials of the Complex Figure Test.

In support of the findings of Barth and colleagues, results of the Leininger et al. investigation revealed unequivocal evidence of neuropsychological impairment in minor head injury patients. Furthermore, linear comparisons determined there was no significant difference between the test performance of persons with or without concussion. A statistically uncorrected analysis revealed that persons in litigation did significantly poorer on the copy performance of the Complex Figure test ($p < .05$). However, this difference disappeared with Bonferroni correction (a statistical procedure that reduces the probability of obtaining a significant finding by chance). There was no significant difference in performance between patients tested within or beyond three months of the injury suggesting a protracted course for neuropsychological deficits.

As was found by the Barth et al. study,[15] neuropsychological deficits were greater in persons age 30 or above, and were not related to whether the person lost consciousness. Likewise, problems were most obvious on tests of reasoning and information processing. A unique finding was that MHI persons demonstrated trouble with verbal learning.

The above studies clearly demonstrate that many persons with MHI will exhibit persistent neuropsychological deficits after the first post trauma month. An investigation conducted by Ettlin and colleagues revealed that such problems are obvious even during the first week following injury.[7]

Neuropsychological evaluation was conducted within 3 to 7 days on 21 patients. Attention was measured with simple reaction time (see below), counting backwards from 20 to 1, reciting the ABCs, and the WAIS-R Digit Forwards subtest, Corsi's block tapping forward, and the Stroop Test II. Concentration was tested with Brickenkamp's "d2" (see the previous chapter). Verbal and visual memory were tested with the WAIS-R Digit Backwards subtest and the learning and recall of a story. Additional tests included Corsi's block tapping backwards, Benton's labyrinth, and recall of the Complex Figure. Higher cognitive functions were examined through mental arithmetic, the WAIS-R Picture Arrangement and Picture Completion subtests, the Stroop Test III, and two tests of visuospatial integration.

Over 95% of the patients showed a significantly higher simple motor reaction time ($p < .01$) and poorer performance in reciting the ABCs ($p < .05$). Patients also demonstrated inferior Digit Span recall ($p < .05$), poorer sustained attention on the Stroop II ($p < .05$), and impaired ability to recall a story ($p < .05$) following a timed delay. Verbal and nonverbal learning were similar in patients and controls, as was higher cognitive functions. These findings suggest that the initial neuropsychological deficits experienced by MHI patients are limited to problems with motor speed, attention, and concentration. That other studies show that higher cognitive processes are also hindered by MHI point to the effects of time and other intervening variables on neuropsychological functioning. It may be that functional CNS changes worsen and continue to reveal themselves during the first month post trauma and beyond. Furthermore, the impact of psychological variables such as depression and anxiety can negatively impact abstract higher reasoning abilities.

Ettlin et al. acknowledge that it is difficult to account for the neuropsychological deficits shown by MHI patients.[7] They speculate that etiological factors include a confluence of the effects of medication, pain and distress, and depression. Initial problems with attention, concentration, sleep disturbances, and emotional changes suggest possible damage to basal frontal and upper brain stem structures, sites of limbic and hypothalamic connections. Because their findings revealed deficits that were restricted to neuromotor functioning, the authors do not believe that secondary gain or malingering played a role. Ettlin et al.[7] argue that it would be expected that persons seeking secondary gain would present a less consistent test profile that would include feigned higher cognitive function deficits.

Effects of Trauma Across Functional Domains

Intelligence

The intellectual functioning of minor head injury and whiplash patients has primarily been assessed with the Wechsler Adult Intelligence Scale-Revised (WAIS-R [see the previous chapter]). Some argue that patients demonstrate little if any IQ deficits on the WAIS-R.[14] Contrarily, Parker estimated that the average post trauma IQ of the sample he examined was 14 points below the pre-injury Full Scale score.[11] When deficits are evident, they are usually specific and reflected in the distribution of subtest scale scores. For instance, a person may show problems with those tests that include a strong attentional component (e.g., Digit Span, Arithmetic), but do well on the remainder of the battery. Regardless, the WAIS-R performance of post traumatic patients generally improves over time, especially for those subtests that measure verbal IQ (e.g., Vocabulary, Comprehension, Similarities).[14] As discussed in the last chapter, verbal IQ is either less influenced by head trauma, or it recovers more quickly than nonverbal IQ, because it reflects "crystallized" or deeply ingrained and well-rehearsed knowledge and abilities. Jones and colleagues reported that verbal WAIS-R performance often returns to essentially premorbid levels within ten months of the injury.[14] Contrarily, nonverbal, or performance IQ, has been shown to be significantly lower than premorbid levels three years after the trauma.

Memory

Among the most common complaints following head injury are memory problems. Jones et al. reported that the degree of memory deficit is related to the severity of injury, associated complications such as premorbid psychiatric conditions, and demographic factors such as education and employment.[14]

Rimel et al. hypothesized that minor head injury leads persons to adopt an inappropriate "semantic encoding strategy" that results in defective memory recall.[6] In other words, the approach that MHI patients use to remember something by associating it with relevant cues is inefficient. To test this hypothesis, the investigators examined 11 MHI patients who were matched with 9 control participants on age, sex, education, and handedness. Each participant was administered the California Verbal Learning Test (CVLT) and the Rey-Osterreith Complex Figure (see the previous chapter).

While no significant difference was noted on the Complex Figure performance of the two groups, the post trauma participants exhibited important verbal deficits. The MHI group remembered significantly fewer words during each of the CVLT learning trials. MHI patients also produced fewer words during the interference, short-, and long-term free recall, and short and long-term cued trials.

While Rimel et al.[6] found that post traumatic verbal memory problems were more obvious, Crossen and Wiens[13] demonstrated that memory deficits are common across both the verbal and nonverbal domains. A group of 20 closed head injury patients were compared against 20 control participants matched on sex, language, handedness, years of education, and WAIS IQ scores. The mean age of both groups was about 29 years. Approximately one half of the patients were in the mild to moderate range of head injury. None of the patients had a previous history of neurologic, psychiatric, or medical disorder, nor did any have a history of alcoholism.

Despite good recovery, every patient continued to present post traumatic symptoms such as difficulty in concentrating, fatigue, irritability, and an overall decrease in premorbid level of performance. Testing revealed significant differences between the head injury and control group on a number of subtests across several instruments. On the Wechsler Memory Scale (WMS), patients had greater difficulty identifying nonverbal stimuli (WMS associates, delay), reproducing visual stimuli (WMS reproductions), and recalling verbal material (WMS story delay).

Findings of this study further indicated that these patients' neuropsychological problems were not limited to the area of memory. They also demonstrated slowed Finger Tapping performances with their dominant hand, slowed Stroop color time, and a greater number of perseverative errors on the Wisconsin Card Sorting Test (WCST). Of importance is that the severity of deficits exhibited by the head injury patients was not related to whether a person was in litigation.

The indication that memory problems accompany other neuropsychological deficits, especially within the domain of psychomotor functioning, was further demonstrated by Arcia and Gualtieri in 1993.[17] The investigation studied the association between specific sets of post traumatic symptoms and specific areas of neurobehavioral functioning. The sample consisted of 32 outpatients, with a mean age of 35.7 years and mean level of education of 12.66 years, who had experienced less than one hour of unconsciousness. Almost one half of the patients were merely dazed. None of the participants showed focal brain injuries. The neuropsychological battery consisted of standard tests (e.g., Finger Tapping, Continuous Performance Test [CPT]), as well as measures developed for the study, including tests of complex perceptual-motor performance, memory, and learning (e.g., symbol-digit substitution, pattern comparison, pattern memory, serial digit learning, switching attention).

Complaints of memory problems were significantly associated with performance on all the simple motor tests (e.g., finger tapping $r = -0.48$), the reaction time and attention tasks (CPT $r = 0.48$, switching attention $r = 0.77$), as well as those measuring complex-perceptual motor abilities (symbol-digit substitution $r = 0.42$, pattern comparison $r = 0.52$) and immediate memory (pattern memory $r = 0.52$). The more severe the memory problems, the slower were the reaction times to both simple and complex stimui.

Arcia and Gualtieri found that memory problems were the most common complaint among their patients and were most closely associated with neuropsychological performance.[17] The memory problems appeared to lie in difficulties with the ability to rapidly process information rather than actual deficits of recall. The investigators argued that support for this finding came from observed deficits in simple and complex reaction time and complex perceptual-motor performance, but not in visual learning. These results suggest that while post traumatic patients report memory problems, the source of these difficulties may come from a general slowing of the nervous system that impedes the ability to concentrate and process information.

Attention and Information Processing

Attention is often broken down into sustained attention or vigilance and divided attention.[14] Vigilance is the ability to attend to a specific task for a period of time. Divided attention entails attending to two or more tasks simultaneously. Information processing is the ability to synthesize and use sequential information over time.

Attention is often measured through *reaction time tasks*. These tests ask the participant to respond to a particular target stimulus as quickly as possible, for instance, when a light turns on. The length of time it takes the person to respond (usually by pressing a button) is then measured (usually in milliseconds). Tests that involve responding to just one stimulus are called *simple reaction time tasks*. A *choice reaction time task* is when the participant is asked to respond to a specific stimulus within a group of stimuli (e.g., responding just to the yellow light and ignoring the red and green lights). Information processing tasks are usually more demanding and often require the participant to engage in a joint-attention. One of the most widely applied tests of information processing has been the Paced Auditory Serial Addition Test (PASAT-R [see above and previous chapter]).

In an early study of reaction time, Macflynn et al.[18] showed significant response slowing in minor head injury patients. The test was a four-choice reaction time task that required the participant to press one of four buttons that corresponded to four colored lights that turned on in random sequence. The task was administered to 45 minor head injury patients and a matched control group (mean age = 30.9 years, 28 men). The MHI patients were tested within 24 hours of admission into the hospital and at 6 weeks post trauma.

MHI patients exhibited significantly slower reaction time than the control participants at both the immediate and 6 week testings. At 24 hours post trauma, the MHI patients' mean reaction time was approximately one third slower than matched control participants (MHI M = 999.3 milliseconds, control M = 671.4 milliseconds). While the MHI patients did show improvement at the six-week follow-up, their performance was still about 20% slower than the control group (MHI M = 827.9 millisecond). These findings continue to support the notion that even minor head injury has a substantial impact on the nervous system, particularly with respect to a generalized slowing of psychomotor functioning.

Language

Because MHI is suspected to result in diffuse brain injury, language deficits are often part of a sequela that reflects general left hemisphere dysfunction.[14] The most common language symptom following head injury is word and name finding problems (i.e., word retrieval). Recovery of language function following head injury is good and often surpasses the recovery of memory and other cognitive functions.

Visual Functions

Some form of visual deficit may appear in as many as 50% of minor head injury patients and is one of the most commonly reported long-term symptoms. Jones et al. reported that such deficits often arise not from damage to the visual cortex, but from injury to the eye itself, or to the peripheral pathway leading to the brain.[14]

The Role of Pain in Neuropsychological Functioning

The relationship between pain and a person's neuropsychological functioning is complex and it represents a bidirectional phenomenon:[19] pain can impact a person's psychological functioning through its effect on behaviors such as sleep, libido, and job performance. The consequences of these effects, in themselves, contribute to emotional reactions, such as anxiety and depression, which then make the person more vulnerable to the pain.

Parker argues that the prognosis of MHI patients is affected by "distractors."[19] A distractor is "an unpleasant symptom that reduces adaptive functioning through distracting the patient's attention, thereby interfering with control of ongoing activity, reducing concentration upon tasks, lowering stamina, or clouding awareness" (p. 14). Distractors are persistent symptoms that last beyond six months. Such symptoms can alter a person's self perception and lead to feelings of reduced capacity, and of being less attractive physically and socially.

Whiplash and MHI distractors include headaches, somatic pain, and hyperarousal from post traumatic stress. Parker argues that distractors may be a major reason why MHI produces neuropsychological symptoms greater than would be expected with the degree of brain damage.[19]

Pain is an important distractor whose etiology can range from entirely neurophysiological to entirely psychological.[19] The global effect of pain is that it produces disorganization. As indicated above, pain interacts with cognition, depression, anxiety, and anger, affecting the severity and nature of such symptoms.

Parker maintains there are a variety of pain classifications, including neuropathic (aberrant somatosensory processing in the peripheral or central nervous system); myofascial (palpable tender modules or bands of muscles [i.e., trigger points] associated with pain, stiffness, limitation of motion, and weakness); fibromyalgia (nonpalpable multiple tender points often associated with depression, anxiety, and sleep disturbances); perceptual (dependent on the person's level of arousal, attention, and past experience); and suffering (whose intensity is dependent on the person's mood, previous life experience, SES factors, and social support).[19] Each pain experience has a learned component. The intensity and quality of pain can be affected by emotional problems which, in turn, may influence how the patient copes with discomfort. Pain may be used to gain attention, and with some patients, can represent an emotional conversion of depression. Pain increases with chronic stress. Expecting pain increases anxiety, and if chronic, leads to depression and feelings of hopelessness. Chronic pain patients can lose insight to the environmental factors affecting pain and become even further depressed. Pain can also increase irritability, impatience, poor treatment compliance, and deteriorates relationships within the family and across social situations.[19] All of these myriad factors interact with cognitive and intellectual processes to hinder neuropsychological functioning.

Headache with neck and shoulder pain is probably the most common form of post traumatic pain.[19] Parker argues that post traumatic headache has a significant psychological effect that stems from the interaction between the pain the patient is experiencing and its effect upon the person's life style and economic predicament. Post traumatic headache has been found to be worse in patients with preexisting emotional distress and concerns about ability to work. Psychological factors can initiate or exacerbate head or neck pain which, in turn, impact the psychological factors in the vicious circle.[19]

Summary

There is strong convergence across many studies that persons with minor head injury experience significant neuropsychological impairment that is evident through testing. Deficits range across a number of functional domains, including attention, information processing, and higher cognitive processes. Symptoms begin almost immediately following the trauma and can persist for months or even years. Neuropsychological dysfunction appears greater in persons over the age of 30 and who have less education.

Findings from a number of investigators suggest that the source of many of the post traumatic cognitive deficits is a decrease in the patient's ability to attend to and process information. It appears that following the injury, the patient's entire nervous system slows down and is less able to focus upon and process the level of information that was possible prior to the trauma. That this general slowing occurs within both the peripheral and central nervous systems (see the previous chapter) is evident by reduced performance on simple motor tasks such as finger tapping and lower scores on more complex tests such as the PASAT-R, TPT, and Trails B. Over time, the symptoms of decreased attention and concentration persist and are accompanied by more global neuropsychological deficits that entail higher cognitive functions such as abstract thinking, language, and memory. It is not currently known whether the decreased attentional and information processing abilities underlie the generalized neurocognitive deficits observed in MHI patients. Certainly, there are mediating and modifying variables which contribute to the process: Depression and anxiety arise from the awareness of decreased information processing abilities and the effect such deficits have upon a person's functioning. Both depression and anxiety, of themselves, are widely known to hinder cognitive abilities. Chronic pain is also an important distractor which impinges upon a person's ability to function across most of life's situations.

MALINGERING IN MINOR HEAD INJURY AND WHIPLASH PATIENTS

Overview

DSM-IV describes malingering as a condition whereby the patient intentionally exaggerates physical or psychological symptoms for personal gain.[5] The diagnosis of malingering is seldom made, predominately because the behavior is so difficult to detect. Furthermore, mis-assigning the diagnosis can have very negative consequences for a patient.

It is widely acknowledged that the occurrence of malingering in MHI patients is unknown. Binder has stated that estimates range from 1% to 50% of patients.[31] The extremes of this range probably reflect gross under- and overestimates. While malingering with malice is probably rare, some exaggeration of post traumatic symptomatology is not uncommon, but no more so than with other chronic injuries.

In their review, Millis and Putnam[30] proposed a number of reasons why the post traumatic syndrome has been linked to interest in malingering:

1. Since chronic post traumatic symptoms are influenced by psychosocial factors, symptom exaggeration may be more common.
2. Neuropsychological test findings are more often used to validate MHI symptoms.
3. Failure to detect malingering has important clinical, financial, and legal consequences.

While these authors acknowledge that there is no fool-proof test for malingering, they suggest a "multivariate approach to the diagnosis of malingering" that includes the following strategies:

1. Quickly establish the severity of the patient's injury at the time of the trauma.
2. When evaluating neuropsychological test findings, consider the pattern of scores in relation to others who have similar injuries (see the previous chapter).
3. Consider how other medical and psychiatric diagnoses may contribute to assessment findings.
4. Use test norms (see the previous chapter) that are adjusted for the particular demographic group of which the patient is a member.
5. Use specific and general neuropsychological tests that aid in detecting malingering.

Specific Tests Used for Detecting Malingering

Neuropsychological tests used to detect malingering focus upon the faking of cognitive symptoms. The malingering of psychiatric symptoms is usually assessed through interview, observation, and personality inventories such as the MMPI.

The strategy behind tests of malingering is that patients are given the impression that the task is difficult. Furthermore, the tasks themselves appear challenging on cursory observation. In fact, they are quite simple: even persons with significant brain trauma can do well.

Rey's 15-Item Visual Memory Test

Perhaps the most widely used screen for malingering, the Rey Visual Memory Test consists of a card on which is printed 15 figures (consisting of letters, numbers, and shapes). The card is presented to the patient for 10 seconds, is then taken away, and he or she is asked to draw as many figures as remembered.

In their study of persons feigning memory problems, Schretlen and colleagues found that patients with mild brain injuries, with at least a borderline premorbid IQ, are expected to perform well on Rey's 15-Item Memory Test.[33] Lee et al.[32] studied the Rey Memory Test in patients with temporal lobe epilepsy and neurological disorders and found that a score of 7 or below indicates malingering.

Dot Counting

The instrument consists of presenting the patient with series of grouped and nongrouped dots to count. Evaluation of performance is based upon the expected time periods it should take patients to complete the tasks. For instance, grouped dots should be counted more quickly than nonpaired groups, and response times should lengthen as the number of dots increase.[30] Boone et al. found that scores should not exceed 180 seconds total for the ungrouped dots and more than 130 seconds for the grouped dots.[30]

Forced-Choice Tests (Symptom Validity Testing)

These methods assess symptom exaggeration by asking patients to recognize previously seen items from two alternatives. Most often strings of digits are used as the stimuli. For instance, the *Digit Memory Test* (DMT) consists of a set of stimulus and test cards. For each trial, the patient is presented a stimulus card on which is printed five numbers. Each stimulus card is presented for five-seconds and is then followed by a test card on which appears the stimulus digit set and another set of five numbers. The patient is asked to chose the previously seen stimulus digit set.

In a study of the DMT, Prigantano and Amin[34] found that even patients with severe cerebral dysfunction correctly identified between 95% and 100% of the target stimuli during the test trials. Contrarily, patients suspected of malingering correctly identify, on average, 74% of target stimuli.

This brief section introduced the most popular tests used to detect the malingering of neurocognitive symptoms. Most agree that the current approaches for detecting malingering leave much to be desired. Detecting who is, or is not, feigning cognitive and/or psychiatric symptoms, relies upon a skilled clinician who triangulates findings from tests, previous history, and behavioral observations. This process always involves clinical judgment based upon past experience, objective findings, and intuition.

PSYCHIATRIC CONSIDERATIONS OF THE POST TRAUMATIC SYNDROME

Introduction

As has been demonstrated above, the post traumatic syndrome significantly impacts the emotional well-being of the individual. Symptoms of anxiety, depression, irritability, and even personality change occur in at least 40% of patients at some point during their post trauma experience. Few clinicians or researchers deny that MHI and whiplash patients experience psychological distress: the point of contention has been whether preexisting character traits or psychopathology is why some patients experience symptoms, and others do not. This section will explore this issue and offer an alternative conceptualization for the psychological distress associated with the post traumatic syndrome.

Psychiatric Symptoms Associated with the Post Traumatic Syndrome

In 1996, Parker examined the medical records of 33 patients with whiplash resulting from motor vehicle accidents.[11] On average, this sample was about 39 years old, had average IQs, and were well educated. Findings suggested that the majority of these post traumatic patients suffered from significant symptoms of psychological distress. Thirty-one of the patients (93.94%) were assigned a secondary psychiatric diagnosis by their attending physician. The distribution of psychiatric diagnoses included post traumatic stress disorder — 48.48% (PTSD [see below]), depression — 36.36%, dementia — 9.09%, affective disorder — 6.06%, mixed neurotic reaction — 3.03%, anxiety reaction — 3.03%, and conversion reaction — 3.03%.

Other investigators have also examined the breath of psychiatric symptoms in post traumatic syndrome patients. Commonly, psychological evaluation has included administration of the Minnesota Multiphasic Personality Inventory (MMPI).

In a preliminary study, Novack, Daniel, and Long[21] found that nearly 60% of minor head injury patients demonstrated clinical elevations above 70 on either MMPI scales 1 (Hypochondriasis), 2 (Depression), or 3 (Hysteria). Forty-six percent of the patients had simultaneous elevations on all three scales.

Leininger et al.[16] examined MMPI profiles from 73 head injury persons (29 minor and 44 severe) without a pretrauma history of psychiatric disorder, substance abuse, or antecedent head trauma. Minor head injury persons had a Glasgow Coma Score of 12 or less, or experienced altered consciousness for less than 20 minutes. The mean ages, level of education, and months since injury were similar across the two groups. On average, patients were in their early thirties and had slightly above a high school education.

In general, minor head injury persons exhibited a significantly greater degree of psychopathology. MHI patients demonstrated clinical elevations above 70 on scales 1, 2, 3, 7 (Psychasthenia), and 8 (Schizophrenia). Only scale 2 was clinically elevated in severe head injury patients; scale 8 approached clinical significance. While the severe head injury group demonstrated fewer clinical elevations, the profile of the two groups were similar: both groups exhibited L and K scores between 50 and 55, and a F scale around 65. Scales 1 (Minor M = 74.1, Severe M = 64.3), 2 (Minor M = 77.1, Severe M = 71.4), and 3 (Minor M= 72.9, Severe M = 64.3) showed an inverted "V" pattern, with scale 2 being greater than scales 1 and 3. Scales 5 (Male-Female) and 9 (Hypomania) were lower in relation to the rest of the profile, and scales 7 (Minor M = 70.2, Severe M = 63.9) and 8 (Minor M = 74.2, Severe M = 68.9) showed elevations comparable to those found on scales 1, 2, and 3. Statistical tests demonstrated that MHI patients scored higher than severe head injury patients on scales 1 ($p < .01$), 3 ($p < .01$), and 7 ($p < .05$). Leininger et al.[16] reported that psychiatric patients who exhibit MMPI profiles similar to those of minor head injury patients are often described as dysphoric, anxious, ruminative, confused, egocentric, and preoccupied with physical symptoms. That MHI patients exhibited a greater degree of psychological symptoms than severe head injury patients is probably related to at least two factors. First, MHI patients have more intact cognitive abilities which permit greater awareness of their current level of functioning, especially as it compares to premorbid levels. Second, because MHI patients are more functional, they attempt to live life as it was prior to the trauma, thus setting up and maintaining the biopsychosocial vicious cycle outlined in earlier sections of this chapter.

In an extensive investigation of MMPI profiles across the accepted headache diagnoses, Dieter and Swerdlow found similarities and important differences in their group of post head trauma patients.[23] All of the 58 post concussive patients in the study had minor head injuries. Table 21.2 provides the mean MMPI scale scores broken down by gender.

Table 21.2 Mean Scale t Scores of Male and Female Headache Patients with Post Concussive Syndrome

	L	F	K	1Hs	2D	3Hy	4Pd	5Mf	6Pa	7Pt	8Sc	9Ma	0Si
Male	49.54	57.69	51.31	76.62*	70.23*	71.23*	59.54	57.31	56.88	61.31	63.54	62.69	54.77
Female	52.16	58.53	53.44	73.41*	65.03	71.81*	59.50	48.31	58.38	60.06	62.72	59.53	56.69

Adapted from Dieter, J.N., Swerdlow, B., *Headache*, 28, 212–222, 1988.

With the exception of scale 2, the profiles of men and women MHI patients were similar. In general, elevations were observed on those scales that measure physical symptoms, somatic overconcern, and depression (i.e., scales 1, 2, and 3). Contrary to the findings of Leininger and his colleagues, no clinically significant elevations were observed on scales 7 or 8.

In consideration of their findings, Dieter and Swerdlow addressed some important issues with respect to how representative MMPI findings are of psychopathology across minor head trauma patients. While the mean scores of MHI patients on scales 1, 2, and 3 reflected significant clinical elevations, the standard deviation associated with each of these means was fairly large. *Standard deviation* is essentially the average number of points that the range of scores, for a particular test, deviate from the mean (i.e., the arithmetic average). The standard deviations observed in the scale 1, 2, and 3 scores of post trauma patients were, respectively, 11.98, 14.75, and 11.74. These standard deviations indicate considerable variability in the range of scores across the patients. In other words, it was common to observe post trauma patients with completely normal profiles, as well as those whose MMPIs suggested substantial psychological distress. Examination of the standard deviations of the mean MMPI scores obtained in the Leininger et al. study also revealed considerable and comparable variability.

Another important issue is to what degree the MMPI elevations demonstrated by MHI patients reflect true psychopathology, rather than merely measuring the patient's physical complaints and realistic concerns. The possibility of this is evident in many of the questions that compose scales 1, 2, and 3: for instance, "Much of the time my head seems to hurt all over", "I hardly ever feel pain in the back of my neck", and "I have few or no pains". Unless scoring corrections are made, acknowledging such symptoms contributes to elevations in the 1, 2, and 3 scales, regardless of whether the patient's complaints are real (i.e., arising from an actual injury), or are the result of hypochondriasis, hysteria, malingering, or conversion reaction. In fact, Dieter and Swerdlow found that when only nine items, which addressed symptoms common to the post concussive syndrome and chronic headache, were removed from the entire set of over 500 MMPI questions, clinical elevations (i.e., 70 or above) were eliminated in 24 of 25 randomly selected MMPI profiles.

Are Post Traumatic Patients Especially Neurotic?

While MMPI findings from individuals with MHI and whiplash are questionable, Parker clearly demonstrated that clinicians still commonly assign psychiatric diagnoses to post trauma patients.[11] Although the labels of several of these diagnoses are not longer widely applied, each does have a DSM-IV (see the previous chapter) counterpart. As a whole (with the exception of dementia), the group of diagnoses falls under the rubric of what many mental health professionals refer to as *neurotic*. A neurosis is a *functional* mental disorder (i.e., not arising from brain disease) in which reality testing is intact (as opposed to *psychosis* where the person may hallucinate or maintain delusions) and the person is plagued by unpleasant psychological symptoms such as anxiety, depression, obsessions, or phobias.[20] Using the rubric of neurosis, one might speculate that persons who experience the greatest neuropsychological and psychiatric symptoms following minor head injury or whiplash might be prone towards *neuroticism* (a tendency to experience neurotic symptoms, particularly in response to psychosocial stress).

The notion that post traumatic syndrome patients may be more neurotic was recently tested by Radanov and colleagues.[4] The authors maintained that two psychosocial factors particularly affected patients' post trauma recovery: *negative affectivity*, defined as a propensity towards aversive mood states such as anger, disgust, scorn, guilt, fearfulness, and depression, and *neuroticism*, defined as a tendency to experience negative distressing emotions and to possess associated behavioral and cognitive traits.

The predictive value of these traits, as well as psychosocial factors, and self-reported somatic and cognitive complaints was examined in 78 consecutive whiplash patients who were referred for assessment at a mean of 7.2 days post-MVA. On presentation, and at six months, a semi structured interview and several standardized tests were administered. The Freiburg Personality Inventory (FPI), was used to assess psychological functioning. The FPT measures 12 personality traits including neuroticism, calmness, nervousness, spontaneous aggressiveness, depression, excitability, and depression. Head and neck pain was assessed with a self-report scale ranging from 0 to 10 points. Self-reported measures of well-being (Well-being Scale — 25 pairs of polarized positive and negative adjectives) and cognitive ability (Cognitive Failures Questionnaire — 25 questions addressing real-life circumstances) assessed the patients' subjective perception of their current functioning.

Findings indicated that neck pain was the most common symptom on presentation (86% in persons recovered at six months and 95% in persons with persistent symptoms at six months). The group with persistent symptoms (i.e., lasting at least six months) had significantly higher frequencies of irritability, sleep disturbance, and forgetfulness on presentation. There was only a low correlation ($r = 0.24$) between severity of neck pain and level of neuroticism on presentation; furthermore, there was little relationship between severity of headache and psychopathology. There was no significant relationship between level of neuroticism and severity of head or neck pain at six months, regardless of prognosis. On presentation, there were no significant differences between the patients who were fully recovered at six months and those who had persistent symptoms with respect to life history or current psychosocial stress. The entire patient sample fell within the normal range of FPI personality functioning. There was no significant difference in the Well-Being scale scores between the good and poor prognosis groups on presentation.

The results obtained by Radanov et al.[4] failed to demonstrate significant personality psychopathology in their sample of whiplash patients. Furthermore, there was little relationship between character traits and how quickly a patient recovered. In a more recent investigation, Fenton and colleagues[24] also found little evidence for global premorbid psychopathology in their sample of 45 MHI patients. Using the Katz Adjustment Scale, no significant difference was observed between the MHI patients and matched control participants on chronic social difficulties, psychological adjustment, and quality of social interactions. An important within-group finding among MHI patients was the relationship between persistent post concussive symptoms and chronic social difficulties: patients who exhibited persistent symptoms, six months post trauma, reported twice as many chronic social difficulties (social difficulties were not specifically defined in the study; it is presumed they reflected predicaments such as financial and occupational problems). This suggests that the patient's environment does have a significant impact on post traumatic symptoms. An important consideration is that these chronic social problems need not be overwhelming. Support for this comes from the fact that, in general, there was no significant difference across the control and MHI groups with respect to the occurrence of life troubles. It is presumed that the biopsychological changes evoked by the patients' injuries were sufficient to increase their vulnerability to chronic life stressors. Those patients who did not demonstrate persistent post traumatic symptoms probably had fewer chronic social difficulties than many of the control participants.

A recent investigation has challenged not only the notion that post traumatic symptoms reflect underlying psychopathology, but that even social factors are not the predominate cause of psychological distress. In an intriguing experiment, Wallis et al.[27] examined 17 whiplash patients who suffered from chronic neck pain and psychological distress. Patients were randomly assigned to receive either an actual or placebo-control surgical procedure. The procedure, *precutaneous radiofrequency neurotomy*, involved inserting an electrode adjacent to the cervical nerves that were causing the patient pain, and administering stimulation that led to coagulation of the affected nerves. Control patients underwent all aspects of the procedure, except no lesions were made to their painful nerves. Prior to surgery, the psychological status of patients was assessed with the Symptoms Checklist-90, Revised (SCL-90-R), a self-report, multidimensional instrument that yields nine clinical subscales similar to those found on the MMPI (e.g., depression, anxiety, psychoticism). Three months after surgery, each patient was assessed by a psychologist who was "blind" as to whether the patient received the actual surgery or just the placebo procedure. Pre- and postoperative SCL-90-R scores were then compared across the two groups. Of the nine patients who underwent the actual surgery, six (66.67%) demonstrated complete relief of both their pain and psychological distress. Of the eight patients who were administered the placebo procedure, only three reported some pain relief. Interestingly, these patients also demonstrated significant reductions in psychological distress. None of the control patients who continued to experience pain exhibited any significant resolution of psychological distress.

The results of this investigation suggest that the most important contributor to psychological distress is physical pain. While these findings are important, they should not be accepted to the exclusion of other etiological contributors to the suffering associated with MHI and whiplash. The collective research across disciplines, and findings obtained from MHI and whiplash patients whose injuries are of varying severity, continue to support a model whereby emotional and cognitive changes interact with preexisting psychological traits, social situations, and individual life stressors.

The Psychodynamics of Post Traumatic Syndrome

Despite findings that indicate that the majority of post trauma patients do not have excessive psychopathology, or suffer from preexisting personality problems, this group of persons does experience significant psychological distress that is related to the impact of injury on their lives. As described throughout this chapter, this distress reflects a confluence of biological, psychological, and social factors. A number of investigators have focused upon those psychological processes that may contribute to distress as the post trauma patient responds to the somatic and social stressors.

Parker (1996) proposes a number of psychosocial dimensions that affect adaptive capacity and prognosis following minor head trauma:[11]

1. *The social context*: The impaired head injury victim is perceived differently by family, employer, and friends. Loss of social interest is common, and is consequent to pain, embarrassment, communication problems, lack of money, etc. The social network is reduced through deliberate withdrawal, loss of others' interest and social mishaps.
2. *Information processing:* Beside cognitive processes, social monitoring can become impaired. The ability to learn from experience and modify behavior can be hindered.
3. *Identity:* The patient's experience of feeling impaired reduces morale and social interest initiative. This can produce significant changes in the patient's sense of self and how they view themselves in relation to the world.
4. *Unconscious psychodynamic processes:* Dynamics can shape the meaning that the injury has for the patient. Preexisting psychological conflicts may be exacerbated. Patients may rely more heavily upon their specific psychological defense mechanisms.
5. *Affective changes:* Emotional reactions can be disproportional to an event, or essentially unrelated to it (e.g., increased irritability, anger, and impulsivity).
6. *Reduced motivation:* Impairs efforts at rehabilitation, social interest, and social desirability.

O'Hara[25] has proposed that persons with MHI manifest psychological distress within a number of symptom clusters. In her experience, MHI patients who are referred for psychotherapy (see below) typically present with one or two of the following:

1. *Depression/paralysis:* Fostered by the failure of health care providers to assign the patient with an early diagnosis; as well as the patient's perception of the difference in his or her level of functioning, pre- and post-morbidity.
2. *Anger/blame:* Related to the first cluster, the onset of anger and blame may be directed towards health care professionals who are perceived to have failed in providing an early diagnosis. Behavioral manifestations include hostility, rejection or refusal of assistance, as well as angry outbursts. Anger and blame can also arise in the patient's family members.
3. *Denial/defensiveness:* A tendency to remain overly optimistic, to deny the significance of symptoms, and to appear normal to others. Over-reliance on denial can impede recovery when the patient ignores symptoms or fails to seek treatment.
4. *Somatization:* This defense arises when physical symptoms become exaggerated or replace any acknowledgment of emotional distress. Persons who somatize, post trauma, may have a predisposition towards this defensive posture.
5. *Regression/dependency:* Post trauma patients may develop "learned helplessness" as a result of becoming fearful of further loss and/or having encountered failure in situations where they were

successful pre-injury. Family members may step in and provide excessive caretaking, which only fosters further dependency.

6. *Psychotic disintegration:* Although very rare, some MHI patients experience total psychological decompensation which includes a disruption in reality testing. Psychotic disintegration is marked by gradually escalating depression, paranoia, and suspiciousness that ultimately requires psychotropic medication and possibly hospitalization.

Is the Psychological Distress Experienced by MHI and Whiplash Patients Akin to Post Traumatic Stress Disorder?

Most investigators propose that the psychological distress that arises post trauma is related to the difficulties that patients have with adjusting to emotional and cognitive changes that are secondary to brain injury. An important alternative account for the psychological reactions of MHI patients has recently been proposed by Wright and Telford (1996).[26]

The authors' position is that symptoms exhibited by MHI patients are consistent with the psychological trauma model and the DSM-IV diagnosis of post traumatic stress disorder (PTSD).[26] PTSD symptoms include reexperiencing the traumatic event, avoiding reminders of the trauma, and increased physiological and behavioral arousal when encountering similar events or associated stimuli. Wright and Telford argue that while PTSD is usually thought to arise from an event that is outside of normal experience, traffic accidents and other traumas can elicit PTSD symptoms. For instance, patients are often phobic about driving following an MVA, or they encounter heightened arousal and over-reactivity while driving. Furthermore, the accident may alter how the person usually views life, particularly through a weakening of his or her sense of security that the world is a predictable and safe place.

To test their hypothesis, Wright and Telford interviewed 50 people admitted to the hospital with MHI at six months and three years, post trauma. During both follow-up assessments, MHI patients exhibited considerable PTSD symptomology, including reexperiencing phenomena (e.g., intrusive imagery = 58%/65% [6 months/3 years], intensification of distress by reminder = 63%/74%, nightmares = 10%/22%), avoidance/numbing phenomena (e.g., avoidance of thoughts or feelings related to trauma = 47%/61%, diminished interest = 58%/39%, fears of further catastrophe = 37%/17%), and symptoms of increased arousal (e.g., sleep difficulties = 47%/61%, hypervigilance = 37%/39%, physiological reactivity = 35%/17%).

The authors concluded that events causing head injury can be significantly traumatic experiences which challenge the patient's assumptions about themselves and reality.[26] MHI patients appear to perceive themselves and the world differently following their injuries, and this altered perception instills great psychological distress.

The notion that MHI and whiplash patients experience a form of PTSD further complicates the clinical picture of the post traumatic syndrome. That this group of individuals is left to cope with such a complex biopsychosocial predicament sends an important message to health care providers that interventions which address the emotional and cognitive consequences of this disorder should be initiated as quickly as possible following the traumatic injury.

Psychological Intervention with Post Traumatic Syndrome Patients

Neuropsychological Counseling

Bennett[28] describes neuropsychological counseling as "a variant of psychotherapy within a neurological framework" (p. 10). Global goals of neuropsychological counseling include helping patients deal with their losses; facilitating patients' abilities to cope with the difficulties that cognitive deficits have upon their personal and professional lives; educating them about the normal symptoms of post traumatic syndrome; and validating the symptoms patients are experiencing. Practitioners who wish to effectively undertake the counseling of MHI persons must have a good knowledge of neuropsychological assessment, neuroanatomy and physiology, and the cognitive and emotional predicament of minor head injury.

The focus of neuropsychological counseling is on the present and the future. Bennett argues that greater patient progress is often made through group sessions.[28] Patients find it easier to express their concerns in a group of persons who are presently experiencing the same symptom spectrum. He reports that it is also validating to patients when they discover that they are not alone in their predicament.

Counseling Cognitive Deficits

Education is the predominant strategy for assisting MHI patients with cognitive deficits.[28] Just learning about the syndrome can be very therapeutic to most patients. Teaching focuses upon what the patient can expect during recovery and how to develop adaptive strategies for dealing with attentional, memory, and cognitive problems. Specific interventions include: enhancing the patient's self-monitoring of disruptive or maladaptive behaviors; homework assignments (e.g., self-management and planning tasks) to promote adaptation and ameliorate apathy; stress management and relaxation exercises for anger control; working with the patient's family to structure the home environment, promote autonomy, and lessen dependency. Longer-term approaches include *cognitive retraining* or *rehabilitation*. This area of specialization often uses computers to retrain patients in areas where they demonstrate weaknesses. In addition, the demands of the patient's job must be evaluated to determine whether he or she can cope. Sometimes patients will have to pursue a less demanding career. Intervention then includes occupational rehabilitation.

Individual Psychotherapy

For some patients, individual psychotherapy is appropriate, particularly if psychological or cognitive problems are more entrenched, or the individual has a greater degree of psychopathology. Bennett argues that patients must meet three criteria if psychotherapy is to be effective:[29] (1) they must have the capacity to communicate and form a therapeutic relationship; (2) there must be some awareness of cognitive deficits and emotional problems, as well as the impact they have on life; and (3) patients must have some motivation to participate in the therapeutic process.

When engaging in individual psychotherapy, the therapist must be able to distinguish premorbid personality from the postinjury psychological functioning.[29] Furthermore, the therapist must contend with an increase in concrete thinking that can accompany even minor head trauma. He or she must be vigilant about using more direct language, easily understood interpretations, and practical interventions, as well as remembering what has transpired across sessions, since patients are likely to have attentional and memory problems.

The goals of individual psychotherapy are essentially the same as with neuropsychological counseling (see above). The approach towards treatment taken by the therapist is more akin to that of behavioral therapists in that an active goal-oriented role is assumed. A realistic framework must be adopted that is neither too optimistic nor too pessimistic.[29] Patients must often "work through" the losses entailed through their injuries and learn to rise to the challenges that accompany coping with the post traumatic syndrome.

REFERENCES

1. Kwentus, J.A., Hart, R.P. et al., Psychiatric complications of closed head trauma, *Psychosomatics*, 26, 8–17, 1985.
2. Alves, W.M., Colohan, A.R.T., O'Leary, T.J. et al., Understanding posttraumatic symptoms after minor head injury." *Journal of Head Trauma and Rehabilitation*, 1, 1–12, 1986.
3. Berg, R., Franzen, M., Wedding, D., *Screening for Brain Impairment: A Manual for Mental Health Practice,* 1987.
4. Radanov, B.P., Di Stefano, G., Schnidrig, A., Ballinari, P., Role of psychosocial stress in recovery from common whiplash, *Lancet*, 338, 712–715, 1991.
5. *Diagnostic and Statistical Manual of Mental Disorders,* 4th ed., American Psychiatric Association, Washington, D.C., 1994.
6. Rimel, R.W., Giordani, F. et al., Disability caused by minor head injury, *Neurosurgery*, 9, 221–228, 1981.
7. Ettlin, T.M., Kischka, U., Reichmann, S. et al., Cerebral symptoms after whiplash injury of the neck: a prospective clinical and neuropsychological study of whiplash injury, *Journal of Neurology, Neurosurgery and Psychiatry*, 55, 943–948, 1992.
8. Keshavan, M.S., Channabasavanna, S.M., Narayanna Reddy, G.N., Post traumatic psychiatric disturbances: Patterns and predictors of outcome, *British Journal of Psychiatry*, 138, 157–160, 1981.
9. Klonoff, P.S., Snow, W.G., Costa, L.D., Quality of life in patients 2 to 4 years after closed head injury, *Neurosurgery*, 19, 735–743, 1986.
10. Levin, H.S., Grossman, R.G., Behavioral sequelae of closed head injury, *Archives of Neurology*, 35, 720–727, 1978.
11. Parker, R.S., The spectrum of emotional distress and personality changes after minor head injury incurred in a motor vehicle accident, *Brain Injury*, 10, 287–302, 1996.
12. *Diagnostic and Statistical Manual of Mental Disorders,* 3rd ed. Rev., American Psychiatric Association, Washington, D.C.
13. Crossen, J.R., Wiens, A.N., Residual neuropsychological deficits following head-injury on the Wechsler Memory Scale-Revised, *Clinical Neuropsychologist*, 2, 393–399, 1988.
14. Jones, R.D., Anderson, S.W. et al., Neuropsychological sequelae of traumatic brain injury, in *Head Injury and Postconcussive Syndrome,* Rizzo, M., Tranel, D., Eds., Churchill Livingstone, New York, 1996.
15. Barth, J.T., Macciocchi, S.N. et al., Neuropsychological sequelae of minor head injury, *Neurosurgery*, 13, 529–533, 1983.
16. Leininger, B.E., Kreutzer, Hill, M.R., Comparison of minor and severe head injury emotional sequelae using the MMPI, *Brain Injury*, 5, 199–205, 1991.
17. Arcia, E., Gualtieri, Association between patient report of symptoms after mild head injury and neurobehavioral performance, *Brain Injury*, 7, 481–489, 1993.
18. Macflynn, G., Montogomery, E.A. et al., Measurement of reaction time following minor head injury, *Journal of Neurology, Neurosurgery, and Psychiatry*, 47, 1326–1331, 1984.
19. Parker, R.S., The distracting effects of pain, headaches, and hyper-arousal upon employment after "minor head injury", *Journal of Cognitive Rehabilitation,* May/June, 14–22, 1995.
20. *Dorland's Illustrated Medical Dictionary,* 27th ed., W.B. Saunders, Philadelphia.
21. Novack, T.A., Daniel, M.S., Long, C.J., Factors related to emotional adjustment following head injury, *International Journal of Clinical Neuropsychology*, 6, 139–142, 1984.
22. Leininger, B.E., Kreutzer, Hill, M.R., Comparison of minor and severe head injury emotional sequelae using the MMPI, *Brain Injury*, 5, 199–205, 1991.
23. Dieter, J.N., Swerdlow, B., A replicative investigation of the reliability of the MMPI in the classification of chronic headaches, *Headache*, 28, 212–222, 1988.
24. Fenton, G., McClelland, R., Montgomery, A. et al., The postconcussional syndrome: social antecedents and psychological sequelae, *British Journal of Psychiatry*, 162, 493–497, 1993.
25. O'Hara, C., Emotional adjustment following minor head injury, *Cognitive Rehabilitation*, March/April, 26–33, 1988.
26. Wright, J.C., Telford, R., Psychological problems following minor head injury: a prospective study, *British Journal of Clinical Psychology*, 35, 399–412, 1996.

27. Wallis, B.J., Lord, S.M., Bogduk, N., Resolution of psychological distress of whiplash patients following treatment by radiafrequency neurotomy: a randomized, double-blind, placebo-controlled trial, *Pain*, 73, 15–22, 1997.
28. Bennett, T.L., Neuropsychological counseling of the adult with minor head injury, *Cognitive Rehabilitation*, January/February, 10–16, 1987.
29. Bennett, T.L., Individual psychotherapy and minor head injury, *Cognitive Rehabilitation,* September/October, 10–16, 1987.
30. Millis, S.R., Putnam, S.H., Detection of malingering in postconcussive syndrome, 1996.
31. Binder, L.M., Malingering following minor head trauma, *Clinical Psychologist*, 4, 25–36, 1990.
32. Lee, G.P., Loring, D.W., Martin, R.C., Rey's 15-item visual memory test for the detection of malingering: normative observations on patients with neurological disorders, *Psychological Assessment*, 4, 43–46, 1992.
33. Schretlen, D., Brandt, J. et al., Some caveats in using the Rey 15-Item Memory Test to detect malingered Amnesia, *Psychological Assessment*, 3, 667–672, 1991.
34. Prigantano, G.P., Amin, K., Digit Memory Test: Unequivocal cerebral dysfunction and suspected malingering, *Journal of Clinical and Experimental Neuropsychology*, 4, 537–546, 1993.

CASE HISTORIES*

CLAUDE
Category: Psychological conditions

This was a 64-year old man who was in an auto accident. He was a passenger with a seatbelt and there was a rear-ended four-car pileup. He states that he does not remember hitting his head, but thinks he was momentarily unconscious and he denies having any headache problem of any sort prior to the accident.

His headaches are somewhat unusual in that they started several weeks after the accident, but this can happen with some people. Often when there are other injuries that are more acute, the patients do not complain of headache in the beginning because they are focused more on the other major complications. In this case, it was only the headaches that he was bothered with after the accident.

Incapacitating headaches: These started $2^1/_2$ weeks after his accident and he was getting two to three attacks a day. When he saw me, the last one was a month ago. They would last anywhere from ten minutes to an hour and a half. It was severe sharp pain, and a burning on the top of his head in the right frontal region. There were associated features such as lacrimation (running of the eye), rhinorrhea (running of the nose), and he would have to go to bed. He had numbness in his hands and feet after the headache.

Interfering headaches (moderate to severe): These also started $2^1/_2$ weeks after the accident, and he was getting two to three a week. They were constant when he came to see me. There was also severe sharp pain and burning on the top of his head. There were no other associated features.

He had seen other physicians before he saw me, and had a good neurological workup, CT scan, and also an MRI of both the head and neck, and all were normal. On my examination, I found multiple myofascial trigger points in the upper neck region.

This is one of the few patients that you will see who looked like he had a post traumatic cluster-type headache, rather than a migraine-like headache. An attempt was made to treat him as an outpatient with trigger point injections and various medications; however, the patient continued to get worse and he was placed in the hospital and started with intravenous DHE (dihydroergotamine), and other medications. While in the hospital, he became headache-free.

After discharge the patient did well for a very short period of time, and then started getting headaches again. At the same time, he became very depressed as a result of his headaches. He had been on some antidepressant medication, which was not helping his headaches, and eventually the headaches became a daily occurrence and he became extremely depressed. I referred the patient to a psychiatrist for pharmacological treatment, but he continued to spiral downwards, both with depression an daily headaches.

As a result of this and his not responding to treatment, I was asked to evaluate his condition and because of the combination of the depression and the terrible pain that was cluster-like, he was given a 15 to 20% disability of the total body.

This is an example of how a post traumatic headache problem can eventually lead to a significant psychiatric problem and depression is one of the symptoms that comes secondarily with chronic pain.

* On the headache assessment forms that accompany these case histories, incapacitating headaches are indicated with solid black lines, interfering headaches with dotted lines, and irritating headaches with gray shading.

MEDICAL HEADACHE HISTORY

Name: Claude **Age:** 64 **Sex** M **Date:** 12/20/90

Date of Birth: 00/00/26 **Birthplace:** KY **Race:** W **Education:**__________

Occupation: Retired **Accident:** 8/16/90

Armed Services & Type of Discharge: 1944-1946 – Air Force; Honorable Discharge

PAST HISTORY:

1.	Did you have a normal birth?		Yes	No
	a) forceps used?		Yes	No
	b) cesarean section?		Yes	No
2.	Did you have problems with bedwetting?		Yes	No
	a) If yes, age bedwetting stopped		______	
3.	Were you car sick as a child (motion)?		Yes	No
	a) If yes, how severe?	Slight	Moderate	Severe
4.	Did you have unexplained abdominal cramps as a child?		Yes	No
5.	Did you have any of the following illnesses in childhood?			
	a) meningitis		Yes	No
	b) encephalitis		Yes	No
	c) scarlet fever		Yes	No
	d) rheumatic fever		Yes	No
6.	Did you have any head injuries as a child?		Yes	No
	a) If yes, please explain:__________			
7.	Were you treated for emotional illness as a child?		Yes	No

HABITS:

8.	Do you drink alcohol?	Yes	No
	a) If yes, what kind and how much? Wine, maybe 10 times a year		
	b) Does alcohol bring on or aggravate a headache?	Yes	No
9.	Do you smoke?	Yes	No
	a) If yes, how much?__________		
	b) Does smoking or smoke-filled rooms cause or aggravate headaches?	Yes	No
10.	Do you drink caffeinated beverages?	Yes	No
	a) If yes, how much?__________		

MENSTRUAL HISTORY:

At what age did menses begin?______ Were they regular or irregular?__________

How were they related to your headache?__________

Are you or were you ever on Birth Control Pills?______ Did they affect your headache? ______

Have you had a hysterectomy, partial or total, and why?__________

Are you in menopause, and if yes, how long?__________

Are you on hormones, and if yes, which ones?__________

HEADACHE ASSESSMENT FORM

HA PROFILE	INCAPACITATING #3	INTERFERING #2	IRRITATING #1
ONSET (Years ago and frequency)	8/90 – 2 to 3 every day	8/90 - 2 to 3 every week	N/A
CURRENT FREQUENCY	Last one was one month ago	Every day, Constant	N/A
TIME OF ONSET	Anytime	Can awaken with	N/A
DURATION	10 minutes to 1 hour, 3 or 4 attacks	Constant	N/A
CHARACTER	Severe sharp pain Burning on top of head	Same, less intense	N/A
PRODROME OR AURA	N/A	N/A	N/A
ASSOCIATING FEATURES	Nausea; Vomiting; Sensitivity to Light? Noise? Odors? Do you get pale or flush? Do your eyes or nose run? Does your nose get stuffy? Does the white of your eyes get red? Does your eyelid droop? Do you pace, or go to bed?	Nausea; Vomiting; Sensitivity to Light? Noise? Odors? Do you get pale or flush? Do your eyes or nose run? Does your nose get stuffy? Does the white of your eyes get red? Does your eyelid droop? Do you pace, or go to bed?	Nausea; Vomiting; Sensitivity to Light? Noise? Odors? Do you get pale or flush? Do your eyes or nose run? Does your nose get stuffy? Does the white of your eyes get red? Does your eyelid droop? Do you pace, or go to bed?
PRECIPITATING OR AGGRAVATING FEATURES	Has numbness in hands and feet after headache	N/A	N/A

LOCATION: Mark the location for each type of headache with a different color pen.

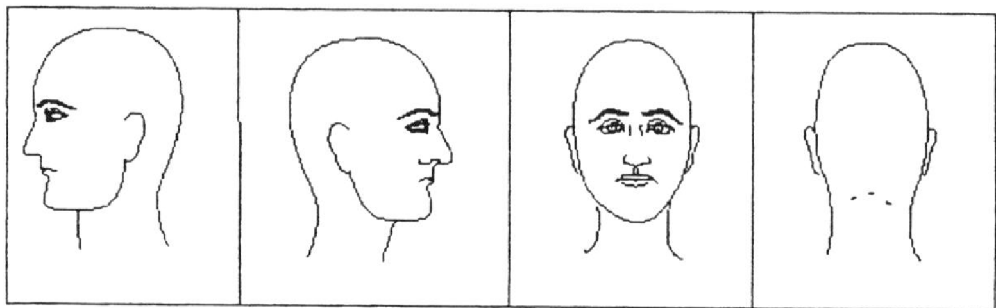

MEDICAL HISTORY:

Have you ever been or are you currently being treated for any of the following?

	Yes	No
a) high blood pressure	Yes	<u>No</u>
b) stomach ulcers	<u>Yes</u>	No
c) asthma	Yes	<u>No</u>
d) allergies	<u>Yes</u>	No
e) pneumonia	Yes	<u>No</u>
f) kidney problems	Yes	<u>No</u>
g) low blood sugar	Yes	<u>No</u>
h) glaucoma	Yes	<u>No</u>
i) diabetes	Yes	<u>No</u>
j) heart problems	Yes	<u>No</u>

If you answered yes to any of the above, please describe: Ulcers diagnosed 1953, resolved.
Environmental allergies.

List all other medical problems you have had in the past. Include date diagnosed and treatment.
DO NOT LIST OPERATIONS

None

SURGICAL HISTORY (List operations and dates performed)

Appendectomy, 1943.

PSYCHIATRIC HISTORY (List visits with counselors, psychologists, etc., and type of treatment)

None

ACCIDENTS IN ADULT LIFE (Briefly describe any accident that caused any blow to the head or that you feel is related to your headache)

7/16/90 – Passenger with seatbelt. Rearended in 4-car pile up. Don't remember hitting head. Momentarily unconscious. Not taken to emergency room. No headache until September, 1990. No headache before accident.

FAMILY HISTORY:

		Yes	No
1.	Is your father living?	Yes	<u>No</u>
	Age ______		
	Cause of death Tuberculosis, 29		
	Was there a headache history?	Yes	<u>No</u>
2.	Is your mother living?	<u>Yes</u>	No
	Age 88		
	Cause of death ______		
	Was there a headache history?	<u>Yes</u>	No

3. Ages of brothers---Circle the ones with headache
   66 63
4. Ages of sisters---Circle the ones with headache
   None
5. List any other blood relatives with a history of severe headaches.
   None

MARITAL HISTORY:

List marriages:

1st marriage age 21 to 63	Did spouse have headaches?	Yes	No
2nd marriage age _____ to _______	Did spouse have headaches?	Yes	No
3rd marriage age _____ to _______	Did spouse have headaches?	Yes	No

Age of current spouse: Widower

List ages and sex of all children:

Age 41	Sex F	Headaches?	Yes	No
Age 38	Sex F	Headaches?	Yes	No
Age 35	Sex M	Headaches?	Yes	No
Age 30	Sex M	Headaches?	Yes	No
Age _____	Sex ______	Headaches?	Yes	No

STRESS FACTORS:

List any factors that may be affecting your headaches (money, loneliness, sexual problems, work, etc.)

____

____

VEGETATIVE SIGNS:

1.	Do you have trouble falling asleep?	Yes	No
2.	Do you have trouble staying asleep?	Yes	No
3.	Has your appetite decreased?	Yes	No
4.	Have you gained or lost weight in the past year?	Yes	No
5.	Have you felt tearful or depressed lately?	Yes	No
6.	Have you had any thoughts of wanting to die?	Yes	No
7.	Have you been forgetful lately?	Yes	No
8.	Any other changes in your normal day-to-day living?___________		

Please list any medications you are allergic or sensitive to: Penicillin (rash).

____

____

Please list any medications you are currently taking (including dosages and frequency per day):

Indocin 50 mg. Darvocet 100 mg.

____

PREVIOUS CARE:

1, List doctors who have treated you for headaches: Dr. H. Dr. S. Dr. T.

2, List any tests you have had for your headache (e.g., EEG, CT scan, MRI, X-Ray, etc.):
CAT scan, 9/90 (without contrast) – normal.
X-rays. MRI, 11/90 – normal.

3, List any other treatment you have had for your headache (e.g., biofeedback, acupuncture, chiropractic, or any other treatment you had):
None.

CYNTHIA
Category: Psychological conditions

Although this was not a whiplash patient, this is an example of what may result from an accident.

The patient was injured at work about a year before I saw her. She was working for a large company and was unloading boxes from a truck. She felt achiness in her shoulder and neck that evening. She continued to work, but found she was unable to lift things. She began to have severe muscle spasms. She went to a walk-in clinic and was examined and given medication. Six months prior to seeing me, she had a laminectomy at C6, and her headaches began while she was hospitalized after surgery. She rarely had any headaches prior to that, but when she did she would take several aspirin and they would go away. The surgery she had at that time did not correct her problem with the pain, and she was operated on again five months later. She feels now that she has more mobility in her neck and shoulders, but has an ongoing headache problem.

Incapacitating headaches: These started approximately nine months before I saw her, after her surgery, and she had them every day for five days a week in the hospital. She would have them daily when she did not have Demerol, Valium, or Fiorinal. They now seemed to start as a moderate to severe headache and work themselves into being incapacitating. It is a constant headache. The character of the pain is throbbing and pressure. The pain is in the periorbital regions and the frontal region. There is no aura. Associated features are nausea, vomiting, photophobia, sonophobia, lacrimation, and she would have to go to bed.

Irritating headaches (annoying): These started in her thirties. They were rare. She was able to abort them in one hour with over-the-counter medication. It was a dull ache at the frontal part of her head. She has not had these headaches since her operation.

It appears that these migraine-like headaches started after her surgical procedure and she could be considered to have a post traumatic "surgical" migraine-like headache. She had seen many doctors prior to seeing me, but still continued to ask for narcotic medication. She was having these incapacitating headaches on a daily basis, demanding more medication.

An MMPI (Minnesota Multiphasic Personality Inventory) was done and this was grossly abnormal, showing that there were many areas in which the patient was suffering psychological stress. After multiple attempts to correct her headaches and to reduce her medication, it became obvious to me that these headaches appeared to be primarily subjective, in the sense that I feel that the need for medication was far greater than the intensity of her headaches. I referred the patient to a psychiatrist, but did not give the patient any impairment rating because I could not see the relationship between the original accident and the current status of her headache. It is also interesting to note that the area of her surgery, C5-6, discussed in the chapter on anatomy, is not related to the nerves that are coming from C1 to C3, which would be responsible for the cervicogenic and the occipital headaches. Therefore, the area of the surgery was also questionable as to whether this precipitated that type of headache problem.

MEDICAL HEADACHE HISTORY

Name: Cynthia **Age:** 41 **Sex** F **Date:** 1/16/91

Date of Birth: 00/00/49 **Birthplace:** CA **Race:** C **Education:** 2 yrs college

Occupation: Unemployed **Accident:** 2/90

Armed Services & Type of Discharge: N/A

PAST HISTORY:

1.	Did you have a normal birth?		Yes	No
	a) forceps used?		Yes	No
	b) cesarean section?		Yes	No
2.	Did you have problems with bedwetting?		Yes	No
	a) If yes, age bedwetting stopped			
3.	Were you car sick as a child (motion)?		Yes	No
	a) If yes, how severe?	Slight	Moderate	Severe
4.	Did you have unexplained abdominal cramps as a child?		Yes	No
5.	Did you have any of the following illnesses in childhood?			
	a) meningitis		Yes	No
	b) encephalitis		Yes	No
	c) scarlet fever		Yes	No
	d) rheumatic fever		Yes	No
6.	Did you have any head injuries as a child?		Yes	No
	a) If yes, please explain:			
7.	Were you treated for emotional illness as a child?		Yes	No

HABITS:

8.	Do you drink alcohol?	Yes	No
	a) If yes, what kind and how much?		
	b) Does alcohol bring on or aggravate a headache?	Yes	No
9.	Do you smoke?	Yes	No
	a) If yes, how much?		
	b) Does smoking or smoke-filled rooms cause or aggravate headaches?	Yes	No
10.	Do you drink caffeinated beverages?	Yes	No
	a) If yes, how much? Pepsi every other day		

MENSTRUAL HISTORY:

At what age did menses begin? 16 Were they regular or irregular? WNL

How were they related to your headache? N/A

Are you or were you ever on Birth Control Pills? No Did they affect your headache? N/A

Have you had a hysterectomy, partial or total, and why? No

Are you in menopause, and if yes, how long? No

Are you on hormones, and if yes, which ones? No

HEADACHE ASSESSMENT FORM

HA PROFILE	INCAPACITATING #3	INTERFERING #2	IRRITATING #1
ONSET (Years ago and frequency)	3/90 – Every day for 5 days in hospital	N/A	In 30's, rare
CURRENT FREQUENCY	Every day without Demerol, Valium, Fiorinal	N/A	None since surgery
TIME OF ONSET	Better in a.m., increases during day	N/A	Anytime
DURATION	Constant	N/A	1 hour with OTC medication
CHARACTER	Throbbing, pressure	N/A	Dull ache
PRODROME OR AURA	N/A	N/A	N/A
ASSOCIATING FEATURES	Nausea; Vomiting; Sensitivity to Light? Noise? Odors? Do you get pale or flush? Do your eyes or nose run? Does your nose get stuffy? Does the white of your eyes get red? Does your eyelid droop? Do you pace, or go to bed?	Nausea; Vomiting; Sensitivity to Light? Noise? Odors? Do you get pale or flush? Do your eyes or nose run? Does your nose get stuffy? Does the white of your eyes get red? Does your eyelid droop? Do you pace, or go to bed?	Nausea; Vomiting; Sensitivity to Light? Noise? Odors? Do you get pale or flush? Do your eyes or nose run? Does your nose get stuffy? Does the white of your eyes get red? Does your eyelid droop? Do you pace, or go to bed?
PRECIPITATING OR AGGRAVATING FEATURES	Movement	N/A	N/A

LOCATION: Mark the location for each type of headache with a different color pen.

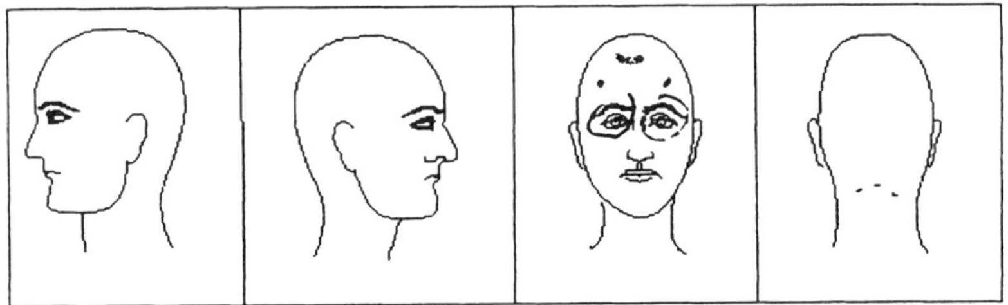

MEDICAL HISTORY:

Have you ever been or are you currently being treated for any of the following?

a) high blood pressure	Yes	No
b) stomach ulcers	Yes	No
c) asthma	Yes	No
d) allergies	Yes	No
e) pneumonia	Yes	No
f) kidney problems	Yes	No
g) low blood sugar	Yes	No
h) glaucoma	Yes	No
i) diabetes	Yes	No
j) heart problems	Yes	No

If you answered yes to any of the above, please describe:____________________

List all other medical problems you have had in the past. Include date diagnosed and treatment.
DO NOT LIST OPERATIONS

None.

SURGICAL HISTORY (List operations and dates performed)

3/90 - Laminectomy. 10/90 - Laminectomy. 1982 - Tubal ligation.

PSYCHIATRIC HISTORY (List visits with counselors, psychologists, etc., and type of treatment)

Dr. B.

ACCIDENTS IN ADULT LIFE (Briefly describe any accident that caused any blow to the head or that you feel is related to your headache)

2/90 – Unloading UPS boxes from a truck. Achiness in shoulder and neck that evening. Continued to work. Was unable to life. Then began to have severe muscle spasms. Went to walk-in clinic, examined; medication given. Surgery 3/90 (laminectomy). Headaches began while hospitalized after surgery. Had rare #1 headaches before this.

FAMILY HISTORY:

1. Is your father living? — Yes — No
   - Age________
   - Cause of death Accident, 58
   - Was there a headache history? — Yes — No
2. Is your mother living? — Yes — No
   - Age 62
   - Cause of death________________
   - Was there a headache history? — Yes — No

3. Ages of brothers---Circle the ones with headache
   44 38 21
4. Ages of sisters---Circle the ones with headache
   37
5. List any other blood relatives with a history of severe headaches.
   None

MARITAL HISTORY:
List marriages:

1st marriage age 18 to 20	Did spouse have headaches?	Yes	No
2nd marriage age 22 to 23	Did spouse have headaches?	Yes	No
3rd marriage age _____ to _____	Did spouse have headaches?	Yes	No

Age of current spouse:__________

List ages and sex of all children:

Age 23 Sex F	Headaches?	Yes	No
Age 20 Sex M	Headaches?	Yes	No
Age 14 Sex M	Headaches?	Yes	No
Age _____ Sex _____	Headaches?	Yes	No
Age _____ Sex _____	Headaches?	Yes	No

STRESS FACTORS:

List any factors that may be affecting your headaches (money, loneliness, sexual problems, work, etc.)

VEGETATIVE SIGNS:

1.	Do you have trouble falling asleep?	Yes	No
2.	Do you have trouble staying asleep?	Yes	No
3.	Has your appetite decreased?	Yes	No
4.	Have you gained or lost weight in the past year?	Yes	No
5.	Have you felt tearful or depressed lately?	Yes	No
6.	Have you had any thoughts of wanting to die?	Yes	No
7.	Have you been forgetful lately?	Yes	No
8.	Any other changes in your normal day-to-day living?__________		

Please list any medications you are allergic or sensitive to: Codeine, Darvon, Darvocet, Dilantin

Please list any medications you are currently taking (including dosages and frequency per day):
Bellergal, twice a day.

PREVIOUS CARE:

1. List doctors who have treated you for headaches: Dr. J. Dr. R.

2. List any tests you have had for your headache (e.g., EEG, CT scan, MRI, X-Ray, etc.):

CAT scan - 1990, with and without contrast (normal).

EEG - 1990 (normal)

MRI - 1990 (normal)

3. List any other treatment you have had for your headache (e.g., biofeedback, acupuncture, chiropractic, or any other treatment you had):

None.

Chapter 22

Psychiatric Considerations of the Post Traumatic Patient: Malingering, Factitious Illness, and Other Confusing Diagnoses

As reported in Chapter 14, in 1989 the National Safety Council estimated 12,800,000 motor vehicle accidents in the U.S. and of these, over 3,280,000 were rear-ended collisions. There were an estimated 1,000,000 to 3,000,000 whiplash injuries. Almost 10 years later and with an expanding population, the number of auto accidents, rear-end collisions, whiplash and post trauma head injuries will increase significantly.

In addition, in a country where a system of tort law exists, there will be an increase in litigation. Treating physicians will be asked to report as to the condition of the patient, the maximum medical improvement, the impairment, the disability, and the prognosis of that patient in relationship to the accident.

As reported in previous chapters (see Chapters 13, 14, 20 and 21), there are many symptoms other than headache, neck pain and other physical complaints that are reported after the accident. Symptoms considered psychological, such as anxiety and nervousness, sleeping problems, depression, fatigue, diminished concentration, irritability, impatience, restlessness, feeling disorganized, loss of interest, confusion, memory problems, dizziness, sexual problems, speech problems and others are also reported by the chronic sufferer.

Chapters 20 and 21 by Dieter have given a thorough description of the neuropsychology and neuropsychological testing concerned with these symptoms. Despite the evidence to support the validity of post traumatic symptoms, the question always arises as to whether the patient contrives these symptoms for financial gain.

Psychiatric conditions that either existed before or developed as result of the accident can confuse the clinician in an objective evaluation of how much the particular accident caused the patient's symptoms. That is, was there a significant psychiatric condition that preexisted the accident, and is the patient now using this accident as an excuse to maintain those symptoms?

The second problem is whether the patient who is not really suffering has contrived a condition for secondary gain, such as money or job changes.

Some of the illnesses that may add to the confusion of this problem are: *somatoform disorders*, *factitious illness*, and *malingering*. The clinical and psychological testing of these conditions are discussed in this chapter.

If the clinician is not aware that the patient being examined has suffered from *somatization disorder* before the accident, then the clinician may feel the accident was responsible for the present post trauma condition. Therefore, his or her opinion regarding maximum medical improvement (MMI), impairment, disability, and the patient's prognosis will be incorrect.

Somatization disorder 300.81, as described by the diagnostic criteria of the *Diagnostic and Statistical Manual* (DSM-IV) of the American Psychiatric Association, is a disorder that must be excluded before post traumatic symptoms from the accident are found responsible for the patient's complaints.

This disorder begins before age 30 and the patient seeks ongoing treatment. Symptoms usually impair social, occupational, and other functioning.

To meet the criteria of somatization disorder the following conditions must be met:

1. Four pain symptoms: there should be a history of pain in at least four sites or functions (e.g., head, abdomen, back, joints, extremities, chest, rectum, during menstruation, during sexual intercourse, or during urination).
2. Two gastrointestinal symptoms: other than pain there should be at least two other symptoms (e.g., nausea, bloating, vomiting, diarrhea, or intolerance of several foods).
3. One sexual symptom other than pain: (e.g., sexual indifference, erectile or ejaculatory dysfunction, irregular menses, excessive menstrual bleeding, vomiting throughout pregnancy).
4. One pseudoneurological symptom: a history of at least one symptom or deficit suggesting a neurological condition not limited to pain (conversion symptoms such as impaired coordination or balance, paralysis or localized weakness, difficulty swallowing or lump in throat, aphonia, urinary retention, hallucinations, loss of touch or pain sensation, double vision, blindness, deafness, seizures; dissociative symptoms such as amnesia; or loss of consciousness other than fainting).
   a. These symptoms following appropriate investigation cannot be explained by a known general medical condition or direct effects of medication or substance abuse.
   b. Even if there is a medical condition, the intensity of the physical symptoms or resulting social or occupational impairment are in excess of what should be from the history, physical examination, or laboratory findings.

The symptoms are not intentionally produced or feigned (as in factitious disorders or malingering).

Other disorders that may be confused with post traumatic injury that are not intentionally produced or feigned (as in factitious disorder or malingering) are

Undifferentiated Somatoform Disorder 300.81
Conversion Disorder 300.11
Hypochondriasis 300.7
Body Dysmorphic Disorder 300.7

An explanation of these disorders may be found in the Quick Reference to the Diagnostic Criteria, in DSM-IV.

The next group of illnesses that may interfere with the proper assessment of post traumatic or cervical acceleration/deceleration (whiplash) are factitious disorders. The *Diagnostic and Statistic Manual of Mental Disorders,* 3rd edition of the American Psychiatric Association, or DSM-III, defines factitious disorders as the following:[2]

> "Factitious" means not real, genuine, or natural. Factitious Disorders are therefore characterized by physical or psychological symptoms that are produced by the individual and are under voluntary control. The sense of voluntary control is subjective and can only be inferred by an outside observer. The judgment that the behavior is under voluntary control is based, in part, on the patient's ability to simulate illness in such a way that he or she is not discovered. This involves decisions as to timing and concealment that require a degree of judgment and intellectual activity suggestive of voluntary control. However, these acts have a compulsive quality, in the sense that the individual is unable to refrain from a particular behavior, even if its dangers are known. They should therefore be considered "voluntary" in the sense that they are deliberate and purposeful but not in the sense that the acts can

be controlled. Thus, in Factitious Disorders, behavior under voluntary control is used to pursue goals that are involuntarily adopted.

The judgment that a particular behavior is under voluntary control is made by the exclusion of all other possible causes of the behavior. For example, an individual presenting with hematuria (blood in the urine) is found to have anticoagulants in his possession; he denies having taken them, but blood studies are consistent with the injection of the anticoagulants. A reasonable inference is that the individual may have voluntarily taken the medication. A single episode of such behavior could be accidental rather than intentional. Repeated episodes would justify an inference of voluntary production of the symptoms — a factitious disorder. The presence of factitious psychological or physical symptoms does not preclude the coexistence of true psychological or physical symptoms.

Factitious disorders are distinguished from acts of malingering. In malingering, the patient is also in voluntary control of the symptoms, but it is for a goal that is obviously recognizable with the knowledge of the individual circumstances, rather than of his or her psychology. For example, a claim of physical illness in order to avoid jury duty, standing trial, or conscription into the military, would be classified as malingering. Similarly, for a patient in a mental hospital to simulate an exacerbation of his or her illness in order to avoid transfer to another less desirable facility, would be an act of malingering. In contrast, in a factitious disorder, there is no apparent goal other than to assume the patient role. If the patient mentioned above were being transferred to an obviously more desirable facility, his or her simulated exacerbation of symptoms would be a factitious disorder. Whereas an act of malingering may, under certain circumstances, be considered adaptive, by definition the diagnosis of factitious disorder always implies psychopathology, most often a severe personality disturbance.

Because symptoms of both chronic post concussive syndrome and cervical acceleration-deceleration (whiplash) syndrome are similar, reference will not be made to these two entities specifically, but will be used as one major syndrome in determining the problems of malingering.

The problem of dealing with a chronic factitious disorder with physical symptoms after these auto accidents is far less than having to deal with a malingerer. The reason for this is that most people who have factitious disorders seem to be preoccupied with illnesses most of their lives, and have had multiple hospitalizations and constantly try to get admitted to or to stay in hospitals. Most of the symptoms of this particular problem are abdominal symptoms, often with nausea and vomiting, dizziness, blacking out, generalized rashes, and fevers of unknown origin, seizures of undetermined origin, bleeding secondary to injection of anticoagulants, or vomiting blood secondary to taking irritants such as large dosages of aspirin or nonsteroidal anti-inflammatories, and all of their organ systems are potential targets. Because of their sophistication, patients will find various medications or means of having these particular organs act up.

These patients generally have great dramatic flair in presenting their histories, but at the same time are extremely vague, and there is inconsistency when questioned in more detail. There appears to be a great deal of pathological lying and often they will create stories that are intriguing to listen to. This is called pseudologica fantastica. These patients have extensive knowledge of medical terminology and hospital routines, and are often very difficult patients to deal with, especially because of their noncompliance with hospital routines and regulations. When their initial complaints prove to be negative, then they will begin to complain of other organ systems. They seem to enjoy multiple invasive procedures with needles, biopsies, operations, etc. While in the hospital they usually have few visitors, and if presented with the fact that they have a fictitious illness, they often will discharge themselves against medical advice. But they do not hesitate to get themselves admitted to another hospital the same day. They are eventually recognized by people in the medical community who cross their paths and begin to put the picture together. Although this diagnosis of factitious disorder may be one of the differential diagnoses of the doctor following the chronic symptoms of a post concussion syndrome or whiplash syndrome, these patients may be difficult to assess in the early stages of the work up and treatment by the clinician or headache specialist.

Patients with somatoform disorders, factitious disorders or who appear to be exaggerating the symptoms of an accident always seem to be labeled malingerers. Yet the term "malingerer" is very specific and has a distinct classification. DSM-III gives the following definition of malingering:

> The essential feature is the voluntary production and presentation of false or grossly exaggerated physical or psychological symptoms. The symptoms are produced in pursuit of a goal that is obviously recognizable with an understanding of the individual's circumstances rather than of his or her individual psychology. Examples of such obviously understandable goals include: to avoid military conscription or duty, to avoid work, to obtain financial compensation, to evade criminal prosecution, or to obtain drugs.

Under some circumstances, Malingering may represent adaptive behavior, for example, feigning illness while a captive of the enemy during wartime.

A high index of suspicion of malingering should be aroused if any combination of the following is noted:

1. Medical-legal context of presentation, e.g., the person's being referred by his attorney to the physician for examination;
2. Marked discrepancy between the person's claimed distress or disability and the objective findings;
3. Lack of cooperation with a diagnostic evaluation and prescribed treatment regimen;
4. The presence of Antisocial Personality Disorder.

The differentiation of malingering from factitious disorders depends on the clinician's judgment as to whether the symptom's production is in pursuit of a goal that is obviously recognizable and understandable in the circumstances. Individuals with factitious disorders have goals that are not recognizable in light of their specific circumstances, but are understandable only in light of their psychology as determined by careful examination. Evidence of an intrapsychic need to maintain the sick role suggests Factitious Disorders. Thus the diagnosis of Factitious Disorders excludes the diagnosis of the act of malingering.

Malingering is differentiated from conversion and other somatoform disorders by the voluntary production of symptoms and by the obvious, recognizable goal. The malingering individual is much less likely to present his or her symptoms in the context of emotional conflict, and the symptoms presented are less likely to be "symbolic" of an underlying emotional conflict. Symptom relief in malingering is not often obtained by suggestion, hypnosis, or intravenous barbiturates, as it frequently is in a conversion disorder.

Because symptoms of both chronic post concussive syndrome and cervical acceleration-deceleration (whiplash) syndrome are similar, reference will not be made to these two entities specifically, but will be used as one major syndrome in determining the problems of malingering.

When attempting to diagnose malingering, one has to keep in mind the following possibilities that may confuse the diagnosis of malingering:

1. Borderline intellectual functioning: if the IQ of the individual falls in the borderline intellectual functioning span of 71 to 84, this may mislead the clinician into thinking that the patient has the capacity to create a scheme that would take a higher intelligence.
2. Adult antisocial behavior.
3. Childhood or adolescent antisocial behavior.
4. Academic problems.
5. Occupational problems.
6. Uncomplicated bereavement.
7. Noncompliance with medical treatment.
8. Phase of life problem, or other life circumstance problems.
9. Marital problems.

10. Parent-childhood problems.
11. Other specified family circumstances.
12. Other interpersonal problems.

These are all rather sophisticated psychiatric diagnoses, and it is not expected for the average non-trained psychiatrist to be able to recognize this, except for the fact that something does not seem to be right. However, the malingerer still stands out as someone who has the obvious goal of secondary gain. In the case of these particular injuries, one would be money, two would be attention, or three, the opportunity to change a lifestyle that the patient was unhappy with prior to the accident.

Often after a post traumatic/post concussion injury which appears to be a minor accident, or an acceleration-deceleration (whiplash) accident, a neuropsychological examination is not done. After the history is taken and a physical examination is done and treatment is initiated, the examiner will come to a conclusion as to the prognosis of the patient after a period of time of working with that patient based on this approach.

Because the patient appears to be functioning at a "normal" level, it is assumed that there is no neuropsychological sequela or abnormality following the injury. Therefore, the prognosis and the interpretation of malingering or factitious illness are based on what may be a superficial investigation of that patient.

It should be recognized, however, that in certain instances there can be brain injury secondary to these particular accidents, and that this brain injury may cause significant changes in the patient's behavior that the examiner is unaware of. It is to the advantage of the examiner in drawing his or her conclusion to interview someone who is close to the patient to see if there have been any changes in behavior since the accident.

Some of the symptoms following these injuries can affect memory, attention and information processing, intellect, language, visual functions, executive functions, personality, and social outcome.

1. *Memory.* It has been shown that even with mild brain injury there can be chronic memory defects, even though most memory deficits will return to normal or near normal.
2. *Attention and information processing.* This refers to the ability to synthesize and use sequential information on an ongoing basis. Both attention and information processing defects are common after brain injury caused by these accidents.
3. *Intellect.* Studies have shown that following brain injury there are intellectual deficits generally related to the severity of the trauma.
4. *Language.* Generally, difficulties with language such as aphasia (inability to speak or express oneself in writing, or to comprehend spoken or written language), or alexia (loss of reading ability), etc., can result from brain injury. This is mostly seen where patients have had loss of consciousness at least for 10 to 15 minutes.
5. *Visual functions.* It has been shown that impairments of complex visual attention has been seen with mild traumatic brain injury.
6. *Executive functions and personality.* This is an extremely important symptom that may follow brain injury secondary to accidents. The executive function can interfere with cognitive abilities (perceiving, thinking, recognizing, and remembering) which are involved in judgment, decision making, social conduct, planning, and regulation and organization of behavior. A case study is presented at the end of this chapter that describes frontal lobe damage and demonstrates a complete personality change according to a relative of the patient. There have been findings with some consistency that damage to the orbital surface of the frontal lobes can cause severe damage to social conduct, rational judgment, and planning. This must be considered because the frontal lobes in the orbital areas are susceptible to damage in these minor accidents. Unfortunately, patients with this disorder are usually unaware that they have lost these cognitive assets. Some of the common symptoms of this problem are disinhibition, irritability, low frustration tolerance, and lack of motivation. Many of these symptoms are increased abnormalities of a premorbid personality prior to the accident. The ability

for abstract thinking becomes decreased and the patient tends to be more concrete in their thinking ability.

7. *Social outcome.* It has been shown with these traumatic brain injuries that there are impaired social interactional styles and social relationships.

The reason that these post concussion symptoms should be taken into consideration prior to designating someone as a malingerer would be to recognize that these symptoms are not in the control of the patient's consciousness and, as has been defined in malingering, that the expression of the patient's problems is conscious and goal-oriented.

Therefore, if there is any consideration for making the diagnosis of malingerer, and there has been some evidence of the possibility of brain injury, a battery of neuropsychological tests would be essential to perform prior to making the diagnosis of malingering.

Once these psychiatric and neurological conditions are ruled out and the clinician feels that the patient is willfully, deliberately expressing a fraudulent imitation or exaggeration of illness with the conscious intent to deceive others for the purpose of financial compensation, or to avoid legal or other responsibilities, the responsibility for the clinician is to present a case for malingering.

This is not an easy task, and the clinician often has to use his or her experience and knowledge to demonstrate that this patient is exaggerating manufactured symptoms and appears evasive during the interview and the examination. The patient never commits to any definite statements about returning to work, financial gain, or other expectations. They often contradict themselves by relating facts of the injury or symptoms differently to different examiners. The neurotic patient is more sincere about his symptoms, but less affectively concerned about them. Neurotic symptoms remain more constant over time, are more sudden in onset, often follow emotional shock, last longer, and tend to be more profound than those of simulated disorders. In the hysterical patient, often the symptoms will go into remission or disappear with suggestion, hypnosis, or other forms of psychotherapy. This effect is never observed with malingering, unless the malingerer is discovered or the secondary gains that they are seeking are obtained. The experienced clinician is often able to detect inconsistencies in the behavior and contradictions to known symptom complexes, and therefore can easily recognize malingering.

Although exaggeration of symptoms is seen both with the malingerer and the neurotic patient, a careful interview will often reveal the unconscious factor involved in the production of the conversion disorder, anxiety disorder, and so on, with the neurotic patient. The malingerer tends to present a picture that is more confusing, and the clinician can generally uncover the obvious attempts to deceive.

Although the well-trained clinical specialist can accurately detect malingering, relying on clinical judgment in general for all those who may be treating post concussive or whiplash injuries is likely to result in an unacceptably high error of accurately determining a malingerer. The other problem is that even if the specialist is accurate with his clinical assumptions, proving this in the legal system by clinical judgment alone can usually be challenged.

It is interesting that in my own experience, the few true malingerers that I have come across in a practice with thousands of patients, when their cases finally reached court, the juries would often end up by giving them nothing or next to nothing. For some reason or other, when presented in a proper fashion, the juries seem to be able to pick up on the game plan of the malingerer and rule accordingly.

Therefore, it is important when the clinician or the lawyer suspects malingering that neuropsychological testing be ordered to support the clinical diagnosis. Although there does not appear to be a specific test for malingering, abnormalities in existing tests that are done with the neuropsychological battery can often support the clinical diagnosis. One looks for excessively poor neuropsychological test scores after mild head injury. Although excessively poor neuropsychological test performances or excessive disability does not necessarily establish proof of malingering, it can provide an indication to the clinician that motivational and psychosocial factors need be carefully considered in the differential diagnosis.[3]

As stated before, it is important to rule out other medical conditions before arriving at the conclusion that malingering is the diagnosis from the post traumatic injury; that is, that the poor neuropsychological test performances may be part of other disorders, but existed previously to the accident. As an example, endocrine, hepatic (liver), renal (kidney), pulmonary, cerebrovascular, and substance abuse disorders have all been associated with impairment through neuropsychological tests. The chronic use of prescription medication such as narcotics, tranquilizers, and sedatives or hypnotic medications may also impair neuropsychological testing.

One has to be aware that many people with lifetime psychiatric disorders have never received professional treatment. Therefore, premorbid psychiatric vulnerabilities have a profound impact on how an individual adapts to a mild head injury. Keep in mind then that the absence of a documented psychiatric history does not automatically rule out a preexisting psychiatric disorder that may be associated with protracted post concussive symptoms.

Some tests have been devised that are seemingly difficult, but are actually simple tests that can be completed successfully by persons with mild brain impairments. However, it has been found that malingerers will misjudge the level of actual difficulty of a test and perform more poorly than the severely impaired patients. It has also been found that some malingerers attempt to perform all tests poorly, which would lead to defective performances on the simple procedures as well as the more difficult ones.

Packard and Hamm[4] have attempted to determine impairment ratings for post traumatic headache, and in the process used several scores. One score is for the impairment itself and the other is for the modifiers in which there is a score. The modifiers can be information from relatives that increase the patient's impairment that both the patient and the family are always concerned whether contacts were made with the patient's attorney, the affect of the patient in which they may be somewhat flippant, or inappropriate to the interview at that time, and that these affects are not part of a psychotic disease. Although these modifiers are used as part of the impairment rating, they certainly can be looked on as additional information for the diagnosis of malingering.

Although the number of actual malingerers seen in a headache practice may be small, the amount of time, energy, and finances involved is often enormous. As a result of these few patients, the term "malingering" has become universal. There are many patients whose symptoms may be exaggerated, but for unconscious reasons which were previously mentioned, such as neurosis, mild brain damage, or preexisting conditions, which have only been exacerbated by the present accident.

One interesting problem that arises out of an attempt to find methods to accurately diagnose a malingerer is that, as this information is disseminated in the literature, it can be used by malingerers or those who coach malingerers to prevent themselves from being detected. On the other hand, the ethical question that arises is, do you hold back information that helps to elevate the scientific knowledge that enhances our efforts to be better clinicians?

It is obvious that there is no definitive physical or psychological test to pinpoint the malingerer. Unfortunately, methods such as surveillance tapes or investigators have to be used to uncover the fabrications of some patients. The costs to workers compensation, medical insurance companies, automobile insurance companies, medical malpractice costs, and so on, are driving charges to a premium and bleeding the system, thereby preventing deserving patients from appropriate compensation.

There are disputes between some psychologists and the American Psychiatric Association's diagnostic criteria from the DSM-III-R and IV and suggestions have been made on a somewhat different approach to evaluate the malingering patient. However, there are no disputes that every attempt should be made to recognize with objectivity and weed out those patients who are only interested in the legal struggle and the desire for compensation that they truly do not deserve.

The clinician is unfortunately thrust into the legal arena and needs every instrument necessary to defend his or her position.

There is no question that objective testing to accurately diagnose the malingerer will help not only to identify this type of patient, but will also help to protect those patients who suffer real psychiatric or neurologic disease from being labeled malingerers, and at the same time to be able to give these patients adequate care.

REFERENCES

1. *Diagnostic and Statistical Manual of Mental Disorders*, 4th ed., Washington, D.C., American Psychiatric Association, 1994.
2. *Diagnostic and Statistical Manual of Mental Disorders*, 3rd ed., Washington, D.C., American Psychiatric Association.
3. Rizzo, M., Tranel, D., Detection of malingering in post concussive syndrome, in, *Head Injury and Post Concussive Syndrome*, Mills, S.R., and Putnam, S.H., Eds., Churchill Livingstone, New York, 1996.
4. Packard, R.C., Hamm, L.T., Impairment ratings for post traumatic headache, *Headache Journal*, 33, 359–364, 1993.

CASE HISTORIES*

HELEN
Category: Malingering headache

This case represents some of the difficulties that one has in assessing diagnosis and treatment, prognosis and a disability rating. As you look at the medical headache history form, it appears obvious that this looks like a diagnosis of migraine with aura, or classical migraine, and one that is in a status condition, which means that it is not breaking by itself and needs acute treatment.

When a patient such as this comes into the office, right from the start the doctor knows that this is going to be a very difficult case to correct, just based on the history.

The patient is a 43-year-old woman with some college education, and has been out of work for several months from a large corporation prior to seeing me. She states that she was in the armed forces, but had a medical discharge in 1963 because of a heat stroke.

Her major complaint is that since she was exposed to some chemicals at work several years before in 1987, her headache problem has been aggravated. The headache profile when she comes into the office is the following: She says they started approximately $3^1/_2$ to 4 years ago. The patient would get one every five months. Currently for the past two months she has experienced them on a daily basis. Prior to that time, the patient was having one to two a week for about two years, then they increased as a result of chemical exposure and prior to that she was having them once a month. Duration can last up to five days. The character of her pain is typical of migraine, that is throbbing and is generally on the right side of her head most of the time. There is an aura of scintillating scotomata, for only seconds (scintillating scotomata are little light flashes), and she has nausea, vomiting, photophobia, sonophobia, pallor, lacrimation (eyes running), and she must go to bed. She said exertion would make it worse, and this is typical of migraine.

Interfering headaches (moderate to severe): These started two years ago. They are currently continuous. The patient feels that these headaches may have started with the chemical problems at work and now they're continuing. The duration is constant. The character of the pain is dull, throbbing, which is located in the same area just described, and the headache features are similar except there is no aura.

There is no history of headaches in any member of her family.

Medications: The patient has been treated over the years by various doctors and has various medications that she has been using that have been prescribed for her headache. She is on significant narcotic pain medication called Talwin, taking 8 a day (obviously much too much), and also other pain medications with codeine in them. It was obvious in the beginning that there was a dependency problem, and she had been on various other medications over the years that she had also become dependent on. This was a red flag to start with when she came in. She had all types of treatments prior to seeing me, and various trigger point injections, and treatment with various machines that are used for pain, with no success.

Her psychiatric history was not very significant. She had seen someone eight years ago for some marital problems and her MMPI (Minnesota Multiphasic Personality Inventory) did not show a very distorted psychological distress pattern, but the typical reaction that one sees to chronic pain.

My immediate concern was to see if I could break the cycle of these headaches to give her some relief, and then to work on reducing her medications. She was hospitalized and given intravenous DHE (dihydroergotamine) and some other medications (and an attempt to reduce her narcotic medications was done while she was in the hospital). Also, various types of nerve blocks were done in order to help reduce the headache, which turned out not to be beneficial and they were discontinued.

* On the headache assessment forms that accompany these case histories, incapacitating headaches are indicated with solid black lines, interfering headaches with dotted lines, and irritating headaches with gray shading.

Although the patient states that these chemicals were responsible for her current headache problem, her history indicates that there were so many other traumas that it was difficult to assess the effects of the "chemicals" on her headache problem.

In 1973, the patient was in a rear-ended accident and sustained a cervical strain with headaches for a short period of time. In 1978, the patient was rear-ended again, given a cervical collar, had headaches for awhile and went into remission. In 1982, the patient was hit on the driver's side and hit her head against the window. She had headaches for several days, and then went into remission. In 1985, the front side of the car in which the patient was riding on the passenger side was hit in the front. She had headaches for a short period of time and went into remission. Again, the patient had a cervical strain and upper back muscle problems. In 1987, the patient's car was rear-ended, which resulted in pulled muscles of the neck and she was placed in pelvic-cervical traction, had headaches which went into remission. In 1980, she dove into a pool and hit her head, but the current headaches she said are not related to this. In 1987, she had chemical exposure and feels since that time the headaches have increased in frequency. Again, it is difficult not to consider while all this is going on that the patient is on leave and is applying for disability and there is going to be litigation involved.

In my hospital notes, I ended by saying that she had made moderate progress in the hospital and had only one attack in a five-day period as opposed to having it every day, and that we were withdrawing her from the Talwin and other drugs that cause addiction. After discharge, the patient had only come to the office one time stating that her headaches were back every day. She stopped all the migraine medication because she said it wasn't helping. The patient stopped in the office and was talking to the nurse stating that she was in and out of the hospital since we'd seen her and she still complains of headache. The nurse noted that her speech was slurred and she had a slow, unsteady gait, and she wanted narcotic medication, which we did not give her and we did not see her again.

The problem we were faced with here is that there was a legitimate migraine-type headache that had to be treated. The question is, how much did all of the accidents and problems that she had relate to her headache and has the patient come to a point in her life where she feels that the only way that she is going to survive is by being dependent, be on disability, and be in litigation to recover some income. The doctor knows in advance that he is going to have to be called in deposition or go to court on a case like this. This case is put in the chapter on malingering only because one is not sure which is the chicken, and which is the egg. But, it is an example of what the doctor has to face some patients. My experience over the years is that chemicals will increase migraine attacks if chemicals are one of the triggering mechanisms. However, from the literature that I have studied and the cases I've seen, most of these headache problems go into remission after the exposure is taken away and they are not exposed to this triggering mechanism.

The fact that headaches can last from some chemicals, as seen with Agent Orange in Viet Nam and some of the exposures that our soldiers had in the Persian Gulf war, may have been part of the total syndrome as opposed to just headaches from these agents.

The obvious dilemma here is attempting to tease out what is actually happening with the patient and these become extremely difficult problems to assess. Maintaining one's objectivity while examining a patient like this sometimes can be difficult, but an attempt is made to be fair and honest with all the facts when having to testify as to the findings. This is why this case was presented in this chapter.

MEDICAL HEADACHE HISTORY

Name: Helen **Age:** 43 **Sex** F **Date:** 7/19/89

Date of Birth: 0/00/45 **Birthplace:** OH **Race:** C **Education:** 1 ½ yrs. College

Occupation: On Medical Leave – Manufacturing Co. **Accident:** 1987

Armed Services & Type of Discharge: Marine Corps – Medical Discharge

PAST HISTORY:

1.	Did you have a normal birth?		Yes (underlined)	No
	a) forceps used?		Yes	No
	b) cesarean section?		Yes	No
2.	Did you have problems with bedwetting?		Yes	No (underlined)
	a) If yes, age bedwetting stopped		______	
3.	Were you car sick as a child (motion)?		Yes (underlined)	No
	a) If yes, how severe?	Slight	Moderate	Severe (underlined)
4.	Did you have unexplained abdominal cramps as a child?		Yes	No (underlined)
5.	Did you have any of the following illnesses in childhood?			
	a) meningitis		Yes	No (underlined)
	b) encephalitis		Yes	No (underlined)
	c) scarlet fever		Yes	No (underlined)
	d) rheumatic fever		Yes	No (underlined)
6.	Did you have any head injuries as a child?		Yes	No (underlined)
	a) If yes, please explain: ______			
7.	Were you treated for emotional illness as a child?		Yes	No (underlined)

HABITS:

8.	Do you drink alcohol?	Yes	No (underlined)
	a) If yes, what kind and how much? ______		
	b) Does alcohol bring on or aggravate a headache?	Yes	No (underlined)
9.	Do you smoke?	Yes (underlined)	No
	a) If yes, how much? 10 a day		
	b) Does smoking or smoke-filled rooms cause or aggravate headaches?	Yes	No (underlined)
10.	Do you drink caffeinated beverages?	Yes (underlined)	No
	a) If yes, how much? 16 oz. day		

MENSTRUAL HISTORY:

At what age did menses begin? 14 Were they regular or irregular? Irregular - cramping

How were they related to your headache? In bed 3 days with cramps

Are you or were you ever on Birth Control Pills? Yes Did they affect your headache? ______

Have you had a hysterectomy, partial or total, and why? Partial (1972)

Are you in menopause, and if yes, how long? No

Are you on hormones, and if yes, which ones? ______

HEADACHE ASSESSMENT FORM

HA PROFILE	INCAPACITATING #3	INTERFERING #2	IRRITATING #1
ONSET (Years ago and frequency)	3 ½ to 4 years ago one every 5 months, now daily	2 years ago	N/A
CURRENT FREQUENCY	Now daily	Continuous	N/A
TIME OF ONSET	Anytime	Constant	N/A
DURATION	1 to 60 hours	Constant	N/A
CHARACTER	Throbbing, "flickering lights"	Dull throbbing	N/A
PRODROME OR AURA	90% flickering lights seconds before headache	N/A	N/A
ASSOCIATING FEATURES	Nausea; Vomiting; Sensitivity to Light? Noise? Odors? Do you get pale or flush? Do your eyes or nose run? Does your nose get stuffy? Do the whites of your eyes get red? Does your eyelid droop? Do you pace, or go to bed? darkness	Nausea; Vomiting; Sensitivity to Light? Noise? Odors? Do you get pale or flush? Do your eyes or nose run? Does your nose get stuffy? Do the whites of your eyes get red? Does your eyelid droop? Do you pace, or go to bed?	Nausea; Vomiting; Sensitivity to Light? Noise? Odors? Do you get pale or flush? Do your eyes or nose run? Does your nose get stuffy? Do the whites of your eyes get red? Does your eyelid droop? Do you pace, or go to bed?
PRECIPITATING OR AGGRAVATING FEATURES	Turning head	N/A	N/A

LOCATION: Mark the location for each type of headache with a different color pen.

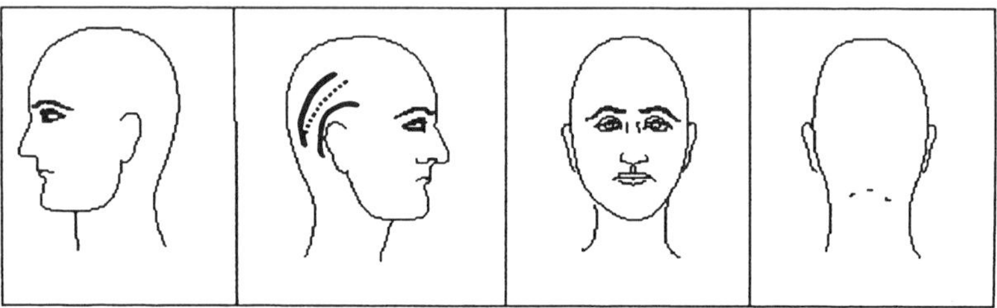

MEDICAL HISTORY:

Have you ever been or are you currently being treated for any of the following?

a) high blood pressure	Yes	<u>No</u>
b) stomach ulcers	<u>Yes</u>	No
c) asthma	Yes	<u>No</u>
d) allergies	Yes	<u>No</u>
e) pneumonia	Yes	<u>No</u>
f) kidney problems	Yes	<u>No</u>
g) low blood sugar	Yes	<u>No</u>
h) glaucoma	Yes	<u>No</u>
i) diabetes	Yes	<u>No</u>
j) heart problems	Yes	<u>No</u>

If you answered yes to any of the above, please describe: Ulcers 1975, 1980 (take Tagamet, Zantac)

List all other medical problems you have had in the past. Include date diagnosed and treatment.
DO NOT LIST OPERATIONS

Food poisoning 1974. Concussion mid-1970's. Auto accidents 1973, 1978, 1982, 1985, 1987. Back injury 1974.

SURGICAL HISTORY (List operations and dates performed)

Hysterectomy, 1972. Ganglions removed from right wrist, 1958, 1972, 1973. Foot surgery, bunion and reconstruction, 1980. Breast surgery (left), 1988.

PSYCHIATRIC HISTORY (List visits with counselors, psychologists, etc., and type of treatment)

Dr. G. – marital problems, 1981.

ACCIDENTS IN ADULT LIFE (Briefly describe any accident that caused any blow to the head or that you feel is related to your headache)

Diving in pool, hit head causing concussion. Car accidents. Possible chemical exposure at work.

FAMILY HISTORY:

1.	Is your father living?	<u>Yes</u>	No
	Age 67		
	Cause of death ______		
	Was there a headache history?	Yes	<u>No</u>
2.	Is your mother living?	<u>Yes</u>	No
	Age 65		
	Cause of death ______		
	Was there a headache history?	Yes	<u>No</u>

3. Ages of brothers---Circle the ones with headache
   None
4. Ages of sisters---Circle the ones with headache
   None
5. List any other blood relatives with a history of severe headaches.
   None

MARITAL HISTORY:

List marriages:

1st marriage age 20 to Present	Did spouse have headaches?	Yes	No
2nd marriage age _____ to _____	Did spouse have headaches?	Yes	No
3rd marriage age _____ to _____	Did spouse have headaches?	Yes	No

Age of current spouse: 54

List ages and sex of all children:

Age 22	Sex F	Headaches?	Yes / No
Age 20	Sex F	Headaches?	Yes / No
Age 18	Sex F	Headaches?	Yes / No

STRESS FACTORS:

List any factors that may be affecting your headaches (money, loneliness, sexual problems, work, etc.)
?

VEGETATIVE SIGNS:

1.	Do you have trouble falling asleep?	Yes	No
2.	Do you have trouble staying asleep?	Yes	No
3.	Has your appetite decreased?	Yes	No
4.	Have you gained or lost weight in the past year?	Yes	No
5.	Have you felt tearful or depressed lately?	Yes	No
6.	Have you had any thoughts of wanting to die?	Yes	No
7.	Have you been forgetful lately?	Yes	No
8.	Any other changes in your normal day-to-day living?		

Please list any medications you are allergic or sensitive to: Codeine; Darvocet; Benzol Peroxide

Please list any medications you are currently taking (including dosages and frequency per day):
Inderal 160 mg. daily; Dilantin 300 mg daily; Talwin 6 to 8 tablets daily.

PREVIOUS CARE:

1. List doctors who have treated you for headaches: Dr. A. Dr. B. Dr. C. Dr. D. Dr. E. Dr. F.

2. List any tests you have had for your headache (e.g., EEG, CT scan, MRI, X-Ray, etc.):
MRI, 1987 and 1989. CAT scan, 1987. X-Rays, 1987. (All normal)

3. List any other treatment you have had for your headache (e.g., biofeedback, acupuncture, chiropractic, or any other treatment you had):
Trigger point injections (no help).

CAROL
Category: Psychological

This is a history of a 28-year-old woman who came to see me nine years after she had been in an accident. She was riding on a motorcycle and collided with a car, slid under the car, lost consciousness and awoke when the paramedics came and took her to the hospital. She does not remember the treatment. Her headaches began several months later. She states there were no headaches prior to the accident.

Interfering headaches (moderate to severe): These started two months after her accident. She was getting 2 to 3 a week. Currently she states that she is getting 3 to 7 a week, coming on at any time. They will last all day. It is constant, severe pressure. The pain is in the bilateral temporal regions. There is no aura and there are some of the associated features of nausea, photophobia, and sonophobia. She says lying down sometimes increases her headache, which is generally the opposite of what most migraine people want. That is, they want to lie down and not move.

There is a history of many psychiatric hospitalizations and going to many crisis centers and state hospitals, etc. She is currently taking Lithium for a bipolar disorder (a psychiatric disorder) and is also taking Tegretol for a seizure disorder.

By history, this appears to be a headache disorder that started following a significant accident; however, the fact again that it took several months before the headaches started puts the question as to the direct effect of the trauma to the headache. There is a great deal of history of headache in the patient's family, which I assume might have been migraine. The patient was treated for vascular headaches; however, she did not return after the first visit, so there was no follow-up. I would suspect that one would have to be very careful before saying that this headache disorder is directly related to the accident, but it is in the realm of possibility that headaches can start later on.

MEDICAL HEADACHE HISTORY

Name: Carol **Age:** 28 **Sex** F **Date:** 8/6/92

Date of Birth: 00/00/63 **Birthplace:** MD **Race:** C **Education:** 11th Grade

Occupation: ____________ **Accident:** 1983

Armed Services & Type of Discharge: N/A

PAST HISTORY:

1.	Did you have a normal birth?		Yes	No
	a) forceps used?		Yes	No
	b) cesarean section?		Yes	No
2.	Did you have problems with bedwetting?		Yes	No
	a) If yes, age bedwetting stopped		______	
3.	Were you car sick as a child (motion)?		Yes	No
	a) If yes, how severe?	Slight	Moderate	Severe
4.	Did you have unexplained abdominal cramps as a child?		Yes	No
5.	Did you have any of the following illnesses in childhood?			
	a) meningitis		Yes	No
	b) encephalitis		Yes	No
	c) scarlet fever		Yes	No
	d) rheumatic fever		Yes	No
6.	Did you have any head injuries as a child?		Yes	No
	a) If yes, please explain: ______			
7.	Were you treated for emotional illness as a child?		Yes	No

HABITS:

8.	Do you drink alcohol?	Yes	No
	a) If yes, what kind and how much? ______		
	b) Does alcohol bring on or aggravate a headache?	Yes	No
9.	Do you smoke?	Yes	No
	a) If yes, how much? A pack a day		
	b) Does smoking or smoke-filled rooms cause or aggravate headaches?	Yes	No
10.	Do you drink caffeinated beverages?	Yes	No
	a) If yes, how much? A liter a week		

MENSTRUAL HISTORY:

At what age did menses begin? 12 Were they regular or irregular? WNL

How were they related to your headache? N/A

Are you or were you ever on Birth Control Pills? Yes Did they affect your headache? N/A

Have you had a hysterectomy, partial or total, and why? No

Are you in menopause, and if yes, how long? No

Are you on hormones, and if yes, which ones? No

HEADACHE ASSESSMENT FORM

HA PROFILE	INCAPACITATING #3	INTERFERING #2	IRRITATING #1
ONSET (Years ago and frequency)	N/A	2 months after accident 2 to 3 per week	N/A
CURRENT FREQUENCY	N/A	3 to 7 a week	N/A
TIME OF ONSET	N/A	Anytime, Can awaken with	N/A
DURATION	N/A	All day	N/A
CHARACTER	N/A	Constant severe pressure	N/A
PRODROME OR AURA	N/A	N/A	N/A
ASSOCIATING FEATURES	Nausea; Vomiting; Sensitivity to Light? Noise? Odors? Do you get pale or flush? Do your eyes or nose run? Does your nose get stuffy? Does the white of your eyes get red? Does your eyelid droop? Do you pace, or go to bed?	Nausea; Vomiting; Sensitivity to Light? Noise? Odors? Do you get pale or flush? Do your eyes or nose run? Does your nose get stuffy? Does the white of your eyes get red? Does your eyelid droop? Do you pace, or go to bed? Sit quietly	Nausea; Vomiting; Sensitivity to Light? Noise? Odors? Do you get pale or flush? Do your eyes or nose run? Does your nose get stuffy? Does the white of your eyes get red? Does your eyelid droop? Do you pace, or go to bed?
PRECIPITATING OR AGGRAVATING FEATURES	N/A	Lying down increases headaches	N/A

LOCATION: Mark the location for each type of headache with a different color pen.

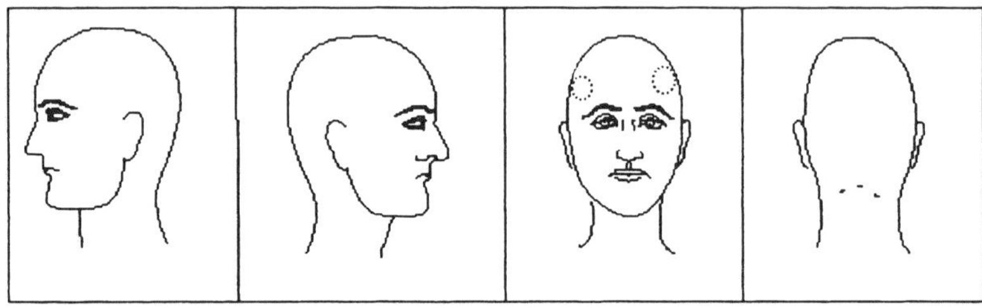

MEDICAL HISTORY:

Have you ever been or are you currently being treated for any of the following?

a) high blood pressure	Yes	No
b) stomach ulcers	Yes	No
c) asthma	Yes	No
d) allergies	Yes	No
e) pneumonia	Yes	No
f) kidney problems	Yes	No
g) low blood sugar	Yes	No
h) glaucoma	Yes	No
i) diabetes	Yes	No
j) heart problems	Yes	No

If you answered yes to any of the above, please describe: Pneumonia as an infant.

List all other medical problems you have had in the past. Include date diagnosed and treatment. DO NOT LIST OPERATIONS

Seizures – 1984. On Tegretol.

SURGICAL HISTORY (List operations and dates performed)

Appendectomy 1968. Tonsillectomy. Knee 1980.

PSYCHIATRIC HISTORY (List visits with counselors, psychologists, etc., and type of treatment)

State Hospital. Crisis Unit. Outpatient.

ACCIDENTS IN ADULT LIFE (Briefly describe any accident that caused any blow to the head or that you feel is related to your headache)

1983 – Motorcycle accident. Driving, collided with a car. Slid under car, lost consciousness. Awake when paramedics came and out on way to hospital. Don't remember being treated. Headaches began 2 months later. No headaches before accident.

FAMILY HISTORY:

1. Is your father living? Yes No
   - Age________
   - Cause of death N/A
   - Was there a headache history? Yes No
2. Is your mother living? Yes No
   - Age 59
   - Cause of death________
   - Was there a headache history? Yes No

3. Ages of brothers---Circle the ones with headache
   Three brothers ______
4. Ages of sisters---Circle the ones with headache
   One sister ______
5. List any other blood relatives with a history of severe headaches.
   ______

MARITAL HISTORY:
List marriages:

1st marriage age _____ to _______ Did spouse have headaches? Yes No
2nd marriage age _____ to _______ Did spouse have headaches? Yes No
3rd marriage age _____ to _______ Did spouse have headaches? Yes No

Age of current spouse:__________

List ages and sex of all children:

Age _____ Sex ______ Headaches? Yes No
Age _____ Sex ______ Headaches? Yes No
Age______ Sex ______ Headaches? Yes No

STRESS FACTORS:
List any factors that may be affecting your headaches (money, loneliness, sexual problems, work, etc.)

______

______

VEGETATIVE SIGNS:

1.	Do you have trouble falling asleep?	<u>Yes</u>	No
2.	Do you have trouble staying asleep?	<u>Yes</u>	No
3.	Has your appetite decreased?	Yes	<u>No</u>
4.	Have you gained or lost weight in the past year?	Yes	<u>No</u>
5.	Have you felt tearful or depressed lately?	<u>Yes</u>	No
6.	Have you had any thoughts of wanting to die?	<u>Yes</u>	No
7.	Have you been forgetful lately?	<u>Yes</u>	No
8.	Any other changes in your normal day-to-day living?______		

Please list any medications you are allergic or sensitive to: No known allergies.

______

______

Please list any medications you are currently taking (including dosages and frequency per day):
Lithium, 900 mg. a day. Tegretol, 800 mg. a day.

______

______

PREVIOUS CARE:

1. List doctors who have treated you for headaches: None.

2. List any tests you have had for your headache (e.g., EEG, CT scan, MRI, X-Ray, etc.):
CAT scan - 1988, with and without contrast (normal).
EEG - 1988 (normal)

3. List any other treatment you have had for your headache (e.g., biofeedback, acupuncture, chiropractic, or any other treatment you had):
None.

STEVEN
Category: Psychological

This is a 27-year-old man with a tenth grade education who was a laborer. His accident occurred two months prior to my seeing him. While he was returning from work, he was sitting in the back of the van and another car cut in front of the van and the van hit that car. He had significant head and neck flexion-extension injuries. He says his headaches started immediately, and he feels they are getting worse. He states he had no headaches prior to the accident.

Incapacitating headaches: These started the day of the accident. He is having them daily. It is a constant, throbbing and burning in his neck, and in the bilateral periorbital (around the eye) region in the front of his head, the back of his head, and the cervical region. He states that since he has had these headaches, he has become violent and unable to tolerate the pain. He has typical features of migraine, with nausea, vomiting, light sensitivity, noise sensitivity, sensitivity to odors, and must sit quietly at all times.

He says that before the accident, he could have a six-pack of beer a week and it did not bother him. But, since the accident, he cannot drink any alcohol because it causes pain. When I saw him, he was in treatment with a psychiatrist. A month before I saw him, he was hospitalized psychiatrically for violent temper and depression. He states that most of it was really due to his headaches and, because the pain is so severe, he has these emotional problems. The patient felt that if he did not have the headaches, he would not have these psychological symptoms.

All of his neurological tests and imaging tests with CT scan, EEG and x-rays were normal. He had a great many severe myofascial trigger points in the area of the back of the neck, the trapezius, the splenius capitis, that radiate to his head and cause severe headache on palpation. Because of the severity and the constant daily headache problem, I placed him in the hospital in order to treat him with intravenous medications for his migraine, and also to have better control of his treatment.

He was a very difficult patient to treat in the hospital. He demanded narcotic medication and I attempted to follow him in the office with little success. It was difficult for any of the physicians to have control of his treatment.

The major problem here was whether this behavior existed prior to the accident, or whether the accident was responsible for both his headache and his psychological behavior. What makes me suspect that there were psychological problems prior to the accident was that the patient would not permit the insurance company to have any medication information prior to the accident that we would need to be able to evaluate his psychological status prior to the accident. I do feel that the headaches are related to the accident, but have to question both the frequency and the intensity of having an incapacitating headache every day, and whether this satisfies a medication need or not is questionable. However, this history was put into this chapter because it certainly is an example of the result of what appears to be a relatively minor injury causing multiple psychological conditions.

MEDICAL HEADACHE HISTORY

Name: Steven **Age:** 27 **Sex** M **Date:** 9/23/91

Date of Birth: 00/00/64 **Birthplace:** NM **Race:** W **Education:** 10th Grade

Occupation: General Laborer (on medical leave) **Accident:** 1991

Armed Services & Type of Discharge: N/A

PAST HISTORY:

1.	Did you have a normal birth?		<u>Yes</u>	No
	a) forceps used?		Yes	<u>No</u>
	b) cesarean section?		Yes	<u>No</u>
2.	Did you have problems with bedwetting?		Yes	<u>No</u>
	a) If yes, age bedwetting stopped		______	
3.	Were you car sick as a child (motion)?		Yes	<u>No</u>
	a) If yes, how severe?	Slight	Moderate	Severe
4.	Did you have unexplained abdominal cramps as a child?		Yes	<u>No</u>
5.	Did you have any of the following illnesses in childhood?			
	a) meningitis		Yes	<u>No</u>
	b) encephalitis		Yes	<u>No</u>
	c) scarlet fever		Yes	<u>No</u>
	d) rheumatic fever		Yes	<u>No</u>
6.	Did you have any head injuries as a child?		Yes	<u>No</u>
	a) If yes, please explain: ______			
7.	Were you treated for emotional illness as a child?		Yes	<u>No</u>

HABITS:

8.	Do you drink alcohol?	<u>Yes</u>	No
	a) If yes, what kind and how much? Past 2 months – 0. Before accident – 6 pack a week.		
	b) Does alcohol bring on or aggravate a headache?	<u>Yes</u>	No
9.	Do you smoke?	<u>Yes</u>	No
	a) If yes, how much? 1½ packs a day		
	b) Does smoking or smoke-filled rooms cause or aggravate headaches?	Yes	<u>No</u>
10.	Do you drink caffeinated beverages?	Yes	<u>No</u>
	a) If yes, how much? ______		

MENSTRUAL HISTORY:

At what age did menses begin? ______ Were they regular or irregular? ______
How were they related to your headache? ______
Are you or were you ever on Birth Control Pills? ______ Did they affect your headache? ______
Have you had a hysterectomy, partial or total, and why? ______
Are you in menopause, and if yes, how long? ______
Are you on hormones, and if yes, which ones? ______

HEADACHE ASSESSMENT FORM

HA PROFILE	INCAPACITATING #3	INTERFERING #2	IRRITATING #1
ONSET (Years ago and frequency)	Since day of accident Every day	N/A	N/A
CURRENT FREQUENCY	Every day	N/A	N/A
TIME OF ONSET	Awakens with	N/A	N/A
DURATION	Constant	N/A	N/A
CHARACTER	Throbbing, burning in neck	N/A	N/A
PRODROME OR AURA	N/A, Has become violent since accident	N/A	N/A
ASSOCIATING FEATURES	Nausea: Vomiting: Sensitivity to Light? Noise? Odors? Do you get pale or flush? Do your eyes or nose run? Does your nose get stuffy? Does the white of your eyes get red? Does your eyelid droop? Do you pace, or go to bed? Sits quietly	Nausea: Vomiting: Sensitivity to Light? Noise? Odors? Do you get pale or flush? Do your eyes or nose run? Does your nose get stuffy? Does the white of your eyes get red? Does your eyelid droop? Do you pace, or go to bed?	Nausea: Vomiting: Sensitivity to Light? Noise? Odors? Do you get pale or flush? Do your eyes or nose run? Does your nose get stuffy? Does the white of your eyes get red? Does your eyelid droop? Do you pace, or go to bed?
PRECIPITATING OR AGGRAVATING FEATURES	Any head movement	N/A	N/A

LOCATION: Mark the location for each type of headache with a different color pen.

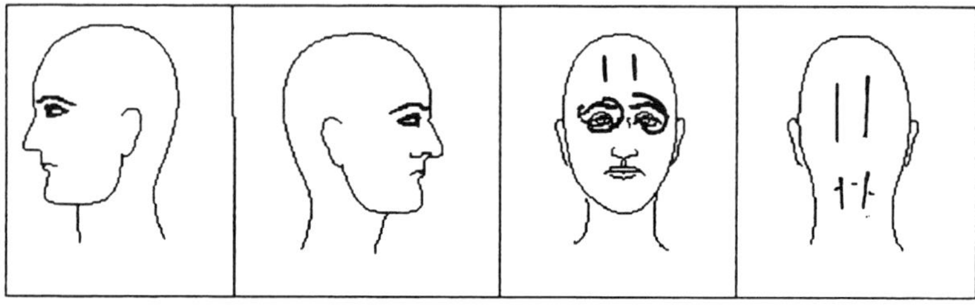

MEDICAL HISTORY:

Have you ever been or are you currently being treated for any of the following?

a) high blood pressure	Yes	No
b) stomach ulcers	Yes	No
c) asthma	Yes	No
d) allergies	Yes	No
e) pneumonia	Yes	No
f) kidney problems	Yes	No
g) low blood sugar	Yes	No
h) glaucoma	Yes	No
i) diabetes	Yes	No
j) heart problems	Yes	No

If you answered yes to any of the above, please describe:_______________

List all other medical problems you have had in the past. Include date diagnosed and treatment.
DO NOT LIST OPERATIONS

Therapy for neck, back, left leg.

SURGICAL HISTORY (List operations and dates performed)

1986, finger amputated.

PSYCHIATRIC HISTORY (List visits with counselors, psychologists, etc., and type of treatment)

Dr. J.

ACCIDENTS IN ADULT LIFE (Briefly describe any accident that caused any blow to the head or that you feel is related to your headache)

1991 – Passenger in back of van. Another car cut in front of the van and we hit that car. Taken to emergency room, treated and released. Headaches began 2 days later. No headaches before accident.

FAMILY HISTORY:

1. Is your father living? Yes No
   - Age 60 something
   - Cause of death_______________
   - Was there a headache history? Yes No
2. Is your mother living? Yes No
   - Age 70 something
   - Cause of death_______________
   - Was there a headache history? Yes No

3. Ages of brothers---Circle the ones with headache
   29 41 38 47
4. Ages of sisters---Circle the ones with headache
   28
5. List any other blood relatives with a history of severe headaches.
   None

MARITAL HISTORY:

List marriages:

1st marriage age _____ to _______ Did spouse have headaches? Yes No
2nd marriage age _____ to _______ Did spouse have headaches? Yes No
3rd marriage age _____ to _______ Did spouse have headaches? Yes No

Age of current spouse:__________

List ages and sex of all children:

Age _____ Sex _____ Headaches? Yes No
Age _____ Sex _____ Headaches? Yes No
Age_____ Sex _____ Headaches? Yes No

STRESS FACTORS:

List any factors that may be affecting your headaches (money, loneliness, sexual problems, work, etc.)
Neck is hurting causing headaches, plus bad nightmares. Daytime and nighttime voices telling me to do weird things.

VEGETATIVE SIGNS:

1.	Do you have trouble falling asleep?	<u>Yes</u>	No
2.	Do you have trouble staying asleep?	<u>Yes</u>	No
3.	Has your appetite decreased?	<u>Yes</u>	No
4.	Have you gained or lost weight in the past year?	<u>Yes</u>	No
5.	Have you felt tearful or depressed lately?	<u>Yes</u>	No
6.	Have you had any thoughts of wanting to die?	Yes	<u>No</u>
7.	Have you been forgetful lately?	<u>Yes</u>	No
8.	Any other changes in your normal day-to-day living?__________		

Please list any medications you are allergic or sensitive to:__________

Please list any medications you are currently taking (including dosages and frequency per day):
Elavil, 50 mg twice a day and 150 mg at bedtime. Lithium, one capsule three times a day.
Thorazine 100 mg in morning, 100 mg in evening, 200 mg at bedtime.

PREVIOUS CARE:

1. List doctors who have treated you for headaches: Dr. O., Dr. E.

2. List any tests you have had for your headache (e.g., EEG, CT scan, MRI, X-Ray, etc.):
CAT scan, 1991.

3. List any other treatment you have had for your headache (e.g., biofeedback, acupuncture, chiropractic, or any other treatment you had):
None.

BRENDA
Category: Factitious disorders and malingering

This history has been put in this chapter because of the way the case developed and also some of the questions that I had when I first saw the patient.

I had seen her a year and a half after she had her accident, in which she was a passenger in a friend's speedboat. They began driving very fast and she states other boats caused a wake, and they hit one of the wakes and, according to her, they went up 70 degrees. She went to grab her daughter and fell forward and then backwards and hit her back and head on the rear seat. She said her headaches started after the accident.

Incapacitating headaches: She said these started two to four months after the accident and when I saw her she was getting one every other week. They would last three to four days. It was a throbbing headache, often in the right periorbital or around the eye region, the frontal region, and the parietal or side of her head. Associated features were nausea, photophobia (light sensitivity), sonophobia (noise sensitivity), and she goes to bed.

Interfering headaches (moderate to severe): These started also two to four a month. They come at any time. She can awaken with them, and the features are similar to the incapacitating headaches. One would have to say that these are typical features of a migraine-like headache, and we have discussed the fact that this is very common after a trauma in which the head is injured, or even a whiplash injury. It is not common that someone will get headaches from an accident that happened several months prior to the symptoms appearing, although it has been reported sometimes as much as 4%. By her last visit, three months after I had seen her, she was seeing other doctors and states that none of the treatment helped her headache. Now she was complaining of memory loss and depression, and feels that she is in a "fog" most of the time. An MRI of the brain was done, which was normal, and that was when I began to find that the symptoms seemed to be increasing as she was becoming more frustrated with her lawsuit. Then she began to add more and more symptoms concerning her whole body as time went on.

There is great difficulty in saying that the patient was not experiencing any of these recent symptoms, but at the same time one hears the same from many patients and especially those in litigation. Those who may be having other psychological problems make one feel that these symptoms may be part of an entire process involving both the litigation or previous psychological problems I am not aware of. If I was called to be in a deposition, I probably would have requested a battery of psychological tests; however, the patient did not come back after that last visit and I do not know what happened to her case.

MEDICAL HEADACHE HISTORY

Name: Brenda **Age:** 29 **Sex** F **Date:** 11/25/91

Date of Birth: 0/00/62 **Birthplace:** NJ **Race:** H **Education:** 1yr. College

Occupation: Real Estate **Accident:** 1990

Armed Services & Type of Discharge: N/A

PAST HISTORY:

1.	Did you have a normal birth?		<u>Yes</u>	No
	a) forceps used?		Yes	<u>No</u>
	b) cesarean section?		Yes	<u>No</u>
2.	Did you have problems with bedwetting?		Yes	<u>No</u>
	a) If yes, age bedwetting stopped		______	
3.	Were you car sick as a child (motion)?		<u>Yes</u>	No
	a) If yes, how severe?	Slight	<u>Moderate</u>	Severe
4.	Did you have unexplained abdominal cramps as a child?		Yes	<u>No</u>
5.	Did you have any of the following illnesses in childhood?			
	a) meningitis		Yes	<u>No</u>
	b) encephalitis		Yes	<u>No</u>
	c) scarlet fever		Yes	<u>No</u>
	d) rheumatic fever		Yes	<u>No</u>
6.	Did you have any head injuries as a child?		Yes	<u>No</u>
	a) If yes, please explain: ______			
7.	Were you treated for emotional illness as a child?		Yes	<u>No</u>

HABITS:

8.	Do you drink alcohol?	Yes	<u>No</u>
	a) If yes, what kind and how much? ______		
	b) Does alcohol bring on or aggravate a headache?	Yes	<u>No</u>
9.	Do you smoke?	<u>Yes</u>	No
	a) If yes, how much? 2 to 3 per night		
	b) Does smoking or smoke-filled rooms cause or aggravate headaches?	Yes	<u>No</u>
10.	Do you drink caffeinated beverages?	<u>Yes</u>	No
	a) If yes, how much? 1 cup of coffee per day		

MENSTRUAL HISTORY:

At what age did menses begin? 8 Were they regular or irregular? WNL

How were they related to your headache? N/A

Are you or were you ever on Birth Control Pills? Yes Did they affect your headache? No

Have you had a hysterectomy, partial or total, and why? No

Are you in menopause, and if yes, how long? No

Are you on hormones, and if yes, which ones? No

HEADACHE ASSESSMENT FORM

HA PROFILE	INCAPACITATING #3	INTERFERING #2	IRRITATING #1
ONSET (Years ago and frequency)	2 to 4 months after accident 1 to 2 a month	2 to 4 months after accident; 1 to 2 a month	N/A
CURRENT FREQUENCY	1 every other week	3 to 4 a month	N/A
TIME OF ONSET	Anytime Can awaken with	Anytime Can awaken with	N/A
DURATION	3 to 4 days	1 day	N/A
CHARACTER	Throbbing	Same, less intense	N/A
PRODROME OR AURA	N/A	N/A	N/A
ASSOCIATING FEATURES	Nausea; Vomiting; Sensitivity to Light? Noise? Odors? Do you get pale or flush? Do your eyes or nose run? Does your nose get stuffy? Do the whites of your eyes get red? Does your eyelid droop? Do you pace, or go to bed?	Nausea; Vomiting; Sensitivity to Light? Noise? Odors? Do you get pale or flush? Do your eyes or nose run? Does your nose get stuffy? Do the whites of your eyes get red? Does your eyelid droop? Do you pace, or go to bed?	Nausea; Vomiting; Sensitivity to Light? Noise? Odors? Do you get pale or flush? Do your eyes or nose run? Does your nose get stuffy? Do the whites of your eyes get red? Does your eyelid droop? Do you pace, or go to bed?
PRECIPITATING OR AGGRAVATING FEATURES	N/A	N/A	N/A

LOCATION: Mark the location for each type of headache with a different color pen.

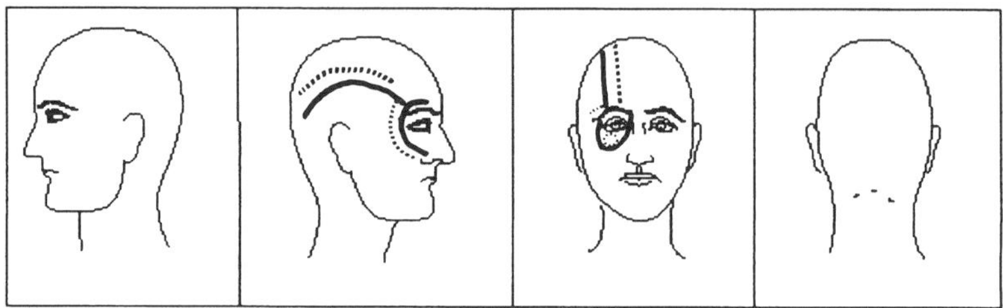

MEDICAL HISTORY:

Have you ever been or are you currently being treated for any of the following?

a) high blood pressure	Yes	<u>No</u>
b) stomach ulcers	Yes	<u>No</u>
c) asthma	Yes	<u>No</u>
d) allergies	Yes	<u>No</u>
e) pneumonia	Yes	<u>No</u>
f) kidney problems	Yes	<u>No</u>
g) low blood sugar	Yes	<u>No</u>
h) glaucoma	Yes	<u>No</u>
i) diabetes	Yes	<u>No</u>
j) heart problems	<u>Yes</u>	No

If you answered yes to any of the above, please describe: <u>Mitral valve prolapse, have palpitations.</u>

List all other medical problems you have had in the past. Include date diagnosed and treatment.
DO NOT LIST OPERATIONS

<u>Fracture of L3 after accident.</u>

SURGICAL HISTORY (List operations and dates performed)

<u>Tonsillectomy & Adenoidectomy, 1965. Appendectomy, 1977. Ovarian cyst, 1977. Ectopic pregnancy, 1986. Cesarean, 1989.</u>

PSYCHIATRIC HISTORY (List visits with counselors, psychologists, etc., and type of treatment)

<u>None.</u>

ACCIDENTS IN ADULT LIFE (Briefly describe any accident that caused any blow to the head or that you feel is related to your headache)

<u>Was riding as a passenger on a friend's speedboat when sudddenly he began driving faster to race other boats. Some other boats caused wakes and we hit one. We went up on a 70° angle. I went to hold my daughter and fell forward then backward and banged my back and head on the rear seat. I passed out.</u>

FAMILY HISTORY:

1. Is your father living?	<u>Yes</u>	No
Age <u>48</u>		
Cause of death ______		
Was there a headache history?	Yes	<u>No</u>
2. Is your mother living?	<u>Yes</u>	No
Age <u>47</u>		
Cause of death ______		
Was there a headache history?	Yes	<u>No</u>

3. Ages of brothers---Circle the ones with headache
   21 4
4. Ages of sisters---Circle the ones with headache
   23
5. List any other blood relatives with a history of severe headaches.
   None

MARITAL HISTORY:
List marriages:

1st marriage age 19 to 23	Did spouse have headaches?	Yes	No
2nd marriage age 25 to Present	Did spouse have headaches?	Yes	No
3rd marriage age ______ to ______	Did spouse have headaches?	Yes	No

Age of current spouse: 32

List ages and sex of all children:

Age 10	Sex F Headaches?	Yes	No
Age 2	Sex M Headaches?	Yes	No
Age ______	Sex ______ Headaches?	Yes	No

STRESS FACTORS:

List any factors that may be affecting your headaches (money, loneliness, sexual problems, work, etc.)
None known.

VEGETATIVE SIGNS:

1.	Do you have trouble falling asleep?	Yes	No
2.	Do you have trouble staying asleep?	Yes	No
3.	Has your appetite decreased?	Yes	No
4.	Have you gained or lost weight in the past year?	Yes	No
5.	Have you felt tearful or depressed lately?	Yes	No
6.	Have you had any thoughts of wanting to die?	Yes	No
7.	Have you been forgetful lately?	Yes	No
8.	Any other changes in your normal day-to-day living? ______		

Please list any medications you are allergic or sensitive to: None known.

Please list any medications you are currently taking (including dosages and frequency per day):
None.

PREVIOUS CARE:

1. List doctors who have treated you for headaches: None.

2. List any tests you have had for your headache (e.g., EEG, CT scan, MRI, X-Ray, etc.):
None.

3. List any other treatment you have had for your headache (e.g., biofeedback, acupuncture, chiropractic, or any other treatment you had):
None.

Chapter 23

Problems in the Courtroom: The Lawyer's Viewpoint

Don McKeever

All potential plaintiffs should be told that there is no such thing as a good lawsuit, particularly when it comes to chronic cervical syndrome, a/k/a whiplash. I tell potential clients that before they will collect the first dime they will have to visit their doctor on a regular basis, spending countless hours in depressing waiting rooms thumbing through old magazines, go through rigorous physical therapy session where their progress will be subjectively evaluated by desensitized therapists, complete volumes of paperwork requiring a meticulous accounting of their medical history (regardless of whether it is related to the problem for which they seek treatment), and undergo scores of tests ranging from inconvenient, at best, to terribly painful at worst. Of course, all of this activity will necessarily require that they miss a substantial amount of time from work and, unless totally medically disabled during this time, there will likely be no compensation for the time missed from work to attend this treatment.

Let's not forget that if the potential plaintiff works in a position that requires physical labor, he or she is not only jeopardizing their current job by missing work, but their future employability because of the stigma associated with someone who suffers from chronic head pain, regardless of the severity. This disclosure invariably separates those who are legitimately injured from those who are motivated by financial gain. The latter will quickly lose interest, whereas the former will endure what has been described above, which is not exaggeration in the typical head and neck injury case.

In head and neck accidents, there are generally common and critical issues which prove to be decisive to the success or failure of the case. From the prospective of the average juror, one of the most compelling factors in assessing the degree of injury to the plaintiff is the extent of property damage to the vehicles involved in the accident. Little or no damage to one or both vehicles is often an insurmountable obstacle to recovering any more than just economic damages, such as medical bills and lost wages. Generally, a jury will award these elements of damages to an injured person even in a minor impact case. Convincing a jury, however, that the person involved in what appears to be a minimal impact accident is entitled to pain and suffering damages is an uphill and costly battle. Direct testimony on this point is imperative. For this reason, it is paramount that the lawyer for the injured person impress upon the testifying doctor the importance of explaining that there is not always a direct correlation between the damage to the vehicle and the injury to the occupant of the vehicle. Once an experienced doctor testifies that the extent of property damage to a 3000 pound automobile is not necessarily indicative of the forces that are applied to the spine of the 150 pound occupant, the presumption of no damage/no injury should begin to dissipate. This point should be made by all the doctors, if possible.

It is also extremely beneficial to get the defense expert to concede that in fact one person may walk away from a major collision, whereas another may be seriously injured in an accident involving little impact between the vehicles. The jurors cannot be reminded of this enough.

Offering an analogy is often quite effective in painting the picture that will stay with a jury. I sometimes mention in my closing argument to the jury that if a person wearing a football helmet is struck in the back of the head by someone swinging a baseball bat, the helmet will probably show no sign of damage. Does this mean that the head and neck of the person receiving the unexpected blow did not suffer injury? I don't know if this has been helpful, but it certainly suggests that things aren't always what they appear to be.

Generally, contrary to popular opinion, most accident victims do not seek the advice of a lawyer until long after critical information surrounding the accident and resultant injuries has been, frequently and most unfortunately, recorded in a haphazard fashion. There is probably nothing more important than fully and completely disclosing to the initial medical care provider, whether it be the hospital or the treating physician, a complete medical history pertaining to the part of the body for which the patient is seeking treatment.

I was painfully reminded of the importance of this disclosure just recently when I tried the lawsuit of a 68-year-old female client whose car was rear-ended while she was stopped for traffic. The impact was moderate, and although she declined treatment at the scene, she drove herself to the hospital two hours after the collision. She had been involved in another auto accident five years earlier and treated for similar injuries. Unknown to her, her doctor assigned a permanent impairment rating from the injuries she suffered in that accident. However, for the $3^1/_2$ years before the second accident, she received no treatment, took no medication, and experienced no pain. In fact, shortly after the first accident, she returned to her full time job doing physically demanding custodial work.

The problem arose after the second accident when at the hospital she was asked the question, "Did you have back problems before the collision?" Understanding the question to mean immediately before the accident, rather than at any time in her 68 years, she innocently replied, "No." This statement was documented by the hospital personnel and, subsequently, by the initial treating doctor as "no history of back problems."

It was no surprise to me that the entire defense at trial pivoted on this simple misunderstanding, which the defense characterized as dishonesty on the part of the plaintiff. It was argued by the defense that my client knowingly withheld this information about her preexisting condition from her doctors because she was afraid it would adversely affect her claim for damages in the second accident. And, it was further argued, if the plaintiff was not being honest with her doctors, could she be trusted on the issue of subjective complaints of pain and suffering? Although the medical causation between her injuries and the second accident was easily established, the jury had a difficult time believing that the miscommunication was simply a misunderstanding. Unfortunately, this issue proved to be fatal to the plaintiff's recovery of damages for pain and suffering.

This incident exemplifies how an innocent mistake by an unsophisticated client can be devastating to a legitimate claim. In any head and neck injury case, the entire case hinges on the credibility of the plaintiff and, if it can be effectively assailed, the case will be lost.

Another important area of concern is the history the initial doctor takes from the patient regarding the facts of the occurrence which brings them together. An inexperienced doctor might feel that it is in the best interest of the patient to record an extensive, comprehensive and detailed account of the event. For the most part, details about the facts of the occurrence have absolutely no medical significance. Unfortunately, however, such details can have fatal legal repercussions.

For instance, I represented a young man in his early twenties who was a passenger in a car which was struck from behind. When describing the impact to the doctor (long before he retained me), and said it "felt like" they got hit at 70 mph. Unfortunately, the doctor failed to note the qualifying language in his report and, having no independent recollection of the conversation, had to stand by his notes. His testimony therefore was that the patient said his vehicle was struck from behind at 70 mph. The actual impact was more like 15 to 20 mph. The defense attorney, very effectively, capitalized on this simple and innocent miscommunication to suggest that from the onset the patient was being dishonest and had ulterior motives. This theory cast doubt on the legitimacy of the claim from the outset.

In essence, the doctor, who thought he was doing the patient a favor by recording this extensive history, was unwittingly creating evidence which proved devastating to the patient's eventual claim for fair compensation.

The attorney's initial interview with the client is generally the most important contact with the client, particularly in a neck injury case. The old axiom, "there is one thing about a first impression, you never get another one," is particularly true in these cases.

The first hour of the interview is critical in terms of assessing the likability and believability of the plaintiff. This is the time a decision is made by the attorney whether or not he wants to one day put this client on the witness stand. My philosophy is that if I don't like the person, a jury won't either. Of course, we can all be fooled and I learned this the hard way.

Years ago, however, I has humbly reminded otherwise in the middle of trial. I represented an 83-year-old widow who sustained a soft tissue neck injury after her car was rear-ended. Since our first interview, I always thought what a great witness she would make and how she would melt a jury! Well, the day came when I had the opportunity to test my intuition. I saved her for my last witness, knowing she would charm the jurors and they would handsomely compensate this sweet old lady.

During the direct examination, she looked at the jury and spoke sweetly and softly about her ongoing pain which necessitated extensive doctors' visits, as many as 85 in the two years after the accident. By the time I finished my direct examination, I was feeling rather smug because I knew she had the jury eating out of her hand. She handled cross-examination beautifully, being extremely respectful and courteous to the defense attorney. He had not scored any points and was about to sit down when, as a final question, he very gently inquired whether many of the visits to her doctor were perhaps occasioned by loneliness rather than pain.

Wow! You would have thought he dipped her Depends in Tabasco sauce! I have never seen such a sudden transformation. She jerked her glasses off, leaned forward in her seat, glared at him for what seemed an eternity, and venomously growled, "Mister, don't you be so presumptuous to tell me that I need attention. You don't know what it's like to lose a spouse, and if I want to continue going to the doctor, I'll do what I damn well please."

I immediately realized where Stephen King came up with the title to his book, *Cujo*. Evidently, the jury did, too, because they found this woman 35% at fault for getting struck in the rear and awarded only her past medical bills.

I also make it a rule that if, during the first meeting, the client asks what his case is worth, I decline to represent the person. This generally is the best indictor of someone who is more interested in a financial gain rather than physical recovery, assuming they are truly injured.

In most cases, it is at least six months between the time of the accident and the time when the case is in a settlement posture, i.e., the client is at maximum medical improvement and has returned to work. I have found, however, that it is generally closer to a year before the treating doctor feels comfortable offering final opinions about the patient's prognosis. During this time, the patient has probably returned to work and the lawyer should have in his possession verification from the employer of the patient's earnings and the amount of time the patient missed from work. While obtaining this information, the lawyer is also collecting all other pertinent medical records, including medical records of treatment for preexisting injuries or conditions. These records should be furnished to the treating doctor prior to his forming any opinions about the casual relationship between the patient's complaints and subject accident.

After the patient reaches maximum medical improvement (MMI), it is important to obtain from the treating doctor an opinion about the diagnosis and, more importantly, the prognosis. Generally, this information is obtained before a lawsuit is instituted. It is extremely important that the plaintiff's lawyer meet personally with the doctor.

Some attorneys send the doctor a standard form letter which outlines specific questions which should be addressed by the doctor. If the doctor fails to respond to a certain issue, it will be necessary to do a follow up letter. This will generally be resented by the doctor who is more interested in practicing medicine than answering medicolegal questions posed by an attorney. A personal visit to the doctor shows not only that the attorney is personally interested in the case, but it enables the doctor to give a recorded statement in a question-and-answer format which should encompass all issues that need to be addressed. When the doctor is reminded that giving a recorded statement will increase the likelihood of settlement and perhaps obviate the need for a subsequent deposition, he or she is usually more than willing to cooperate.

Ideally, after the audiotape is transcribed, the statement and a copy should be mailed to the doctor for his signature. Therefore, it is not likely the doctor will change his opinions. This approach often facilitates settlement because the defendant's insurance carrier is provided with a comprehensive statement signed by the doctor.

Once the above information has been collected, it should be forwarded to the adjuster for the insurance company representing the defendant. It typically takes the adjuster less than one month to review the claim and respond. If negotiations fail, a lawsuit is filed against the insured.

Once the claim moves to litigation with the filing of a lawsuit, the chances of settlement generally diminish until some discovery is completed. The defendant usually sends legal documents to the plaintiff (via his attorney, of course) known as interrogatories. These are written questions which inquire into many areas, including the plaintiff's accident and medical history. Generally, the purpose of interrogatories is to learn, *from the plaintiff*, if he or she has previously sustained injuries similar to those for which he or she is claiming compensation, and the identity of the medical providers.

With this information, the defense attorney retrieves these records in preparation of the plaintiff's deposition. Additionally, after being provided the plaintiff's name, address and social security number, the defense attorney will independently obtain and verify this information through the claims index bureau. This is a network used by insurance companies to record all medical claims made by individuals, however minor. A problem can arise if, for whatever reason, the plaintiff has failed to disclose prior treatment, even for the mot superficial of injuries, or a prior accident, even if no treatment was received.

Since the interrogatories' answers must be sworn to by the plaintiff, failure of the plaintiff to identify the places where or persons who have treated him in the past can be used to impeach him at trial. In view of the importance of the plaintiff's credibility in these cases, an oversight in this regard, whether intentional or not, can prove to be devastating.

A deposition of the treating physician is generally taken by the defense attorney. The patient's attorney should always meet with the doctor before the deposition and educate the doctor about the legal issues in the case. It is incumbent upon the patient's attorney to discuss in detail with the doctor all accidents, injuries (however minor), or treatment experienced by the patient before the accident in question. If the doctor is unaware of the pertinent history, irreparable damage can occur to the case.

A good defense lawyer who is aware of the patient's medical history will get the doctor to unwittingly commit himself on the issue of causation, then blind-side the doctor with additional facts about the patient's history. In most cases, the doctor cannot extricate himself without looking like an advocate for the plaintiff. Furthermore, the doctor usually looks with disfavor upon the plaintiff's attorney because he feels that he has been manipulated by the nondisclosure of material facts. If it can be avoided, never let the doctor first become aware of the patient's history through the mouth of the defense attorney. Enlightening the doctor about the patient's relevant medical history may not change the doctor's opinions, but it will give him or her the whole picture of the plaintiff's medical history, and will certainly facilitate rehabilitating the damaging testimony on redirect examination.

If the plaintiff intends to call the doctor at trial, the plaintiff generally does not ask the doctor any questions at the deposition unless it is necessary to clear up any misunderstandings during the examination by the defense counsel. As mentioned earlier, this should all be explained to the doctor at the predeposition conference between the plaintiff's attorney and the doctor. If the doctor is the treating physician, he probably will be called to tesify at trial, if he is available. If he is not available or simply will not testify, the plaintiff's attorney should take the deposition by video, unless the doctor for some reason makes a poor appearance. Again, the plaintiff's attorney should meet with the doctor well before the deposition to discuss the testimony.

The plaintiff's attorney must know in advance of all of the doctor's opinions. If there is any suspicion by the plaintiff's attorney that the doctor is not going to be supportive of his patient and the issues in the case, have the patient attend the meeting and the deposition. It is less likely the treating doctor will testify unfavorably in the presence of the patient and, if he does, let him look the patient in the eye while doing so. This technique is generally unnecessary, but should certainly be considered when warranted.

During the trial testimony of the doctor, whether by video or in person, it is important that the doctor look at the jury while testifying.

I recently tried a case in which the anesthesiologist refused to testify at trial. I therefore took his videotaped deposition. While asking him questions on direct examination, I was not necessarily paying attention to where he was looking while answering the questions. Instead, I was reviewing my notes and preparing for the next question. His testimony was particularly important because he was rendering opinions on the necessity and costs of future care. As a matter of fact, his opinions in this regard were undisputed. I read the transcript of his testimony before trial and felt confident his testimony would be compelling. I did not, however, view the actual videotape of the deposition.

During the trial, I played the videotape for the jury and, since my table was not in view of the monitor, I simply followed his testimony by reading his deposition transcript as the video played.

After a disappointing result and no award for future care, I had the fortune to run into one of the jurors. She volunteered that the doctor was not believable because he never looked up from his chart. Obviously, even if I had seen this before trial, there would not have been anything I could have done (since he wouldn't appear at trial). However, it was another important lesson on the need to remind the doctor that it is important to look at the jury while testifying.

On the other hand, I tried a case last year where the treating doctor testified extensively on direct examination and looked at the jury the entire time. However, before answering *every* opinion question, he would pause and crinkle his face as if struggling to find an elusive answer. A friend and seasoned defense attorney who happened to be sitting in the courtroom during both the direct and cross examination, commented afterwards that the doctor's testimony, on both direct examination and cross examination, was the finest he had ever seen. We obtained a great result, and following trial had an opportunity to talk to a juror. She remarked that our doctor came across somewhat disingenuous because of this very performance. This simply illustrates that what lawyers believe is impressive and effective testimony presented at trial may not necessarily be how the same is perceived or received by the jury.

The doctor should have available charts, anatomic models, and any other demonstrative aids which help the jury better understand the testimony about the patient's injuries. In a soft tissue case, objective signs of the injury are of the utmost importance. The most common objective signs are muscle spasms. Most good plaintiffs' attorneys will not go over every office visit in direct examination of the treating physician. They will, however, ask the doctor early in the testimony to explain the involuntary nature of a muscle spasm and then point out all of the different times throughout the treatment muscle spasms are noted.

If the patient has undergone any type of injections, it is compelling to have the doctor bring to trial the types of needles used to perform the treatment. The doctor should approach the jury and demonstrate in painstaking detail the procedure involved in administering the injection. If epidural injections have been used, bring the entire kit and have the doctor unravel it before the jurors' eyes. The doctor should also vividly describe the reaction of the patient to this procedure, particularly if the patient is resistant to injection therapy.

I tried a case years ago involving a woman who had been sitting at a table in a restaurant eating lunch. The restaurant was busy and the waitress was scrambling to not only serve my client and her three friends at the table, but another dozen customers at various tables in the restaurant. In her haste, the waitress accidentally spilled a cup of scalding coffee down my client's back. My unsuspecting client reacted by violently jerking her head backwards causing a self-inflicted hyperflexion extension injury. She treated with an osteopathic physician who performed cervical adjustments.

At the trial, I had my client wear slacks and asked the judge if the doctor could come down from the witness stand and perform an adjustment on the plaintiff. The judge reluctantly agreed and we had the doctor do the adjustment with the client laying on plaintiff's table within ten feet of the jury. The procedure demonstrated to the jury the obvious discomfort the plaintiff experienced while undergoing this treatment. The demonstration concluded with a loud "crack" emanating from the cervical region which, in turn, resulted in a "scream" and near mistrial.

The scream did not come from the plaintiff, not did it come from a juror. It was a scream from my new legal assistant who, unknown to me, had a phobia about such matters. Anyway, the jury found in favor of the plaintiff and awarded her compensation. I found in disfavor of my legal assistant and awarded her a new job.

The bottom line is that the doctor could have talked all day about manipulations and adjustments, but until they viewed the actual procedure, the jury could not appreciate the nature of treatment and how much the plaintiff must have been suffering to endure this treatment.

In cross examination of the doctor at trial, a good defense attorney will laboriously and in detail emphasize all of the doctor's normal findings throughout his course of treatment of the patient, comments in the records made by the patient when same felt he or she was doing better, and any appointments missed or canceled by the patient.

In the typical neck and head injury case, the defense attorney will also get the doctor to agree that, in the absence of muscle spasms and objective signs, the doctor would have no objective basis to find anything wrong with the patient. This is obviously a very effective strategy in most head and neck injury cases because the entire case usually revolves on the believability of the patient. If the defense attorney can cast doubt on the sincerity of the plaintiff's complaints, the jury usually will not generally resolve the doubt in favor of the plaintiff.

Another typical means of attacking the plaintiff's case is by exposing any ongoing relationship between the plaintiff's attorney and the doctor. Although this testimony is not relevant to any of the medical issues, it implies collusion and can certainly taint the credibility of the doctor's testimony.

Whether the jury listens to the medical testimony is usually not entirely in the hands of the testifying physician. I do not care how charming, gregarious and captivating the doctor presents, if he is called to testify at traditionally dull points in the trial, it is not likely he will have the full attention of the jury. The most effective time to present medical testimony is during the beginning of the case on any particular day. The last witness of the day is also generally a very memorable witness. The least effective time to offer testimony is in the middle of the afternoon when the jurors have returned from lunch and might have trouble staying awake. If it can be avoided, a videotape should never be played during this time.

In the final analysis, regardless of the appearance, demeanor and substance of the testimony of the doctor, the jury is always instructed that they can accept, reject, or give the medical testimony whatever weight they feel it deserves. Even when the doctor has treated the patient over an extended period of time and vouches for the patient's credibility, the doctor cannot change the jury's perception of the plaintiff. Except on rare occasions, the jury and only the jury has the final word on whether the plaintiff will be compensated for an invisible injury that only the plaintiff can feel.

In soft tissue cases, the entire case rests with the believability and likability of the patient. There is probably nothing more devastating than surveillance film which depicts the plaintiff performing an activity which is directly or indirectly inconsistent with his testimony.

My most memorable experience involving surveillance films came at the conclusion of a personal injury trial. I represented Barney, who worked for a local sanitation company. He would stand on the rear of a garbage truck and empty garbage cans into the rear of the truck.

One morning the truck was hit broadside by a car and Barney was thrown from the truck and struck the curb. He suffered neck and back injuries and was treated in the emergency room of the local hospital.

He was out of work for a couple of weeks and, upon returning, found he was unable to perform his job without significant pain. Consequently, he remained off work for several months. During his deposition, Barney testified that there were a number of activities he could not perform, including lifting heavy objects, particularly if it involved lifting above the shoulder.

Subsequently the insurance company for the defendant hired an investigator to perform surveillance on Barney and immediately thereafter withdrew all offers of settlement. The case proceeded to trial and, as the rules of civil procedure require, I was shown the videotape before trial. When the video was offered at trial, I objected to the relevance of the film and argued that the video did not depict the pain and discomfort Barney was experiencing when he appeared in the film. The judge overruled my objection and permitted the film to be shown to the jury.

For 30 minutes, the camera followed the activities of a very healthy man diligently working under the hood of a car in the parking lot of an auto parts store. The limber subject repeatedly squatted down and effortlessly crawled under the car. He would painlessly jump to his feet and resume bending and stretching under the hood. After feverishly working on the car for what seemed like days, he finally emerged with the car battery. He then effortlessly raised it into the air over his head with one hand and lazily strutted into the auto parts store.

As you can imagine, the defense attorney was relishing the moment, having exposed a fraud by catching the lying plaintiff red-handed. And, of course, the jury was incredulous, having just heard three days of riveting testimony after the plaintiff's disabilities.

After the film was shown, I proceeded to cross examine the individual who operated the video camera. He was an enormous man weighing probably 300 pounds, 200 of which were covered with vulgar tattoos. His unattractiveness was surpassed only by his arrogance. Setting him up, I asked him questions about the importance of his role in the trial and if he know how devastating his film could be on the plaintiff's case. I then had Barney stand and asked the video operator if he was certain that it was in fact the plaintiff who was working on the car in the video and carrying the battery into the auto parts store. As I expected, my questions were met with adamant absolute, unequivocal answers.

After asking a few more questions to get him inextricably committed that it could be no one on the film other than the plaintiff, I gave the signal to bring Barney's younger brother into the courtroom to stand behind Barney. I then directed the attention of Mr. Absolutely Certain to Barney's younger brother, the star of the surveillance film, and asked if he had ever seen this witness. The operator, who had turned crimson red, looked like a deer caught in the proverbial headlights.

By this time, the defense attorney was going berserk screaming incoherent objections. The verdict in favor of the plaintiff was substantial and I imagine it was in no small part due to this little episode.

Unfortunately, most surveillance film stories do not have such a happy ending. To the contrary, most videos that are played at trial present compelling damaging evidence which cannot be easily overcome. Had the above video actually depicted my client engaging in those activities, the case would have been lost, and rightfully so.

There is no specific amount of time it takes a personal injury claim to progress from filing the lawsuit to trial. I have cases that have been tried within five months of filing suit, and others that have taken over four years to get to trial. Each case is as unique as the individual plaintiff.

I have had many cases prepared for trial when I got a call from the plaintiff informing me that the doctor has just tried trigger point injections or epidural blocks. This sort of problem is generally due to a lack of communication between the plaintiff's lawyer and the treating physician. Nevertheless, a new treatment plan changes the entire complexion of the case. If the treatment is not completed by the time the case is tried, the doctor offering the prognosis can be challenged. Furthermore, the cost of future medical treatment cannot be approximated. Uncertainly about the effectiveness of treatment also gives the jury a reason, particularly if they dislike the plaintiff, not to award future damages. This is one type of problem which can prolong the trial of a case.

Cases involving neck and back injuries are long, expensive, and both physically and mentally stressful on the plaintiff. If the plaintiff is not likeable and believable, the obstacles generally encountered in these types of cases are magnified tenfold.

Unfortunately, most juries have been poisoned by propaganda disseminated by the insurance companies and other large corporations about the impossibility of serious injury in neck and back cases involving minor impact between vehicles. Consequently, even when there has been a legitimate loss and damages, many deserving plaintiffs receive no compensation and sometimes end up paying the attorney's fees and costs of the defendant.

The best advice I can offer anyone who has suffered a neck and back injury is get better and get on with your life. Unless there is a substantial and permanent injury, the legal arena is not where you want to end up.

The opinions expressed in this chapter are those of the author based on experience and do not necessarily reflect the opinions of others in the legal community.

CASE HISTORY

This is a report written to a lawyer who asked for an independent evaluation on a patient who was going to court. This report was written several years ago. The passages printed in **bold** and marked with an asterisk (*) have recently been added to the original report based on our current knowledge of cervicogenic headache.

BERNARD SWERDLOW, MD
Diplomate, American Board of Psychiatry and Neurology (p)

Medical Headache Consultation — Mr. Steven X

This is a consultation and evaluation done on Mr. Steven X, requested by Mr. John Z, attorney.

This patient was originally seen and treated by [...], MD, at the clinic at [...]. He was originally seen on [date] and since that time Dr. [...] has moved from this area and I have retired from this office.

As a headache expert, I have been asked to review various records on this patient and also to evaluate his current status secondary to an injury that he had in 1993.

The patient was born [...], and has an Associate degree and some classes for a Bachelor's degree in Engineering.

Currently, he is working as a [...] for [...], which is a firm, and Mr. X currently works as a [...]. He has been with this firm for almost [...] years.

The patient was never in military service.

The patient states that he was in an automobile on [...], 1993, heading south in a long line of cars on [...] Avenue when a woman headed north turned left into the side rear quarter of his car. He only had a fraction of a second "before impact" and tried to veer to the right. The patient states that he thinks he was going approximately 30 to 35 miles per hour at that time.

The patient was in a convertible with the top down and states that when he was hit he was wearing a lap seatbelt and struck his head on the left side of a beam that was supporting the convertible roof. The patient states that he is not sure that he was unconscious momentarily, but does know that he was dazed as a result of the accident. He states that he thought there might be a loss of consciousness, because he had thought that he hit his head once, but found out later that he had hit his head more than once. He was taken to [...] Hospital, where he had a CT scan of his head at that time which was reported as "normal." He was released with apparent scalp contusions in the left frontal region. He was asked whether there was any alteration in his mental state at the time of the accident, as an example, feeling dazed, disoriented, or confused, and the patient stated that reports from his wife and others revealed that they noticed he was confused and dazed. He also states that right after the accident, he felt a tingling in his legs and also in his right arm from time to time.

The patient states that since the accident he has been suffering headaches, irritability, insomnia for which he currently takes Elavil 50 mg at bedtime to help him sleep, has some anxiety at times, and has some concentration problems. He also complains of pain in his back and legs. He states that since the accident and being put on the Elavil, his depression has been reduced, his dizziness has improved; but he still has problems in carrying out plans because of his pain.

OTHER ACCIDENTS

In [...] of 1980, while working as a machine operator splitting steel rolls, he had to bend down to crank a lever and hurt his back. He states he was treated for that and this pain was resolved by the end of 1987 or early 1988, and he has not had any pain in his back until this current accident.

In 1981, at about age [...], he states that he was in an automobile accident in which someone pulled in front of the patient and he was hit on the driver's side of the car and the car went over the curb. There was no physical injury to him and there were no headaches.

There was another auto accident in [...] in which he was driving down a "freeway" and hit a car-towing truck and the truck kept going. Again, there was no physical injury to the patient and no history of headaches.

The patient was given forms to fill out to evaluate his headaches on the basis of the intensity of the headaches, and these intensities in the future will be identified. A #3 headache, or incapacitating headache, limits your function to having to either sit still or lie in bed. A #2 headache, or interfering headache, is a moderate to severe headache which generally permits you to perform essential tasks, but with a great deal of discomfort, and you are not able to do pleasurable tasks. A #1 headache, or an irritating headache, is an annoying headache that is generally relieved with over-the-counter medications, massage, or similar types of treatment.

Incapacitating or #3 headaches: They started with the accident on [...] 1993, and were daily for several weeks. He would have these attacks about three times a week since the accident until this current time. On May [...], 1994, and June [...], 1994, the patient had epidural blocks and after the June [...], 1994 block, he had a cerebrospinal leak and was having an incapacitating headache for a three-week period of time, and then the headaches again became a three-times-a-week problem. He states that these attacks seem to come in the morning and later in the evening, and sometimes during the day. The duration of the headache will last for days without any medications, and during this time he will put himself into traction and take Flexeril, a muscle relaxant, three times a day, and Naprosyn, a nonsteroidal anti-inflammatory, twice a day, and his Elavil 50 mg at night.

He describes the character of this pain as either a crushing of his skull or a feeling like a knife is current from inside of his skull to the outside. There is no prodrome, or warning sign of the headache, and no aura either official or sensory.

Associated features of this headache will be nausea at times, sensitivity to light, noise, odors, and he has been told that he gets pale or flushed when he gets these headaches. He has been told that his eyelid droops, and he has to go to bed.

Precipitating or aggravating factors are lights, noise, driving, and activity, and as soon as he gets this headache, he will put himself in traction and go into a dark room. The location of the headache is mostly in the frontal and parietal, or sides, of his head and radiates to the occipital portion of his head. There is also some pain in the posterior cervical region.

Interfering or #2 headaches: These seem to come on after his daily incapacitating headaches reduced from daily to three times a week. He states that he gets this headache every day and that this headache basically is no different from the #3 or incapacitating headache, except with slightly less intensity. He states that the onset of these headaches, like his incapacitating headaches if he is not having them, is in the morning and at night.

He states that the duration of these headaches without medications will last two to four hours and he will have these several times a day; with medications, one to three hours.

The character of pain is also a stabbing, crushing, or cutting, with somewhat less intensity than the incapacitating headache. There is no prodrome or aura.

Associated features include sensitivity to light, noise, and odors, like in the incapacitating headaches.

The location of headaches is in the posterocervical region radiating up to the parietal and frontal regions of his head.

Irritating or #1 Headaches: He has had this type of headache since the accident, and again he described this headache as a decrease in intensity of the #2 or interfering headache. Therefore, the patient states that he has headaches every day ranging in intensity from irritating to interfering (moderate to severe) to incapacitating.

He states that prior to the accident, he would have this irritating headache as a youngster if he were sick or did not eat all day, or did not sleep for long periods of time. These headaches seemed to stop after his teenage years, until the accident.

Location of this headache is in the posterocervical occipital region and parietal frontal regions of his head.

PAST HISTORY

The patient was most probably a normal delivery. There is no history of enuresis or unexplained abdominal cramps pre-puberty. There is no history of car sickness as a child. There is no history of meningitis, encephalitis, scarlet fever, or rheumatic fever. There were no head injuries as a child.

HABITS

He states that he rarely drinks. Once in four or five months he may have a gin and tonic or a glass of wine, but does not get headache with it, and he smokes a pack of cigarettes a day.

MEDICAL HISTORY

His is essentially normal and there is no history of any pulmonary, cardiovascular, gastrointestinal, or urogenital problems.

SURGICAL HISTORY

He had a tonsillectomy in [...].

PSYCHIATRIC HISTORY

He has no history of psychotherapy.

FAMILY HISTORY

His father is living, age approximately 75, with no headache history. Mother is living, age 68, with no headache history. There are two brothers, one 46 and one 44. The younger one has some headaches. There are two sisters, 43 and 42, with no headaches. He has been married from age [...] to present and there are five children, girls 12, 9, and 3, and two boys, 7 and 4, and none of them have headache histories.

The patient has been on multiple medications since he has been in treatment and has been on muscle relaxants such as Soma and Parafon Forte and currently Flexeril.

He currently is on Amitriptyline or Elavil. He also has been on Pamelor and Desyrel in the past. He currently is taking Bellergal-S daily, which he said seems to help because if he stops it, his headaches will become worse. He also takes Midrin, which also seems to help reduce the number of these incapacitating headaches.

He has taken multiple analgesics in the past, such as Darvocet-N 100, Fiorinal with Codeine, Lorcet Plus, and currently on occasion he takes Ultram.

He has seen multiple practitioners in the past since his accident. He has seen [...], DDS, and is being treated with a centric splint and cervical traction, and physical therapy for a TMJ (temporomandibular joint) problem since his accident. He has seen a Dr. [...], who is his family physician, and has been treated since the accident by this physician.

After the accident, he was taken to the emergency room at [...] Hospital where his complaints were moderate amounts of dizziness and left-sided frontal head pain. At that time, he did not complain of neck or back pain, which he states started later that day or the following day. He was diagnosed with a forehead hematoma.

He had also seen on, [...], 1994, [...] MD, a neurologist, and was diagnosed as having post-traumatic headaches. He has also seen Dr. S. [...], orthopedic doctor, on [...], 1994, for his back, and Dr. M. [...] in [...], 1996, and had an MRI of his back, which the patient states showed a protruding disk. Also, on [...], 1994, he had seen Dr. [...] at the [...] Clinic, and was diagnosed as: 1) "post-traumatic cervicogenic headache, 2) cervical strains/sprains secondary to motor vehicle accident, and 3) lumbar sprain/strain secondary to motor vehicle accident." On May [...], 1994, the patient had a cervical steroid epidural block, and another one on June [...], 1994. It appears that he had a "wet tap," and then had a severe incapacitating headache for several weeks. He returned on June [...], 1994, and stated that he felt "considerably improved," and can stand 15 to 20 minutes up to an hour before his headaches become symptomatic.

On June [...], 1994, Dr. [...] at the [...] Clinic felt that the patient had reached his MMI (maximum medical improvement), and was given an impairment rating based on the Minnesota guidelines that would be 5% for his headaches, and 3.5% for cervical complaints, for a total of 8.5% as an impairment rating.

The patient returned to see Dr. [...] on December [...], 1994, and it appears that his headaches were about the same or "a little better" and he was currently working; however, Dr. [...] felt he still remained as a maximum medical improvement with the same impairment and was to be seen in three to six months for medication management.

PHYSICAL EXAMINATION

Blood pressure 120/80, pulse 78. The patient is six feet tall and weighs approximately 220 pounds. The lungs were clear to auscultation and percussion. There was no asymmetry to the face, and eyes appeared normal. Conjunctivae were clear and pupils reacted equally to light and accommodation. Retinal fundus examination revealed no papilledema and no abnormalities of the arteries or veins.

In reviewing all the reports of the different physicians who have examined the patient, the neurological examinations all seemed to be within normal limits, and therefore another neurological examination of the patient's body was not done.

However, I did pay attention to the muscles and myofascial aspects of the neck and face and found some abnormal findings. In palpating the posterocervical region of the patient's neck bilaterally, I found two active trigger points on the right upper neck region in the area of the upper trapezius and the splenius capitis muscles, and found some tender points on the left side all along the scapula, trapezius, splenius capitis, etc. In palpating the trigger points on the right side, which are felt as taut bands, I could induce an increase in headache pain by pressing on these bands, which caused referred pain by definition of an active trigger point. He also demonstrated a "jump sign" as described by Travell and Simons in their textbook, *Myofascial Pain and Dysfunction, The Trigger Point Manual.* Also, in palpating the lateral (external) pterygoid muscles, I was able to elicit increased pain in both posterior and anterior aspects of these trigger points. The pain was in the frontal region of his face and also in the posterior region in front of his ear. This also began to increase the pain of his headache.

DIAGNOSES

1. Automobile injury [...], 1993, of an acceleration/deceleration type accident.
2. Continued post traumatic/concussion cervicogenic headache.
3. Cervicogenic headache with vascular features (migraine-like).
4. Chronic active trigger points in the posterior cervical region and area of the temporomandibular joint, increasing both muscular and vascular type headaches.
5. Secondary to automobile accident on [...], 1993, chronic, ongoing, continuous headaches varying in intensity from irritating to incapacitating.
6. Previous in early life, teenage years, irritating headaches which went into remission.
7. Previous lumbar strain/sprain secondary to a work accident in 1980, which was resolved by late 1987.
8. By previous examinations and histories of other physicians since his accident interviewed lumbar sprain/strain secondary to motor vehicle accident.

IMPRESSION

This pleasant 35-year-old gentleman and his wife were interviewed for one hour and a half after I had reviewed all the records that were available to me from other physicians.

The patient and his wife were very cooperative and seemed to give a history that was consistent with his problems, and there did not seem to be symptoms that were added extraneously to increase the depth of his problems. I was impressed by the fact that both patient and his wife were more concerned about the means of treating and ending this problem, rather than continuing to talk about the symptoms.

The fact that these headaches did not clear and resolve after six months would make this then a chronic condition. Significant literature studies have shown that those who continue to have these headaches past that period of time, whether or not litigation was resolved, continued after five years to the extent of 30% of the cases.

The fact that this was a side-impact or broadside collision, from a biomechanical point of view, the chances of more severe alterations of these soft tissue injuries have a greater propensity than a rear or frontal type of accident. The reason is, in side impact there is little protection to lateral acceleration forces by either seat back or restraint systems. This explains why there is a high incidence of low back pain in this type of collision. The initial response to impact is lateral flexion toward the striking vehicle, with compression of the spinal structures on the concave side, and stretching of myofascial and other structures on the convex side. The lap belt will serve as an anchor for the pelvis, thus reducing the potential for serious injury related to ejection trauma. But, the anchoring may intensify bending movements in the lumbosacral or thoracolumbar spine, thus increasing the likelihood of soft tissue injury. In the case of a broadside collision, the resulting vectors of deceleration for the occupants will be oblique. In the case of a car that is struck on the driver's side, the occupant will decelerate in a vector that is forward and toward the striking car. It has been shown that the oblique rear-impact collisions hold much greater potential for injury than pure rear-impact collisions. The impact is not only extension and then flexion, but also ramping, which is an upward spiraling effect, that adds to the injury.

On examination of the patient, multiple *trigger points* were found. Trigger points are a focus of hyperirritability in a tissue that, when compressed, are locally tender and are officially hypersensitive, and give rise to referred pain and tenderness. A trigger point is felt as a taut or palpable band or nodule, and these are a group of taut muscle fibers that are associated with the myofascial trigger point and are identifiable by a tactile examination of the muscle. Both a latent and myofascial trigger point are painful when palpated. With this hyperirritability, one will see a "jump sign" in which there is a general pain response of the patient who winces and may cry out, and he may withdraw in response to pressure applied to a trigger point. An active trigger point is one in which on palpation there is referred pain and the pain is felt at a distance from the palpation. This distribution of a referred third trigger point pain does not necessarily coincide with the distribution of the peripheral nerve, or dermoterminal segment. Oftentimes with an active trigger point, you can also get a referred autonomic response or phenomenon which is also at a distance from the palpation of the trigger point, which produces vasoconstriction (blanching), coldness, sweating, ptosis, or hypersecretion. That is caused by activity of a trigger point in a region separate from the trigger point. In palpating the various trigger points in the posterocervical muscles, such as the trapezius, the splenius capitis, and the sternocleidomastoid muscle, I could produce pain in the top of the head and frontal region of the head. Also, in palpating the area of the temporomandibular joint around the masseter muscle, and the pterygoid muscles, I was able to increase the patient's headaches and have pain in areas referred further from the area of palpation.

I feel that the headaches are precipitated from the ongoing active trigger points and the inflammation of the tendons attached from these muscles to the skull and the bodies of the vertebrae. Because of this inflammation, the nerve becomes irritated and this begins a pain process through the nervous pathways to the brain. I also feel that the migraine headaches are a result of these continuous inflamed areas and the trigger points, and that one type of headache feeds the other. It is interesting to note that the patient tends to get some relief when he puts himself in traction on the floor to immobilize the cervical region of his neck, and also when he stays in a dark, quiet room, which is typical for people who have migraine-like headaches.

***One also has to consider the diagnosis of cervicogenic headache based on the chronicity and the type of headache and the fact that the patient gets relief when he puts himself in traction. Therefore, special studies should be done with MRI of the zygapophyseal joint and a nerve block into that joint should be carried out. If the patient gets relief from this block over a period of time, weeks to months, then a radiofrequency neurotomy should be considered.**

Therefore, as long as the inflammation and trigger points remain, he will continue to have these types of headache. I feel that as long as he continues to have these painful areas, starting from irritating to incapacitating intensities, this will continue to interfere with his ability to function and take on the responsibilities of increasing his workload and also going to school to complete his degree in engineering. Therefore, I feel that it is the pain of these cervicogenic and vascular headaches that has created a disability. Utilizing the Minnesota guidelines, I feel this patient, for his hidden ache, neck only, has an impairment rating of 8.5%, that is 5% for the headache because of the association of nausea which is associated with vascular headache, and 3.5% for the cervical spine, because of the pain associated with the rigidity (loss of motion or postural abnormality) or chronic spasm. The chronic muscle spasm or rigidity is substantiated by objective clinical findings. These objective findings were the palpation of the active trigger points and this is 3.5%.

I do not feel that there is a cure for this problem, but there may be several methods to reduce the discomfort to permit the patient a greater latitude to work and to be less incapacitated. These methods would be the use of various medications, such as beta-blockers, or calcium channel blockers, to help reduce some of the vascular headaches, and regional nerve blocks of C1, 2, and 3, or about the greater occipital and lesser occipital and also the spinal segment of the trigeminal nerve. This spinal segment of the trigeminal nerve will be affected by the absorption of the medications for the regional block. If the regional blocks utilizing an anesthetic such as lidocaine and Marcaine and steroids such as DepoMedrol are effective for any period of time, then I would suggest the substitution of Sarapin, which is a nonsteroid, and may give the patient some relief in the cervical region for longer periods of time, hopefully three to six months at a time. *** Again, if there are positive findings for zygapophyseal joint disease, then these joints should be injected before long and palliative treatment procedures carried out.**

For many reasons associated with my background and years of experience with these problems, I do not see any malingering or other types of psychological mechanisms for secondary gain, but rather one who sincerely wants to be better and wants to be more productive and in a higher position to care for his wife and five children. The only psychological factors involved would be some depression and frustration because of the continuous pain. I feel that if the pain is relieved or reduced significantly, these other symptoms would also be decreased.

Sincerely,

BERNARD SWERDLOW, MD

CHAPTER 24

Examination of the Patient

The headache intake form has been discussed in Chapter 4. I cannot overstate the importance of a detailed comprehensive history in establishing the diagnosis of the headache condition. Whether the headache is the result of an insidious condition or the result of an accident, or a combination, it is the history that is going to direct the examiner in determining any other workup that will be considered. If the patient is being seen as a result of an accident and litigation may be involved then the pre-accident history is also essential.

When completing the headache intake form, it is important to list key factors for the examiner to review. Remember the examiner is attempting to differentiate between physiological, psychological, pathological, non-accident, accident, and any reasons for the headache problem from which the patient is suffering. It is the patient who is going to cue the examiner on what direction should be followed in working up the disorder.

Important information to report concerning the headache includes:

1. Abruptness of onset
2. Progression of headache pattern
3. Any abnormal physical problems
4. Any abnormal neurological findings
5. Alleviating factors
6. Provoking factors:
    - Hormonal changes
        - Oral contraceptives
        - Menstruation
        - Hormonal replacement
        - Amenorrhea
    - Medications
    - Exertion
    - Changes in position
    - Changes in weather
    - Lack of, or excessive, sleep
    - Stress, exhilaration, let-down, over-demand, anger, depression, etc.
    - Bright lights
    - Loud noises
    - Smoke
    - Missed meals
    - Certain foods

Table 24.1 demonstrates certain foods that may provoke a headache and foods that can be used to avoid vascular headaches.

A mental status examination, at least in a cursory manner, is done to rule out any major psychiatric disease and to make sure there is no organic reason for abnormal behavior, such as chemical abuse or work-related chemical causes. Orientation is also important in the diagnosis of aging diseases and pathological processes taking place. After an accident or head injury, it is extremely important to look for "soft neurological signs" that may demonstrate themselves as psychiatric symptoms.

There are many people who may appear to respond to questions in an appropriate way and then are totally incapable of producing answers concerning recent memory. Confabulation is a symptom of an organically induced brain dysfunction. When an affected patient does not have the capacity to answer the question, they will confabulate by filling in material that is irrelevant to the question. Unfortunately, the patients do not realize that they are confabulating. Sometimes the mental status examination is the only clue that an intracranial condition is occurring, such as an infection, tumor, bleeding, brain cell deterioration, or any condition that is slowly altering the brain's ability to function. Interestingly, headache that often is considered a benign disease may actually be the first sign of a malignant disease.

If the headaches are related to an accident, then documentation is essential. Once this becomes part of the legal system, then anything that is not written down can be considered nonexistent. Anything that existed before the accident is used as a base line. Were there headaches existing before the accident? Were there any medical illnesses that preceded the accident that caused headaches? Was there any emotional illness that necessitated psychological treatment before the accident? Were there any doctors' office visits or emergency room visits where headache was discussed, even if headache was not the primary reason for the visit? Did the accident cause or aggravate the current headache condition? Since the accident, is there a different type of headache, different frequency, different duration? Everything that existed before the accident and all the symptoms that followed the accident must be reported.

I cannot emphasize enough that the worst approach the patient can take is to purposely omit any of the above information. Lawyers are excellent investigators. They will do a thorough examination of the patient's background, and any information that appears to be withheld will be held against the patient. This holds true for the defense as well as for the plaintiff. If the examining physician finds during a legal conference or a deposition that the patient has not been honest, then that physician will no longer feel confident in supporting his or her assessment of the case. It might also appear that the treating physician is attempting to hide this information and any previous episodes of trauma. If the independent medical examiner has the same information, then he or she will hold that against the patient and either way the patient will lose their credibility. The chances of a deception not being found out after the patient has been examined by the multiple examiners and the records scrutinized by the insurance companies and law offices are at least slim and probably close to impossible.

If the headache syndrome is secondary to a vehicular trauma, then all the information regarding that accident should be brought to the examiner in order to understand the biomechanics of the injury. Police reports of the accident will also help in understanding the physical forces involved and to clarify the shearing forces that promote the injury. Information as to whether seat belts were worn, or whether they were lap or shoulder or both; was the head struck on any stationary item; were the patient's glasses knocked off or were dentures knocked out; was the patient aware that an accident was imminent, or was it a total surprise?

Besides the information filled in on the headache intake form, other complaints from the accident should also be noted, such as loss of consciousness, seizures, visual disturbances, pain other than headache, weakness in any other parts of the body, and any other symptoms that are being treated by another physician or any medical personnel.

After the history the examiner proceeds with the physical examination. Other than head and neck injuries that may cause headache, there are hundreds of other reasons that may also cause

Table 24.1

Food	Foods Allowed	Foods to Avoid
Beverages	Decaffeinated coffee, fruit juices, club soda, noncola sodas. *Caffeine sources to be limited to 2 cups per day.	Caffeine sources*: coffee, tea, cola-type soda, in excess of 2 cups, no chocolate or cocoa. Alcoholic beverages: none.
Meat, fish, poultry	Fresh or frozen: turkey, chicken, fish, beef, lamb, veal, pork, egg as meat substitute (limit 3 eggs a week), tuna, tuna salad.	Aged, canned, cured or processed meats, canned or aged ham, pickled herring, salted dried fish, chicken liver, aged game, hot dogs, fermented sausages (no nitrates or nitrites): bologna, salami, pepperoni, summer sausage; peanut and peanut butter; any meat prepared with meat tenderizer, soy sauce or yeast extracts.
Dairy	Milk: homogenized, 2%, or skim. Cheese: American, cottage, farmer's, ricotta, cream cheese, Yogurt: limit to $^1/_2$ cup.	Cultured dairy, such as buttermilk, sour cream, chocolate milk. Cheese: bleu, Boursault, brick, Brie types, camembert types, cheddar, Swiss, gouda, roquefort, Stilton, mozzarella, parmesan, provolone, romano, Emmentaler.
Breads and cereals	Commercial breads: white, whole wheat, rye, French, Italian, English muffin, melba toast, crackers, rye krisp, bagel. All hot and dry cereals: cream of wheat, oatmeal, cornflakes, puffed wheat, rice, all-bran, etc.	Hot, fresh, homemade yeast breads, breads and crackers with cheese. Fresh yeast coffee cake, doughnuts, sour dough breads. Any containing chocolate or nuts.
Potato or substitute	White potato, sweet potato, rice, macaroni, spaghetti, noodles.	
Vegetables	Asparagus, string beans, beets, carrots, spinach, pumpkin, tomatoes, squash, corn, zucchini, broccoli, green lettuce, etc. All except those to avoid.	Pole or broad beans, lima or Italian beans, lentils, snow peas, fava beans, navy beans, pinto beans, pea pods, sauerkraut, garbanzo beans, onions except for flavoring, olives, pickles.
Fruits	Any juice, such as prune, apple, applesauce, cherries, apricots, peach, pear, fruit cocktail. Limit intake to $^1/_2$ cup: orange, grapefruit, tangerine, pineapple, lemon, lime.	Avocados, banana (1/2 allowed per day), figs, raisins, papaya, passion fruit, red plums. Nuts and seeds: peanut butter, sunflower, sesame, and pumpkin seeds, peanuts.
Soups	Cream soups made from foods allowed. Homemade broths.	Canned soups: soup cubes, bouillon cubes, soup bases with autolyzed yeast or monosodium glutamate (MSG) (read labels).
Desserts	Fruit listed above, sherbets, ice cream, cakes and cookies made without chocolate or yeast, jello.	Chocolate type: ice cream, pudding, cookies, cakes, mincemeat pies.
Sweet	Sugar, jelly, jam, honey, hard candy.	Chocolate candies, chocolate syrup, carob.
Miscellaneous	Salt in moderation, lemon juices, butter or margaine, cooking oils; whipped cream.	Pizza, cheese sauce, soy sauce, MSG in excessive amounts, yeast, yeast extracts, Brewer's yeast, meat tenderizers, seasoned salt.
	White vinegar and commercial salad dressing in small amounts.	Mixed dishes: macaroni and cheese; beef stroganoff; cheese blintzes, lasagna; frozen TV dinners.
		Nuts and seeds: peanut butter, pumpkin, sesame.
		Some snack items to be avoided. Read all labels. Any pickled, preserved, or marinated foods.

From Diamond, S., Dalessio, D.J., *The Practicing Physician's Approach to Headache,* 4th ed., Williams & Wilkins, Baltimore, 1986. With permission.

this type of pain. Therefore, an attempt must be made to find any cause of headache that might be organically induced.

In ruling out physical disease, the vital signs, heart, lungs, abdomen, eyes, ears, and mouth are examined. A neurological examination is done of the cranial nerves, the brain (motor sensory and cerebellar systems), the reflexes, and the vascular pulses.[2] The muscular system of the head and neck is also examined and must be evaluated after any accident. The outline of the physical examination is presented as part of the headache intake form in Chapter 4.

If, after the history and physical, the examiner needs further validation for a medical or neurological condition, the laboratory, radiology department, or other medical specialties may be called upon. These approaches were discussed in Chapter 12 (How to Diagnose Headaches) and should be referred to.

After a whiplash (cervical acceleration/deceleration) accident or a post concussion/trauma accident where headache is the presenting symptom, the examiner must evaluate whether there are any other symptoms that may have been caused by this injury. Therefore, examination of the muscles and their attachments, the bones, and the nervous system of the head and neck must be carried out.

Palpation of the muscles may reveal active or latent trigger points, atrophy, swelling, tenderness or spasms. Palpation may also reveal abnormal lymph glands and any abnormality in the size of the thyroid gland. Inspection of the temporomandibular joints may reveal tenderness or asymmetry of mandibular motion.

Range of motion: In examining the neck, the range of motion may give information as to the integrity of the bones, ligaments, and the musculature. If there is a restriction of the range of motion there may be a fracture or a dislocation of bone or compression of the facet joints. Tears or spasms of the ligaments or muscles may also restrict motion.

Coordination test: Any accident that causes shearing forces to the neck and head may cause neurological injury to the spinal cord or the brain. Damage to the dorsal columns of the spinal cord or to the cerebellum will affect coordination, gait, and equilibrium.

The walking test done with the eyes closed and heel-to-toe reveals information about the patient's ability to walk smoothly and execute turns with balance and no aid.

The Romberg test is performed by instructing the patient to place his feet together, close his eyes, and maintain a normal balance. If the patient sways or falls, then this test is considered positive (Figure 24.1).

The finger test requires the patient to close his or her eyes and touch the tip of the nose with the index finger, with the arm starting outstretched from the side of the body and moving smoothly in the direction of the face (Figure 24.2).

The finger movement test requires the patient to touch each finger with the thumb rapidly and also to be able to touch the tip of a pen with the thumb and index finger. The inability to do this is called dysdiadokinesia (Figure 24.3).

The rebound phenomenon test (Holmes test) requires the patient to stop strong active movements. If the examiner holds the contracted arm and then quickly releases it, the patient will strike his/her shoulder if there is cord or cerebellar damage.

Motor strength: If there was damage to the neck, especially in the area of C5 to T1, and the nerve root was involved, various muscles could be affected, which can be demonstrated by examination. The table lists nerves that affect involved muscles:[3]

Level	Nerve	Muscles
C5	Axillary	Deltoid [Figure 24.4A]
C6	Musculocutaneous	Biceps [Figure 24.4B]
C7	Radial	Triceps [Figure 24.4C]
C8	Median	Finger flexors [Figure 24.4D]
T1	Ulnar	Finger abductors

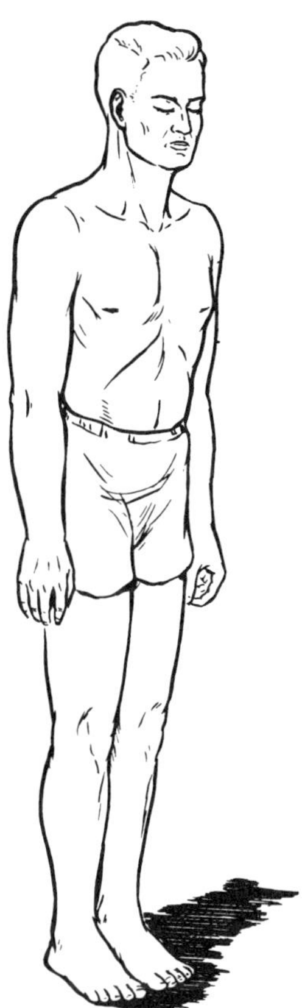

Figure 24.1 The Romberg test. (From Van Allen, M.W., *Pictorial Manual of Neurologic Tests*, Mosby-Year Book, Chicago, 1969. With permission.)

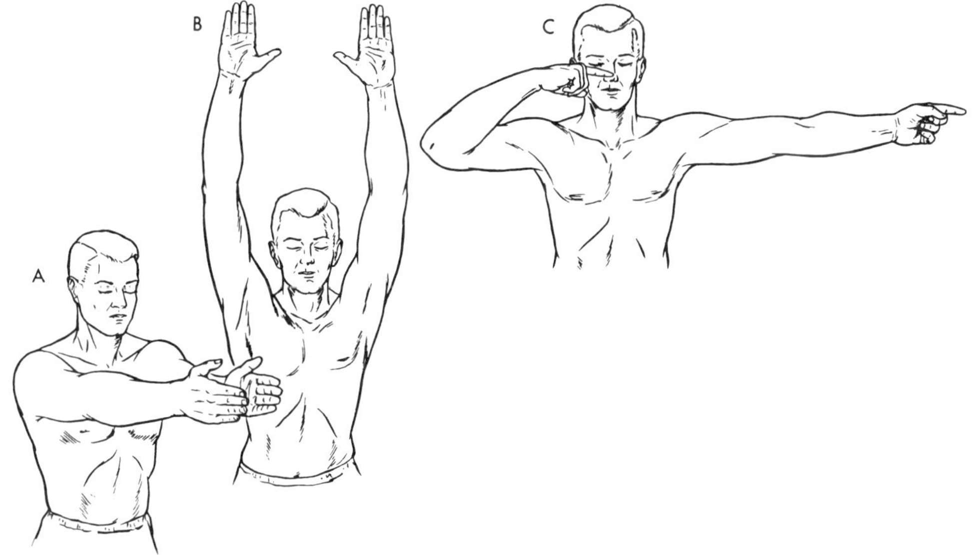

Figure 24.2 Posture of arms and hands. (From Van Allen, M.W., *Pictorial Manual of Neurologic Tests*, Mosby-Year Book, Chicago, 1969. With permission.)

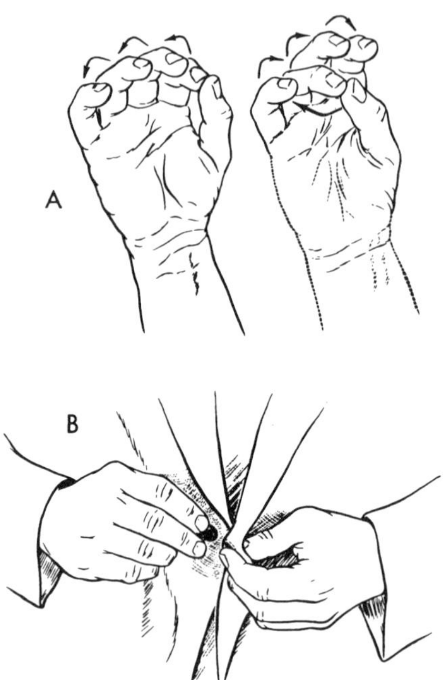

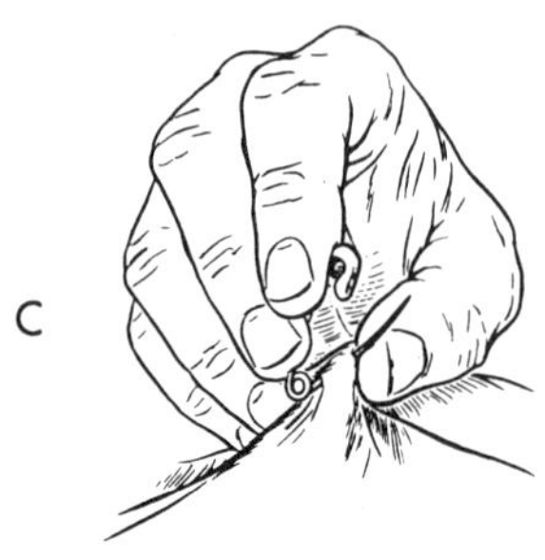

Figure 24.3 Finger movement tests. (From Van Allen, M.W., *Pictorial Manual of Neurologic Tests*, Mosby-Year Book, Chicago, 1969. With permission.)

Examining the endurance or strength of the muscle may offer evidence of nerve root damage. The grades are numbered 0 to 5, with 5 considered normal, to 0 where there is no evidence of muscle contraction.

Sensory examination: Whenever the examiner finds any suspicious symptoms on a cursory sensory evaluation, the patient should be referred to a neurologist for a complete examination. Sensory alterations may be caused by injuries to specific peripheral nerves or spinal nerve roots (Figure 24.5).

These injuries may cause alterations in:

1. Pain perception, and may be detected by complete loss of sensation (anesthesia), diminished sensation (hypesthesia), increased sensibility to touch (hyperesthesia), and increased sensibility to pain (hyperalgesia) (Figure 24.6).
2. Temperature sensibility may be altered by damage to the peripheral nerves or the lateral spinothalamic tract of the spinal cord. The patient loses the perception of hot or cold (Figure 24.7).
3. Two point discrimination is a test where two pins are placed closely together on the patient's skin and gradually moved farther apart until the two separate points are felt. The distance at which it is felt varies on different parts of the body. This discrimination is determined by specialized tactile receptors using the dorsal columns and the lemniscal system in the brainstem (Figure 24.8).
4. Vibratory perception is perceived by special cells called Meissner and Pacini corpuscles and is transmitted in the dorsal column. A testing tuning fork (128-cycle/second) is placed on a bony prominence and it is determined if the vibration is felt. (Figure 24.9).
5. Sense of position tests both the static and kinesthetic (perception of position) of the joints or extremity in relation to the body. With eyes closed, the patient attempts to determine the direction of the movement of the joint (i.e., the great toe). There are many nerve endings that are responsible for interpreting these joint movements (Ruffini endings, Golgi tendon receptors, Pacini corpuscles), which then are transmitted to the dorsal column of the spinal cord.

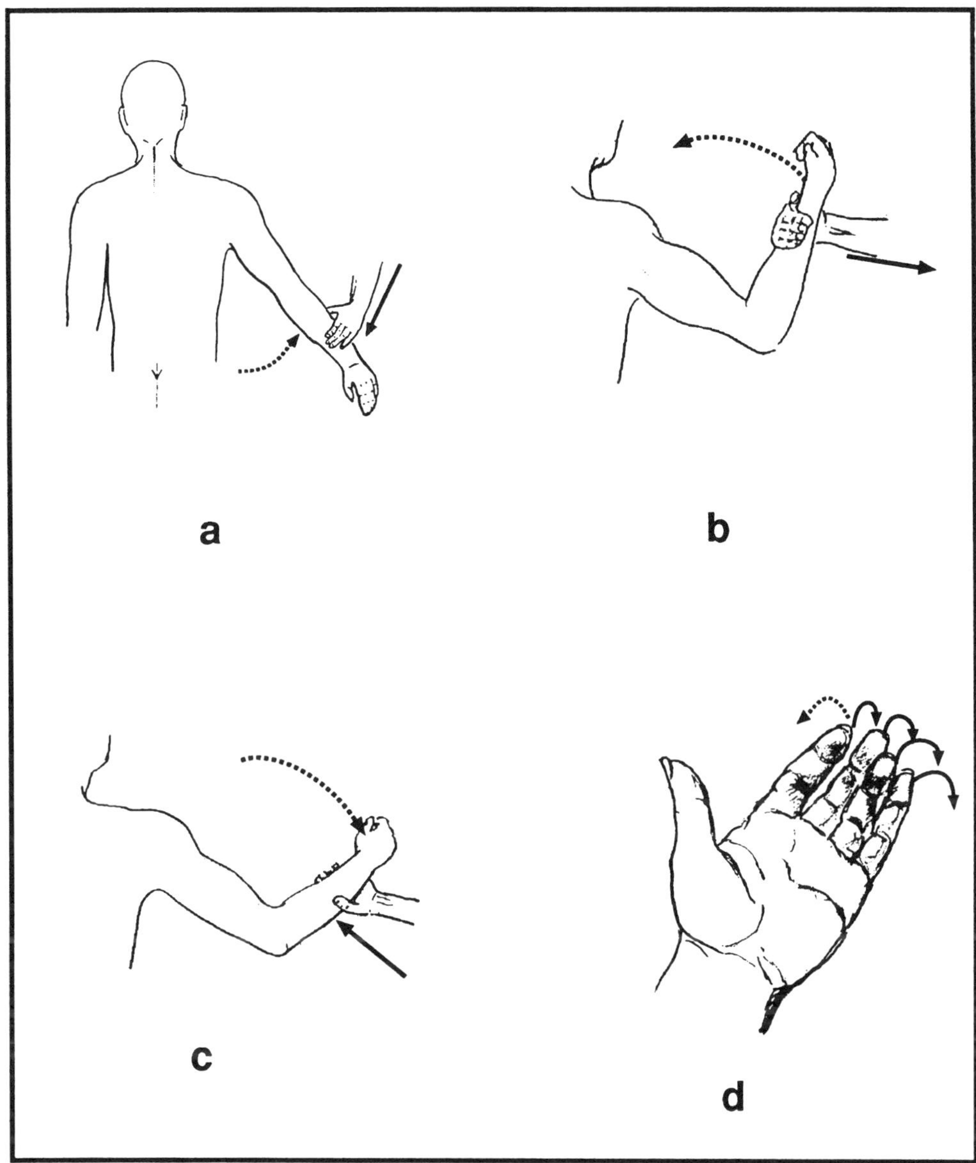

Figure 24.4 Illustrations to demonstrate strength of the following muscles: (a) Deltoid, C5-6; (b) biceps, C5-6; (c) triceps, C6-8; and (d) finger flexors, C7, 8, and T1.

6. Stereognosis is the brain's ability to interpret weights and forms of objects held in the hand. With the eyes closed, the patient is asked to recognize and identify objects like a key or coin, etc., when placed in the hand (Figure 24.10).
7. Light touch is that ability to perceive sensation on the skin like the stroke of a thread.
8. Topogenosis is the ability of the patient to recognize with eyes closed the spot where the examiner touched the skin.

Circulatory tests: Just as sensations such as numbness and parathesias arise from neurological disorders, they may also arise from circulatory disorders as a result of cervical acceleration/deceleration (whiplash disorders) which may decrease the vascular supply.

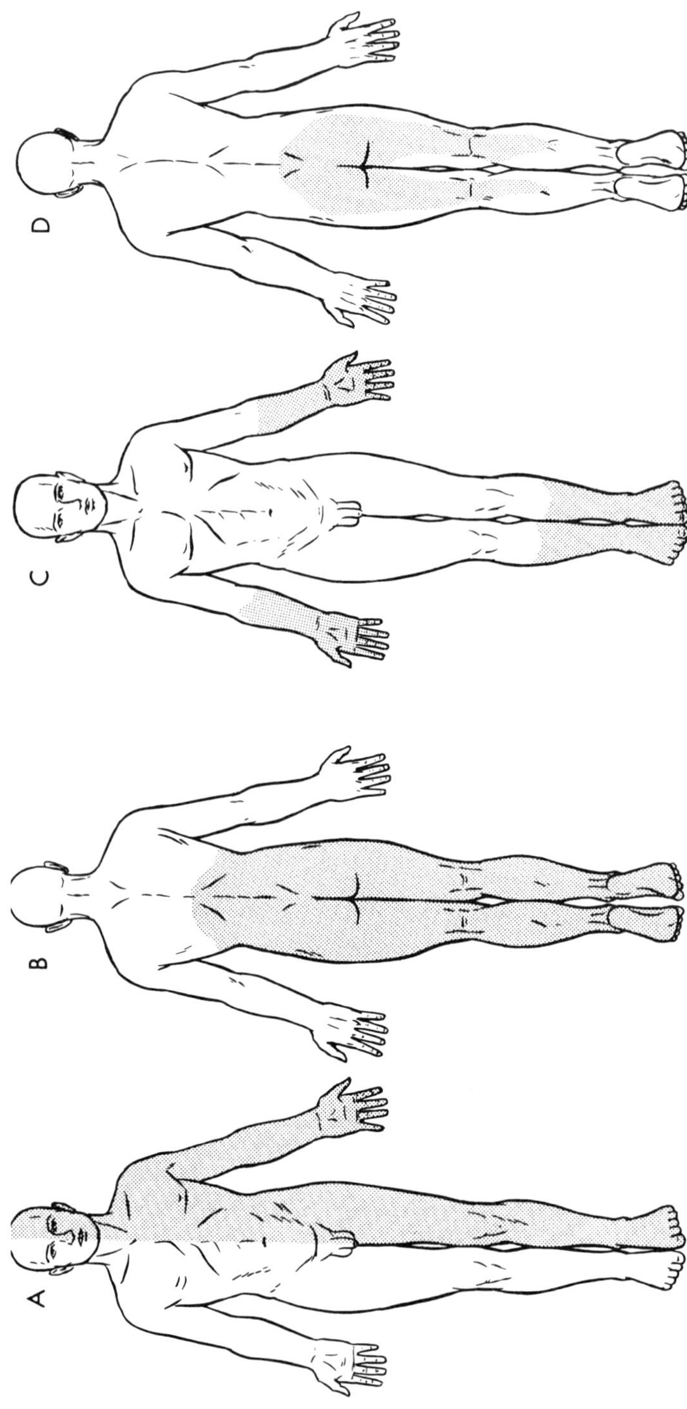

Figure 24.5 Patterns of sensory loss. (From Van Allen, M.W., *Pictorial Manual of Neurologic Tests*, Mosby-Year Book, Chicago, 1969. With permission.)

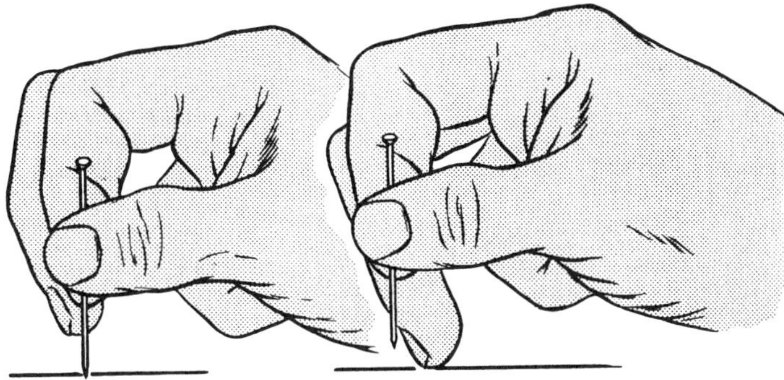

Figure 24.6 Testing for pain sensation. (From Van Allen, M.W., *Pictorial Manual of Neurologic Tests*, Mosby-Year Book, Chicago, 1969. With permission.)

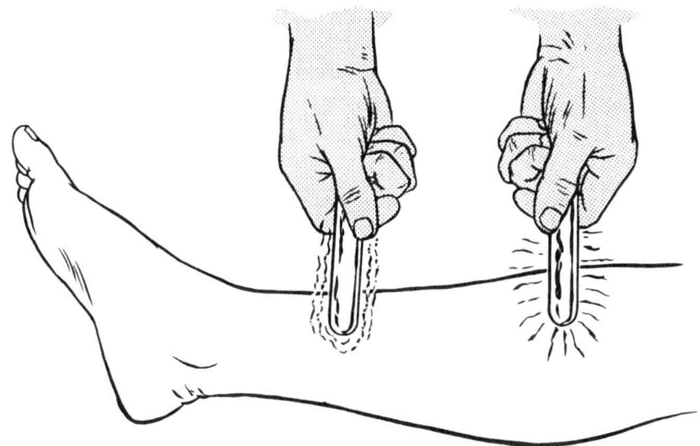

Figure 24.7 Testing for temperature sensation. (From Van Allen, M.W., *Pictorial Manual of Neurologic Tests*, Mosby-Year Book, Chicago, 1969. With permission.)

Adson's test will be the only test described in this book because one of the injuries from a cervical acceleration/deceleration (whiplash) may cause a thoracic outlet syndrome (see Chapter 14) with symptoms of parathesias and pain to the arm, forearm, and fourth and fifth fingers. The examiner palpates the patient's radial pulse and establishes the rate, force, and amplitude. The patient then rotates the head toward the side being tested, raises the chin, and takes a deep breath for twelve seconds. The examiner will try to detect an alteration in the radial pulse as a result of neurovascular compression of the subclavian artery.

Blood pressure testing is always done in any physical examination.

Reflex examination: A reflex is an involuntary motor response to sensory stimuli. It starts from the extremity through the spinal cord and back to the extremity. If there is a disruption in this lower neuron, then the reflex is disrupted. Injury in the central nervous system may cause an increase in the reflex by causing a loss of inhibition to the reflex. Reflexes are graded from 0 to 4. A grade of 2–, 2, or 2+ is considered normal. Less than 2– is hypoactive, and 3 or more is hyperactive.

It is beyond the scope of this book on headaches to describe neuropathology of abnormal reflexes, but a list of common reflexes will be mentioned in the event the name appears on the medical report.

1. Maxillary or jaw reflex
2. Biceps reflex (C5)

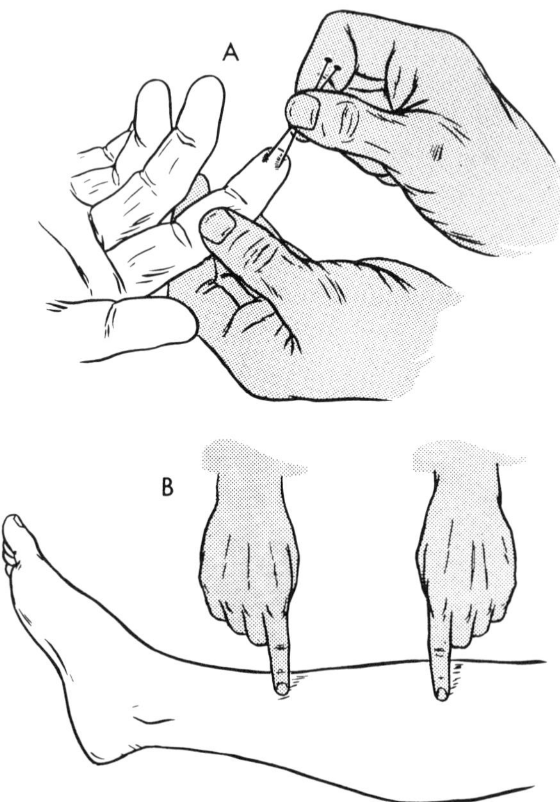

Figure 24.8 Two-point discrimination (see text). (From Van Allen, M.W., *Pictorial Manual of Neurologic Tests*, Mosby-Year Book, Chicago, 1969. With permission.)

3. Brachioradialis reflex (C6)
4. Triceps reflex (C7)
5. Patellar or knee reflex (L4)
6. Achilles reflex (S1)
7. Other upper extremity reflexes (Figure 24.11)
   - Chaddock's wrist sign
   - Hoffmann's sign
   - Gordon's finger sign
   - Tromners sign
   - Forced grasping sign
   - Souques' sign
8. Other Lower Extremity Reflexes (Figure 24.12)
   - Babinski's sign
   - Schaffer's sign
   - Oppenheims's sign
   - Gordon's sign
   - Rossolimo's sign
   - Gonda reflex
   - Ankle clonus
   - Patellars clonus (treidation sign)

As a result of a whiplash injury, cervical levels from C5 to T1 (thoracic) may be involved. The following levels of nerves may affect the motor innervation of different muscles and the sensory innervation in specific areas of the arm.[3]

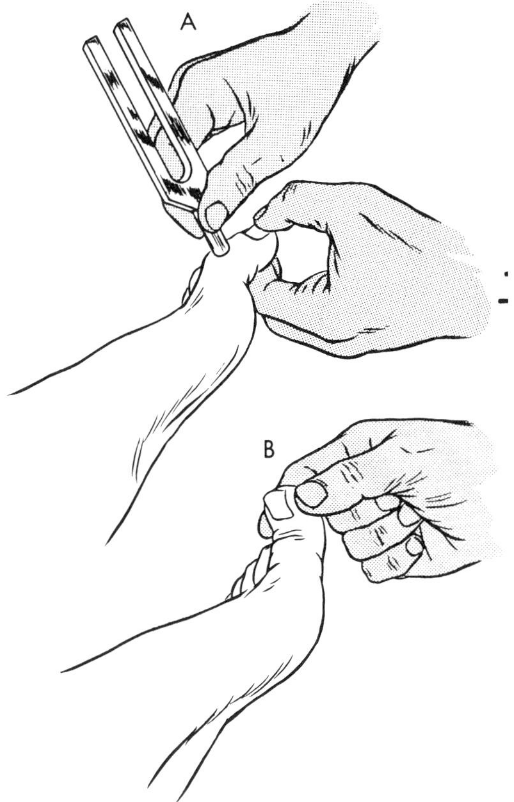

Figure 24.9 Vibratory and position sense (see text). (From Van Allen, M.W., *Pictorial Manual of Neurologic Tests*, Mosby-Year Book, Chicago, 1969. With permission.)

C5 neurological level. The C5 nerve root is the uppermost level of the brachial plexus. It supplies motor innervation to the deltoid and the biceps as well as many other muscles. It also supplies the sensory innervation via the axillary nerve to the lateral arm. This level is tested with the biceps reflex (Figure 24.13).

C6 neurological level. The upper trunk of the brachial plexus is made up of both the C5 and C6 nerve root. It supplies motor innervation to the biceps and wrist extensor muscles. The sensory innervation to the lateral forearm comes from the musculocutaneous nerve receiving some of its supply from C-6. The brachioradialis muscle, although it receives sensory innervation from the radial nerve, is largely a function of C6 (Figure 24.14).

C7 neurological level. The C7 nerve root is the primary supplier of motor innervation to the triceps, finger extensors, and wrist flexor muscles. Branches of the ulnar, radial, and median nerves receive input from C7. The triceps reflex is the primary indicator of C7 neurological function. The third finger on each hand receives its sensory supply from the C7 level (Figure 24.15).

The neuroanatomy, neurophysiology, and neuropathology of the cervical nerves from C5 to T1 is an extensive topic and exceeds the scope of this book. Various books containing information on this subject are listed in the Bibliography.

Once an individual is in an accident and proceeds with medical treatment, the likelihood is that there will be involvement with an insurance company for at least the cost of the treatment. If headache and pain persist and become chronic, the likelihood is that there is going to be litigation. Once that process begins, then the medical record becomes the essential ingredient that both the plaintiff and defense team use to make their case.

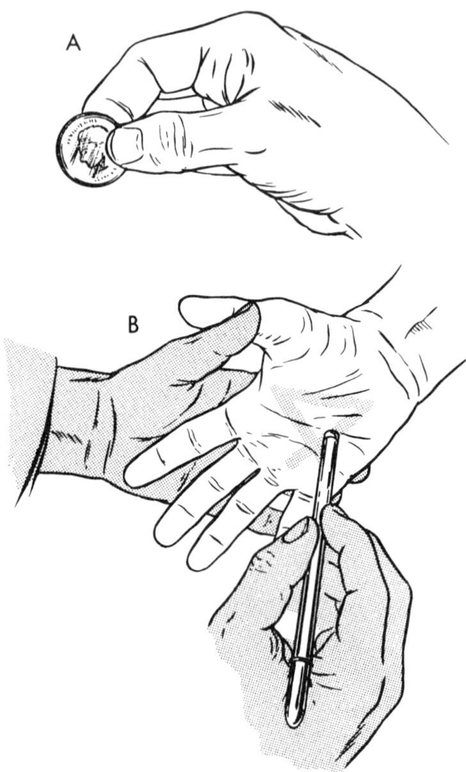

Figure 24.10 Stereognosis and graphesthesia. This tests whether the individual can identify small objects without visualization, hold an object without dropping it, and recognize letters and numbers written on the skin. (From Van Allen, M.W., *Pictorial Manual of Neurologic Tests*, Mosby-Year Book, Chicago, 1969. With permission.)

Those professionals involved in the diagnosis and treatment of the patient have been trained to correct the cause of the pain, whatever their specialty may be. Few of these professionals have ever been trained in the area of tort law. Most of the people involved in these treatments not only are not trained in the legal system, but wish to avoid it like the plague. Medical language, theories, and prognosis do not fit comfortably with legal language and probabilities. Medical personnel often feel attacked and misunderstood in cross examination.

One way to ease the discomfort of these confrontations is to not have to use recall from memory in attempting to explain an answer to the examiner. Conferences, depositions and court appearances take place months to years after the patient is seen. This is why complete notes are essential. Taking a complete history, physical, and all other measures to work up the patient, plus summarizing all these notes to come to a conclusion, plus keeping complete progress notes, will save the professional time and aggravation. Most lawyers who will oppose the medical professional will look for

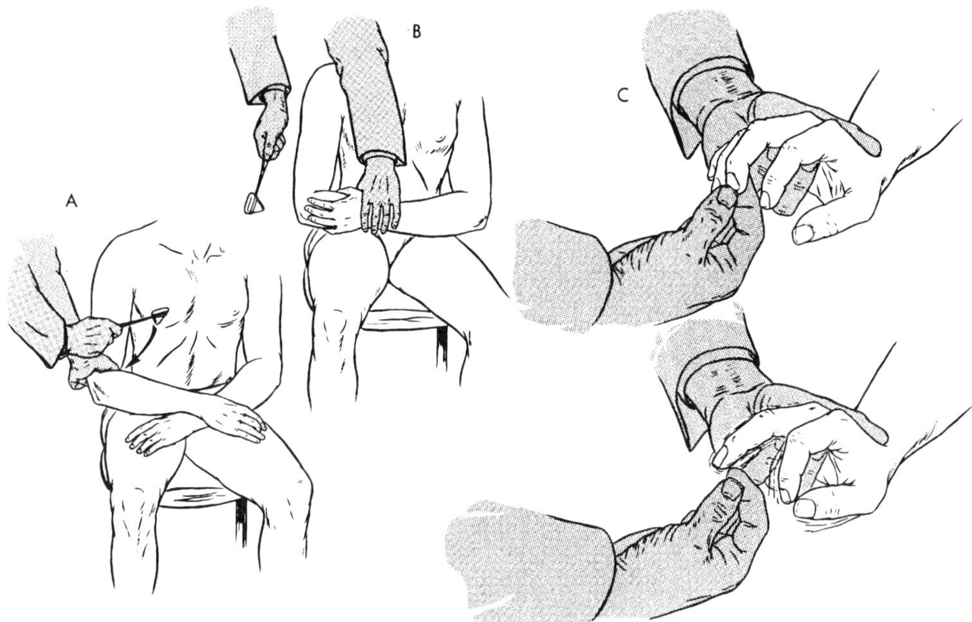

Figure 24.11 Reflexes in the upper extremities. These reflexes demonstrate the biceps (A), triceps (B), and the Hoffman sign (C). If the finger does not reflex properly, this would be an indication of spinal (corticospinal dysfunction) damage. (From Van Allen, M.W., *Pictorial Manual of Neurologic Tests*, Mosby-Year Book, Chicago, 1969. With permission.)

weaknesses in the reports and they will also look for contradictions using other medical professional's reports. Whether the lawyer represents the plaintiff or the insurance company the same tactic will be used.

No sample is ever complete; however, the headache intake form presented in Chapter 4 and the information given in this chapter should help to reduce much of the difficulties often encountered.

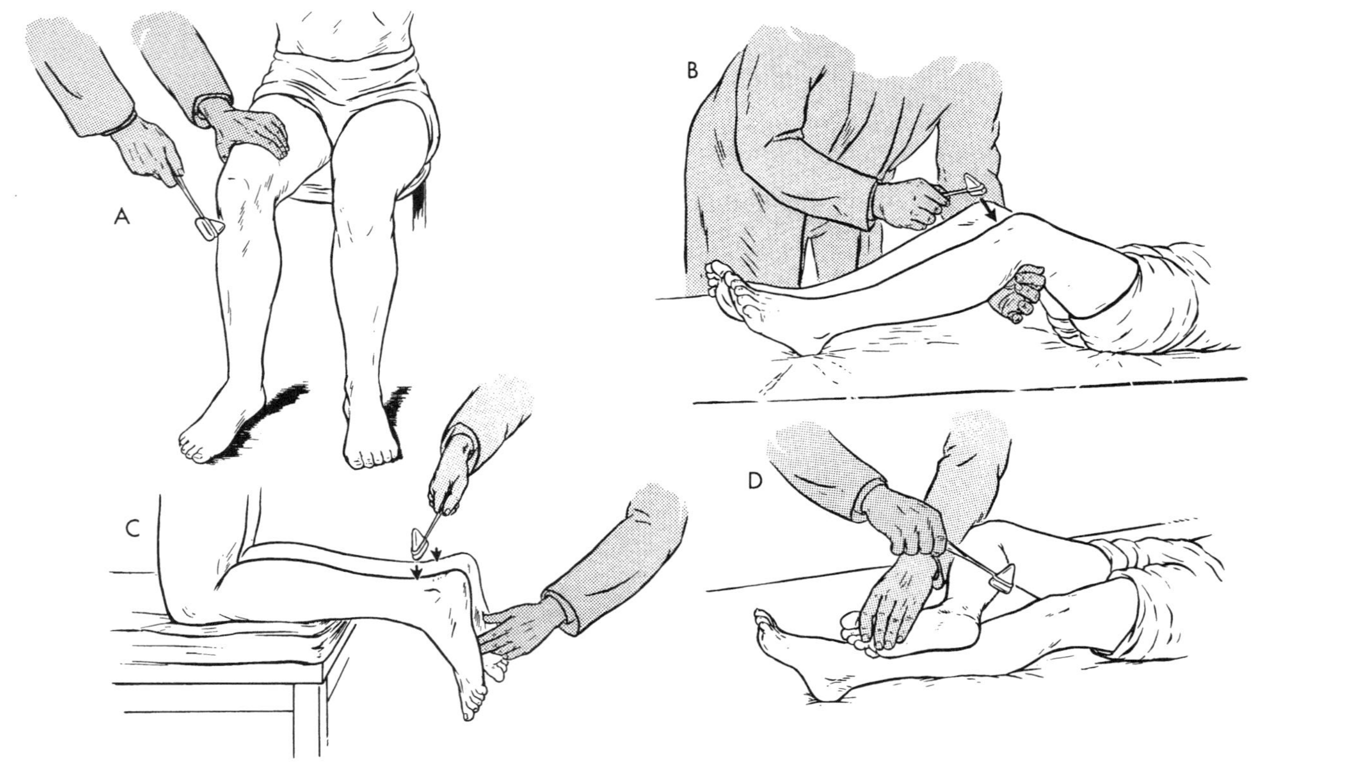

Figure 24.12 Reflexes in the lower extremities. This demonstrates the patellar reflex, both in a sitting (A) and lying (B) position, and the Achilles reflex in two different positions (C and D). (From Van Allen, M.W., *Pictorial Manual of Neurologic Tests*, Mosby-Year Book, Chicago, 1969. With permission.)

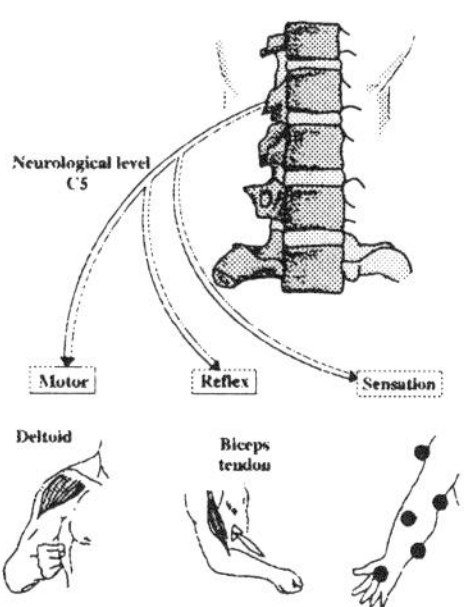

Figure 24.13 The distribution in muscles from the C5 neurological level.

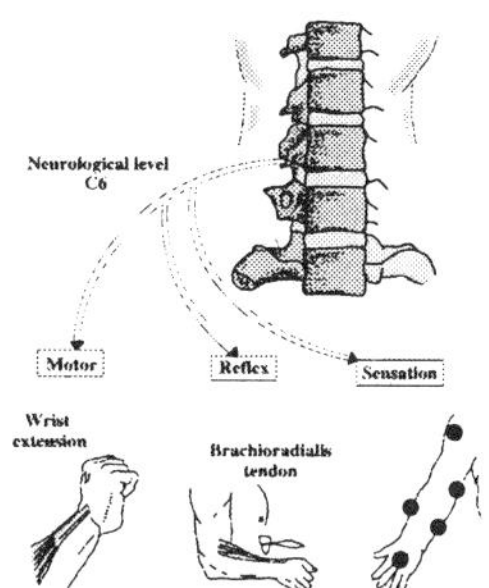

Figure 24.14 The distribution from the C6 neurological level.

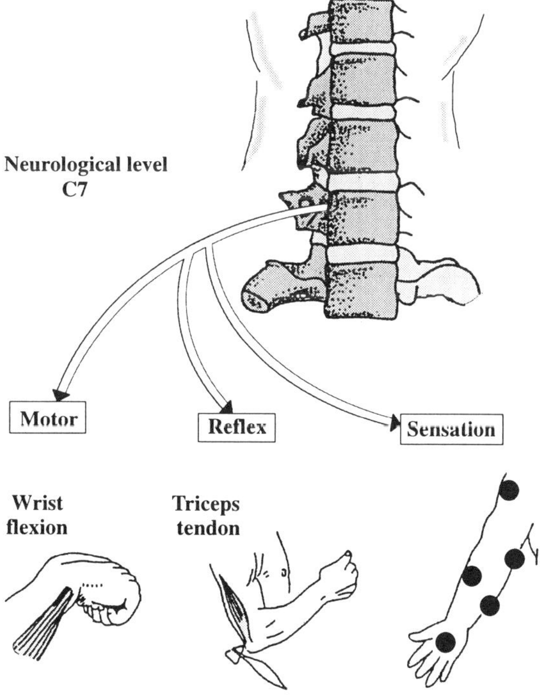

Figure 24.15 The distribution from the C7 neurological level.

REFERENCES

1. Diamond, S., Dalessio, D.J., *The Practicing Physician's Approach to Headache,* 4th ed., Williams & Wilkins, Baltimore, 1986.
2, Van Allen, M.W., *Pictorial Manual of Neurologic Tests,* Mosby-Year Book, Chicago, 1969.
3. Foreman S.M., Croft A.C., *Whiplash Injuries: The Cervical Acceleration/Deceleration Syndrome,* 2nd ed., Williams & Wilkins, Baltimore, 1995.

CHAPTER 25

Headache Treatments

As I mentioned in Chapter 3 on the theories of pain, regardless of the causal factor, the neuromechanisms of the pain in headache are the same. Therefore, if the pain was caused by stress, hormones, food sensitivities, exercise, allergies, fatigue, hunger, a blow to the head, whiplash or any other cause, the final neural pathway for the actual headache is most likely the same.

The treatments are usually directed toward the pain itself, the cause of the headache, or both. I do not know of any condition that has more treatment modalities that have been documented over the past 10,000 years than headache. As soon as one person tries something that works, the message is communicated around the world as a new panacea to rid this misery from the human race. It doesn't matter whether we use the Internet in today's electronic super highway or passed the information by drum thousands of years ago, somehow the word gets out that a new cure has been found and all the sufferers seek someone who will give them this new and miraculous treatment.

The interesting aspect of all this is that many of the scientifically logical treatments may not work, while some illogical approaches may be successful, and that may be the reason sufferers will try anything for relief.

Although this book is directed toward the headache that is caused by an accident of head or neck injury, the eventual headache will be vascular (migraine-like) or tension-like, or a combination type. Therefore, treatments of these types of headache, whether or not they are caused by an accident or trauma, will be similar. There are some treatments that will be mentioned that are specific for the post trauma patient. The type of treatment, and variations of treatment types is determined by the headache specialist, for the specialist knows that often the treatment varies and is altered to suit a particular patient. This comes from enormous experience and the knowledge that the "patient's body often doesn't read or follow the doctor's book."

It would be impossible to list all the treatments that are performed and, although some variations of treatment will be mentioned, the emphasis in this book will be the pharmacology, nerve blocks and physical applications of treatment. Besides the references that will be mentioned in the text, a list of other references that have been reviewed will be provided at the end of the chapter.

In Chapter 1 of this book, I referred to Papua-New Guinea where for thousands of years people used headbands to scarify their foreheads for treatment of recurrent headaches. There is evidence dating back to the Neolithic and Bronze ages in Europe, Mexico and the American continent, and until recently in the Melanesian communities on the islands of the South Pacific, that the custom of trephining was used to cure headaches. Trephining is an operation in which a hole is made in the skull with some sharp object to let the evil spirits out. Evidence of this dates back 10,000 years and it is certain that this treatment was going on long before the trephining of the skulls we found.

During the middle ages, rags soaked with vinegar and cow dung were applied to the painful area. Bloodletting, with and without vacuum cups, and anything that could be used to rid the body of evil spirits or any type of toxin was used. Unfortunately some of the "successful" treatments that eliminated the pain did so by killing the patient.

Considering that we are convinced, as a result of much scientific investigation, that migraine and headache in general are products of alterations of our neurochemistry that affect the neuropathways in our brain and result in the production of chemical pain mediators, then the purpose of any treatment should be to bring these alterations of neurochemicals back to normal (homeostasis). Therefore, any treatment using medicines or non-medicines will be successful if the brain chemistry is brought back to equilibrium and the inflammation of the nervous system and the vascular system subsides.

Lance reported that attacks may be initiated in the hypothalamus, whether due to a built-in periodicity or a response to sensory stimuli from the cerebral cortex. Wherever the stimuli come from (triggering factors), the mechanism follows a course of action in which impulses are generated that descend from the hypothalamus to the periaqueductal gray matter, thence to the raphe nuclei that affect the cortical microcirculation, initiating a "spreading depression" in the cortex (producing the aura phase of the attack) and at the same time closing the (enkephalinergic) "gate" in the spinal cord.

This phase depends on the hyperactivity of both the noradrenergic and the serotonergic brainstem systems, causing the "pain gate" in the cord to open, flooding the head with previously inhibited pain. This mechanism opens the afferent gate to the special senses producing the characteristic and intolerable affects to light, sound and smells.

Now other areas come into operation. The convergence in the spinal cord of afferent fibers from the upper three cervical nerves with the descending tract of the trigeminal nerve means that pain can be referred from the neck to the temples, and back again. The trigeminal impulses by a neurovascular reflex further increase intracranial blood flow. This activation alters the physiology of neurons, glia, and blood vessels in such a way that pain provoking and neuroinflammatory mediators are generated within the cerebral cortex and supporting tissues.

These mediators activate nociceptors (nerve centers that perceive painful stimuli) on the trigeminal afferent terminals within the meninges (brain coverings), which in turn stimulate neurons in the brainstem, thalamus, and cerebral cortex to create the awareness of pain.

When this happens, the perivascular terminals are activated and the following mediators are released: substance P, neurokinin A, and calcitonion gene related peptide, which sensitize nerve endings, causing hyperalgesia (increased pain) and sustaining the pain long after the initial trigger has disappeared. This leads to more pain and still more vasodilatation and the process becomes a vicious circle. The goal of stopping or reducing the pain is not only to relieve the suffering, but also to prevent this self-perpetuation by normalizing this trigeminovascular reflex (Figure 25.1).

Understanding the principle of these major elements in the production of migraine or migraine-like headaches, we then can understand how it might be possible, by interfering with a *critical link* in the primary pathogenic process in the brainstem, to prevent or greatly modify the course of this headache.[2]

It is with this understanding of the mechanism for migraine or migraine-like headaches that one has to consider that any type of treatment that aborts, prevents, or minimizes the pain may be interfering with this critical link.

Once again, I must emphasize that no treatment should be instigated until a diagnosis is made. No diagnosis should be made unless a complete history is taken and a physical and appropriate testing are done. The idea that all headaches are benign and are not to be investigated until other symptoms present themselves is a very dangerous one. Headache may be the first symptom of a major medical problem, and waiting for other symptoms to develop may put the patient in a compromising position. Infections, circulatory problems, hypertension, eye problems, ear problems, dental problems, brain tumors, cancer, etc. (see Chapter 10) have to be diagnosed.

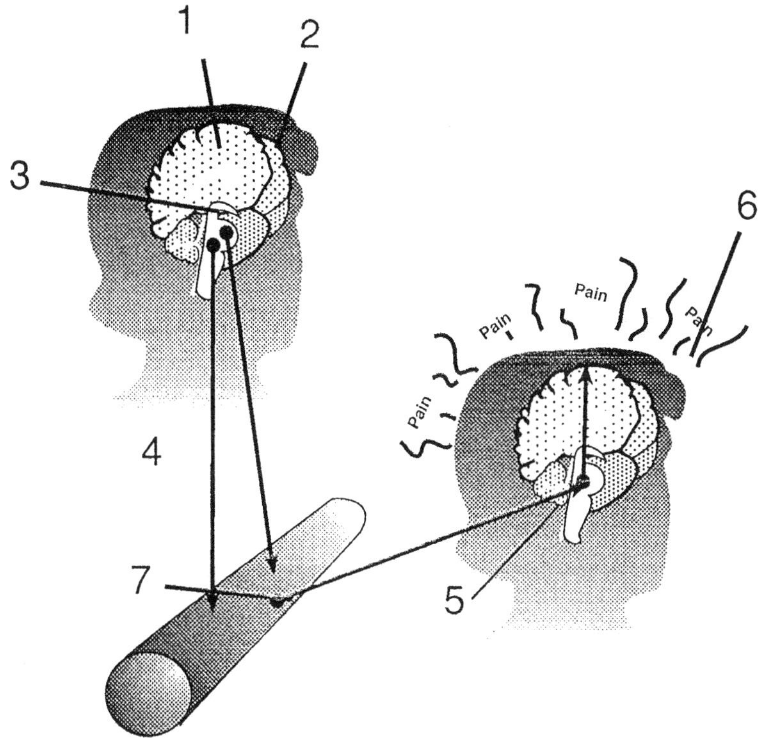

1. Triggering factors: Hunger, fatigue, hormones, stress, senses.
2. Threshold
3. Locus Ceruleus and Dorsal Raphe Nuclei
4. Activates Neuro- Inflammatory Mediators
5. Meninges
6. Awareness of pain
7. Pain chemicals

Figure 25.1 The neurovascular hypothesis of migraine or vascular headaches. (**1**) There are external or internal triggering factors that exceed (**2**) a threshold that different individuals have, and when the threshold is exceeded, there is activation of (**3**) 5-HT (5-hydroxytryptamine) and norepinephrine containing neurons in the locus ceruleus and dorsal raphe nuclei in the brainstem. (**4**) This activation alters the physiology of these neurons and eventually the blood cells, and generates pain-provoking chemicals (neuroinflammatory mediators) within the cerebral cortex and the supporting tissues. (**5**) These mediators activate pain receptors in the trigeminal vascular terminals within the coverings of the brain (meninges), which then stimulate neurons in the (**6**) brainstem and the thalmus and cerebral cortex that creates awareness of pain. (**7**) The activation by the pain chemicals substance P, neurokinin A, and CGRP (calcitonin gene related peptide) causes a sterile inflammation that sensitizes nerve endings and causes dilatation of the arteries of the head and increased pain. If the migraine is not treated immediately, and these chemicals are permitted to stay around the nerve and blood vessels, then this may add to the length of time of the headache pain.

Once the diagnosis is made, the course of treatment may start. If the headache is the secondary symptom of a medical disease, then it is obvious that the primary disease should be treated; and if that is the reason for the headache, no further steps have to be taken. There are several hundred medical conditions that may contribute to headache.

However, the greatest number of headaches are not secondary to major medical diseases and these are the conditions that will be addressed in this chapter. There are many non-medication treatments that headache sufferers feel have been successful for their particular problem and as long as there is no danger to their general health, I certainly have no objection to these treatments. Most of these treatments are not part of any experimental design and the results are anecdotal presentations. The danger comes from persons who claim that these treatments are specific for migraine or a specific diagnostic category because of the marketing value. All too often package inserts make claims that these substances cure migraine. Interestingly enough, these claims cannot even be made with well-developed and researched medications.

Some of the more common nonprescription treatments are :

1. Changing your diet and eliminating any foods that may precipitate a headache.[3] Table 24.1 in the previous chapter is a list of foods that may help prevent headache, and those that may trigger headache.
2. Relaxation techniques:[4] deep breathing, progressive relaxation, overall body relaxation, guided relaxation, relaxation by the numbers, autogenic training, creative imagery, color imagery, affirmation, meditation, etc.
3. Biofeedback:[5] biofeedback is a method of using electronic equipment to monitor your physiological responses while using guided relaxation exercises. Children and adults who are capable of focusing will often benefit from this exercise.
4. Massage, warm baths, hot tubs and yoga.
5. Hypnosis:[6] patients who have good focusing ability may use this technique to abort pain.
6. Reducing stress or triggering factors by various types of psychotherapy. There are many different approaches to therapy, including psychoanalysis, based on the work of Sigmund Freud; modifications of Freudian psychoanalysis of Adler, Jung, Horney, Rank, Sullivan and others; analytically oriented therapy; psychobiological therapies of Adolf Meyers; hypnosis, hypnotherapy, hypnoanalysis; conditioning, operant conditioning, and learning theory using desensitization, Wolpe's reciprocal inhibition, reinforcement, shaping, aversive control, assertive training and others; client-centered therapy (nondirective counseling of Carl Rogers); logotherapy of Victor Frankl; primal therapy of Arthur Janov; rational-emotive therapy of Albert Ellis; reality therapy of William Glasser; group psychotherapy; transactional analysis; Gestalt therapy of Fritz Perls; psychodrama; Adlerian family counseling; and conjoint family therapy. There are many other types of psychotherapy and all make the assumption that if an underlying conflict causes anxiety or depression, it is essential to uncover this cause and resolve it to eliminate the secondary symptom of migraine. Although this appears to be a logical approach, in many cases even with successful treatment of the psychological condition, the headaches may not alter.
7. Exercise therapy. We have learned over the years that exercise is beneficial for the prevention and treatment of many illnesses. Many patients with migraine fear exercise because movement of the neck may sometimes initiate a headache response, like running or stair climbing, etc. However, I have found that if one can do various maneuvers without jarring the neck, the benefits of exercise can be accomplished without precipitating a migraine. Stationary or regular bicycling often is successful. Water exercise seems to have many excellent results. Wearing a floating device and jogging in a pool at a comfortable temperature has many beneficial effects. Besides the cardiopulmonary benefits, there seems to be a very relaxing effect that water has on the individual. I recall that many of my patients feel they have had positive results and this has also been reported by patients with post traumatic headaches. One book I highly recommend is *The Complete Waterpower Workout Book*, by Lynda Huey and Robert Forster (Random House).[7]

Over the years, many of my patients have tried many alternative therapies for which they have claimed some or a great deal of relief of their headache problems. In evaluating their headache logs over a period of time, I have not found a consistent pattern of improvement; that is to say, there seemed to be periods when they appeared to be improved and then there were exacerbations of the headache problem. This is also seen with medication therapy, and may be due to the complex nature of the intricate neural and chemical pathways that are responsible for migraine and headache in general. As long as I do not feel that these alternative therapies are masking an underlying medical condition and this therapy is not medically a threat to the patient's health, then I do not discourage alternative therapies. Migraine is an incapacitating disease and any treatment that will prevent the debilitating effects of its symptoms should be considered.

MEDICATIONS USED FOR THE TREATMENT OF HEADACHE

Although many medications are mentioned here, the reader should understand this is not a complete list. The reader should also understand that there are no universal medications or combinations of these medications that guarantee success. It is also possible that some treatments that seem successful may not last, and returning to these medicines does not mean they are going to be successful again. Many of these treatments have not been approved by the FDA specifically for treatment of headaches but have been used by experts who have reported "success" with these medications. Only those who understand the pharmacology and are experienced in using these drugs should prescribe them, and they should be given only to those patients who understand the instructions and are compliant with the doctor's orders. The physician must make it rather clear that "a little makes it feel better" does not mean "a lot is going to make it that much better." Many pain medications and tranquilizers may be addicting and strict control and cooperation is essential. Some of this control comes from patient education, laboratory testing and periodic visits.

It has been observed by headache specialists that often medication treatment for migraine headaches that may be successful does not seem to work or work as well with headaches caused by accidents. Other treatments will be mentioned after this segment.

Treatment of headaches is divided into three categories: abortive, preventive, or a combination of both. Abortive therapy is directed toward eliminating or reducing the pain at the time of the headache attack. Preventive therapy uses medications on an ongoing basis to prevent attacks or diminish the intensity of the attack. A combination of these two types of treatments is used when neither of the above two treatments is able to accomplish those goals.

The manner of selecting the above treatments is based on criteria agreed upon by headache specialists.

When using abortive therapy, the treatment should be successful within hours to two days. The attacks should be infrequent, certainly not more than two a week, and there should be breaks where there are no attacks for longer periods of time. Sometimes abortive medications are used more frequently when preventive medications are contraindicated or when patients are not able to follow instructions.

Preventive therapy is considered when attacks are more frequent (two or more a week), when the duration of a single attack may last several days or the attack does not respond to abortive therapy, when abortive medication is contraindicated, when it is not effective as an abortive medication, or to enhance the abortive medication.

The combination of abortive therapy and preventive therapy is used to increase the effectiveness of the abortive therapy and also to reduce future attacks. Because severe pain reduces absorption in the stomach, abortive medication is often used sublingually (under the tongue), as a nasal spray, rectally, by patch, creams, and by injections.

Medications used to abort headache include[8] analgesics and analgesic combinations, nonsteroidal anti-inflammatory medications, ergotamine derivatives, isomethepene, corticosteroids, phenothiazines/neuroleptics, and the tripans.

Medications used to prevent headache include[8] beta-adrenergic blockers, calcium channel antagonists, antidepressants, ergot derivatives, anticonvulsants, antihistamines, lithium carbonate, pizotofen, captopril, clonidine, baclofen, muscle relaxants, capsaicin.

Medications Used to Abort Headaches

Analgesics and Analgesic Combinations[8]

Analgesics may be used to abort irritating (mild), interfering (moderate to severe), and incapacitating headaches. It is customary to use other abortive medications for severe migraine, with the addition of analgesic drugs to rapidly reduce the intensity and the duration of the pain. Table 25.1 is a list of frequently used analgesics.

Table 25.1

- Analgesics (simple and combination)
  - Aspirin
  - Tylenol
- Analgesics (combination containing barbiturates)
  - Fiorinal — aspirin 325 mg, caffeine 40 mg, butalbital 50 mg
  - Fioricet, Esgic — acetaminophen 325 mg, butalbital 50 mg
  - Phrenilin — acetaminophen 325 mg, butalbital 50 mg
- Analgesics (combination containing codeine)
  - Fiorinal w/codeine — aspirin 325 mg, caffeine 40 mg, butalbital 50 mg, codeine 30 mg
  - Tylenol w/codeine — acetaminophen 325 mg, codeine 30 mg
  - Phrenilin w/codeine — acetaminophen 325 mg, codeine 30 mg, butalbital 50 mg
- Narcotic Analgesics (analgesics containing narcotics)
  - Darvon CPD-65 — propoxyphene HCl 65 mg, aspirin 389 mg, caffeine 32.4 mg
  - Darvocet-N — propoxyphene napsylate 50/100 mg, acetaminophen 325 mg
  - Vicodin — hydrocodone 5 mg, acetaminophen 500 mg
  - Percocet — oxycodone 5 mg, acetaminophen 325 mg
  - Percodan — oxycodone 4.5 mg, acetaminophen 325 mg
  - Demerol — meperidine 50/100 mg tablet; injectable
  - Dilaudid — hydromorphone $^{1}/_{2}$/$^{3}/_{4}$ mg tablet; 3 mg suppository; 2 mg/ml injections
  - Stadol — butorphanol 10 mg/mL (IM, IV, or nasal spray)

From Saper, J.R. et al., *Handbook of Headache Management*, Williams & Wilkins, Baltimore, 1993. With permission.

The major disadvantage of narcotic medication is habituation and addiction. Another frequent problem is the overuse of non-narcotic medication, which may lead to rebound headaches, countering the purpose of the therapy.

The advantage of analgesics is that there are multiple mechanisms of action. By using caffeine there is a more rapid absorption of the analgesic medication. Some of the analgesics with and without combination will reduce the anxiety accompanying the pain by offering tranquilization.

Prostaglandin, a pain mediator in the body's chemistry, is inhibited in its synthesis by aspirin. Acetaminophen does the same in the central nervous system and may affect the endorphin/opiate system. Narcotics will enhance the effect of the body's endorphin system by stimulating the endogenous (in the body) opiate receptors. Caffeine will increase gastrointestinal absorption and enhances analgesia.

With so much information verifying that overuse of analgesics will actually cause more headaches by the rebound phenomenon, it is best to use these medications on a limited basis. Our clinic sets a limit of 30 pills a month as a standard. Narcotic medication orally has the same limit, taking into account that some narcotics are more powerful, in relation to both the pain and the addiction process. With migraine there are often accompanying gastrointestinal symptoms of nausea and vomiting, and therefore injections of the medications or rectal suppositories may be necessary. Injections are limited to twice a month and the narcotic is generally combined with an anti-vomiting medication.

Aspirin is not recommended for children because of its relationship to Reye's syndrome.

Some of the adverse effects of these medications are

Aspirin: asthma, rash, gastrointestinal irritation, and effects on coagulation
Acetaminophen: liver toxicity, kidney or renal disease
Narcotics: nausea, vomiting, respiratory depression, sedation, constipation, addiction, and effects on coagulation

Consult the *Physician's Desk Reference* or other references for a more complete list of untoward reactions.

Table 25.2 lists the caffeine content of common foods and drugs.

Table 25.2

Product	Example	Caffeine Content (mg)
Cocoa and chocolate	Baking chocolate (1 oz)	35
	Chocolate candy bar	25
	Cocoa beverage (6 oz mixture)	10
	Milk chocolate (1 oz)	6
Coffee	Decaffeinated (5 oz)	2
	Drip (5 oz)	146
	Instant, regular (5 oz)	53
	Percolated (5 oz)	110
Over-the-counter drugs	Anacin	32
	Excedrin	65
	No-Doz tablets	100–200
	Vanquish	33
	Vivarin tablets	200
Prescription drugs	Darvon	32.4
	Esgic	40
	Fioricet	40
	Fiorinal	40
	Norgesic	30
	Norgesic Forte	60
	Supac	33
	Synalgos-DC	30
Soft drinks (12 oz)	7-Up/Diet 7-Up	0
	Coca-Cola	34
	Diet Pepsi	34
	Dr. Pepper	38
	Fresca	0
	Ginger Ale	0
	Hires Root Beer	0
	Mountain Dew	52
	Pepsi-Cola	37
	Tab	44
Tea	1-minute brew (5 oz)	9–33
	3-minute brew (5 oz)	22–46
	5-minute brew (5 oz)	20–50
	Canned ice tea (12 oz)	22–36

From Saper, J.R. et al., *Handbook of Headache Management*, Williams & Wilkins, Baltimore, 1993. With permission.

Nonsteroidal anti-inflammatory medications (NSAIDs) can be used both as preventive or abortive drugs. Often, in order to prevent addiction, these drugs are used instead of narcotic medication to abort headache pain. Emergency rooms will often use these medications as an injectable for the same reason. But, in general, patients do not feel they have the same effect in reducing the pain as a narcotic. Table 25.3 lists NSAIDs used in the treatment of headache.

Table 25.3 Nonsteroidal Medications Used in the Treatment of Headache

Type	Available Size (mg)
Carboxylic acids	
Acetylated	
Aspirin	
Nonacetylated	
Choline magnesium trisalicylate (Trilisate)	500/750/1000
Salsalate (Salflex, Disalcid)	500/750
Propionic acids	
Ibuprofen (Motrin, Advil)	200/400/600
Naproxen (Naprosyn)	250/375/500
Fenoprofen (Nalfon)	200/300/600
Naproxen sodium (Anaprox)	275/375
Aryl and heterocyclic acids	
Tolmetin (Tolectin)	200/400/600
Indomethacin (Indocin)	25/50/75; 50 (Rectal)
Diclofenac (Voltaren)	25/50/75
Sulindac (Clinoril)	150/200
Fenamic acids	
Mefenamic acid (Ponstel)	250
Meclofenamate (Mecloment)	50/100
Enolic acids	
Phenylbutazone (Butazolidine)	100
Piroxicam (Feldene)	10/20
Pyrrolo-pyrrole	
Ketorolac (Toradol) (IM)	15/30/60
Ketorolac (Toradol) (PO)	10

From Saper, J.R. et al., *Handbook of Headache Management*, Williams & Wilkins, Baltimore, 1993. With permission.

Their effectiveness seems best in the following conditions: mild to moderate migraine, exertional and menstrual headache, benign orgasmic cephalgia, chronic paroxysmal hemicrania (indomethocin), "ice pick" headaches, incapacitating migraine attack.[8] NSAIDs are often used after whiplash or trauma that may cause headaches because of the inflammatory condition of the muscles and ligaments. Prolonged and frequent use should be avoided.

The mechanism of action of the nonsteroidal anti-inflammatory drugs is that it interferes, through a series of complex reactions, with the production of prostaglandins (a pain mediator produced in the body) and therefore reduces the pain of this inflammatory response.

There are many different agents in this category and often if one seems not to help, other agents may be effective. There are also injectables which frequently are used in the emergency room. Although these drugs are effective in pain management, there are significant adverse reactions with constant use. Therefore, it is not recommended that this type of medication be taken indiscriminately. The following reactions should be monitored: gastrointestinal ulcers and bleeding, oral ulcers, colitis (caused by or aggravated), headache, lightheadedness, dizziness, tinnitus (ringing in ears), fluid retention, asthma aggravation, aggravation of high blood pressure, aggravation of kidney disease.

NSAIDs should not be taken if the following medical problems exist, unless the patient is monitored carefully by a physician: active ulcer disease, gastritis, renal (kidney) disease, bleeding disorders, aspirin sensitive asthma, severe hypertension, and colitis.

For a more complete list of adverse reactions and contraindications refer to the *Physician's Desk Reference* or other standard references.

Ergotamine and Ergotamine Derivatives

Since 1925, the ergot fungus has been found to be useful for the treatment of migraine and vascular headaches, and a derivative dihydroergotamine (DHE) has been used since 1945. The ergot alkaloids are derived from the ergot fungus or rye fungus (*Claviceps purpurea*). The ergotamines and ergotamine derivatives can be used both for abortive and preventative approaches for migraine and migraine-like headaches. It is used for both nontraumatic and the post traumatic headache treatment. Its use as a preventative will be discussed later in this chapter.

Ergotamine tartrate antagonizes the 5-HT2 (5-hydroxytryptamine) postsynaptic receptor site and agonizes the 5-HT1 presynaptic receptor site. It causes a constriction of the arteries by a reduction of both the vasogenic and neurogenic inflammation. Reducing the inflammation reduces the pain.

Ergotamine tartrate is used in moderate to severe to incapacitating migraine and migraine-like headaches. It is also used in cluster headaches. It is prepared in oral, sublingual, nasal spray, rectal and injectable forms (see Table 25.4).

Table 25.4 Ergotamine Derivatives Used in the Treatment of Headache

Drug	Strength
Cafergot suppositories/tablets	Ergotamine tartrate 1 mg, caffeine 100 mg
Wigraine suppositories/tablets	Ergotamine tartrate 1 mg, caffeine 100 mg
Ergomar sublingual tablets	Ergotamine tartrate 2 mg
Ergostat sublingual tablets	Ergotamine tartrate 2 mg
Migrogot tablets	
DHE (dihydroergotamine) nasal spray, suppository	1 mg/ml (IM, IV, SC) capsules
Contraindications	
Age over 60 years (relative contraindication)	
Pregnancy	
Breast feeding	
Bradycardia	
Cardiac valvular disease (moderate to severe)	
Collagen vascular disease, vasculitis	
Coronary artery disease	
Hypertension (moderate to severe)	
Impaired hepatic or renal function (moderate to severe)	
Infection or fever/sepsis (enhances vasoconstriction)	
Peptic ulcer disease	
Peripheral vascular disease	
Cerebral vascular disease	
Severe pruritus	

From Saper, J.R. et al., *Handbook of Headache Management*, Williams & Wilkins, Baltimore, 1993. With permission.

Although very effective, there are limiting factors for using this drug. The drug is capable of producing nausea, vomiting, paresthesias, muscle cramping, and chest pain in sensitive people. There is also the potential to become dependent and abuse of the drug could cause ergotism, which is a poisoning by the drug, leading to spasms, cramps, and dry gangrene of the feet, which could result in amputation. In defense of this medication, I have never seen any patient have any permanent problem if they were compliant. To correct any problems with nausea or vomiting the dosage is usually reduced and/or administered with an antiemetic drug. It is the least expensive drug to take to abort a migraine.

The contraindications to using the drug are the following: pregnancy, breast feeding, slow heart rate (bradycardia), cardiac valvular disease, peripheral vascular disease, coronary artery disease, hypertension, liver disease, kidney disease, infection or fever, peptic ulcer disease, cerebral vascular disease, and collagen vascular disease.

For a more complete list of adverse reactions or contraindications it is best to use the *Physician's Desk Reference* or other standard references.

Dihydroergotamine (DHE)

Dihydroergotamine or DHE is a derivative of ergotamine and was developed by Sandoz Pharmaceuticals. It entered the therapeutic market around 1945 and was labeled DHE-45.

It was much less severe in its secondary unpleasant reactions then ergotamine tartrate. Compared to ergotamine, it is a weaker vasoconstrictor, has selective venoconstricting properties, and has much less emetic (nauseating and vomiting) properties. It also has less contracting effects on the uterus.

During the mid-1980s when Glaxo Pharmaceuticals was developing sumatriptan or Imitrex (to be discussed later in this chapter), the mechanism for DHE was also investigated and those of us who had been using it for many years now were enlightened to its neuropharmacology. After Professor Neil Raskin of the University of California at San Fransico made his landmark announcement of using DHE on a continuous basis to abort intractable migraine in the early 1980s, an entirely new and relatively safe approach was ushered in for this most difficult medical problem. My headache inpatient unit at Winter Park Memorial Hospital, Winter Park, Florida was filled for years with patients from Florida and the southeastern United States who sought this new and exciting treatment for their debilitating condition. These patients, who would normally spend days or weeks in a hospital bed, unable to function because of pain and sedation with narcotics and tranquilizers, were now able to ambulate within hours or a day, involved in exercise and a headache program with little or no pain while a tiny needle was taped to their arms.

DHE and ergotamine have similar mechanisms of actions, but DHE has significantly fewer unpleasant side reactions; it has become the drug of choice. However, there are cases where ergotamine is much more effective in aborting the migraine attack.

DHE usually comes in an ampule of 1 mg/ml that can be given intramuscularly, subcutaneously, or intravenously. I was able to have a compounding pharmacy (Thayer's Colonial Pharmacy, Orlando, FL) prepare DHE in capsules (short acting and long acting), as a nasal spray, sublingual and suppositories (Table 25.5).

Table 25.5 Compounded Medications Used for Treatment of Headaches

Brand Name	Generic
Ergo-Pac suppositories	Ergotamine/pentobarbital/atropine/caffeine
Ergo-Pac + Pmz	Ergotamine/pentobarbital/atropine/caffeine/promethazine
Ergo-Cap tablet	Ergotamine/pentobarbital/atropine/caffeine/promethazine
Ergo-Cap + Pmz	Ergotamine/pentobarbital/atropine/caffeine/promethazine
DHE Nasal Spray	Dihydroergotamine
DHE SR caps	Dihydroergotamine
Oxycodone suppositories	Oxycodone

DHE is effective for severe migraine, cluster, or any "vascular" headache that responds to this medication. This may also be effective for post traumatic migraine-like headaches. This treatment may be used in the doctor's office, the emergency room, or even by the patient injecting himself.

There are some patients who may have an adverse reaction, while other patients may just need an adjustment in dosage.

Adverse reactions may be the same as ergotamine but usually are less frequent, less likely and less intense.

When a patient is hospitalized in order to deal with a condition known as status migrainous (a continuous migraine attack that does not respond to the usual abortive treatment), then the treatment of choice is to use intravenous therapy. This is usually a 3 to 7 day treatment. In 1992, with the help of Rotech Medical Corporation and Thayer's Colonial Compounding Pharmacy, Orlando, FL, I was able to develop an outpatient protocol for treating these difficult patients without having to hospitalize them.

A very small catheter that was originally developed for premature infants was inserted into the suffering patient and the catheter was then connected to a small computerized pump the size of a Walkman radio, which contained the DHE medication. In this manner the patient could function at home or work while being treated and when the migraine attack went into remission, the treatment was discontinued and the catheter was removed. I found this method successful for both nontraumatic and post traumatic migraine-like headache.

We found that while the patient was being treated, he or she could function in almost any capacity, homemaker to laborer. I was able treat a lawyer who was suffering from a cluster headache attack who had to appear in Denver at an important trial. By inserting the catheter and hooking the catheter to the computer that was attached to the back of his pants, no one was able to see the pump and he was able to conduct his duties without ever having an attack. This was also done with a horse trainer the same way.

Isometheptene

Midrin is an older and well-known medication. It is a drug that I frequently use as a first line of defense. Another drug is called Isocom. There are three active ingredients: isometheptene mucate 65 mg, acetaminophen 325 mg, and dichloralphenazone 100 mg.

Isometheptene mucate may act on the vascular system through the central nervous system, while acetaminophen is an analgesic, and dichloralphenazone has mild tranquilizing properties.

It is recommended with mild to moderate migraine and tension-type headache. This medication may also be used in combination with some of the stronger analgesics and also with the NSAIDs. I do not recommend more than 10 per week.

Rare instances of dizziness and sedation have been reported.

Do not use this drug, or use with caution, with: glaucoma, kidney disease, severe high blood pressure, severe heart or liver disease, and with spinal cord lesions. *These drugs should never be used with monomine oxidase inhibitors (MAO) and patients with spinal cord lesions. This combination may cause severe hypertensive reactions.*

Refer to the *Physician's Desk Reference* or other standard references for a complete list and explanations of untoward reactions, guidelines, contraindications and warnings.

Corticosteroids

The corticosteroids probably act as anti-inflammatories on the neurogenic system and reduce the swelling of the vascular system.

The steroids are usually not the first line of defense and are used when the NSAIDs are not successful. They are often used with success with cluster headache, intractable migraine, headaches with intracranial pressure and swelling (edema).

These drugs should only be used under the guidance of a physician. Some of the contraindications are gastrointestinal ulcers, osteoporosis, diabetes, hypertension, myopathy (disease of the muscles), and necrosis of the bone. However, in some instances under supervision and if necessary, these drugs may be the drug of choice for very short periods of time.

See the *Physician's Desk Reference* or other standard references for untoward reactions, guidelines, contraindications and warnings.

Phenothiazines/Neuroleptics

These medications are often classified as tranquilizers. However, they are often used as antiemetics and sometimes may offer some pain relief. Some emergency room physicians have claimed that they sometimes relieve migraine pain with injections of these medications. This has not been a successful therapy in my attempts to use this type of treatment.

They certainly help to control nausea and vomiting. When a patient is already suffering from nausea and vomiting, these drugs are given by injection intravenously or rectally.

Some of these drugs are chlorpromazine (Thorazine), prochlorperazine (Compazine), perphenazine (Trilafon), metoclopramide (Reglan), promethazine (Phenergan), and trimethobenzamide (Tigan).

See the *Physician's Desk Reference* or other standard references for additional untoward reactions, guidelines, contraindications, and warnings.

Sumatriptan (Imitrex)

Work began on this project in 1972 by Humphrey and colleagues. In 1984 Glaxo Pharmaceuticals synthesized the drug and it was approved in 1992. I was privileged to be involved in three of their studies.

Its mechanism is via its action as an agonist on the presynaptic nerve 5-HT1. This is a selective serotonin (5-hydroxytryptamine) receptor site. The 5-HT1 receptors are known to mediate vasoconstriction of certain cranial vessels and the highly selective stimulation of these receptors by sumatriptan may be responsible, at least in part, for the antimigraine action. It is also thought to have an effect on the neurovascular system and, like the ergotamine derivatives, may reverse neurogenic inflammation.

Imitrex may be used for acute moderate to severe migraine and migraine-like headaches, as well as cluster headache. The drug comes with an auto-injector with which the patient may take his or her own medication once educated in dispensing the drug. There is an oral Imitrex that now eliminates having to use the injection route. However, my experience is that the injectable route is more effective.

The medication is contraindicated in patients with (1) ischemic heart disease, (2) symptoms or signs consistent with ischemic heart disease, (3) Prinmetal's angina, (4) uncontrolled hypertension, as well as (5) those who have used ergotamine within 24 hours, and (6) pregnant women (because no controlled studies have been done).

Some of the adverse events are injection-site reaction, tingling sensation, dizziness, vertigo, nausea/vomiting, chest heaviness, breathing difficulties, flushing, neck pain and/or stiffness, lightheadedness, fatigue, feeling of heaviness, and increase in the migraine attack. These symptoms are produced in a minority of patients, and by and large this medication is an excellent abortive drug.

It is very important that the first injection should be done in a doctor's office and that the doctor's staff should be prepared to care for the patient in the event of an adverse reaction.

These medications fall into a class of drugs called triptans. Currently other pharmaceutical companies are preparing new versions of this medication.

Medications Used to Prevent Headaches

The major drug groups used for the prevention of headaches include:[8]

1. Beta-adrenergic blockers
2. Calcium channel antagonists

3. Antidepressants
4. Ergot derivative (methysergide and related)
5. Anticonvulsants
6. Nonsteroidal anti-inflammatory
7. Lithium
8. Others

Both headache sufferers and their treating physicians must be patient while awaiting results. Often these medications take time and sometimes it is necessary to change medications within the same family of drugs, or sometimes it may be necessary to combine various groups. Many of these patients have headaches with frequencies of several times a week to daily. The physician must follow these patients, maintaining a headache log, in order to calculate the progress of the drug or drugs they are taking. Just having the patient tell you that he or she feels better or worse is not enough, since appropriate alterations cannot be made unless the percentages based on frequency, intensity, and duration are measured.

Beta-Adrenergic Blockers

This group of drugs has been used for well over thirty years and has had a great deal of success in both reducing the frequency, intensity, and duration of chronic migraine and mixed daily headaches.

The action of these drugs appears to be to inhibit norepinephrine release, and they may also interfere with the synthesis of norepinephrine. They also may reduce the firing of information in the locus ceruleus in the brain, which was discussed in Chapter 3 on the mechanism of headache pain.

These drugs are generally given in small divided doses. Enough time should be allowed to elapse before the medication is elevated. However, under-dosing may be a reason for therapeutic failure. Headache specialists often have a clinical feel of the quantity to start with.

Some adverse responses are: (1) fatigue, (2) depression, (3) memory disturbance, (4) impotence, (5) reduced tolerance for physical activity, (6) low blood pressure (hypotension), (7) slow heart rate (bradycardia), (8) weight gain, (9) constriction of peripheral arteries, and (10) elevation of cholesterol and lipid metabolism.

Contraindications include: (1) congestive heart failure, (2) asthma, (3) significant diabetes or hypoglycemia, (4) bradycardia (slow heart rate), (5) low blood pressure (hypotension), (6) increased blood fat (hyperlipidemia), (7) moderate to severe peripheral vascular disease, and (8) significant cerebrovascular disease.

For a more complete list of adverse responses and contraindication and guidelines, see the *Physician's Desk Reference* or a standard reference.

Calcium Channel Antagonists[8]

Some of the drugs in this group are verapamil (Calan, Isoptin), nifedipine (Procardia), nimodipine (Nimotop), diltiazem (Cardizem), flunarazine (Sibelium) (not available in the United States).

Some of the untoward reactions are constipation, heart block (A-V block), congestive heart failure, hypotension (verapamil); hypotension, reflex tachycardia, headache, nausea, and vomiting (nifedipine); hypotension, A-V block, headache (diltiazem); weight gain, somnolence, dizziness, hypotension, and extrapyramidal reactions (postural abnormalities; flunarizine).

Some contraindications are (1) congestive heart failure, (2) heart block, (3) bradycardia, (4) hypotension, (5) atrial flutter or fibrillation, (6) constipation.

The mechanism of action may be interference with neurovascular inflammation, inhibition of contraction of vascular smooth muscle, influences on the serotonin systems and others.

Recommended use is with migraine, daily chronic headache and they are also very effective with cluster headache.

See the *Physician's Desk Reference* or standard references for additional information regarding untoward reactions, contraindications and warnings.

Antidepressants

Antidepressants can be broken down into three groups: tricyclics, MAO inhibitors, and serotonin uptake inhibitors.

Tricyclics

Although the tricyclic antidepressants have been used for depression for well over 40 years, it was recognized over 20 years ago that this group of drugs seems to have many anti-pain features. Their use in the treatment of chronic headaches has added a significant alternative in this treatment by reducing pain without creating addiction problems. These drugs also seem to be effective in the treatment of atypical facial pain and neck pain disorders. There is also some benefit for intermittent migraine and other headache forms.

It also seems that the action of the tricyclics begins to be effective more rapidly for pain problems than for depression. Some of the actions are due to increasing the availability of synaptic norepinephrine or serotonin, inhibition of 5-HT and norepinephrine reuptake, enhancement of opiate mechanisms, and others.

The drugs are recommended for: migraine and related headaches, episodic and chronic daily "tension-type" headache, neck pain, facial pain syndromes, and pain syndromes with sleep disturbance and/or anxiety.

The various drugs in this group are: amitriptyline (Elavil, Endep), nortriptyline (Pamelor, Aventyl), doxepin (Sinequan, Adapin), desipramine (Norpramin), protriptyline (Vivactyl) and others.

Some of the untoward reactions are (1) weight gain, (2) dizziness, (3) tremors, (4) confusion, (5) anticholinergic symptoms (drowsiness, dry mouth, constipation, urinary retention, blurred vision, tachycardia, and others).

Some of the contraindications for taking these drugs are cardiac arrhythmia, glaucoma, urinary retention, severe hypotension and others.

The use of this group of drugs will be determined by the specialist. Experience often permits the physician to make an appropriate choice of which drug to use and the dosage.

For a more complete list of untoward reactions, guidelines, contraindications, warnings, plus dosages, see the *Physician's Desk Reference* or any other standard guideline references.

MAOI (Monoamine Oxidase Inhibitors)

This group of drugs has been used for moderate to severe depression with a great deal of success. They have also been found to be successful for the treatment of chronic daily headache. However, there are adverse reactions with this group when combined with certain other drugs and certain foods. This medication should only be used by patients who understand these pitfalls and who are compliant patients. However, it has been reported that they appear to be successful with refractory recurring headaches that have not responded to other treatments.

The two most common MAOI (monoamine oxidase inhibitors) are phenelzine (Nardil) and tranylcypromine (Parnate).

The mechanism of action is similar to the other antidepressants. It prevents the breakdown of norepinephrine and 5-hydroxytriptamine and therefore enhances the quantity of synaptic catacholamines.

These drugs are recommended with severe resistant migraine, severe resistant non-neurologic facial pain syndromes, severe resistant chronic daily headache and severe headache in the presence of depression, panic disorder, and obsessive-compulsive disorder.

Some of the untoward reactions are (1) orthostatic hypotension, (2) severe hypertension (when combined with a contraindicated substance — see Tables 25.6 to 25.9), (3) reduced libido, (4) constipation, (5) insomnia, (6) weight gain, (7) peripheral edema, (8) agitation, (9) anticholinergic effects (see tricyclics).

Table 25.6 Guidelines for Combined MAOI and TCA Usage

1. Begin both phenelzine and TCA (amitriptyline, nortriptyline, or doxepin only) simultaneously, or
2. Add phenylzine to existing program of the above.
3. Do not add TCA to existing treatment of phenelzine.
4. Avoid MAOI usage with imipamine, desipramine, or fluoxetine, and certain others. MAOI must be discontinued for at least 3 weeks before any one of these agents is administered; fluoxetine must be discontinued for at least 5 weeks prior to the administration of MAOI.
5. When switching from one MAOI to another, at least 3 weeks must separate the administration of the second agent from the discontinuation of the first.
6. Informed consent is advisable.

From Saper, J.R. et al., *Handbook of Headache Management*, Williams & Wilkins, Baltimore, 1993. With permission.

Some contraindications when considering the use of MAOI are (1) pheochromocytoma, (2) certain drugs (meperidine [Demerol], isometheptene [Midrin], some of the serotonin uptake inhibitors, carbamazepine [Tegretol]), (3) severe liver disease, (4) severe cardiac disease, (5) closed angle glaucoma, (6) severe prostatic disease. See Tables 25.7 to 25.9 for lists of foods and other medication to avoid while taking these drugs.

Table 25.7 Foods To Avoid While on MAO Inhibitors

1. Foods that have a high tyramine content (most common in foods that are aged, fermented, or smoked to increase their flavor), such as cheeses, sour cream, yogurt, pickled herring, chicken livers, bananas, avocadoes, soy sauce, broad bean pods (fava bean pods), yeast extracts, meats prepared with tenderizers, or dry sausage
2. Alcoholic beverages, including beer and wines (especially Chianti and other hearty red wines)
3. High caffeine-containing foods or beverages, such as coffee, chocolate, tea, or cola

From Saper, J.R. et al., *Handbook of Headache Management*, Williams & Wilkins, Baltimore, 1993. With permission.

Table 25.8 Selected Categories of Medications to Be Avoided With MAOI

• Appetite suppressants	• Most other antidepressants, particularly fluoxetine, imipramine, desipramine, others
• Certain asthma medications	
• Decongestant cold medications (including those with dextromethorphan)	• Nasal sprays (except steroids only)
	• Stimulants and weight-reducing preparations
	• Anticonvulsants (specifically carbamazepine)
• L-tryptophan-containing preparations	• Opiate preparations containing meperidine
• Isometheptene-containing drugs	• Mixed allergy drugs (except simple antihistamines)
• Other MAOIs	

From Saper, J.R. et al., *Handbook of Headache Management*, Williams & Wilkins, Baltimore, 1993. With permission.

Table 25.9 Selected Over-the-Counter Products Containing Either Pseudoephedrine, Phenylephrine, or Phenylpropanolamine

Pseudoephedrine	
Actifed	Robitussin-PE
Contac	Sine-Aid
CoTylenol	Sinutab
Vicks Formula 44M	Tylenol Maximum Strength
Vicks Formula 44D	Sinus Medication
Vicks Nyquil	
Phenylephrine	
Dimetane decongestant	Nostril
Dristan Advanced Formula	Vicks Sinex
Tablets and Coated Caplets	Robitussin Night Relief
Neo-Synephrine	
Phenylpropanolamine	
Alka-Seltzer Plus	Coricidin
Acutrim	Dexatrim
Allerest	Sine-Off
Cheracol Plus	Triaminic

From Saper, J.R. et al., *Handbook of Headache Management*, Williams & Wilkins, Baltimore, 1993. With permission.

See standard references or the *Physician's Desk Reference* for a more complete guide to adverse reactions, contraindications, warnings and treatment guidelines.

Serotonin Uptake Inhibitors

These drugs are antidepressants that are chemically unrelated to the tricyclic antidepressant agents. They generally have fewer side effects than the tricyclics and may even cause loss of weight. The oldest drug in this group is fluoxetine (Prozac); some of the newer ones are sertraline (Zoloft), paroxetine (Paxil), venlafaxine (Effexor), and fluvoxamine (Luvox).

The mechanism of action is a potent 5-HT reuptake inhibitor and similar actions of the other antidepressants.

These drugs may be used with migraine, daily chronic headache, facial pain syndromes, and any of these pain problems associated with psychiatric symptoms that would respond to this group of drugs.

Some untoward reactions are (1) agitation, (2) tremor, (3) nausea, (4) headache, (5) hypomania and/or other psychiatric symptoms, (6) insomnia, (7) lower seizure threshold, (8) neurological symptoms (akathesia/tremor/extrapyramidal reactions), (9) nausea, (10) diarrhea, (11) sexual dysfunction, (12) unlikely suicidal preoccupation, (13) impulsive behavior, and others.

Some contraindications are seizure disorder, history of neurological symptoms that have been demonstrated with other antidepressant or other psychoactive drugs.

There have been reported deaths when fluoxetine and MAOIs have overlapped. Therefore, it is strongly recommended that MAOIs be discontinued for at least 3 weeks before fluoxetine is added and fluoxetine discontinued for 5 weeks before MAOIs are added. Fluoxitine has had behavioral and neurological effects when combined with lithium, haloperidol, trytophan, and carbamazepine.

It is always important that an experienced clinician be involved whenever any of these medications are used.

See the *Physician's Desk Reference* or standard references for additional untoward reactions, guidelines, contraindications and warnings.

Ergot Derivatives: Methysergide, Methylergonovine[8]

The drugs in this group are methysergide (Sansert), methylergonovine (Methergine), and ergonovine maleate (Ergotrate), no longer commercially available.

The proposed mechanisms are (1) 5-HT2 receptor antagonist, (2) 5-HT1 agonist, (3) other central effects.

The conditions that these drugs are recommended for are resistant migraine, resistant cluster headache, resistant daily chronic headache, and resistant atypical facial pain syndromes. Recommended dosages are methysergide (Sansert), 2 mg two to five times a day, maximum daily dose 8 to 14 mg a day, preferably plus or minus 8 mg/day; methylergonovine (Methergine), 0.2 to 0.4 mg three to four times a day. Neither of these drugs should be used for more than six months without a one-month interruption and an appropriate examination for fibrotic reactions.

Sansert (methysergide) entered the clinical arena about 1959 and was considered the wonder drug for resistant migraine. It was considered to have remarkable anti-serotonin effects and it was claimed that improvement was seen in 90% of migraine patients. Today, however, the major benefits appear to be about 35% of this difficult type of migraine.

Besides many side effects, the one problem that contributed to the clinician's fear of using the drug is a condition called fibrotic induration. This is where tissue will grow in certain areas causing severe medical conditions. Although very rare, the tissue has grown in pleural or pericardial spaces and over 100 cases have been reported of fibrotic lesion in the retroperitoneal space. If the lesion is in the pleural or pericardial space, the symptoms may present as breathlessness, pleuritic pain, chest pain, coldness, and numbness of the fingers, etc. There can also be severe kidney disease called hydronephrosis (collection of urine in the pelvis of the kidney).

However, there is still a great deal to say in favor of this drug. When the drug was first introduced over 40 years ago there were few guidelines and both patients and physicians over-used and over-prescribed the drug. Once this situation was controlled and the drug was discontinued, many of these conditions were reversed, and since the drug was given one month's holiday every five to six months, there have been very few problems. I have been prescribing this drug since 1980, and with periodic examinations and drug holidays, I have never had any fibrotic lesions with my patients.

The major problem among my patient population was that about 35% of the patients could not tolerate the drug and it had to be discontinued. Adverse reactions are severe chest pain, painful urination, dizziness, fever, flank or groin pain, leg cramps, lower back pain, appetite and weight loss, cold hands or feet, shortness of breath, swelling of hands or ankles. Less severe reactions include itching, numbness and tingling of fingers, toes or face, weakness of toes, changes in vision, difficulty in thinking, hallucinations, nightmares.

Other nonmedical emergencies include diarrhea, some dizziness upon getting up, drowsiness, trouble sleeping, nausea, vomiting or stomach pain.

However, of the 65% of my patients who tolerated the drug, about 70% were much improved and it was difficult having them stop for the one month holiday.

The medical conditions that would be considered contraindications to using this drug are (1) peripheral, cerebral, or cardiovascular disease, (2) thrombophlebitis, (3) severe hypertension, (4) pregnancy, (5) significant renal or hepatic disease, (6) previous fibrotic reactions.

Any physician treating these resistant cases of headache should have a thorough knowledge of these drugs. If by history every six months there is a suspicion of fibrotic changes, then further studies should be done. Saper et al. suggest the following monitoring for patients on continuous ergot therapy for six months or more:[8]

1. Cardiac and carotid auscultation for new murmurs or bruits or change from known abnormalities (echocardiogram, carotid ultrasound testing recommended if suspected abnormality)

2. Palpation of peripheral vascular and carotid pulsations (ultrasound testing recommended if abnormality suspected)
3. Abdominal CT scanning (with and without contrast) for retroperitoneal fibrosis
4. Chest x-ray for pleuropulmonary fibrosis

Consult the *Physician's Desk Reference* or standard references for additional untoward reactions, guidelines, contraindications and warnings.

Anticonvulsants

Anticonvulsants are used and may be effective in treating some selected cases of migraine, cluster, and facial pain.

The drugs discussed here are phenytoin (Dilantin) and carbamazepine (Tegretol). The mechanism of these drugs may be membrane stabilization on pain control through reduction of electrical discharge in the brain.

These drugs may be used in migraine, cluster, daily chronic headache, facial pain, atypical facial pain syndromes, and headaches with associated neurologic conditions. The dosages are generally phenytoin 200 to 400 mg per day, carbamazepine (Tegretol) 100 to 200 mg two to three times a day.

Untoward reactions to Phenytoin include dizziness, rash, insomnia, ataxia, psychosis.[9] Adverse reactions to carbamazepine include leukopenia, dizziness, ataxia, drowsiness, diplopia, and severe drug reactions. Neither of these drugs should be used in pregnancy, and they also should not be used with calcium channel antagonists, oral contraceptives or combined with MAOI.

Valproate (Depakene, Depakote): although this is one of the anticonvulsants, it has been used and written about as a significant medication for refractory headache patients.

This medication has been recommended for use with: (1) difficult migraine, (2) daily chronic headaches, (3) cluster headache, (4) atypical facial pain.

The mechanisms of valproate are complex and may help headaches by: (1) inhibiting "firing" of 5-HT (5-hydroxytryptamine) neurons of the dorsal raphe, (2) increasing GABA (gamma-aminobutyric acid) in the synaptosomes, (3) enhancing postsynaptic response to GABA, (4) increasing potassium conductance producing neuronal hyperpolarization.

Untoward reactions include nausea and gastrointestinal upset, sedation, platelet dysfunction, hair loss, tremor, hepatotoxicity, and weight gain.

Contraindications are pregnancy, hepatic disease, children under 10, concurrent barbiturate and benzodiazepam use.

This is a relatively good drug for refractory headaches but should only be used by a specialist who is well aware of the potential dangers and complications.

See the *Physician's Desk Reference* or standard references for additional untoward reactions, guidelines, contraindications and warnings.

Antihistamines

Certain antihistamines have been helpful both for the symptomatic and preventive treatment of head pain.[8] The drugs in this group that are most often used are cyproheptadine (Periactin), hydroxyzine (Vistaril, Atarax).

Recommended uses are (1) migraine (cyproheptadine may be particularly useful in children, both symptomatic and preventive), (2) combined with other medications to eliminate addicting medication, (3) atypical facial pain.

Cyproheptadine may work as an antagonist at 5-HT2, and also has histamine H-1 and muscarine receptor influence.

Untoward reactions include sedation, weight gain, and anticholinergic effects.

Contraindications are closed angle glaucoma and prostatic hypertrophy. See the *Physician's Desk Reference* or standard references for additional untoward reactions, guidelines, contraindications and warnings.

Lithium Carbonate

Lithium carbonate made its mark in the mid-1960s for the treatment of manic depressive illness, a cyclic disorder. As the years progressed, it was thought that because cluster headache appeared to be cyclic, it may well respond to lithium. Interestingly enough, cluster headache in many cases did respond, but later on the thinking was that it was not because it may be a cyclic disorder but perhaps due to the neurochemical actions of this drug. Perhaps it is because the drug affects the hypothalamus and also may affect the distribution of ions in the central nervous system that cluster responds.

The conditions that lithium is used for are (1) cluster headache, (2) cyclic migraine, (3) atypical facial pain, (4) headache syndromes with significant psychiatric mood disorders.

Untoward reactions include (1) tremors, (2) polyuria, (3) thirst, (4) edema, (5) mental changes, (6) increase in the white blood count.

When the drug is used for a long period, the clinician must monitor the levels of the drug and look for secondary hypothyroidism, oliguric renal failure, and diabetes insipidus. Sodium depletion may lead to some of the problems associated with side effects of lithium.

Contraindications for using this drug are (1) renal or cardiac disease, (2) dehydration, (3) sodium depletion, (4) hypothyroidism. See the *Physician's Desk Reference* or standard references for additional untoward reactions, guidelines, contraindications, and warnings.

Table 25.10 provides a list of selected drugs used in the pharmacotherapy of head, neck, and face pain.

NON-MEDICATION TREATMENTS

Although the headaches that are a result of whiplash and post head trauma are similar to non-accident headaches (migraine-like, tension-type, headache-like, cluster-like, etc.), they do not seem to respond as well to medications as the non-accident headaches. Therefore, other non-medication treatments are often added to the medications to be more effective in helping the patients.

Some of these treatments are

1. Biofeedback
2. Neuromuscular therapy
3. Spinal manipulation
4. Acupuncture
5. Trigger point injections
6. Nerve blocks
7. Physical therapy

Biofeedback

Biofeedback is a method that teaches the patient to control certain functions of the autonomic (involuntary) nervous system, including brain wave activity, heart rate, blood pressure, skin temperature, and muscle tension. It has been reported that biofeedback was practiced on the space shuttle to control brain wave activity that might be producing motion sickness. A patient who learns biofeedback is able to reduce his overall headache frequency, as well as his medical expenses by:

1. Less consumption of expensive medicine
2. Fewer visits to the emergency room

Table 25.10 Selected Drugs Used in the Treatment of Head, Neck and Face Pain

Symptomatic treatment
Analgesics
Nonsteroidal anti-inflammatory drugs (NSAIDs)
  Naproxen sodium (p.o.)
  Indomethacin (p.o.)
  Indocin SR
  Indomethacin suppositories
  Meclofenamate
  Ibuprofen
  Ketorolac (p.o. and IM)
Special Migraine Drugs
  Isometheptene combinations
  (Midrin, etc.)
  Ergotamine tartrate (ET)
    Oral (Cafergot, Wigraine, etc.)
    Suppositories (Cafergot, Wigraine)
    Sublingual (Ergomar, Ergostat)
  Dihydroergotamine (DHE)
    Intramuscular
    Intravenous
Phenothiazine/neuroleptic
  Chlorpromazine (p.o., supp., IM, IV)
  Metoclopramide (p.o. [tablet and syrup]; parenteral)
  Promethazine (p.o., IM)
  Perphenazine (p.o., IM)
Antihistamines
  Hydroxyzine (p.o.)
  Cyproheptadine (p.o.)
Steroids
  Prednisone
  Hydrocortisone (IV)
Preventive Drugs
Tricyclic antidepressants
  Amitriptyline
  Nortriptyline
  Doxepin
Other Antidepressants
  Fluoxetine
MAO Inhibitors
  Phenelzine
Beta-adrenergic blockers
  Propranolol
  Inderal LA
  Atenolol
  Timolol
  Metopolol
  Nadolol

From Saper, J.R. et al., *Handbook of Headache Management*, Williams & Wilkins, Baltimore, 1993. With permission.

3. Fewer visits to the doctor's office
4. No drug side effects (with resultant medical expenses)

Although clinicians and biofeedback therapists have different approaches to therapy our clinic averaged six one-hour sessions. We found that if the patient would utilize the strategy we taught and practiced properly at home, six sessions seemed to work well and periodically the patient would return for a booster session.

Neuromuscular Therapy

Neuromuscular therapy uses additional aids in helping to reduce pain and muscle spasm. Some of these therapies have been reported by patients to be as effective as medications. Other patients have said the combination of neuromuscular therapy plus the medications has been more effective than using just one or the other therapy.

Neuromuscular therapies include the use of electrical stimulator devices, hot packs, ultrasound stimulation, and vapocoolant sprays.

Spinal Manipulation[10,11]

This treatment is generally done by chiropractors and some osteopaths. If the proper patient is selected and the headache is triggered by some "alterations" of the cervical spine, then spinal manipulation may be an alternative method in the treatment of cervicogenic headache or other headaches resulting from this "alteration." Foreman and Croft list contraindications to spinal manipulation.

Relative contraindications are (1) patients with prior stroke, (2) women on oral contraceptives, (3) abdominal aortic aneurysm, (4) vertebrobasilar syndrome, (5) metastatic disease, (6) disc herniation, (7) spondylarthopathy, (8) severe spondylosis, (9) moderate to severe osteoporosis, (10) osteomyelitis, (11) discitis, (12) stable spinal fracture, (13) osteogenesis imperfecta, (14) clotting disorders, (15) intersegmental instability.

Absolute contraindications are (1) unstable spinal fracture, (2) acute spinal cord injury, (3) lack of formal training in spinal manipulation.

There is no reason if a patient is receiving spinal manipulation that conventional treatment has to be sacrificed. Sometimes the combination of these two therapies can enhance the therapeutic effect.

Acupuncture

Acupuncture has played a traditional role in Chinese medicine for well over 2000 years. It was introduced in this country and to Western medicine within the past 40 years. The mechanics of acupuncture are that it is supposed to have an effect on the endogenous opiate systems in the body. The argument is that, like many other treatments that claim success, it basically has a placebo effect related to therapeutic attention. What is needed is a controlled, double-blind study, but this may not be as easy as with a drug.

Many headache specialists' observations are that while the migraine may improve during treatment, there is a relapse shortly after treatment stops. This relapse may be seen equally with a specific or a placebo effect.

Trigger Point Therapy

I recommend that anyone involved in treating myofascial trigger points read and have at their finger tips at least volume one of *Myofascial Pain and Dysfunction: The Trigger Point Manual,*[12] Figures 25.2 and 25.3 demonstrate techniques for the treatment of trigger points.

Nerve Blocks

Nerve blocks play the roles of diagnosis and treatment and often accomplish relief where medication may not be effective. In the chapter on cervicogenic headache it was pointed out that

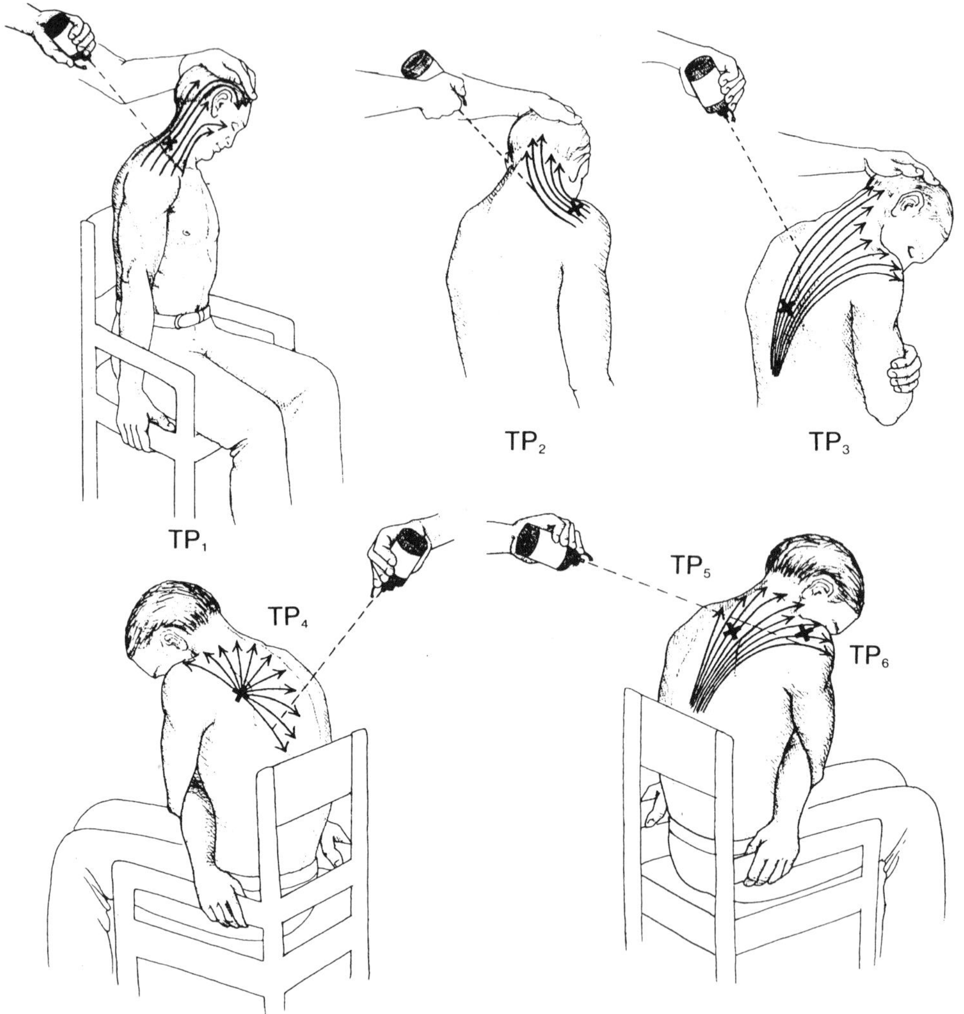

Figure 25.2 Vapocoolant spray therapy for trigger points, as suggested by Travell and Simons.[12] (From Travell, J.G., Simons, D.G., *Myofascial Pain and Dysfunction: The Trigger Point Manual*, Williams & Wilkins, Baltimore, 1983. With permission.)

Bogduk was able to diagnose this headache by blocks to the zygapophyseal joints in the cervical vertebrae even though radioimaging techniques were not able to visualize this pathology. Not only was he able to confirm the diagnosis, but he was also able to give the patient relief.

Unfortunately, the positive results of a nerve block are short-lived and repeat procedures are necessary. It is difficult to predict how long the effectiveness of a nerve block will last. It is not unusual that a particular block in one patient may only last a few days while the same block in another patient may last for months. However, when a nerve block works, the dramatic effect is startling. The patient enters the block room in excruciating pain, pale, red-eyed, and terribly sick, and minutes after the block, the pain, the red eyes, and sickness are gone and the patient is able to leave on his or her own and return to work or to do home chores. I have had lawyers, operating room nurses, and construction workers leave their jobs disabled, come in, and an hour after treatment return to their work at full capacity.

Anesthetic blocks are divided into those that most physicians can do and those that are done by specialists.[13] Trigger points (previously discussed), sphenopalatine ganglion, temporomandibular

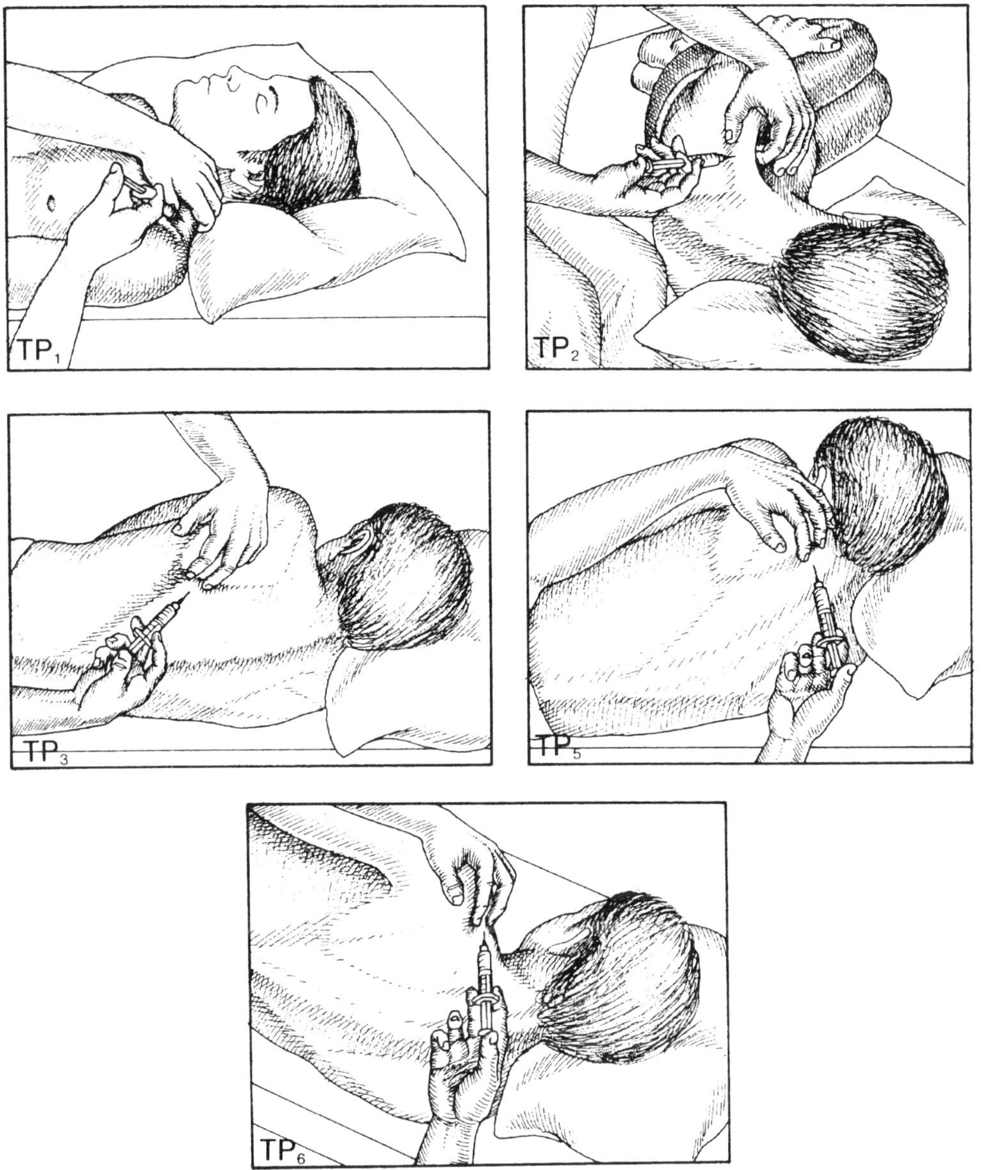

Figure 25.3 Injection techniques for treatment of trigger points, as suggested by Travell and Simons.[12] (From Travell, J.G., Simons, D.G., *Myofascial Pain and Dysfunction: The Trigger Point Manual*, Williams & Wilkins, Baltimore, 1983. With permission.)

joint (TMJ), anterior ethmoid nerve, cranial nerve branches, and occipital nerve blocks can be taught to the general physician without the concern of having to use general anesthesia.

Blocking the TMJ can be done by blocking the auriculotemporal nerve posterior to the mandibular condoyle and branches of the fifth nerve anterior to the TMJ, or an anesthetic can be injected directly into the TMJ. Relief from jaw pain may come by blocking the auriculotemporal nerve which blocks part of the sensation to the temporalis muscle.

Sphenopalatine ganglion (SPG) block is done through the nose using four cotton-tipped, wired applicators dipped in 0.4 ml of a 10% cocaine solution or sarapin, while the patient is in a sitting position. Once the applicators reach the ganglion the patient is placed on his or her back in a quiet room for half an hour, and then the applicators are removed. This is a relatively painless procedure and can be quite effective in aborting a migraine or cluster attack. Although some patients feel it has some lasting qualities, there is no evidence that this is an effective preventive treatment.

If there is a nasal-septal deviation which then prevents the above approach, an ENT specialist or a dental surgeon may do this through the palatine canal using a curved wire. The anterior ethmoid nerve can be blocked with a cotton-tipped wire soaked in 5% Xylocaine.

Many patients will complain that their headache pain originates in the neck or cervical area, regardless of whether it is of traumatic or nontraumatic origin. The cause or etiology of this pain is rarely identified by x-ray or other imaging techniques, and medication therapy, physical therapy, and manipulation therapy do not seem to give patients very much relief. Blocking the greater and lesser occipital nerves can serve as both diagnostic and therapeutic procedures.

If the patient had relief from the diagnostic block, a series of three blocks are done in a week's time and the patient then keeps a headache log and returns in one month for evaluation. Successful blocks give the patient relief for weeks to months. Most of the time the blocks are combined with medication therapy and it is felt that the blocks help interrupt the pain cycle. The posterior head pain is most likely reduced by interrupting the pain coming from C1, C2, and C3, while the anterior head pain is reduced by the interruption of the spinal segment of the trigeminal nerve.

The following is a generic progress note from *Headache and Pain Management* describing the paravertebral nerve block.

Paravertebral Block — Regional of C1, C2, C3 Generic Form

The procedure of a regional block of C1, C2 and C3 of the posterior neck was explained to the patient including possible complications, and the appropriate consent form was signed. The patient was placed in the examining room and after examination of the posterior neck and after pressing on the various vessels and muscles, it was determined to do this block on the ___ and/or ___ side. The patient was hurting worse in the _____ side and the posterior neck was scrubbed with Betadine. Using a 25 gauge by $1^1/_2$" needle, a mixture of 4.5 cc's of 2% Xylocaine without epinephrine and 4.5 cc's of 0.5% Marcaine 4 mg of Dexamethasone Suspension was mixed in a 10cc thumb ring syringe. The needle was introduced over the occipital ridge 1" lateral to the occipital protuberance and the needle was simply pressed through the skin down to the bone.

At this point, 1 cc of the mixture was injected. Then the needle was "marched" across the occipital ridge to the occipital protuberance medially and about three places were injected with a total of 1.5 cc's mixture. The needle was withdrawn then reinjected again about 1" lateral to an occipital protuberance and the needle was "marched" down 1/4" below the ridge toward the deep neck structures and 3 cc's of the mixture was injected. The needle was then withdrawn and again the needle was marched along the occipital ridge and then about 1" out it was aimed just inferior to the posterior mastoid bone and the needle left contact of the bone to avoid hitting the occipital artery. One cc to two cc's were introduced in this area. Then the needle was again withdrawn and redirected down into the *paravertebral*, cervical vertebral muscles mainly to the belly of the semispinalis capitis, and the rest of the anesthetic material was injected into this area to the depth of the needle. When the needle was withdrawn, pressure was applied to the injection site to prevent any bleeding or oozing, and then the patient was placed on an ice pillow with pressure to reduce swelling, bleeding and pain.

The patient tolerated the procedure well and was kept for observation to see what conclusions could be drawn based on the results, as to whether the pain decreased or not.

The other anesthetic blocks require a specialist, who is usually an anesthesiologist trained in the area of pain.

Stellatate Ganglion Block

The sympathetic nervous system (responding for flight or fight) also affects blood flow and pain transmission from the head, tissues covering the brain, and blood vessels in the head. The major "control center" is called the stellate ganglion, located in the neck at the level of the Adam's Apple. This procedure consists of injecting a local anesthetic near the stellate ganglion to temporarily interrupt the transmission of nerve impulses.

This can be effective in aborting a vascular headache when other approaches fail.

Epidural Block

The intervertebral discs are covered by a tough outer fibrocartilaginous ring. The cervical joints are further strengthened by anterior and posterior ligaments, which attach to the intervertebral discs.

Injury to the cervical spine may cause a painful inflammatory reaction affecting the head and neck region. Injecting local anesthetics or saline with corticosteroids (anti-inflammatory) to reduce the inflammation in the epidural space at the back of the neck may help to reduce or eliminate this pain.

Facet Blocks

Pain syndromes may arise from the cervical facets. Each cervical vertebra has a superior and inferior articular facet and there are anterior and posterior articular facets of the odontoid process of the axis. Both head and neck pain may be caused by disease of any of the articular surfaces. Pain may come as a result of limited motion of the neck or by muscle splinting (rigidity to avoid pain).

The C1–2 zygapophyseal joint (facet) can be blocked with a C2 ganglion block, but this is not specific for just that facet. The C2–3 joint (facet) can be blocked with a C3 ganglion block which is specific for that joint. Other zygapophyseal joints (facets) can be blocked directly.

In Chapter 19, on cervicogenic headache, I discussed Bogduk's work on making a specific diagnosis by doing this type of block. The importance of this work is that it has verified the whiplash syndrome even when imaging has not been able to visualize the problem. This block can help differentiate cervical headaches from migraine and tension-type headache. The block can be used to identify C1 ganglion pain syndrome. The C2 ganglion pain syndrome means that the pain impulse travels through the C2 ganglion to get to the brain. According to Bogduk, there are three nerve branches entering the C2 nerve to the C2 ganglion.

Sinuvertebral nerves innervate the dura matter of the posterior fossa, the median atlantoaxial joint, and the cruciate ligament complex. The dorsal ramus supplies sensory sensation to the semispinalis capits, longissimus capitis, and splenius capitis muscles. The ventral ramus innervates the lateral atlantoaxial joint, the prevertebral muscles, trapezius, and sternocleidomastoid.

C3 ganglion pain syndrome is caused by disease in the C2–3 zygapophyseal joint (facet). A branch of this nerve supplies the joint with sensory innervation. For structures innervated by the third cervical nerve, only the C2–3 zygapophyseal joint is the source of chronic pain, except for cases in which the nerve is contused from injury. As a diagnostic test, the C3 nerve root is easier to block than the C2–3 zygapophyseal joint.

Physical Therapy

Many patients after an accident are diagnosed with cervical sprain as the cause of their headaches. This diagnosis is often made because the physician is not trained in headaches. The patients are then referred to physical therapy and the results seem to be dependent on whether the patients will go into their own remission or become chronic.

Those patients who go into remission in weeks or months seem to benefit from physical therapy by reducing their pain while they are healing. Those patients who are going to become chronic will get palliative treatment but will find that the treatment is often good for only hours to a day. The following is a list of physical therapy modalities.

Thermal
1. Pool therapy
2. Whirlpool therapy
3. Fluidotherapy
4. Paraffin bath
5. Moist air units
6. Hot packs (Hydrocullator)
7. Electric heating pads
8. Contrast baths

Cold
1. Cold packs
2. Ice bags
3. Ice slush, ice towels
4. Compressive cryotherapy
5. Vapocoolant sprays

Electrotherapy
1. High frequency currents — deep penetration — Diathermy, microthermy
2. Electrical stimulation
   Total fiber response
   Increased circulation
   Increased phagocystosis
   Mild heating experienced
   Increased beta-endorphin released — analgesia
   Osteogenic stimulation — bone healing
   Enhances open wound healing
   Indications are spasm with subsequent relaxation, exercise, as in disuse atrophy, pain, as associated with the above, and as an adjunct in the healing process

Transcutaneous electrical nerve stimulation (TENS): interrupts pain interpretation by the thalamus; stimulates A fibers, not motor C fibers; increases beta-endorphins

Iontophoresis — ionic transfer through the skin — 10 to 45 minutes
- Epsom salts — magnesium
- Mechoyl (chloride ointment)
- Hydrocortisone
- Zinc
- Copper
- Calcium
- Lithium
- Acetate (acetic acid)
- Salicylates
- Chloride (nacl)
- Lidocaine

Ultrasound — 2 to 4 minutes 2 to 3 times per week

Therapy for Intractable Migraine and Migraine-Like Headaches

Although, most migraine and migraine-like headaches are usually self-limited (<72 hours), and with abortive therapy last for even shorter periods, there are a number of patients who have continuous debilitating migraine who will not respond to outpatient treatment and need a different therapeutic approach.

These headache situations are called intractable (persistent) migraine and migraine-like headaches. It is this group of patients who are in need of hospitalization on a headache unit or pain unit that understands how to deal with chronic pain and the medical situation.

As a result of the incapacitating nature of this type of headache and the debilitating result of the pain, many of these patients are now dangerously over-medicated, dehydrated from vomiting, severely depressed and most often have to be withdrawn from addiction to narcotic pain medications.

The Michigan Head-Pain and Neurological Institute in Ann Arbor, and Blue Cross/Blue Shield of Michigan set criteria for admission to a hospital.[8] The following are the criteria (modified):

1. Moderate to severe, intractable headache failing to respond to appropriate and aggressive outpatient or emergency department measures and requiring repetitive, sustained parenteral treatment (e.g., DHE, etc.).
2. The presence of continuing nausea, vomiting, or diarrhea.
3. The need to detoxify and treat toxicity, dependency, or rebound phenomena and/or monitor carefully against withdrawal symptoms, including seizures.
4. The presence of dehydration, electrolyte imbalance, and prostration, requiring monitoring and intravenous fluids.
5. The presence of unstable vital signs.
6. The presence of repeated, previous emergency department treatments.
7. The likely presence of serious disease (e.g., intracranial infection, cerebral ischemia, severe hypertension).
8. The need to simultaneously develop an effective pharmacological prophylaxis in order to sustain improvement achieved by parenteral therapy (aggressive daily drug level evaluation).
9. The need to acutely address other comorbid conditions contributing to or accompanying the headache, including medical or psychological illness.
10. Concurrent medical and/or psychological illnesses requiring careful monitoring in high-risk situations.

In order for the patient to receive the best and most cost-efficient therapy, a program should be established that would be able to accomplish all these goals in five to twelve days.

An immediate work up should be done to rule out any other medical condition that might be contributing to this intractable headache. Proper laboratory, cardiological, neurological and radiological testing should be done if necessary the day of admission, plus establishing an IV line with a heparin lock.

All previous pain medication should be discontinued as rapidly as possible to eliminate the effect of rebound headache. Unless contraindicated, dihydroergotamine (DHE) should be started and given through the heparin lock three to four times a day in small doses. This should be preceded with metoclopramide to avoid any nausea or vomiting. If necessary, IV fluids may be administered if the patient is dehydrated. Corticosteroids should be given with the DHE for the first four days in decreasing dosages. Oral preventative medications should be started with the IV medications, to be effective when the IV medications are discontinued.

As part of the treatment, the patient should start an exercise, diet, drug education, relaxation, and intensive psychotherapy program immediately. At our headache treatment program, the patient would be awakened early and would be showered, dressed and ready for the doctor's rounds by 7:30 a.m., and would begin the day's program immediately after breakfast. Our staff would take the patients for an early morning walk to start the day. The patients would lose their fear of having headaches with motion because the IV DHE was preventing a migraine attack. By eliminating the rebound effect of the previous analgesic medication they were taking, their remission was quite rapid. Most patients were ready for discharge in five to seven days.

We compared our patients with other headache patients who were admitted in other parts of the hospital where the conventional treatments (bed rest and narcotic pain medications) were given, and found that our patients went into remission much more rapidly, and almost all were discharged headache-free.

When managed care began to regulate care for patients, I no longer was able to maintain our headache treatment center and unfortunately we had to close down.

In an attempt to accomplish some of these treatments, I was able to develop an outpatient medical treatment program that would give the patient an opportunity to have the IV DHE and still be able to function at home. With the help of Rotech Medical Corporation, I was able to insert a tiny catheter into the patient's arm and attach a computerized medicine delivery system that would measure the exact amount of DHE I wanted the patient to have so the patient would be able to resume his normal functions without losing time.

Because this treatment was unique to our clinic, the entire protocol is included here for any physician who may be interested in this technique as developed by Headache and Pain Management Center Inc. I used this method with many of our post traumatic headache population that had intractable migraine-like headaches and were addicted to narcotic medication. Unfortunately, as I was preparing to do a study of this method of treatment, we ran into the same problems with managed care.

I wish to thank H. D. Bangert, III, R.N., for his assistance in preparing this protocol and helping to set up this infusion technique for Headache and Pain Management Center Inc., Winter Park, Florida.

DIHYDROERGOTAMINE (DHE) INFUSION TECHNIQUE FOR CHRONIC INTRACTABLE MIGRAINE

Peripherally Inserted Central Catheter (PICC)

Indications for Placement and Infusion of Dihydroergotamine

1. Daily and continuous headache — intractable and unresponsive to multiple appropriate outpatient therapies
2. Pain accompanied by excessive medication use to the extent that alleviation of both the pain and the medication overuse cannot be achieved without invasive intervention
3. Pain in the presence of ergot or analgesic toxicity
4. Pain in the presence of suspected drug abuse
5. Pain in the presence of significant emotional disturbance such that successful management by less invasive means has been inadequate
6. Pain requiring frequent parenteral medication or ER visits
7. Status migrainus — A disabling migraine which has not responded to other abortive treatment in last 40 hours
8. Status cluster headache — A cluster headache that has not responded to other abortive treatments in last 72 hours
9. Status vascular headache — A vascular headache that has not responded to other abortive treatments in last 72 hours, e.g.
   A. post traumatic headache
   B. metabolic headache
   C. allergic headache
   D. etc.

Contraindications to Infusion of Dihydroergotamine

1. Ergot hypersensitivity or prior allergic response to dihydroergotamine
2. History of frequent phlebitis or solitary episode of deep vein thrombosis

3. History of coronary artery disease or vasospastic angina
4. History of renal or hepatic insufficiency
5. History or peripheral vascular disease either arterial or venous
6. Significant dehydration prior to correction
7. Pregnancy
8. Symptomatic bradycardia or hypotension

Dihydroergotamine Protocol

1. **Day one**
   - A. Stop all nonessential medications*
   - B. Begin infusion at 0.5 mg/day**
   - C. Ibuprofen 600 mg t.i.d. X 48 hr.
2. **Day two**
   - A. Increase to 1 mg/day**
3. **Day three**
   - A. Increase to 1.5 mg/day**
4. **Day four**
   - A. Increase to 2 mg/day**
5. **Day five**
   - A. Increase to 2.5 mg/day**
6. **Day six**
   - A. Increase to 3 mg/day**
7. Once headache free, begin oral prophylactic treatment
8. Once doing better overall, taper by 0.5 mg/day to 1 mg/day
9. Stop IV therapy at 1.0 mg/day; start oral DHE if patient responded to IV DHE
10. Heparin lock to ensure improvement for 72 hours
11. Give 0.5 mg bolus — 1.0 mg bolus when pulling line
12. If no improvement at 3.0 mg/day, then stop, or consider short trial at 4.0 mg/day

Dihydroergotamine Protocol (A)

- Initial dosing
  - .5 mg/24 hours
  - Increase by .5 mg/24 hours as necessary
  - Do not go above total dosing 3 mg/24 hours
- Adverse reactions
  - Nausea — regain 10 mg p.o. t.i.d. p.r.n.
  - Peripheral vascular involvement — decrease dosage until symptoms subside
- Headache breakthrough
  - Analgesics as required
  - Prednisone — 10 mg q.i.d. p.o., reduced by 10 mg daily
- Headache abortion
  - 4 mg dexamethasone IV
- Phlebitis
  - 4 mg dexamethasone IV
- Concurrent medications
  - Acceptable
    - Beta-blockers (Inderal)
    - Calcium channel blockers (Procardia, Calan, etc.)
  - Caution:
    - Sansert — decrease after 2 days by 2 mg

* See protocol for use of concurrent medications
** Change/stop based on side effects or stay at given dose if headache free

Every 2–3 days
Contraindicated:
Ergotamine (Caffergot)
Vasoconstrictors

DHE Calculation Sheet

Cassette Conc.	Rate (ml/hour)	Dose/Day (mg/day)	Days
2.6 mg/NS 55 ml	0.3	0.338	7
	0.4	0.452	5
	0.5	0.564	4
	0.6	0.677	3.5
	0.7	0.790	3
	0.8	0.902	2
3.5 mg/NS 55 ml	0.3	0.454	7
	0.6	0.907	3.5
7.0 mg/NS 55 ml	0.2	0.610	10
	0.3	0.914	7
	0.4	1.22	5
	0.5	1.55	4
	0.6	1.63	3.5
10.5 mg/NS 55 ml	0.2	0.917	10
	0.3	1.38	7
	0.4	1.83	5
	0.5	2.29	4
	0.6	2.75	3.5
14 mg/NS 55 ml	0.3	1.84	7
	0.6	3.67	3.5

Peripherally Inserted Central Catheter (PICC) Policy

1. Standardized procedure for the insertion and maintenance of PICC
2. Registered nurses must meet all educational and skill requirements
   A. Demonstration of competency in placement and care of PICC lines
   B. Successful completion of educational courses on PICC lines
   C. Successful completion of written examination 85% or better score
   D. Annual evaluation and recertification by qualified PICC instructor
3. Registered nurses qualified to do this procedure may do so only under the following conditions:
   A. A written physician's order for the procedure has been obtained indicating catheter tip placement
   B. The patient's written consent for the insertion procedure has been obtained
4. Physicians must be notified if any of the following occur:
   A. Complications arising during the performance of the procedure
      1. Excessive bleeding
      2. Change in vital signs
      3. Respiratory distress
      4. Chest pain
      5. Numbness or tingling of the affected arm/hand
   A. Unsuccessful attempt at catheter insertion

C. Procedure is contraindicated if the nurse determines previously unrevealed medical contraindications (e.g. severe coagulopathies, valvular heart disease, etc.)

Dihydroergotamine Infusion Protocol Via PICC Line

1. Proper patient selection (see guidelines)
2. Proper insertion (see guidelines)
3. Initial dosage (always communicate total 24 hour dosage)
   - A. Administer 5 mg Reglan followed by 0.5 mg DHE over 5 min
     1. Observe for 5 min
     2. If no adverse reactions noted, repeat
     3. If still no adverse reaction noted begin dosing of 24 hour cassette at 1–2 mg per 24 hour, per physician direction
     4. Observe for 60–120 minutes
     5. Reinforce patient education
   - B. Increase following day to 2–3 mg per 24 hour per physician direction
     1. Patients should be seen daily for 2–3 days
     2. Patients should then be followed weekly
   - C. Maximal daily dosage is 3 mg per 24 hours
   - D. Continue the infusion if tolerated and if effective
     1. Taper when patient is pain free and oral program is in place
     2. Continue for 2–6 weeks in refractory patients
        - a. Simultaneous behavioral program
        - b. Simultaneous oral pharmacologic options
   - E. Nausea is common
     1. Options (medications)
        - a. Reglan 5–10 mg q 8 hours
          - (1) toxicity limits use
          - (2) hepatic and extrapryrimidal toxicities
        - b. Vistaril 25–50 mg q 8 hours
          - (1) sedation is major adverse reaction
          - (2) not as effective as Reglan
     2. If DHE causes nausea it is less effective
     3. Consider dosage reduction
4. Adverse reactions to DHE (see physician guidelines)
   - A. Hypotension
   - B. Bradycardia
   - C. Diarrhea
   - D. Leg aching/cramping
   - E. Chest ache
   - F. Phlebitis — manual should be reviewed
5. Patient Management
   - A. Before institution, education must be thorough
     1. Assess if patient is capable
     2. Nursing input is helpful
     3. Must document completion of study course
   - B. Patients chosen according to guidelines — document as part of quality assurance
   - C. Procedures performed according to guidelines
   - D. Follow-up care per guidelines — full case documentation
6. Patient Management — Head Pain
   - A. Concurrent medications that are acceptable
     1. Beta-blockers
     2. Calcium channel blockers
     3. Tricyclic antidepressants
     4. Depakote

5. Prozac and Zoloft
6. Dilantin
7. Tegretol
8. Phenobarbital
9. Non-rebounding analgesics (nsaids)
10. Antihistamines
11. Phenothiazines
12. Abortive meds — rebounding (rarely needed for pain control)
    a. Narcotics
    b. Midrin
    c. Acetominophen
    d. Benzodiazepines
    e. Steroids

B. Concurrent medications that are UNACCEPTABLE
   1. Sansert
   2. Ergotamine
   3. Methergine
   4. Ergonovine
   5. Caffeine
   6. Vasoconstrictors — sympathomimetics

7. Principles of management
   A. Abort pain as needed as DHE increased
      1. Avoid narcotics or rebounders
      2. Use antihistamines, NSAIDs (Toradol), etc.
   B. Begin daily preventative program when patient is pain free
      1. Increase dosage as applicable at each visit
      2. Occasional adjustment upward at home
   C. If DHE is ineffective, steroid burst simultaneously (hydrocortisone 100 mg q 8 h × 6 doses)
   D. Taper when pain free and oral program is stable
   E. Concurrent behavioral program is essential (see guidelines)

Peripherally Inserted Central Catheter (PICC) Protocol

1. Database
   A. Documentation of presence of need for PICC line for continuous infusion of DHE (see medical policy)
   B. Documentation of current EKG, echocardiogram, CBC, chemistry panel, and coagulation profile
   C. Confirmation of line placement via CXR immediately after placement
2. Insertion
   A. Qualified inserters
   B. Procedure
      1. Avoid kinking and coiling of catheter on itself
      2. Identify correct flow rate per manufacturer's prescription and physician's prescription
      3. Heparization
      4. Troubleshooting
   C. Infection control
   D. Cassette changes
3. Documentation
   A. Informed consent
   B. Insertion procedure must be documented in patient chart
      1. Date of insertion

2. Site of insertion
3. Sterilization technique
4. Location of catheter tip
5. Length of catheter
6. Complications of insertion

C. Assessment of site following insertion and with each dressing change

Peripherally Inserted Central Catheter (PICC) Informed Consent

Patient Name____

Your physician ________________________ has recommended that you are a candidate for a peripherally inserted central catheter to administer dihydroergotamine on a continuous basis via an ambulatory infusion device. This means that you will have a specifically trained, certified registered nurse who will insert a small needle into an arm vein through which will be placed a very small tube (catheter). This catheter will remain in your vein and the needle will be removed. The tube will be secured to your arm with a transparent adhesive dressing and tape.

This procedure will be performed under sterile conditions in your doctor's office. While the nurse is placing the needle, you will experience a needle stick at the insertion site (similar to the feeling of having blood drawn at a lab). Some patients may have bleeding at the site, a feeling of flushing or coolness with the beginning of the medication or soreness of the arm. Your nurse has been trained to remedy these possible events with simple measures.

Some of the complications of this type of IV therapy may be:

- Weakness in legs
- Vein irritation
- Redness at the site of catheter entry
- Movement of the catheter (in or out)
- Leaking at the site
- Excessive soreness at the site

Some medication side effects may be:

- Slow pulse
- Low blood pressure
- Nausea or vomiting
- Tingling sensation
- Chest discomfort
- Pain in thighs or calves or legs
- Diarrhea

If any of these things should happen to you (*chills, fever, redness in your arm, tenderness in your arm, drainage from the insertion site, portable pump alarms*), you should immediately inform the nurse. Side effects of medications can occur at any time and it is important that you call the nurse so that your physician can decide about the best dose of medication for you.

The benefit to you of the above described therapy is to gain better control of your headache condition while allowing you to remain at home, work, or recreation.

The risks of the described therapy include infection, heart infection requiring surgery, breaking of the catheter, blood clot formation, loss of an arm, or death.

Your physician knows your individual medical history as you have described it to him/her. Medical conditions that would prevent you from being a candidate for this therapy would include but are not limited to: a history of bleeding problems, a history of clotting problems, any heart condition, a history of frequent infections, or your unwillingness to follow your physician's instructions.

Your physician can determine with you any alternative and appropriate treatment for your headache disorder if you should decide that you cannot follow your physician's instructions.

The above procedure has been described to me to my satisfaction, my questions have been answered, and I understand all of the above. I am giving my permission for Dr. __________________________ and staff to perform this procedure.

Patient Signature __________________________ Date _______________
Nurse Signature __________________________ Date _______________
Physician Signature __________________________ Date _______________

Peripherally Inserted Central Catheter (PICC)

PRE-PLACEMENT PHYSICIAN CHECKLIST

	Y	N
Are placement indications met	______	______
Are there any contraindications to PICC placement	______	______
Are there any contraindications to DHE infusion	______	______
Complete general history done	______	______
Complete general physical done	______	______
CBC done	______	______
Chemistry panel done	______	______
PT, PTT done	______	______
U/A done	______	______
EKG done	______	______
2D, M mode echocardiogram done (optional)	______	______
Patient education done	______	______
Informed consent signed	______	______
Physician/nurse conference done	______	______

Peripherally Inserted Central Catheter (PICC) Procedure

1. Equipment
   - A. 2 - pair sterile gloves
   - B. 4 - sterile towels
   - C. 2 - sterile 4 × 4 gauze
   - D. 2 - sterile 2 × 2 gauze
   - E. 1 - tourniquet
   - F. 3 - Povidone iodine scrub swabsticks
   - G. 6 - alcohol swabsticks
   - H. 1 - nonsterile waterproof pad
   - I. 1 - 5 cc sterile syringe with 21 gauge needle
   - J. 1 - 10 cc sterile syringe with 21 gauge needle
   - K. 1 - injection cap
   - L. 1 - 10 cc vial normal saline for injection
   - M. 1 - 5 cc vial Hep-Lok solution 100 u/ml
   - N. 1 - percutaneous catheter

O. 1 - face mask with shield
P. 1 - gown (non-sterile)
Q. 1 - 4 × 6 Tegaderm dressing
R. 1 - set sterile Steri-strips
S. 1 - sterile pickups
T. 1 - sterile scissors
U. 1 - breakaway insertion needle
V. 1 - 1" Transpore tape roll

2. **Vein selection** — the PICC line may be inserted in (dominant side preferred):
   A. Basilic vein (preferred site)
   B. Median cubital vein
   C. Cephalic vein
3. Procedure and key points for insertion

	Procedure	**Key Points**
A.	Explain procedure to the patient.	A patient teaching session prior to insertion reduces anxiety.
B.	Wash hands with antiseptic soap.	
C.	Select an appropriate vein by placing the tourniquet firmly around the upper arm approx. 4"–6" above the antecubital fossa. After selecting the vein, release the tourniquet. Patient should be flat with head turned away from insertion site. Measure the distance from the proposed insertion site to the proposed termination of the catheter tip. The arm selected for placement should be positioned 90 degrees to the trunk.	
D.	Place the nonsterile waterproof pad under the patient's arm.	
E.	Open and arrange sterile field using aseptic technique. Drop syringes, injection cap, ext. tubing on sterile field. Swab with alcohol tops of both saline and heparin vials, place next to sterile field. Don mask, gown, and sterile gloves.	
F.	Prep insertion site from the mid upper arm to the mid lower arm with: 1. 3 alcohol swabsticks. 2. 3 iodine swabsticks (1 min. ea.)	Begin the venipuncture point and expand in concentric circular fashion from mid upper arm to mid lower arm and on side to drape surface.
G.	Open sterile towels and drape access site.	
H.	Reapply tourniquet firmly around the upper arm near the axilla region approx. 4"–6" above the antecubital area.	
I.	Remove gloves — open PICC tray, don second pair sterile gloves.	
J.	Fill sterile syringes with saline and heparin separately.	
K.	Place syringe with catheter, introducer needle sterile 4 × 4, sterile gauze, and sterile forceps on sterile drape next to patient.	

L.	Using the introducer needle, perform venipuncture.	Enter the skin approx. 1 cm below the proposed entrance site of the distended vessel. CAUTION: never withdraw the introducer catheter while the needle is still in place.
M.	Insert the catheter through the introducer needle and advance it approximately 2"–3".	At this point, instruct the patient to turn head toward insertion site and place chin on chest to pinch off ext. jugular vein to prevent catheter from advancing in wrong vein.
N.	Using sterile 4 × 4, release tourniquet.	
O.	Flush catheter with small amount of Hep-Lok solution as catheter advances to verify patency.	This helps float the catheter up the vein and prevents clotting at tip.
P.	Continue to advance catheter until the redistend predetermined length is reached.	If resistance is met, have patient rotate arm vessel, or raise arm to rearrange venous vasculature.
Q.	Hold catheter with forceps 1" from introducer threading site, withdraw needle.	This secures catheter during needle removal.
R.	Press needle wings together, break and peel away needle.	
S.	Hold pressure over insertion site for approx. 15 seconds.	
T.	Place sterile Steri-Strips over exposed catheter near insertion site to secure catheter.	Suturing is contraindicated.
U.	Cover site with Tegaderm, anchor hub to Tegaderm with Transpore tape, place gauze under hub to prevent pressure to tissue.	
V.	Attached flushed extension tubing and injector site to catheter.	
W.	Dispose of all equipment properly.	
X.	Verify position of catheter with chest x-ray.	
Y.	Document procedure in chart.	

Line Dressing Change Procedure

1. **Equipment**
   A. 2 - pair sterile gloves
   B. 2 - sterile 4 x 4 gauze
   C. 3 - Povidone iodine swabsticks
   D. 3 - alcohol swabsticks
   E. 1 - set sterile Steri-Strips
   F. 1 - 4 × 6 Tegaderm dressing
   G. 1 - bottle hydrogen peroxide
   H. 1 - injection site cap
2. **Dressing change** will occur each week with office visit and routine inspection of insertion site

3. **Procedure for dressing change**

A. Explain the procedure to the patient. Use opportunity to teach patient to observe site daily and preserve intact dressing.

B. Remove transparent dressing by stabilizing. Never use a mechanical clamp hub, then gently pull away from the hub toward device (hemostat) to secure the injection site parallel to the skin. Go slowly as this may inflict damage to the catheter from the patient.

C. Inspect the insertion site for any signs of infection. If purulent drainage is present, may need to culture drainage.

D. To clean insertion site and surrounding area:

i. Don sterile gloves.

ii. Defat skin and remove dried blood with alcohol swabsticks (hydrogen peroxide on sterile 4 × 4 may help).

iii. Using sterile technique, use a circular inside to out concentric circle motion from insertion site outward for 2 in. Do not return to center. Repeat with next two swabsticks.

iv. Clean site with betadine swabs using the same technique as above and allow to dry completely.

v. Lay exposed catheter against skin.

vi. Verify exposed length.

vii. Secure catheter hub with Steri-Strips.

viii. Apply Tegaderm transparent dressing.

ix. Check entire IV tubing system and pump to ensure the system is free flowing at the prescribed rate.

x. Chart the procedure, observations, and patient status.

Line Declotting Procedure

I. **Equipment**

A. 2 - 10 cc luer-lok syringes

B. 1 - sterile 3-way stopcock

C. 1 - vial UROKINASE

D. 1 - pair sterile gloves

E. 1 - sterile mask

F. 1 - sterile central line dressing tray kit

G. 1 - Povidone-iodine swabsticks

H. 1 - vial sterile water

II. **Procedure and key points**

	Procedure	**Key Points**
A.	Reconstitute UROKINASE per manufacturer's recommendation.	
B.	Remove the current dressing only enough to expose the catheter hub/extension tubing connection.	Maintain sterile and keep catheter securely in place.
C.	Keeping the arm below the level of the heart, remove the extension and swab the catheter hub with iodine swab. Using sterile technique, attach 3-way stopcock to catheter hub making sure catheter is in off position.	Decrease the risk of air embolism. The off position maintains a closed central line system.

D. Swab one port of the stopcock with iodine swab and attach empty 10 cc syringe. After remaining port of stopcock has been swabbed with iodine, the other 10 cc syringe UROKINASE is attached.	Use of 2 syringes allows contents of catheter to be aspirated without risk of contamination.
E. Turn the stopcock off to the syringe containing UROKINASE and open to the empty 10 cc syringe.	
F. Gently aspirate the catheter until the plunger is pulled back to the 8–9 cc mark.	Allows evacuation of any substance that may lie between the hub and clot formation. Allows a clear pathway for medication delivery.
G. When the plunger reaches the 8–9 cc mark, stopcock is turned off to the aspirated syringe and on to the UROKINASE.	Medication will be drawn by negative pressure into catheter.
H. Stopcock is turned to off position toward the catheter. UROKINASE is allowed to remain in catheter per manufacturer's recommendation. Stopcock may be opened and the line aspirated to check for blood return; if blood noticed, aspirate 3–5 cc waste then flush line with 20 cc normal saline. If no blood return, repeat above procedure.	Wait 5 minutes before attempting to aspirate the drug and residual clot. Repeat aspiration attempts every 5 min. If catheter is not open within 30 min, catheter may be capped, allowing UROKINASE to remain in catheter for 30–60 min before attempting to aspirate. The 3–5 cc waste will ensure removal of all UROKINASE as well as particles of clot that may still remain.
I. After restoring catheter patency, remove the stopcock and attach a new preflushed extension tubing. Entire line should be thoroughly flushed and heparinized. New sterile dressing may now be applied.	Flushing and heparinization maintains catheter patency. Dressing change maintains sterility and prevents catheter migration.

III. Important Points

A. Never use a tuberculin syringe or sub-Q syringe for the administration of UROKINASE with PICC lines. Small bore syringes exert approx. 120–150 psi of pressure. PICC lines are tested to 40–60 psi of pressure. Additional pressure will rupture PICC line.

B. UROKINASE is supplied in a vial containing 250,000 IU in powdered form. This may be reconstituted ONLY with 5 cc sterile water. Add 1 cc of reconstituted drug to 9 cc of sterile water. This equals a final dilution of 5000 IU per ml. Only 1 cc is required for catheter clearance.

C. Priming volumes for PICC catheters:

1. 9fr. catheter 0.04 ml
2. 2.8fr catheter 0.11 ml
3. 3.8fr catheter 0.25 ml
4. 4.8fr catheter 0.34 ml

Complication Management: Physician Options

1. Bleeding/compartment syndrome secondary to hematoma

A. Elevate extremity.
B. Apply "iced pressure."
C. Check CBC, PT, PTT, platelet count, bleeding time as indicated.
D. Assess peripheral nervous system compromise (i.e. symptoms of compressive neuropathy).
E. Assess the likelihood of control and management without removal of the PICC line. This will be determined by the etiology of the bleeding.

Note: Most often, this complication is acute and mechanical, and can be managed without loss of site. If it occurs later in treatment, the proposed mechanism must be carefully assessed.

2. Tendon/nerve damage

A. Immobilize affected extremity in a position of comfort.
B. Examine to include a full neurologic exam of the affected area.
C. X-rays as appropriate.
D. Assess potential mechanism of the complication.
E. Define diagnosis and treatment.

Note: Most often mechanical; can be managed without a loss of site. Persistent local pain or progressive neurologic symptoms, even without objective signs, should be carefully addressed.

3. Sinus bradycardia secondary to DHE

A. Usually asymptomatic and can be managed by dose reduction.
B. EKG should be performed to exclude other varieties of bradycardia (i.e., conduction block with nodal pacing).
C. If symptomatic, DC DHE, stabilize patient to a supine position with oxygen, if warranted.
D. If pulse is less than 40 bpm or if the patient is symptomatic, then Atropine 0.5mg IV push via separate peripheral line or via PICC line after flushing with nominal saline. May repeat every 5 to 10 minutes up to 2 mg total dose.
E. Move to ACLS protocol if required.

Note: If vital signs are measured frequently while the patient is followed, bradycardia will be apparent as dosage of DHE is increased. Would suggest maintaining the pulse over 50 bpm to avoid compromise. Symptomatic bradycardia is rare and usually occurs in the individual with baseline bradycardia (often secondary to beta blockers) after their initial dosing with DHE. It is possible that continuous infusion may minimize this complication compared to bolus dosing.

4. Chest pain/tightness

A. Stabilize patient — supine, comfortable position, oxygen, check vital signs and temperature.
B. EKG.
C. Cardiac enzymes if indicated.
D. Antacid of choice to exclude esophageal pathology.
E. Sublingual nitroglycerin 1/100, if warranted.
F. If EKG is WNL and if there is no suspicion of cardiac or esophageal pathology, consider warm soak/moist heat and NSAID administration.
G. If W/U is negative, DHE dose reduction.

Note: Muscular cramping is common with DHE administration and will improve with dosage reduction. It is crucial to assess for angina and/or esophagitis. Often and especially in older patients, a cardiology consultation with Thallium stress test will be needed.

5. Leg aching/cramping

A. Stabilize patient in supine position.
B. Assess peripheral pulses; examine for signs of superficial or deep venous thrombosis. Evaluate for muscle tenderness.
C. If exam is not suggestive of vascular compromise, only DHE dosage reduction is needed.
D. Warm soaks.

Note: Muscular aching/cramping is common with DHE administration and responds to dosage reduction, but this may take several hours.

6. Phlebitis

A. Thorough patient assessment to exclude signs or symptoms of local or systemic infection.
B. Follow temperature TID while inflammation is active.
C. CBC, ESR, blood cultures (two separate sites).
D. If there are no signs of infection (i.e., fever, increased WBC, drainage, adenopathy, obvious cellulitis, etc.):
   1. Warm/moist compresses
   2. Elevation
   3. Consider 4 mg dexamethasone IV push
E. If sterile inflammation persists past 48 hours, line should be discontinued and the distal tip (2 mm) cultured.

Note: Labs are optional if the patient is without obvious infection or is afebrile. Close daily observation with physician supervision is mandatory for all cases of phlebitis. HMC policy for phlebitis will be an ongoing quality assurance parameter for all patients.

7. Diarrhea secondary to DHE

A. Exclude dehydration.
B. Lomotil 1–2 p.o. q 8 h p.r.n.
C. Sitz baths.
D. Reduction in DHE dosage.
E. Exclude alternate pathology if indicated.

Note: Diarrhea is a very common problem with IV DHE. It is seldom a major problem and can usually be easily managed.

8. Hypotension Secondary to DHE

A. Stabilize patient if symptomatic:
   1. Supine position.
   2. TED hose.
   3. Increase p.o. fluids.
B. More aggressive therapies (i.e. intravenous fluid bolus or pressors) are rarely needed.
C. Dosage reduction of DHE.
D. Reduce concurrent meds (i.e. diuretic) as needed.

Note: Reduction of DHE dosage alone should suffice to deal with this problem.

9. Cellulitis

A. Thorough patient assessment for signs or symptoms of systemic infection — daily patient visit.
B. Temperature q 6 h.
C. CBC, ESR, blood cultures (two separate sites).
D. Local evaluation and management of insertion site, including consideration of topical antimicrobials.
E. Broad spectrum antibiotics p.o.

F. At any sign of systemic infection, discontinue the PICC line and culture the catheter tip (distal 2 mm).

Note: Careful maintenance of the insertion site is the best way to minimize this complication. This will be an ongoing quality assurance issue.

10. Air embolism

A. Stabilize the patient on the left side with feet elevated.
B. Start oxygen.
C. Immediate transfer to acute care facility.
D. ACLS intervention as required.

Note: This is a complication that is avoided with proper technique. Education of staff and, most importantly, patients is crucial.

11. Catheter tip fracture with migration

A. May be asymptomatic and only defined at catheter withdrawal.
B. May cause acute chest pain, SOB, diaphoresis.
C. Immediate CXR.
D. Cardiology consult.

Note: Fortunately, this is quite rare and usually is asymptomatic. Procedures vary from institution to institution. We would not recommend line removal if fracture is suspected until there is x-ray confirmation.

12. Stuck catheter/blocked catheter

A. Follow nursing manual procedures initially.
B. Consider UROKINASE procedure (see manual).
C. Carefully assess clinically for signs of phlebitis or cellulitis.
D. If catheter is stuck and refractory, surgical consult.
E. If catheter is blocked and refractory, discontinue line and culture tip (distal 2 mm).

Complication Management: Nursing

The nurse evaluating the PICC patient must be instructed in the recognition and management of complications of the PICC line. Insertion complications are best avoided through development of excellent insertion techniques and complete patient screening.

Insertion complications include:

1. **Bleeding/compartment syndrome**
   S/S:
   - Hematoma at site or adjacent to site
   - Numbness/tingling of extremity distal to site
   - Coldness pallor of skin in accessed extremity
   - Limited range of motion of accessed extremity

   Nurse action:
   - Cold pack to site for active bleeding
   - Elevate extremity to promote venous return
   - Notify physician immediately
2. **Tendon/nerve damage**
   S/S:
   - Pain in accessed arm
   - Limited range of motion of accessed extremity

- Numbness/tingling of extremity

  Nurse Action:
- Stabilize affected extremity
- Notify physician

3. **Cardiac arrhythmias**

   S/S:
   - c/o palpitations, dizziness, diaphoresis
   - Change in level of consciousness
   - Change in blood pressure and pulse

   Nurse action:
   - Document bp and hr (rate, rhythm, regularity)
   - Provide supplemental oxygen p.r.n.
   - Notify physician immediately
4. **Chest Pain/Respiratory Distress**

   S/S:
   - c/o chest tightness, pressure
   - c/c dyspnea
   - Change in respiratory rate/rhythm
   - Pallor, diaphoresis, labored respirations

   Nurse action:
   - Assist patient to position of comfort
   - Supplemental oxygen p.r.n.
   - Notify physician immediately

Post-insertion complications may include:

1. **Phlebitis**

   S/S:
   - c/o pain, erythema, swelling
   - Induration
   - Palpable venous cord at or around IV site

NOTE: Sterile mechanical phlebitis usually occurs in the first 48 to 72 hours after insertion, occurs more often in women than in men, occurs more often on non-dominant insertion extremity, occurs more often on large gauge catheters.

Nurse action:
- Warm moist compresses to the upper arm (between the insertion site and the shoulder) for 20 minutes q.i.d.
- Elevation of the affected extremity
- Mild exercise

NOTE: If phlebitis progresses beyond a grade 3+ (see Table 25.11, criteria for infusion phlebitis) or pain becomes severe, continuation of the catheter must be evaluated by the physician. Dexamethasone may be required (see DHE infusion protocol).

2. **Cellulitis**

   S/S:
   - c/o pain, tenderness, and erythema at insertion site
   - Observed spread of erythema in a diffuse circular pattern in the surrounding subcutaneous tissue may indicate phlebitis

Nurse action:
- Notify physician

- Antibiotics as prescribed
- Continued evaluation of the insertion site

3. **Catheter sepsis**
   S/S:
   - c/o chilling, sweats, general lassitude, documented fever, purulent drainage

   Nurse action:
   - Notify physician
   - Blood cultures as ordered
   - Culture catheter tip when removed
   - Antibiotics as prescribed

4. **Air embolism**
   S/S:
   - c/o chest pain, dyspnea, substernal pain, nausea
   - Observed hypoxia, apnea, hypotension, confusion

   Nurse action:
   - Immediate positioning of patient on left side with feet elevated
   - Notify physician immediately

5. **Catheter tip migration**
   S/S:
   - c/o pain in jaw, ear, or teeth
   - c/o flushing sensation during infusion

NOTE: Occurrence may be precipitated by frequent nausea and vomiting or severe coughing d/t changes in interthoracic pressure

   Nurse action:
   - Notify physician
   - Catheter can be withdrawn and manually secured

6. **Stuck catheter**
   S/S:
   - Catheter appears to be held firmly within vessel (vasospasm, vasoconstriction, phlebitis, valve inflammation, thrombophlebitis are all potential causes)

   Nurse action:
   - Notify physician
   - Place tension on the catheter with tape securing catheter for steady pressure
   - Redress the catheter site
   - Warm compresses
   - Attempt removal in 24 hours

7. **Occluded line**
   S/S:
   - c/o portable pump alarming high pressure
   - c/o blood backflow into tubing

   Nurse action:
   - Look for kinked tubing or catheter
   - Look for closed clamp
   - Verify that dressing is not occluding fluid flow
   - Attempt gentle aspiration with syringe

- If blood return, continue to draw back 1 cc of blood and discard. Follow with 1 cc heparinized saline solution flush
- If no blood return, line may be gently irrigated with 1 cc heparinized saline flush solution. Never force an irrigation when severe resistance is encountered
- Notify physician and prepare for UROKINASE procedure

Quality Assurance Data

Patient Date of Birth
Drug Diagnosis
Dosage
Frequency
Method of delivery
Pump SN#
Catheter manufacturer
Catheter lot #
Catheter gauge
Catheter total cut length
Catheter inserted length
Catheter insertion site
Verification of placement (distal tip)
Patient performance scale
Catheter related problems

1. Phlebitis
2. Infiltration
3. Infection at entry site
4. Cellulitis
5. Pain access extremity
6. Limited ROM in accessed extremity
7. Pain or unpleasant sensation during infusion
8. Leakage or drainage from entry site

Catheter removed due to:

1. Successful completion of therapy
2. Catheter complications (describe)
3. Other problems

Total catheter days
Date of insertion
Date of removal
Signature of patient on informed consent form, complication and adverse reaction forms
Signature of person inserting catheter

Patient Information — Dihydroergotamine (DHE) Therapy

You have been diagnosed as having migraine headaches. As you know, many attempts to provide you the relief you desire have been performed. At this time your physician has decided that you are a candidate for an intravenous infusion (IV) solution that has afforded headache relief to a vast majority of migraine sufferers.

Table 25.11 Severity Grade Criteria for Infusion Phlebitis

Grade of Severity	Criteria
0	No pain, erythema, swelling, induration, or palpable venous cord at or around IV site
1+	Pain at IV site, no erythema, swelling, induration, or palpable venous cord
2+	Some erythema or swelling or both at IV site, no induration or palpable venous cord
3+	Erythema and swelling at IV site, induration and palpable venous cord <3 inches above site
4+	Erythema and swelling at IV site, induration and palpable venous >3 inches above site

Thanks to the use of computer technology, this IV solution no longer has to be administered within the confines of the hospital. You will be provided with a small ambulatory infusion device (pump) that will be programmed with your individualized dosage of medication that your physician has developed specifically for you. This means that you will be provided headache relief, be able to stay at home (no hospitalization), and resume work. This will create a savings for your insurance company and help maintain your personal life intact.

Your physician's nurse will place a very small, flexible catheter (tube) into the large vein located on the inside of your arm. This special catheter can stay in place for a very long time without the need for replacement or site change. The nurse will then begin administration of your medication. You will be asked to stay in the office for an appropriate amount of time to allow the doctor to observe your response to the medication. During this time the nurse will provide you with any information needed to help make you comfortable with the infusion pump, the IV, and the medication. A nurse and/or pharmacist will be available to you 24 hours a day in case questions or problems arise.

Medication Side Effects to be Alert for

Contact the nurse if these adverse reactions should occur while at work or home. This will help the doctor determine the correct dosage that will provide you optimal relief.

- Nausea/vomiting
- Pain in thighs/calves
- Weakness in legs
- Chest discomfort
- Diarrhea
- Dizziness
- Slow pulse

IV Complications to be Alert for

- Redness at insertion site
- Catheter migration (in or out)
- Leakage at site of catheter insertion
- Excessive soreness at site or involved arm
- Fever

DHE Visitation Record

HISTORY:
Past Medical History Brief:
Medical Diagnosis(es):
IV access device type and size: Insertion site: Insertion date:
Last Dressing Change: Last extension change: Infusion device in use:
TODAY: Date: Ht. Wt. Temp. Pulse Resp.
BP:

Chief Complaint:
Pain Assessment:
How much, often, and what types of p.r.n. pain medications were used since last visit?

Percent pain relief from pre-DHE level:
Objective/subjective observations and comments:
Intravenous infusion assessment:
Site Condition:
Describe any problems with infusion pump/device:
Describe any untoward effects of medication:

MEDICATION PRESCRIPTION:
Pump type:

Pump serial number:

Medication:
1.
2.
3.
4.
5.

Prescription Changes:
( ) Discontinue medication and remove venous access.
( ) Heparin lock the venous access and DC medication.
( ) No change in current prescription

Procedures done today:
( ) Patient education/reinforcement of education
( ) First hour on infusion observation
( ) IV dressing change
( ) PICC line insertion
( ) Mid line insertion
( ) Peripheral IV insertion
( ) Pump maintenance and/or filling
( ) Additional infusion observation
( ) Declotting of venous access
( ) Repair of venous access
( ) Removal of venous access
Others:

Next Appointment: Doctor: Vital Care
I, the physician, have/have not examined this patient on this date and feel that the continued use of DHE ambulatory infusion therapy is necessary in this care.

Physician Signature:

( ) See page 2 for additional notes
Place of visit: ( ) Doctors Office ( ) Pt.
( ) Phone ( ) Other:
Visit Date: Time:
Nurse/technician:

Patient:

DHE Ambulatory Infusion Nursing Documentation

NAME____DATE______________
HT.______WT.______B/P(L)____/____(R)____/____TEMP______PULSE______RESP______
Chief Complaint____
Brief History____
Start Date____________________________Venous Access________Arm________Vein________
Venous Access Device_____________________Size____________Length, Lot #_____________
Site Appearance____
Dressing__________Last Changed__________Changed Today
Extension/Hub_____Last Changed__________Changed Today
Infusion Device SN# CADD + ____________Medfusion_____________Other_______________
Current Infusion Rate
Dosage_________mg/24 Hour Rate_____________ml/hr
Side Effects
______No______Yes (Describe)____
____

Headache Relief: ___N.R. ___10% ___25% ___50% ___75% ___100%
Adjustments
Increase Dose To ________mg/24 Hours Decrease Dose to _____ mg/24 Hours
No Change in Dosage, Maintain _____________mg/24 Hours

Comments____
____
____

Diagnosis____
I, the physician, feel that the continued use of DHE ambulatory infusion therapy is necessary for this patient.

Physician Signature____Date________________

PICC/DHE Ambulatory Infusion Consent Form

PATIENT:_____________________________________DATE__________TIME____________
DOCTOR_____________________________________NURSE_________________________
have discussed my medical condition with me and have explained the PICC Line insertion and ambulatory infusion procedure via ambulatory infusion pump for which I have been scheduled as well as the risks involved in the insertion of the PICC Line and the administration of intravenous____________________. It is my understanding that the physician and nurse indicated above will be solely responsible for activities in their respective areas of training and expertise.

1. I hereby authorize the above mentioned physicians and nurses, and whomever they may designate as their assistants, to perform the insertion of a PICC Line as it was explained to me.
2. I hereby consent to treatment by physicians and nurses other than the primary physician or nurse listed above in the event that either or any of these individuals should be unavailable at the scheduled time for my PICC Line insertion.
3. The nature of this treatment, purpose, attendant risks, discomforts, and complications which may result from this procedure (which are explained to me to my understanding), and other methods of alternative treatments have been fully explained to me. I understand that no guarantees can be made regarding the outcome of the procedure to be performed or any of the available alternatives.

4. One of the alternatives available to me is to refuse the proposed procedure should I desire to do so. I am aware of the risks of refusing the procedure and hold neither my physician(s) nor nurse(s) responsible for any consequences suffered by myself as a result of such a refusal.
5. I recognize that unforeseen conditions at the time when the procedure begins may require additional or different techniques, etc., be performed, and I authorize the above listed physicians and nurses to perform these procedures.
6. I am aware that the practice of medicine and nursing are not exact sciences, and acknowledge that no guarantees have been made to me concerning the results of the proposed procedures.
7. Other professionals may be present during the performance of the above mentioned procedure for learning or consultation.
8. I CERTIFY THAT I HAVE READ, AND FULLY UNDERSTAND, THE CONTENTS OF THIS DOCUMENT AND AM AWARE OF THE POSSIBLE CONSEQUENCES OF THE PROCEDURE DESCRIBED ABOVE AS THEY WERE EXPLAINED TO ME. ALL BLANKS WERE FILLED IN AND ANY INAPPLICABLE PARAGRAPHS WERE STRICKEN FROM THIS FORM BEFORE I SIGNED IT.

SIGNATURE OF PATIENT_______________________________Date_____________
WITNESS____Date_____________

Physician PICC Order

*PATIENT NAME*____
*ADDRESS*__________________*CITY*__________________*STATE*______*ZIP*________
*PHONE*_____________________________*ALT. PHONE*__________________________

The following orders pertain to the above patient:

1. Registered Nurse to perform PICC insertion procedure.
2. Pre-insertion diagnostic studies requested:
   ________NONE_________CBD W/DIFF________SMAC {# } _____PT/PTT ______EKG
   OTHER:
3. Desired catheter tip location: _______SUBCLAVIAN VEIN_______SUPERIOR VENA CAVA
   Other:____
4. Catheter size: ____2 fr ____3 fr _____4 fr
5. EMLA CREAM if needed: _____YES _____NO
6. Flushing procedure:
   After insertion, flush PICC with SALINE for injection, 5 cc, followed by HEPARIN 100 u/ml, 1 ml
   Other:____
7. Chest X-Ray to determine tip placement: ____YES ____NO
   Radiographic Technique:

Male:	Female:	Contrast medium may be used
KV: 65-75	KV: 54-65	After x-ray, follow flushing
MAS: 100	MAS: 100	procedure
Exp. Time: 0.5–1.0 sec	Exp. Time: 0.2–0.5 sec	

8. Medication
   Orders:____

____

Physician's Signature______________________ Date____________________________

____

Typed or printed name of physician

Instruction Sheet

Preventive Medications

_____ Keep headache log and bring with you when you return.
_____ Doxepin (Sinequan): _____mg_____tab(s) ______times per day
_____ Amitriptyline (Elavil): _____mg_____tab(s) ______times per day
_____ Bellergal S_____ tab(s) ______ times per day
Beta blockers: _______________ _____mg_____tab(s) ______times per day
Ca. channel blockers:_________ _____mg_____tab(s) ______times per day
____

Abortive Medications (To Stop Headaches)

First Line of Defense

_____Midrin. Take two tablets when headache starts. May repeat one tablet every 30 minutes three times if needed. Maximum 5 tablets in one day, but not more than 10 tablets a week.

_____Ergostat. Please take one tablet under the tongue to dissolve. May repeat one tablet every 30 minutes 2 times if needed. Maximum: 3 tablets in 5 days.
____
____

Second Line of Defense

_____ Phenergan suppositories: ____mg. Take _____suppository as soon as you get a #3 headache. If nausea persists, may repeat_____suppository in _____ hours. Maximum: 4 in one day.
______ Ergo Pac suppositories: Insert _____Ergo Pac Suppository. May repeat _____Ergo Pac every 30 minutes _____times if needed. Maximum 3 whole suppositories in 5 days.

PICC Quality Assurance

Patient Calls and Problems

Total Patients + ________________Month____________Date________to________

PROBLEM/CALLS	#	%	Comments
Blood from site			
Blood in line			
Cassette change			
Catheter migration			
Chest and or leg pain			
Dosage change			
Dressing changes			
Extremity pain			
Extremity sore and red			
Hep-lok			
Infection at site			
Infiltrated			
Line acc. Pulled out			
Line broken			
Line occluded			
Nausea			
Pain med. required			
Pump malfunction			
Shoulder pain			
Stomach pains			

Patient Information

What Is a PICC Line?

A PICC (peripherally inserted central catheter) line is a special IV (intravenous) that was originally developed for use in premature infants. The PICC is made of soft material (hypoallergenic silastic) that will not irritate or harm your vein. The PICC is much longer than the normal type of IV catheter (peripheral angiocath or butterfly) you may be used to: the end will be in a large vein (subclavian) under your collarbone (clavicle).

Why a PICC Line?

There are many reasons to use a PICC line; most of them are for your comfort and safety. Since the tip is in a very large vein, past your shoulder, any medication ordered by your doctor will not burn or hurt as the peripheral IV will sometimes do. Because of its length, the PICC line cannot come out of your vein and leak medication into the surrounding tissue causing much pain and possible harm as the peripheral IV can. Hospital and "regular" nursing agencies are forced to change the peripheral IV every 2 to 3 days, the smaller catheters and medications are so damaging to the small veins. However, the PICC line may be left in place for 6 months or longer if needed. This means only one needle stick for your IV therapy instead of multiple sticks (every 2 to 3 days of therapy).

How is a PICC Line Inserted?

Usually a PICC line is inserted into the large vein located near the inside of your elbow. We prefer to use your dominant arm (the right if you are right-handed). The vein is selected and the area is cleaned and a large sterile field is set up under and around the arm where the insertion will take place. We take care to maintain a sterile environment for your IV insertion to protect you from the possibility of infection. The specially trained RN (registered nurse) will then place a needle into the selected vein. The needle is larger than one used by a laboratory to draw blood, but smaller than the needle used to donate blood. It will hurt about as much as a peripheral IV insertion or as in giving blood. If appropriate, the nurse will apply "numbing cream" at the insertion site to reduce the amount of discomfort. When blood comes out of the needle, the RN will thread the PICC line through the center of the needle and into your vein. The RN will then gently guide the PICC line up the vein, past the shoulder until the end tip is in the subclavian vein. The flow of blood in the vein will actually "float" the catheter to its destination. Since there are no nerve endings in the vein you will have no feelings or sensations of the PICC line being threaded to its appropriate location. The RN will then remove the needle and dispose of it. The only thing left in your arm will be the soft and thin PICC line. A transparent waterproof barrier (like sticky Saran Wrap) will be placed over the insertion site to keep it clean. The entire procedure should take no more than 30 minutes.

What Are My Limitations During Activity/Work?

You will have very few limitations. If it is medically approved by your doctor, you may go back to work or school. The dressing MUST STAY DRY to prevent infection of your site, tub baths are preferable to showers, and obviously no swimming. There are to be no blood pressures taken or right bands placed around the arm that has the PICC line. ABSOLUTELY NO BLOOD DRAWING or INJECTIONS may take place in the arm that has the PICC line. You MAY run, drive, bicycle or carry out any other of your usual activities as long as it does not involve getting the IV site wet and your doctor approves of the activity during your illness. Unlike the peripheral IV, the PICC line is very durable.

After Insertion of the PICC Line, Then What?

Immediately after the insertion of your PICC line, your doctor may order a chest x-ray. This is so that the PICC line may be visualized to determine its exact location. Then your RN will go over the exact details of your treatment. The RN will not send you home until you have had all your questions answered and you have demonstrated an understanding of your problem and therapy requirements. You will be given instructions on how to reach the RN for help that is available 24 hours a day. The nurse may then schedule to see you the next day to review what you have been taught as well as to check your PICC line and insertion site. The doctor will make appointments with you for follow up at intervals he feels are appropriate for your current condition. He may change your treatment plan during these visits, depending on how you are doing. Your IV nurses will make every effort to be with you at each of your follow up visits with the doctor to see you and answer any questions that may have come up.

What Can Go Wrong with the PICC Line?

Potential complications of a PICC line are similar to those of peripheral IVs. Following is a list of complications; most are very rare. The potential consequences of PICC Line Therapy are similar to that of any intravenous therapy.

1. Bleeding
2. Phlebitis — an inflammation of the vein
3. Catheter sepsis — an infection caused by the patient's reaction to the catheter
4. Air embolism — an air bubble within the blood vessels
5. Catheter migration — the catheter moving in or out of the body
6. Thrombosis/embolism — a blood clot that has broken loose and has traveled to a different location within the body
7. Pain during infusion
8. Catheter tip embolism — the catheter breaks within the blood vessel, and travels to a different location within the body
9. Arrhythmias — abnormal heart beat pattern, similar to palpitations
10. Stuck catheter
11. Nerve and tendon damage
12. Cellulitis — inflammation or infection of cellular or connective tissue
13. Perspiration under the transparent bio-occlusive dressing
    a. Moisture, in the form of perspiration under the dressing, may provide an ideal environment for pathogenic organisms to flourish. This increases the patient's risk of infection.
    b. Under the most benign circumstances, moisture under the dressing can cause the dressing to fail to adhere to the patient's skin. This causes an inconvenience for the patient, who has to interrupt his or her schedule to have the dressing changed.

Guidelines of Care for the Patient With a PICC Line or Midline

General Instructions

1. If you have any problems or concerns, call ______________ 24 hours/day.
2. Most medications should be stored in your refrigerator. Please check your label.
3. Protect your infusion pump from falls, hard bumps, freezing cold, and direct sunlight.
4. If your one-way valve leaks when your tubing is disconnected, put a red cap on the end and call your nurse.
5. Please DO NOT allow anyone to draw blood, start IVs, or give you shots in the arm with the IV.
6. Keep your dressing dry. Baths are preferable to showers.
7. Do not use your IV for any medications other than those your nurse has instructed you to use.

Changing Clothes

We do not recommend disconnecting your tubing from the catheter to change clothes.

1. Slip the pump down your sleeve and out the bottom of your shirt or blouse. Then place the pump in your fanny pack with the excess tubing coiled inside.
2. If you have a button-up shirt or blouse the tubing will automatically thread itself through the sleeve as you slide your arm into the sleeve.

Disconnecting the Catheter and Tubing

If you must disconnect the catheter and tubing for any reason:

1. Stop the pump.
2. Disconnect the tubing and catheter with a twisting motion, as if unscrewing a bolt.

Never disconnect anywhere other than the one-way valve.

3. Before allowing the end of the tubing to touch anything, put a new sterile red cap on the end.
4. Please do not leave your pump off very long. A delay of several minutes could lead to clots in your catheter that will not harm you, but could ruin the catheter.
5. When reconnecting, remove the red cap and throw it away.
6. Reconnect the tubing and catheter with a gentle twisting motion.
7. Restart the pump.

Traveling With Your Infusion Pump

If you are going to be a long way from home, it is a good idea to take enough supplies with you to flush your line and cap it. You may put these items in your glove box in a clean zip lock bag. Be sure to have your nurse's phone number ________________, with you and carry the Emergency Instructions for Health Care Personnel form on your person. (This will be given to you at the time the PICC line is inserted, describing the type of line, length, location and proper maintenance instructions.)

If you need to travel out of town, please contact your nurse a week ahead of time, if possible. Usually nursing coverage and medications can be arranged for you with appropriate notification.

Problems that Need to be Reported Immediately

1. A high fever.
2. Sudden shortness of breath and/or chest pain.
3. Pain at your IV site or up your arm.
4. Red streaks or hard long knots running up your arm.
5. Swelling of your arm or neck.
6. Pus underneath your dressing around the insertion site.
7. If water or perspiration should loosen your dressing so that air can get to the catheter insertion site.

Trouble Shooting the CADD Plus Infusion Pump

How to Start and Stop Your Pump

1. To start the pump: Push and hold the STOP/START button until three dashes appear then disappear. The pump will beep several times as it displays its program setting and the "STOP" will disappear from the lower right hand corner of the display.
2. To stop the pump: Push and hold the STOP/START button until the three dashes appear then disappear. The word "STOP" will blink in the lower right hand corner. There will be three "beeps" every 5 minutes as a reminder that the pump is stopped.
3. To turn the power on or off: You must insert or remove the battery. There is no ON/OFF button.

Alarms

1. LOW RESERVOIR VOLUME
   If a variable tone beeps and 003, 002, or 001 shows in the "RES VOL". Medication is running low; time to change the medication cassette as your nurse has instructed you.
2. OUT OF MEDICATION
   If you hear 2 beeps every second and "000" shows in the display. Call your nurse immediately; you are out of medication.
3. LOW BATTERY

The display "LO BAT" appears and blinks. Three beeps sound every 5 minutes. Read the section of your patient information booklet on how to change the battery and do so immediately.

4. DEAD BATTERY
   The display "LO BAT" appears and stays on without blinking and a continuous tone is emitted. The battery is dead. Change immediately.
5. OCCLUSION
   The display "HI P" appears and a continuous tone sounds indicate that there is a block in the line. Try these things:
   - Straighten out the arm.
   - Check the tubing between the pump and the IV insertion site for kinks, pinching, or closed clamps.
   - Try moving the arm all around and in full circles so that the shoulder joint is moved in every direction it can. Shrug and wiggle the shoulder as well.
   - If you fix the problem, the alarm will stop and the pump action will resume.
   - If the alarm continues, stop the pump and call your nurse immediately.
6. Pump Failure
   A continuous variable tone sounds and an "E" followed by two numbers or "OFF" appears on the display.
   - A possible internal pump failure has occurred. Please make a note of the numbers.
   - Clamp or disconnect the IV tubing from your catheter, remove the battery from the pump.
   - Call your nurse immediately. Do not attempt to restart the pump.
7. "STOP" reminder
   Three beeps are heard every five minutes and "STOP" will blink on the display. The pump is reminding you that it has been stopped and the battery is still in place. When you are finished with what you are doing with the pump, be sure to restart.

Changing the Battery

Your battery will not suddenly go dead. The pump will warn you several hours before. It will beep three times every three minutes and "LO BAT" will appear on the display screen. Your nurse will change the battery periodically (the battery will last about 10 to 14 days) so you will probably never have to.

- Stop the pump.
- Turn the pump over and slide the battery cover off.
- Lift out the old battery and insert the new one (bottom end of the battery is put in first).
- Be sure that the polarity is correct ("+" and "–") by matching the battery to the markings in the battery well.
- Replace the battery cover.
- The pump will beep several times as it displays its previous programming. When it stops beeping BE SURE TO START THE PUMP AGAIN. The pump holds the programming in memory with the battery out so that you will not have to reprogram.

Trouble Shooting and Care of IV Lines

Blood Backing Up Into Tubing or Fluid Leaking

1. Check to be sure that the pump is on. The word "STOP" should NOT be displayed in the upper right corner of the screen. If the pump is stopped, restart it now.
2. If the pump is running, look for any leaks. Check all tubing connections carefully by retightening.
3. If the dressing is wet and you believe that the catheter or catheter site may be leaking under the dressing, call the nurse immediately.
4. If there is enough blood in the tubing that you cannot see light through it, the line must be "flushed" immediately. Instructions are as follows.

Flushing the Line

1. Prepare a saline (sodium chloride) syringe as instructed by your nurse.
2. Stop the pump.
3. Disconnect the tubing from the catheter and place a needle or cap on the end of the tubing before laying it down.
4. Connect the saline syringe to the catheter with gentle twisting motion.
5. Start by SLOWLY injecting the saline. As the blood starts to move down the tubing you may push faster. DO NOT PUSH HARD! IF YOU MEET RESISTANCE, DO NOT FORCE IT. CALL THE NURSE IMMEDIATELY!
6. You may repeat the flushing as many times as necessary to clear out the blood, once or twice is usually enough.
7. Reconnect the tubing to the catheter.
8. Restart the pump. Then discard the syringe and needles into the needle box.

Drawing Medication from a Vial

1. Wash your hands and gather your supplies. Check the medication vial to make sure it matches your instructions. Do not have more than one vial at a time near your work area.
2. Remove the cover from the top of the medication vial, if applicable. Wipe the top with an alcohol pad and leave the pad resting on top of the vial.
3. Remove a syringe from its wrapper. Check to be sure that the needle is twisted on tight.
4. Check your instructions carefully and pull the plunger back until the top of the plunger is even with the mark for the amount of medication that is to be drawn up.
5. Remove the alcohol pad from the vial of medication, check again that it is the correct medication to be used.
6. Remove the needle cover from the syringe. Insert the needle straight down through the middle of the rubber vial stopper.
7. Leaving the needle and syringe in the vial, turn the syringe and vial upside down and inject the air from the syringe into the vial.
8. Making sure that the end of the needle is well below the medication level, pull back on the plunger and withdraw the proper amount of medication that your physician has ordered. If you have air bubbles within the syringe, tap the syringe sharply so that the bubbles will rise to the top of the syringe. Push the air back into the vial and again withdraw the medication until the proper amount is in the syringe.
9. Pull the syringe and needle from the vial and set the vial down.
10. You may carefully recap the needle and then use the medication as directed. Use the drawn up medication very soon. Do not let it sit around.

SUMMARY

Treating difficult headaches requires two major components, one, a clinician who specializes in, or devotes a significant amount of his/her practice to, headaches, and two, a compliant patient. The clinician who is not prepared to take the time to evaluate the history of the patient (see Chapter 4) and to understand the variables that are part of this complex problem not only will miss the diagnosis, but may treat incorrectly. As you have read in all these chapters, *a headache is not just a headache*, and treating them requires an in-depth understanding of the patient, the diagnosis, and the wide assortment of treatments that are available. Snap decisions and pain pills are the sufferer's worst nightmare and only lead to worse problems. Too often a clinician will become frustrated and refer the patient to a psychiatrist or a psychologist, which may relieve the practitioner's anxiety but does nothing for the patient unless the psychotherapist is a headache specialist. Therefore, a patient who is suffering chronic headaches should find someone who meets the qualifications of having taken courses in the treatment of headches. Information of this nature can be gotten from the National Headache Foundation and The American Association for the Study of Headache (addresses in the back of this book).

The second component is a compliant patient. Headaches are difficult medical problems and usually do not respond to "rapid cures." It may take many different approaches to find help. Patients must learn to follow instructions carefully and keep records of their progress. The headache log (an example is shown following the References) is essential for both the clinician and the patient to evaluate treatments. The headache log is simple to keep, but complex in the information it gives out and I was always astounded at what the patient thought was going on and what was really happening. From the headache log, one can see patterns of the headache, and evaluating percentages of each type of headache (incapacitating, interfering, and irritating) helps to decide how to change medications or any other treatment that is in progress. The headache specialist can often zero in on the problem by just evaluating the log. Therefore, the patient must take an active role in his or her own therapy.

An attempt was made in this chapter to cover a wide assortment of treatments for headaches. Obviously, there are many reported treatments that were not covered, and treatments that have not been reported. This book is primarily written for an educated reader and is not a text or a doctor's treatment manual.

There are many references made to books and other publications that were intended for medical practitioners in the back of this book.

REFERENCES

1. Lance, J.W., *Mechanism and Management of Headaches,* 4th ed., Butterworth, London, 1982.
2. Sacks, O., *Migraine,* University of California Press, Berkeley, 1992.
3. Diamond, S., Dalessio, D.J., *The Practicing Physician's Approach to Headache*, Williams & Wilkins, Baltimore, 1986.
4. Rapoport, A.M., Sheftel, F.D., *Headache Relief*, Simon & Schuster, New York, 1990.
5. Robbins, L., Lang, S.S., *Headache Help,* Houghton Mifflin, Boston, 1995.
6. Swerdlow, B., A rapid hypnotic technique in a case of atypical facial neuralgia, *Headache*, 24(2), 104–109, 1984.
7. Huey, L., Forster, R., *The Complete Waterpower Workout Book*, Random House, New York.
8. Saper, J.R., Silberstein, S.D., Gordon, C.D., Hamel, R.I., *Handbook of Headache Management,* Williams & Wilkins, Baltimore, 1993.
9. Swerdlow, B., Acute brain syndrome associated with sodium diphenylhydantoin intoxication, *American Journal of Psychiatry*, 126(1), 100–101, 1965.
10. Vernon, H., Spinal manipulation and headaches, an update, *Topics in Clinical Chiropractic,* 2(3), 33–47, 1995.
11. Foreman, S.M., Croft, A.C., *Whiplash Injuries: The Cervical Acceleration/Deceleration Syndrome,* 2nd ed., Williams & Wilkins, Baltimore, 1995.
12. Travell, J.G., Simons, D.G., *Myofascial Pain and Dysfunction: The Trigger Point Manual,* Williams & Wilkins, Baltimore, 1983.
13. Francis, J.H., *Acute and Chronic Headaches: A Guide for the Primary Physician and Headache Specialist,* Aadvark Publishers, 1992, 109–112.

Headache Log – 19___

	S	M	T	W	TH	F	SA
Jan							
Feb							
Mar							
Apr							
May							
Jun							

	S	M	T	W	TH	F	SA
Jul							
Aug							
Sep							
Oct							
Nov							
Dec							

Mark each day for the most extreme headache experienced: "1" for irritating, "2" for interfering, "3" for intractable. Mark "m" on each day for menstruation.

Chapter 26

Long-Term Outlook for the Whiplash Patient

The first part of this book was written in an attempt to educate the reader about the various types of headaches and their mechanisms. Part two aimed to explain headaches as a result of trauma, whether the accident created a blow to the head or not.

It is unfortunate that this medical problem has become a legal issue resulting in drawn out settlements and continued suffering for the patient. Much of this is the result of a small percentage of malingerers and physicians not understanding this medical problem. Physicians recognize that a rear-end collision that causes a hyperextension followed by flexion of the neck can cause acute pain and suffering and have diagnosed these injuries as cervical sprain, cervical acceleration-deceleration injuries, hyperextension injury, whiplash and others.[1] Croft suggests the term hyperextension/hyperflexion, a term commonly used may be inaccurate. His studies and research indicate the injury can occur to muscle, ligament, and disc well within the physiologic range of motion. Hence, the term cervical acceleration-deceleration (CAD). In some cases, the suffering is short, lasting days to several months, and then the pain subsides, while 30% to 55% have continued pain, leading to disability in almost 10%.[1]

It is when the pain continues beyond this time period and other symptoms persist that the physician becomes skeptical because of the lack of objective findings, such as neurological deficits, abnormal x-ray, CT, or MRI findings. Coupled with the fact that these accidents are generally the result of low speed collisions and end up in litigation, the physician becomes weary of being able to defend the patient's complaints. It also doesn't help when the physician comes across some people who are obviously feigning their symptoms for financial reward. In this regard, the legal system and the term "whiplash" becomes a turn-off for the treating physician.

Hopefully, with education, continued research, and a method of weeding out the malingerers, attention will be paid to those who suffer from a medical disease.

Considering the fact that in 1989 there were 12,800,000 motor vehicle accidents in the United States, with over 3,280,000 of them being rear-end collisions currently estimated from 1,000,000 to 3,000,000 whiplash injuries, it certainly appears that we have to take this problem seriously. The fact that billions of dollars are spent each year and there is the potential of reducing these costs considerably if we understood this disease makes it essential that we don't continue to wave our hands shouting "psychological or malingering" and treat this problem as an organic disease.

What we know about these injuries from experimental and cadaver studies is that there are certain anatomical injuries that have been demonstrated. These injuries include (see Chapters 14, 15, 16, 17 and 19) muscle tears, hemorrhages, rupture of the anterior longitudinal ligament and other ligaments between C4 to C7, tears of the disc from the vertebral bodies, and disc herniations.

There can be bleeding in the esophagus and around the structures of the internal neck (retropharyngeal and intralaryngeal), and damage to the sympathetic nervous system. There can also be nerve root damage, cervical spinal contusions, and hemorrhages and contusions over surfaces of the cerebral hemispheres, brain stem, and cerebellum. Now, there is evidence that apophyseal joint injuries can lead to chronic pain.

Other studies indicate that there are risk factors that may lead to the chronicity of this disease. The risk factors include older age of the patient, interscapular or upper back pain, occipital headache, multiple symptoms or parathesias at presentation, reduced range of movement of the cervical spine, objective neurologic deficit, preexisting degenerative osteoarthritic changes, cervical stenosis, upper middle occupational category, and abnormal cervical spine curves.

As stated in earlier chapters, even in patients involved in medicolegal cases, 79% returned to work by one month, 86% by three months, 91% by 6 months, and 94% by one year.

What then are some of the factors that may lead to chronic pain and headache symptoms?

Elderly patients, especially those older than sixty, may be more vulnerable to fractures and may heal more slowly than younger patients. Older patients prior to the accident will have had arthritic changes, loss of flexibility, and generally be less capable of healing as well as a younger person.

Alterations in the size of the spinal canal may have a significant relationship in the continuing problems following a whiplash injury.[2] Patients with narrow spinal canals are at far greater risk of suffering neurological deficits than those with large spinal canals. The spinal canal size classifications have been labeled relative and absolute.[2] Absolute spinal stenosis refers to canals that have midsagittal diameters of 10 millimeters or less. Here the bony canal is placing direct pressure on the spinal cord, and minor injury may cause cord swelling that may result in a partial or complete neurological deficit. Relative stenosis refers to spinal canals with midsagittal diameters of 13 millimeters. In this case moderate hyperextension injuries may produce sufficient spinal cord swelling to cause neurological deficits. As the spinal canal increases in size, the chances of neurological deficits decrease and studies indicate that at C4 to C5, 19 mm was a size that had relatively small chance to cause neurological deficits. The narrowing of the canal may be due to congenital malformation, overgrowth of the posterior facets, ossification of the posterior ligament, infolding of the yellow ligaments on the posterior aspect of the spinal canal, and other reasons.

Other conditions that may preexist the accident that may contribute to a chronic state following the accident are osteoarthritis, degeneration of vertebral body joints, disc degeneration and inflammatory processes.

Osteoarthritis: Most physicians agree that arthritic changes begin as early as the late thirties, but do not necessarily demonstrate any symptomatic changes and the patient is unaware of these changes. The degeneration is seen in the facet joints and the changes are similar to the changes that take place in the digits of the fingers. Eventually these degenerative changes could cause radiculopathy (disease of the roots of the spinal nerves) and pain. Therefore, degenerative changes probably preexisted the accident, and radiographic changes have little correlation with subjective pain. It is difficult to predict whether these changes will translate into future pain. There have been studies that demonstrated that these arthritic changes have resulted from whiplash accidents and those patients who had normal radiographic studies before the accident developed osteoarthritic changes after the accident. Other studies indicate that preexisting osteoarthritic changes contributed to alter the prognosis adversely.

These conditions are often examined legally. The medical expert will be asked to determine how this disease will affect future degenerative changes as a result of the accident.

Disc degeneration: As we get older there is a degeneration of the intervertebral disc. This degeneration affects the height of the disc. When there is loss of disc height, then this may cause a decrease of motion of the posterior facets and lead to restriction of motion at that level. Therefore the biomechanical function of these vertebrae are affected. If there is restricted motion and a cervical acceleration/deceleration accident takes place, an insult to the facet joint and disc is more probable and can lead to the chronicity of the pain.

Inflammatory diseases include:

1. Ankylosing spondylitis (fixation of the vertebral joint because of inflammation), which may lead to fracture of the joint in CAD because of osteoporosis and atrophy of the muscles due to the immobilization of the vertebrae.
2. Rheumatoid arthritis, which may also affect the bony and ligamentous structures of the cervical spine. The disease weakens the ligamentous structures and because 85% of the motion in the cervical spine occurs in the upper cervical spine, dislocation may be more likely to occur as a result of high-force trauma.
3. Klippel-Feil syndrome (congenital fusion of multiple cervical levels), which reduces the motion of the cervical spine and also presents stenosis of the spinal canal, especially in the C2 to C3 area. Even minor trauma may cause disastrous cord symptoms.

Foreman and Croft[3] have attempted to set up a classification that could, on the basis of early examination, predict with some accuracy the prognosis of the patient after a cervical acceleration/deceleration accident. The concern is that there is a considerable amount of time between the accident and the settlement and this leads to abusive medical and legal charges. As a result of this, these authors feel the following problems result:

1. Excessive medical charges accumulate in an attempt to relieve symptoms that will not resolve.
2. Attorneys request large monetary settlements in an attempt to pay the unreasonable medical charges. Generally, there is a lack of objective data to prove the patient's injury.
3. Insurance carriers deny payment for unnecessary medical charges and force the claim to litigation.

Therefore, Foreman and Croft[3] have devised a numerical scale to "spot the problem cases" on the days the injuries occur. They feel the advantages of using such a scale include the following:

1. The physician can predict, with some accuracy, the probability of future problems, such as development of neurological deficits or failure to respond to conservative care.
2. The attorney can monitor the patient's progress, knowing in advance the approximate degree of probable clinical complications.
3. The insurance carrier can establish accurate settlement reserves and decrease the number of litigated cases.
4. The patient can better understand what future problems may result from the injury.

The classification is called MIC (major injury category) and is based on physical examinations, radiographic examinations, and patient questionnaires which provide the data to forecast the clinical prognosis.

MIC 1. "MIC 1 is used for patients who present with symptoms directly relating to their injuries. On physical examinations, however, there are no objective signs of loss of motion or neurological deficit with the patients' complaints."

MIC 2. "Patients who present with decreased range of motion of the cervical spine in addition to MIC 1. Subjective symptoms are placed in MIC 2. A measurable increase in cervical muscular diameter also may be expected. MIC 2 patients do not present with neurological deficit signs."

MIC 3. "MIC 3 patients present with MIC 1 and MIC 2 symptoms plus objective neurological loss (either sensory or motor). These losses should be objectified by a neurologist because of the clinical decisions that will be made with this information."

Residual pain in MIC 1 is 56%, MIC 2 is 86%, and MIC 3 is 90% and the symptoms remaining are neck pain, headache, and paresthesias. The authors point out that 41% of MIC 1 patients go into total remission.

As discussed before, there are modifiers that affect the prognosis. They are the size of the spinal canal, straight cervical spine, kyphotic cervical curve, fixated segments, preexisting degenerative changes, and loss of consciousness. These modifiers are given points:

Modifiers	Point Value
Canal size of 10–12 mm	20
Canal size of 13–15 mm	15
Kyphotic curve	15
Fixated segment of flexion and extension films	15
Loss of conciousness	15
Straight cervical curve	10
Preexisting degeneration	10

Points are also assigned to each MIC group (see above for definition of these groups). For example, MIC 1 is assigned 10 points, MIC 2 50 points and MIC 3 90 points.

Although the initial points will give a patient's prognosis, alterations of the factors may modify the course of treatment and perhaps the prognosis.

Prognosis group 1 (10–30 points). These patients have an excellent prognosis and usually recover fully.

Prognosis group 2 (35–70 points). This group may be composed of MIC 1 or MIC 2. The prognosis here is generally good, and long-term risk of dependence on medications, neurological deficits, and possible surgery is low.

Prognosis group 3 (75–100 points). Prognosis group 3 is primarily composed of MIC 2 patients who have several modifiers. The remainder of the group is composed of MIC 3 patients. The prognosis for patients in this group is fair, and a number of these patients develop neurological deficits.

Prognosis group 4 (105–125 points). The probability of future or persistent neurological deficits is likely, so prognosis for patients in this group is poor.

Prognosis group 5 (130–165 points). Prognosis group 5 is composed of patients whose prognosis is termed "unstable." Foreman and Croft[3] report that these patients will not benefit from conservative care and future care will probably necessitate surgical intervention. These patients will probably become medication-dependent.

The authors state these scales concentrate on identifying patients that may develop dependence on medications, neurological deficits, or the possibility for surgical intervention. They point out that these scales do not take into account frequency and duration of treatment and should not be used in this manner. "Any attempt to use this scale for purposes other than intended should be condemned."

I commend the authors for attempting to logically set up guidelines prognosticating the patient's future in the adversarial medicolegal arena. The difficulty with the headache patient is that there are no anatomical structures that can be used for modifiers that can be identified initially after the accident. If the patient already suffers migraine or migraine-like headaches prior to the accident, these headaches may increase in frequency and intensity regardless of the modifiers they use. Secondly, migraine-like headaches may be initiated from the accident without alterations of spinal canal size, kyphotic curves or even loss of consciousness.

Now that Barnsley et al.[4] have made a landmark case for headache that may be a result of pathology of the zygapophyseal joints (see Chapters 14 and 19), previous arthritic conditions of these joints may be exacerbated by the accident. However, this problem is often not recognized until the headache symptoms are chronic, and at this point the most reliable test is an intra-articular injection of corticosteroids. X-ray, CT and MRI have not been helpful in identifying this pathology and certainly these tests done at the time of the accident would not reveal the information necessary to make this diagnosis. The intra-articular injection would have to be in the hands of a well-trained specialist who is usually not available in the emergency room and it is not a procedure that is part of the training of a neurologist.

Because about 40% to 60% of whiplash patients improve or actually go into remission within six months, the prognostic scale would serve to identify those patients who become chronic headache sufferers, or about 20% to 40%. Considering that there are about 4 million rear-end collisions annually, and over 1 million to 3 million are whiplash injuries, we are looking at 200,000 to 500,000 patients a year that may become chronic headache sufferers. Therefore, any means of identifying the patients early would serve to reduce expenditures significantly.

The fact that Foreman and Croft report that 56% of MIC 1 patients suffered residual pain (neck pain, headache, and paresthesias) may indicate that the initial evaluation is not complete and other modifiers should be considered. Considering that there are many triggering mechanisms for headache and some of these mechanisms are a result of trauma, I would suggest that other modifiers should be added to their list, e.g., (1) preexisting migraine or other headache problems, (2) family history of migraine, and (3) history of enuresis, motion illness, pre-puberty abdominal cramps (seen in 65% of migraine sufferers).

It has been demonstrated that there may be brain damage during a whiplash accident without direct contact of the skull to an immovable object. Experimental whiplash on rhesus monkeys has produced gross hemorrhages and contusions over the surface of the brain and upper cervical cord with rotational displacement of the head on the neck. These injuries have also been detected on postmortem examinations on humans. If the patient complains of retrograde or post traumatic amnesia or other symptoms that follow a closed head injury, such as incapacitating headache and/or stiff neck that may resemble subarachnoid hemorrhage, an EEG (electroencephalogram) or spinal tap should be considered as a modifier in the examination. A neuropsychological battery may also be in order to determine "soft neurological" signs or damage.

Another modifier may be a TMJ (temporomandibular) dysfunction as a result of the shearing forces of the accident. This TMJ displacement may cause trigger points and nerve irritation that may continue the ongoing headaches. Early examination and correction of this problem may eliminate unnecessary ongoing and extensive treatment.

There have been enough studies to document that pre-traumatic headache coupled with injury to the cervical spine increases the likelihood of post traumatic headache and this information may also be a modifier.

Psychological symptoms preceding the accident or as a result of the accident may account for a delayed recovery and add to the chronicity of the symptoms. This certainly should be taken as a modifier that might add to the score that decreases a good and rapid prognosis. A rapid and inexpensive psychological test, such as the MMPI (Minnesota Multiphasic Personality Inventory) may give information as to depression, psychopathic traits, schizophrenia, hysteria, hypochondriasis, validity of test taking, etc. If the validity scales are abnormal, there may be clues that this is a patient who is contriving symptoms for secondary gain.

Foreman and Croft[3] did not publish their questionnaire and I would be interested in whether they considered multiple accidents and previous litigation as well as the patient's work status, marital status, type of discharge from military service, previous incarcerations, psychiatric hospitalizations, history of abuse as a child, etc., as warning signs for poor prognosis. These problems may also be considered as modifiers. Although the literature suggests that psychological symptoms improve as the somatic complaints improve, my clinical impression from treating patients with significant pre-accident "psychosomatic disorders," or severe personality disorders, is that they have a poor prognostic course.

However, their attempt to objectify this major and costly process must be applauded.

Another important study written was "Whiplash-Associated Disorders," a scientific monograph of the Quebec Task Force published in the *Spine*.[5] They reviewed more than 10,000 publications and found only 346 worthwhile. The papers turned down were biographical and were scientifically neither reliable nor valid. They questioned papers that were anecdotal and reported only on papers that were proven scientifically.

During 1989 to 1990 the Quebec Automobile Insurance Society (Societe d'assurance automobile du Quebec or SAAQ) approached Dr. W. O. Spitzer of the Department of Epidemiology and Biostatistics, McGill University, and inquired about an in-depth analysis of clinical, public health, social, and financial determinants of "the whiplash problem."

The summary findings of the WAD (whiplash-associated disorders) cohort study were the following:

1. The population-based overall annual incidence rate of compensated insurance claims for whiplash injury in Quebec in 1987 was 70 per 100,000 inhabitants. The incidence rate was higher among female subjects and people aged 20–24 years. The overall incidence rate was generally comparable with that of other countries, but much lower than that found in Saskatchewan where the rate may be as high as 700 per 100,000. A possible explanation for this difference between the two provinces may be because of the contrasting no-fault insurance system in Quebec and tort system in Saskatchewan.

2. Female gender, older age, married/cohabital status, and a greater number of dependents were the socio-demographic factors associated with a longer time of absence for whiplash. Being in a severe collision, in a vehicle other than a car or taxi, in a collision other than rearend, and not using a seatbelt were the collision-related factors associated with a longer time of absence. The presence of multiple injuries was also an important prognostic factor.

3. Rearend collisions and having one or more dependents were associated with higher rate of relapse or recurrence of symptoms of whiplash subjects.

4. Of the more than 18 million Canadian dollars paid out by the SAAQ to the 1987 cohort of 4757 whiplash subjects, over 70% was paid for the replacement of regular income. Thus, the main portion of the total cost incurred by the SAAQ for whiplash is directly related to the duration of compensation.

5. The 26% of subjects with only a whiplash injury whose absence lasted between 2 and 6 months accounted for 39.5% of the costs, whereas the remaining 12.5% of patients still compensated 6 months after the collision accounted for 46% of the total costs paid out by SAAQ. For the patients with multiple injuries besides whiplash, 15.3% of patients were still compensated 6 months after the event, and they accounted for 60.4% of the total costs. Therefore, the financial burden of whiplash injury to the SAAQ results from the small number of persons who became chronic.

The Quebec Task Force adopted the term whiplash-associated disorders (WAD) and proposed a classification of WAD on two axes: (1) a clinical anatomic axis, and (2) a time axis.

The clinical-anatomic axis has five grades that correspond to severity.

Grade	Clinical presentation
0	No complaint about the neck No physical sign(s)
I.	Neck complaint of pain, stiffness, or tenderness only No physical signs Presumed pathology: microscopic or multimicroscopic lesion Lesion is not serious enough to cause muscle spasm
II.	Neck complaint and musculoskeletal signs (<motion, tenderness) Presumed pathology: neck sprain and bleeding around soft tissue (articular capsules, ligaments, tendons, and muscles) Muscle spasm secondary to soft tissue injury
III.	Neck complaint and neurological sign(s) <deep tendon reflexes, weakness and sensory deficits Presumed pathology: neurologic system injured by irritation secondary to bleeding or inflammation
IV.	Neck complaint and fracture or dislocation

Symptoms that can manifest in all grades include deafness, dizziness, tinnitus, headache, memory loss, dysphagia, and TMJ pain.

The time axis is classified within each grade from the time of injury as those (1) less than 4 days, (2) 4–21 days, (3) 22–45 days, (4) 46–180 days, and those (5) more than 6 months.

The task force evaluated specific treatments regarding the studies of efficacy and effectiveness and left little choice of treatments for these patients. The following is a summary of their conclusions.

Immobilization collars. Soft foam collar, the Philadelphia collar, and the Queen Anne collar have little effect on cervical range of motion in healthy adults. Soft collars do not restrict the range of motion of the cervical spine. Collars may promote inactivity, which can delay recovery in patients with WAD.

Prescription of rest. Although this is common recommendation for WAD, all the studies the Task Force evaluated suggest that prolonged periods of rest are detrimental to recovery.

Cervical pillows. There were no studies found regarding cervical pillows for WAD.

Activation manipulation (adjustment). Other than improvement lasting only minutes, they felt that although this a common treatment in WAD, its value must be established in randomized controlled trials.

Mobilization. The cumulative evidence suggests that mobilization techniques can be used as an adjunct to strategies that promote activation. In combination with activating interventions, they may appear to be beneficial in the short term, but long-term benefit has not been established.

Exercise. The independent effect of exercise has not been evaluated. The cumulative evidence suggests that active exercise as part of a multimodal intervention may be beneficial in the short and long term. This suggestion should be confirmed in future studies.

Traction. There was no research found regarding the independent benefit of traction in any grade of WAD.

Postural alignment and advice. There was no research found regarding postural alignment.

Spray and Stretch. There were no studies found regarding spray and stretch.

Passive modalities and electrotherapies: transcutaneous electrical nerve stimulation (TENS). There were no accepted studies regarding TENS.

Pulsed electromagnetic treatment. The treatment course was 12 weeks, adding physiotherapy after 4 weeks. The treatment group appeared to show greater improvement than the control group, but after 4 weeks more there was no difference between the control and the treatment group. At 12 weeks there was more improvement in the control group. Because the pulse electromagnetic treatment device is a soft collar, which tends to encourage inactivity, it cannot be recommended until it is shown to be superior or at least equivalent to mobilizing interventions.

Electrical stimulation. There were no accepted studies regarding electrical stimulation.

Ultrasound. There were no accepted studies regarding ultrasound in WAD.

Laser, short wave diathermy, heat, ice, massage. There were no accepted studies regarding the independent effect of any of these treatments for WAD or neck pain.

Surgical treatment. There were no accepted studies of disc surgery or nerve block in managing WAD or cervical disorders. No research was found concerning the benefit of rhizolysis in WAD.

Injections. No accepted studies were found addressing epidural or intrathecal steroid injections for management of WAD. Accepted studies were found addressing intra-articular steroid injections for chronic WAD and subcutaneous sterile water trigger point injections for chronic neck and shoulder pain (each was one study).

Intra-articular steroid injection. The short duration of pain relief overall, and the lack of a substantial difference in duration of efficacy between steroid and local anesthetic, leads to the conclusion that intra-articular steroid injection is not justified in the management of cervical zygapophyseal joint pain after whiplash injury.

Subcutaneous sterile water injection. One paper reported improvement in pain and cervical range of motion; however, the pain associated with the injection is so severe that a blind study could not be done.

Pharmacologic interventions. No research was found regarding the benefit of narcotic analgesics or psychopharmacologic therapeutics in WAD. Analgesics and nonsteroidal anti-inflammatory drugs combined with other treatment modalities were associated with short-term benefit for WAD Grades I and II in the acute phase or less than 72 hours post collision. No accepted studies were found regarding muscle relaxants in management of WAD.

Psychosocial interventions. No research was found regarding the psychosocial interventions in the management of WAD.

Prescribed function. Prescribed function in the first 72 hours of WAD I and II (advice to mobilize, exercise, limit inactivity, and avoid dependence on collars and analgesics) was effective short-term in improving cervical range of motion and more effective long term in improving symptoms than physiotherapy.

Acupuncture. No research was found concerning acupuncture in the management of WAD.

Magnetic Necklace. There was one accepted study regarding the efficacy of the management of chronic neck pain, but not in any studies concerning WAD.

After reading this report, one finds that there is little to offer the patient who comes to the clinic with daily or almost daily severe headache and pain and is looking for relief of this pain in order to function once again as he or she did before the accident.

The Task Force on Whiplash-Associated Disorders (WAD) base their findings on what they conclude as insufficient in the research of the various treatment modalities. They list the following as deficiencies in the research design:

Lack of clarity in statement of study purpose, research question, or hypothesis
Lack of appropriate denominator
Lack of controls or suitable reference group for comparisons
Inappropriate study design to test research questions or form conclusions
Inappropriate statistical analysis
Absent or unclear statement of inclusion-exclusion criteria
Absent or unclear statement of interval between collision and study entry, or wide variability of interval
Sources of subjects that introduce intrinsic selection biases
Substantial losses to follow-up resulting in potential for biased estimate of outcome frequencies and determinants
Ascertainment of outcomes subject to investigator and patient reporting biases
Measurement methods whose reliability and validity are not established
Inadequate statistical power (small sample sizes)

The Quebec Task Force concluded that CAD injuries are self-limiting and that pain is not harmful. However, as a clinician, the major disability of the CAD patients that I treated was the pain. Not only does pain restrict the patient physically, but it creates significant psychiatric symptomatology, ranging from anger and withdrawal to severe depression. Therefore, the elimination of pain is essential to remobilize the patient into a productive individual.

In order to conduct research that meets the standards that the Task Force is suggesting requires a great deal of money and time. The clinicians who see most of these patients have neither and must use whatever resources they have to help reduce the suffering of these people. The specialty of the clinician will determine the type of treatment that will be used. If the patient responds to the particular treatment, then the clinician will use that modality again and again. If the clinician feels comfortable with the results, then he or she will report a positive result regardless of scientific design.

In the area of headache, many drugs are used that were not originally researched for headache and were accidentally discovered to help headache pain. The whole group of beta-blockers, calcium channel blockers, anticonvulsants, antidepressants, etc., are used for headache and none of them are listed as headache medications because they were not originally researched for headache. Today pharmaceutical companies must spend hundreds of millions of dollars to design and research a medication to gain approval from the U.S. Food and Drug Administration. Because the various treatments mentioned in the Task Force's report are not financially sound for medical corporations to invest in, money to support these investigations is not going to be forthcoming. Therefore, the type of investigation they are calling for will not take place and another method of investigation will have to be sought after.

A suggestion I propose is that university centers sponsor an investigation. Several centers in this country and other countries develop a protocol of scientific design that they agree would meet the criteria for valid and relevant scientific investigation. Once this protocol is agreed upon, then send the questionnaires to all clinicians in every discipline who treat whiplash patients. The clinicians would fill in these questionnaires as to their history-taking, physical examination, radiography, laboratory, and all other methods used to make a diagnosis. They should then fill in the diagnosis and how they came to that conclusion. Then all treatment modalities should be entered, in a way that can be interpreted statistically by the research centers. In this manner, all the criteria that the Task Force reports are missing in good scientific reporting will be available for accurate investigation by these university centers who have agreed upon this protocol. Then let these centers blindly interpret the evidence and come to the conclusion of what works and what doesn't and where, how, and when different types of treatment should be used.

Although I appreciate the Task Force's monumental task, I do not feel that the "soldiers" in the trenches will be able to fulfill the research they are asking for.

Another area that needs development is an instrument that will identify, with a high degree of certainty, the identification of the malingerer or secondary gainer. Although their number is small, they have had a negative impact on attempts to help those who truly are suffering. In a country where we practice a tort system, there is going to be litigation and those who have been hurt unjustifiably deserve compensation. Most patients I have treated would prefer to be well and continue with their lives as they were before the accident and the idea of litigation is anathema to them. Unfortunately, litigation seems to be the only way to recover medical costs, lost work wages, and be compensated for pain and suffering. However, because of those who are looking for "that big reward," the majority suffer at the hands of the few. It is for this reason that we need to identify this group.

Another group that has to be identified is those who purposely are bilking the system. All medical practitioners would have to justify their treatments according to approved standards; however, we must never deny new treatments if they can be rationally justified and then those treatments would be added to the data bank to be later evaluated.

A third group are lawyers who contribute to the costs by defending obvious malingerers and continuing to have these patients run up extensive bills for no medical improvement.

By eliminating this minority of people from escalating the cost of treatment, billions of dollars would be saved.

There is a small percentage of patients with whiplash injuries who will end up with a chronic condition that causes long term disability. It is the obligation of the clinician to find a means of treatment that will eliminate or decrease the pain and suffering of that patient. To dismiss a patient because a treatment has not met the scientific validity of a double blind study, or to point a finger and cry malingerer without justification is a violation of the Hippocratic Oath.

REFERENCES

1. Croft, A.C., A proposed classification of cervical acceleration-deceleration (CAD) injuries with a review of prognostic research, *Palmer Journal of Research*, submitted.
2. Veriest, H., Neurogenic intermittent claudication in cases with absolute and relative stenosis of the lumbar vertebral canal (ASLC & RSLC) in cases with narrow lumbar intervertebral foramina and in cases with both entities, *Clinical Neurosurgery*, 20, 204–214, 1972.
3. Foreman, S.M., Croft, A.C., *Whiplash Injuries: The Cervical Acceleration/Deceleration Syndrome*, 2nd ed, Williams & Wilkins, Baltimore, 1995, 435–442.

4. Barnsley, L., Lord, S., Bogduk, N., Clinical review: whiplash injury, *Pain,* 58, 283–307, 1994.
5. Spitzer, W.O., Skovron, M.L., Salmi, L.R., Cassidy, J.D., Duranceau, J, Suissa, S., Zeiss, E., Scientific monograph of the Quebec Task Force on Whiplash-associated Disorders: redefining "whiplash" and its management, *Spine,* 20(85), 43S, 1995.

Glossary

Abduction: Movement away from the midline.

Adduction: Movement toward the midline.

Adrenergic: Indicating a relationship to epinephrine, its release or its actions, especially in association with the sympathetic nervous system; also called sympathomimetic.

Apophysis: Any outgrowth or swelling, especially a bony outgrowth that has never been entirely separated from the bone of which it forms a part, such as a process, tubercle, or tuberosity.

Arachnoid membrane: Thin delicate membrane that is the middle of the three Membranes (meninges) enclosing the brain and spinal cord; the outer membrane is the dura mater, the inner the pia mater.

Ataxia: Lack of coordination in muscle action, manifested as unsteady movements and staggering gait.

Ateriography: Using x-ray and a contrast medium to study the patency of the artery.

Aura: Sensation, e.g., flickering lights, halos, etc., that may be a signal of an impending migraine attack.

Axonal injury: Fracture of brain tissue when the nerve filaments are stretched or separated by rotational or translational forces.

Basilar migraine: Originating from the brainstem or from the occipital lobes.

Benign: Mild, not recurrent, not malignant.

Bruxism: Grinding or gnashing of the teeth when not masticating or swallowing.

Centric occlusion: The position of jaw closure with full tooth contact.

Choroid plexus: Vessels that lie within the ventricles of the brain producing cerebrospinal fluid to protect the brain.

Cognition: The mental faculty of knowing, including perceiving, thinking, recognizing, and remembering.

Concussion: A violent jarring or shaking, as from a severe blow or shock, especially one to the head. A concussion may cause a limited period of unconsciousness.

Contrecoup: Injury to one side that results from a blow to the opposite side (e.g., a blow to the forehead causing damage to the back of the skull or rear part of the brain).

Contussion: A bruise caused by a superficial, nonlacerating injury from a blow, e.g., a bruise to the brain.

CT: Computed tomography uses x-rays with the beam passing repeatedly (scanning) through a body part, and a computer calculating tissue absorption at each point scanned, from which a visualization of the tissue is developed.

Diplopia: Double vision in which a single object is seen as two objects. If one eye is covered, diplopia often disappears.

Dura mater: Thickest and outermost of the three membranes (meninges) that enclose the brain and spinal cord (others are the pia mater and arachnoid membrane).

Dysarthria: Difficulty in pronouncing words clearly or correctly, usually because of poor control over the speech muscles.

Dystonic: Abnormal muscle tone.

Edema: Abnormal collection of fluid in spaces between cells, especially just under the skin or in a given cavity.

Electrocardiogram, (EKG or ECG) A graphic recording of the electrical activity of the heart.

Electroencephalography (EEG): A device for receiving and recording the electrical activity of the brain. Electrodes are attached to various areas of the head and the electrical activity is recorded.

EMG (electromyogram): Recording of electrical activity occurring when voluntary (skeletal) muscles work; it is helpful in diagnosing muscle and nerve abnormalities.

Enuresis: Passing urine without control, especially during sleep (bedwetting).

Ependyma: Very thin membrane that lines the ventricles of the brain and helps form cerebrospinal fluid.

Evoked potential: An electrical response produced in the central nervous system by an external stimulus (e.g. flash of light). The response is monitored on recording equipment and used to verify the integrity of nerve connections.

Facial nerve: One of a pair of mixed sensory and motor nerves, the seventh cranial nerves, that innervate much of the face, with sensory fibers extending from taste buds in the tongue and motor fibers extending to the scalp muscles of facial expression, and some of the lacrimal (tear) and salivary glands.

Glossopharyngeal nerve: One of a pair of mixed sensory and motor nerves, the ninth cranial nerves, essential to taste, sensation to the palate, secretion of the parotid glands, and swallowing.

Hemiplegic: Paralysis of only one half of the body.

Hemisensory: Loss of sensation to one half of the body.

IHS: The International Headache Society.

Jump sign: A general pain response of the patient who winces, may cry out, and may withdraw in response to pressure applied on a trigger point.

Ligaments: These are bands of fibers that connect bones or cartilage, serving to support and strengthen joints.

Lumbar puncture: Insertion of a hollow needle into the subarachnoid space of the lumbar region of the spinal cord for diagnostic (to obtain a sample of cerebrospinal fluid for analysis) or therapeutic (to remove blood, pus, or inject drugs) purposes.

Migrainous infarction: Area of dead tissue resulting from diminished or stopped blood flow to the tissue area.

MRI or NMR: Magnetic resonance imaging or nuclear magnetic resonance. A diagnostic technique in which an electromagnetic field stimulates atomic nuclei within the patient's body, causing those nuclei to release energy that is recorded with sensitive receivers.

Neurotransmitter: A chemical that affects or modifies the transmission of an impulse across a synapse between nerves or between a nerve and a muscle.

NINDB: 1962 Ad Hoc Committee on Classification of Headache of the National Institute of Neurological Disease and Blindness.

Oculomotor nerve: One of a pair of motor nerves, the third of the cranial nerves, essential for eye movements.

Ophthalmoplegic migraine: Headache associated with paresis of one or more of the ocular nerves without an intracranial lesion (tumor).

Organic disease: Observable or detectable changes in the body.

Palpable band (taut band): The group of taut muscle fibers that is associated with a myofascial trigger point and is identifiable by tactile examination of the muscle.

Paresis: Partial or incomplete paralysis.

Paresthesia: Sensation, such as tingling or pins and needles.

Phonophobia: Abnormal intolerance to sound.

Photophobia: Abnormal intolerance to light.

Physiology: Science dealing with the functioning of living matter and organisms.

Pia mater: Innermost of the three meninges covering the brain and the spinal cord (others are dura mater and arachnoid); it is highly vascularized and closely applied to the brain and spinal cord, nourishing the nerve cells.

Prodrome: Earliest sign of a disease or a developing condition.

Ptosis: Drooping of one or both eyelids; it may be congenital or result from damage or irritation to the oculomotor nerve.

Ramping: Vertical displacement during the acceleration phase in a whiplash accident.

Rhinitis: Inflammation of the mucous membrane lining of the nose, usually associated with a nasal discharge.

Serotonin: A chemical widely distributed in the body, especially in the brain, where it acts as a neurotransmitter; in the blood platelets upon an injury, it acts as a vasoconstrictor; and in the small intestine it stimulates smooth muscle to contract.

Sinusitis: Inflammation of one of the paranasal sinuses occurring as a result of an upper respiratory infection, an allergic response, a change of atmospheric pressure, or a defect of the nose.

Spasm: Increased tension with or without shortening of a muscle due to nonvoluntary motor activity. Spasm cannot be stopped by voluntary relaxation.

Spondylitis: An inflammation of a joint of the spinal column, usually characterized by pain and stiffness. May occur after injury, arthritis, or infection.

Spondylolisthesis: Forward dislocation of one vertebra over the one below it causing pressure on the spinal nerves.

Spondylosis: A condition in which vertebral joints become fixed or stiff, causing pain and restricted mobility.

Status migrainous: A migraine attack that lasts more than 72 hours.

Thermography: A technique for sensing (by means of an infrared detector) and recording the heat produced by different parts of the body. It can be used to study blood flow and nerve damage.

Tinnitus: Ringing in ears.

Trigeminal nerve: One of a pair of motor and sensory nerves, the fifth and largest cranial nerves; involved in facial sensibility, chewing, and other muscular actions of the face.

Trigger point (active): A focus of hyperirritability in a muscle or its fascia that is symptomatic with respect to pain; it refers to a pattern of pain at rest and/or on motion that is specific for the muscle. An active trigger point is always tender, prevents full lengthening of the muscle, causes weakness of the muscle, usually refers pain on direct compression, mediates a local twitch reponse of muscle fibers when adequately stimulated, and often produces specific referred autonomic phenonema, generally in its pain reference zone.

Trigger point (myofascial): A hyperirritable spot, usually within a taut band of skeletal muscle or in the muscle's fascia, that is painful on compression and that can give rise to characteristic referred pain, tenderness, and autonomic phenomena.

Trigger point (latent): A focus of hyperirritability in muscle or its fascia that is clinically quiescent with respect to spontaneous pain. It is painful only when palpated.

Trigger point: A hyperirritable locus within a taut band of skeletal muscle and/or its associated fascia. The spot is painful on compression and can evoke characteristic referred pain and autonomic phenomena.

Ultrasound: A process by which the reflection of high-frequency sound waves is used to develop an image (sonogram) of a structure. This helps in the study of fetal growth and can detect abnormalities of the heart and many other organs.

Vagus nerve: One of a pair of motor and sensory nerves, functioning in swallowing, speech, breathing, heart rate, and many other body functions.

Vascular headaches: Pertaining to or composed of blood vessels, primarily arteries in headaches.

Venous sinus: Any of several sinuses that collect blood from the dura mater covering the brain and drain it into the internal jugular vein.

Vertigo: Sensation of unsteadiness, faintness, or whirling in space, often with the inability to maintain balance (dizziness).

Zygapophysis: An articular process of a vertebra.

Bibliography

The following is a list of scientific articles reviewed. An attempt was made to put them into various categories. Some of them could be cross-referenced and therefore the categories are not totally specific.

BIOMECHANICS

Ashton-Miller, J.A., McGlashen, K.M., et al., Cervical muscle myoelectric response to acute experimental sternocleidomastoid pain, *Spine*, 15(10), 1006–1012, 1990.

Christian, M.S., Non-fatal injuries sustained by seatbelt wearers: a comparative study, *British Medical Journal*, 2, 1310–1311, 1976.

Grunsten, R.C., Gilbert, N.S., Mawn, S.V., The mechanical effects of impact acceleration on the unconstrained human head and neck complex, *Contemporary Orthopaedics*, 18(2), 1989.

Hamilton, J.B., Seat-belt injuries, *British Medical Journal*, 4, 485–486, 1968.

Insurance Institute for Highway Safety, Head Restraints. *Status Report*, Vol. 32, No. 4, April 12, 1997.

Insurance Institute for Highway Safety, Crashworthiness Evaluation of Midsize Utility Vehicles. March, 1997.

Insurance Institute for Highway Safety, Air Bags. Status Report, Vol. 32, No. 2, February 15, 1997.

Insurance Institute for Highway Safety, Highway Loss Data Institute. Addressing the risks from airbag inflation for infants, children, and short drivers. Advisory, No. 20, November, 1996.

Insurance Institute for Highway Safety, Saving our necks in car crashes. Status Report, Vol. 30, No. 8, September 16, 1995.

Jeffery, R.S., Cook, P.L., Seat belts and reclining seats, *Injury: the British Journal of Accident Surgery*, 22(3), 1991.

Mackay, M., Mechanisms of injury and biomechanics: vehicle design and crash performance, *World Journal of Surgery*, 16, 420–427, 1992.

Mimura, M., Moriya, H. et al., Three-dimensional motion analysis of the cervical spine with special reference to the axial rotation, *Spine*, 14(11), November, 1989.

Morris, F., Do head-restraints protect the neck from whiplash injuries?, *Archives of Emergency Medicine*, 6, 17–21, 1989.

National Highway Traffic Safety Administration, Office of Crashworthiness Standards, Light Duty Vehicle Division, Head Restraints — Identification of Issues Relevant to Regulation, Design, and Effectiveness. November 4, 1996.

Osterman, A.L., The double crush syndrome, *Orthsopedic Clinics of North America*, 19(1), January, 1988.

Panjabi, M., Dvorak, J. et al., Three-dimensional movements of the upper cervical spine, *Spine*, 13(7), July 1988.

Rutledge, R., Thomason, M. et al., The spectrum of abdominal injuries associated with the use of seat belts, *Journal of Trauma*, 31(6), 1991.

Warfield, C.A., Biber, M.P. et al., Epidural steroid injection as a treatment for cervical radiculitis, *Clinical Journal of Pain*, 4(4), 1988.

White, A.A. III, Johnson, R.M. et al., Biomechanical analysis of clinical stability in the cervical spine, *Clinical Orthopaedics and Related Research*, No. 109, June, 1975.

Yoganandan, N., Sances, A. Jr. et al. Injury biomechanics of the human cervical column, *Spine*, 15(10), 1031–1039, 1990.

BRAIN INJURY

Adams, J.H., Graham, D.I. et al., Diffuse axonal injury due to nonmissile head injury in humans: an analysis of 45 cases, *Annals of Neurology*, 12(6), December 1982.

Anderson, J.M., Kaplan, M.S., Felsenthal, G., Brain injury obscured by chronic pain: a preliminary report, *Archives of Physical Medicine Rehabilitation*, 71, 703–708, 1990.

Bovim, G., Jenssen, G. et al., Orbital phlebography: a comparison between cluster headache and other headaches, *Headache*, 32, 408–412, 1992.

Cantu, R.C., Cerebral concussion in sport: management and prevention, *Sports Medicine*, 14(1), 64–74, 1992.

Dalessio, D.J., Some reflections on the etiologic role of depression in head pain, *Headache*, 28–31, April, 1968.

Davis, R.W., Phantom sensation, phantom pain, and stump pain, *Archives of Physical Medicine Rehabilitation*, 74, January 1993.

Denker, P.G., The postconcussion syndrome: prognosis and evaluation of the organic factors. *New York State Journal of Medicine*, February 15, 379–384, 1944.

Elkind, A.H., Headache and head trauma, *Clinical Journal of Pain*, 5(1), 77–87, 1989.

Evans, R.W., The postconcussion syndrome and the sequelae of mild head injury, *Neurology of Trauma*, 10(4), November 1992.

Feinstein, B., Langton, N.J.K. et al., Experiments on pain referred from deep somatic tissues, *Journal of Bone and Joint Surgery*, 36-A(5), October 1954.

Friedman, A.P., Brenner, C., Denny-Brown, D., Post-traumatic vertigo and dizziness, *Journal of Neurosurgery*, 2, June 1945.

Gelberman, R.H., Woo, S.L.-Y. et al., Effects of early intermittent passive mobilization on healing canine flexor tendons, *Journal of Hand Surgery*, 7(2), March 1982.

Gellman, H., Keenan, M.A.E. et al., Reflex sympathetic dystrophy in brain-injured patients, *Pain*, 51, 307–311, 1992.

Gennarelli, T.A., Thibault, L.E., Adams, J.H. et al., Diffuse axonal injury and traumatic coma in the primate, *Annal of Neurology*, 12(6), December 1982.

Gennarelli, T.A., Mechanisms of brain injury, *Journal of Emergency Medicine*, 11, 5–11, 1993.

Gibson, P.H., A method for determining tentorial herniation in closed-head injury from a quantitative estimation of cerebral trauma, *Neuropathology and Applied Neurobiology*, 8, 489–493, 1982.

Grande, P.O., The effects of dihydroergotamine in patients with head injury and raised intracranial pressure, *Intensive Care Medicine*, 15, 523–527, 1989.

Grigsby, J., Kaye, K., Incidence and correlates of depersonalization following head trauma, *Brain Injury*, 7(6), 507–513, 1993.

Gualtieri, C.T., The problem of mild brain injury, *Neuropsychiatry, Neuropsychology, and Behavioral Neurology*, 8(2), 127–136, 1995.

Hardy, M.A., The biology of scar formation, *Physical Therapy*, 69(12), December 1989.

Hart, R.G., Miller, V.T., Cerebral infarction in young adults: a practical approach, *Current Concepts of Cerebrovascular Disease — Stroke*, 17(4), July-August 1982.

Jane, J.A., Steward, O., Gennarelli, T., Axonal degeneration induced by experimental noninvasive minor head injury, *Journal of Neurosurgery*, 62, 96–100, 1985.

Karpman, R.R., Weinstein, P.R. et al., Observation of the alert, conscious patient with closed head injury, *Arizona Medicine*, 37(11), 772–775, 1980.

Katz, R.T., Deluca, J., Sequelae of minor traumatic brain injury, *American Family Physician*, 46(5), 1491–1498, 1992.

Kay D.W.K., Kerr T.A., Lassman L.P., Brain trauma and the postconcussional syndrome, *Lancet*, p. 1052, Nov. 13, 1971.

Kelly, R., The post traumatic syndrome, *Pahlavi Medical Journal*, 3, 530–547, 1972.

Kerr, F.W.L., A mechanism to account for frontal headache in cases of posterior-fossa tumors.

Kraus, J.F., Nourjah, P., The epidemiology of mild, uncomplicated brain injury, *Journal of Trauma*, 28(12), 1988.

Lance, J.W., Curran, D.A., Treatment of chronic tension headache, *Lancet*, June 6, 1964.

Levi, L., Guilburd, J.N. et al., Diffuse axonal injury: analysis of 100 patients with radiological signs, *Neurosurgery*, 27(3), 429–432, 1990.

Light, K.E., Nuzik, S. et al., Low-load prolonged stretch vs. high-load brief stretch in treating knee contractures, *Physical Therapy*, 64(3), March 1984.

Manzoni, G.C., Terzano, M.G. et al., Cluster headache — clinical findings in 180 patients, *Cephalalgia*, 3, 21–30, 1983.

Minderhoud, J.M., Boelens, M.E.M., Huizenga, J., Saan, R.J., Treatment of minor head injuries, *Clinical Neurology and Neurosurgery*, 82(2), 127–140, 1980.

Mokri, B., Houser, O.W. et al., Spontaneous dissections of the vertebral arteries, *Neurology*, 38, 880–885, 1988.

Oppenheimer, D.R., Microscopic lesions in the brain following head injury, *Journal of Neurology, Neurosurgery, and Psychiatry*, 31, 299–306, 1968.

Overgaard, J., Christensen, S. et al., *Lancet*, 22, September 1973.

Paxson, C.L. Jr., Brown, D.R., Post-traumatic anterior hypopituitarism. *Pediatrics*, 57, (6), June 1976.

Payne-Johnson, J.C., Evaluation of communication competence in patients with closed head injury, *Journal of Communication Disorders*, 19(4), 237–249, 1986.

Povlishock, J.T., Becker, D.P. et al., Axonal change in minor head injury, *Journal of Neuropathology and Experimental Neurology*, 42(3), 225–242, 1983.

Povlishock, J.T., Becker, D.P., Fate of reactive axonal swellings induced by head injury, *Laboratory Investigation*, 52(5), 540–552, 1985.

Povlishock, J.T., Pathobiology of traumatically induced axonal injury in animals and man, *Annals of Emergency Medicine*, 22(6), June 1993.

Pozzati, E., Grossi, C., Padovani, R., Traumatic intracerebellar hematomas, *Journal of Neurosurgery*, 56, 691–694, 1982.

Russell, W.R., Amnesia following head injuries, *Lancet*, October 5, 1935.

Ryan, G.B., Spector, W.G., Macrophage turnover in inflamed connective tissue, *Proceedings of the Royal Society of London Series B*, 175, 269–292, 1970.

Sackellares, J.C., Giordani, B. et al., Patients with pseudoseizures: intellectual and cognitive performance, *Neurology*, 35, 116–119, 1985.

Savino, P.J., Glaser, J.S., Schatz, N.J., Traumatic chiasmal syndrome, *Neurology*, 30, 963–970, 1980.

Siesjo, B.K., Basic mechanisms of traumatic brain damage, *Annals of Emergency Medicine*, 22, 959–999, 1993.

Simons, D.J., Wolff, H.G., Studies on headache: mechanisms of chronic post-traumatic headache, *Psychosomatic Medicine*, Vol. 8, 1946.

Sokoloff, L., Mapping of local cerebral functional activity by measurement of local cerebral glucose utilization with [\s\up2(14) C] deoxyglucose, *Brain*, 102, 653–668, 1979.

Sokoloff, L., The deoxyglucose method: theory and practice, *European Neurology*, 20, 137–145, 1981.

Starkstein, S.E., Mayberg, H.S. et al., Mania after brain injury: neuroradiological and metabolic findings, *Annals of Neurology*, 27(6), June 1990.

Suzuki, N., Hardebo, J.E., Anatomical basis for a parasympathetic and sensory innervation of the intracranial segment of the internal carotid artery in man; possible implication for vascular headache, *Journal of Neurological Science*, 104, 19–31, 1991.

Symonds, C., Concussion and its sequelae, *Lancet*, 6 January 1962.

Takahashi, H., Manaka, S., Sano, K., Changes in extracellular potassium concentration in cortex and brain stem during the acute phase of experimental closed head injury, *Journal of Neurosurgery*, 55, 708–717, 1981.

Taylor, A.R., Bell, T.K., Slowing of cerebral circulation after concussional head injury, *Lancet*, 178–180, July 23, 1966.

Taylor, A.R., Post-concussional sequelae, *British Medical Journal*, 3, 67–71, 1967.

Tysvaer, A.T., Head and neck injuries in soccer: impact of minor trauma, *Sports Medicine*, 14(3), 200–213, 1992.

Van Zomeren, A.H., Deelman, B.G., Long-term recovery of visual reaction time after closed head Injury, *Journal of Neurology, Neurosurgery, and Psychiatry*, 41, 452–457, 1978.
Wei, E.P., Dietrich, W.D. et al., Functional, morphological, and metabolic abnormalities of the cerebral microcirculation after concussive brain injury in cats, *Circulation Research*, 26(1), January 1980.
Windle, W.F., Groat, R.A., Fox, C.A., Experimental structural alterations in the brain during and after concussion, *Surgery, Gynecology and Obstetrics*, 79(6), December 1944.

CERVICAL SPINE AND NECK

Batzdort, U., Batzdorff, A., Analysis of cervical spine curvature in patients with cervical spondylosis, *Neurosurgery*, 22(5), 1988.
Birney, T.J., Hanley, E.N., Traumatic cervical spine injuries in childhood and adolescence, *Spine*, 14(12), 1989.
Bland, J.H., Boushey, D.R., Anatomy and physiology of the cervical spine, *Seminars in Arthritis and Rheumatism*, 20(1), August 1990.
Braaf, M.M., Rosner, S., Trauma of cervical spine as cause of chronic headache, *Journal of Trauma*, 15(6), May 1975.
Brian Lord., Some unsolved problems of cervical spondylosis, *British Medical Journal*, 771–777, March 23, 1963.
British Medical Journal, Incidence and duration of neck pain among patients injured in car accidents, 292(11), January 1986.
Conry, B.G., Hall, C.M., Cervical spine fractures and rear car seat restraints, *Archives of Disease in Childhood*, 1987.
Craig, J.B., Hodgson, B.F., Superior facet fractures of the axis vertebra, *Spine*, 16(8), 1991.
Davis, S.J., Teresi, L.M. et al., Cervical spine hyperextension injuries: MR findings, *Radiology*, July 1991.
Edmeads, J., Soyka, D., Headache associated with disorders of the skull and cervical spine, in *The Headaches*, Olesen, J., Ed., Raven Press, New York, 1993.
Epstein, N., Epstein, J.A. et al., Traumatic myelopathy in patients with cervical spinal stenosis without fracture or dislocation: methods of diagnosis, management, and prognosis, *Spine*, 5(6), November/December 1980.
Evans, D.K., Anterior cervical subluxation, *Journal of Bone and Joint Surgery*, 58-B(3), August 1976.
Farbman, A.A., Neck sprain: associated factors, *Journal of the American Medical Association*, 223(9), February 26, 1973.
Fielding, J.W., Cochran, G.V.B., Tears of the transverse ligament of the atlas, *Journal of Bone and Joint Surgery*, 56-A(8), December 1974.
Gargan, M.F., Bannister, G.C., Long-term prognosis of soft-tissue injuries of the neck, *Journal of Bone and Joint Surgery*, 72-B, 901–903, 1990.
Garvey, T.A., Marks, M.R., Wiesel, S.W., A prospective, randomized, double-blind evaluation of trigger-point injection therapy for low-back pain, *Spine*, 14(9), 1989.
Gore, D.R., Sepic, S.B., Gardner, G.M., Roentgenographic findings of the cervical spine in asymptomatic people, *Spine*, 11(6), 1986.
Graff-Radford, S.B., Reeves, J.L., Jaeger, B., Management of chronic head and neck pain: effectiveness of altering factors perpetuating myofascial pain, *Headache*, April 1987.
Green, J.D., Harle, T.S., Harris, J.H. Jr., Anterior subluxation of the cervical spine: hyperflexion sprain, *AJNR*, 2, 243–250, 1981.
Harata, S., Tohno, S., Kawagishi, T., Osteoarthritis of the atlanto-axial joint, *International Orthopaedics*, 5, 277–282, 1981.
Hildingsson, R., Toolanen, G., Outcome after soft-tissue injury of the cervical spine: a prospective study of 93 car-accident victims, *Acta Orthopaedica Scandinavica*, 61(4), 357–359, 1990.
Hohl, M., Soft tissue injuries of the neck, *Clinical Orthopaedics and Related Research*, No. 109, June, 1975.
Hohl, M., Soft-tissue injuries of the neck in automobile accidents, *Journal of Bone and Joint Surgery*, 56-A(8), December 1974.
Huelke, D.F., Kaufer, H., Vertebral column injuries and seat belts, *Journal of Trauma*, 15(4), April 1975.
Journal of the American Medical Association, Animals riding in carts show effects of "whiplash" injury, 194(3), October 18, 1965.

Kellett, J., Acute soft tissue injuries — a review of the literature, *Medicine and Science in Sports and Exercise*, 18(5), 1986.

Lancet, Neck injury and the mind, 338, 728–729, 1991.

Macnab, I., Acceleration extension injuries of the cervical spine, in *The Spine*, Vol. 2, Rothman, R.H., Simeone, F.A., Eds.,W.B. Saunders, Philadelphia, 1982, 654.

Macnab, I., Acceleration injuries of the cervical spine, *Journal of Bone and Joint Surgery*, 46-1(8), December 1964.

Macnab, I., Cervical spondylosis, *Clinical Orthopaedics and Related Research*, No. 109, June 1975.

Miles, K.A., Maimaris, C. et al., The incidence and prognostic significance of radiological abnormalities in soft tissue injuries to the cervical spine, *Skeletal Radio*, 17, 493–496, 1988.

Norris, S.H., Watt, I., The prognosis of neck injuries resulting from rear-end vehicle collisions, *Journal of Bone and Joint Surgery*, 65-B(5), November 1983.

Robinson, D.D., Cassar-Pullicino, V.N., Acute neck sprain after road traffic accident: a long-term clinical and radiological review, *Injury: The British Journal of Accident Surgery*, 24(2), 1993.

Rosomoff, H.L., Fishbain, D.A. et al., Physical findings in patients with chronic intractable benign pain of the neck and/or back, *Pain*, 37, 279–287, 1989.

Scher, A.T., Anterior cervical subluxation: an unstable position, *American Journal of Roentenology,* 133, August 1979.

Schutt, C.H., Dohan, F.C., Neck injury to women in auto accidents, *Journal of American Medical Association*, 206(12), December 6, 1968.

Sloop, P.R., Smith, D.S. et al., Manipulation for chronic neck pain: a double-blind controlled study, *Spine*, 7(6), 1982.

Smythe, H., The "repetitive strain injury syndrome" is referred pain from the neck, *Journal of Rheumatology*, 15, 1604–1608, 1988.

Sumchai, A., Eliastam, M., Werner, P., Seatbelt cervical injury in an intersection type vehicular collision, *Journal of Trauma*, 28(9), September 1988.

Tamura, T., Cranial symptoms after cervical injury: aetiology and treatment of the Barré-Lieou Syndrome, *Journal of Bone and Joint Surgery*, 71-B(2), March 1989.

Webb, J.K., Broughton, R.B.K. et al., Hidden flexion injury of the cervical spine, *Journal of Bone and Joint Surgery*, 58-B(3), August 1976.

Whitley, J.E., Forsyth, H.F., The classification of cervical spine injuries, *American Journal of Roentgenology*, 83, 633, 1960.

Wolfe, F., Simons, D.G. et al., The fibromyalgia and myofascial pain syndromes: a preliminary study of tender points and trigger points in persons with fibromyalgia, myofascial pain syndrome and no disease, *Journal of Rheumatology*, 19(6), 944–951, 1992.

Yarnell, P.R., Rossie, G.V., Minor whiplash head injury with major debilitation, *Brain Injury*, 2(3), 255–258, 1988.

Youdas, J.W., Garrett, T.R. et al., Normal range of motion of the cervical spine: an initial geometric study, *Physical Therapy*, 72(11), November 1992.

CERVICOGENIC

Aprill, C., Bogduk, N., The prevalence of cervical zygapophyseal joint pain: a first approximation, *Spine*, 17(7), 1992.

Aprill, C., Dwyer, A., Bogduk, N., Cervical zygapophyseal joint pain patterns. II. A clinical evaluation, *Spine*, 15(6), 1990.

Arnér, S., Lindblom, U. et al., Prolonged relief of neuralgia after regional anesthetic blocks. A call for further experimental and systematic clinical studies, *Pain*, 43, 287–297, 1990.

Bansevicius, D., Sjaastad, O., Cervicogenic headache: the influence of mental load on pain level and EMG of shoulder-neck and facial muscles, *Headache*, June 1996, p. 372–378.

Barnsley, L., Bogduk, N., Medial branch blocks are specific for the diagnosis of cervical zygapophyseal joint pain, *Regulations in Anesthesia*, 18(6), 1993.

Barnsley, L., Lord, S., Bogduk, N., Comparative local anaesthetic blocks in the diagnosis of cervical zygapophysial joint pain, *Pain*, 55, 99–106, 1993.

Barnsley, L., Lord, S., Wallis, B., Bogduk, N., False-positive rates of cervical zygapophyseal joint blocks, *Clinical Journal of Pain*, 9, 124–130, 1993.

Barnsley, L., Lord, S.M., Wallis, B.J., Bogduk, N., Lack of effect of intraarticular corticosteroids for chronic pain in the cervical zygapophyseal joints, *New England Journal of Medicine*, 330(15), 1994.

Barnsley, L., Lord, S.M., Wallis, B.J., Bogduk, N., The prevalence of chronic cervical zygapophysial joint pain after whiplash, *Spine*, 20(1), 20–26, 1995.

Blau, J.N., Path, E.A., MacGregor, M.B., Migraine and the neck, *Headache*, February 1994, p. 88-90.

Blume, H.G., Rothbart, P. et al., Greater occipital nerve block: methodology of diagnosis and treatment of cervicogenic headaches: an international authoritative determination, *International Spinal Injection Society*, 1995.

Bogduk, N., Aprill, C., On the nature of neck pain, discography and cervical zygapophysial joint blocks, *Pain*, 54, 213–217, 1993.

Bogduk, N., Corrigan, B. et al., Cervical headache, *Medical Journal of Australia*, 143(5), 1985.

Bogduk, N., Lambert, G.A., Duckworth, J.W., The anatomy and physiology of the vertebral nerve in relation to cervical migraine, *Cephalalgia*, 1981.

Bogduk, N., Marsland, A., On the concept of third occipital headache, *Journal of Neurology, Neurosurgery and Psychiatry*, 49, 775–780, 1986.

Bogduk, N., Marsland, A., The cervical zygapophysial joints as a source of neck pain, *Spine*, 13(6), June 1988.

Bogduk, N., Windsor, M., Inglis A., The innervation of the cervical intervertebral discs, *Spine*, 13(1), 1988.

Bogduk, N., An Anatomical Approach to Cervical Pain Syndromes. Division of Neurology, Prince Henry Hospital and School of Medicine, University of New South Wales.

Bogduk, N., Headaches and the cervical spine. An editorial, *Caphalalgia*, 4, 7, 1984.

Bogduk, N., Neck pain: an update, *Australian Family Physician*, 17(2), February 1988.

Bogduk, N., The argument for discography, *Neurosurgery Quarterly*, 6(2), 1996.

Bogduk, N., The clinical anatomy of the cervical dorsal rami, *Spine*, 7(4), 1982.

Bovim, G., Berg, R., Dale, L.G., Cervicogenic headache: anesthetic blockades of cervical nerves (C2-C5) and facet joint (C2/C3), *Pain*, 49, 315–320, 1992.

Bovim, G., Fredriksen, T.A. et al., Neurolysis of the greater occipital nerve in cervicogenic headache. A follow up study, *Headache*, April, 1992, p. 175–179.

Bovim, G., Sand, T., Cervicogenic headache, migraine without aura and tension-type headache. Diagnostic blockage of greater occipital and supra-orbital nerves, *Pain*, 51, 43–48, 1992.

Bovim, G., Sjaastad, O., Cervicogenic headache: responses to nitroglycerin, oxygen, Ergotamine and morphine, *Headache*, May 1993, p. 249–252.

Bovim, G., Cervicogenic headache, migraine, and tension-type headache. Pressure-pain threshold measurements, *Pain*, 51, 169–173, 1992.

Collins, J., Sinu-vertebral nerve, *Lumbar Discography*, 1965.

D'Amico, D., Leone, M., Bussone, G., Side-locked unilaterality and pain localization in long-lasting headaches: migraine, tension-type headache, and cervicogenic headache, *Headache*, October 1994, p. 526–530.

Dwyer, A., Aprill, C., Bogduk, N., Cervical zygapophyseal joint pain patterns. I: A study in normal volunteers, *Spine*, 15(6), 1990.

Ehni, G., Benner B., Occipital neuralgia and the C1-2 arthrosis syndrome, *Journal of Neurosurgery*, 61, 961–965, 1984.

Gawel, M.J., Rothbart, P.J., Occipital nerve block in the management of headache and cervical pain, *Cephalalgia*, 12, 9–13, 1992.

Gore, D.R., Sepic, S.B. et al. Neck pain: a long-term follow-up of 205 patients, *Spine*, 14(1), 1987.

Jaeger, B., Are "cervicogenic" headaches due to myofascial pain and cervical spine dysfunction?, *Cephalalgia*, 9, 157–64, 1989.

Jonsson, H. Jr., Bring, G. et al., Hidden cervical spine injuries in traffic accident victims with skull fractures, *Journal of Spinal Disorders*, 4(3), 251–263, 1991.

Kerr, F.W.L., Olafson, R.A., Trigeminal and cervical volleys, *Archives of Neurology*, 5, August 1961.

Kidd, R.F., Nelson, R., Musculoskeletal dysfunction of the neck in migraine and tension headache, *Headache*, Nov-Dec 1993, p. 566–569.

Leone, M., D'Amico D. et al., Possible identification of cervicogenic headache among patients with migraine: an analysis of 374 headaches, *Headache*, September 1995, p. 461–464.

Lord, S.M., Barnsley, L. et al., Percutaneous radio-frequency neurotomy for chronic cervical zygapophyseal-joint pain, *New England of Journal Medicine*, 335(23), 1996.

Lord, S.M., Barnsley, L., Wallis, B.J., Bogduk, N., Third occipital nerve headache: a prevalence study, *Journal of Neurology, Neurosurgery, and Psychiatry*, 57, 1187–1190, 1994.

Lord, S.M., Barnsley, L., Wallis, B.J., McDonald, G.J., Bogduk, N., Percutaneous radio-frequency neurotomy for chronic cervical zygapophyseal-joint pain, *New England of Journal Medicine*, Dec 5, 1996.

Lord, S.M., Barnsley, L., Bogduk, N., Percutaneous radiofrequency neurotomy in the treatment of cervical zygapophysial joint pain: a caution, *Neurosurgery*, 36(4), April 1995.

Lord, S.M., Barnsley, L., Wallis, B.J., Bogduk, N., Third occipital nerve headache: a prevalence study, *Journal of Neurology, Neurosurgery, and Psychiatry*, 57, 1187–1190, 1994.

Michler, R.-P., Bovim, G., Sjaastad. O., Disorders in the lower cervical spine. A cause of unilateral headache? A case report, *Headache*, September 1991, p. 550–551.

Nilsson, N., The prevalence of cervicogenic headache in a random population sample of 20-59 year olds, *Spine*, 20(17), 1884–1888, 1995.

North American Cervicogenic Headache Society, Proposed Taxonomical Definition of Cervicogenic Headache, North York, ON, Canada.

Pearce, J.M., Cervicogenic headache: an early description, *Journal of Neurology, Neurosurgery, and Psychiatry*, 58(6), 1995.

Phillips, J.M., Characteristics of patients successfully treated for cervicogenic headache by surgical decompression of the second cervical root, *Headache*, Nov/Dec 1995, p. 621–629.

Poletti, C.E., Proposed operation for occipital neuralgia: C-2 and C-3 root decompression, *Neurosurgery*, 12(2), 1983.

Poletti, C.E., Sweet, W.H., Entrapment of the C2 root and ganglion by the atlanto-epistrophic ligament: clinical syndrome and surgical anatomy, *Neurosurgery*, 27(2), 1990.

Radanov, B.P., Dvorak, J., Valach, L., Cognitive deficits in patients after soft tissue injury of the cervical spine, *Spine*, 17(2), 1992.

Radanov, B.P., Sturzenenegger, M., DiStefano, G., Long-term outcome after whiplash injury: a 2-year follow-up considering features of injury mechanism and somatic, radiologic, and psychosocial findings, *Medicine*, 74(5), 1995.

Rothbart, P., Unilateral headache with features of hemicrania continua and cervicogenic headache — a case report, *Headache*, October 1992, p. 459–460.

Rothbart, P.J., Chronic tension-type headache with cervical spine pathology, unpublished.

Saadah, H.A., Taylor, F.B., Sustained headache syndrome associated with tender occipital nerve zones, *Headache*, April 1987, p. 201–205.

Saper, J.R., Occipital neuralgia with symptoms of orofacial pain, *Topics in Pain Management*, 12(3), October 1996.

Schonstrom, N., Twomey, L., Taylor, J., The lateral atlanto-axial joints and their synovial folds: an *in vitro* study of soft tissue injuries and fractures, *Journal of Trauma*, 35(6), 1993.

Sjaastad, O., Fredricksen, T.A., Pfaffenrath, V., Cervicogenic headache: diagnostic criteria, *Headache*, November 1990, p. 725–726.

Sjaastad, O., Cervicogenic headache: the controversial headache, *Clinical Neurology and Neurosurgery*, 94 (Suppl.), S147, 1992.

Taren, J.A., Kahn, E.A., Anatomic Pathways Related to Pain in Face and Neck. Section of Neurosurgery, Department of Surgery, University of Michigan Hospital, Ann Arbor, Michigan.

Vernon, H., Spinal manipulation and headaches: an update, *Topics in Clinical Chiropractic*, 2(3), 1995.

Wilson, P.R., Chronic neck pain and cervicogenic headache, *Clinical Journal of Pain*, 7, 5–11, 1991.

Zwart, J.-A., Sand, T., Exteroceptive suppression of temporalis muscle activity: a blind study of tension-type headache, migraine, and cervicogenic headache, *Headache*, June 1995, p. 338–343.

CHILDREN

Brink, J.D., Imbus, C., Woo-Sam, J., Physical recovery after severe closed head trauma in children and adolescents, *Journal of Pediatrics*, 97(5), 721–727, 1980.

Chaplin, D., Deitz, J., Jaffe, K.M., Motor performance in children after traumatic brain injury, *Archives of Physical Medicine and Rehabilitation*, 74, February 1993.

Del Bene, E., Poggioni, M., Typical and atypical cluster headache in children, *Cephalalgia*, 7(Suppl. 6), 1987.

Dillon, H., Leopold, R.L., Children and the post-concussion syndrome, *Journal of the American Medical Association*, Jan. 14, 1961.

Donders, J., Memory functioning after traumatic brain injury in children, *Brain Injury*, 7(5), 431–437, 1993.

Glassman, S.D., Johnson, J.R., Holt, R.T., Seatbelt injuries in children, *Journal of Trauma*, 33(6), 882–886, 1992.

Gulbrandsen, G.B., Neuropsychological sequelae of light head injuries in older children 6 months after trauma, *Journal of Clinical Neuropsychology*, 6(3), 257–268, 1984.

Haas, D.C., Pineda, G.S., Lourie, H., Juvenile head trauma syndromes and their relationship to migraine, *Archives of Neurology*, 32, November 1975.

Harrington, J.A., Letemendia, F.J.J., Persistent psychiatric disorders after head injuries in children.

Hashimoto, I., Nemoto, S., Sano, K., Hyperexcitable state of the brainstem in children with post-traumatic vomiting as evidenced by brainstem auditory-evoked potentials, *Neurology Research*, 6, March/June, 1984.

Jaffe, K.M., Fay, G.C., Polissar, N.L., Martin, K.M. et al., Severity of pediatric traumatic brain injury neurobehavioral recovery at one year — a cohort study, *Archives of Physical Medicine and Rehabilitation*, 74, June 1993.

Klonoff, H., Clark, C., Klonoff, P.S., Long-term outcome of head injuries: a 23 year follow up study of children with head injuries, *Journal of Neurology, Neurosurgery, and Psychiatry*, 56, 410–415, 1993.

Klonoff, H., Low, M.D., Clark, C., Head injuries in children: a prospective five-year follow-up, *Journal of Neurology, Neurosurgery, and Psychiatry*, 40, 1211–1219, 1977.

Lewis, R.J., Yee, L., Inkelis, S.H., Gilmore, D., Clinical predictors of post-traumatic seizures in children with head trauma, *Annals of Emergency Medicine*, 22, 7, 1993.

Michaud, L.J., Rivara, F.P., Jaffe, K.M., Fay, G., Dailey, J.L., Traumatic brain injury as a risk factor for behavioral disorders in children, *Archives of Physical Medicine and Rehabilitation*, 74, April 1993.

Ruijs, M.B.M., Keyser, A., Gabreëls, F.J.M., Long-term sequelae of brain damage from closed head injury in children and adolescents, *Clinical Neurology and Neurosurgery*, 92(4), 323–328, 1990.

Simpson, D.A., Blumbergs, P.C., McLean, A.J., Scott, G., Head injuries in infants and children, measures to reduce mortality and morbidity in road accidents, *World Journal of Surgery*, 16, 403–409, 1992.

LITIGATION

Bagger-Sjöbäck, D., Perols, O., Bergenius, J., Audiovestibular findings in patients with vestibular neuritis: a long-term follow-up study, *Acta Otolaryngology (Stockh)*, 503(Suppl.) 16–17, 1993.

Barnat, M.R., Post-traumatic headache patients. I. Demographics, injuries, headache, and health status, *Headache*, 26, 271–277, 1986.

Blakely, T.A. Jr., Harrington, D.E., Mild head injury is not always mild; implications for damage litigation, *Medical Science and Law*, 33(3), 1993.

Cornfeld, R.S., Help stamp out junk science: a practical approach, *For the Defense*, April 1993.

Denker, P.G., Perry, G.F., Postconcussion syndrome in compensation litigation: analysis of 95 cases with electroencephalographic correlations, *Neurology*, 4, 1954.

Epstein, C.M., Editorial: Computerized EEG in the courtroom, *Neurology*, 44, 1556–1569, 1994.

Galasko, C.S.B., Murray, P.M., Pitcher, M. et al., Neck sprains after road traffic accidents: a modern epidemic, *Injury: the British Journal of Accident Surgery*, 24(3), 1993.

Goldstein, M., Editorial: Traumatic brain injury: a silent epidemic, *Annals of Neurology*, 27(3), 1990.

Hendler, N.H., Kozikowski, J.G., Overlooked physical diagnoses in chronic pain patients involved in litigation, *Psychosomatics*, 34(6), 1993.

Jennett, B., Who cares for head injuries?, *British Medical Journal*, 2 August 1975.

Kelly, R., The post-traumatic syndrome: an iatrogenic disease, *Forensic Science*, 6, 17–24, 1975.

Matarazzo, J.D., Psychological assessment versus psychological testing: validation from Binet to the school, clinic, and courtroom, *American Psychologist*, September 1990.

McKinlay, W.W., Brooks, D.N., Bond, M.R., Post-concusional symptoms, financial compensation and outcome of severe blunt head injury, *Journal of Neurology, Neurosurgery, and Psychiatry*, 46, 1084–1091, 1983.

Mendelson, G., Not "cured by a verdict," *Medical Journal of Australia*, 2, 132–134, 1982.

Miller, H., Accident neurosis, *British Medical Journal*, April 1, 1961, 919–925.

Packard, R.C., Posttraumatic headache: permanency and relationship to legal settlement, *Headache*, 32, 496–500, 1992.

Packard, R.C., Ham, L.P., Impairment ratings for posttraumatic headache, *Headache*, 33, 359–364, 1993.

Packard, R.C., Ham, L.P., Posttraumatic headache: determining chronicity, *Headache*, 33, 133–134, 1993.

Packard, R.C., Weaver, R., Ham, L.P., Cognitive symptoms in patients with posttraumatic headache, *Headache*, 33, 365–368, 1993.

Parmar, H.V., Raymakers, R., Neck injuries from rear impact road traffic accidents: prognosis in persons seeking compensation, *Injury: British Journal of Accident Surgery*, 24(2), 1993.

Rimel, R.W., Giordani, B., Barth, J.T. et al., Disability caused by minor head injury, *Neurosurgery*, 9(3), 1981.

Saper, J.R., Chronic posttraumatic headache: often a myth?, *Topics in Pain Management*, 12(1), 1996.

Scheinberg, P., Editorial: The hidden costs of medicolegal abuses in neurology, *Archives of Neurology*, 51, July 1994.

Silvain, P.B., Psychological injury claims: a primer for defense counsel, *For the Defense*, July 1986.

Speed, W.G. III., Closed head injury sequelae: changing concepts, *Headache*, 29, 643–647, 1989.

Strugar, J., Sass, K.J., Buchanan, C.P. et al., Long-term consequences of minimal brain injury: loss of consciousness does not predict memory impairment, *Journal of Trauma*, 34(4), 1993.

Uomoto, J.M, Esselman, P.C., Traumatic brain injury and chronic pain: differential types and rates by head injury severity, *Archives of Physical Medicine and Rehabilitation*, 74, January 1993.

Youngjohn, J.R., Burrows, L., Erdal, K., Brain damage or compensation neurosis? The controversial post-concussion syndrome, *The Clinical Neuropsychologist*, 9(2), 112–123, 1995.

Ziegler, D.K., Editorial: Are headache patients disabled?, *Headache Quarterly*, 3, 2, 1992.

MYOFASCIAL PAIN SYNDROME

Campbell, S.M., Regional myofascial pain syndromes, *Rheumatic Disease Clinics of North America*, 15(1), February 1989.

Graff-Radford, S.B., Reeves, J.L., Jaeger, B., Management of chronic head and neck pain: effectiveness of altering factors perpetuating myofascial pain, *Headache*, 27, 186–190, 1987.

Simons, D.G., Myofascial pain syndromes: Where are we? Where are we going?, *Archives of Physical Medicine and Rehabilitation*, 69, 207–212, 1988.

NEUROPSYCHOLOGICAL

Adams, K.M., Putnam, S.H., Coping with professional skeptics: reply to Faust, *Psychological Assessment*, 6(1), 5–7, 1994.

Adams, K.M., Putnam, S.H., Book review: what's minor about mildhead injury?, *Journal of Clinical and Experimental Neuropsychology*, 13(2), 388–394, 1991.

Alafano, D.P., Neilson, P.M., Fink, M.P., Long-term psychosocial adjustment following head or spinal cord injury, *Neuropsychiatry, Neuropsychology, and Behavioral Psychology*, 6(2), 117–125, 1993.

Alves, W., Macciocchi, S.N., Barth, J.T., Postconcussive symptoms after uncomplicated mild head injury, *Journal of Head Trauma and Rehabilitation*, 8(3), 48–59, 1993.

Amadio, P.C., Current concepts review: pain dysfunction syndromes, *Journal of Bone and Joint Surgery*, 70-A(6), July 1988.

Arcia, E., Gualtieri, C.T., Association between patient report of symptoms after mild head injury and neurobehavioural performance, *Brain Injury*, 7(6), 481–489, 1993.

Barth, J.T., Macciocchi, S.N., Giordani, B. et al., Neuropsychological sequelae of minor head injury, *Neurosurgery*, 13(5), 1983.

Baubrey, J., Dobbs, A.R., Rule, B.G., Laypersons' knowledge about the sequelae of minor head injury and whiplash, *Journal of Neurology, Neurosurgery and Psychiatry*, 52, 842–846, 1989.

Ben-Porath, Y.S., The ethical dilemma of coached malingering research, *Psychological Assessment*, 6(1), 14–15, 1994.

Bennett, T., Post-traumatic headaches: subtypes and behavioral treatments, *Cognitive Rehabilitation*, March/April 1988.

Berry, D.T.R., Lamb, D.G., Weter, M.W. et al., Ethical considerations in research on coached malingering, *Psychological Assessment*, 6(1), 16–17, 1994.

Binder, L.M., Villanueva, M.R. et al., The Rey AVLT recognition memory task measures motivational impairment after mild head trauma, *Archives of Clinical Neuropsychology*, 8, 137–147, 1993.

Brown, S.J., Fann, J.R., Grant, I., Postconcussional disorder: time to acknowledge a common source of neurobehavioral morbidity, *Journal of Neuropsychiatry and Clinical Neurosciences*, 6, 15–22, 1994.

Blumer, D., Heilbronn, M., The pain-prone disorder: a clinical and psychological profile, *Psychosomatics*, 22(5), May 1981.

Cohen, R.J., Suter, C., Hysterical seizures: susggestion as a provocative EEG test, *Annals of Neurology*, 11(4), April 1982.

Crane, M., Malpractice, lies, and videotape, *Medical Economics*, 71, June 13, 1994.

Davidoff, D.A., Kessler, H.R., Laibsain, D.F., Mark, V.H., Neurobehavioral sequelae of minor head injury: a consideration of post-concussive syndrome versus post-traumatic stress disorder, *Cognitive Rehabilitation*, March/April 1988.

De Benedittis, G., De Santis, A., Chronic post-traumatic headache: clinical, psychopathological features and outcome determinants, *Neurosurgical Science*, 27, 1983.

DeGood, D.E., Cundiff, G.W., Adams, L.E., Shutty, M.S. Jr., A psychosocial and behavioral comparison of reflex sympathetic dystrophy, low back pain, and headache patients, *Pain*, 54, 317–322, 1993.

Desai, B.T., Porter, R.J., Penry, J.K., Psychogenic seizures: a study of 42 attacks in six patients, with intensive monitoring, *Archives of Neurology*, 39, April 1982.

Dicker, B.G., Focus on clinical research: preinjury behavior and recovery after a minor head injury: a review of the literature, *Journal of Head Trauma Rehabilitation*, December 1989.

Dicker, B.G., Profile of those at risk for minor head injury, *Journal of Head Trauma and Rehabilitation*, 7(1), 83–91, 1992.

Dikmen, S., McLean, A., Temkin, N., Neuropsychological and psychosocial consequences of minor head injury, *Journal of Neurology, Neurosurgery, and Psychiatry*, 49, 1227–1232, 1986.

Dikmen, S.S., Levin, H.S., Methodological issues in the study of mild head injury, *Journal of Head Trauma and Rehabilitation*, 8(3), 30–37, 1993.

Dikmen, S., Reitman, R.M., Emotional sequelae of head injury, *Annals of Neurology*, 2(6), December 1977.

Dikmen, S.S., Reitman, R.M., Temkin, N.R., Machamer, J.E., Letter to the Editors. Minor and severe head injury emotional sequelae, *Brain Injury*, 6(5), 477–478, 1992.

Dikmen, S.S., Temkin, N.R., Machamer, J.E. et al., Employment following traumatic head injuries, *Archives of Neurology*, 51, 177–186, 1994.

Drommond, L.M., Gravestock, S., Delayed emergence of obsessive-compulsive neurosis following head injury: case report and review of its theoretical implications, *British Journal of Psychiatry*, 153, 839–842, 1988.

Erickson, R.C., Forum: two views of malingering. View I: A muddle to avoid, *Clinical Neuropsychologist*, 4(4), 379–389, 1990.

Faust, D., Hart, K., Pediatric malingering: the capacity of children to fake believable deficits on neuropsychological testing, *Journal of Consulting and Clinical Psychology*, 56(4), 578–582, 1988.

Faust, D., Guilmette, T.J., Hart, K. et al., Neuropsychologists' training experience, and judgment accuracy, *Archives of Clinical Neuropsychology*, 3, 145–163, 1988.

Fioravanti, M., Ramelli, L., Napoleoni, A., Lazzari, S. et al., Post-traumatic headache: neuropsychological and clinical aspects, *Cephalalgia*, Suppl. 1, 1983.

Gensemer, I.B., Walker, J.C., McMurry, F.G., Brotman, S.J., IQ levels following trauma, *Journal of Trauma*, 29(12), 1989.

Gould, R., Miller, B.L., Goldbert, M.A., Benson, D.F., The validity of hysterical signs and symptoms, *Journal of Nervious and Mental Disease*, 174(10), 1986.

Gouvier, W.D., Uddo-Crane, M., Brown, L.M., Base rates of post-concussional symptoms, *Archives of Clinical Neuropsychology*, 3, 272–278, 1988.

Gronwall, D., Wrightson, P., Delayed recovery of intellectual function after minor head injury, *Lancet*, 14, September 1974.

Guilmette, T.J., Giuliano, A.J., Taking the stand: issues and strategies in forensic neuropsychology, *Clinical Neuropsychologist*, 5(3), 197–219, 1991.

Heaton, R.K., Smith, H.H. Jr., Lehman, R.A.W., Vogt, A.T., Prospects of faking-believable deficits on neuropsychological testing, *Journal of Consulting and Clinical Psychology*, 46(5), 892–900, 1978.

Jennett, B., Teasdale, G., Braakman, R. et al., Prognosis of patients with severe head injury, *Neurosurgery*, 4(4), 1979.

Johnson, M.H., Magaro, P.A., Effects of mood and severity on memory processes in depression and mania, *Psychological Bulletin,* 101(1), 28–40, 1987.

Jones, R.D., Anderson, S.W., Cole, T., Hathaway-Nepple, J., Neuropsychological sequelae of traumatic brain injury, *Head Injury and Postconcussive Syndrome*, Rizzo, M., Tranel, D., Eds., Churchill Livingstone, New York, Chap. 20.

Katz, D.I., Neuropathology and neurobehavioral recovery from closed head injury, *Journal of Head Trauma and Rehabilitation,* 7(2), 1–15, 1992.

Kessler, R.C., McGonagle, K.A., Zhao, S., Nelson, C.B. et al., Lifetime and 12-month prevalence of DSM-III-R psychiatric disorders in the United States: results from the National Comorbidity Study, *Archives of General Psychiatry*, 51, January 1994.

Klonoff, P.S., Snow, W.G., Costa, L.D., Quality of life in patients 2 to 4 years after closed head injury, *Neurosurgery*, 19, 724–732, 1986.

Kreutzer, J.S., Gordon, W.A., Rosenthal, M., Marwitz, J., Neuropsychological characteristics of patients with brain injury: preliminary findings from a multicenter investigation, *Journal of Head Trauma and Rehabilitation* 8(2), 47–59, 1993.

Kwentus, J.A., Hart, R.P., Peck, E.T., Kornstein, S., Psychiatric complications of closed head trauma, *Psychosomatics,* 26(1), January 1985.

Jakobsen, J., Baadsgaard, S.E., Thomsen, S., Henriksen, P.B., Prediction of post-concussional sequelae by reaction time test, *Acta Neurologica Scandinavica*, 75, 341–345, 1987.

Lavin, J.H., Everyone believed the plaintiff — except his doctor, *Medical Economics,* 68, November 4, 1991.

Lees-Haley, P.R., English, L.T., Glenn, W.J., A fake bad scale on the MMPI-2 for personal injury claimants, *Psychological Reports*, 68, 203–210, 1991.

Lees-Haley, P.R., Williams, C.W., Brown, R.S., The Barnum effect and personal injury litigation, *American Journal of Forensic Psychology*, 11(2), 1993.

Lees-Haley, P.R., Brown, R.S., Neuropsychological complaint base rates of 170 personal injury claimants, *Archives of Clinical Neuropsychology,* 8, 203–209, 1993.

Levin, H.S., Eisenberg, H.M., Benton, A.L., *Mild Head Injury,* Oxford University Press, New York, 1989.

Levin, H.S., O'Donnell, V.M., Grossman, R.G., The Galveston Orientation and Amnesia Test: a practical scale to assess cognition after head injury, *Journal of Nervous and Mental Disease*, 167(11), 1979.

Levin, H.S., Mattis, S., Ruff, R.M., Eisenberg, H.M. et al., Neurobehavioral outcome following minor head injury: a three-center study, *Journal of Neurosurgery,* 66, 234–243, 1987.

Lipowski, Z.J., Somatization: the concept and its clinical application, *American Journal of Psychiatry,* 145, 11, November 1988.

Livingston, M.G., Brooks, D.N., Bond, M.R., Three months after severe head injury: psychiatric and social impact on relatives, *Journal of Neurology, Neurosurgery, and Psychiatry,* 48, 870–875, 1985.

MacFlynn, G., Montgomery, E.A., Fenton, G.W., Rutherford, W., Measurement of reaction time following minor head injury, *Journal of Neurology, Neurosurgery and Psychiatry*, 47, 1326–1331, 1984.

Martin, R.C., Boltcr, J.F., Tgodd, M.E. et al., Effects of sophistication and motivation on the detection of malingered memory performance using a computerized forced-choice task, *Journal of Clinical and Experimental Neuropsychology*, 15(6), 867–880, 1993.

Matarazzo, J.D., Psychological assessment versus psychological testing: validation from Binet to the school, clinic, and courtroom, *American Psychologist*, 45(9), 999–1017, 1990.

McCaffrey, R.J., Lynch, J.K., A methodological review of "Method Skeptic" reports, *Neuropsychology Review,* 3(3), 1992.

McLean, A., Dikmen, S.S., Temkin, N.R., Psychosocial recovery after head injury, *Archives of Physical Medicine and Rehabilitation*, 74, October 1993.

McNairy, S.L., Maruta, T., Ivnik, R.J. et al., Prescription medication dependence and neuropsychologic function, *Pain*, 18, 169–177, 1984.

Mendelson, G., Guest Editorial: Compensation and chronic pain, *Pain*, 48, 121–123, 1992.

Merskey, H., Editorial: Psychiatry and the cervical sprain syndrome, *Canadian Medical Association Journal*, 130, May 1, 1984.

Middleboe, T., Anderson, H.S., Birket-Smith, M., Friis, M.L., Minor head injury: impact on general health after 1 year. A prospective follow-up study, *Acta Neurologica Scandinavica,* 85, 5–9, 1992.

Millis, S.R., The recognition memory test in the detection of malingered and exaggerated memory deficits, *Clinical Neuropsychologist*, 6(4), 406–414, 1992.

Millis, S.R., Dijker, M., Use of the recognition memory test in traumatic brain injury: preliminary findings, *Brain Injury,* 7(1), 53–58, 1993.

Millis, S.R., Putnam, S.H., The recognition memory test in the assessment of memory impairment after financially compensable mild head injury: a replication, *Perceptual and Motor Skills*, 79, 384–386, 1994.

Mitchell, K.R., Wallis, B.J., Patterns of illness behavior and perceived coping in chronic low back and chronic neck pain patients, *Psychiatric Med.*, 5(2), 1987.

Montgomery, E.A., Fenton, G.W., McClelland, R.J. et al., The psychobiology of minor head injury, *Psychological Medicine*, 21, 375–384, 1991.

Nadler, J.D., Mittenberg, W., DePiano, F.A., Schneider, B.A., Effects of patient age on neuropsychological test interpretation, *Professional Psychology: Research and Practice*, 25(3), 288–295, 1994.

Newcombe, F., Rabbitt, P., Briggs, M., Minor head injury: pathophysiological or iatrogenic sequelae?, *Journal of Neurology, Neurosurgery, and Psychiatry*, 57, 709–716, 1994.

Pankratz, L., A new technique for the assessment and modification of feigned memory deficit, *Perceptual and Motor Skills*, 57, 5367–5372, 1983.

Pankratz, L., Forum: two view of malingering. View II: a necessary assessment enterprise, *Clinical Neuropsychologist,* 4(4), 384–389, 1990.

Pankratz, L., Fausti, S.A., Peed, S., Case study: a forced-choice technique to evaluate deafness in the hysterical or malingering patient, *Journal of Consulting and Clinical Psychology*, 43(3), 421–422, 1975.

Perr, I.N., Cross-examination of the psychiatrist, using publications, *Bulletin of the American Academy of Psychiatry and The Law*, Vol. 5, 1977.

Radanov, B.P., DeStefano, G., Schnidrig, A., Sturzenegger, M., Common whiplash: psychosomatic or somatopsychic?, *Journal of Neurology, Neurosugical and Psychiatry*, 57, 486–490, 1994.

Rogers, R., Harrell, E.H., Liff, C.D., Feigning neuropsychological impairment: a critical rview of methodological and clinical considerations, *Clinical Psychology Review*, 13, 255–274, 1993.

Ruesch, J., Intellectual Impairment of Head Injuries, Office of Scientific Research and Development and Harvard University, Cambridge, MA.

Ruff, R.M., Levein, H.S., Marshall, L.F., Neurobehavioral methods of assessment and the study of outcome in minor head injury, *Journal of Head Trauma and Rehabilitation*, 1(2), 43–52, 1986.

Rogers, R., Models of feigned mental illness, *Professional Psychology Research and Practice*, 21(3), 182–188, 1990.

Snook, S.H., The costs of back pain in industry, *Occuptional Medicine*, 3(1), 1–5, 1988.

Stewart, D.P., Kaylor, J., Koutanis, E., Cognitive deficits in presumed minor head-injured patients, *Academic Emergency Medicine*, 3(1), January 1996.

Tarsh, M.J., Royston, C., A follow-up study of accident neurosis. *British Journal of Psychiatry*, 146, 18–25, 1985.

Tranel, D., The release of psychological data to nonexperts: ethical and legal considerations, *Professional Psychology: Research and Practice*, 25(1), 33–38, 1994.

Wedding, D., Faust, D., Clinical judgment and decision making in neuropsychology, *Archives of Clinical Neuropsychology*, 4, 233–265, 1989.

Weighill, V.E., "Compensation Neurosis": a review of the literature, *Journal of Psychosomatic Research*, 27(2), 97–104, 1983.

Weintraub, M.I., Regional pain is usually hysterical, *Archives of Neurology*, 45, August 1988.

PAIN

Davis, K.D., Treede, R.D., Raja, S.N., Meyer, R.A., Campbell, J.N., Topical application of clonidine relieves hyperalgesia in patients with sympathetically maintained pain, *Pain*, 47, 309–317, 1991.

Hoehn-Saric, R., Neurotransmitters in anxiety, *Archives of General Psychiatry*, 39, June 1982.

Kantor, T.G., Proceedings of a Symposium: Evolving trends in the management of chronic pain, *American Journal of Medicine*, 101 (1A), July 31, 1996.

Shea, J.D., Ed., Pain medicine: is there relief in sight? Part I, *Journal of the Florida Medical Association*, 83(10), December 1996.

Shea, J.D., Ed., Pain medicine: is there relief in sight? Part II, *Journal of the Florida Medical Association*, 84(1), January 1997.

Yaksh, T.L., *Basic Pharmacology and Physiology of Pain Processing: A Review*, University of California, San Diego, CA.

POST CONCUSSION SYNDROME

Carlsson G.S., Svärdsudd, K., Welin, L., Long-term effects of head injuries sustained during life in three male populations, *Journal of Neurosurgery*, 67, 197–205, 1987.

Feinsod, M., Hoyt, W.F., Wilson, W.B., Spire, J.-P., Visually evoked response: use in neurological evaluation of postraumatic subjective visual complaints, *Archives of Ophthalmology*, 94, 237–240, 1976.

Frazee, J.G., Head Trauma, *Emergency Medicine Cinics of North America*, 4(4), November, 1986.

Goldstein, J., Posttraumatic headache and postconcussion syndrome, *Medical Clinics of North America*, 75(3), May 1991.

Lee, S.-T., Lui, T.-N., Early seizures after mild closed head injury, *Journal of Neurosurgery*, 76, 435–439, 1992.

Khurana, R.K., Nirankari, V.S., Bilateral sympathetic dysfunction in post-traumatic headaches, *Headache*, 26, 183–188, 1986.

Matthews, W.B., Footballer's migraine, *British Medical Journal*, 2, 326–327, 1972.

Ommaya, A.K., Gennarelli, T.A., Cerebral concussion and traumatic unconsciousness: correlation of experimental and clinical observations on blunt head injuries, *Brain*, 97, 633–654, 1974.

Rizzo, P.A., Pierelli, F., Pozzessere, G., Floris, R., Morocutti, C., Subjective postraumatic syndrome: a comparison of visual and brain stem auditory evoked responses, *Neuropsychobiology*, 9, 78–82, 1983.

Schlageter, K., Gray, B., Hall, K., Shaw, R., Sammet, R., Incidence and treatment of visual dysfunction in traumatic brain injury, *Brain Injury*, 7(5), 439–448.

Vijayan, Y., Dreyfus, P.M., Posttraumatic dysautonomic cephalalgia: clinical observations and treatment, *Archives of Neurology*, 32, October 1975.

Waddell, P.A., Gronwall, D.M.A., Sensitivity to light and sound following minor head injury, *Acta Neurologicsa Scandinavica*, 69, 270–276, 1984.

POST TRAUMATIC MIGRAINE

Balla, J., Karnaghan, J., Whiplash Headache, *Clinical and Experimental Neurology*, 23, 1987.

Bennett, D.R., Fuenning, S.I., Sullivan, G., Weber, J., Migraine precipitated by head trauma in athletes, *American Journal of Sports Medicine*, 8(3), 1980.

Haas, D.C., Lourie, H., Trauma-triggered migraine: an explanation for common neurological attacks after mild head injury, *Journal of Neurosurgery*, 68, 181–188, 1988.

Olesen, J., Clinical and pathophysiological observations in migraine and tension-type headache explained by integration of vascular, supraspinal and myofascial inputs, *Pain*, 46, 125–132, 1991.

Truong, D.D., Dubinsky, R., Hermanowicz, N. et al., Posttraumatic torticollis, *Archives of Neurology*, 48, 221–223, 1991.

Weil, A.A., EEG findings in a certain type of psychosomatic headache: dysrhythmic migraine, *EEG Clinical Neurophysiology*, 4, 181–186, 1952.

Weiss, H.D., Stern, B.J., Goldberg, J., Post-traumatic migraine: chronic migraine precipitated by minor head or neck trauma, *Headache*, 31, 451–456, 1991.

REFLEX SYMPATHETIC DYSTROPHY

Bruehl, S., Carlson, C.R., Predisposing psychological factors in the development of reflex sympathetic dystrophy, *The Clinical Journal of Pain*, 8, 287–299, 1992.

Schwartzman, R.J., Reflex sympathetic dystrophy, *Current Science*, 1993.

Van Houdenhove, B., Vasquez, G., Onghena, P. et al., Etiopathogenesis of reflex sympathetic dystrophy: a review and biopsychosocial hypothesis, *Clinical Journal of Pain*, 8, 300–306, 1992.

Veldman, H.J.M., Reynen, H.M., Arntz, I.E., Goris, J.A., Signs and symptoms of reflex sympathetic dystrophy: prospective study of 829 patients, *Lancet*, 342, October 23, 1993.

TEMPOROMANDIBULAR JOINT

Bohnen, N., Jolles, J., Neurobehavioral aspects of postconcussive symptoms after mild head injury, *Journal of Nervous and Mental Disease*, 180, 683–692, 1992.

Brooke, R.I., LaPointe, H.J., Temporomandibular joint disorders following whiplash, *Spine: State of the Art Review*, 7(3), September 1993.

Deutsch, P.M., Sawyer, H.W., A Guide to Rehabilitation. Vol 2, Matthew Bender, Times Mirror Books, 1990.

Howard, R.P., Benedict, J.V., Raddin, J.H. Jr., Smith, H.L., Assessing neck extension-flexion as a basis for temporomandibular joint dysfunction, *Journal of Oral Maxillofacial Surgery*, 49, 1210–1213, 1991.

Kryzer, T.C., Lambert, P.R., Herniation of temporomandibular joint contents into the external ear canal, *Otolaryngology — Head and Neck Surgery*, 23(10), 1992.

McKenzie, J.A., Williams, J.F., The dynamic behavior of the head and cervical spine during "whiplash," *Journal of Biomechanics*, 4, 477–490, 1971.

Morgan, D.H., Commentary, the great imposter: diseases of the temporomandibular joint, *Journal of the American Medical Association*, 235(22), 1976.

Ommaya, A.K., Hirsch, A.E., Tolerances for cerebral concussion from head impact and whiplash in primates, *Journal of Biomechanics*, 4, 13–21, 1971.

Ranawat, C.S., O'Leary, P., Pellicci, P. et al., Cervical spine fusion in rheumatoid arthritis, *Journal of Bone and Joint Surgery*, 61-A(7), October 1979.

Roydhouse, R.R., Letter to Editor: Whiplash and temporomandibular dysfunction, *Lancet*, 1394–1395, June 16, 1973.

Schneider, K., Zernicke, R.F., Clark, G., Modeling of jaw-head-neck dynamics during whiplash, *Journal of Dental Research*, 68(9), 1360–1365, 1989.

Sessle, B.J., Hu, J.W., Amano, N., Zhong, G., Convergence of cutaneous, tooth pulp, visceral, neck and muscle afferents onto nociceptive and non-nociceptive neurones in trigeminal subnucleus caudalis (medullary dorsal horn) and its implications for referred pain, *Pain*, 17, 219–235, 1986.

Smith, R.G., Cherry, J.E., Traumatic eagle's syndrome: report of a case and review of the literature, *Journal of Oral Maxillofacial Surgery*, 46, 606–609, 1988.

Torg, J.S., Vegso, J.J., Sennett, B., Das, M., The National Football Head and Neck Injury Registry: 14-year report on cervical quadriplegia, 1971 through 1984, *Journal of the American Medical Association*, 254, 3439–3443, 1985.

Torg, J.S., Epidemiology, pathomechanics, and prevention of athletic injuries to the cervical spine, *Medicine and Science in Sports and Exercise*, 17(3), 1985.

Walter, J., Doris, P.E., Shaffer, M.A., Clinical presentation of patients with acute cervical spine injury, *Annals of Emergency Medicine*, 13, 7, 1984.

Webb, J., March, L., Tyndall, A., The neck-tongue syndrome: occurrence with cervical arthritis as well as normals, *Journal of Rheumatology*, 11, 4, 1984.

Weinberg, S, LaPointe, H., Cervical extension-flexion injury (whiplash) and internal derangement of the temporomandibular joint, *Journal of Oral Maxillofacial Surgery*, 45, 653–656, 1987.

THORACIC OUTLET SYNDROME

Carroll, R.E., Hurst, L.C., The relationship of thoracic outlet syndrome and carpal tunnel syndrome, *Clinics in Orthopaedics and Related Research*, No 164, April 1982.

Cherington, M., Cherington, C., Thoracic outlet syndrome: reimbursement patterns and patient profiles, *Neurology*, 42, May 1992.

Hawkes, C.D., Neurosurgical considerations in thoracic outlet syndrome, *Clinics in Orthopaedics and Related Research*, No. 207, June 1986.

Leffert, R.D., Thoracic outlet syndromes, *Hand Clinics*, 8(2), May 1992.

Lindgren, K.-A., Leino, E., Subluxation of the first rib: a possible thoracic outlet syndrome mechanism, *Archives of Physical Medicine and Rehabilitation*, 68, September 1988.

Novak, C.B., Mackinnon, S.E., Patterson, G.A., Evaluation of patients with thoracic outlet syndrome, *Journal of Hand Surgery*, 18A(2), March 1993.

Razi, D.M., Wassel, H.D., Traffic accident induced thoracic outlet syndrome: decompression without rib resection, correction of associated recurrent thoracic aneurysm, *International Surgery*, 78, 25–27, 1993.

Roos, D.B., The thoracic outlet syndrome is underrated, *Archives of Neurology*, 47, March 1990.

Sanders, R.J., Pearce, W.H., The treatment of thoracic outlet syndrome: a comparison of different operations, *Journal of Vascular Surgery*, 10, 626–34, 1989.

TREATMENTS

Ballerini, R., Casini, A., Chinol, M. et al., Study on the absorption of ketoprofen topically administered in man: comparison between tissue and plasma levels, *International Journal of Clinical Pharmacology Research*, 69–72, 1986.

Burry, H.C., Accident compensation: gates and gatekeepers, *Medical Journal of Australia*, 152(9), May 7, 1990.

Byrn, C., Borenstein, P., Linder, L.-E., Treatment of neck and shoulder pain in whiplash syndrome patients with intracutaneous sterile water injections, *Acta Anaesthesiologica Scandinavica*, 1991, 35, 52–53, 1991.

Catchlove, R.F.H., Braha, R., The use of cervical epidural nerve blocks in the management of chronic head and neck pain, *Canadian Anaesthesiology Society Journal*, 31(2), 188–191, 1984.

Chi, S., Jun, H.W., Anti-inflammatory activity of ketoprofen gel on carrageenan-induced paw edema in rats, *Journal of Pharmaceutical Sciences*, 79(11), November 1990.

Choi, H.-K., Flynn, G.L., Some general influences of *n*-decylmethyl sulfoxide on the permeation of drugs across hairless mouse skin, *Journal of Investigative Dermatology*, 96(6), June 1991.

Choi, H.-K., Flynn, G.L., Amidon, G.I., Transdermal delivery of bioactive peptides: the effect of *n*-decylmethyl sulfoxide, pH, and inhibitors on enkephalin metabolism and transport, *Pharmacology Research*, 7(11), 1990.

Flechas, J.D., Fibromyalgia: A Neuro Endocrine Disorder, Clinical Evaluation and Treatment, unpublished report.

Flechas, J.D., DHEA and Fibromyalgia, unpublished report.

Flouvat, B., Roux, A., Delhotal-Landes, B., Pharmacokinetics of ketoprofen in man after repeated percutaneous administration.

Graff-Radford, S.B., Reeves, J.L., Baker, R.L., Chiu, D., Effects of transcutaneous electrical nerve stimulation on myofascial pain and trigger point sensitivity, *Pain*, 37, 1–5, 1989.

Mazzocco, M.W., Lynn, J.M., Comparison of percutaneous ketoprofen and iontophoresis in the treatment of myositis/myalgia associated with headache, Pittsburgh Headache Institute.

Planas, M.E., Gonzalez, P., Rodriguez, L. et al., Noninvasive percutaneous induction of topical analgesia by a new type of drug carrier, and prolongation of local pain insensitivity by anesthetic I liposomes, *Anesthesia and Analgesia (Cleveland)*, 75, 615–21, 1992.

Singh, P., Roberts, M.S., Skin permeability and local tissue concentrations of nonsteroidal anti-inflammatory drugs after topical application, *Journal of Pharmacology and Experimental Therapeutics*, 258(1), 1994.

Willimann, H., Walde, P., Luisi, P.L. et al., Lecithin organogel as matrix for transdermal transport of drugs, *Journal of Pharmaceutical Sciences*, 81(9), September 1992.

TRIGEMINAL AND OCCIPITAL NEURALGIA

Denny-Brown, D., Yanagisawa, N., The function of the descending root of the fifth nerve, *Brain*, 6, 783–814, 1973.

Ehni, G., Bener, B., Occipital neuralgia and the C1-2 arthrosis syndrome, *Journal of Neurosurgery*, 61, 962–965, 1984.

Graff-Radford, S.B., Jaeger, B., Reeves, J.L., Myofascial pain may present clinically as occipital neuralgia, *Neurosurgery*, 19(4), 1986.

Kerr, F.W.L., Structural relation of the trigeminal spinal tract to upper cervical roots and the solitary nucleus in the cat, *Experimental Neurology*, 4, 134–148 1961.

Mealy, K., Brennan, H., Fenelon, G.C.C., Early mobilisation of acute whiplash injuries, *British Medical Journal*, 92(8), March 1986.

Phero, J.C., Raj, P.P., McDonald, J.S., Transcutaneous electrical nerve stimulation and myoneural injection therapy for management of chronic myofascial pain, *Dental Clinics of North America*, 31(4), October 1987.

Saadah, H.A., Taylor, F.B., Sustained headache syndrome associated with tender occipital nerve zones, *Headache*, 27, 201–205, 1987.

Sluijter, M.E., Koetsveld-Baart, C.C., Interruption of pain pathways in the treatment of the cervical syndrome, *Anesthesia*, 35, 302–307, 1980.

Vijayan, N., Dreyfus, P.M., Posttraumatic dysautonomic cephalalgia, *Archives of Neurology*, 32, October 1975.

WHIPLASH

Barnsley, L., Lord, S., Bogduk, N., Clinical review: whiplash injury, *Pain*, 58, 283–307, 1994.

Barnsley, L., Lord, S.M., Wallis, B.J., Bogduk, N., The prevalence of chronic cervical zygapophysial joint pain after whiplash, *Spine*, 20(1), 20–26, 1995.

Barnsley, L., Lord, S.M., Wallis, B.J., Bogduk, N., Lack of effect of intraarticular corticosteroids for chronic pain in the cervical zygapophyseal joints, *New England Journal of Medicine*, 330(5), April 14, 1994.

Carette, S., Whiplash injury and chronic neck pain, *New England Journal of Medicine*, 330(15), April 14, 1994.

Dieter, J.N., Swerdlow, B., A replicative investigation of the reliability of the MMPI in the classification of chronic headaches, *Headache*, 28(3), April 1988.

Evans, L., Frick, M.C., Car size or car mass: which has greater influence on fatality risk?, *American Journal of Public Health*, 82(8), August 1992.

Evans, R.W., Some observations on whiplash injuries, *Neurology of Trauma*, 10(4), Nov. 1992.

Fisher, C.M., Whiplash amnesia, *Neurology*, 1982, 32, 667-668, 1982.

Gershon-Cohen, J., Budin, E., Glauserm F., Whiplash fractures of cervicodorsal spinous processes, *Journal of the American Medical Association*, 155(6), June 5, 1954.

Gibbs, F.A., Objective evidence of brain disorder in cases of whiplash injury, *Clinical Electroencephalography*, 2(2), 1971.

Gotten, N., Survey of one hundred cases of whiplash injury after settlement of litigation, *Journal of the American Medical Association*, 162(9), October 27, 1956.

Graff-Radford, S.B., Jaeger, B., Reeves, J.L., Myofascial pain may present clinically as occipital neuralgia, *Neurosurgery*, 19(4), 1986.

Hirsch, S.A., Hirsch, P.J., Hiramoto, H., Weiss, A., Whiplash Syndrome: fact or fiction?, *Orthopedic Clinics of North America*, 9(4), October 1988.

Jacome, D.E., Basilar artery migraine after uncomplicated whiplash injuries, *Headache*, 26, 515–516, 1986.

Keith, W.S., "Whiplash" — Injury of the 2nd cervical ganglion and nerve, *Canadian Journal of Neurological Science*, 13, 133–137, 1986.

Lamer, T.J., Ear pain due to cervical spine arthritis: treatment with cervical facet injection, *Headache*, 31, 682–683, 1991.

Liu, Y.K., Chandran, K.B. et al., Subcortical EEG changes in rhesus monkeys following experimental hyperextension-hyperflexion (whiplash), *Spine*, 9(4), 1984.

Livingston, M., Whiplash injury: misconceptions and remedies, *Australian Family Physician*, 21(11), November 1992.

Macnab, I., The "whiplash syndrome," *Orthopedic Clinics of North America*, 2(2), July 1971.
Martinez, J.L., Garcia, D.J., A model for whiplash, *Journal of Biomechanics*, 1, 23–32, 1968.
McKenzie, J.A., Williams, J.F., The dynamic behaviour of the head and cervical spine during whiplash, *Journal of Biomechanics*, 4, 477–490, 1971.
McNamara, R.M., O'B M.C., Davidheiser, S., Post-traumatic neck pain: a prospective and follow-up study, *Annals of Emergency Medicine*, 17, 906–911, 1988.
Newman, P.K., Whiplash injury, *British Medical Journal*, 301, 1 September 1990.
Ommaya, A.K., Faas, F., Yarnell, P., Whiplash injury and brain damage, *Journal of the American Medical Association*, 204(4), April 22, 1968.
Ommaya, A.K., Hirsch, A.E., Tolerances for cerebral concussion from head impact and whiplash in primates, *Journal of Biomechanics*, 4, 3–21, 1971.
Ommaya, A.K., Yarnell, P., Subdural hematoma after whiplash injury, *Lancet*, August 2, 1969.
Oosterveld, W.J., Kortschot, H.W. et al., Electronystagmographic findings following cervical whiplash injuries, *Acta Otolaryngology (Stockholm)* 111, 201–205, 1991.
Pearce, J.M.S., Whiplash injury: a reappraisal, *Journal of Neurology, Neurosurgery, and Psychiatry*, 52, 1329–1331, 1989.
Pearce, J.M.S., Editorial: Polemics of chronic whiplash injury, *Neurology*, 44, 1993–1997, 1994.
Pennie, B., Agambar, L., Patterns of injury and recovery in whiplash, *Injury*, 22(1), 57–59, 1991.
Porter, K.M., Neck sprains after car accidents, *British Medical Journal*, 298, 15 April 1989.
Radanov, B.P., Di Stefano, G., Schnidrig, A. et al., Cognitive functioning after common whiplash: a controlled follow-up study, *Archives of Neurology*, 50, January 1993.
Radanov, B.P., Sturzenegger, M. et al., Factors influencing recovery from headache after common whiplash, *British Medical Journal*, 307, 11 September 1993.
Riley, L.H. III, Long, D., Riley, L.H. Jr., Commentary: The science of whiplash, *Medicine*, 74(5), 1995.
Schneider, K., Zernicke, R.F., Clark G., Modeling of jaw-head-neck dynamics during whiplash, *Journal of Dental Research*, 68(9), 1360–1365, 1989.
Severy, D.M., Mathewson, J.H., Bechtol, C.O., Controlled automobile rear-end collisions, an investigation of related engineering and medical phenomena, *Canadian Services Medical Journal*, 11, November 1955.
Spitzer, W.O., Skovron, M.L., Salmi, L.R. et al., Scientific monograph of the Quebec Task Force on Whiplash-Associated Disorders: redefining "whiplash" and its management, *Spine*, 20(8S), 1995.
Sturzenegger, M., DiStefano, G., Radanov, B.P., Schnidrig, A., Presenting symptoms and signs after whiplash injury: the influence of accident mechanisms, *Neurology*, 44, April 1994.
Toglia, J.U., Rosenberg, P.E., Ronis, M.L., Posttraumatic dizziness: vestibular, audiologic, and medicolegal aspects, *Archives of Otolaryngology*, 92, November 1970.
Torres, F., Shapiro, S.K., Electroencephalograms in whiplash injury, *Archives of Neurology*, 5, July 1961.
Winston, K.R., Whiplash and its relationship to migraine, *Headache*, 27, 452–457, 1987.

RECOMMENDED READING

Text Books – Recommended

Diamond, S., *Diagnosing and Managing Headaches*, Professional Communications, Inc., Caddo, OK, 1994.
Diamond, S., Dalessio, D.J., *The Practicing Physician's Approach to Headache*, 4th ed., Williams & Wilkins, Baltimore, 1993.
Elkind, A.H., *Handbook of Headache Disorders*, 2nd ed., Essential Medical Information Systems, Inc., Durant, OK, 1994.
Foreman, S.M., Croft, A.C., *Whiplash Injuries: The Cervical Acceleration/Deceleration Syndrome*, 2nd ed., Williams & Wilkins, Baltimore, 1995.
Francis, J.H., *Acute and Chronic Headaches*, Aardvark Publishers, Irving, TX, 1992.
Francis, J.H., Pennal, B.E., *Headache Classification System*, Aardvark Publishers, Irving, TX, 1990.
Goadsby, P.J., Silberstein, S.D., *Headache*, Butterworth-Heinemann, Newton, MA, 1997.
Kudrow, L., *Cluster Headache Mechanisms and Management*, Oxford University Press, Oxford, 1980.
Lance, J.W., *Mechanism and Management of Headache*, 4th ed., Butterworths, Kent, England, 1982.
Raskin, N.H., *Headache*, 2nd ed., Churchill Livingstone, New York, 1988.

Rizzo, M., Tranel, D., *Head Injury and Postconcussive Syndrome*, Churchill, Livingstone, New York, 1996.

Saper, J.R., Silberstein, S., Gordon, C., Hamel, R.L., *Handbook of Headache Management*, Williams & Wilkins, Baltimore, 1993.

Travell, J.G., Simons, D.G., *Myofascial Pain and Dysfunction, The Trigger Point Manual*, Williams & Wilkins, Baltimore, 1983.

Non-Text Books: Recommended

Diamond, S., *A Pain Specialist's Approach to the Headache Patient*, International Universities Press, Madison, CT, 1993.

Diamond, S., *Hope For Your Headache Problem*, International Universities Press, Madison, CT, 1988.

Lance, J.W., *Headache: Understanding — Alleviation*, Charles Scribner's Sons, New York, 1975.

Murphy, W., *Dealing With Headaches*, Time-Life Books, Chicago, 1982.

Rapoport, A.M., Sheftell, F.D., *Headache Relief*, Simon & Schuster, New York, 1990.

Robbins, L., Lang, S.S., *Headache Help*, Houghton Mifflin, New York, 1995.

Sacks, O.W., *Migraine*, University of California Press, Berkeley, CA, 1992.

Saper, J.R., *Help for Headaches*, Warner Books, New York, 1987.

Saper, J.R., Mage, K.R., *Freedom From Headaches*, New York, 1981.

Swerdlow, B., *The Headache Handbook*, Mayfield Press, Winter Park, FL, 1985.

Text Books: Reviewed

Anderson, J.E., *Grant's Atlas of Anatomy*, 7th ed., Williams & Wilkins, Baltimore, 1978.

Appenzeller, O., *Pathogenesis and Treatment of Headache*, Spectrum Publications, New York, 1976.

Blau, J.N., *Migraine: Clinical and Research Aspects*, The Johns Hopkins University Press, Baltimore, 1987.

Cesarani, A., Alpini, D., Boniver, R., Claussen, C.F., Gagey, P.M., Magnusson, L., Ödkvist, L.M., *Whiplash Injuries: Diagnosis and Treatment*, Springer-Verlag Italia, Milano, Italy, 1996.

Chusid, J.G., *Correlative Neuroanatomy and Functional Neurology*, 18th ed., Lange Medical Publications, Los Altos, CA, 1982.

Dalessio, D.J., *Wolff's Headache and Other Head Pain*, 4th ed., Oxford University Press, New York, 1980.

Edmeads, J., *Headache*, Sandoz (Canada), Toronto, 1980.

Evans, R.W., Baskin, D.S., Yatsu, F.M., *Prognosis of Neurological Disorders*, Oxford University Press, New York, 1992.

Gray, H., *Gray's Anatomy*, Lea & Febiger, Philadelphia, 1973.

Heyck, H., *Headache and Facial Pain*, Year Book Medical Publishers, Chicago, 1981.

Kapandji, I.D., *The Physiology of the Joints*, Churchill Livingstone, New York, 1974.

Levine, R.S., *Head and Neck Injury*, Society of Automotive Engineers, Warrendale, PA, 1994.

Netter, F.H., *The Ciba Collection of Medical Illustrations, Vol. 1: Nervous System*, CIBA Pharmaceutical Company, Summit, NJ, 1962.

Netter, F.H., *The Ciba Collection of Medical Illustrations, Vol. I: Nervous System, Part II: Neurologic and Neuromuscular Disorders*, CIBA Pharmaceutical Company, West Caldwell, NJ, 1986.

Netter, F.H., *The Ciba Collection of Medical Illustrations, Vol. 8: Musculoskeletal System, Part I: Anatomy, Physiology and Metabolic Disorders*, CIBA Pharmaceutical Company, West Caldwell, NJ, 1987.

Olesen, J., Tfelt-Hansen, P., Welch, K.M.A., *The Headaches*, Raven Press, New York, 1993.

Raskin, N.H., Appenzeller, O., *Headache*, W. B. Saunders, Philadelphia, 1980.

Rose, F. C., *The Management of Headache*, Raven Press, New York, 1988.

Sances, A. Jr., Thomas, D.J., Ewing, C.L., *Mechanisms of Head and Spine Trauma*, Aloray, Inc., Goshen, NY, 1986.

Symposium on Headache and Related Pain Syndromes, *Medical Clinics of North America,* W. B. Saunders, Philadelphia, 1978.

Van Allen, M.W., *Pictorial Manual of Neurologic Tests,* Year Book Medical Publishers, Chicago, 1969.

White, A.A., Panjabi, M.M., *Clinical Biomechanics of the Spine*, J.B. Lippincott, Philadelphia, 1990.

Non-Text Books: Reviewed

American Council for Headache Education, *Migraine: The Complete Guide*, Dell Publishing, New York, 1994.
Bircher-Benner Clinic, *Nutrition Plan for Headache and Migraine Patients*, Pyramid Books, New York, 1972.
Cady, R., Farmer, K., *Headache Free*, Bantam Books, New York, 1996.
Diamond, S.M.D., *The Hormone Headache: New Ways to Prevent, Manage, and Treat Migraines and Other Headaches*, Macmillan, New York, 1995.
Duckro, P.N., Richardson, W.D., Marshall, J.E., *Taking Control of Your Headaches: How to Get the Treatment You Need*, The Guilford Press, New York, 1995.
Ford, N.D., *Eighteen Natural Ways to Beat a Headache*, Keats Publishing, New Canaan, CT, 1990.
Gronwall, D. and Wrightson, P., *Head Injury: The Facts: A Guide for Families and Care-Givers*, Oxford University Press, New York, 1990.
Hanington, E., *Migraine*, Technomic Publishing Co., Westport, CT, 1973.
Hanington, E., *The Headache Book*, Technomic Publishing Co., Inc., Westport, CT, 1980.
Inlander, C., Shimer, P., *Headaches: 47 Ways to Stop the Pain*, Walker and Company, New York, 1995.
Kandel, J., Sudderth, D.B., *Migraine: What Works!*, Prima Publishing, Rocklin, CA, 1996.
Lipton, R.B., Newman, L.C., MacLean, H., *Migraine: Beating the Odds*, Addison-Wesley, Reading, MA, 1992.
Solomon, S., Fraccaro, S., *The Headache Book*, Consumer Reports Books, Mount Vernon, NY, 1991.
Stromfeld, J., Weil, A., *Free Yourself from Headaches*, Frog Ltd., Palm Beach Gardens, FL, 1995.
Theisler, C., *Migraine — Winning the Fight of Your Life*, Starburst, Lancaster, PA, 1995.
Wilkinson, M., *Migraines and Headaches*, Arco Publishing, New York, 1982.
Wyckoff, B., *Overcoming Migraine*, Staton Hill Press, Barrytown, NY, 1994.

Appendix

HEADACHE ORGANIZATIONS FOR ADDITIONAL INFORMATION

The American Association for the Study of Headache
875 Kings Highway
Suite 200
Woodbury, NJ 08096-3172
Phone: 609-845-0322
Fax: 609-384-5811

The National Headache Foundation
467 W Deming Place
Chicago, IL 60614-1726
Phone: 312-388-6390
Fax: 312-907-6278

North American Cergicogenic Headache Society
York Mills Centre
16 York Mills Road
Unit #125, Box 129
North York, ON, Canada
M2P 2ES
Phone: 416-512-6407
Fax: 416-512-6375

The American Council for Headache Education [ACHE]
875 Kings Highway
West Deptford, NJ 08096
Phone: 800-255-ACHE

INDEX

D

E

F

G

N

O

P

R

S

T

U

V

W

X

Z